Pocket Companion
to the Fourth Edition
of
TEXTBOOK
of
VETERINARY
INTERNAL
MEDICINE

i

Compiling Editors

STEPHEN J. ETTINGER, D.V.M.

DAVID G. FELDMAN, D.V.M.
California Animal Hospital
Drs. Ettinger, Lusk, Feldman and Associates, Inc.
Los Angeles, California
Diplomate, American College of Veterinary Internal Medicine
Internal Medicine

JENIFER LUNNEY BRAYLEY, D.V.M.
Veterinary Medical Specialists of Houston
Houston, Texas
Diplomate, American College of Veterinary Internal Medicine
Cardiology and Internal Medicine

KYLE A. BRAYLEY, D.V.M.
Veterinary Medical Specialists of Houston
Houston, Texas
Diplomate, American College of Veterinary Internal Medicine
Cardiology and Internal Medicine

Pocket Companion
to the Fourth Edition
of
TEXTBOOK
of
VETERINARY
INTERNAL
MEDICINE

STEPHEN J. ETTINGER, D.V.M.

California Animal Hospital
Drs. Ettinger, Lusk, Feldman and Associates, Inc.
Los Angeles, California

Diplomate, American College of Veterinary Medicine
Cardiology and Internal Medicine

W.B. SAUNDERS COMPANY
A Division of Harcourt Brace & Company

Philadelphia / London / Toronto / Montreal / Sydney / Tokyo

W.B. SAUNDERS COMPANY

A Division of Harcourt Brace & Company

The Curtis Center
Independence Square West
Philadelphia, Pennsylvania 19106

Library of Congress Cataloging-in-Publication Data

Ettinger, Stephen J.
    Pocket companion to the fourth edition of Textbook of
veterinary internal medicine / Stephen J. Ettinger.—2nd ed.
        p.   cm.
    Includes index.
    ISBN 0-7216-5766-4
    1. Dogs—Diseases.   2. Cats—Diseases.   3. Veterinary
internal medicine.   I. Ettinger, Stephen J.   Textbook of
veterinary internal medicine.   II. Title.
SF991.E87   1995
636.7'0896—dc20   95-23426

POCKET COMPANION TO THE
FOURTH EDITION OF TEXTBOOK
OF VETERINARY INTERNAL MEDICINE   ISBN   0–7216–5766–4

Printed in the United States of America.

Last digit is the print number: 9   8   7   6   5   4   3   2   1

PREFACE

The first edition of the *Pocket Companion to Textbook of Veterinary Internal Medicine* (third edition) was published late in the life of the parent book. We were uncertain when we began the process of redacting the parent text what reception a condensed version would have. We have been very pleased with the acceptance and use of the "Cliff Notes version" by students and practitioners alike. Therefore, we undertook the effort to produce a pocket version early in the life of the fourth edition of the parent textbook.

Your comments and constructive critique of the first edition provided us with helpful hints for continuing the production of this pocket version. You requested a book that would still be concise, inexpensive, immediately clinically relevant, even more user friendly and with an expanded drug index.

As before, the redactors have worked to keep the material clinically relevant and immediately useful. Wherever possible, referencing back to the parent book has been done to give the reader direction for more in-depth reading. Algorithms, abundantly present in the parent text, were left out because they would not be readable in this format with the reduced page size and print. The reader should make use of these clinically informative guides in the parent textbook. Pictures, radiographs, and references have been omitted to save space and keep the format simple. Included charts and figures were chosen to help the student quickly identify problems while not confusing the subject material.

In the last edition, we introduced the drug formulary, a compilation of data taken from the parent text, my clinical experience and that of my colleagues, and other sources listed in the introduction to that section. This format continues with more than fifty new drugs added to the list, some newly introduced and others that have found clinical relevancy in other clinics. Drugs are identified both by trade and generic names with cross referencing for ease of use. Canine and feline dosaging at times varies. Such differences are very important and warrant separation, thus two columns, one for the dog and one for the cat.

We have attempted to sort out and present that material which will, at the examination table, be useful in defining clinical syndromes and making clinical decisions. Throughout, the reader is referenced back to the parent text for further help.

Once again, kudos to the editorial and production staff at WB Saunders. Ray Kersey, Dave Kilmer, and Lorraine Kilmer are to be congratulated for their efforts in moving this book along smoothly, efficiently, and with great accuracy. Each has participated in the process admirably and each deserves a vote of appreciation from the editor.

STEPHEN J. ETTINGER, DVM
Los Angeles, CA
1995

NOTICE

Companion animal practice is an ever-changing field. Standard safety precautions must be followed, but as new research and clinical experience grow, changes in treatment and drug therapy become necessary or appropriate. The authors and editors of this work have carefully checked the generic and trade drug names and verified drug dosages to assure that dosage information is precise and in accord with standards accepted at the time of publication. Readers are advised, however, to check the product information currently provided by the manufacturer of each drug to be administered to be certain that changes have not been made in the recommended dose or in the contraindications for administration. This is of particular importance in regard to new or infrequently used drugs. Recommended dosages for animals are sometimes based on adjustments in the dosage that would be suitable for humans. Some of the drugs mentioned here have been given experimentally by the authors. Others have been used in dosages greater than those recommended by the manufacturer. In these kinds of cases, the authors have reported on their own considerable experience. It is the responsibility of those administering a drug, relying on their professional skill and experience, to determine the dosages, the best treatment for the patient, and whether the benefits of giving a drug justify the attendant risk. The editors cannot be responsible for misuse or misapplication of the material in this work.

THE PUBLISHER

CONTENTS

SECTION XI
THE ENDOCRINE SYSTEM

SECTION XII
THE REPRODUCTIVE SYSTEM

SECTION I
MANIFESTATIONS OF CLINICAL DISEASE

CHAPTER 1
CHANGES IN BODY WEIGHT
(pages 2–5)

Changes in body weight result when metabolic utilization and/or nutrient loss exceeds or falls short of energy intake. Documentation should be based on serial body weight measurements or on standard body weight charts. *Weight loss* refers to a decrease in body weight (>10 per cent of body weight). *Weight gain* refers to an increase in body weight (>10 per cent of body weight).

WEIGHT LOSS (pp. 2–4)

HISTORICAL FINDINGS

Weight loss can be caused by inadequate food intake, increased energy demand, malassimilation of food, or loss of nutrients, fluids, and electrolytes. Weight loss associated with polyphagia is suggestive of malassimilation, excessive nutrient loss, hypermetabolism, inadequate feeding, or adverse environmental conditions. Weight loss associated with anorexia may indicate infectious, inflammatory, neoplastic, toxic, neurologic, or metabolic abnormalities. Weight loss associated with malnutrition can be identified by a complete and detailed dietary history. A thorough dietary history includes calculation of the animal's caloric needs and careful questioning as to the amount and frequency of feeding. Weight loss associated with gastrointestinal signs indicates caloric intake that is inadequate to meet the energy expenditure of the body.

WEIGHT LOSS: PHYSICAL FINDINGS

Weight loss associated with fever can be attributed to (1) infectious, (2) inflammatory, (3) neoplastic, and (4) toxic causes. Depending on the site and extent of involvement, infectious agents may cause weight loss via both fever and anorexia. Weight loss without fever is often caused by metabolic disorders such as renal, hepatic, and cardiac disease, which may affect both appetite (usually decreased) and energy demands (increased). Immune-mediated neuromuscular disorders and degenerative joint disease can cause loss of muscle mass. Weight loss can be caused by the loss of nutrients through the gastrointestinal tract (as in parasitism or protein-losing enteropathy) or secondary to the

---

Original chapter written by Deborah S. Greco

exudative skin conditions (e.g., burns, pyoderma) or urinary loss of nutrients (such as protein or glucose).

WEIGHT LOSS: DIAGNOSTIC PLAN

A complete blood count, serum chemistry profile, urinalysis, fecal examination, thoracic and abdominal radiography, and thyroid concentrations should be evaluated as needed. Serologic tests (viral, rickettsial, fungal, dirofilariasis, ANA) may be warranted. Contrast radiology, echocardiography, ultrasonography, gastrointestinal endoscopy, exploratory laparotomy with biopsies, and other diagnostic procedures (nuclear studies, such as liver scans) may be necessary to determine the exact etiology of the weight loss.

WEIGHT GAIN (pp. 4–5)

Caloric intake that exceeds metabolic demands and nutrient loss results in weight gain and possible obesity.

HISTORICAL FINDINGS

Weight gain associated with polyphagia can be caused by overeating, boredom, drug therapy, reduced physical activity, and endocrine disorders. Weight gain associated with anorexia or normal appetite can be caused by overfeeding, genetic predisposition, or hypometabolism. Decreased activity can contribute to obesity. Labrador retrievers, cocker spaniels, collies, and certain terriers may have a genetic predisposition to weight gain. Endocrine disorders, such as panhypopituitarism, hypogonadism, and hypothyroidism, can result in hypometabolism and weight gain.

WEIGHT GAIN: PHYSICAL FINDINGS

Weight gain associated with ascites and/or peripheral edema may be caused by hypoproteinemic states, cardiac disorders, infectious or inflammatory abdominal disorders, hepatic disorders, or posthepatic disorders. Hypertensive patients may exhibit weight gain as a result of sodium and fluid retention. Weight gain associated with an increase in lean body mass may result from increased exercise and caloric intake, endocrine disorders such as insulinoma and acromegaly, and drug therapy (e.g., anabolic steroids).

Weight Gain Associated with Organomegaly. Dogs and cats suffering from hyperadrenocorticism exhibit hepatomegaly. Organomegaly in an otherwise poorly controlled diabetic cat on insulin therapy is strongly suggestive of feline acromegaly.

WEIGHT GAIN: DIAGNOSTIC PLAN

A complete blood count, serum chemistry profile, and urinalysis should be collected. Endocrine testing may be indicated (TSH stimulation test, ACTH simulation test, insulin:glucose ratios) to refine the diagnosis.

CHAPTER 2

THE SKIN AS A SENSOR OF INTERNAL MEDICAL DISORDERS
(pages 6–10)

CONGENITAL-HEREDITARY SYNDROMES (GENODERMATOSES) (p. 6)

Dermatomyositis has been reported primarily in collies and Shetland sheepdogs. Cutaneous changes include crusts, ulcerations, vesicles, and/or alopecia around the mucocutaneous junctions, front legs, ear tips, and tail. Muscular atrophy may be generalized or may be selective, often affecting the temporal and masseter muscles. The onset of clinical signs usually occurs before the age of 6 months. Vitamin E or immunosuppressive doses of prednisolone have been tried as therapy.

Cyclic Neutropenia.   Oral and lip ulcerations may lead to severe necrotizing stomatitis.

Enzyme Deficiencies.   Mucopolysaccharidoses have been reported only in the cat. Affected kittens have broad, flat faces, small ears, and corneal clouding. Occasionally cutaneous nodules may be seen.

Chédiak-Higashi symdrome is reported in Persian cats that have partial oculocutaneous albinism.

ENDOCRINOPATHIES (pp. 6–8)

Hypothyroidism.   Cutaneous lesions may consist of alopecia; seborrhea; hyperpigmentation; a dry, easily epilated hair coat; or secondary pyoderma. Pruritus may be present.

Hyperadrenocorticism.   Alopecia, hyperpigmentation, seborrhea, pyoderma, dermatophytosis or demodicosis, thin skin, easy bruising, and calcinosis cutis may be seen. Skin lesions may be the *only* abnormality noted.

Gonadal Hormone Abnormalities.   Sertoli cell tumors of the testes in dogs may cause alopecia and feminization. Seminomas and interstitial cell tumors may (rarely) cause the same clinical signs. Testosterone- and estrogen-responsive alopecias and castration- and spay-responsive dermatoses are much less common.

Growth-Hormone-Dependent Syndromes.   In dwarf dogs this is usually seen in the German shepherd or Carnelian beardog. Adult onset deficiency usually occurs in Pomeranians, poodles, chow chows, and keeshonden.

Diabetes Mellitus.   Cutaneous lesions have been reported as pyoderma, seborrhea, thin skin, alopecia, demodicosis, and xanthomatosis.

Pheochromocytoma.   This disease should be included in the differentiation of erythema without pruritus.

Original chapter written by Stephen D. White

BACTERIAL INFECTIONS (p. 8)

Staphylococcal Infections.　Always attempt to rule out an underlying cause, e.g., allergy, endocrine disease, or immunosuppressive condition.

Brucellosis canis may cause a scrotal swelling or dermatitis.

FUNGAL INFECTIONS

Sporotrichosis causes a cutaneous infection characterized by nodular, draining, suppurative lesions. It may become generalized, affecting internal organs.

Deep or Systemic Mycoses.　Cutaneous lesions may be varied and may be the first signs noted by the client.

PARASITIC DISEASES (p. 8)

Demodicosis.　Generalized demodicosis is thought to occur in dogs with an underlying immunosuppressive disorder. Hyperadrenocorticism, diabetes mellitus, hypothyroidism, or internal neoplasia should be considered. Therapy consists of the miticidal dip amitraz.

Leishmaniasis.　Alopecia, erythema, and especially scaling and ulceration of the ears and mucocutaneous junctions may occur.

Rickettsial Diseases.　Ehrlichiosis and Rocky Mountain spotted fever may both present with petechiae of the mucous membranes or skin. Edema of the extremities, and acral necrosis have been reported with RMSF.

Heartworms.　*Dirofilariasis immitis* has been implicated in causing a scabies-like eruption.

Intestinal Nematodes and Cestodes.　Hookworms may cause a papular, inflammatory eruption on the parts of the body in contact with infected soil. These intestinal parasites may rarely cause pruritus, papules, erythema, and/or seborrhea.

Babesiosis may be associated with edema, petechiae, urticaria, and erythema.

NUTRITIONAL DISORDERS (pp. 8–9)

Zinc-responsive dermatosis is seen as two syndromes. The first occurs primarily in Siberian huskies and Alaskan malamutes. Crusts, scale, erythema, and alopecia occur around the mucocutaneous junctions, face, footpads, and abdomen. These dogs are on balanced diets with adequate levels of zinc. Syndrome II occurs in pups of any breed fed an oversupplemented (especially a high-calcium) diet. Hyperkeratotic plaques and crusts may occur on the head, trunk, extremities, and footpads.

Diagnosis is based on skin biopsy. Therapy for syndrome I is zinc supplementation. For syndrome II, changing to a balanced dog food is indicated.

Vitamin A–responsive dermatosis has been seen primarily in cocker spaniels. The dermatosis is characterized by a seborrhea. Diagnosis is by elimination of other causes of seborrhea and by skin biopsy.

Pansteatitis is a deficiency of vitamin E and its antioxidant property. It has been reported only in cats, usually those eating diets containing red fish or excessive cod liver oil. Subcutaneous and abdominal fat may feel firm or lumpy. Draining tracts may be present. Diagnosis is based on history and biopsy.

Food Hypersensitivity.　Clinical signs in dogs are generally pruritus, papules, and erythema. In cats, pruritus is often prominent on the face, head, and neck.

AUTOIMMUNE DISORDERS (pp. 9–10)

Systemic lupus erythematosus (SLE) exhibits cutaneous lesions with crusts, ulcers, or depigmentation affecting the mucocutaneous junctions and footpads.

Cold Agglutinin Disease. At the extremities erythema, cyanosis, ulceration, and necrosis may all be present when these dogs are exposed to cold (usually 0 to 4°C).

Drug eruption may occur with long- or short-term usage. Lesions may mimic almost any skin condition.

Toxic Epidermal Necrolysis (TEN) is characterized by a multifocal or generalized vesiculobullous eruption. Pain is moderate to severe. TEN often seems to be associated with various diseases, such as neoplasia, bacterial infection, drug eruption, or liver disease.

Erythema multiforme is an accute eruption of the skin and mucous membranes. It is characterized clinically by annular ("target") lesions. The lesions may be secondary to another disease.

MISCELLANEOUS DISEASE (p. 10)

Thallium Toxicosis. In chronic thallium poisoning, alopecia, erythema, crusts, and ulceration occur on the axillae, ears, genitalia, posterior abdomen, paws, and mucocutaneous junctions. "Brick-red" mucous membranes may be noted.

Hepatic Disease. *Superficial necrolytic dermatitis* (hepatocutaneous syndrome, diabetic dermatosis) is a rare condition in old dogs. The cutaneous lesions include erythema, crusting, oozing, and alopecia of the face, genitals, and distal extremities, as well as hyperkeratosis and ulceration of the footpads. This disease resembles the glucagonoma syndrome of humans.

Renal disease has been reported to cause oral ulcerations.

Neoplasia may cause nonspecific clinical signs related to the skin, such as a sparse, dull, or dry haircoat, mild seborrhea, or possibly pruritus.

CHAPTER 3
TABLES OF ABNORMAL VALUES AS A GUIDE TO DISEASE SYNDROMES
(pages 11–17)

Original chapter written by Lon J. Rich and Embert H. Coles

HEMOGRAM CHANGES

TABLE 3-1. NEUTROPHILIA

CAUSE	NEUTROPHIL RESPONSE	OTHER LEUKOCYTES*	MECHANISM
Physiologic—exercise, hypoxia, excitement	Mature—moderate absolute increase	Lymphocytosis, particularly in cats	MGP to CGP† (neutrophils); altered recirculation (lymphocytes)
Increased glucocorticoids (endogenous, exogenous)	Mature—moderate absolute increase	Lymphopenia, eosinopenia, monocytosis (dogs, sometimes cats)	Decreased migration of neutrophils from blood, increased removal from marrow storage pool; altered recirculation of lymphocytes; sequestration of eosinophils in bone marrow
Early inflammation	Left shift with increase in absolute neutrophil count	Variable	Increased tissue demand with excess release from storage pool of bone marrow
Acute intense inflammation	Marked left shift neutrophilia; often toxic neutrophils	Variable	Continued stimulation and tissue demand for same
Established inflammation	Increase in absolute neutrophil count; slight to no left shift	Variable	Increased neutrophil production and release to meet established tissue demand

*A stress pattern may be present.
†MGP = marginal granulocyte pool; CGP = circulating granulocyte pool.

TABLE 3-2. NEUTROPENIA

CAUSE	NEUTROPHIL RESPONSE	OTHER LEUKOCYTES*	MECHANISM
Overwhelming bacterial infection	Neutropenia usually with left shift (immatures exceed matures; degenerative left shift)	Normal	Increased tissue demand with depletion of peripheral blood and marrow pools
Decreased production of neutrophils	Neutropenia, no left shift	Normal	Decreased marrow production
Sequestration	Sudden neutropenia, no left shift	Normal	CGP to MGP† (as in shock)
Ineffective granulopoiesis	Neutropenia, no left shift	Increased marrow granulopoiesis	Abnormal maturation and release from marrow pools

*A stress pattern may be present.
†MGP = marginal granulocyte pool; CGP = circulating granulocyte pool.

TABLE 3–3. OTHER BLOOD CELL CHANGES

ERYTHROCYTES

Causes of Absolute Erythrocytosis
Non-erythropoietin driven
    Primary (polycythemia vera)
Erythropoietin driven (secondary)
    Hypoxia (cardiovascular disorder—especially right-to-left shunting of blood;
        chronic pulmonary disease; living at high altitudes)
    Renal neoplasia (carcinoma, lymphosarcoma, fibrosarcoma)
    Extrarenal fibrosarcoma (pulmonary, nasal)
    Non-neoplastic renal disease (cysts, hydronephrosis)

Causes of Relative Erythrocytosis
Decreased fluid compartment of blood secondary to dehydration

MONOCYTES

Causes of Monocytosis
Inflammation and tissue necrosis
Increased glucocorticoids (dog)
Suppuration (body cavity)
Granulomatous disorders
Moncytic or myelomonocytic leukemia

LYMPHOCYTES

Causes of Lymphocytosis
Physiologic: Cats, uncommon other species
    Increased epinephrine activity (e.g., exercise, anxiety)
    Temporary following some vaccinations (reactive lymphocytes frequently present)
Pathologic:
    Autoimmune disease
    Lymphosarcoma (not in all patients)
    Feline leukemia virus (not in all cases)
    Hypoadrenocorticism (rarely an absolute increase, but counts may be normal
        in an obviously ill patient)

Causes of Lymphopenia
Excess glucocorticoids
    Endogenous
        Stress
        Debilitating disease
        Hyperadrenocorticism
        Surgery
        Shock
        Trauma
        Heat or cold exposure
    Exogenous
        Glucocorticoid therapy
Lymphocyte loss
    Protein-losing enteropathy (lymphangiectasia)
    Chylothorax with repeated drainage
Reduced lymphopoiesis
    Prolonged corticosteroid therapy
    Congenital T-cell immunodeficiency
Viral infections (acute stages)
    Canine distemper
    Feline panleukopenia
    Infectious canine hepatitis
    Coronavirus enteritis
    Feline leukemia virus (thymic atrophy)

EOSINOPHILS

Causes of Eosinophilia
Hypersensitivity
    Parasitism in sensitized hosts (gastrointestinal parasites and heartworm are
        common)

Immediate hypersensitivity reactions
Specific eosinophilic diseases
  Eosinophilic enterocolitis
  Eosinophilic granuloma (cat)
  Hypereosinophilia syndrome
  Eosinophilic pneumonitis (dog, cat)
  Eosinophilic leukemia (rare)
Other associations
  Carcinoma
  Lymphosarcoma
  Mast cell tumor
  Myeloproliferative disease (cat)
  Uterine inflammation
  Hypoadrenocorticism: normal numbers in a "stressed" patient inappropriate

Causes of Eosinopenia
Excess corticosteroids
  Endogenous: hyperadrenocorticism; inflammation with stress
  Exogenous: corticosteroid therapy

BASOPHILS

Causes of Basophilia
Heartworms (eosinophilia usually also present)
Hookworms (eosinophilia usually also present)
Concurrent with eosinophilia in hypersensitivity
Hypothyroidism (occasional)
Basophilic leukemia (rare)
Mast cell tumor (rare)

ENZYMES

TABLE 3–4. SERUM ENZYME ABNORMALITIES

ALKALINE PHOSPHATASE (ALP)

Causes of Increased ALP
Induced isoenzyme by glucocorticoids (dog only); steroid therapy
Bone growth in young animals
Cholestasis secondary to liver disease or pancreatic inflammation
Isoenzyme induced by anticonvulsant drugs (phenobarbitol, primidone; dog)
Increased osteolytic activity (hyperparathyroidism)
Neoplasia: mixed mammary tumor, sarcoma, carcinoma
False increase—severe lipemia, bilirubin >8.0 mg/dl

Cause of Decreased ALP
False decreases due to contamination with EDTA, fluoride, oxalate, phosphate,
    zinc, arsenate, citrate

AMYLASE AND LIPASE

Causes of Hyperamylasemia and/or Hyperlipasemia
Pancreatic inflammation, necrosis, and neoplasia
Obstruction of pancreatic ducts
Renal insufficiency
Slight increase with glucocorticoids (lipase only)
Intestinal perforations (minor increase)
Liver cancer (rare case—minor increase)

TRANSAMINASE

Causes of Increased Serum Glutamic-Oxaloacetic Transaminase
    (AST or SGOT)
Muscle damage (also an increase in creatine kinase [CK])
Hemolysis of RBC
Hepatic disease (when mitochondria are damaged)

Table continued on following page

TABLE 3–4 *Continued*

***Causes of Increased Serum Glutamate Pyruvate Transaminase
(ALT or SGPT)***
Hepatocellular damage
Hepatocellular regeneration
Muscle damage (slight increase only)

CREATINE KINASE

Causes of Increased CK
Myositis
    Infectious (toxoplasmosis)
    Immune mediated systemic lupus erythematosus (SLE)
    Endocrine (hypothyroidism, hyperadrenocorticism)
    Nutritional
Muscle trauma
    Prolonged exercise
    Intramuscular injection
    Recumbency
    Hypothermia
    Bruising
    Myocardial infarction
    Cardiomyopathy (thromboembolic)

LACTATE DEHYDROGENASE (LDH)

Causes of Increased LDH
Handling artifact–serum standing on erythrocytes
Hemolysis of erythrocytes
Cell necrosis of liver, kidney, muscle, and other cells
Neoplasia

PROTEINS

TABLE 3–5. SERUM PROTEIN ABNORMALITIES

ALBUMIN

Causes of Hypoalbuminemia
Decreased production
    Intestinal malabsorption (primary or secondary)
    Maldigestion (exocrine pancreatic insufficiency)
    Malnutrition (parasitic or dietary)
    Chronic liver disease (atrophy or fibrosis)
Increased loss
    Renal disease with chronic proteinuria
    Protein-losing enteropathy (globulins may also be decreased)
    External hemorrhage (globulins may also be decreased)
    Exudative skin lesions (globulins may also be decreased)
    Blood loss (globulins may also be decreased)
Compensatory
    With hyperglobulinemia
    Body cavity effusions

Causes of Hyperalbuminemia
Dehydration (globulins also increased)
Laboratory error

GLOBULIN

Causes of Hypoglobulinemia
Lack of colostrum in newborn
Blood loss
Protein-losing enteropathy
Protein-losing nephropathy
Combined immunodeficiency

Causes of Hyperglobulinemia
Monoclonal
  Plasma cell myeloma
  Ehrlichiosis
  Lymphosarcoma (rarely)
  Feline infectious peritonitis (rarely)
  Idiopathic
Polyclonal
  Feline infectious peritonitis (usually)
  Chronic bacterial infection
  Parasites (*Demodex, Dirofilaria*, scabies)
  Neoplasia
  Immune-mediated disease (SLE, pemphigus, rheumatoid arthritis, AIHA, ITP, immune complex disease)
  Dehydration (also hyperalbuminemia)

FIBRINOGEN

Causes of Hypofibrinogenemia
Severe liver disease
Disseminated intravascular coagulopathy
Congenital afibrinogenemia (St. Bernard)

Causes of Hyperfibrinogenemia (total protein may be normal)
Inflammatory disease

MINERALS

TABLE 3–6. SERUM MINERAL ABNORMALITIES

CALCIUM

Causes of Hypercalcemia
Hyperalbuminemia
Hypercalcemia of malignancy (lymphosarcoma, myeloproliferative disease, multiple myeloma, solid tissue tumors)
Primary hyperparathyroidism
Hypoadrenocorticism
Hypervitaminosis D
Renal disease (uncommon; occurs with familial renal dysplasia and chronic renal failure)
Osteolytic bone lesions (e.g., septic osteomyelitis)
Plant toxicity (jasmine in dogs and cats)
Calciferol-containing rodenticides
Certain granulomatous diseases (e.g., canine blastomycosis)
Severe hypothermia
Disuse osteoporosis

Causes of Hypocalcemia
Hypoalbuminemia
Primary hypoparathyroidism
Secondary renal hyperparathyroidism
Primary renal disease (ethylene glycol toxicity, acute and chronic renal disease)
Necrotizing pancreatitis
Dietary imbalance (hypovitaminosis D, excess phosphorus)
Eclampsia (puerperal tetany)
Intestinal malabsorption (dog)
Hypercalcitonism (neoplasia of parafollicular cells in thyroid)
Factitious (sample run on EDTA plasma)
Iatrogenic—following thyroidectomy (bilateral)
Following excessive use of high phosphate containing (Fleet) enemas or intravenous phosphate administration
Rhabdomyolysis—soft tissue damage

Table continued on following page

TABLE 3–6 *Continued*

PHOSPHATE

Causes of Hyperphosphatemia

Reduced glomerular filtration rate (renal, prerenal, or postrenal azotemia from any cause)
Factitious—sample held too long before analysis (phosphorus released from RBC)
Growing animals
Dietary phosphorus excess
Phosphorus enema or administration of phosphorus-containing fluids
Hypervitaminosis D
Osteolytic bone disease (neoplasia)
Jasmine toxicity
Soft tissue trauma
Hypoparathyroidism with normal glomerular filtration
Hyperthyroidism in cats without renal insufficiency
Drug treatment (anabolic steroids, furosemide, minocycline, hydrochlorothiazide occasionally cause slight increases)

Causes of Hypophosphatemia

Diabetes mellitus with ketoacidosis
Hypercalcemia of malignancy (early stages before renal calcinosis)
Primary hyperparathyroidism (about one-third of dogs with disorder)
Hypovitaminosis D
Respiratory alkalosis due to hyperventilation
Malabsorption or starvation
Canine Fanconi-like syndrome
Vitamin D intoxication
Following insulin administration in diabetics
Hypothermia

ELECTROLYTES

TABLE 3–7. SERUM ELECTROLYTE ABNORMALITIES

SODIUM

Causes of Hyponatremia

Gastrointestinal loss (vomiting, diarrhea)
Congestive heart failure (edema)
Hypoadrenocorticism (aldosterone deficiency)
Diuretic treatment
Syndrome of inappropriate antidiuretic hormone secretion (SIADH)
Administration of hypotonic fluid (e.g., 5% dextrose in water)
"Third space" loss (pancreatitis, peritonitis, uroperitoneum)
Diabetes mellitus
Renal disease (polyuric acute renal failure)
Persistent polyuria if water replaced but not electrolytes
Factitious

Causes of Hypernatremia

Increased insensible water loss (fever, high environmental temperature, hyperthermia)
Gastrointestinal loss (vomiting, diarrhea)
Renal failure (acute and chronic)
Diabetes insipidus
Diabetes mellitus (following insulin treatment)
Diuretic treatment
Polyuria without adequate water intake
Increased salt intake (with limited or no water intake) or intravenous administration
Administration of sodium-containing drugs (e.g., sodium bicarbonate, hypertonic saline)
Primary hyperaldosteronism (rare)
Artifact due to improper sample handling (allowing evaporation of water from serum)

POTASSIUM

Causes of Hypokalemia
Gastrointestinal loss (vomiting, diarrhea)
Intravenous administration of potassium-poor fluids
Bicarbonate therapy
Diuretic treatment
Hyperaldosteronism
Acute renal failure (polyuric phase)
Renal tubular acidosis
Chronic renal failure (especially cats)
Insulin treatment
Alkalosis (translocation)
Factitious (hyperlipidemia, improper sample handling)
Reduced dietary intake (rarely the sole cause)

Causes of Hyperkalemia
Hypoadrenocorticism
Renal failure (including urethral obstruction)
Diffuse cell death secondary to shock, circulatory stasis
Metabolic acidosis
Diabetic ketoacidosis (may be total body K deficit)
Uroperitoneum
Hemolysis (Akita and Sheba breeds)
Delayed separation of clotted blood (Akita and Sheba breeds, excessive leukocytosis or thrombocytosis)
Improper KCl administration
Collection in potassium heparin
Collection from IV tube when potassium administered
High doses of potassium penicillin G
Factitious

TABLE 3–8. GLUCOSE ABNORMALITIES

Causes of Hyperglycemia
Exertional—epinephrine (common in cats)
Diabetes mellitus
    Increased glucocorticoids (stress, hyperadrenocorticism, glucocorticoid or ACTH therapy)
    Acute pancreatitis
    Progesterone elevation (iatrogenic [megestrol acetate] or spontaneous diestrus)
    Excess growth hormone (acromegaly)
    Drug-induced—thiazide diuretics, morphine, intravenous fluids with glucose

Causes of Hypoglycemia
Delayed separation of serum from RBCs
Hepatic diseases
Hyperinsulinism (islet cell neoplasm or insulin therapy)
Extrapancreatic tumors
Idiopathic in toy breeds, puppies
Septicemia/endotoxemia
Endocrine hypofunction (hypopituitarism, hypoadrenocorticism)
Drug-induced (exogenous insulin, salicylates, ethylene glycol, ethanol)
Glycogen-storage disease
Starvation
Severe polycythemia

CHAPTER 4

ANOREXIA AND POLYPHAGIA
(pages 18–21)

Anorexia is loss of the appetite for food and is generally considered to be associated with illness. *Polyphagia* is excessive or voracious eating; it can be associated with disease or can be a physiologic response to increased energy demand.

HISTORICAL FINDINGS (pp. 18–19)

Anorexia from psychologic causes may be associated with *environmental changes* or *changing the diet*. Animals that do not eat because of oral or cranial pain or dysfunction may often *show an interest in food but cannot eat.* There may be a history of *trauma* or oral foreign bodies. Animals with trigeminal neuritis may attempt to eat with their tongues, yet *drop food.* The historical findings of animals with anorexia because of systemic disease will be variable and depend on the disease present. *Pain, vomiting, diarrhea, coughing,* and *dyspnea* may all be signs of diverse diseases that often lead to anorexia. A polyphagic animal that is *gaining weight* consumes more calories than needed. Drugs such as anticonvulsants or corticosteroids may lead to polyphagia with weight gain. Questioning about *drug therapy, dietary changes,* or *addition of pets* to the household is important. Polyphagia associated with *weight loss* leads to a negative nutrient balance. *Hyperthyroid* cats, animals with *diabetes mellitus,* and pancreatic exocrine insufficiency and ingestion of poor quality diet are all examples of polyphagia weight loss. Polyphagia with *no change in body condition* may be associated with a history of exposure to a *cold environment* or *increased exercise demands.*

PHYSICAL FINDINGS (pp. 19–20)

An animal that is willing but unable to eat because of pain or dysfunction of the mouth or head may resist and cry out when the clinician attempts to open the mouth for examination. Evidence of *dental disease* may be evident. Nasal pathology may be noted. *Exophthalmos* is seen with retrobulbar abscesses or tumors. Physical examination findings associated with *systemic diseases* causing anorexia are as varied as the potential causes of disease. Physical findings in animals with polyphagia and weight gain may include a typical Cushingoid appearance. Animals with *insulinoma* may show weakness, seizures, or disorientation. Weight loss in spite of polyphagia indicates a negative caloric balance. Animals with *malassimilation diseases* usually have a diarrheic stool.

DIAGNOSTIC PLAN (pp. 20–21)

Animals that are interested in food but unable to eat should receive a thorough *oral, dental,* and *cranial examination.* A minimum data base to include a (CBC), heartworm test, serum chemistry profile, and urinalysis may aid in the diagnosis of inflammatory, degenerative, endocrine, metabolic, neoplastic, or toxic disorders. Further diagnostic testing should be directed toward abnormalities already identified. The first thing to do with an animal that is polyphagic with weight loss in spite of an adequate diet is to rule out *parasitism.* If negative, a CBC,

---

Original chapter written by William E. Monroe

chemistry profile, and urinalysis should be done. The diagnostic plan for confirmation of causes of *polyphagia with weight gain* should include a minimum data base. The history may often identify most causes of *polyphagia with no change in body condition.*

GOALS OF TREATMENT

See textbook Chapter 4.

CHAPTER 5

PAIN
(pages 21–25)

Pain perception can be defined as the awareness or perception of a noxious stimulus that is potentially damaging to tissue. Such stimuli can be traumatic, chemical, mechanical, inflammatory, ischemic, or thermal (heat or cold).

GENERAL PATHOPHYSIOLOGY (pp. 21–22)

Two basic kinds of pain, superficial and deep, have been recognized. Superficial pain can be subdivided into pricking, bright, sharp, or fast pain (first pain). Deep pain can be subdivided into burning, aching, or slow pain (second pain). Pain mediators such as histamine, serotonin, prostaglandins, substance P, and complement are released during the course of the inflammatory process and the cause initiation and continuation of pain. The pain receptors use A delta and C fibers to transmit this information to the brain so that the organism knows that it hurts somewhere.

DIFFERENTIAL DIAGNOSIS OF PAIN (p. 23)

Traumatic causes of orthopedic pain include projectiles, intervertebral disc disease, cord contusion with dorsal route pain, and vertebral fracture or fracture dislocation. Congenital or genetic lesions include dens disease, C1-C2 subluxation, and cervical vertebral instability. Infection or inflammation includes discospondylitis, vertebral osteomyelitis, spondylitis, meningitis, and spinal arthritis. Neoplastic etiologies and dietary causes must be considered. Pain in the extremities involves a similar differential list. The differential diagnosis of abdominal pain must include trauma, projectiles, inflammation, pancreatitis, infection (peritonitis, hepatic abscess), ischemic disease, and passage of uretral or urethral calculi.

HISTORICAL FINDINGS AND THEIR MEANINGS

See textbook Chapter 5.

PHYSICAL FINDINGS AND THEIR INTERPRETATION
(pp. 23–24)

Original chapter written by Michael J. Kelly

Observation. A most important aspect for localization of pain is observation of the patient at rest and when walking. Reluctance to move the head and neck freely points to the cervical region. Roaching of the back and tucking of the abdomen muscles suggests abdominal or thoracolumbar disease.

Palpation. The single most important part of pain evaluation is palpation. Palpate each limb for periosteal pain (panostitis). Manipulate each joint gently, independent of all other joints. Palpate the shaft of all long bones for lumps and bumps. Painful areas that are warm relative to the surrounding tissue suggest cellulitis, abscess, or osteomyelitis. Feel for crepitation of the joints, laxity, and/or osteoarthritis. The lumbar sacral junction should be palpated for a clue suggesting cauda equina syndrome. Muscle masses should be palpated for cellulitis, abscess, or polymyositis. Palpation of the abdomen must be gentle yet firm. Feel for splinting and/or discomfort. Localize the area of pain. It is important to appreciate the phenomenon of referred pain, caused by excitation of nocioceptors at one site that is sensed as originating from another.

Neurologic Examination. Helps to localize the etiology of pain to the periphery, spinal cord, or skull.

Temperature. Elevated temperature suggests an inflammatory and/or infectious process.

GOALS OF TREATMENT (p. 25)

The goals of treatment are twofold; to bring about relief of pain and to restore function to the affected part or organ if possible. Both the narcotic analgesics and the narcotic antagonists are potent analgesics that increase pain tolerance greatly. The mild analgesics or NSAIDS elevate the pain threshold but have little effect on pain tolerance. Butorphanol tartrate has analgesic properties five times more potent than morphine It is beneficial for both somatic and visceral pain. However, butorphanol seems to reach a ceiling beyond which higher doses fail to increase the depression. A new drug to use in the control of pain secondary to arthritis is the chondroprotective drug Adequan, a polysulfated glycosaminoglycan. It not only alleviates pain, but actually assists in repairing the lesion. Acupuncture has been utilized in the treatment of pain. Its mechanism of action is best explained by the gate theory of pain.

CHAPTER 6

THERMOREGULATION, HYPOTHERMIA, HYPERTHERMIA
(pages 26–30)

Temperature is important to the speed of chemical reactions, and maintenance of normal-range body temperature is critical to the bioenergetics of survival. Thermoregulation is a balance between heat production and heat loss. The thermostatic center is located in the anterior hypothalamus. Immediate thermoregulation is exerted via the

Original chapter written by Steve C. Haskins

TABLE 6–1. CAUSES OF HYPOTHERMIA

Diminished heat production
    Anesthetic drug-induced depression of hypothalamic thermostatic mechanisms
    Anesthetic drug-induced depression of metabolism
    Diminished muscular activity from any cause
    Hypopituitarism, hypoadrenalism, myxedema
Enhanced heat loss
    Conduction
        Immersion in cold water or air
        Infusion of cold solutions
        Room temperature surgical scrub solutions
        Lying on cold, uninsulated surfaces
        Over-aggressive treatment of hyperthermia
    Convection
        Depilation
        Windy days or well-ventilated rooms
    Radiation
        Cold room or environment
        Induced vasodilation
    Evaporation
        Body surface-wetting solutions such as surgical scrub solutions, urine
        Open, exposed body cavities
Impaired thermoregulation
    Phenothiazines, dipyrone
    Organic CNS disease (trauma, neoplasia, edema)
    Endogenous "toxemia" from end-stage visceral organ failure

sympathetic nervous system, and delayed thermoregulation is regulated through the release of thyrotropin-releasing hormone, which causes the release of thyroid-stimulating hormone from the anterior pituitary. Both neuroendocrine mechanisms modulate metabolic rate and therefore heat production.

HYPOTHERMIA (pp. 26–29)

Hypothermia results when heat loss exceeds heat production (Table 6–1). In general, progressive hypothermia causes progressive depression of organ function (Table 6–2). The clinical implication of the inability of a critically ill animal to control its body temperature is impaired hypothalamic function. It is an indication of serious intracranial or extracranial disease. Mild degrees of hypothermia are not, per se, harmful to the patient, and aggressive rewarming techniques are not necessary. Moderate to severe hypothermia may be a component of any emergency presentation or may have been intentionally induced to prolong brain tolerance to intentional cardiac arrest for intracardiac surgery.

Passive rewarming (minimize further heat loss and allow the patient to warm itself metabolically) is only effective in mild to moderate hypothermia (above about 30°C [86°F]) when the patient is capable of metabolic or shivering thermogenesis (Table 6–3). External active rewarming is necessary in moderate to severe hypothermia and is the method most commonly used in hypothermic animals. There are hazards to these techniques. Surface warming may decrease the thermogenesis response. Surface warming may lead to excessive hypotension (see Chap. 6). The greater the hypothermia and the longer its duration, the greater the danger of surface rewarming. The rewarming rate should be limited to less than 1°C (2°F) per hour. Hot water bottles and electric heating blankets are dangerous in that they can burn the skin if they are too hot. Active core rewarming techniques minimize the potential for vascular collapse associated with surface rewarming tech-

TABLE 6-2. CLINICAL IMPORTANCE OF VARIOUS LEVELS OF HYPOTHERMIA

TEMPERATURE		
Centigrade	*Fahrenheit*	**CLINICAL IMPORTANCE**
Above 36	Above 96	Minimal detrimental effect
		Shivering thermogenesis increased
		Nonshivering thermogenesis increased
32 to 34	90 to 94	Cerebral obtundation and reduced anesthetic requirements
		Anesthetic recovery may be prolonged
		Shivering thermogenesis impaired and artificial rewarming may be necessary
28 to 30	82 to 86	Marked obtundation; little or no anesthetic required
		Shivering thermogenesis nonexistent
		Artificial rewarming necessary
		Atrial arrhythmias
25 to 26	77 to 80	Cold-induced ECG changes: prolonged PR interval and widened QRS
		Increased myocardial automaticity
		Inadequate oxygen delivery; lactic acidosis; rewarming acidemia
		Absent reflexes and pain response
		Increased blood viscosity; microcirculatory sludging
22 to 23	72 to 74	Autonomic and endocrine thermogenesis mechanisms are inactive
		Spontaneous ventilation ceases
		Ventricular fibrillation likely
		Coagulation disorders
Below 20	Below 68	EEG silence
		Asystole

TABLE 6–3. TREATMENT OF HYPOTHERMIA

Minimize further conductive, convective, radiant, and evaporative heat loss (passive rewarming)
    Dry the body surface
    Wrap patient in blankets, towels, drapes, or "space blanket"
    Insulate from cold table surface and room objects
Active surface rewarming
    Circulating warm-water blanket
    Infrared heat lamps (75 cm)
    Infant radiant heat warmers
    Surgical lamps
    Warm water baths
    Forced-air hair dryers
    Electric floor heaters
    Hot water bottle–heat tent (avoid contact with skin)
    Electric blanket (avoid contact with the skin)
Active core rewarming
    Warmed intravenous fluids
    Warmed, humidified inspired air
    Flushing the open body cavity with warm, sterile, isotonic, polyionic fluids
    Peritoneal dialysis
    Flushing the stomach or rectum with warm isotonic, polyionic fluids
    Extracorporeal techniques

niques. The efficacy of the intravenous administration of warmed fluids is limited by the volume of fluid that can safely be administered. The breathing of heated, humidified air is a recommended field resuscitation technique in human beings. Moderate to severe hypothermia, particularly if it has existed for some time, may necessitate additional considerations. The electrocardiogram, blood electrolytes and glucose, coagulation, cardiovascular function, and renal function should be assessed.

HYPERTHERMIA (pp. 29–30)

Hyperthermia results when heat production exceeds heat loss (Table 6–4). Fever, as opposed to heat exhaustion/stroke, is associated with an elevated hypothalamic set-point. The endogenous pyrogen is the monokine interleukin-1 from monocytes. Appropriate fevers should not be treated per se; effective management of the underlying infection allows the fever to subside.

Heat stroke is associated with marked elevations in body temperature; control of body temperature is lost. Cell damage starts to occur at (108°F). *Malignant hyperthermia* is a rapid, often relentless, progressive increase in body temperature associated with the metabolic heat

TABLE 6–4. CAUSES OF HYPERTHERMIA

Fever—interleukin-1 released from monocytes following tissue injury, infection, allergic reactions
Factors that inhibit heat losing ability
  Severe cardiac disease
  Dehydration
  Drugs which inhibit skin vasodilation
    Phenothiazines; antihistamines
    Alcohol
  Hot environment
  Humid environment
  Individual tolerance
    Minimized by extremes of age
  Obesity
Excessive environmental temperatures
  Simple exposure
  Enclosed automobile
  In-hospital
    Large dogs in small cages with poor ventilation and high humidity
Intraoperative hyperthermia secondary to light anesthesia (high metabolic activity), in large dogs, heavily draped and insulated, and breathing a fully humidified gas
Excessive muscular activity
  Exercise (field trials)
  Anxiety
    Particularly in dogs with partial upper airway obstructions
  Exaggerated breathing effort
  Seizures
Transient rebound hyperthermia following a hypothermic episode
Dehydration is associated with vasoconstriction (diminishes skin temperature) and may interfere with hypothalamic function
"Unknown origin"
Organic hypothalamic disease
Malignant hyperthermia
  Anesthetic agent or neuromuscular blocking agent–induced
  Emotional or physical stress in predisposed humans
  Neuroleptic syndrome (humans receiving long-term phenothiazines)

TABLE 6–5. TREATMENT OF HYPERTHERMIA

Large-dose crystalloid fluid infusion
Oxygen
Surface cooling techniques
    Fan
    Water (preferably cool, not cold)
    Alcohol
    Ice packs placed over large-vessel areas (neck, axilla, inguinal region)
    Whole-body ice water baths
    Combinations
Antipyretic drugs
    Antiprostaglandins
    Dipyrone
    Aminopyrine
    Dantrolene
Internal cooling techniques
    Cold/iced isotonic, polyionic crystalloids
    Intravenous
    Rectal
    Gastric lavage
    Open body cavity
    Peritoneal dialysis
    Extracorporeal techniques
For moderate to severe hyperthermia, check and recheck all major organ systems; support as necessary. Remove offending agent and administer dantrolene for drug-induced malignant hyperthermia.

production due to disturbed intracellular calcium metabolism. The exact mechanism is unknown. Dantrolene is the specific and highly effective treatment for this syndrome.

Severe hyperthermia causes multiple organ dysfunction and failure: renal failure, hepatic failure, gastrointestinal failure, disseminated intravascular coagulation, hypoxemia, metabolic acidosis, hyperkalemia, myocardial failure, skeletal muscle cytolysis, tachycardia and hypotension, tachypnea and hyperventilation, and cerebral edema. Exertional heat stroke may be associated with widespread rhabdomyolysis, hyperkalemia, myoglobinemia/-uria, and markedly elevated plasma levels of CPK.

Mild hyperthermia (less than 40°C or 104°F) does not normally require treatment. Effective treatment of the underlying disease process should suffice. More severe hyperthermia (temperatures in excess of 106°F) should be treated aggressively (Table 6–5). External and internal cooling techniques should be implemented. The more severe the hyperthermia, the more aggressive the cooling techniques should be. Surface cooling techniques with ice water may impede heat loss via the skin radiator system. The most effective core cooling in humans is achieved by wetting the patient with cool (but not cold) water and keeping convection currents high with a fan. Aggressive cooling should be terminated when the core temperature is still somewhat above the desired end-point.

CHAPTER 7

VAGINAL AND PREPUTIAL DISCHARGE
(pages 31–37)

VAGINAL DISCHARGE (pp. 31–34)

The presence of any vaginal discharge requires a thorough gynecologic or obstetric examination, with special emphasis on vaginoscopy. The appearance of the vaginal discharge and inspection of the abdomen provide the initial assessment of physiologic or pathologic conditions that may underlie the discharge. The vaginal discharge is collected on a white cotton swab and examined for color and consistency. Vaginoscopic inspection provides patterns so characteristic of the different physiologic and pathologic conditions that, in most cases, an immediate diagnosis can be made (Table 7–1). At the same time, specific cytologic and bacteriologic sampling from the cranial part of the vagina can be performed through the scope under direct vision. The most important findings are summarized in Table 7–2. Confirmation, modification, or refutation of the clinical diagnosis will require laboratory studies (hematology, endocrinology, serology, and chromosome examination) as well as x-ray and/or ultrasonography.

TABLE 7–1. INSPECTION OF THE VAGINA AND CERVIX IN THE NONPREGNANT FEMALE ANIMAL

PHYSIOLOGIC OR PATHOLOGIC STATE	VAGINOSCOPIC FINDINGS
Anestrus Postpartum period	Color: rosy pink; no mucosal profile; dorsal vaginal fold
Proestrus	Color: pale pink; high-grade edema; deep folds; bloody discharge
Estrus	Color: anemic; shrivelled mucosa; pale serosanguineous discharge
Metestrus Closed pyometra	Color: rosy pink; longitudinal folds; greyish white discharge
Open pyometra	Color: pale pink, cyanotic; no mucosal profile; brown-red or greyish green-yellow discharge
Acute endometritis	Color of cervix: red; color of vagina: rosy pink; longitudinal folds; greyish green-yellow discharge
Subestrus	Color: pale pink; low-grade edema; small folds; bloody discharge
Prolonged proestrus Granulosa cell tumor	Color: anemic; constricted vaginal lumen; bloody discharge
Urovagina	Color: red; vestibule and vagina tilted cranioventrally; pond-like accumulation of clear watery liquid in cranial vagina
Mating injury	Color: anemic; red wound; ligament of urinary bladder visible; mesometrium visible; bloody discharge
Foreign body	Color: rosy pink; grey-green yellow discharge

Original chapter written by Hans-Klaus Dreier

TABLE 7-2. CELL CONTENT OF VAGINAL SMEAR UNDER SOME IMPORTANT PHYSIOLOGIC AND PATHOLOGIC CONDITIONS

	BC	PBC	IMC	SFC	AC	RBC	WBC	BAC	CD	MUC	BAS	ACI	DIS	SP
Anestrus	+	+	+	–	–	–	+	–	–	(+)	+	–	–	–
Proestrus, early	–	+	+	+	–	+	(+)	–	–	(+)	+	–	–	–
Proestrus, late	–	–	(+)	+	+	+	–	(+)	(+)	–	–	+	–	(+)
Estrus	–	–	–	+	+	(+)	–	(+)	(+)	–	–	+	–	(+)
Mesestrus	+	+	+	–	–	–	+	–	–	+	+	–	–	(+)
Pregnancy	+	+	+	–	–	–	+	–	–	+	+	–	–	–
Pyometra, closed	+	+	+	–	–	–	+	–	–	+	+	–	–	–

BC = basal cells; PBC = parabasal cells; IMC = intermediate cells; SFC = superficial cells; AC = anuclear cells; RBC = red blood cells; WBC = white blood cells; BAC = bacteria; CD = cell detritus; MUC = mucus; BAS = basophilic cells; ACI = acidophilic cells; DIS = discolored cells; SP = sperms.
+ = present; (+) = sometimes present; – = absent.

22

PREPUTIAL DISCHARGE (pp. 34–37)

Small amounts of greyish white or greyish yellow preputial discharge are normal in the dog. Excessive preputial discharge is found in connection with balanoposthitis, irritation by hypersexual behavior, prostatic hypertrophy, prostatitis, trauma and injuries, inflammation by foreign bodies, tumors of the penis, and feminine pseudohermaphroditism. The examination should begin with an inspection of the prepuce and its surroundings for remnants of the discharge, hypoplasia and edema of the prepuce, and swellings of the penis. Edema of the prepuce points to traumatic or inflammatory causes; a nonedematous prepuce relates the discharge to prostatic hypertrophy, prostatitis, balanoposthitis, or a tumor of the penis. After retraction of the prepuce using caution to identify impediments such as adhesions, phimosis, paraphimosis, or a persistent frenulum, the color of the discharge, the glans penis, and preputial mucosa can be evaluated. Rectal palpation of the prostate allows for differentiation between prostatitis and hypertrophy. These diagnoses should be complemented by x-ray and ultrasound examinations as well as hematologic, cytologic, microbiologic, endocrinologic, and serologic examinations.

CHAPTER 8
FAILURE TO GROW
(pages 37–40)

When an animal does not increase in size at the normal rate or to a normal extent, a "failure to grow" is identified. Determination of normal growth is sometimes difficult, because breed sizes vary and mixed breed pets predominate.

HISTORY (pp. 37–38)

The owner of the dog or cat should be questioned as to the size of the pet's parents and littermates, if known.

Duration of the Problem. Congenital defects should be strongly considered when growth has been slow since birth. Acquired disorders must be considered when growth suddenly stops.

Diet. A less palatable or poor-quality diet may not be eaten well by the animal or may be poorly utilized. An owner may be underfeeding the animal.

Concurrent Clinical Signs. Vomiting or regurgitation suggests a gastrointestinal problem or systemic illness, as may diarrhea or voluminous stools. Polyuria, seizures, or exercise intolerance or syncope may add further pertinent information. Administration of glucocorticoids may have slowed the pet's growth.

PHYSICAL FINDINGS (p. 38)

A short animal with a poor body condition is more likely to have a nutritional, nonhormonal, or cardiac abnormality, whereas a short ani-

---

Original chapter written by Sherri L. Ihle

TABLE 8–1. CAUSES OF GROWTH FAILURE IN
DOGS AND CATS

Small size and poor body condition
Dietary problem
  Underfeeding
  Poor-quality diet
Cardiac disorder
  Congenital anomaly
  Endocarditis
Hepatic dysfunction
  Portosystemic vascular anomaly
  Hepatitis
  Glycogen storage disease
Esophageal disease
  Megaesophagus
  Vascular ring anomaly (e.g., persistent right aortic arch)
Gastrointestinal disease
  Parasites
  Inflammatory bowel disease
  Obstruction (e.g., foreign body, intussusception, stricture)
  Histoplasmosis
  Exocrine pancreatic insufficiency
Renal disease
  Renal failure (congenital or acquired)
  Glomerular disease
  Pyelonephritis
Inflammatory disease
Diabetes mellitus

Small size and good body condition
Hypothyroidism
Hyperadrenocorticism
Growth hormone deficiency
Chondrodystrophy

mal with a good body condition is likely to have an hormonal problem
or be chondrodysplastic (Table 8–1). Alopecia or the prolonged presence of a soft puppy haircoat suggests a thyroid or growth hormone
deficiency. Mental dullness can be seen with hypothyroidism, hepatic
encephalopathy, or hydrocephalus.

DIAGNOSTIC PLAN (pp. 38–40)

A brief *feeding trial* can provide information on appetite and caloric
consumption. Multiple *fecal examinations* and possible deworming
should be performed. A *complete blood count* should be evaluated, as
should a *serum biochemical* profile and urinalysis. *Radiographs* may
detect a cardiopulmonary abnormality, organomegaly, small liver or
kidneys, or intestinal foreign body. *Ultrasonography,* an *electrocardiogram, contrast radiographic studies, hepatic function tests, gastrointestinal function tests, biopsy,* or *hormonal assays* can be used to detect
various disease states that may impact growth.

TREATMENT (p. 40)

Treatment varies widely based on the underlying pathology. The
reader is referred to specific sections of the text for complete discussions.

CHAPTER 9
HYPONATREMIA AND HYPOKALEMIA
(pages 40–45)

The sodium (Na) ion is found predominantly in the extracellular fluid (ECF), while the potassium (K) ion is primarily intracellular. In a normal animal the serum Na concentration is approximately 142 to 155 mEq/L and the K concentration is 4 to 5.5 mEq/L. These concentrations are maintained by an (Na-K ATPase) located in the cellular membrane.

HYPONATREMIA (pp. 41–42)

Hypo-osmolar Hyponatremia

Effective Circulating Volume Depletion. The most common cause of hyponatremia in small animal patients is solute loss and volume depletion due to vomiting and diarrhea. Other causes include third space loss (tube drainage, hemorrhage), renal loss (diuretics, hypoadrenocorticism, renal disease), and skin loss. Hyponatremia and hypoosmolality occur if losses are replaced with a hypotonic fluid such as water, and hyponatremia will persist if the ability of the kidneys to excrete free water is diminished. Decreased delivery of solute to the distal renal tubule, volume depletion, and ADH release may occur in renal disease when the GFR decreases to low levels or if additional solute is lost. Hyponatremia may also occur during diuretic therapy due to similar mechanisms. Hyponatremia is common in hypoadrenocorticism. Aldosterone deficiency allows renal Na loss, volume depletion, ADH release, and stimulation of thirst. Hyponatremia is exacerbated by vomiting and diarrhea. Inadequate tissue perfusion occurs in many hypervolemic disease states such as congestive heart failure, severe liver disease, nephrotic syndrome, and oliguric renal failure. These diseases cause activation of the renin-angiotensin system, ADH release, and Na retention. Hyponatremia may develop despite an increased total body Na content.

Inappropriate ADH Secretion. The syndrome of inappropriate ADH secretion (SIADH) is characterized by ADH secretion in the absence of normal osmotic or nonosmotic stimuli. SIADH is rare in small animals but has been reported in dogs with dirofilariasis and hypothalamic neoplasia (see textbook Chap. 9).

Primary (Psychogenic) Polydipsia. If water intake is extremely excessive, the kidneys' ability to excrete free water may be overwhelmed, and a potentially fatal hyponatremia can develop.

Hyperosmolar Hyponatremia

This occurs with severe hyperglycemia and the administration of hypertonic solutions such as mannitol.

Euosmolar Hyponatremia

Serum Na concentration may be artifactually decreased by the presence of severe hyperlipidemia or hyperproteinemia.

Original chapter written by J. Catharine R. Scott-Moncrieff

DIAGNOSIS OF HYPONATREMIA

The cause of hyponatremia can usually be established by documenting resolution of hyponatremia after hydration is normalized and/or the primary disease state is resolved or controlled. Measurement of serum osmolality is required to establish a diagnosis of SIADH. The diagnosis of hypoadrenocorticism requires an ACTH stimulation test.

Severe hyponatremia (<120 mEq/L) may be associated with severe progressive central nervous system dysfunction and weakness due to cerebral overhydration and edema.

TREATMENT PRINCIPLES

If volume depletion is present, the fluid of choice for volume replacement is usually isotonic saline. In severe hyponatremia careful administration of 3 per cent hypertonic saline may be necessary. In patients with hyponatremia due to edematous states, dietary Na restriction and diuretic therapy should be considered. In general, better control of the underlying disease will correct the electrolyte abnormality.

HYPOKALEMIA (pp. 42–45)

CAUSES OF HYPOKALEMIA

Decreased intake alone is an unlikely cause of hypokalemia, but it may be an important contributory cause in debilitated or anorexic animals. Diets deficient in K and high in protein and acid content have been shown to cause hypokalemic nephropathy in cats. Gastrointestinal loss due to vomiting or diarrhea is the most common cause of hypokalemia in dogs and cats.

Transcellular Shifts. Exogenous insulin administration can cause hypokalemia during the initial management of patients with diabetic ketoacidosis. Administration of insulin drives K into cells and unmasks hypokalemia. Catecholamine release or administration of β_2 agonists may also acutely lower serum K concentrations. Alkalosis causes hypokalemia due to movement of K ions intracellularly, whereas acute acidosis causes hyperkalemia due to the reverse effect. However, chronic acidosis causes hypokalemia. Iatrogenic causes include administration of parenteral nutrition solutions, peritoneal dialysis with K-free dialysates, and administration of bicarbonate.

Renal Loss. Causes of hypokalemia due to renal loss in dogs and cats include chronic renal failure and renal tubular acidosis (RTA). Hypokalemia has been reported to occur in 30 per cent of cats with renal disease, but only 10 per cent of dogs. In distal RTA, K loss is caused by increased aldosterone secretion and is usually present before treatment. In proximal RTA, hypokalemia develops during treatment with Na bicarbonate. Additional causes include postobstructive diuresis and loop and thiazide diuretics.

CLINICAL CONSEQUENCES OF HYPOKALEMIA

Clinical signs do not develop until the serum K concentration decreases below 3.0 mEq/L. The clinical consequences relate primarily to the neuromuscular and cardiovascular systems. Profound skeletal muscle weakness, decreased myocardial contractility, decreased cardiac output, and cardiac arrhythmias may occur. Ventroflexion of the neck, forelimb hypermetria, and a broad-based hindlimb stance may be observed. In severe hypokalemia, respiratory paralysis can occur. Characteristic ECG changes include decreased amplitude of the T wave, ST segment depression, U waves, and supraventricular and ventricular arrhythmias. Hypokalemia potentiates digitalis toxicity. Other metabolic effects include hypokalemic nephropathy, metabolic acidosis, and impaired urinary concentration.

DIAGNOSTIC APPROACH TO HYPOKALEMIA

See textbook Chapter 9.

TREATMENT PRINCIPLES

Oral supplementation with potassium gluconate is preferable, if possible, since IV supplementation may initially worsen hypokalemia owing to dilution, increased renal distal flow, and cellular uptake of potassium. Potassium chloride is the supplement of choice for IV supplementation. Potassium chloride should not be administered at rates greater than 0.5 mEq/kg/hour, except in cases of severe life-threatening hypokalemia. Oral K supplementation should be initiated as soon as possible.

CHAPTER 10

HYPERKALEMIA AND HYPERNATREMIA
(pages 46–49)

Hyperkalemia is defined as a serum potassium concentration exceeding 5.5 mEq/L.

CAUSES (Table 10–1)

TABLE 10–1. CAUSES OF HYPERKALEMIA

Pseudohyperkalemia
　　*Hemolyzed blood sample, especially in the Akita dog
　　*Thrombocytosis
　　Extreme leukocytosis

Redistribution of potassium
　　*Metabolic and respiratory acidosis
　　Hypertonic solutions
　　Hyperkalemic periodic paralysis (very rare)
　　Drugs
　　Prostaglandin inhibitors
　　Beta-blocking agents
　　Succinylcholine

Potassium loading
　　Endogenous
　　Hemolysis (rare in the dog and cat)
　　Rhabdomyolysis (rare without renal failure)
　　Exogenous
　　*Potassium salts

Reduced potassium excretion
　　*Acute renal failure (oliguric, anuric)
　　*Hypoadrenocorticism
　　Drugs
　　　　Potassium-sparing diuretics
　　　　Converting enzyme inhibitors
　　　　　　Nonsteroidal anti-inflammatory agents

*Denotes more common causes in the dog and cat.

Original chapter written by Michael Schaer

Oliguria, Anuria, and Urinary Outflow Obstructions. Since the kidney is the main route for potassium excretion from the body, one should anticipate the occurrence of hyperkalemia in these cases.

Adrenocortical Insufficiency. Hyperkalemia will follow when enough destruction of the adrenal zona glomerulosa occurs to cause a major depletion of aldosterone.

Acidosis. This tendency is usually restricted to conditions in which inorganic ion accumulations associated with metabolic acidosis are the main cause.

EFFECTS ON THE PATIENT

Physical Examination Findings. Skeletal muscle weakness is typically diffuse. Hyperkalemic dogs may have bradycardia and palpably weak pulses. Cardiac arrest can occur in advanced stages.

Electrocardiographic Changes. Typical progressive alterations include peaking or depression of the T wave, decreased R-wave and P-wave amplitudes, increased duration of the P wave, prolongation of the PR interval, eventual disappearance of the P wave, widening of the QRS complex, and sine wave-type QRS complexes. When the serum potassium concentration exceeds 8 to 9 mEq/L, impaired conduction can result in heart block, idioventricular complexes, ventricular escape beats, and eventually ventricular fibrillation or asystole.

DIAGNOSIS

An attempt to identify hyperkalemia in any dog or cat should be prompted by the clinical presentation.

Goals in treatment should be aimed at correcting the underlying disorder as well as the immediate reversal of myocardial alterations. If the ECG is normal, treatment with intravenous isotonic saline solution will be sufficient. In more urgent situations additional treatment measures (Table 10–2) may be necessary.

Hypernatremia is defined as a serum sodium concentration exceeding 155 mEq per liter. Hypernatremia will occur most often when hypotonic fluid losses occur in combination with a disturbance in water intake. Hypernatremia can be categorized as hypovolemic, isovolemic, and hypervolemic types (Table 10–3). Extrarenal loss of hypotonic fluid occurs most frequently due to diarrhea and osmotic diuresis due to mannitol, glucose, or urea. Loss of free water without loss of electrolytes such as sodium, as seen in diabetes insipidus (DI), does not result in severe plasma volume contraction unless oral intake of water is restricted. Continued diuresis in the absence of water intake will lead to severe hypernatremia, plasma volume contraction, hypotension, renal ischemia, and renal shutdown. Hypernatremia associated with

TABLE 10–2. PRINCIPLES OF TREATING HYPERKALEMIA

OBJECTIVE	METHOD
1. Enhance potassium excretion	a. Relieve any urinary tract obstruction
	b. Intravenous isotonic saline
	c. Cation exchange resin
	d. Peritoneal dialysis
2. Intercompartmental transfer	a. Intravenous sodium bicarbonate
	b. Intravenous insulin and glucose combination
3. Counteract myocardial cell membrane toxicity	Intravenous 10% calcium gluconate

TABLE 10–3. CAUSES OF HYPERNATREMIA

HYPERNATREMIA ASSOCIATED WITH WATER LOSS	HYPERNATREMIA ASSOCIATED WITH SALT GAIN
Pure Water Loss	*Water Loss with High Urine Sodium*
Normal total body Na$^+$ and normal ECF volume	Increased total body Na$^+$ and increased ECF volume
Pituitary diabetes insipidus	Increased salt intake
Nephrogenic diabetes insipidus	Dietary
Heat stroke	Sea water
Fever	Saline emetics
Inadequate access to water (CNS disease, infirmity)	IV hypertonic fluids
Burns	IV sodium bicarbonate
	Hyperaldosteronism
Hypotonic Water Loss	Hyperadrenocorticism
Decreased total body Na$^+$ and decreased ECF volume	
Diarrhea	
Vomiting	
Oral hyperalimentation	
Osmotic diuresis	
Acute renal failure	
Chronic renal failure	
Diabetes mellitus	
Diuretic use	
IV solute administration (mannitol, glucose, urea)	

Abbreviations: ECF = extracellular fluid; IV = intravenous.
Modified from Hardy R.M.: Hypernatremia. Vet Clin North Am 19:231–239, 1989.

excess sodium intake is usually iatrogenic. In essential hypernatremia, there is a failure of the osmoreceptors to respond appropriately to an increase in serum osmolality; however, there is usually an adequate ADH response to hypovolemia. These patients are adipsic.

EFFECTS ON THE PATIENT

The main sequel is the formation of a hypertonic extracellular fluid environment.

In the brain, shrinkage of cells causes tearing of fine meningeal vessels, resulting in subarachnoid and subcortical hemorrhages. Clinical signs include restlessness, irritability, lethargy, muscular twitching, spasticity, seizures, coma, and death. When the onset of hypertonicity is more gradual, the brain attempts to counteract the osmotic disequilibrium by forming "idiogenic" osmols. This compensatory mechanism is of limited benefit. Hypernatremia caused by sodium loading causes extracellular fluid overload and can result in pulmonary edema due to congestive heart failure.

DIAGNOSIS

The presence or absence of normal skin turgor will vary with the cause. The water-deprived patient with DI retains normal skin turgor until the advanced stages of water depletion.

The animal with essential hypernatremia has gradual-onset hypernatremia and typically has normal skin turgor. Hypernatremia is diagnosed by laboratory sodium quantitation. Serum osmolality (normal, 290 to 310 mOsm/L) can be calculated using the formula:

$$2 \frac{(Na^+ + K^+)}{\text{in mEq/L}} + \frac{\text{Glucose (mg/dl)}}{18} + \frac{\text{BUN (mg/dl)}}{2.8}$$

GOALS IN TREATMENT

When the patient has hypovolemia, isotonic sodium chloride solution should be given until hemodynamic stability is restored. In the patient with central diabetes insipidus, aqueous ADH should be given. Seizure control can be accomplished traditionally. The comatose patient requires meticulous care. Hypernatremia caused by excessive sodium intake should be treated with furosemide. Essential hypernatremia patients require extra water added to their food.

CHAPTER 11
WEAKNESS AND SYNCOPE
(pages 50–57)

WEAKNESS (pp. 50–54)

Lassitude and *fatigue* both refer to a lack of energy. *Lethargy* identifies a state of drowsiness, inactivity, or indifference in which there are delayed responses to external (auditory, visual, or tactile) stimuli. Generalized muscular weakness, or *asthenia,* refers to a true loss of strength. *Syncope,* or fainting, refers to a sudden, transient loss of consciousness due to a deprivation of either oxygen or glucose that briefly impairs cerebral metabolism.

Physical examination may, in itself, identify the cause of the weakness (see textbook Chap. 11).

Laboratory Tests. At a minimum, an animal with signs of weakness or syncope should have a complete blood count, a blood sugar analysis, and a blood urea nitrogen or serum creatinine determination, and the blood electrolytes (sodium, chloride, and potassium) and plasma carbon dioxide levels. A complete urinalysis is also indicated. If the problem warrants additional study, complete serum chemistry profiles, thyroid profiles, radiographs of the abdomen and thorax, and electrocardiography may be run. More specialized laboratory techniques may be indicated.

Anemia. Acutely, syncope is a more likely clinical finding than weakness. Long-standing anemia is associated with chronic weakness. Anemia in the dog usually does not present as weakness until the hematocrit levels are less than 22 to 25 per cent and in the cat 10 or 15 per cent.

Ascites. The reader is referred to Chapter 14 of the textbook.

Cardiovascular Signs. Syncope may be the result of an acute decrease in cardiac output. In more chronic states, both cardiac wasting and weakness can develop. Cardiac rhythm disturbance, bacterial endocarditis, pericardial effusion, valvular heart diseases and congeni-

---

Original chapter written by Stephen J. Ettinger and Kirstie A. Barrett

tal heart diseases, cardiomyopathies, heartworm disease, and causes of pulmonary hypertension must be considered in the diagnosis.

Chronic Inflammation or Infection. Chronic diseases of the liver, pancreas, prostate, skin, oral cavity, pulmonary, anal glands, ears, joints, bones, and muscles all include weakness as a primary sign. It is virtually impossible to describe all the clinical signs that may be associated with this category of disease.

Chronic Wasting. Diseases of the liver terminating in cirrhosis, cardiac cachexia, renal disease, chronic gastrointestinal diseases, and chronic cutaneous disease are examples.

Drug-Related Weaknesses. Chronic low-level organophosphate and carbamate toxicity, barbiturates, antidiarrheals with sedatives, anticonvulant preparations, antihistamines, tranquilizers, antibiotics, diuretic agents, vasodilators, antiarrhythmic preparations, and digitalis are examples.

Electrolyte Disorders. *Hyperkalemia* is associated with listlessness, severe asthenia, and bradycardia. Potassium wasting resulting in *hypokalemia* is an important weakness syndrome in dogs and cats. *Hyponatremia* and *hypernatremia* are important electrolyte disturbances responsible for asthenic states. *Hypocalcemia* is associated with the clinical signs of nervous excitability, tetany, and, in severe cases, convulsive seizures. Weakness is observed between periods of hyperexcitability. *Hypercalcemic states* may result in signs that are variable, but include depression, muscle weakness, and arrhythmias.

Endocrine Disturbances. Cushing's syndrome, hypothyroid disease, hypoadrenocortical activity, hypoglycemia, hyperparathyroidism, hypoparathyroidism, the inappropriate secretion of antidiuretic hormone, and diabetes mellitus are examples.

Fever. See textbook Chapter 6.

Metabolic Dysfunction States. Endocrine diseases, chronic infections and chronic wasting problems, nutritional disorders, and primary or secondary dyslipoproteinemia are examples.

Neoplastic diseases are frequently associated with episodic weakness resulting from an invasive, destructive, or obstructive mass. Chronic unidentified weakness is a cause for a thorough "tumor search" in any patient.

Neurologic Disorders. Infections within the brain or spinal canal, space-occupying lesions such as neoplasia, or granulomas, injury or trauma to the brain or peripheral nerves, vascular accidents, epilepsy, central or peripheral vestibulitis, instability of the atlanto-occipital or atlantoaxial joint are examples.

Polyneuropathies and Neuromuscular Diseases. Tick paralysis, coonhound paralysis, botulism, heavy metals, avitaminoses, and lupus erythematosus and periarteritis are examples. Myasthenia gravis, polymyositis, and muscular dystrophy-like diseases are further examples.

Nutritional Disorders. Long-term nutritional deficiencies may result in generalized weakness. An owner's overindulgence may result in increased body weight and obesity. Poorly designed diets may be incomplete or may simply provide poor-quality nutrients (e.g., taurine, potassium, and others). If underfed, hunting or working dogs exhibit a starvation-like syndrome.

Overactivity, Overwork, and Psychological Factors. These may occur in animals being used for excessive racing or hunting, in those animals who are being deprived of normal rest, and in those animals being stressed by owners with excessive expectations. Pseudocyesis is associated with weakness. Aging pets with blindness, deafness, or senility may present with weakness.

Pulmonary Diseases. Pulmonary emboli, chronic coughing and chronic pulmonary infection, heartworm disease, and laryngeal paralysis are examples.

SYNCOPE (pp. 54–57)

Syncope refers to a sudden, yet transient, loss of consciousness due to a deprivation of energy substrate, either oxygen or glucose, that briefly impairs the cerebral metabolism. Syncope develops with generalized muscle weakness, progressing rapidly to ataxia, which may be followed by collapse and a brief period of loss of consciousness. Initially, the patient is motionless, but this may progress to uncoordinated muscular activity, giving the impression of seizure-like activity. Recovery is usually rapid and complete.

Clinical Summary. With a complete history and physical examination, most cases of syncope can be identified without further study. An electrocardiogram and simple blood chemical analyses are usually all that are required.

Syncope in a Normal Heart but with Peripheral Vascular Dysfunction. Neurocardiogenic (vasovagal or vasodepressor) syncope is associated with a sudden incident of either fright or extreme excitement. Cardiac output fails to rise despite a decrease in peripheral resistance, and vagal overactivity results in bradycardia. Postural hypotension patients develop a fall in both systolic and diastolic pressures with variable changes in the heart rate upon rising. Postural hypotension can be a complication of a number of disease entities and drug therapy. The hyperventilation syndrome is usually associated with anxious or hyperexcitable pets (see Chap. 12).

Carotid sinus sensitivity results in a chain of events that can cause vertigo, lightheadedness, and syncope. This syndrome is observed in cases where neoplasms, inflammatory processes, or tight collars stimulate the carotid sinuses. Glossopharyngeal neuralgia, deglutition syncope, and postmicturition syncope are infrequently recognized.

Syncope Due to Cardiac Dysfunction. Subvalvular and valvular aortic stenosis are associated with syncope and a high incidence of sudden death. Animals with severe pulmonic stenosis with or without right-to-left shunts may similarly (but less commonly) suffer syncope upon exertion. Atrial tumors, dirofilariasis, and ball valve thrombi are examples of obstructive cardiac disease. Cardiac tamponade, pericardial effusion, restrictive pericarditis, and obstructive cardiomyopathy in dogs and cats are further examples. Rhythm disturbances causing syncope may include bundle branch block irregularities as well as the bradyarrhythmias and tachyarrhythmias. In cardiopulmonary dysfunction, syncopal episodes usually occur with physical exertion or shortly thereafter. The duration of unconsciousness varies but is usually brief (1 to 2 minutes). Cyanosis is often present.

Metabolic Disturbances Associated with Syncope. Hypoglycemic coma, hyperventilation states, calcium imbalances, and renal dysfunction are examples.

Iatrogenic Causes of Syncope. Digitalis intoxication, potent diuretics, phenothiazine derivatives, nitroglycerin, propranolol, ACE inhibitors, and quinidine are examples.

Miscellaneous Causes. *Tussive syncope* is the result of an alteration in the normal circulation. Pulseless disease occurs with major obstructions to one or more major vessels supplying the head.

CHAPTER 12
COUGHING
(pages 57–60)

Coughing is an expiratory effort producing a sudden, noisy expulsion of air from the lungs, usually in an effort to free the lungs of foreign material (real or imagined). *Respiratory distress* is a general term referring to difficulty, or a change for the worse, in breathing habits. The coughing reflex is the result of mechanical or chemical irritation of the pharynx, larynx, tracheobronchial tree, and some of the smaller airways. Occasionally, pathology of the pleura, pericardium, diaphragm, nose, and nasal sinuses may cause coughing.

DIAGNOSTIC APPROACH (pp. 57–59)

General Approach. Past medical problems and all current medical activity should be reviewed. A complete physical and radiographic examination of the thorax and cervical region is part of the evaluation. Auscultation and palpation of the larynx, trachea, and thorax for physical deformities or pain are essential in all cases. A complete blood count, fecal flotation examination, heartworm examination, blood chemistry profile, electrocardiogram, bronchial wash, with culture, bronchoscopy, pleural tap, and blood gas analysis may provide the clinician with additional specific information.

Nature of the Cough. Knowing when the cough occurs, what, if anything, brings it about, whether it is moist or dry, and a description of the coughing sound itself may be useful information. The cardiac cough is most prominent at night initially. Pneumonia is likely to be worse initially during the day. Coughing due to infectious, parasitic, allergic, or neoplastic disease most commonly occurs in the daytime. Coughing due to collapse of the trachea and bronchi is stimulated by drinking water. The typical "goose-honk" sound occurs. Coughing that develops while eating or immediately afterward suggests upper airway obstruction, laryngeal paralysis, or an esophageal disorder. Hemoptysis is a sign of heart worms, neoplasia, foreign body, or coagulopathy.

Sound of the Cough. Moist coughing suggests free alveolar or bronchial pulmonary fluid. Inhalation pneumonia, pulmonary emboli, and pulmonary edema are examples.

Dry coughing sounds suggest a cardiac origin (without cardiac failure), bronchitis, tracheobronchitis, tonsillitis, most allergic coughs, diffuse pulmonary parenchymal disease or those associated with neoplasia when free alveolar fluid accumulation is not present. Goose's "honk" sounds are associated with the collapsing trachea main stem bronchi and segmental tracheal injury. Wheezing and rattling are noisy types of sounds often heard with bronchiectasis, chronic obstructive lung disease, and some allergies.

Terminal Retch. It tends to be nonproductive in early cardiac disease, tracheitis, bronchitis, and irritating lesions of the pulmonary tract. In diseases in which mucus, edema, mucopurulent materials, or hemorrhage accumulates, there is likely to be material expectorated following the coughing.

Environmental Factors. (See textbook Chapter 12.)

Original chapter written by Stephen J. Ettinger and Kirstie A. Barrett

TABLE 12–1. CAUSES OF COUGHING IN DOGS AND CATS

Inflammation
    Pharyngitis
    Tonsillitis
    Tracheobronchitis
    Chronic bronchitis
    Bronchiectasis
    Pneumonia—bacterial, viral, fungal
    Granuloma
    Abscess
    Chronic pulmonary fibrosis
    Collapsed trachea
    Hilar lymph node enlargement
    Secondary to achalasia
    Inhalation
Neoplasia
    Primary
    Mediastinal
    Metastatic
    Tracheal
    Laryngeal
    Ribs, sternum, muscle
    Lymphoma
Cardiovascular causes
    Left heart failure
    Enlarged heart (esp. left atrium)
    Heart failure (pulmonary signs)
    Pulmonary emboli
    Pulmonary edema (vascular origin)
Allergic causes
    Bronchial asthma
    Eosinophilic pneumonitis
    Eosinophilic pulmonary granulomatosis
    Pulmonary infiltrate with esoinophilia (PIE)
    Other immune states
    Sinusitis (?)
    Reverse sneeze (postnasal drip?)
Trauma and physical factors
    Foreign body—esophageal; tracheal
    Irritating gases
    Trauma
    Collapsed trachea
    Hypoplastic trachea
    Hepatomegaly
    Inhalation—liquid; solid
Parasites
    Visceral larva migrans
    Filaroides osleri (lung worm)
    Aelurostrongylus (feline lung worm)
    Paragonimus kellicotti (lung fluke—dog; cat)
    Dirofilaria immitis (dog; cat)
    Pneumocystis
    Capillaria aerophilia (dog; cat)
    Crensoma vulpis (dog)
    Filaroides milksi (dog)

TREATMENT GOALS (p. 60)

Accurate knowledge of the nature of the cough usually permits reasonable and accurate classification of the problem (see Table 12–1). In general, drugs that are used to treat the coughing pet include antibiotics for infectious disease, corticosteroids for allergic conditions; digitalis, diuretics, and vasodilators for congestive heart failure; and antispasmodic or antitussive agents for inflammatory, noninfectious lung and tracheal problems.

CHAPTER 13

DYSPNEA AND TACHYPNEA
(pages 61–64

Dyspnea or respiratory distress is an inappropriate degree of breathing effort, based on an assessment of respiratory rate, rhythm, and character. Dyspnea may be exertional, paroxysmal, or continuous. *Tachypnea* refers to an increased rate of breathing but need not be an indication of dyspnea. *Orthopnea* indicates difficulty in breathing while in a recumbent position.

PHYSICAL FINDINGS (pp. 61–62)

A thorough physical examination includes observation, palpation, and auscultation. The patient is observed for any abnormal discharges, for deformities, for whether the dyspnea is inspiratory, expiratory, or both, and for whether there is an obstructive or restrictive breathing pattern. Auscultation may detect the presence of abnormal breath sounds, such as crackles and wheezes, including stridor and cardiac sounds. The larynx and trachea should be carefully palpated, especially if upper airway obstruction is present.

DIAGNOSTIC PLAN (pp. 62–64)

In nasal cavity disease, radiographs are usually indicated. In obstruction of the pharynx or larynx, the patient may need to be anesthetized prior to direct examination of the affected structures. If radiographs suggest evidence of airway disease and/or pulmonary parenchymal disease, and/or if a cough is present, transtracheal aspiration (TTA) may follow. Cytologic examination with aerobic and possibly anaerobic culture should be performed if indicated. Endoscopy is useful, particularly if obstructive disease is present or suspected. Bronchoalveolar lavage may also be useful during endoscopy.

If heartworm disease is suspected, a Knott test, filter test, or serologic test is indicated. Baermann's fecal analysis may diagnose pulmonary and tracheal parasites.

If pleural effusion is present, thoracentesis and fluid analysis with culture are indicated. If ultrasonography is available, it is preferable to evaluate the thorax by this technique prior to removal of fluid.

If the patient has pulmonary parenchymal disease, but a diagnosis has not been obtained by the aforementioned tests, percutaneous pulmonary biopsy is occasionally diagnostic (e.g., blastomycosis, neoplasia). Pulmonary vascular disease usually is apparent radiographically. Occasionally, angiography or nuclear perfusion scans may be required.

In patients with decreased breathing movements, the problem can be

Original chapter written by Grant H. Turnwald

TABLE 13–1. CAUSES OF DYSPNEA

Upper Airway Disorders
  Nasal cavity
  Stenotic nares
  Obstruction (infection, inflammation, neoplasia, trauma, bleeding disorders)
  Pharynx/larynx
  Elongated or edematous soft palate
  Pharyngeal polyp (cat)
  Laryngeal edema, collapse, foreign body, inflammation, trauma, paralysis,
    spasm, neoplasia
  Everted laryngeal saccules
  Cervical trachea
  Collapse, stenosis
  Trauma, foreign body
  Neoplasia, osteochondral dysplasia
  Parasites (*Osleri osleri*)

Lower Airway Disorders
  Thoracic trachea
  (See Cervical trachea)
  Extraluminal compression (lymphadenopathy, heart-based tumors, enlarged
    left atrium)
  Bronchial disease (allergic, infectious, parasitic, chronic obstructive pulmonary
    disease)

Pulmonary Parenchymal Disorders
  Edema (cardiogenic, noncardiogenic)
  Pneumonia (infectious, parasitic, inhalation)
  Neoplasia
  Allergy
  Embolism (dirofilariasis, hyperadrenocorticism, disseminated intravascular
    coagulation)
  Trauma, bleeding disorders
  Pulmonary granulomatosis

Pleural/Body Wall Disorders
  Pneumothorax
  Pleural effusion
  Congenital body wall disorders (pectus excavatum)
  Thoracic wall trauma
  Thoracic wall neoplasia
  Thoracic wall paralysis
  Diaphragmatic hernia (congenital, acquired)

Mediastinal Disorders
  Infection
  Trauma including pneumomediastinum
  Neoplasia

Peritoneal Cavity Disorders
  Organomegaly, obesity
  Effusion
  Gastric torsion

Hemoglobin Disorders
  Anemia
  Methemoglobinemia
  Cyanosis

Miscellaneous
  Central nervous system (brain, spinal cord)
  Peripheral nerve/neuromuscular/muscular
  Metabolic (acidemia)
  Anxiety
  Fear
  Pain

localized to brain disease causing depression of the respiratory center or spinal cord/peripheral nerve disease causing poor ventilation.

A CBC is useful, but rarely diagnostic. In cats, eosinophilia is not helpful in predicting the predominant cell type in bronchial exudates. The appearance of blood (darker and browner than normal) and the concurrent presence of Heinz-body anemia is suggestive of methemoglobinemia.

CHAPTER 14

ASCITES, PERITONITIS, AND OTHER CAUSES OF ABDOMINAL DISTENSION
(pages 64–71)

THE PERITONEAL SURFACE (pp. 64–65)

The purposes of the peritoneum are protection and absorption. It protects the peritoneal cavity by walling off areas of inflammation and permits the absorption, exudation, or transudation of fluids. Increased abdominal and peritoneal pressures result in the cranial displacement of the diaphragm, resulting in increased respiratory activity and venous stasis in the abdomen, diminished arterial blood pressures, and a decrease in renal blood flow.

RECOGNITION OF PERITONEAL DISEASE (pp. 65–68)

Abdominal pain may reflect a disease process involving the peritoneal lining or may be due to a specific process affecting an abdominal organ. Peritonitis, acute abdominal hemorrhage, free urine in the abdominal cavity, abdominal organomegaly, and ascites are the most common conditions to consider. *Abdominal enlargement* usually develops slowly, except when gastric dilation due to traumatic hemoperitoneum, rupture of the urinary bladder, or a neoplastic vascular structure is suspected. Abdominal enlargement is also associated with pregnancy; hydrometra; pyometra; hepatomegaly and renomegaly; growths involving the spleen, liver, lymph nodes, or other abdominal organs; and ascites due to heart failure, hypoproteinemia, and venous obstruction of the posterior vena cava. In addition, Cushing's syndrome, peritonitis, and fluid collection associated with feline infectious peritonitis are other causes.

ABDOMINAL ULTRASONOGRAPHY

A noninvasive technique of great value in the differential diagnosis of abdominal fluid is ultrasonography. Fluid is taken for culture, cytology, chemical analysis and cell counts. Another technique that is occasionally used is diagnostic peritoneal lavage using normal saline and a human dialysis catheter. Fluids should be compared with venous blood

Original chapter written by Stephen J. Ettinger and Kirstie A. Barrett

with respect to clotting time and cell counts. High white counts suggest peritonitis, as do fluids containing bile, urine, and foreign materials.

ABDOMINAL PARACENTESIS AND FLUID EVALUATION

Abdominal paracentesis is usually performed after ultrasound and radiographic examinations confirm the presence of free peritoneal fluid. The simplest form of abdominal paracentesis is midline centesis using a needle and syringe or intravenous polyethylene catheter.

Although frequently mentioned as a hazard, rapid drainage of the abdomen rarely causes shock or other problems. Nevertheless, drainage should be performed over a period of several hours.

Often air is sucked into the abdomen after centesis. This can yield an excellent double contrast study. Fluid should be saved if culture is deemed necessary. Samples should be saved in EDTA tubes (for cell counts), in heparinized tubes (for cytology), and in plain tubes (for chemistry and cytology). Slides should be prepared immediately after withdrawal.

ASCITES (p. 68)

Ascites refers to a collection of serous fluid within the peritoneal cavity. Ascites develops in portal hypertension, hypoproteinemia, inflammatory peritoneal or visceral disease, sodium and water retention states, coagulopathies, trauma, and obstructive or traumatic lymphatic drainage.

Physical Examination. Clinical signs such as a cardiac cough or jaundice may be associated with the primary disease. Patients may be weak, and, with chronic fluid collection, debilitated. Classic wasting occurs with the cardiomyopathies, hypoproteinemic syndromes, and chronic neoplastic diseases. Palpation reveals a dense abdomen, often with organs that cannot be discretely palpated but can be balloted.

Radiographic Examination. A generally hazy, opaque abdominal cavity with the classic "ground-glass" appearance is recognized. The serosal surfaces are nonexistent.

Differential Diagnosis. Hepatomegaly, splenomegaly, obesity, abdominal muscle flaccidity (as occurs with Cushing's syndrome), malignant neoplasms, 6DV, distended uterus, atonic bladder, urethral obstruction with bladder enlargement, and advanced obstipation all may initially be misinterpreted as fluid collection.

Treatment varies with the nature of the primary disease state. The clinician should not assume that diuretic therapy is indicated or helpful whenever ascites is present (see textbook Chap. 14). Abdominal fluid that is causing respiratory distress or abdominal discomfort should be removed.

PERITONITIS (pp. 68–69)

Peritonitis is an inflammatory process that involves all, or a portion of, the peritoneal cavity. Peritonitis may result from traumatic incidents, penetrating injuries, surgically induced lesions, gangrenous obstruction of the gastrointestinal tract, perforation of the bowel, gastrointestinal tract ulcers, incarcerated hernias, or volvulus of a portion of the gastrointestinal tract.

Physical Examination. Generally the pain is diffuse and the abdomen is acutely tender and tympanic. Pyrexia, tachycardia and other arrhythmias, electrolyte disturbances, coagulopathies, and hypotension may develop. Increased peristalsis initially gives way to ileus.

Radiographic and Ultrasound Examinations. Radiographic examination demonstrates loss of serosal surfaces due to loss of intra-abdominal contrast with the "ground-glass" appearance. When rupture of a viscus has occurred, free air in the abdomen may also be apparent. Pulmonary edema may be a complicating associated finding. Ultrasonography often localizes the area of fluid accumulation.

Laboratory Examination. Blood counts usually reveal a marked leukocytosis of which a large percentage are juvenile forms of PMNs. Abdominal paracentesis is likely to result in aspiration of a small amount of a pus-like fluid. Fluids should be examined cytologically and cultured aerobically, anaerobically, and for fungi.

Differential Diagnosis. It is necessary for the clinician to determine the nature and cause of the irritation rather than to attempt to treat only the irritation.

Treatment. The goal is to remove the prime source of contamination and to restore lost plasma volume. The maintenance of normal pulmonary function is also an important consideration. Of paramount importance in the latter stages is the maintenance of adequate cardiac output. To combat sepsis, antimicrobial therapy is recommended initially while awaiting specific culture results. In some cases, surgical exploration of the abdomen is necessary.

PNEUMOPERITONEUM (p. 69)

Pneumoperitoneum results when free air collects in the abdominal cavity. It is often associated with traumatic stab wounds, rupture of a viscus, surgery, or ulceration of the gastrointestinal tract. After surgery, it may persist for 10 or more days.

HEMOPERITONEUM (p. 69)

Hemoperitoneum develops secondary to penetrating or nonpenetrating abdominal trauma, perforation of gastric or intestinal ulcers and abdominal tumors, warfarin poisoning, or other coagulopathies. Abdominal distention develops as fluid collection progresses. If reabsorption occurs and the trauma is not extensive, the symptoms regress rapidly.

Chylous peritonitis results from spontaneous or postoperative trauma to the abdominal cavity; from tumors, especially lymphoma, involving lymphatic channels within the abdominal cavity; from intestinal obstruction that results in rupture of a major lymph channel; and from lymphangiectasia. Therapy may include surgical exploration of the abdomen to ligate a ruptured duct. Specific therapy requires identification of the etiology.

Abdominal carcinomatosis refers to the widespread dissemination of cancer throughout the abdominal cavity. In veterinary medicine, primary abdominal carcinomatosis (mesothelioma) is unusual.

Physical Examination. The most prominent feature is an enlarged abdomen. Debilitation may be present. Radiographic examination of the abdomen and laboratory evaluation of the ascitic fluid are essential to confirm the clinical suspicion. Cytology of fluid is likely to demonstrate malignancy.

FELINE INFECTIOUS PERITONITIS (FIP), WET FORM (pp. 70–71)

Clinical Signs. The outstanding clinical feature is peritoneal effusion. Other features are anorexia, depression, wasting, dehydration, persistent or recurrent fever, unresponsiveness to antibiotics, anemia, and nonspecific gastroenteritis, as well as dyspnea or jaundice.

Radiographic Examination. Serosal surfaces are absent and specific organ recognition is not usually possible.

Laboratory Examination. The effusion has a characteristic thick and tenacious appearance with a golden color. Strands of a white flocculent fibrin material may develop after the fluid is allowed to stand. The fluid has a specific gravity greater than 1.030 and contains large quantities of protein. The peritoneal fluid, like the serum protein, has characteristic electrophoretic pattern. A nonregenerative depression anemia is common. FIP antibody titers rise during the active disease process but are typically not reliable.

OTHER CAUSES OF ABDOMINAL ENLARGEMENT
(p. 71)

Hepatomegaly, Splenomegaly, and Renomegaly. The reader is referred to the individual sections on those organs for a detailed review of the causes of enlargement.

Canine Cushing's Syndrome. Marked abdominal muscle weakness with flaccidity may falsely lead the clinician to a tentative diagnosis of abdominal fluid accumulation.

CHAPTER 15

CARDIOPULMONARY ARREST AND RESUSCITATION
(pages 71–79)

PREDISPOSITION FOR CARDIOPULMONARY ARREST
(pp. 71–72)

Cardiopulmonary arrest is a sudden cessation of ventilation and effective circulation. It may occur as a result of either primary cardiac or primary respiratory dysfunction or secondary to abnormalities that lead to circulatory and ventilatory impairment. Cardiac arrest, the cessation of breathing and the presence of malignant dysrhythmias, is characterized by apnea and an absence of pulses and heart sounds. A failure of circulation may be due to asystole, ventricular fibrillation, or electromechanical dissociation. Severe anemia or blood loss, primary cardiac or pulmonary disease, anesthetics, drug overdoses, or drug interactions are other causes of cardiopulmonary arrest. When primary respiratory arrest occurs, the heart continues to pump blood for several minutes, and prompt ventilatory assistance may avoid secondary cardiac arrest.

TABLE 15–1. COMMON CAUSES OF RESPIRATORY FAILURE

1. Airway obstruction
2. Diseases of the pulmonary parenchyma
3. Diseases of the pulmonary vasculature
4. Disorders of the pleural space
5. Structural disorders of the thorax
6. Neuromuscular disorders

Original chapter written by Mary Anna Labato

TABLE 15–2. CAUSES OF CARDIAC ARREST

1. Cardiac disease
2. Anesthetics
3. Other drugs
4. Acid/base abnormalities (acidosis)
5. Electrolyte abnormalities (hyperkalemia)
6. Hypoxia
7. Severe anemia or blood loss
8. Electrical shock
9. Hypothermia
10. Central nervous system disease
11. Septicemia

SIGNS OF CARDIOPULMONARY ARREST (p. 72)

There is no typical presentation of incipient arrest. Decreases in heart rate and temperature, cyanosis, slow or delayed respirations, dyspnea, or disorientation warrant checking the animal's pulse, respiratory rate, and perfusion (capillary refill time). A peripheral pulse is absent in the dog once the systolic blood pressure falls below 60 torr. Heart sounds in the dog cease at 50 torr. The dilation of the pupils begins within 20 seconds of circulatory arrest and is maximal by 45 seconds. Pupillary dilation is not a reflection of permanent neurologic damage. The size of the pupil should be used as an indicator of effective therapy rather than as an indicator of when to discontinue resuscitation.

CARDIOPULMONARY RESUSCITATION (pp. 73–78)

STEP 1: BASIC LIFE SUPPORT

Airway. The first important step in cardiopulmonary resuscitation is to secure an unobstructed airway. Always check the oral cavity and the oropharynx to remove any foreign material or vomitus either digitally or by suctioning. Ventilatory assistance should be delivered when hypoxemia is suggested by dyspnea, orthopnea, tachypnea, tachycardia, syncope, or cyanosis. Endotracheal intubation is the most desirable means of ensuring a patent airway. If the larynx is obstructed or damaged, an emergency tracheostomy should be performed.

Breathing. Once breathlessness has been determined, breathe for the animal. Ventilations can be administered using an ambu bag. Anesthetic machines are satisfactory alternatives. Recent recommendations suggest breathing techniques that provide for moderate hyperventilation to offset the developing metabolic acidosis. Simultaneous ventilation and chest compression have been under investigation (see Textbook Chap. 15).

Circulation. One should determine the pulselessness of the animal, using either the carotid or femoral pulse. Chest compressions should be delivered at a rate of 80 to 120 compressions per minute, with the higher rates being used for small dogs and cats.

STEP 2: CLOSED CHEST COMPRESSION VERSUS OPEN CHEST COMPRESSION

External chest compression does not require special equipment and is the primary method of providing artificial circulation to animals in cardiopulmonary arrest.

Additions to the closed chest method of cardiopulmonary resuscitation are simultaneous ventilation and compression techniques and interposed abdominal compression. Wrapping the hind legs and caudal abdomen with elastic bandaging material may improve systemic blood pressure and organ perfusion. A single abdominal tourniquet can also be used. Conditions that may lessen the generation or transmission of intrathoracic pressures, such as rib fractures, or conditions that predispose to inadequate ventilation and perfusion, such as pleural effusion or hemorrhage, pneumothorax, or cardiac tamponade may serve as an indication for open chest cardiac massage. Opening the chest and pericardium to allow direct cardiac massage is indicated if external chest compressions are ineffective in producing a palpable femoral or carotid pulse.

Immediate thoracotomy for the treatment of cardiac arrest probably is usually not warranted because closed chest compression is often successful (see textbook Chap. 15). Other indications for open-chest CPR include: if the mucous membrane color does not improve within 5 minutes, or if the heart has not started beating spontaneously within 10 minutes.

STEP 3: ELECTROCARDIOGRAPHY OF CARDIOPULMONARY ARREST

Cardiac arrhythmias commonly associated with cardiopulmonary arrest include sinus bradycardia, sinus tachycardia, electromechanical dissociation, ventricular asystole, ventricular fibrillation, and ventricular tachycardia.

Ventricular asystole generally carries a poor prognosis for resuscitation. The treatment of choice is epinephrine intravenously and continued cardiopulmonary resuscitation methods. With high vagal tone, atropine intravenously is considered the drug of choice.

Electromechanical Dissociation.   Recommendations for treatment include epinephrine intravenously or high doses of dexamethasone sodium phosphate intravenously.

Ventricular Fibrillation.   The treatment is defibrillating shock treatment.

STEP 4: DRUG THERAPY

Epinephrine has both alpha and beta sympathomimetic effects. A strong alpha agonist increases arterial wall stiffness and increases total peripheral resistance. Epinephrine may precipitate ventricular fibrillation when hypoxia has not been corrected by adequate artificial ventilation. *Atropine* is useful in treating sinus bradycardia or frequent ventricular ectopic beats or atrioventricular block. Atropine may potentiate ventricular arrhythmias. *Calcium chloride* improves the excitability of the ventricles and suppresses sinus impulse formation, but many potential pitfalls exist (see Chap 15). The four major indications for the use of calcium chloride during cardiopulmonary arrest are hypocalcemia, calcium channel blocker overdosage, hyperkalemia, and a recent rapid blood transfusion with citrated blood. Calcium chloride may be tried in cases of electromechanical dissociation when all other treatments have been unsuccessful. *Sodium bicarbonate:* During cardiopulmonary resuscitation, acid/base abnormalities should be corrected through the use of adequate ventilation, cardiac compression, and volume expansion. In animals that were not acidotic at the start of cardiopulmonary arrest, no sodium bicarbonate should be administered for the first 10 minutes of the arrest. When administration is necessary, it should be administered carefully (see textbook Chap. 15). *Lidocaine* is a membrane-stabilizing antiarrhythmic drug effective in suppressing ventricular tachyarrhythmias. Animals with ventricular tachycardia and palpable pulses initially should be given lidocaine intravenously as a bolus because of its rapid onset of action. With successful resuscitation, a continuous infusion may be used.

Other Drugs.   *Methoxamine* is a pure alpha agonist which increases diastolic pressure without contributing to myocardial hypoxia and cardiac arrhythmias. It has been advocated in electromechanical dissociation. *Diltiazem* is a calcium channel blocker. Diltiazem has both a membrane-stabilizing effect and a bradycardia effect. *Bretylium* *tosylate* has been used to treat ventricular fibrillation. *Fluid therapy should be used in hypovolemic animals.*

Routes of Drug Administration.   Intravenous drug administration is preferred during advanced life support measures. Intravenous administration through a central vein is probably the best. The intracardiac route of drug administration has previously been advocated in order to get the drugs to the heart quickly. However, this route has many hazards (see Chap. 15). The intratracheal route of drug administration has been advocated because of the tremendous surface for exchange between the alveoli and the pulmonary capallaries. Some studies have indicated that drug uptake is sporadic, undependable, and delayed. Substantially higher doses are required to produce the same effect as intravenously administered drugs. The intraosseous route can be used for drug and fluid administration since the intramedullary space is continuous with the vascular system.

STEP 5: DEFIBRILLATION

The treatment of choice for ventricular fibrillation is immediate defibrillation. The most important factor for determining ease and success of defibrillation is the time delay between onset of fibrillation and the administration of the electrical countershock. There have been reports of spontaneous recovery from ventricular fibrillation in cats.

POST-RESUSCITATION THERAPY (pp. 78–79)

It is of greatest importance to expect secondary arrests and to closely monitor the animal's ECG, ventilatory pattern, electrolytes, acid/base status, central venous pressure, body temperature, and urinary output. There should be frequent assessment of the animal's level of consciousness, body movements, pupillary light reflexes, mucous membrane color, respiratory rate, heart rate, and rhythm. Seizure activity during the post-resuscitation period is common. Cerebral edema may necessitate the use of diuretics and glucocorticosteroids.

CONCLUSIONS AND ETHICAL CONSIDERATIONS
(p. 79)

Cardiopulmonary resuscitation should not be undertaken when the animal is in the terminal stages of an incurable disease or when there is no reasonable chance to regain central nervous system function.

CHAPTER 16

SNEEZING AND NASAL DISCHARGE
(pages 79–85)

Sneezing and nasal discharge are the primary signs of upper respiratory disease in the dog and cat. Sinus, nasal, and nasopharyngeal disorders are common presenting complaints.

Original chapter written by Brendan C. McKiernan

DEFINITIONS AND GENERAL PATHOPHYSIOLOGY
(pp. 79–81)

Sneezing is an involuntary airway protective reflex and as such is an important component of the normal respiratory defense mechanisms. This reflex may be decreased in frequency or lost completely with chronic disease processes. Multiple direct causes of sneezing have been reported, including congenital (e.g., cleft palate, cilial defects), inflammatory (e.g., allergic, parasitic), and infectious (e.g., viral, bacterial, fungal) conditions; mechanical and chemical stimuli (e.g., foreign bodies, environmental dusts, odors or pollutants), and simple trauma.

Reverse Sneezing. Mechanisms that veterinarians have proposed to explain this reflex have included postnasal drip, soft palate flutter (nasopharyngeal spasm), and entrapment of the epiglottis within the laryngeal opening. Grossly, reverse sneezing is associated with violent, *paroxysmal inspiratory efforts.* Mechanical stimuli seem to elicit reverse sneezing, although inhaled allergens have also been reported to cause the reflex.

Nasal Discharge. A number of characteristics are important to consider. The *type* of discharge may be serous, mucoid, mucopurulent, purulent, blood-tinged to overtly bloody (epistaxis), or discharge containing food particles. Most nasal and sinus diseases initially have a serous discharge, which subsequently progresses to mucoid, then to mucopurulent, and finally to purulent discharge. Blood may occur subsequent to focal irritation or mucosal capillary trauma during violent sneezing episodes, or as part of a coagulopathy.

INTERPRETATION OF HISTORICAL FINDINGS (pp. 81–83)

Signalment. When consideration is given to an animal's signalment, various disease categories or specific disease conditions are brought to mind (see textbook Chap. 16).

Previous Medical History. Questions should be asked regarding any past skull *trauma* or *surgery.* Previous *dental problems, vaccination* history, and *response to previous medical treatments* may provide valuable information.

Sneezing. If the owner can determine whether the sneezing episode is *inspiratory* or *expiratory* in nature, reverse sneezing can be differentiated from primary conditions.

Nasal Discharge. Features of the nasal discharge may assist the clinician in narrowing the list of differential diagnoses (see Table 16–1).

Abnormal Sounds. *Wheezing* and *whistling, stertor,* or *stridor* may be noted.

Halitosis. Usually bad breath is a reflection of necrotic tissue (and secondary bacterial infection) in the nasal cavity and/or mouth.

Signs of Sinus Pressure. *Squinting* and holding the head with the *nose upward* have been observed in some cases.

Bony Involvement. Animals suffering from diseases associated with periosteal involvement (tumor, fungal infection) may demonstrate *pain. Gross swelling* or *facial distortion* may be noted.

Tissue Growth. Tissue growth within the nasal cavity may be detected in the oral cavity or at the external nares.

Pawing at Face (see textbook Chap. 16).

INTERPRETATION OF PHYSICAL EXAMINATION FINDINGS (pp. 82–83)

Nasal Discharge. Evidence is usually found upon careful examination of the nares

Air Flow. Various clinical techniques have been used to *see, hear,* or *feel* that there is a difference in *air flow* between the left and right nostrils (see textbook Chap 16).

TABLE 16–1. CHARACTERISTICS THAT ASSIST IN THE INITIAL LOCALIZATION, INTERPRETATION, AND DIFFERENTIAL DIAGNOSIS OF NASAL DISCHARGE IN CATS AND DOGS

Features
    Evidence of dried discharge; unilateral vs bilateral discharge
    Depigmentation of the alar cartilage
    Character—serous, mucoid, mucopurulent, purulent, blood-tinged, epistaxis, food content
    Epistaxis—may be secondary to:
        Nasal disease (trauma, tumor, fungal, foreign body)
        Oral disease (tooth, tumor)
        Systemic disease (platelet, coagulopathy)
Discharge (unilateral when it initially began) may be associated with
    Dental disease in the upper arcade
    Nasal polyps (C)
    Nasal foreign body
    Nasal tumor
    Fungi—*Cryptococcus* (C), *Aspergillus* (D), *Penicillum* (D), *Rhinosporidium* (D), *Sporothrix* (C)
    Parasites—*Pneuminosoides* (D), *Cuterebra* (D, C), *Lingutula* (C), *Capillaria* (D, C)
Discharge (bilateral when it initially began) may be associated with
    Infection—viral, bacterial, *Chlamydia* (C)
    Immunoglobulin deficiency (IgA)
    Hyperplastic rhinitis (Irish wolfhound)
    Cilial dyskinesia
    Allergy
    Lymphoplasmacytic rhinitis
    Environmental agents—dusts, smoke
    Extranasal disease—pneumonia, esophageal stricture, megaesophagus, cricopharyngeal disease
    Nasopharyngeal foreign body
    Parasites—*Pneuminosides* (D), *Cuterebra* (D, C), *Lingutula* (C), *Capillaria* (D, C)
    Trauma

C = cat; D = dog.

Bony Changes. The nasal and sinus regions, as well as the oral cavity, should be palpated and examined for any evidence of *distortion* or *swelling*.

Oral Examination. Attention should be given to the *hard palate* (defect/clefts, swellings, erosions, trauma secondary to malocclusion), *soft palate* (mucosal erosions, ventral depression from nasopharyngeal masses), *tonsils, teeth* and *periodontia* (gingival hyperemia, deep periodontal pockets/root abscesses, fractures, defects in enamel, oronasal fistulas, and abnormal occlusion), and the *oral mucosa* in general.

Regional Lymph Nodes. Unilateral rhinitis may be associated with ipsilateral lymphadenopathy; unilateral tonsillar involvement may be due to tumor.

Ocular Examination. *Chorioretinitis, conjunctivitis,* and *retinal hemorrhage* may be noted.

DIAGNOSTIC PLAN (pp. 83–85)

Clinical Pathologic Testing. CBC, serum chemistries, and a urinalysis are recommended especially prior to anesthesia for skull radiography. Platelet count, coagulation profile, and factor VIIIR:Ag will be of benefit in suspected coagulopathy.

Serologic testing has been used as an aid in diagnosing nasal fungal conditions including *Aspergillus, Penicillium spp,* and *Cryptococcus neoformans.* A positive serology is supportive of a fungal disease but should not be considered absolutely diagnostic.

Nasal Bacterial and Fungal Cultures.   Results of culture must be interpreted cautiously as they may only reflect airway colonization and not actually be the cause of a given disease process. The significance of positive bacterial cultures if cautiously evaluated, is probably acceptable especially if a pure growth is obtained.

Cytologic Evaluation.   Allergic rhinitis (presence of eosinophils) and certain nasal fungal diseases (e.g., *Cryptococcus, Rhinosporidium, Sporothrix*) are most rewarding cytologically. Intracytoplasmic inclusions have been noted in some chronic viral feline herpes rhinitis.

Skull Radiography.   Loss of structural symmetry, changes in nasal cavity density (increased or decreased), bony abnormalities (loss of turbinates, nasal septum erosion, periosteal reaction, tooth root lysis), and the presence of foreign bodies are some of the more typical radiographic findings suggestive of nasal diseases.

Rhinoscopy should be performed on any dog or cat that has been anesthetized for skull radiographs. Both *anterior rhinoscopy* and *posterior rhinoscopy* should be performed. Lesions can undergo direct biopsy, and foreign bodies may be removed with simple rhinoscopy.

Nasal Flushing Techniques   (see textbook Chap. 16).

Oral Examination.   The hard and soft palate should be palpated, tonsils examined, and the gums and teeth checked. A careful and complete dental examination and periodontal probing are a *mandatory* part of all nasal work-ups.

TREATMENT GOALS (p. 85)

The overall goals are to normalize nasal function, to decrease pain and excessive sneezing, and to minimize secretion production. Antibiotic therapy will decrease the amount of purulent nasal discharge, but the underlying cause (e.g., foreign body, tooth root abscess) must be treated as well. Nasal fungal diseases require antifungal therapy, but they may also require surgical curettage. Surgery is indicated for polyps and foreign bodies. Nasal tumors respond better to radiation therapy than to surgery or chemotherapy alone.

CHAPTER 17
ABNORMAL HEART SOUNDS AND HEART MURMURS
(pages 86–89)

Heart sounds are created by turbulent blood flow and associated vibrations in adjacent tissue during the cardiac cycle.

ALTERATIONS IN NORMAL TRANSIENT SOUNDS (S_1 AND S_2)

Causes of a loud S_1 include high sympathetic tone, tachycardia, and shortened P-R interval. Causes of diminished intensity of S_1 include

---

Original chapter written by Wendy A. Ware

pericardial or pleural effusion, dilated cardiomyopathy, and hypovolemia. A split S_1 may be normal, or it may result from bundle branch blocks. An increase in the intensity of S_2 can result from pulmonary hypertension of any cause. Pathologic splitting of S_2 can result from delayed ventricular activation or ejection secondary to premature contractions, right bundle branch block, and pulmonary hypertension.

ABNORMAL TRANSIENT SOUNDS

Gallop Sounds. The third (S_3) and fourth (S_4) heart sounds are not normally audible. The S_3 and S_4 are usually heard best with the bell of the stethoscope. An audible S_3 usually indicates ventricular dilation with myocardial failure. An audible S_4 is usually associated with increased ventricular stiffness and hypertrophy (e.g., hypertrophic cardiomyopathy). At fast heart rates, differentiation of S_3 from S_4 is difficult. If both sounds are present, this is called a "summation gallop."

Other Transient Sounds. The most common are *systolic clicks.* sudden checking of a portion of the valve as it balloons into the atrium during systole is thought to cause the click(s). The click itself is not of great concern. Early systolic, high-pitched "ejection sound" at the left base may occur with valvular pulmonic stenosis and other diseases causing dilation of a great artery.

CARDIAC MURMURS (p. 87)

Murmurs are caused by turbulent blood flow in the heart or adjacent blood vessels. The development of turbulent blood flow is directly related to the velocity of blood flow and inversely related to blood viscosity.

ABNORMAL HEART SOUNDS (pp. 87–89)

PHYSICAL FINDINGS

Cardiac Auscultation. Patient cooperation and a quiet environment are important during auscultation. If possible, the patient should be standing. All areas of both sides of the chest should be carefully ausculted, focusing special attention to the areas overlying cardiac valves.

Systolic Murmurs. The murmur of mitral insufficiency is heard best at the left apex in the area of the mitral valve. Mitral insufficiency characteristically causes a plateau or regurgitant murmur (holosystolic); however, it may be protosystolic. Sometimes this murmur sounds like a musical "whoop." Systolic ejection murmurs are most often heard at the left base and are caused by ventricular outflow obstruction (textbook Chaps. 93 and 96). The most common causes include congenital (sub)aortic or pulmonic stenosis and hypertrophic obstructive cardiomyopathy. The murmur of subaortic stenosis is heard well low on the left base and at the right base. This murmur also radiates up the

TABLE 17–1. GRADING OF CARDIAC MURMURS

Grade I	Very soft murmur; heard only in quiet surroundings after intently listening
Grade II	Soft murmur, but easily heard
Grade III	Moderate-intensity murmur
Grade IV	Loud murmur, but not accompanied by a precordial thrill
Grade V	Loud murmur with a palpable precordial thrill
Grade VI	Very loud murmur that can be heard with the stethoscope off the chest wall; accompanied by a precordial thrill

carotid arteries. The murmur of pulmonic stenosis is best heard high on the left base. Functional murmurs are nonpathologic and are of soft to moderate intensity. They include innocent murmurs (no apparent cardiovascular cause), which are common in puppies, and physiologic murmurs (where the heart is normal but an altered physiologic state exists). The tricuspid insufficiency murmur sounds similar to mitral insufficiency and is loudest at the right apex. Ventricular septal defect also causes a holosystolic murmur, which usually is loudest at the right sternal border.

Diastolic Murmurs. Uncommon in dogs and cats, these murmurs are usually associated with incompetence of a semilunar valve. Aortic insufficiency from bacterial endocarditis is the most frequent cause. Clinically significant pulmonic insufficiency is rare. These murmurs are heard best at the left base.

Continuous Murmurs. Continuous (also called "machinery") murmurs occur throughout the cardiac cycle. Patent ductus arteriosus is the most common cause.

Concurrent Systolic and Diastolic Murmurs. The most common cause is the combination of (sub)aortic stenosis with aortic insufficiency.

DIAGNOSTIC APPROACH

Careful auscultation should permit identification of the most likely causes. Diagnostic tests that can help to further define the patient's abnormality include electrocardiography, thoracic radiography, and echocardiography.

CHAPTER 18
PULSE ALTERATIONS
(pages 89–93)

Hyperkinetic pulse refers to an arterial pulse that is abnormally strong. *Hypokinetic pulse* refers to a weak arterial pulse. The most important factor in determining the perceived strength of an arterial pulse is the *pulse pressure,* the difference between systolic and diastolic pressures. *Pulse deficit* refers to an absence of arterial pulse when corresponding heart sounds are ausculted.

Arterial pulse is most prominent and best evaluated at the femoral arteries. Differences in pulse quality between left and right femoral arteries occasionally exist. The clinician should take into account the patient's body condition when assessing pulse strength.

Genesis of the Arterial Pulse. There are three physiologic factors important in determining arterial pressure: (1) heart rate, (2) peripheral vascular resistance, and (3) stroke volume (see textbook Chap. 18). The overall pulse strength is a function of the difference between peak systolic pressure and diastolic pressure. With significant loss of diastolic pressure, such as aortic valvular insufficiency or patent ductus arteriosus, pulse pressure becomes high and pulses become hyperkinetic, or bounding.

Arterial Pulse Alterations. Hypokinetic pulses may be present with hypovolemia, left ventricular failure, cardiac tamponade, and subaortic stenosis. Pulses can become hyperkinetic in cases of mitral insufficiency, hyperthyroidism, fever, or anemia as well as PDA and aortic valve insufficiency.

Pulse Deficits. When cardiac rhythm is irregular the pulse rhythm is correspondingly irregular. This occurs when an arrhythmia interferes with diastolic filling and causes insufficient filling of the ventricle. Following an isolated pulse deficit, the next pulse is often accentuated, pulse deficits are present in atrial fibrillation, and frequent atrial and/or ventricular premature contractions are present.

Pulsus Paradoxus and Pulsus Alternans (see textbook Chap. 18).

Absent Arterial Pulsations. Arterial thromboembolism in feline hypertrophic cardiomyopathy is an example.

VENOUS PULSE (p. 92)

Assessment of the Venous Pulse. Adequate visualization of the jugular veins requires the clipping of overlying hair. Jugular pulsations should not extend more than one-third the distance up the neck. Distention of jugular veins indicates that right-sided heart failure is present.

Components of the Normal Venous Pulse. Jugular venous pressures correlate with right atrial (RA) pressure. Jugular pulsations occur when tricuspid regurgitation is present. Accentuation of jugular venous distention through the hepatojugular reflux will result in increased venous return, which, in the presence of underlying right heart disease, elevates right atrial pressure and impedes jugular venous return.

Venous Pulse Alterations. Causes for jugular venous distention include pericardial effusion, pulmonic stenosis, pulmonary hypertension, and cardiomyopathy. Tricuspid insufficiency causes venous distention as well as jugular pulsations. The combination of weak arterial pulses and jugular venous distention is highly suggestive of cardiac tamponade.

CHAPTER 19

HYPERTENSIVE AND HYPOTENSIVE DISORDERS
(pages 93–100)

HYPERTENSION (pp. 93–97)

Most investigators agree that systemic BP in awake, untrained dogs and cats should not normally exceed 180/100 mm Hg systolic/diastolic with borderline or mild HT up to 200/110 mm Hg. Hypertension may be *secondary* to certain underlying diseases (usually renal or endocrine abnormalities) or may be primary (also known as *essential* or idiopathic HT).

Original chapter written by Meryl P. Littman and Kenneth J. Drobatz

GENERAL PATHOPHYSIOLOGY

The systemic BP is proportional to the cardiac output (CO) and the total peripheral resistance (TPR):BP = CO × TPR (see textbook Chap. 19 for a detailed discussion).

HISTORICAL FINDINGS AND THEIR MEANINGS

Signalment. *Age:* Middle-aged to geriatric (dogs, 8.9 ± 3.6, range 2 to 14; cats, 15.1 ± 3.8, range 7 to 20 years are most common). *Sex:* Male dogs may be at higher risk. *Other:* Obese animals have higher valves than normal animals. The most common complaint is *blindness,* often due to retinal hemorrhage and/or detachment. In hypertensive dogs, PU/PD is often associated with renal insufficiency or Cushing's. In hypertensive cats, PU/PD is often associated with renal insufficiency or hyperthyroidism. Signs of *renal insufficiency,* such as vomiting, anorexia, and weight loss may exist; signs of *glomerulonephropathy* may include ascites, edema, or thromboembolic events. The owner may relate historical signs of Cushing's or pheocromocytome or *congestive heart failure. Epistaxis* may be due to high pressure blow-outs in the nasal epithelium. *Neurologic signs* (e.g., seizures, syncope, decorticate posturing, hindleg paresis, collapse) and cerebrovascular accidents or "strokes" from hemorrhage, infarcts, or arteriolar spasm may occur.

PHYSICAL FINDINGS AND THEIR MEANINGS

The strength of peripheral pulses does not help to detect systemic HT. A strong or bounding pulse is palpable because of a large difference discernible between the systolic and diastolic pressure, not because of HT. *Retinal hemorrhages and detachments* are common in moderate to severe hypertension in dogs. Old hemorrhages or scars may be seen. Other intraocular exudation such as hyphema or closed-angle glaucoma can be found. Many old hypertensive cats have *small kidneys. Dehydration* may be suspected. *Ascites* or *edema* may be noted in animals with glomerulonephropathy. Low-grade *mitral murmurs* are often ausculted. *Pulmonary edema* or *pleural effusion* may be ausculted. *Hyperthyroid* cats may pant or have *tachycardia* and *gallop rhythm.*

DIAGNOSTIC PLAN

Multiple measurements may be necessary to support the diagnosis of HT. When HT is confirmed, diagnostic tests seek a possible cause for HT and end-organ involvement. When no underlying cause is found, essential HT is suspected. The data base, including *CBC, biochemical profile, and urinalysis* may suggest renal failure, Cushing's, HAC, hypothyroidism, or HTHYR glomerulonephropathy. The *urine protein/creatinine ratio* helps to quantify proteinuria. *Serologic tests* may be done for lupus or infectious diseases. *Coagulation profile, nasal series, CSF analysis,* and/or *brain scan* may be indicated to help rule out other causes of epistaxis and retinal or neurologic signs. *Chest and abdominal radiographs* and *ultrasonography* may disclose neoplasia, abnormal kidney size/infrastructure, adrenal masses, ascites, or hepatomegaly associated with diseases that can cause HT. *Echocardiography and electrocardiogram* may show LVH. A *serum T₄* may show HTHYR. The *low-dose dexamethasone suppression test* screens for HAC. The diagnosis of PHEO may be supported by abdominal ultrasonography or provocative tests. A *serum aldosterone assay* may detect hyperaldosteronism.

GOALS OF TREATMENT

It is not known whether the mild hypertension commonly noted in many diseases is clinically significant. It seems prudent though, with moderate to severe HT (BPM >200/110 mmHg), to reduce the BPM to

TABLE 19–1. CAUSES OF HYPERTENSION

Essential or primary hypertension (described in dogs and possibly cats)
Secondary hypertension
  Renal (described in dogs and cats)
    Glomerulonephritis
    Amyloidosis
    Glomerulosclerosis
    Chronic interstitial nephritis
    Pyelonephritis
    Polycystic renal disease
  Hyperadrenocorticism (described in dogs)
    Pituitary-dependent
    Adrenal neoplasia
    Exogenous steroids
  Hyperthyroidism (described in cats)
  Pheochromocytoma (described in dogs)
  Hyperaldosteronism (described in dogs)
  Hyperkinetic heart syndrome
    Anemia (described in cats)
    Hyperviscosity
    Polycythemia
    Fever
    Arteriovenous fistula
  Renovascular
    Renal arterial stenosis
    Thromboembolism
    Renal infarct
  Intracranial disease
    Neoplasia
  Hypothyroidism (atherosclerosis)
  Coarctation of the aorta
  Hypercalcemia
  Hyperestrogenism
  Pregnancy toxemia

normal or at least by 20 per cent. Concurrent illnesses should be treated. Extra salt is removed from the diet. Obese animals should lose weight. Antihypertensive regimens may include diuretics, α_1-adrenergic blockers, β-adrenergic blockers, (ACE) inhibitors, and calcium channel blockers. In one regimen, the most commonly used antihypertensives are atenolol and enalapril (alone or in combination). Monitoring of BPMs and reassessment of end-organ changes is initially done every 1 to 2 weeks. Animals with acute blindness lasting a day or two may recover sight with antihypertensive medication. Most patients with blindness of longer duration remain blind. Prognosis for life expectancy depends on concurrent disease processes.

HYPOTENSION (pp. 97–100)

The numeric definition of hypotension may be different for different patients. As a general rule, systolic BP less than 80 mmHg or mean arterial pressure less than 60 mmHg indicates hypotension.

HISTORY

The signalment and history of the hypotensive patient may give clues to the underlying etiology. For example, a young female standard poodle with hypoadrenocorticism may present with hypotension and poor perfusion. Large-breed dogs may have dilated cardiomyopathy and poor tissue perfusion owing to diminished CO.

PHYSICAL EXAMINATION (PE)

Clinical signs consistent with poor perfusion include pale mucous membranes, prolonged capillary refill time, weak arterial pulses, decreased urine output, hypothermia, cold extremities, depressed mental state, muscle weakness, and hyperventilation. With severe hypotension, cardiac arrhythmias may also occur as well as hemorrhagic diarrhea. Patients with hypotension and PE findings such as hyperemic mucous membranes, bounding pulses, and an elevated body temperature should be assessed for an underlying infectious cause. Specific PE findings may suggest the underlying cause. For example, muffled heart sounds are associated with pericardial effusion, pleural space diseases, or severe hypovolemia. Palpation of the abdomen may reveal a distended abdomen suggesting hemoperitoneum, gastric dilatation, or a third-space fluid accumulation.

DIAGNOSTIC AND THERAPEUTIC PLAN

Hypotension causing poor tissue perfusion often requires immediate therapy before a definitive diagnosis has been reached. In the unstable hypotensive patient an intravenous catheter should be placed and blood should be drawn for immediate evaluation of packed cell volume, total solids, estimate of BUN by azostick, and blood glucose. Cardiopulmonary abnormalities demand further diagnostic tests. If cardiac disease is not suspected on the basis of PE and history, then rapid intravenous infusion of crystalloids, colloids, and/or blood products may be required to improve BP. If adequate vascular volume replacement has been administered and hypotension persists, the use of pressor agents such as epinephrine, phenylephrine, or dopamine should be considered. Routine and sophisticated diagnostic studies may be required to identify the etiology of the hypotension. A thorough search for the etiology is warranted.

CHAPTER 20

PERIPHERAL EDEMA
(pages 100–103)

Edema refers to the accumulation of excessive amounts of extracellular fluid in the interstitial space. *Peripheral edema* is a term used to distinguish edema occurring in any of the peripheral (systemic) vascular beds. *Anasarca* refers to severe, generalized edema.

MICROCIRCULATORY PHYSIOLOGY AND MECHANISMS OF EDEMA FORMATION (pp. 100–101)

Forces responsible for exchange of fluid between the capillaries and interstitium are related mathematically by the *Starling law*:

$$K [(P_c - P_{IF}) - \sigma (\pi_{pi} - \pi_{IF})] = Q_{lymph}$$

where K = permeability coefficient; P_c = mean intracapillary pressure; P_{IF} = mean interstitial fluid pressure; σ = reflection coefficient of macromolecules; π_{IF}

Original chapter written by Janice McIntosh Bright

= oncotic pressure of interstitial fluid; π_{pi} = oncotic pressure or the plasma; Q_{lymph} = lymphatic flow

Equilibrium is achieved by a balance of the Starling forces exerted across the capillary membranes and by lymphatic flow. Practically speaking, four mechanisms are responsible for edema formation: (1) increased capillary hydrostatic pressure, (2) decreased plasma oncotic pressure, (3) lymphatic obstruction, and (4) increased vascular permeability. The most important causes of increased capillary hydrostatic pressure include intravascular thrombosis or tumor or extravascular compressive lesions such as a tumor, granuloma, abscess, gastric dilation, bandage, or collar. Less commonly an arteriovenous fistula may be the cause. The most frequent cause of a generalized increase in venous pressure is right heart failure or impairment of right heart filling. This may also result from rapid expansion of the blood volume by administration of a large volume of fluid. A decrease in concentration of plasma proteins can result in generalized, noninflammatory edema. Albumin is responsible for the greatest portion of the plasma oncotic pressure. Hypoalbuminemia may be caused by inadequate synthesis or by excessive loss. Edema due to lymphatic obstruction is nearly always localized because the obstruction is usually focal. Lymphatic obstruction may result from trauma, surgical interruption, congenital malformation, and various inflammatory or neoplastic processes. Primary lymphedema is an important differential diagnosis. Endothelial damage will result in edema via an inflammatory phenomenon or less frequently from toxins, chemicals, or infectious agents.

HISTORICAL FINDINGS (p. 101)

Noninflammatory edema is usually insidious in onset and begins in the dependent parts of the body. Edema of an inflammatory nature is often acute and may begin in nondependent areas.

PHYSICAL FINDINGS (pp. 101–103)

Weight gain usually precedes other manifestations of edema. Other specific clinical signs will depend on the severity, extent, and anatomic location of the abnormal fluid accumulation which, in turn, reflect the underlying cause. Dependent portions of the body should be closely inspected for the presence of subcutaneous edema. A finger pushed against the edematous tissue produces a lasting indentation called *pitting edema* in the presence of noninflammatory subcutaneous edema. This edema is typically painless with no associated lameness or heat. If the edema is due to an arteriovenous fistula, palpation may reveal hyperdynamic pulses and a fremitus ("thrill"). Examination of the lymph nodes may reveal enlargement that is suggestive of neoplasia or lymphangitis. Lymph nodes may be absent in patients with primary lymphedema.

DIAGNOSTIC PLAN (p. 103)

Distribution is an important diagnostic aid. Edema of one rear leg or of one or both front legs is generally due to venous and/or lymphatic obstruction. Obstruction of the cranial vena cava causes subcutaneous edema of the neck, the thoracic limbs, and occasionally the neck and face. Edema that results from hypoalbuminemia is usually dependent first and then generalized. In dogs, congestive heart failure tends to cause ascites with or without hydrothorax, whereas cats experience clinical hydrothorax prior to ascites. Survey radiographs, sonographic evaluation, radiographs of the affected anatomic region, a complete blood count, a serum biochemical profile, urinalysis. and analysis of fluid removed from body cavity effusions will distinguish between inflammatory and noninflammatory processes and may also reveal an etiologic agent. A complete cardiac evaluation may be warranted. Biopsy of the affected skin and subcutaneous tissues may be needed to obtain a definitive diagnosis.

CHAPTER 21
VOMITING, REGURGITATION, AND DYSPHAGIA
(pages 103–111)

VOMITING (pp. 103–108)

Vomiting refers to a forceful ejection of gastric and occasionally proximal small intestinal contents through the mouth. The vomiting act involves three stages: nausea, retching, and vomiting. *Nausea* is recognized as a premonitory sign and is clinically manifested by a state of depression, salivation, licking of the lips, and increased swallowing motions. *Retching* is a preparatory maneuver during which forceful respiratory movements overcome natural anti-reflux characteristics of the abdominal esophagus and cardia. Vomiting then occurs as the high intra-abdominal pressure expels gastric contents through a relaxed cardia. It is essential that the clinician make a clear differentiation between *regurgitation* and *vomiting* at the outset. *Regurgitation* is defined as *passive,* retrograde movement of ingested material.

CLINICAL FEATURES OF VOMITING

Vomiting may be the first indication of intestinal obstruction, renal failure, pancreatitis, addisonian crisis, drug toxicity, neoplasia, and others. A complete historical review with emphasis on all body systems is essential for determining a realistic and effective initial work-up plan and treatment protocol. All too often concentration on only the gastrointestinal tract leads to a misdiagnosis and inappropriate treatment.

Duration of Signs and Systems Review. It should be determined whether any nonsteroidal anti-inflammatory drugs have been used. Gastric and intestinal erosions and potentially serious ulceration may develop in conjunction with their use. Chemotherapeutic agents, erythromycin and tetracycline, and cardiac glycosides may cause vomiting. Specific information regarding diet, vaccinations, travel history, and environment is obtained in all cases.

Time Relation to Eating. Vomiting shortly after eating most commonly suggests dietary indiscretion or food intolerance, overeating, stress or excitement, gastritis, or a hiatal disorder. Vomiting of undigested or partially digested food more than 6 to 7 hours after eating usually indicates a gastric motility disorder or gastric outlet obstruction. Causes include foreign bodies, hypertrophic gastritis, pyloric mucosal hypertrophy, and antral or pyloric neoplasia or polyps.

Content of the Vomitus. Bile is often present when vomiting is due to inflammatory bowel disease, bile reflux syndromes, idiopathic or

---

TABLE 21–1. CAUSES OF VOMITING

DIETARY PROBLEM

Sudden diet change
Ingestion of foreign material (garbage, grass, plant leaves, etc.)
Eating too rapidly
Intolerance to specific foods
Food allergy

DRUGS

Intolerance (e.g., antineoplastic drugs, cardiac glycosides, antimicrobial drugs
 [e.g., erythromycin, tetracycline], arsenical compounds)
Blockage of prostaglandin biosynthesis (nonsteroidal anti-inflammatory
 drugs)
Injudicious use of anticholinergics
Accidental overdosage

TOXINS

Lead
Ethylene glycol
Zinc
Others

METABOLIC DISORDERS

Diabetes mellitus	Hyperkalemia
Hypoadrenocorticism	Hypokalemia
Renal disease	Hypercalcemia
Hepatic disease	Hypocalcemia
Sepsis	Hypomagnesemia
Acidosis	Heat stroke

DISORDERS OF THE STOMACH

Obstruction (foreign body, pyloric mucosal hypertrophy, external compres-
 sion, etc.)
Chronic gastritis (superficial, atrophic, hypertrophic)
Parasites (*Physaloptera* spp—dog and cat, *Ollulanus tricuspis*—cat)
Gastric hypomotility
Bilious vomiting syndrome
Gastric ulcers
Gastric polyps
Gastric neoplasia
Gastric dilatation
Gastric dilatation-volvulus

DISORDERS OF THE GASTROESOPHAGEAL JUNCTION

Hiatal hernia (axial, paraesophageal, diaphragmatic herniation, gastroesophageal intussusception)

DISORDERS OF THE SMALL INTESTINE

Parasites
Enteritis
Intraluminal obstruction (foreign body, intussusception, neoplasia)
Inflammatory bowel disease—idiopathic
Diffuse intramural neoplasia (lymphosarcoma)
Fungal disease
Intestinal volvulus
Paralytic ileus

DISORDERS OF THE LARGE INTESTINE

Colitis
Obstipation
Irritable bowel syndrome (IBS)

Table continued on following page

TABLE 21–1 *Continued*

ABDOMINAL DISORDERS

Pancreatitis
Zollinger-Ellison syndrome (gastrinoma of pancreas)
Peritonitis (any cause, including FIP)
Inflammatory liver disease
Bile duct obstruction
Steatitis
Prostatitis
Pyelonephritis
Pyometra
Urinary obstruction
Diaphragmatic hernia
Neoplasia

NEUROLOGIC DISORDERS

Psychogenic (pain, fear, excitement)
Motion sickness (rotation or unequal input from the labyrinths)
Inflammatory lesions (e.g., vestibular)
Edema (head trauma)
Autonomic or visceral epilepsy
Neoplasia

MISCELLANEOUS CAUSES OF VOMITING

Heartworm disease (feline)
Hyperthyroidism (feline)

---

secondary gastric hypomotility, intestinal foreign bodies, and pancreatitis. Large clots of blood or "coffee grounds" usually indicate a significant degree of erosion or ulceration. A fecal odor suggests intestinal obstruction.

Intermittent Chronic Vomiting. The clinician should strongly consider chronic gastritis, inflammatory bowel disease, irritable bowel syndrome, and gastric motility disorders as leading differential diagnoses. It is a *common* clinical sign of inflammatory bowel disease in both dogs and cats.

PHYSICAL EXAMINATION

The mucous membranes are evaluated for evidence of blood loss, dehydration, sepsis, shock, and jaundice. An oral examination may reveal a foreign body that may extend to the stomach or intestine. The cervical region should be palpated for thyroid nodules. A careful assessment is made for abdominal pain, either generalized or more localized. Other factors to evaluate include abnormal organ size, small or large kidneys, presence of a mass, degree of gastric distention, and altered bowel sounds. Bowel sounds are often absent in peritonitis and increased in acute inflammatory disorders. A rectal examination is always doen to evaluate mucosal texture, stool characteristics, melena, foreign material and to obtain a fresh sample for parasite examination.

DIAGNOSTIC PLAN

If reasonable concern is established, a mimimum data base of *CBC, biochemical profile, urinalysis,* and *fecal examination* is essential. *Survey abdominal radiographs* are indicated if thorough abdominal palpation is not possible or suggests an abnormality. Ancillary tests include *ACTH stimulation, complete barium series* (for gastric or intestinal foreign body, gastric hypomotility, gastric outflow obstruction, partial or complete intestinal obstruction), and *serum bile acids assay. Barium swallow with fluoroscopy* is often necessary for diagnosis of hiatal hernia disorders and gastroesophageal reflux disease. Vomiting is a *fre-*

quent presenting sign in cats with heartworm disease. *Serologic tests* should be done in endemic areas. *Thyroid testing* should also be done on vomiting cats over 5 years of age. *Serum gastrin levels* are tested if a gastrinoma is suspected. *Ultrasonography* may be useful in the diagnostic work-up. Disorders of the liver, gallbladder and bile ducts, GI foreign bodies, intestinal and gastric wall thickening, intestinal masses, intussusception, kidney disorders, pancreatitis, and other disorders may be identified. *Fiberoptic endoscopy* is considerably more reliable than barium series for diagnosis of gastric erosions, chronic gastritis, gastric neoplasia, and inflammatory bowel disease. Biopsy samples should always be obtained from the stomach and, whenever possible, the small intestine regardless of gross mucosal appearance. *Abdominal exploratory* surgery is indicated for foreign body removal, intussusception, gastric mucosal hypertrophy syndromes, and procurement of biopsies and for resection of neoplasms.

TREATMENT

Goals of therapy include (1) removing the initiating cause, (2) controlling the vomiting episodes, and (3) correcting the fluid, electrolyte, and acid-base abnormalities that are a frequent consequence. Antiemetics such as phenothiazines (for example, chlorpromazine) are the safest and most effective. Fluid administration is based on replacing daily maintenance and dehydration requirements and on the replacement of continued fluid losses.

REGURGITATION (pp. 108–110)

Regurgitation refers to a passive, retrograde movement of ingested material to a level proximal to the upper esophageal sphincter. *Reflux* refers to movement of gastric or duodenal contents into the esophagus without associated eructation or vomiting.

TABLE 21–2. CAUSES OF REGURGITATION

Megaesophagus—idiopathic
Megaesophagus—secondary
    Myasthenia gravis (focal or generalized)
    Hypoadrenocorticism
    Polyneuropathy (giant axonal neuropathy—canine; Key-Gaskell syndrome—
        feline)
    Canine distemper
    Systemic lupus erythematosus
    Polymyositis
    Hypothyroidism
    Lead toxicosis
    Organophosphate toxicity
    Thallium toxicosis
Motility disorder—segmental
Foreign body
Stricture
    Intraluminal lesion
    Extraluminal compression (vascular ring anomaly, anterior mediastinal mass,
        other intrathoracic tumors, hilar lymphadenopathy, abscess)
Esophagitis
Hiatal disorder
Neoplasia of esophagus
    Primary
    Metastatic
Granuloma (e.g., *Spirocerca lupi*)
Esophageal diverticulum

CLINICAL FEATURES

Many animals with disorders causing regurgitation are presented by owners who incorrectly interpret the problem as vomiting.

Coughing and dyspnea suggest aspiration secondary to regurgitation. Many patients with megaesophagus have radiographic evidence of aspiration pneumonia.

Weakness in association with regurgitation suggests myasthenia gravis, hypoadrenocorticism, or polymyositis. Dogs with *focal* myasthenia gravis of the esophagus often do not show any signs of weakness.

Weight loss in association with regurgitation indicates insufficient nutrient uptake.

Post-ingestion distress is characterized by extension of the head, frequent swallowing attempts, and then regurgitation. This most often indicates an acquired esophageal stricture. A puppy or kitten with vascular ring anomaly may show signs as soon as feeding of solid foods is initiated.

Ravenous appetite indicates hunger due to inadequate nutrient transfer.

PHYSICAL FINDINGS

Many megaesophagus patients are thin and in poor condition. Thoracic auscultation may reveal aspiration pneumonia. Physical findings such as weakness (myasthenia gravis), weakness and bradycardia (hypoadrenocorticism), muscle pain (polymyositis), and signs that may include joint pain, shifting limb lameness, erosive glossitis, and others (systemic lupus erythematosus) often occur with systemic disorders. Cats that regurgitate secondary to an anterior mediastinal mass often have a noncompressible cranial chest cavity. In cats with Key-Gaskell syndrome, persistent pupillary dilation, decreased nasal and lacrimal secretions, bradycardia, and constipation may occur.

DIAGNOSTIC PLAN

Thoracic radiography for survey evaluation of the esophagus is the first and most important step in the diagnosis of a regurgitation disorder. A *barium esophagram* (with fluoroscopy if available) should be performed to evaluate the cervical and thoracic esophagus if necessary. A CBC, biochemical profile, thyroid tests, CPK, and urinalysis should be done as part of the initial evaluation in all patients with megaesophagus. Specific tests such as ACTH stimulation, antinuclear antibody, and serum AChR antibody titer, Tensilon test are done if indicated. If esophageal stricture, foreign body, mass, or diverticulum is suspected, *fiberoptic endoscopy* provides the most rapid definitive diagnosis.

TREATMENT

The main objectives are to remove the initiating cause, minimize chances for aspiration, and maximum nutrient intake to the GI tract. Idiopathic megaesophagus is usually incurable, and treatment involves an individually tailored feeding regimen with the patient eating in an elevated position. Esophageal foreign bodies can often be removed and intraluminal strictures dilated with fiberoptic endoscopy techniques and bougienage or balloon dilation, respectively. Medical management is indicated for secondary causes.

DYSPHAGIA (p. 110)

Dysphagia refers to difficulty in swallowing, which may be due to obstruction, motility disturbance, or pain.

Clinical findings include acute gagging, increased frequency of swallowing, salivation, ravenous appetite, rarely inappetence, and coughing (due to laryngotracheal aspiration). Abnormal eating habits may also be noted.

DIAGNOSTIC PLAN

The initial diagnostic step involves *survey cervical and thoracic radiography* (e.g., mass, foreign body, evidence of a penetrating wound). A *barium contrast study* with *fluoroscopic examination* of the swallowing process is indicated for more difficult cases. *Esophagoscopy* and *manometry* are recommended if radiographic studies are unremarkable.

CHAPTER 22

DIARRHEA
(pages 111–114)

Diarrhea is the most consistent clinical manifestation of intestinal disease in dogs and cats. It is defined as an abnormal increase in the frequency, fluidity, or volume of feces resulting from excessive fecal water content. Diarrhea may be classified by duration, anatomic site, pathophysiology, and, when possible, etiology.

HISTORICAL FINDINGS (pp. 112–113)

Young animals are prone to dietary, infectious, and parasitic causes of diarrhea. The clinician should consider metabolic, inflammatory, and neoplastic diseases as causes of diarrhea in older animals. Adverse reactions to food (food intolerance or allergy) are common causes of diarrhea. Diarrhea that ceases when the animal is not fed suggests osmotic diarrhea.

Environment. Animals that roam are more likely to develop parasitic, toxic, and infectious disorders. Antibiotics, anti-inflammatory agents and cardiac glycosides can cause diarrhea.

Vomiting may occur as a consequence of small intestinal inflammation. It may occur in up to 30 per cent of dogs with colitis.

Loose to watery feces that contain fat droplets, undigested food, melena, and variable colors suggest small bowel disease. Loose to semi-solid feces containing excess mucus and fresh blood (hematochezia) indicate large bowel disease.

Frequency of defecation is normal to slightly increased with small bowel diarrhea but greatly increased with large bowel disease.

Quantity of feces is always increased with small bowel diarrhea. The volume of feces is variable with large bowel disease.

Tenesmus (straining) and dyschezia (painful defecation) are the hallmarks of large bowel disease.

Weight loss in animals with diarrhea may result from decreased caloric intake (anorexia), decreased nutrient assimilation (maldigestion/malabsorption), or excessive caloric loss (protein-losing enteropathy or nephropathy). Weight loss is uncommonly observed with large bowel disorders.

Original chapter written by Albert E. Jergens

TABLE 22–1. GENERAL CAUSES FOR ACUTE AND CHRONIC DIARRHEA

Dietary
    Food allergy/intolerance
    Ingestion of "toxins"
Gastrointestinal inflammation
    Inflammatory bowel diseases
    Parasitism
    Infectious enteritis
    Hemorrhagic gastroenteritis
    Infiltrative neoplasia
    Bacterial overgrowth
    Ulceration/erosion
Intestinal lymphangiectasia
Functional/mechanical ileus
Exocrine pancreatic insufficiency
Acute pancreatitis
Liver disease
Kidney disease
Systemic disorders
    Drugs
    Hypoadrenocorticism
    Hyperthyroidism
    FeLV/FIV infection
Irritable bowel syndrome

PHYSICAL FINDINGS (p. 113)

General Examination. Watery diarrhea contributes to dehydration and electrolyte depletion. Animals often are depressed, emaciated, and malnourished. Edema and ascites are observed with protein-losing enteropathy. Fever suggests severe mucosal breakdown or transmural inflammatory disease. Animals having large bowel diarrhea are typically alert, active, and well-fleshed. Abdominal palpation should be performed to detect pain, mass lesions, thickened bowel loops, or mesenteric lymphadenopathy. Rectal palpation provides information on rectal masses, strictures, and the presence of anal diseases.

DIAGNOSTIC PLAN (p. 113)

A *hemogram, serum biochemistries,* and *urinalysis* should be performed in animals with chronic diarrhea to rule out systemic diseases. *Serologic tests* for FeLV, FIV, and hyperthyroidism are warranted in cats.

TABLE 22–2. DIFFERENTIATION OF SMALL AND LARGE BOWEL DIARRHEA

SIGN	SMALL BOWEL	LARGE BOWEL
Quality of feces	Loose to watery	Loose to semi-solid
Fecal volume	Usually increased	Normal to decreased
Frequency of defecation	Mildly increased	Greatly increased
Tenesmus	Absent	Present
Fecal blood	Melena	Hematochezia
Excess mucus	Absent	Present
Weight loss	Common	Uncommon
Vomiting	May be seen	May be seen

Fecal Studies. Intestinal parasites must be ruled out in all cases of diarrhea by *fecal flotation* for parasitic ova and *direct fecal smears* for protozoa. *Fecal cytology* may detect the presence of infectious agents (histoplasmosis, clostridia spores) or inflammatory disease (fecal leukocytes). In patients whose diarrhea is severe and bloody, consider *fecal serology* for parvovirus or *fecal cultures* for enteropathogenic bacteria such as *Campylobacter* and *Salmonella.*

Radiographic Studies. Foreign bodies, obstructive lesions, and masses may be diagnosed with *survey abdominal radiographs.* Barium contrast upper gastrointestinal series enhance the sensitivity for detecting mucosal lesions of infiltrative disease. *Abdominal ultrasonography* may delineate mass lesions and intestinal mural thickenings.

Gastrointestinal Function Tests. *Assays for trypsin-like immunoreactivity* are simple and highly sensitive for the diagnosis of canine exocrine pancreatic insufficiency. *Breath hydrogen excretion* and *serum* assays of folate and *cobalamine* are useful in the diagnosis of intestinal bacterial overgrowth.

Intestinal Biopsy. Biopsies are required in many cases of chronic diarrhea to document the presence of morphologic injury and to provide prognostic information. *Endoscopy* is preferred since it is inexpensive, fast, and minimally invasive. *Laparotomy* should be performed to obtain full-thickness intestinal biopsies when endoscopy is unavailable.

THERAPEUTIC GOALS (pp. 113–114)

The objectives of symptomatic therapy include (1) bowel rest, (2) maintenance and restoration of fluid and electrolyte balance, and (3) minimizing ongoing fluid losses. Rest the gastrointestinal tract by withholding food for at least 24 hours. When signs abate, resume feeding with controlled diets of chicken or cottage cheese combined with boiled rice. Lactated Ringer's solution is an appropriate replacement fluid in most cases of diarrhea. To prevent hypokalemia, the clinician should supplement fluids with potassium chloride. Oral rehydration therapy has proved beneficial in patients that can ingest oral fluids. Motility modifiers (opioids) are principally used in the management of secretory diarrheas. Opioids are contraindicated in diarrhea resulting from invasive bacteria. Routine administration of antibiotics for the treatment of acute diarrhea is *not* recommended. Legitimate indications include the presence of specific enteropathogens and clinical conditions associated with severe mucosal injury. Parasitic diseases should be treated appropriately.

OUTCOME (p. 114)

Most cases of acute diarrhea are transient and mild, and they readily respond to symptomatic therapy. Patients with chronic diarrhea should receive a guarded prognosis. A definitive diagnosis, often requiring intestinal biopsy, will be necessary prior to initiating specific treatment.

CHAPTER 23

CONSTIPATION, TENESMUS, DYSCHEZIA, AND FECAL INCONTINENCE
(pages 115–122)

CONSTIPATION, TENESMUS, AND DYSCHEZIA
(pp. 115–118)

Constipation is defined as infrequent or absent passage of feces and is characterized by straining to defecate and by retention of hard dry feces in the colon and rectum. *Obstipation* is intractable constipation in which fecal impaction throughout the rectum and colon is so severe that defecation cannot occur. *Tenesmus* refers to straining associated with either defecation or urination. Alimentary tenesmus is characterized by frequent and often unproductive attempts to defecate following a bowel movement. *Dyschezia* is painful and difficult defecation usually caused by diseases of the rectum or anus. Tenesmus and dyschezia often occur together, and differentiation between the two is of little diagnostic value.

HISTORY

Constipation. Lack of defecation for several days is the usual owner complaint regarding the constipated dog or cat. An owner who reports that a pet is constipated may actually be observing tenesmus from disorders other than constipation. Inflammatory colorectal diseases cause tenesmus accompanied by scant, soft feces with blood or mucus. Hard dry feces or no feces are observed with constipation. Some chronically constipated animals have episodes of liquid diarrhea, giving the false impression that diarrhea is the primary problem. Idiopathic megacolon occurs most frequently in adult male cats. Sacral spinal deformity of Manx cats and English bulldogs can result in both constipation and fecal incontinence. Diet, recently administered medications, and ingestion of foreign material must be questioned.

Tenesmus and Dyschezia. A careful history must be obtained to differentiate urinary tenesmus and dysuria from alimentary tenesmus and dyschezia. It is important to determine whether tenesmus occurs prior to or following defecation. Straining prior to defecation is suggestive of an obstructive lesion or of diminished colonic motility. Tenesmus after defecation is more consistent with irritative or inflammaory colorectal disease.

PHYSICAL EXAMINATION

Constipation. Chronically constipated or obstipated animals are often weak and dehydrated and may have a distended and painful abdomen. A firm and distended colon is easily detected by abdominal palpation. The anus and rectum should be examined digitally for the presence of pain, blood, foreign material, masses, prostatic size, conformation of the pelvic canal, and anal sphincter tone. Neuromuscular status should be evaluated.

Tenesmus and Dyschezia. Abdominal and digital rectal palpation help to determine the cause. A firm or distended urinary bladder may indicate straining to urinate. The urethra, prostate, penis, and

---

Original chapter written by Robert C. DeNovo

TABLE 23–1. CAUSES OF CONSTIPATION IN THE DOG AND CAT

Dietary	Foreign material in feces (hair, bone, cloth, cat litter, etc.) Lack of adequate fiber*
Environmental/behavioral	Hospitalization Dirty litter pan Inactivity
Rectal-colonic obstruction Extraluminal	Pseudocoprostasis Perirectal/perianal tumor Prostatic hypertrophy, cyst, abscess, tumor Perineal hernia Healed pelvic fracture
Intraluminal	Congenital imperforate anus Stricture Neoplasia Granuloma Diverticulum/prolapse Foreign body
Neuromuscular dysfunction	Lumbosacral spinal cord disease Bilateral pelvic nerve injury Paraplegia Dysautonomia CNS disease (lead) Idiopathic megacolon*
Fluid and electrolyte imbalances	Dehydration Hypokalemia Hypercalcemia
Painful defecation	Anal sac abscess Perianal fistula Anorectal stricture/tumor Proctitis Spinal injury Pelvic injury
Drug-induced	Anticholinergics Opiates Diuretics Sucralfate Barium sulfate Aluminum hydroxide antacids Antihistamines Phenothiazines Kaopectate Vincristine Oral iron supplements
Metabolic disease	Hypothyroidism Hyperparathyroidism-pseudohyperparathyroidism Pheochromocytoma

*Classification uncertain

vagina should be examined for pain, inflammation, calculi, and masses. A distended colon and rectum impacted with feces indicate that constipation is the cause of tenesmus. Dyschezia is most prominent with inflammatory diseases of the distal rectum and anus. Gentle digital rectal examination should be done to detect enlarged or abscessed anal sacs, anal fissures or fistulas, rectal masses or strictures, and foreign material in the feces.

TABLE 23–2. CAUSES OF TENESMUS AND DYSCHEZIA IN THE DOG AND CAT

Colonic/rectal disease
    Constipation (Table 23–1)
    Colitis/proctitis
        Infectious-bacterial fungal
        Inflammatory bowel disease
    Neoplasia/polyps
    Foreign body (e.g., bones, food wrapping)
    Irritable bowel syndrome
    Rectal diverticula
Perineal/perianal disease
    Anal sac abscess
    Anal sac neoplasia
    Perianal fistula
    Perineal hernia
Urogenital disease
    Cystitis/urethritis/vaginitis
    Cystic—urethral calculi
    Prostatitis/abscess
    Parturition
    Neoplasia of urethra, bladder, prostate, vagina
Miscellaneous
    Caudal abdominal cavity mass
    Pelvic fracture/neoplasia

DIAGNOSIS

Constipation. Diagnosis of constipation is straightforward, based primarily on history and clinical evaluation. Additional tests including a complete blood count, biochemical profile, and urinalysis should be done on all chronically constipated, obstipated, or systemically ill patients to detect complicating conditions. Abdominal radiographs may identify predisposing causes such as foreign material in the bowel, abdominal masses, megacolon, peritonitis, or pelvic narrowing. Endoscopic examination is helpful to identify tumors and obtain biopsies to detect strictures and inflammatory lesions.

Tenesmus and Dyschezia. Diagnostic procedures are similar to those suggested for the diagnosis of constipation. Response to dietary restriction for 24 to 72 hours and anthelmintic treatment for occult trichuriasis is a logical approach to acute disease. Tenesmus and dyschezia lasting for several days and not responding to symptomatic therapy require additional diagnostic measures as for constipation (see textbook Chap. 24).

TREATMENT

Constipation. Treatment of constipation includes correction of metabolic abnormalities, removal of the fecal mass, identification of predisposing causes, and prevention of recurrence. Fluid, electrolyte, and metabolic abnormalities must be corrected initially to restore intestinal secretions and motility. Simple constipation with no systemic illness is easily treated with enemas and/or oral or suppository laxatives. Treatment of the obstipated patient is difficult and usually requires manual removal of the feces. This procedure is best accomplished using general anesthesia once the patient is metabolically stable (see textbook Chap. 24 for precautions). If medical management fails to relieve the fecal mass, a colotomy or subtotal colectomy may be necessary.

Tenesmus and Dyschezia. Most patients will benefit from a 24- to 72-hour fast. Cleansing the perineum with iodine soap, clipping matted hair, and hydrotherapy are of benefit if anusitis, fistulas, abscess, or proctitis is present. Anal sac abscesses should be drained. Deep infection from fistulas and abscesses should be treated with systemic antibiotics. Topical antibiotic, steroid, or anesthetic preparations are helpful to decrease anal inflammation. Motility-modifying drugs symptomatically relieve tenesmus and dyschezia. In most instances, symptomatic therapy should be limited to 3 to 5 days.

FECAL INCONTINENCE (pp. 118–122)

Fecal incontinence is the inability to control defecation and retain feces until defecation is desired. Loss of voluntary control of defecation accompanied by urgency and tenesmus can be caused by inflammatory colorectal disease. Incontinence characterized by lack of con-

TABLE 23–3. CAUSES OF FECAL INCONTINENCE IN THE DOG AND CAT

Neurologic disease

Sacral spinal cord	Congenital vertebral malformation
	Spina bifida/meningomyelocele
	Sacrococcygeal hypoplasia of Manx cats
	Trauma
	Sacral fracture
	Sacrococcygeal subluxation
	Lumbosacral instability compression
	Infection
	Viral meningomyelitis (e.g., distemper)
	Discospondylitis
	Degenerative myelopathy
	Neoplasia
	Vascular compromise
Peripheral neuropathy	Trauma
	Perineal hernia repair
	Perineal urethrostomy
	Penetrating wounds
	Dysautonomia
	Polyneuropathy*
	Hypothyroidism
	Diabetes mellitus
	Drug-induced (e.g., vincristine)

Non-neurologic disease

Colonic/rectal	Inflammatory bowel disease
	Neoplasia
	Infectious
	Constipation (Table 23–1)
Anorectal	Trauma/Surgery
	Anal sac/tumor removal
	Perineal hernia repair
	Rectal resection
	Perianal fistula
	Rectovaginal fistula
	Neoplasia

Miscellaneous

	Severe diarrhea
	Anuria in the Carin Terrier
	Altered mentation
	Irritable bowel syndrome
	Old age

*Classification uncertain

scious posture to defecate and uncontrolled passage of feces is more suggestive of a neurologic or muscular abnormality of the rectum or anal sphincter.

HISTORY

The owner should be questioned about previous spinal disease, pelvic trauma, dystocia, chronic constipation, or anorectal surgery; all are conditions that could have damaged the mechanisms of fecal continence. Severe diarrhea caused by either small or large bowel disease can cause symptoms of fecal incontinence, whereas normal feces in the incontinent patient suggests presence of a neurologic lesion. Frequent and conscious defecation is usually caused by inflammatory, infectious, and neoplastic diseases of the bowel. Failure to posture to defecate accompanied by uncontrolled passage of feces suggests neurogenic disease or anal sphincter damage. Concurrent fecal incontinence and abnormal micturition suggest neurologic disease.

PHYSICAL EXAMINATION

Inspection of the perineum and a digital examination of the anorectum for deformity, fistulas, perineal hernia, abscess, fecal impaction, rectal masses, or strictures should be done. Patulous anal canal is easily recognized and suggestive of neuromuscular dysfunction. An empty colon occurs with inflammatory bowel disease. A distended and flaccid bladder is consistent with neurologic disease. A complete neurologic examination should be done. Hyperesthesia of the lumbosacral muscles, or evidence of self-induced trauma to the hind limbs, may indicate an irritative lesion involving the sacral spinal cord. Perianal sensation and sacral spinal cord function are best assessed by the anal reflex and the pudendal-anal (bulbocavernosus) reflex. Lesions of the sacral spinal cord, the sacral nerve roots, or the pudendal nerves can abolish these reflexes and cause a dilated anal sphincter, loss of sensation to the sacral and coccygeal dermatomes, and loss of the micturition reflex.

DIAGNOSIS

Proctoscopy or colonoscopy with biopsy is indicated to identify primary colorectal disease. If neurologic disease is suspected, vertebral radiographs and special imaging using myelography, epidurography, magnetic resonance imaging, and cerebral spinal fluid analysis should be considered. Laboratory evaluation is of limited use in most instances except to screen for immune-mediated or endocrine disease. Electrodiagnostics and manometric tests should be considered if available.

TREATMENT AND OUTCOME

Non-neurogenic incontinence caused by loss of reservoir function or overflow incontinence caused by constipation usually resolves with treatment of the primary disease. Neurogenic incontinence is difficult to manage and often not treatable. Symptomatic management of non-neurogenic and mild neurogenic incontinence can be attempted. Frequent small meals of a low-residue diet will decrease fecal volume. Opiates will slow intestinal transit, allowing absorption of more water from the fecal mass, and may also increase anal sphincter tone. Phenylpropanolamine may be effective in some instances to improve sphincter tone.

CHAPTER 24

MELENA AND HEMATOCHEZIA
(pages 123–125)

Melena describes black, tarry stools resulting from digested blood. Hematochezia refers to the presence of fresh red blood adherent to the stool. The presence of melena suggests large volume hemorrhage from the upper gastrointestinal tract and is a warning sign of serious disease. Hematochezia is usually due to large bowel disease, in particular colitis and is less frequently associated with life-threatening diseases.

CLINICAL EXAMINATION (pp. 123–124)

The owner should be asked whether nonsteroidal anti-inflammatory drugs or glucocorticoids have been used, since these drugs are a com-

TABLE 24–1. CAUSES OF MELENA

Swallowed blood
    Hemoptysis
    Nasal and oropharyngeal neoplasia
Esophagus
    Neoplasia
Stomach
    Severe gastritis
    Ulcers (drugs, stress, uremia, liver failure, mastocytosis, gastrinoma)
    Neoplasia (adenocarcinoma, leiomyosarcoma, lymphosarcoma)
    Upper small intestine
    Severe duodenitis
    Duodenal ulcers (drugs, stress, uremia, liver failure, mastocytosis, gastrinoma)
    Neoplasia (mast cell neoplasia, lymphosarcoma, adenocarcinoma)
    Severe hookworm burden
Lower small intestine and large bowel
    Neoplasia
    Polyps
Gastrointestinal ischemia
    Shock
    Volvulus
    Intussusception
    Mesenteric avulsion
    Gastrointestinal infarction
Drug administration
    Nonsteroidal anti-inflammatory drugs
    Glucocorticoids
Miscellaneous
    Coagulopathies (especially DIC)
    Gastrointestinal blood vessel malformations (varices, arteriovenous fistulas)
    Severe acute pancreatitis
    Hemobilia
    Liver failure
    Rocky mountain spotted fever
    Uremia

Abridged from Strombeck, D. R., and Guilford, W. G.: Approach to clinical problems in gastroenterology. In Small Animal Gastroenterology. 2nd ed. Davis, Stonegate Publishing, 1990, pp 56–89. With permission.

Original chapter written by W. Grant Guilford

mon cause of gastroduodenal ulceration. The risk of exposure to anti-coagulant rodenticides should be assessed and the likelihood of trauma determined. Clinical signs usually pertain primarily to anemia and hypovolemia. Concomitant regurgitation suggests esophageal or pharyngeal disease, cough raises the likelihood of hemoptysis, and jaundice with ascites implies liver disease. Hematemesis strongly suggests gastric or duodenal bleeding. Concurrent signs of tenesmus, dyschezia, frequent defecation, and/or increased stool mucus suggest that hematochezia or melena is due to large bowel disease. Hepatic encephalopathy may be precipitated by gastrointestinal hemorrhage. The physical examination should include careful inspection for the presence of bleeding disorders. Abdominal palpation may reveal abdominal pain or an abdominal mass.

DIAGNOSIS (pp. 124–125)

The diagnostic evaluation of hematochezia is similar to that described for the evaluation of tenesmus and dyschezia (Chap. 23). The first step in the diagnostic evaluation of melena is the objective confirmation of the problem. The classic appearance of melena is of coal-black, shiny, sticky, foul-smelling feces of tar-like consistency. It can become important to confirm the presence of digested blood by use of tests for fecal blood, such as the orthotolidine and guaiac tablet tests. False-positive results can occur in animals ingesting large quantities of raw meat or iron. A complete blood count helps to determine the severity and chronicity of the melena. Microcytic hypochromic anemias are common following prolonged gastrointestinal blood loss. Reticulocytosis is usually present after a few days except in those animals with iron-deficiency or neoplastic infiltrates in the bone marrow. Buffy coat examination for mast cell neoplasia and lymphoma can be useful. Coagulation tests may be required if a bleeding problem is suspected. The serum chemistry panel allows detection of renal and liver failure, which can result in melena. A fecal flotation for hookworms should not be neglected. The procedure of most value in localizing the site of bleeding and in determining the cause is upper gastrointestinal endoscopy. If no upper gastrointestinal lesions are found, the nasopharynx should be examined. Contrast radiography is usually of less value than endoscopy and does not provide a definitive (histologic) diagnosis. Exploratory surgery may be required, but bleeding mucosal lesions can be missed. In difficult cases, ^{99m}Technetium-labeled red blood cells or arteriography may be required to diagnose the problem.

TREATMENT (p. 125)

Symptomatic management may include treatment trials with parasiticides effective against whipworms, sulfasalazine (the drug of choice for idiopathic colitis), and sulfa drugs in young animals suspected of having coccidiosis. Symptomatic management of melena due to severe upper gastrointestinal hemorrhage can include crystalloids, colloids, and/or blood transfusions. Administration of cimetidine or omeprazole or sucralfate may be useful. Surgical resection of the bleeding lesion may be required.

CHAPTER 25

PTYALISM
(pages 125–128)

Ptyalism refers to the excessive production of saliva. Pseudoptyalism is the dribbling or drooling of saliva that has accumulated in the oral cavity.

Age, Breed. Megaesophagus and portosystemic shunts should be considered in young animals. Congenital portosystemic shunts have been reported in certain purebred dogs. Puppies and kittens are more likely to have ingested a foreign body, bitten an electric cord, or ingested caustic compounds or toxins.

Diet. Signs of hepatic encephalopathy may be precipitated by a diet high in protein including ptyalism.

Eating Behavior. With a unilateral lesion the animal may not chew on the affected side, may take a bite of food and then release it because of pain on chewing, or may hold the head in unusual positions. Anorexia, weight loss may occur with acute or chronic oral lesions.

Medication, Topical Products. Adverse reactions, including hypersalivation, can occur with the oral administration of cholinergic drugs (e.g., bethanechol) or anticholinesterase drugs (e.g., pyridostigmine). Cholinesterase inhibitors may result in cholinergic signs (i.e., ptyalism) if an overdose is given, as may pyrethrin insecticides. Ivermectin toxicity in dogs may cause increased salivation. Cats administered benzyl alcohol as a preservative have developed clinical signs including hypersalivation. Oral ulceration may occur along with cutaneous lesions in animals with drug eruption.

Environment. Exposure to household cleaning products that may be caustic or toxic. Household cleaning products may cause irritation to the tissues in the oral cavity. House plants (e.g., dieffenbachia, poinsettia, Christmas tree) may cause oral inflammation with increased salivation. Illicit drugs and toxins resulting in CNS stimulation may cause excessive salivation. Caffeine toxicosis causes ptyalism. Increases in environmental temperature result in increased salivation in dogs and cats. Foreign bodies may become lodged and cause ptyalism. Venom from black widow spiders, gila monsters, and North American scorpions may cause salivation. Pseudorabies should be considered in any dog with acute ptyalism that has been exposed to swine.

Anesthesia. Reflux esophagitis symptoms (e.g., hypersalivation, regurgitation) usually develop 1 to 4 days following the anesthetic procedure.

Swallowing Difficulty. Rabies should be included in the differential diagnosis in any animal with difficulty in swallowing. Regurgitation is a classic sign of esophageal disease, and animals may salivate excessively.

Vomiting. Nausea may be accompanied by increased salivation.

Behavioral Changes. Dogs or cats with oral pain may become aggressive or become more reclusive. Changes may be associated with hepatic encephalopathy and may occur in rabid dogs or cats.

Hepatic Encephalopathy. Ptyalism is a common clinical sign in cats with portosystemic shunts. Signs, which may be intermittent, may be precipitated by foods with a high level of protein or in association with gastrointestinal bleeding.

Original chapter written by Linda J. DeBowes

Seizure.   Autonomic discharge may occur during a seizure and result in salivation, urination, and defecation.

PHYSICAL FINDINGS AND THEIR INTERPRETATION
(p. 127)

Halitosis.   Animals with oral, esophageal or gastric lesions may have mild to severe halitosis.

Periodontal Disease.   Increased salivation may occur as a result of pain and inflammation.

Stomatitis.   Inflammation and ulceration of the oral mucosa may cause significant discomfort resulting in excessive salivation. Irritants, foreign bodies, trauma, periodontal disease, and immune-mediated diseases may cause inflammation of the oral mucosa.

Oral Masses.   Neoplasms, eosinophilic granulomas, and granulomatous lesions may be present in the oral cavity. Lesions that ulcerate and become painful may cause excessive salivation. The saliva may be dark or blood-tinged if the lesions become ulcerated or necrotic.

Glossitis.   Lingual ulcers may occur as a result of trauma (e.g., chemical irritants), systemic infections (viral), metabolic disorders (uremia), immune-mediated disease (e.g., pemphigus vulgaris), and tumors.

Base of Tongue.   Masses and foreign objects beneath the tongue may cause ptyalism secondary to pain.

Ulcerations at Mucocutaneous Junctions.   Immune-mediated skin disorders may cause ulceration at the mucocutaneous junctions.

Dysphagia.   Animals that are drooling excessively should be evaluated for dysphagia, which may be caused by anatomic neuromuscular problems in the oral cavity or pharynx.

Cranial Nerve Deficits.   Lesions of cranial nerves IX and X often cause dysphagia and a weak or absent gag reflex. Dysfunction of cranial nerve XII may also cause difficulty in swallowing. Animals with facial nerve paralysis may drool from the affected side.

Dropped Jaw.   An animal with trigeminal nerve paralysis will not be able to close its mouth and will drool.

Muscle Atrophy.   This may be secondary to cranial nerve deficits or myositis that result in a swallowing problem.

Lymph Nodes.   Lymphadenopathy may cause dysphagia.

DIAGNOSTIC PLAN (pp. 127–128)

A complete *history* and *physical examination* should be performed. Sedation or anesthesia may be required if the animal is in too much pain or difficult to examine. The animal should be observed while eating and drinking so that the examiner can observe evidence of dysphagia. The source of the problem may be apparent after careful examination. Oral or cervical masses should be evaluated either by *fine-needle aspiration* and *cytologic study* or by *biopsy* and *histopathologic study*. *Thoracic radiographs* are indicated when oral neoplasia is suspected. Immune-mediated disease is evaluated by histologic and immunofluorescence examinations of biopsies. If oral lesions are accompanied by signs of systemic disease, a *minimum data base* (e.g., CBC, chemistry profile, UA) should be collected so that the systemic disease can be evaluated. If regurgitation is identified, the dog or cat should be evaluated for a primary esophageal problem (textbook Chap. 102). With nausea or vomiting, the patient should be evaluated for a gastric disorder (textbook Chap. 103). If behavioral changes occur, the diagnostic work-up should include tests of liver function.

CHAPTER 26

GAGGING AND RETCHING
(pages 129–131)

GAGGING (p. 129)

Gagging generally indicates that the neurologic pathways associated with a normal gag reflex are intact (Chapter 82). Most neurologic disorders result in reduced gag reflex and therefore an absence of gagging. A list of causes of gagging is presented in Table 26–1.

TABLE 26–1. CAUSES OF GAGGING IN THE DOG AND CAT

A. Nasal sinus
1. Cleft palate
2. Nasal parasites
3. Nasal tumors
4. Severe rhinitis
5. Nasal foreign body

B. Pharynx
1. Morphologic
   a. Neoplasia
   b. Foreign body
   c. Tonsilar enlargement
   d. Abscess
   e. Overlong soft palate
   f. Nasopharyngeal polyps
   g. Pharyngeal salivary mucocele
   h. Stylohyoid disarticulation
2. Functional
   a. Cricopharyngeal incoordination
   b. Cricopharyngeal achalasia
   c. Pharyngitis
   d. Neuromuscular disease
      (1) Infectious disease (Rabies)
      (2) Hypocalcemia

C. Respiratory tract
1. Upper airway
   a. Morphologic
      (1) Foreign body
      (2) Neoplasia
      (3) Tracheal collapse
   b. Functional
      (1) Laryngeal paralysis
      (2) Laryngitis
      (3) Tracheobronchitis
2. Lower airway
   a. Morphologic
      (1) Neoplasia
      (2) Parasitic granuloma
   b. Functional
      (1) Feline asthma
      (2) Canine tracheobronchitis
      (3) Fungal pneumonitis

D. Esophagus
1. Morphologic
   a. Stricture
   b. Neoplasia
2. Functional
   a. Esophagitis
   b. Megaesophagus
      (1) Neuropathy
         (a) Central
         (b) Peripheral
      (2) Junctionopathy
         (a) Myasthenia gravis
         (b) Organophosphate intox
      (3) Myopathy
         (a) Polymyositis
         (b) Myotonia
         (c) Glycogen storage disease
      (4) Neuromyopathy
         (a) Pylorospasm
         (b) Endocrine disorders (e.g., hypoadrenocorticism, hypothyroidism)

E. Stomach
1. Acute and chronic gastritis
2. Proximal gastric neoplasia

F. Miscellaneous
1. Pericardial effusion
2. Neoplasm of middle ear
3. Familial progressive nephropath

Original chapter written by Mark J. Kopit

RETCHING (p. 131)

Retching by definition is an involuntary and ineffectual attempt at vomiting and is caused by the same motor events that cause vomiting. Retching is discussed in Chapter 21

CHAPTER 27

FLATULENCE AND BORBORYGMUS
(pages 132–133)

Borborygmus and flatulence usually result from dietary intolerances. Maldigestion due to exocrine pancreatic insufficiency or malabsorption resulting from small intestinal diseases often leads to excessive intestinal gas.

CLINICAL EXAMINATION FINDINGS (pp. 132–133)

Historical findings of importance include the presence of concurrent vomiting and diarrhea, either of which suggests more serious gastrointestinal disease. An extensive dietary history is essential. Spoiled diets and diets high in protein or fat are particularly likely to yield odoriferous gases.

MANAGEMENT (p. 133)

The management of borborygmus and flatulence begins with a change to a highly digestible, low-fiber diet of moderate protein and fat content (for instance, Prescription Diet i/d). Charcoal is the most commonly used adsorbent antiflatulent in people but is of questionable effectiveness. Simethicone (25 to 200 mg q6h) is frequently used as a treatment for borborygmus, gaseous colic, and flatulence in human beings. Anecdotal reports suggest that these enzyme supplements can reduce the severity of flatulence in cats and dogs.

Original chapter written by W. Grant Guilford

CHAPTER 28

JOINT EFFUSION
(pages 133–136)

Effusions are classified as inflammatory or noninflammatory; monarticular, pauciarticular (two to five joints), or polyarticular (more than five joints); and proximal or distal in distribution. The nature of the effusion depends on the inciting cause. Tables 28–1 and 28–2 show the causes and clinical pathology of joint effusion.

Rapidity of Onset. Development of noninflammatory joint disease can be insidious (e.g., DJD, chronic anterior cruciate tear, hip dysplasia) or acute (e.g., trauma, hemarthrosis). Primary infectious etiolo-

TABLE 28–1. CAUSES OF JOINT EFFUSION

I. Noninflammatory effusions
    A. Degenerative joint disease
    B. Trauma
    C. Developmental arthropathies
    D. Neoplasia
    E. Coagulopathy
    F. Genetic disease

II. Inflammatory effusions
    A. Primary infectious
        1. Bacterial
        2. Mycoplasmal
        3. Fungal
        4. Protozoal
        5. Viral
    B. Noninfectious
        1. Immunologic
            a. Erosive arthropathy
                (1) Rheumatoid arthritis
                (2) Polyarthritis of Greyhounds
                (3) Feline chronic progressive polyarthritis
            b. Nonerosive arthropathy
                (1) Idiopathic polyarthritis
                (2) Systemic lupus erythematosus
                (3) Drug-induced
                (4) Polyarteritis nodosa
                (5) Arthritis secondary to chronic disease
                    (a) Discospondylitis
                    (b) Pyometra
                    (c) Deep pyoderma
                    (d) Disseminated fungal disease
                    (e) Chronic inflammatory bowel disease
                    (f) Chronic active hepatitis
                    (g) Ehrlichia
                    (h) Lyme disease
                    (i) Neoplasia
                    (j) Other
        2. Nonimmunologic
            a. Crystal-induced arthritis
                 (1) Pseudogout
                 (2) Gout

Original chapter written by David G. Feldman

TABLE 28–2. CLINICAL PATHOLOGY OF JOINT EFFUSION

DISEASE	APPEARANCE	MUCIN CLOT	WBC	% PMN	FEATURES
Normal	Straw colored/clear	Firm	0–2900	0–12	Protein <2.75 gm/dl
Trauma	Bloody, xanthochromic, or clear	Firm	>3000	<25	Few to many RBC, crenated RBC, elevated protein and volume
Degenerative joint disease	Yellow/clear	Firm	1000–3000	<25	Debris, cartilagenous plaques; volume and protein up in acute phase
Nonerosive arthritis (all types)	Yellow/slightly turbid	Firm to friable	4400–371,000	15–95	Increased volume and protein in acute phase; occasional LE cell in patients with SLE
Erosive arthritis	Cloudy	Friable	8000–38,000	20–80	Poor viscosity, inclusion-bearing PMNs; synovial glucose 10–30% lower than serum; rice bodies present (fibrin particles or budded synovium); volume up if acute
Septic arthritis	Grey or green murky. Occasionally bloody	Friable	40,000–262,000 (may be toxic)	>90	Poor viscosity, synovial glucose 50–70% lower than serum; volume increased

gies are often acute. Inflammatory, noninfectious joint swellings are often insidious.

Age, Breed, and Gender.   Breed and age predilections for dogs with joint dysplasias and other developmental diseases are reviewed in Chapters 149 and 150.

DIAGNOSIS (pp. 135–136)

Imaging.   Effusions, especially if the fluid accumulation is slight in volume, may be difficult to visualize radiographically. *Magnetic resonance imaging* is more sensitive than radiography.

Arthrocentesis.   Joint taps, performed under strict asepsis, serve as the definitive tool for diagnosing pathologic effusion. The joints to be tapped include either those with obvious swelling or, if systemic disease is suspected, multiple (even palpably normal) joints.

Ancillary Tests.   Additional diagnostic tests that may be useful in classifying the effusion, particularly in the presence of systemic signs, include a CBC, chemistry panel, urinalysis with culture and sensitivity, coagulogram, blood cultures, serum microbial titers, and titers for antinuclear antibody and rheumatoid factor.

TREATMENT AND OUTCOME (p. 136)

Septic joints are usually treated with systemic antibiotics. More advanced cases may require arthrotomy with lavage and drainage. Primary immunologic diseases are treated with corticosteroids and/or immunosuppressive agents. Traumatic effusions are treated either conservatively (i.e., with rest, support wraps, analgesics) or with surgery if indicated. Joints with DJD should not be therapeutically tapped. Control of the DJD will limit the effusion.

CHAPTER 29

LAMENESS
(pages 136–143)

Tables 29–1 and 29–2 list the most common causes of lameness recognized in dogs and cats respectively. The reader is referred to the appropriate chapters for further reading on specific subjects. In a weightbearing lameness the dog shifts its weight away from the affected limb and therefore extends the stance phase of a stride on the sound limb. The stride of the affected limb is usually shorter than that of the opposite normal limb. Lesions of the shoulder and hip may result in a markedly shortened stride, as these joints normally have the greatest range of motion. A sensory disturbance causing abnormalities in gait is seen clinically as ataxia.

LOCAL EXAMINATION

Signs of pain elicited by hyperextension or hyperflexion of a joint are the most reliable indication of joint disease. Restricted or excessive

Original chapter written by Jean-François Bardet

TABLE 29–1. CAUSES OF LAMENESS IN DOGS

Congenital disorders
  Radial agenesis
  Ectrodactyly; syndactyly
  Chondrodysplasia
  Congenital hyperextension of the
    stifle
  Vertebral abnormalities
  Spina bifida
Degenerative disorders
  Degenerative joint disease
  Degenerative myelopathy
Developmental disorders
  Physeal disorders
  Limb shortening
  Congenital elbow luxation
  Osteochondrosis
  Hip dysplasia
  Patellar luxation
  Legg-Perthes disease
Genetic disorders
  Hemophilic arthropathy
  Mucopolysaccharidosis
  Periarticular calcinosis
Infectious disorders
  Bacterial, viral, fungal, mycoplas-
    mal and protozoal arthritis
  Bacterial and fungal osteomyelitis
  Infectious polymyositis
  Cellulitis and soft tissue abscess
  Bacterial or mycotic granulomas of
    the foot pads
Immunologic disorders
  Canine rheumatoid arthritis
  Idiopathic nondeforming
    polyarthritis
  Systemic lupus erythematosus
  Pemphigus of the footpads
  Polyneuropathies
  Polymyopathies

Metabolic disorders
  Hyperparathyroid bone disease
  Rickets
  Osteomalacia
  Polymyopathies
  Polyneuropathies
Neoplasia
  Bone: primary and secondary
  Synovium
  Spinal cord
  Nerve roots and peripheral nerves
  Connective tissues of a limb
Traumatic disorders
  Fracture
  Luxation
  Contusion
  Strain
  Muscular contusion, laceration rup-
    ture, and contracture
  Tendinous laceration, avulsion
  Traumatic neuropathy
  Intervertebral disc herniation
Vascular disorders
  Fibrocartilaginous infarct of the
    spinal cord
  Bone infarct
Unknown etiology
  Panosteitis
  Multiple cartilaginous exostoses
  Myositis ossificans
  Hypertrophic osteodystrophy
Others
  Bone cyst
  Hypertrophic osteoarthropathy

---

movements, crepitus, pain, and abnormal relationship of bony structures are the hallmarks of fracture and luxation.

DIAGNOSTIC PLAN (pp. 138–143)

Radiography. Once the affected bone and/or joint is localized, the area should be radiographed if bony lesions are expected. Radiographic examinations often require adequate sedation.

Complete Blood Count, Biochemical Profile, and Urinalysis. The hemogram, biochemical profile, and urinalysis provide useful help in the diagnosis, but they are also an important part of the pre-anesthesia evaluation of the patient.

Arthrocentesis and Synovial Fluid Analysis. Arthrocentesis should be performed whenever joint effusion is present or when an inflammatory arthropathy is suspected.

Cultures and Antibiotic Sensitivity Testing. Cultures are more useful in the selection of a proper antibiotic than in making a diagnosis.

Biopsies. Biopsies of suspect tissue are indicated when other tests are negative. They are required if a bone tumor is suspected.

TABLE 29–2. CAUSES OF LAMENESS IN CATS

Congenital disorders
  Radial and tibial agenesis
  Ectrodactyly
  Polydactyly
  Syndactyly
  Congenital hyperextension of the
    stifle
  Spina bifida
Degenerative disorders
  Degenerative joint disease
  Degenerative myelopathy
Developmental disorders
  Physeal disorders
  Limb shortening
  Hip dysplasia
  Patellar luxation
Genetic disorders
  Mucopolysaccharidosis
Infectious disorders
  Bacterial, viral, fungal and
    mycoplasmal arthritis
  Bacterial and fungal osteomyelitis
  Infectious myositis
  Cellulitis and soft tissue abscess
  Feline osteochondromatosis
Immunologic disorders
  Feline progressive polyarthritis
  Feline chronic progressive poly-
    arthritis
  Systemic lupus erythematosus

Metabolic disorders
  Hypervitaminosis A
  Hyperparathyroid bone disease
  Primary
  Secondary
Neoplasia
  Bone
  Synovium
  Connective tissues of a limb
  Spinal cord
Traumatic disorders
  Fracture
  Luxation
  Contusion
  Strain
  Sprain
  Intrameniscal calcification
  Muscular contusion, laceration rup-
    ture, and contracture
  Tendinous laceration, avulsion
  Traumatic neuropathy
  Intervertebral disc herniation
Vascular disorders
  Thromboembolism of caudal aorta
    and/or its branches
  Necrotizing myelopathy
Unknown etiology
  Fibrodysplasia ossificans
Others
  Hypertrophic osteoarthropathy

Immune Tests. The reader should refer to Chapter 149.

Serum Titers. Specific titers are required in infectious arthritis.

Blood Culture. Blood cultures are indicated when lameness is associated with a persistent fever of unknown origin.

Arthroscopy. Arthroscopy provides an effective diagnostic technique with minimal invasiveness and tissue morbidity, and it permits rapid postoperative recovery.

Electromyographic Studies. Electromyographic studies help to differentiate neurologic from orthopedic causes of lameness. The details are discussed in Chapters 85 and 86.

CT Scan and Magnetic Resonance Imaging (MRI). The expense and availability of MRI equipment have limited the use of MRI in veterinary medicine.

Bone Scintigraphy. Bone scintigraphy, which provides a functional rather than structural assessment of the skeleton, has several clinical applications in small animal medicine: detection of osseous tumor metastasis; evaluation of distant metastasis from primary skeletal osteosarcomas; detection of early joint diseases such as degenerative joint disease or polyarthritis; diagnosis of early osteomyelitis or discospondylitis; and evaluation of impairment of the blood supply to bone from trauma, infection, thrombosis, infarction, or vascular compression.

GOALS OF TREATMENT (p. 143)

First, priority should be given to the recognition and treatment of the primary condition. Second, since pain is most often a major component of lameness, analgesic drugs should be used.

CHAPTER 30

SHIVER AND TREMBLE
(pages 143–145)

In the dog, myoclonus is almost pathognomonic of canine distemper.

PHYSIOLOGIC CAUSES OF SHIVERING AND TREMBLING (pp. 143–144)

Temperature Regulation. Shivering may be induced by a reduction in canine skin temperature.

Fear. Fear induces a general increase in muscle tone that may result in trembling.

Fatigue. Trembling and weakness may occur in muscle groups that have been heavily exercised. Such trembling is evident in postural muscles when the animal is standing.

PATHOLOGIC CAUSES OF TREMBLING (pp. 144–145)

CONDITIONS IN WHICH TREMBLING IS ACCOMPANIED BY OTHER SIGNS

Exposure to Toxins. Hexachlorophene, metaldehyde, organophosphates, fenthion, and droperidol with fentanyl citrate are the most frequent offenders (Chapter 61).

Metabolic Diseases. Hyperkalemia, hypocalcemia, and hypoglycemia are three of a number of metabolic diseases (Chapter 3).

Cerebellar Diseases. (Chapter 82).

Nerve Root Diseases. (Chapter 83).

CONDITIONS IN WHICH TREMBLING OR TREMOR IS THE ONLY SIGN

Senile Tremors. The condition primarily involves the pelvic limbs. Trembling is accentuated when the animal stands or moves. Treatment is generally not necessary and not helpful.

Shaker Dogs (Acquired Tremor in Young Adult Dogs). This condition is most common in small breeds, especially those with white hair coats. A sudden onset at 1 or 2 years of age is expressed as a constant tremor involving the entire body. The tremor is exaggerated during excitement. Immunosuppressive doses of corticosteroids administered early in the course of the disease usually result in improvement. Diazepam may improve the clinical signs.

Cerebrospinal Hypomyelinogenesis and Dysmyelinogenesis. These conditions may be seen in puppies as young as 10 days old. Tremors involving the head, neck, body, and limbs are present when the puppy is awake and are virtually absent when it is at rest or asleep. The condition may be hereditary in chows, springer spaniels, Samoyeds, and Weimaraners. It has also been described in Bernese mountain dogs and a Dalmatian. No treatment is necessary in milder cases, as the clinical signs improve with time.

Original chapter written by Robert W. Carithers

CHAPTER 31
ATAXIA, PARESIS, AND PARALYSIS
(pages 145–148)

ATAXIA (pp. 145–146)

Sensory Ataxia.   Sensory ataxia results from a disruption of proprioceptive pathways from the limbs and, occasionally, the trunk (*truncal ataxia*).

Vestibular Ataxia.   Vestibular ataxia results from lesions involving the central or peripheral portions of the vestibular system. Ataxia resulting from a unilateral vestibular lesion can be characterized by an ipsilateral head tilt, tight circling toward the side of the lesion, nystagmus with a fast phase away from the side of the lesion, and a tendency to fall to the ipsilateral side.

Cerebellar Ataxia.   Cerebellar diseases are typically diffuse, producing a symmetric syndrome characterized by some or all of the following: broad-based stance, ataxia in all limbs with preservation of strength, dysmetria (usually hypermetria), truncal ataxia, intention tremors, delayed postural reactions with exaggerated responses, and menace deficits unassociated with visual loss.

PARESIS AND PARALYSIS (pp. 146–148)

Paresis and paralysis imply voluntary motor dysfunction and result from disorders affecting the brain stem, spinal cord, peripheral nerves, or myoneural junction. Tetraparesis/-plegia (quadriparesis/-plegia) describes the animal with voluntary motor dysfunction in all four limbs. Paraparesis/-plegia describes the animal with a partial or complete loss of voluntary motor function in the pelvic limbs. Hemiparesis/-plegia involves the right or left side. For localization of a lesion based on the neurologic exam, see Chapters 82 and 83.

Peripheral Nerve Dysfunction.   Generalized lower motor neuron diseases result in flaccid tetraparesis/-plegia and reduced or absent reflexes in all limbs. Generalized lower motor neuron diseases include tick paralysis, polyradiculoneuritis (coonhound paralysis), metabolic polyneuropathies, botulism, and dysimmune polyneuropathies. Some muscle diseases also produce weakness that can be interpreted as paresis (e.g., myasthenia gravis, steroid myopathy). Diseases that produce paresis or paralysis can also originate in the cardiovascular system. Aortoiliac thromboembolic disease (*saddle thrombi*) has been associated with feline cardiomyopathy.

DIFFERENTIAL DIAGNOSIS (p. 148)

Ancillary diagnostics include radiologic studies, electrodiagnostics, cerebrospinal fluid analysis, muscle and nerve biopsies, and serology.

TREATMENT OF ACUTE SPINAL CORD INJURIES (p. 148)

Methylprednisolone succinate and sodium prednisolone succinate have been shown to improve outcome when administered at a prescribed dosage beginning at ≤8 hours postinjury.

Original chapter written by Andy Shores

The recommended treatment protocol for acute spinal cord injury is as follows:

Initial Dose:	T_o.	15 mg/lb (30 mg/kg) IV
at	$T_{3 hr}$.	7.5 mg/lb (15 mg/kg)IV
at	$T_{6 hr}$.	7.5 mg/lb (15 mg/kg) IV
at $T_{9 hr}$ through	$T_{33 hr}$.	1 mg/lb/hr (2 mg/kg/hr) IV*

This regimen should be used in acute spinal cord injuries with *profound* neurologic effects and caused by trauma (external, blunt trauma; fracture/luxations of the spine; intervertebral disc extrusions) or an ischemic myelopathy (fibrocartilaginous embolization).

---

*By continuous infusion or as 3 mg/lb (6 mg/kg) IV boluses every 3 hours.

CHAPTER 32

ALTERED STATES OF CONSCIOUSNESS: COMA AND STUPOR
(pages 149–152)

Stupor and coma are considered neurologic emergencies.

GENERAL PATHOPHYSIOLOGY (pp. 149–150)

Pathophysiologic aspects such as cerebral edema, increased intracranial pressure, and herniation of brain tissue must be considered when a comatose or stuporous patient is being evaluated.

HISTORICAL AND EXAMINATION FINDINGS
(pp. 150–151)

The first step is to identify and correct any life-threatening non-neural problems such as hemorrhage, shock, and obstructed airway.

Consciousness. Diffuse cerebral disease or midbrain disease can cause stupor, coma, or other changes in consciousness. Lesions of the medulla oblongata can also cause stupor or coma.

Pupil Size. As a general rule, lesions of the brain stem can produce nonresponsive unilateral or bilateral pupil constriction or dilation, whereas lesions of the cerebrum can produce normal or constricted pupils that respond to both light and darkness.

Eye Movements. If the oculocephalic response is absent in a comatose patient, severe brain stem injury is a likely diagnosis, and the prognosis is poor for return of brain function.

Respiratory Character. Any change in normal respiratory patterns suggests a grave prognosis.

Original chapter written by Linda Shell

DIAGNOSTIC PLAN (p. 151)

The majority of the disorders causing coma and stupor are discussed in Chapter 82.

Two of the least invasive means of evaluating intracranial disease are awake electroencephalography (EEG) and brain stem auditory evoked responses (BAER), both of which can be performed without sedation or anesthesia in most patients. Spinal fluid analysis in cases of neoplasia may show an elevation of protein. Increased numbers of cells suggest encephalitis. Computerized tomography and MRI can be rewarding in diagnosing brain tumors, hydrocephalus, and vascular injuries.

GOALS OF TREATMENT (pp. 151–152)

First, establish a patent airway and ensure proper breathing and cardiac function. Second, place an intravenous catheter and collect blood samples prior to any treatment. If the animal is in shock, intravenous fluids are administered at the shock dose. Excessive fluids can contribute to cerebral edema.

There are three main treatments for cerebral edema: corticosteroids, osmotic diuretics, and hyperventilation. Corticosteroids reduce the edema associated with brain tumors, but their benefits in cases of head trauma have been questioned. Osmotic agents, such as mannitol, reduce intracranial pressure by decreasing brain water content. They are short-lived in their therapeutic effect and should never be administered when the animal is hypovolemic. If active brain hemorrhage is present, the reduction of intracranial pressure or the size of the brain may allow more hemorrhage to occur. Hyperventilation is probably the best emergency treatment for increased intracranial pressure. Seizures should be controlled with injectable diazepam. Craniotomy is indicated to remove depressed fractures that are compressing the brain or to control hemorrhage.

CHAPTER 33

SEIZURES
(pages 152–156)

HISTORICAL FINDINGS (pp. 153–155)

German shepherds, Irish setters, miniature poodles, Siberian huskies, beagles, cocker spaniels, Labrador retrievers, keeshonden and miniature schnauzers are examples of purebred dogs with inherited epilepsy. Seizures typically begin between 9 and 36 months of age. Animals under 9 months or over 36 months of age are more likely to have an active disease process. The differential diagnosis of disease based on age range is listed in Table 33–1.

Partial seizures or partial seizures which secondarily generalize are usually associated with structural disease such as an acquired epileptic focus, encephalitis, neoplasia, injury, or vascular insult.

Original chapter written by Cheryl L. Chrisman

TABLE 33–1. DIFFERENTIAL DIAGNOSIS OF SEIZURES IN DOGS AND CATS

YOUNG (UNDER 9 MONTHS OF AGE)

1. Congenital hydrocephalus
2. Lissencephaly
3. Lysosomal storage disorders
4. Distemper or feline infectious peritonitis (FIP) virus encephalitis
5. Other viral, fungal, protozoal or bacterial encephalitis
6. Trauma
7. Toxicity—lead, organophosphates, others
8. Hypoglycemia
9. Hepatic encephalopathy—portosystemic shunt
10. Other congenital defects with associated metabolic disorders
11. Thiamine deficiency

ADULT (9 MONTHS TO 5 YEARS)

1. Distemper and FIP virus encephalitis
2. Other viral, fungal, protozoal, or bacterial encephalitis
3. Steroid-responsive meningoencephalitis
4. Granulomatous meningoencephalitis
5. Trauma
6. Toxicity—lead, organophosphates, others
7. Hypoglycemia
8. Hepatic encephalopathy—portacaval shunt, acquired hepatopathy
9. Other acquired metabolic disorders
10. Inherited epilepsy (9–36 months typically)
11. Acquired epilepsy
12. Cerebral neoplasia—rare

OLD (5 YEARS AND OLDER)

1. Distemper and FIP virus and other causes of encephalitis
2. Steroid-responsive meningoencephalitis
3. Granulomatous meningoencephalitis
4. Trauma
5. Toxicity—lead, organophosphates, others
6. Hypoglycemia—insulinoma
7. Hepatic encephalopathy—acquired hepatopathy
8. Other acquired metabolic disorders
9. Acquired epilepsy
10. Cerebral neoplasia

PHYSICAL FINDINGS (p. 155)

The ocular fundus is evaluated for evidence of recent or past chorioretinitis, which may be associated with encephalitis. A complete neurologic examination is performed. If abnormalities are found during the interictal period, active nervous system disease is considered more likely than idiopathic epilepsy.

DIAGNOSTIC PLAN (p. 155)

A complete blood count, fasting serum chemistry, and urinalysis should be obtained. Fasting and postprandial bile acid determinations are necessary to evaluate liver function. Serum cholinesterase and lead determinations should be performed if exposure to toxicity is suspected. Chest and abdominal radiographs should be obtained, especially in dogs over 5 years of age, to detect neoplasia. If the animal has frequent seizures or other neurologic signs, the diagnostic evaluation should also include electroencephalography (EEG), cerebral spinal fluid (CSF) examination, computerized axial tomography (CAT), and magnetic resonance imaging (MRI).

GOALS OF TREATMENT (pp. 155–156)

Treatment of specific diseases of the brain that can cause seizures is discussed in Chapter 82. The management of status epilepticus is outlined in Table 33–2. Oral anticonvulsant administration for management of seizures is usually begun if seizures occur more frequently than once monthly or in clusters, and an overview is presented in Table 33–3. Oral diazepam is an effective anticonvulsant in cats, but not in dogs. Primidone is toxic to cats.

OUTCOME (p. 156)

The majority of animals with idiopathic epilepsy can lead a normal life and have a normal life span. Periodic evaluation of serum anticonvulsant levels and liver and renal function tests are necessary. If the animal has had no seizures for 6 to 9 months and was not difficult to control, the anticonvulsant dose may be reduced by 10 to 20 per cent every 3 to 6 months, if the seizures do not return. Anticonvulsant therapy may eventually be discontinued in some dogs who have been epileptic for years.

TABLE 33–2. MANAGEMENT OF STATUS EPILEPTICUS

1. Immediate anticonvulsant therapy
   a. Diazepam   2 mg IV to a 5 kg dog or cat
                           5 mg IV to a 10 kg dog
                           10 mg IV to a 20 kg dog
        Each dose can be repeated 2 or 3 times over several minutes in an attempt to stop the seizures.
   b. Sodium pentobarbital IV to effect, usually not to exceed 3–15 mg/kg (watch for respiratory depression)
2. Evaluate respirations, establish a patent airway, and give oxygen if needed. (Monitor for neurogenic pulmonary edema.)
3. Place intravenous catheter and flush with heparinized saline to keep patent for future use if needed.
4. Collect a blood sample and analyze for glucose. If low, administer 50% dextrose IV or orally as needed to correct hypoglycemia. Maintain on 5% dextrose IV, if insulinoma suspected.
5. Monitor vital signs
   a. If temperature is elevated over 105°F after 10 minutes, give cool water bath until temperature is 102°F.
   b. If cerebral edema is suspected, give oxygen and mannitol 1 gm/lb (2.2 gm/kg) and methylprednisolone sodium succinate 4.5–13.5 mg/lb (10–30 mg/kg) IV.
6. Maintenance anticonvulsant therapy
   a. Phenobarbital IV or IM 1–2 mg/lb (2.2–4.4 mg/kg) q6h for 24 hours, if seizures are persistent, to produce effective anticonvulsant levels more rapidly.
   b. Resume or initiate oral anticonvulsants every 8–12 hours, if indicated, as soon as the animal can swallow.
7. Collect data base (history, physical and neurologic examinations, complete blood count, serum chemistry profile, and urinalysis). Animal may be sedated and ataxic for several days.

TABLE 33–3. BASIC GUIDE TO ANTICONVULSANT THERAPY FOR EPILEPSY IN DOGS AND CATS

1. If seizures occur once a month or more or in clusters, begin phenobarbital 1–2 mg/lb (2–4 mg/kg) orally q12h.
2. If the animal is sedated after 24–48 hours and has no seizures, reduce the dose by 10–20%.
3. If the seizures continue after 48 hours on 2 mg/lb (4.4 mg/kg) q12h, increase dosage to 3 mg/lb (6.6 mg/kg) q12h.
4. If periodic seizures continue, measure serum phenobarbital level (2 hours after and 2 hours before oral phenobarbital is given). It takes 7–10 days for phenobarbital to reach steady-state serum levels.
5. If the serum phenobarbital level is below 20 μg/ml, increase the phenobarbital dose by 10–20% and repeat serum phenobarbital levels every 7–10 days until the serum level is between 20 and 30 μg/ml. Increase the dose to q8h if serum level varies greatly during the day.
6. If the serum phenobarbital level goes over 30 μg/ml, liver damage may occur, so decrease the dosage until a serum level of 20–30 μg/ml is obtained. Evaluate fasting and 2-hour postprandial bile acids.
7. If a cat is still having seizures, begin diazepam 1–2 mg q12h and slowly reduce the phenobarbital dose over 7 days and discontinue. Combine drugs only if seizures return.
8. If the serum phenobarbital level is between 20 and 30 μg/ml and the dog still has periodic or clusters of seizures, begin potassium bromide (KBr) 10 mg/lb (22 mg/kg) once daily with food and continue the current dose of phenobarbital. (Owner must wear gloves and sign a release form.)
9. If the seizures are controlled and the dog is sedated on the combination of drugs, reduce the phenobarbital dose by 10–20% every 2–3 days as needed until sedation disappears.
10. If seizures continue, increase the KBr dose by ¼–½ ml depending on the size of the dog and keep the phenobarbital dose constant.
11. Measure KBr serum level in 3–4 months. It should be 500–1500 μg/ml. (This level is toxic in humans and so the laboratory will report this as toxic.)
12. If serum phenobarbital and KBr levels are adequate and the dog is still having seizures, reconsider the diagnosis of epilepsy.
13. If epilepsy is still most likely and seizures are still uncontrolled, refer for acupuncture for seizure control. You may consider acupuncture initially before drug therapy. See Table 33–4 in the textbook for alternative anticonvulsant therapy.

CHAPTER 34

SLEEP DISORDERS
(pages 157–158)

Cataplectic collapses are usually precipitated by excitement associated with play, eating or drinking, greeting owners, being let out of cage, and the like. The collapse is characterized by a sudden loss of tone in voluntary muscles. The duration of the collapse may range from seconds to several minutes. Petting the patient or making loud noises can often terminate the collapse. The patient is aware of its sur-

Original chapter written by Linda Shell

**TABLE 34–1. REPORTED BREEDS OF
DOGS WITH NARCOLEPSY**

Toy poodle	Saint Bernard
Miniature poodle	Cocker spaniel
Doberman pinscher	Irish setter
Labrador retriever	Rottweiler
Dachshund	Cockapoo
Beagle	Welsh corgi
Wire-haired griffon	Mixed breeds

roundings unless hypersomnia is also present. The breeds of dogs reported to have narcolepsy are listed in Table 34–1.

DIAGNOSTIC PLAN (p.158)

The diagnosis of narcolepsy is based on the history, clinical signs, and absence of other diseases. A thorough description of the signs should help to rule out seizures. Syncope and collapse caused by intermittent cardiac arrhythmias are somewhat more difficult to define. Review of a hemogram and blood chemistry profile will help to eliminate metabolic disorders. Worsening of the clinical signs may occur after an edrophonium chloride (Tensilon test) injection if the animal is narcoleptic.

A food-elicited cataplexy test can confirm the diagnosis of cataplexy. This test is based on the amount of time it takes a dog to eat ten half-inch–sized (1 cm) pieces of food placed in a row 14 inches (30.5 cm) apart for small breeds and 23 inches (50 cm) apart for larger breeds. Normal dogs take less than 45 seconds. The test is best performed in the dog's home environment.

TREATMENT GOALS (p. 158)

At present narcolepsy is an incurable disorder. The anticholinergic properties of the tricyclic antidepressants—such as imipramine, protriptyline, amitriptyline, and chlorimipramine—may improve cataplectic signs.

CHAPTER 35
POLYURIA AND POLYDIPSIA
(pages 159–163)

Polyuria (PU) is defined as a daily urine output of greater than 25 ml/lb (50 ml/kg) body weight per day; polydipsia (PD) is defined as fluid intake exceeding 50 ml/lb (100 ml/kg) body weight per day.

ETIOLOGY (pp. 159–162)

See Table 35–1 for a list of the main differential diagnoses for PU/PD.

Original chapter written by Susan M. Meric

TABLE 35–1. DIFFERENTIAL DIAGNOSES FOR POLYURIA AND POLYDIPSIA

Primary Polyuria
  Osmotic diuresis
    Diabetes mellitus
    Primary renal glucosuria, Fanconi syndrome
    Postobstructive diuresis
  ADH deficiency—central diabetes insipidus
    Idiopathic
    Trauma-induced
    Neoplastic
    Congenital
  Renal insensitivity to ADH—nephrogenic diabetes insipidus
    Primary nephrogenic diabetes insipidus
    Secondary nephrogenic diabetes insipidus
      Renal insufficiency/failure
      Pyelonephritis
      Pyometra
      Hypercalcemia
      Hypokalemia
      Hyperadrenocorticism
      Hyperthyroidism
      Hypoadrenocorticism
      Hepatic insufficiency
      Renal medullary solute washout
      Drugs/diet

Primary Polydipsia
  Psychogenic (behavioral)
  Encephalopathy
  Neurologic
  Fever
  Pain

DIAGNOSTIC APPROACH TO THE PATIENT WITH PU/PD (pp. 162–163)

Physical Examination. Lymph nodes and anal sacs should be palpated carefully as common sources for malignancy-associated hypercalcemia. Cataracts may be noted in diabetes mellitus, symmetric truncal alopecia in hyperadrenocorticism, a thyroid mass in hyperthyroidism, vaginal discharge and/or uterine enlargement in pyometra, painful kidneys in pyelonephritis, or small irregular kidneys in chronic renal failure.

DIAGNOSTIC PLAN

Confirm/Quantify. Have the owner *measure the water* the dog is drinking at home for 3 to 5 days to document the PD before committing to a complete diagnostic evaluation.

Evaluate for Common Causes of PU/PD. Recommended initial diagnostic tests include a *complete blood cell count, urinalysis,* and *serum biochemistry profile*. In an adult cat, *serum thyroxine* should also be measured. *Culture of a urine sample* obtained by cystocentesis should also be considered. *Abdominal radiographs* and/or *ultrasound* may be warranted to evaluate liver, kidney, uterus, and adrenals. Tests for hyperadrenocorticism should be considered as part of the initial diagnostic plan for dogs >8 years of age. Physical findings or initial laboratory results may prompt further diagnostic testing including thoracic radiographs, lymph node aspiration, bone marrow biopsy, and liver function tests.

Modified Water Deprivation/ADH Response Test. This test should be used to differentiate between CDI, NDI, and PP. Phases 1 and 2 of this test should not be initiated in animals that appear to be clinically dehydrated or have a plasma osmolality greater than 320 mOsm/kg. These animals are already sufficiently dehydrated to begin phase 3. The test is also contraindicated in patients known to have diabetes mellitus, renal disease, or most of the conditions causing secondary NDI.

TABLE 35–2. PROTOCOL FOR THE MODIFIED WATER DEPRIVATION/ADH RESPONSE TEST*†

PHASE I. PREPARATION—to decrease renal medullary solute washout. This phase should be initiated 5 days (120 hours) before water deprivation begins.
  A. Days 5, 4 and 3 preceding water deprivation: limit water intake to 55 ml/lb (120 ml/kg)/day in small allotments.
  B. Day 2 preceding the test: limit water to 40 ml/lb (90 ml/kg)/day in small allotments.
  C. 24 hours prior to water deprivation: limit water intake to 30 ml/lb (60 ml/kg)/day in small allotments.
  D. Beginning on day 5 preceding water deprivation lightly salt all meals.
  E. Withdraw all food 12 hours prior to initiating water deprivation.
PHASE II. WATER DEPRIVATION—to dehydrate the patient, stimulate endogenous ADH release and monitor ability to concentrate urine.
  A. In the morning:
    1. Completely empty the bladder.
    2. Obtain exact body weight.
    3. Obtain serum osmolality.
    4. Obtain BUN, PCV, total protein.
    5. Check urine specific gravity and/or osmolality.
    6. Withdraw and withhold all food and water.
  B. Every hour:
    1. Completely empty the bladder.
    2. Check exact body weight.
    3. Check CNS status, clinical hydration, BUN, PCV, total protein.
    4. Check urine specific gravity and/or osmolality.
  C. Phase II is ended when:
    1. Patient has lost >5% of body weight or appears clinically dehydrated. Whenever possible dehydration should be documented by a measured increase in serum osmolality.
    2. Patient becomes ill or depressed.
    3. Patient produces concentrated urine (>1.030 dogs, >1.035 cats).
PHASE III. RESPONSE TO EXOGENOUS ADH—ADH is administered to an already dehydrated patient and urine concentration is measured. Response indicates inadequate endogenous ADH release.
  A. Completely empty the bladder.
  B. Continue withholding food and water.
  C. Administer aqueous vasopressin IM (0.25U/lb [0.5U/kg], maximum 5 U).
  D. Every 30 minutes for 120 minutes:
    1. Completely empty the bladder.
    2. Check urine specific gravity and/or osmolality.
    3. Check CNS status, clinical hydration, BUN, PCV, total protein.
PHASE IV. END OF TEST— slowly reintroduce the patient to water to prevent overdrinking.
  A. Offer small amounts of water (10 ml/lb [20 ml/kg]) every 30 minutes for 2 hours.
  B. Continue to monitor hydration, CNS status.
  C. After 2 hours return to ad lib water.

---

*Phases I and II are contraindicated in patients which are clinically dehydrated or who have not been evaluated for diabetes mellitus or the common etiologies of secondary NDI.
†Modified with permission from Feldman EC and Nelson RW (ed): Canine and Feline Endocrinology and Reproduction. Philadelphia: WB Saunders Company, 1987.

CHAPTER 36
INCONTINENCE, ENURESIS, NOCTURIA, AND DYSURIA
(pages 164–169)

ABNORMAL MICTURITION (pp. 164–165)

Storage phase disorders generally are manifested by urinary incontinence. Emptying phase disorders usually produce some degree of incomplete bladder emptying and urinary retention.

Neurogenic Disorders. Neurologic lesions that disrupt the upper motor neuron segments of the micturition reflex arc impair voluntary control of urination and produce a spastic neuropathic bladder (see Chapter 83). Neurologic lesions that disrupt the lower motor neuron segment of the micturition reflex arc produce a flaccid or atonic neuropathic bladder (see Chapter 83).

Non-neurogenic Disorders. A variety of anatomic abnormalities of the lower urinary tract may cause urinary incontinence. The most common congenital disorder is ectopic ureter, which is usually seen in young female dogs (see Chapter 141). Chronic cystitis and urethritis, neoplasia, urolithiasis, and prostatic diseases are frequent causes of such problems (see Chapters 128, 136, 137, 140, and 141).

Many disorders of micturition are associated with excessive outlet resistance during voiding efforts. Such obstruction to urine flow typically produces dysuria, strangury, and urinary retention rather than incontinence (see Chapters 37 and 38).

Complications of Urinary Incontinence. The most common complication of urinary incontinence is development of urinary tract infection. Except in instances of urge incontinence, urinary tract infection is more likely to be a complication of urinary incontinence than it is to be the cause of incontinence. With incontinent animals, development of skin disorders such as rashes or decubital ulcers often is a problem.

HISTORICAL FINDINGS AND THEIR MEANINGS (p. 165)

Indications of polyuria, pollakiuria, strangury, dysuria, and nocturia may be mistaken for urinary incontinence, and a detailed review of the history from the owner should help to differentiate these. Whether urination is voluntary also should be established. Ability to voluntarily initiate and maintain urination suggests that the detrusor muscle is capable of normal reflex activity. When an animal has intermittent dribbling of urine, strangury, and incomplete bladder emptying, excessive outlet resistance is suggested. Leakage of urine during recumbency or sleep is suggestive of sphincter mechanism incompetence.

PHYSICAL FINDINGS AND THEIR INTERPRETATION (pp. 165–166)

Non-neurogenic causes of incontinence often are identified by abdominal palpation combined with digital rectal palpation and examination of the vagina or male external genitalia. Palpation of the bladder should be performed before and after urination. Manual expression of the bladder should then be performed to induce bladder emptying and evaluate outlet resistance.

Original chapter written by Philippe M. Moreau and George E. Lees

Measurement of postmicturition residual urine volume is performed by urethral catheterization (normal values are 0.2 to 0.5 ml/kg). Passing a urinary catheter also helps to detect mechanical obstructions of the urethral lumen.

Neurologic examination is the key to detection of all neurogenic disorders of micturition because neurologic lesions rarely affect only the bladder and urethra. The bulbospongiosus reflex, perineal reflex, anal tone, and sensation over the caudal portion of the back and tail should be carefully evaluated (see Chapter 82).

DIAGNOSTIC PLAN (pp. 166–168)

Routine hemogram and *serum biochemistry* tests generally do not indicate the cause of incontinence, but they help to determine the animal's overall physiologic status. Metabolic complications may require immediate medical attention. *Urinalysis* findings are especially important. Identification of hematuria, proteinuria, and/or pyuria suggests the presence of pathologic changes in the urinary tract.

Radiography is an important diagnostic aid for patients with urinary incontinence. *Spinal radiographs*, sometimes including myelography, often are necessary to identify the cause of a neurogenic disorder of micturition. *Survey abdominal radiographs* may detect radiodense calculi and some neoplasms or prostatic disorders, but contrast radiographic studies usually are necessary to diagnose anatomic abnormalities contributing to urinary incontinence. *Positive contrast urethrography* or *vaginourethrography* and *double contrast cystography* ordinarily are the most informative studies. However, *excretory urography* is used to investigate suspected ureteral ectopia and may be used to evaluate the bladder. *Ultrasonography* may be used to evaluate the bladder, urethra, and surrounding structures. *Cystoscopy* can be performed in some dogs, especially females. Without endoscopy, *bladder wash* and *catheter biopsy* techniques can be used to acquire specimens containing cells or small fragments of tissue for microscopic examination. *Exploratory laparotomy* also may be performed to examine and obtain biopsies. In animals with neuropathic bladders, *electromyography* may be used. The anal sphincter works in synchrony with the external urethral sphincter, and electrical activity of the anal sphincter can be used as a crude index of external urethral sphincter function.

Urodynamic studies measure pressure, volume, and flow relationships within the bladder and urethra during various phases of micturition. A micturition study may be necessary for definitive diagnosis of reflex dyssynergia.

GOALS OF TREATMENT (pp. 168–169)

First, priority should be given to alterations requiring immediate care, such as fluid deficits, electrolyte disturbances, acid-base imbalances, and azotemia. Second, normal micturition should be restored as soon as possible. When urge incontinence associated with urinary tract infection is diagnosed, antibiotic treatment alone might be sufficient, but when morphologic abnormalities are responsible for urinary incontinence, surgical correction usually is indicated. Specific recommendations for pharmacotherapy of disorders of micturition appear in Chapters 140 and 141.

OUTCOME (p. 169)

Prognosis frequently is poor for animals with neurogenic disorders of micturition, whether they are caused by brain, spinal cord, or peripheral nerve lesions.

CHAPTER 37
URINARY OBSTRUCTION AND ATONY
(pages 169–172)

URINARY OBSTRUCTION (p. 170)

Mechanical causes of urinary obstruction include intraluminal masses, calculi, or plugs; intramural neoplasia, inflammation, or fibrosis/stricture of the bladder trigone or urethra; extramural intrapelvic masses compressing the outflow tract; or abnormal placement of the bladder (e.g., retroflexed bladder associated with perineal hernia).

Functional causes of urinary obstruction include causes of increased urethral tone, such as reflex dyssynergia, UMN bladder, or urethral pain/spasm.

BLADDER ATONY (p. 170)

Neurologic causes of bladder atony include LMN disease, UMN diseases with increased urethral tone leading to bladder overdistention, and dysautonomia. *Muscular* causes of bladder atony include inflammation/infection/infiltration of the detrusor, diseases causing muscle weakness, intrapelvic bladder, or bladder overdistention.

If animals present with a history of *failure to urinate,* the clinician must determine whether (1) urine is not being produced (oliguria/anuria), (2) rupture of the urinary tract has caused pooling of urine in the abdominal or retroperitoneal cavity, or (3) urine is being abnormally retained in the urinary bladder.

PHYSICAL FINDINGS AND THEIR INTERPRETATION
(p. 171)

Bladder palpation may determine size, tone, ease or difficulty of manual expression, calculi, or masses associated with the bladder. Manual expression of the bladder may be easy in the case of LMN diseases. Manual expression is difficult with a UMN bladder.

In the male, the *urethra* should be examined by palpation, especially caudal to the os penis, perineally, and rectally, for the presence of calculi or masses. In the female, the urethra may be examined by rectal or vaginal palpation. *Neurologic examination* is important in the differentiation of causes of urinary obstruction or bladder atony.

DIAGNOSTIC PLAN (pp. 171–172)

Blood tests, including CBC and biochemical profile, help to show the degree of systemic involvement due to urinary obstruction or bladder atony. *Urine tests,* including complete urinalysis and urine culture and sensitivity, should be done whenever animals have urinary retention. *Abdominal radiography,* including survey and contrast radiography (cystogram/urethrogram/vaginogram), may show urinary calculi, masses, or bony pelvic or vertebral abnormalities. *Abdominal ultrasonography* helps in the detection of nonradiopaque urinary calculi. Intraluminal and intramural masses of the bladder, prostate, and proxi-

---

Original chapter written by Meryl P. Littman

mal urethra may be studied. Other abnormalities, such as hydroureter and hydronephrosis, renal lesions, and intra-abdominal lymphadenopathy may be seen by ultrasonography. *Pressure profiles,* including urethral pressure profile and cystometrography, may help to define urethral and detrusor tone, respectively.

GOALS OF TREATMENT (p. 172)

Complications of severe urinary retention such as *azotemia* and *infection* must be treated aggressively. The bladder should be kept empty. If urethral tone is increased, alpha-adrenergic antagonists (e.g., phenoxybenzamine) and skeletal muscle relaxants (e.g., diazepam, dantrolene) may be used to help decrease urethral tone. Once the bladder is emptied and when there is no urinary obstruction, cholinergic drugs (e.g., bethanechol) may be used to stimulate the detrusor muscle. If necessary, *catheterization* may be used to keep the bladder empty. The medication of choice for *detrusor atony* is the cholinergic drug bethanechol. Chapters 83, 140, and 141 deal with specific disease entities.

CHAPTER 38

DISCOLORED URINE
(pages 173–174)

Table 38–1 shows potential causes of discolored urine.

RED URINE (pp. 173–174)

Red urine color suggests blood, myoglobin, or hemoglobin contamination of the urine. The presence of red blood cells in the sediment confirms hematuria. A negative occult blood reaction in the supernatant and the absence of red blood cells in the sediment suggest hemoglobin and/or myoglobinuria. To further differentiate the etiology of red colored urine, a plasma capillary tube should be examined. Myoglobinemia does not discolor plasma (it remainds clear), whereas hemoglobinemia discolors plasma pink.

BROWN URINE (p. 174)

Brown or reddish brown urine develops when bilirubin, myoglobin, or heme products are present in an acid urine. Bilirubin tests negatively for occult blood reaction in both the supernatant and urinary sediment. One plus reaction levels for bilirubinuria in the cat are always abnormal.

MILKY URINE (p. 174)

A milky urine sample is likely to be related to pyuria.

Original chapter written by Robert H. Lusk, Jr.

TABLE 38–1. POTENTIAL CAUSES OF DISCOLORED URINE IN DOGS AND CATS

URINE COLOR	CAUSES
Deep yellow	Quinacrine
Yellow-orange	Bilirubin
	Fluorescein
	Concentrated urine
	Sulfasalazine
Yellow-green	Bilirubin
	Biliverdin
Yellow-brown	Bilirubin
	Biliverdin
Brown-black	Methemoglobin
	Methocarbamol
	Phenols
Brown or rust-yellow	Nitrofurantoin
	Furazolidone
	Metronidazole
	Sulfonamides
Red-brown	Methemoglobin
	Myoglobin
	RBCs
	Hemoglobin
	Dilantin
	Dinitrophenol
	Chronic lead or mercury intoxication
Red-purple	Porphyrins
	Phenolphthalein
Red-orange	Rifampin
	Phenazopyridine
Red	RBCs
	Hemoglobin
	Myoglobin
	Dyes
	Porphyrins
	Phenazopyridine
	Phenolsulfonphthalein
	Beets
Blue	Methylene blue
Blue-green	Urinary tract infection due to *Pseudomonas aeruginosa*
	Indicanuria due to intestinal bacterial overgrowth
Dark green	Phenols
Milky	Pyuria
	Lipiduria
Colorless	Dilute

CHAPTER 39

BEHAVIORAL SIGNS OF ORGANIC DISEASE
(pages 175–178)

Associating the behavioral signs with the environment, events, and past medical history and searching for current disease are vital diagnostic steps. Neurologic examination is mandatory on any animal with a behavioral sign.

TYPES OF BEHAVIORAL SIGNS (pp. 175–177)

Aggression. Aggression is a common behavioral sign, but is rarely of pure organic origin. Find out against whom the aggression is directed, under what circumstances it takes place, how often, for how long, and what event triggers it.

Fear, Disorientation, Lethargy. This group of signs is frequently caused by systemic metabolic diseases.

Personality Changes. Descriptions of the signs, their frequency, and/or their progression may become important in identifying diffuse versus focal CNS disease or systemic metabolic disease.

Changes in Urinary or Bowel Habits. Does the animal dribble or void in its sleep or try to get to the appropriate place to relieve itself (polyuria, pollakiuria)? Does the animal adopt an elimination posture (true behavioral) or does it drip or drop stool (organic)? Does it eliminate in a particular spot (territory)?

Repetitive Behaviors. Fly snapping, head bobbing, tail chasing, episodic circling, flank staring, face rubbing, and flank-sucking activities are usually nonorganic in origin.

Pacing and Circling. Diffuse degenerative CNS diseases or focal brain lesions such as tumor, stroke, or encephalitis are likely.

CLIENT RELATIONS (p. 177)

The clinician must become accustomed to using the expression "*We don't know why* an animal does this" or "*We can't explain how* an animal starts or learns this activity." The clinician should not underestimate the ability of stress or change (environmental, population, emotional, pain, irritation, disease) to produce or affect the frequency of a behavioral sign.

Learned attention-getting phenomena (tail chasing, paw chewing) can develop rapidly in some dogs after development of a lesion. Most cases of severe self-mutilation are not attributable to organic disease; they are usually behavioral responses even if originally triggered by a temporary organic lesion (e.g., anal glands, fleas).

SPECIFIC DISEASE STATES (p. 178)

A *brain tumor* and *CNS reticulosis* usually produce a slow progression from dulling of the personality, aimless and constant pacing, circling, and nonrecognition of familiar people and objects to lethargy, obtundation, and seizures. *Toxic agents* can collectively cause any behavioral sign(s), either episodic or continuous. Worthy of note are

Original chapter written by Alan J. Parker

lead and some rawhide dog chews (if bleached by agene). Both are capable of producing hysterical episodes, often leading to seizures. *Encephalitis* can also produce the entire spectrum of behavioral signs. *Hepatic encephalopathy* tends to lead to episodes lasting several hours, including signs of depression, pacing, disorientation, blindness, coma, and seizures.

Cases of *brain trauma* and episodes of *cerebral hypoxia* are not usually diagnostic problems, but clients should be warned that changed bowel habits, disorientation, and loss of owner recognition may be permanent deficits even after the pet exhibits motor recovery. *Hydrocephalus* can result in signs at any age, and they may be insidious in onset or acute and progressive, including dullness, lethargy, disorientation, and coma.

The *feline hyperesthesia syndrome* (FHS) is characterized by episodes of either excessive grooming, sometimes to the point of bilaterally symmetric baldness from the neck caudally (psychogenic alopecic dermatitis), and/or excessive twitching of the back, hissing, sudden body jerks, running wildly, apparent disorientation and fear, irritability, intolerance of being petted, and occasionally attacking the owners. True *hyperkinesis* is rare in dogs, unreported in cats, and characterized diagnostically by a paradoxic calming response to amphetamines.

Mental lapse aggression syndrome (unprovoked and unexplained attacks without prodromal warnings), *sleep disorientation aggression* (waking in an aggressive threat display), and *springer rage syndrome* are all highly dangerous syndromes; euthanasia should be recommended. *Dancing Doberman syndrome* is said to occur when a dog, usually a Doberman, constantly picks up one or both hind legs in turn while standing still. *Flank-sucking, head-bobbing/head-weaving,* and *jaw-champing* are common Doberman behavioral traits, aggravated by stress. They may be responsive to anxiolytics, antidepressants, antiobsessive agents, or sedatives.

CHAPTER 40

BEHAVIORAL DISORDERS
(pages 179–187)

CANINE BEHAVIORAL DISORDERS (pp. 179–183)

Aggression Toward Owner

Dominance-Related Aggression. This is typically exhibited by young adult males. Dominant-aggressive dogs growl, snap, or bite when certain critical resources are threatened: food, a place of rest (especially furniture), and a favored human "mate." They also respond aggressively to perceived challenges such as prolonged direct stares, punishment, physical manipulations, and even being petted. The greatest success lies in "reconditioning" the dog to accept the owner's dominance by using reward-based (food or toy) obedience training. Progestins have reduced aggression in dominant-aggressive dogs. Phenobarbital may be effective in cases of seizure-related aggression.

Original chapter written by Katherine A. Houpt and Ilana R. Reisner

Aggression Toward Children. Dogs exhibiting aggression toward a crawling infant or a toddler may be defensive rather than dominant. If the aggression is mild, behavior modification emphasizes positive interactions. Pronounced aggression is obviously dangerous; it may be advisable to remove the dog from the home.

Aggression Toward Strangers

Territorial Aggression. The behavior may be worsened by regularly tying the dog outdoors for long periods. Treatment of moderate to severe territorial aggression always begins with prevention: the outdoor dog should be brought indoors; the indoor dog should be leashed. Positive reinforcement (food) is used for good behavior.

Fear-Based Aggression. Fear-based aggression is more likely to be directed toward strangers than toward familiar people. Fearful dogs should be on a lead at all times. Treatment involves an emphasis on reduction of fear or anxiety, and gradual desensitization to whatever is eliciting the fear.

Predatory Aggression. In general, predatory behavior, whether toward people or animals, is best stopped by restraint.

Aggression Toward Animals

Aggression Toward Other Dogs in Household. Household dogfights often are conflicts of dominance, typically between dogs of the same sex. If one dog clearly acts dominant over the other *and* is the initiator of fights, treatment can center on reinforcement of dominance. If, however, the status between dogs is unclear, treatment involves general restructuring of the dogs' lives.

Aggression Toward Unfamiliar Dogs. Such behavior is more likely to be rooted in discomfort or fear than in dominance. Prevention is most important here; a leash is essential.

Aggression Toward Other Animals. Dogs attacking cats, squirrels, and other animals are likely to be exhibiting predatory behavior. The treatment of choice is prevention.

PROBLEMS IN THE OWNER'S ABSENCE

Owners frequently complain that destructiveness, vocalization, and inappropriate elimination occur when they are not at home. Treatment for these problems has a general component as well as a specific component that varies with the type of problem and the owner's abilities and desires. The general component consists of increasing the dog's exercise and training so that destructive dogs are adequately exercised and absolutely obedient. The specific component includes pharmacologic intervention, behavior modification, environmental enrichment, occasional restraint, and, rarely, punishment.

Destructiveness

Dogs that exhibit barrier frustration ·or direct their attention to the owner's odors appear to be misbehaving due to anxiety. These dogs usually respond to treatment with antidepressant or antianxiety drugs. The drugs of choice are amitriptyline or clomipramine. (Table 40–1 lists canine and feline psychoactive drugs.)

Barking

Barking occurring for long periods with no apparent cause should not be punished with electric shock collars. If barking is caused by separation anxiety, such punishment may simply redirect the anxiety to destructiveness. The solution can sometimes be as simple as bringing a dog that barks in the yard indoors where it cannot see or hear

TABLE 40-1. PSYCHOACTIVE DRUGS

GENERIC/TRADE NAME	DOSAGE	ROUTE	FREQUENCY	CLASS
Feline				
Medroxyprogesterone acetate (Depo provera)	50–100 mg/cat	IM or SQ	q 4 months	Progestin (aggression)
Megestrol acetate (Ovaban, Megase)	5–10 mg/cat	PO	q24h*	Progestin (aggression)
Diazepam (Valium)	1–2.5 mg/cat	PO	q12–18h†	Antianxiety (spraying)
Cyproheptadine (Periactin)	0.1 mg/cat (0.22 mg/kg)	PO	q24h	H[cf15]1 antagonist (pica)
Amitriptyline (Elavil)	5–10 mg/cat	PO	q24h	Antidepressant (spraying)
Buspirone (BuSpar)	2.5–5 mg/cat	PO	q12h	Antianxiety (aggression and spraying)
Acetylpromazine (Acepromazine)	0.5–1 mg/lb (1–2.2 mg/kg)	PO	pm	Tranquilizer
Canine				
Medroxyprogesterone acetate (Depo provera)	5 mg/lb (11 mg/kg)	IM or SQ	q 4 months	Progestin (aggression)
Megestrol acetate (Ovaban, Megase)	1–2 mg/lb (2.2–4.4 mg/kg)	PO	q24h*	Progestin (aggression)
Amitriptyline (Elavil)	1 mg/lb (2.2 mg/kg)	PO	q12–24h	Antidepressant (destruction)
Diazepam (Valium)	0.2–1 mg/lb (0.5–2.2 mg/kg)	PO	pm	Antianxiety (phobia)
Clorazepate dipotassium (Tranxene)	0.2–1 mg/lb (0.5–2.2 mg/kg)	PO	q12h	Antianxiety (destruction)
Clomipramine (Anafranil)	0.2–0.7 mg/lb (0.5–1.5 mg/kg)	PO	q12h	Antidepressant (destruction)
Phenobarbital	0.5–2 mg/lb (1–4.4 mg/kg)	PO	q12h	Anticonvulsant (aggression)

*After 2 weeks this dose should be reduced by half and after 4 weeks reduced again. Treatment should be discontinued after 6 weeks.
†Sedation and ataxia should abate within several days.

the stimuli. In some cases vocal cordectomy (debarking) is the only solution.

Soiling

Elimination only in the owner's absence can be treated as are other separation problems. Meals and availability of water should be adjusted so that a full stomach (gastrocolic reflex) or bladder does not stimulate elimination. In contrast to separation-based problems, dogs that housesoil whether or not owners are home may be insufficiently housetrained.

PHOBIAS

Thunder and Other Loud Noise Phobias

Fear of loud noises is a normal behavioral reaction, but in some dogs the usual signs of fear—panting and pacing—escalate to frantic attempts to escape. At the moment, the best approach is to try to mask outside noise and use one of the drugs recommended for destructiveness.

Place- or Person-Specific Phobias

Dogs often act afraid of unfamiliar people or people who differ in color, size, or facial hair from their owners. Progressive desensitization is the treatment of choice.

INGESTIVE PROBLEMS

Anorexia

In many cases in which anorexia is presented as a behavior problem, the dog will refuse to eat dog food but will eat treats or human food. The solution is simple: eliminate all calories except those in dog food.

Polydipsia

Psychogenic polydipsia must be differentiated from the many pathophysiologic causes of polydipsia. The best approach is to limit water intake gradually, provide ice so that the dog can moisten and cool its mouth, and increase the dog's exercise and training time.

Pica

This behavior decreases with age in most dogs. Eating grass is normal behavior for dogs.

Hyperphagia

The most common behavioral cause of hyperphagia is addition of another dog to the environment.

SEXUAL PROBLEMS

Urine Marking

Owners usually do not object to urine marking outside and will let their dogs stop and leg-lift a dozen times, but they do object to urine marking in the house. If the dog is intact, castration is usually successful in eliminating the misbehavior. Some dogs may scent mark sporadically even after castration. These dogs could be treated with the progestin megestrol acetate for 2 weeks and then with tapering doses.

Mounting

Young dogs mount in play. Dogs should not be allowed to mount people because of the implied dominance. Counter-conditioning the dog is probably the best approach.

Poor Libido

The most common cause of poor libido in males is fear of the bitch, which occurs if she is dominant to him. It is best to bring the bitch to the dog's environment.

FELINE BEHAVIORAL DISORDERS (pp. 183–187)

HOUSESOILING

The most common medical cause of failure to urinate in the litterbox is urinary tract infection and/or calculi. Medical problems must be successfully treated in order for the behavioral problem to be resolved. More frequent replacement of litter will solve many problems. The type of litter can be a problem if the owner has recently changed litters. The site of the litterbox can be a problem if it has been changed recently. The site of soiling can also be instructive. Soiling immediately outside the box indicates that the box or its contents are being rejected, whereas soiling far away may indicate a preference for that area or that substrate.

Psychoactive drugs are the most effective treatment for spraying. The drug of choice is diazepam. Other drugs that have been used successfully are amitriptyline and buspirone. The oral progestin megestrol acetate may also be effective. Provision of a second litterbox (or maybe more) often helps cats that defecate outside their box. The contents of the box should be discarded daily if the cat has used it at all (except for clumping litters, which can be scooped of urine and feces twice daily). Punishment is apt to make the cat more upset and therefore more likely to eliminate outside the box.

INGESTIVE PROBLEMS

Anorexia

The first step in treating anorexia is to assess the medical condition of the cat. If all is well, consider increasing the palatability, particularly the odor, of the food. The next step is chemical stimulation of appetite. The benzodiazepine diazepam has been successful. Cyproheptadine has also been used.

Pica and Woolchewing

Oropharyngeal problems, especially gingivitis, must be ruled out before the problem is considered behavioral. Woolsucking or woolchewing is sometimes improved by increasing fiber in the diet, by access to grass, or by feeding raw chicken.

Hyperphagia

A simple solution is to hide or scatter pieces of dry food so that the cat must forage. Hyperphagia without weight gain may be a sign of hyperthyroidism or diabetes mellitus.

MATERNAL BEHAVIOR PROBLEMS

Maternal Aggression

Queens are protective of their kittens. Infrequently this behavior is extreme. Removing the kittens from the environment, not simply weaning them, appears to be necessary.

SEXUAL BEHAVIOR PROBLEMS

Masturbation

Few owners are overly concerned about this behavior, and so it is best ignored.

AGGRESSION

Aggression Toward People

Play Aggression.   Such cats may stalk and pounce on the owner's legs and arms, biting or clawing uninhibitedly. Most will outgrow this behavior. Treatment involves redirecting play to an appropriate outlet, such as a toy.

Redirected (Displaced) Aggression Toward People.   If no stimulus is identified, the cat may be exhibiting idiopathic aggression. If identified, the initiating stimulus should be removed. Drug therapy may be indicated in cases of refractory or severe aggression. Unless fearfulness is clearly the cause, benzodiazepines should be avoided because of the potential for disinhibition.

Idiopathic Aggression.   Euthanasia may be the only safe option for severe, refractory cases.

Aggression Toward Cats

Redirected (Displaced) Aggression Toward Cats.   Such cats should be separated for a week or more while litter pans and food bowls are traded. Reintroduction should be gradual and conservative.

Territorial Aggression.   Territorially aggressive cats tend to seek out their targets. Treatment of territorial aggression is difficult; for severe problems the best solution may be to rehome one of the cats.

Aggression Toward Other Animals

Predatory Aggression.   Remains are often brought inside the home and presented to the owner. To prevent predation in the home, precautions must be taken so that the cat has no access to other pets. Outdoor hunting is prevented by keeping the cat indoors.

CHAPTER 41
ANEMIA
(pages 187–191)

A simple measure of bone marrow activity in the dog and cat is a reticulocyte count. However, it must be remembered that the bone marrow needs adequate time to respond to blood loss: 2 to 3 days in cats and 4 to 5 days in dogs.

SIGNIFICANCE OF PHYSICAL EXAMINATION CHANGES (p. 189)

Signs of oxygen deficiency such as dyspnea and tachypnea may be present at rest in severe anemias, but slight exertion may be necessary to produce these signs with an anemia of moderate severity. A soft systolic murmur may develop in animals with severe or acute anemia.

Original chapter written by Kenita S. Rogers

HELPFUL DIAGNOSTIC TESTS (pp. 189–190)

The most important laboratory data to collect in the anemic dog or cat are a CBC with an assessment of RBC morphology, calculation of red cell indices, and a reticulocyte count.

Spherocytes, if prominent on the smear, strongly suggest immune-mediated hemolysis. Autoagglutination of red cells also provides presumptive evidence for immune-mediated hemolysis. Fragmented erythrocytes (schistocytes) can occur with DIC, vascular neoplasia, and caval syndrome in dogs. The presence of nucleated RBCs, in the absence of reticulocytosis, is not considered evidence of a regenerative response.

The mean cell volume (MCV) is a relatively useful estimate of erythrocyte size. An increased MCV is generally associated with larger "young" RBCs that are released during intensified erythropoiesis (regeneration). However, an increased MCV has also been recognized in cats infected with FeLV despite the presence of a nonregenerative anemia. A decreased MCV is most often secondary to iron deficiency. The mean cell hemoglobin concentration is usually decreased in a regenerative anemia.

Bone marrow examination (aspirate or biopsy) is of value when one is trying to understand unexplained nonregenerative anemias. Erythrocyte number and size and hemoglobin concentration are not good indicators of iron adequacy. A reliable indicator of body iron stores in many species is serum ferritin, which is low in iron deficiency and increased during acute inflammatory processes.

DIFFERENTIAL DIAGNOSIS (pp. 190–191)

REGENERATIVE ANEMIAS

The two categories of disease processes that characteristically lead to a regenerative response are excessive blood loss and hemolysis. Hemolytic disease can be divided into intravascular and extravascular sites of hemolysis. Intravascular hemolysis usually represents a more severe disease process. With both types of hemolysis, hemoglobin is degraded, with bilirubin being one of the by-products. Hyperbilirubinemia (icterus) and bilirubinuria result.

NONREGENERATIVE ANEMIAS

1. *Primary failure of erythropoiesis* (pure red cell aplasia). The criteria for diagnosis include documenting a severe, chronic, normocytic, normochromic nonregenerative anemia, with a cellular bone marrow that retains active granulopoiesis and thrombopoiesis.

2. *Secondary failure of erythropoiesis.* Examples include inflammatory disease, neoplasia, chronic renal and liver disease, and certain endocrine disorders. Bone marrow examination is normal or shows mild erythroid hypoplasia.

3. *Nuclear maturation defects* are primarily associated with deficiencies of folate and/or vitamin B_{12}. Macrocytic, normochromic anemia results. The bone marrow is characterized by erythroid hyperplasia with maturation arrest at the rubricyte stage.

4. *Hemoglobin synthesis defects* are primarily associated with iron deficiency but can also be seen with copper deficiency, vitamin B_6 deficiency, and lead intoxication. Microcytic, hypochromic anemia results.

5. *Aplastic anemia* is characterized by an acellular or hypocellular marrow which results in pancytopenia. Aplastic anemia is usually due to chemicals, physical agents, or infectious agents.

6. *Marrow infiltration* can be associated with neoplasia (myelophthisis), myelofibrosis, or osteopetrosis.

CHAPTER 42

CYANOSIS
(pages 192–197)

Cyanosis is determined by the absolute amount of deoxygenated hemoglobin. It is generally less apparent in patients with severe anemia because the absolute amount of hemoglobin is reduced. Clinically, cyanosis may be classified as either central or peripheral (Table 42–1).

HISTORICAL FINDINGS (pp. 193–194)

SIGNALMENT

Central cyanosis in a young patient (less than one year) is suggestive of congenital heart disease.

PATTERN OF RESPIRATION

Stridor. Its presence suggests upper airway obstructive diseases.

Dyspnea. A history of dyspnea provides strong evidence of severe respiratory disease, usually of the lower airway or pleural space.

Cough. Persistent coughing is a common manifestation of cardiac or pulmonary disease.

PHYSICAL FINDINGS (pp. 194–195)

EXAMINATION OF MUCOUS MEMBRANES

Arterial hypoxemia causes cyanosis of all mucous membranes with one notable exception: right-to-left shunting patent ductus arteriosus (PDA) may cause cyanosis of caudal mucous membranes (vagina, penis) but not oral mucous membranes.

PATTERN OF RESPIRATION

Stridor. Stridor is the hallmark of upper airway obstruction.

TABLE 42–1. CAUSES OF CYANOSIS

Central cyanosis
    Arterial hypoxemia
        Reduction of inspired PO_2
        Alveolar hypoventilation
        Diffusion impairment
        Ventilation-perfusion mismatching
        Anatomic shunts
    Methemoglobinemia

Peripheral cyanosis
    Vasoconstriction
        Cold exposure
        Heart failure
        Shock
    Arterial obstruction
    Venous obstruction

Original chapter written by Gilbert Jacobs

Dyspnea.   Dyspnea usually indicates severe lower airway or pleural disease.

Other.   Poor excursions of the thoracic wall during breathing in a cyanotic patient may indicate respiratory muscle weakness from neuromuscular disease.

DIAGNOSTIC PLAN (pp. 195–196)

HEMOGRAM

Gross inspection of the venous blood can be helpful since with methemoglobinemia the blood is usually very dark with a brownish tinge or, in some cases, chocolate-colored. Polycythemia accompanied by hypoxemia is most marked and common in congenital heart diseases due to anatomic shunts.

THORACIC RADIOGRAPHY

Since most causes of central cyanosis and some causes of peripheral cyanosis involve disease of the cardiopulmonary system, thoracic radiography is critical.

ARTERIAL BLOOD GAS ANALYSIS

If you are unsure whether it is central or peripheral cyanosis, determining the Pa_{O_2} is helpful. Decreased Pa_{O_2} (hypoxemia) is associated with all causes of central cyanosis, whereas Pa_{O_2} is generally normal in patients with peripheral cyanosis. Arterial partial pressure of CO_2 is always elevated (hypercarbia) in alveolar hypoventilation. Hypercarbia is not present with the other causes of hypoxemia except for severe ventilation-perfusion mismatching. However, most patients with ventilation-perfusion mismatching are able to maintain a normal Pa_{CO_2}. The Pa_{CO_2} is usually not raised in anatomic shunts.

Hypoxemia associated with most respiratory conditions (alveolar hypoventilation, diffusion impairment, or ventilation-perfusion mismatching) is usually eliminated by breathing 100 per cent oxygen. (The exception is severe ventilation-perfusion mismatching.) With an anatomic shunt (e.g., congenital heart disease), hypoxemia cannot be eliminated by raising the inspired oxygen concentration to 100 per cent.

ELECTROCARDIOGRAPHY

A right ventricular hypertrophy pattern is most consistent with congenital heart disease in young cyanotic patients.

GOALS OF TREATMENT (pp. 196–197)

In the *hypoxemic patient,* symptomatic treatment in the form of *increasing inspired oxygen concentration* is appropriate and often life-saving. If the cause of cyanosis is alveolar hypoventilation, the clinical significance of hypoxemia is usually minimal compared to the CO_2 retention. In these patients, *increasing alveolar ventilation* (relieving airway obstruction or intubating and ventilating) is mandatory in order to eliminate retained CO_2.

Mild sedation may be helpful in patients with distress due to collapsing trachea of upper airway syndrome. In certain instances when methemoglobinemia is severe and life-threatening, methylene blue has been advocated in dogs. Acetaminophen toxicosis in cats can result in life-threatening methemoglobinemia. Gastric lavage and oral administration of activated charcoal to reduce absorption soon after acetaminophen ingestion and N-acetylcysteine orally or intravenously have been advocated as treatments (Chapter 61).

Treatment of *peripheral cyanosis* depends entirely upon the cause. Symptomatic treatment of the cyanosis is not indicated, and efforts should be directed at identifying and correcting the underlying cause.

CHAPTER 43
POLYCYTHEMIA
(pages 197–199)

CLINICAL FINDINGS (p. 199)

Patients with relative polycythemia secondary to dehydration will evidence clinical signs of the initiating cause and symptoms reflecting the severity of the problem. Patients with absolute polycythemias often have signs and symptoms directly referable to polycythemia and increased blood viscosity (polydipsia, polyuria, erythema of skin and mucous membranes, vomiting, diarrhea, anorexia, weakness, seizures, dilated and tortuous retinal vessels) in addition to signs and symptoms referable to the cause of the polycythemia. Patients with polycythemia vera will only have signs and symptoms that are subsequent to polycythemia.

DIAGNOSIS (p. 199)

A diagnosis of polycythemia is based on increased numbers of red cells in blood as determined by an erythrocyte count. It is always important to distinguish between relative and absolute polycythemia by a careful assessment of hydration and response to fluid therapy. Androgen or corticosteroid administration as a cause of polycythemia can be evaluated with a complete history.

The causes of appropriate secondary polycythemia can be established after it is determined that arterial PO_2 is low and the history and the cardiopulmonary system are carefully evaluated. Inappropriate secondary polycythemias are usually associated with renal neoplasia or renal parenchymal disease. Polycythemia vera is diagnosed by determining that the patient has an increased total red cell mass, no causes of secondary polycythemia, normal arterial PO_2, and a normal to low serum erythropoietin concentration.

TREATMENT (p. 199)

Relative polycythemia is symptomatically treated with intravenous fluid replacement and electrolyte supplementation as needed. Mild absolute polycythemias, such as those associated with cortisol or androgen excess, require no special treatment other than that directed against the underlying problem. Polycythemia that is severe enough to result in clinical signs and symptoms (higher than mid 60 per cent range) initially can be treated with a phlebotomy and fluid replacement with a volume of a balanced electrolyte solution equal to the amount of blood removed. The most satisfactory treatment of polycythemia vera in dogs and cats is hydroxyurea (40 to 50 mg/kg divided into two daily doses as a starting dose and titrated to response and toxicity).

Original chapter written by Wallace B. Morrison

CHAPTER 44

BLEEDING DISORDERS: EPISTAXIS AND HEMOPTYSIS
(pages 200–204)

EPISTAXIS (pp. 200–203)

DIFFERENTIAL DIAGNOSES

Systemic Processes

Bleeding disorders are important causes of epistaxis. Defects of primary hemostasis (platelet plug formation) are much more common causes of epistaxis than defects of secondary hemostasis (coagulation cascade). Disorders of primary hemostasis include quantitative and qualitative platelet defects (Chapters 145 and 146). In the absence of other abnormalities, thrombocytopenia is unlikely to result in bleeding until the count is less than 50 to 75,000/µl. Polycythemia occasionally causes epistaxis, and hypertension has been recognized as a cause of epistaxis in people.

Local Processes

Epistaxis secondary to neoplastic, infectious, and inflammatory processes is usually preceded by a chronic mucopurulent discharge (Chapter 80).

Neoplasia. Malignant nasal tumors, especially adenocarcinomas, are much more common in dogs than in cats.

Fungal Rhinitis. *Aspergillus fumigatus* is the most common fungus isolated in dogs, whereas *Cryptococcus neoformans* is most common in cats.

Parasitic Rhinitis. *Linguatula serrata* parasitizes the nasal cavity of dogs. Leishmaniasis is a protozoal disease that causes epistaxis in 10 percent of dogs.

Bacterial Rhinitis. Bacteria usually require predisposing inflammation or damage in order to become established.

Viral Rhinitis. This rarely causes a blood-tinged nasal discharge.

Inflammatory Rhinitis. Lymphoplasmacytic rhinitis is an immune-mediated, corticosteroid-responsive disease of unknown etiology.

Foreign Body Rhinitis. See textbook.

DIAGNOSTIC PLAN

Complete Blood Count. The CBC provides data regarding the presence of anemia, polycythemia, thrombocytopenia, leukocytosis, or leukopenia.

Chemistry Profile. This helps to rule out systemic diseases.

Urinalysis. Hematuria can occur with platelet problems.

Hemostatic Studies. A coagulation profile (prothrombin time, partial thromboplastin time, fibrinogen, and fibrin degradation products) evaluates the intrinsic and extrinsic coagulation pathways (Chapter 145). If the platelet count is over 100,000/µl, platelet function can be evaluated with buccal mucosal bleeding time (Chapter 146). Older tests, such as platelet factor 3 release, lack both sensitivity and specificity.

Serology. This is helpful in the diagnosis of canine ehrlichiosis, RMSF, feline leukemia virus (FeLV) and FIV (feline immunodeficiency virus).

Original chapter written by Orla M. Mahony and Susan M. Cotter

Electrophoresis. This distinguishes between monoclonal and polyclonal gammopathies.

Parasitology. In rare instances, *Linguatula serrata* ova are found in fecal swabs or fecal flotations.

General Anesthesia. This is required for thorough evaluation of the nasal and oral cavities once coagulation has been assessed to be normal. Initial radiographic evaluation involves ventrodorsal, open-mouth, lateral, and frontal sinus views. Rhinoscopy may allow visualization of foreign bodies, tumors, necrotic tissue, and fungal plaques.

Nasal Flushing. Through an endoscope or a red rubber catheter. Nasal flushing with sterile saline can be used to dislodge foreign bodies, or the fluid can be collected and submitted for cytologic evaluation.

Nasal Biopsy. The forceps must not be inserted beyond the level of the medial canthus of the eye.

Blood Pressure. Indirect blood pressure measurements are indicated.

GOALS OF TREATMENT

Moderate epistaxis is usually controlled with cage rest. Sedatives (e.g., butorphanol or oxymorphone, with or without valium) may be required. Drugs such as phenothiazines, which cause hypotension, should be avoided. Fresh whole blood will provide red cells, platelets, and coagulation factors. Persistent epistaxis may necessitate general anesthesia with packing of the external nares and posterior nasal pharynx with gauze soaked in dilute epinephrine (1:100,000).

HEMOPTYSIS (pp. 203–204)

DIFFERENTIAL DIAGNOSIS

If hemoptysis is seen, it suggests either serious disease of the lower respiratory tract or a bleeding disorder. Heartworm disease can cause hemoptysis in both dogs and cats. Pulmonary thromboembolism caused by other diseases, such as Cushing's disease, is rarely associated with hemoptysis. Acute pulmonary edema sometimes results in expectoration of frothy pink sputum. Primary lung tumors have been associated with hemoptysis. Metastatic lung tumors are less likely to be a cause. Examples of infectious cavitary lesions include lung abscesses and parasitic cysts. Hemorrhage into the pulmonary parenchyma secondary to coagulopathies is rare but can result in hemoptysis.

DIAGNOSTIC PLAN

The minimum data base includes a CBC with platelet count, a chemistry profile, urinalysis, and thoracic radiographs. Thoracic radiography is essential. Evaluation of hemostasis is an important component of the initial evaluation and would be carried out in a manner similar to that described for epistaxis.

GOALS OF TREATMENT

Hemoptysis may be life-threatening—not from exsanguination but from asphyxiation—and would therefore require intubation, suctioning, and ventilation.

CHAPTER 45

JAUNDICE
(pages 205–207)

DIAGNOSTIC PLAN (pp. 206–207)

The first diagnostic test should be a *complete blood count* or *packed cell volume/total solids. Severe anemia in the face of jaundice supports hemolysis as a prehepatic cause. With hemolysis, the erythron will be reduced while total plasma solids remain within normal range, making blood loss a less likely cause of anemia. A* serum biochemical analysis should be performed next. Determination of direct and indirect bilirubin (which identify conjugated versus unconjugated bilirubin) is seldom useful in small animals. *Urinalysis* may also confirm jaundice.

In cats, bilirubinuria is always an abnormal finding. Methylene blue, onions, copper, zinc, and lead are toxins likely to induce hemolysis in dogs, whereas propylene glycol, benzocaine, and acetaminophen are more common offenders in cats. A *coagulation profile* may be helpful in ruling out disseminated intravascular coagulopathy (DIC), and a *Knott's test and adult heartworm antigen enzyme-linked immunosorbent assay (ELISA)* would rule out heartworm disease with associated vena caval syndrome. Intrahepatic and posthepatic jaundice are differentiated based on a structural evaluation of the biliary system. Structural integrity of the biliary tract is optimally evaluated via *abdominal ultrasonography.* Two major causes of intrahepatic cholestasis associated with metabolic disease include bacterial septicemia and feline hyperthyroidism.

GOALS OF TREATMENT (p. 207)

The treatment of posthepatic jaundice caused by biliary tract obstruction or rupture is usually surgical. Therapy for intrahepatic jaundice must be based on the underlying hepatic pathology.

Original chapter written by Donna S. Dimski

CHAPTER 46

ACUTE VISION LOSS
(pages 208–210)

EVALUATION OF VISION

Obstacle Course. We usually place the obstacles between the animal and the owner, and have the owner call the animal's name. If the room lights can be dimmed, comparative evaluation of day and night vision can be made.

Original chapter written by Susan A. McLaughlin and Holly L. Hamilton

Motion Detection. This can be evaluated by dropping cotton balls or rolling a cylinder of tape through its visual field and observing eye or head movements.

Menace Reaction. This protective reaction is a learned response that should be present in all dogs and cats over 10 to 12 weeks of age. The palpebral reflex should be evaluated before the menace response is tested.

Visual Placing Postural Reaction. The animal is suspended nearly horizontally, but with the forelimbs lower than the hindlimbs, and the forelimbs brought to the edge of a table. A sighted animal will elevate a foreleg and place it on the table's surface before the leg touches the table.

PUPILLARY LIGHT REFLEXES AND ELECTRORETINOGRAPHY

Pupillary light reflexes (Chapter 84) and electroretinography do not test vision but may be helpful in localizing lesions. Unfortunately, the pupillary light reflex requires much less photoreceptor function than is required for normal vision. Animals with retinal detachment or extensive retinal degeneration may retain enough photoreceptor function to produce a fairly normal PLR. See the textbook for a complete differential list of lesions causing acute blindness.

CHAPTER 47

ALOPECIA
(pages 211–214)

CLINICAL FEATURES (pp. 211–213)

SIGNALMENT

Age. Alopecia in younger animals is more likely to be caused by infectious agents, ectoparasites, or genodermatoses.

PHYSICAL FINDINGS

Distribution of the Alopecia. Patchy alopecia tends to indicate follicular disease, whereas diffuse to symmetric alopecia is more typical of endocrine or genetically determined alopecias.

Hair Integrity and Structure. In patients with diffuse or patchy alopecia, a few hairs should be plucked and examined under low magnification for evidence of structural disturbances and to determine the predominant stage of hair growth.

DIAGNOSTIC PLAN (pp. 213–214)

The minimum data base for any dermatologic disorder is a skin scraping and fungal culture. *Intradermal skin testing* or *in vitro allergy testing* is indicated if the patient has features of atophy. Additional testing for ectoparasite or *therapeutic administration of acaricidal agent* is appropriate to eliminate occult ectoparasitism. *Fecal flotation* is rec-

---

Original chapter written by James O. Noxon

ommended to identify internal parasites that occasionally cause hypersensitivity reactions and is always indicated in pruritic dermatoses to identify ectoparasites that may have been ingested. *Bacterial cultures* are indicated when pustules or papules are present. *Cytologic evaluation of impression smears* may also be helpful.

If the alopecia is not related to pruritus, *hematologic evaluation* is indicated to identify systemic conditions. Specific *endocrine tests* can be used. Measurement of sex hormone concentrations for sex hormone imbalances is generally unrewarding, and surgical neutering is recommended as a diagnostic procedure when the animal is not used in a breeding environment. *Skin biopsy* may provide key diagnostic information but should not be expected to provide a definitive diagnosis.

CHAPTER 48

PRURITUS
(pages 214–219)

DIAGNOSIS OF PRURITUS (pp. 215–219)

SIGNALMENT

Age. Pruritic skin diseases diagnosed frequently in the puppy include flea allergy dermatitis, scabies, demodicosis with or without secondary pyoderma, and intestinal parasitism hypersensitivity. Atopy, food allergy, pyoderma, and exfoliative diseases such as keratinization defects are seen more commonly in adult animals.

Breed. See the appendix in the textbook for breed predilections of many skin diseases.

HISTORICAL FINDINGS

Diet. Food allergy frequently coexists with other allergic skin diseases such as atopy and flea allergy dermatitis.

Environment and Exposure. The likelihood of contagious ectoparasitic skin diseases is affected by environmental exposure.

Site, Onset, and Progression. Knowledge of the initial site of the skin lesions may be useful if the disease has generalized before veterinary care is sought. For example, canine scabies often begins on the margins of the pinnae. Rapid-onset pruritus should increase suspicion for flea allergy dermatitis, canine or feline scabies, cheyletiellosis, chiggers, and drug hypersensitivity. Pruritus of insidious onset is more suggestive of atopy, food allergy, pyoderma, *Malassezia* dermatitis, and seborrhea.

Intensity. Most animals will not exhibit pruritus in the examination room. Canine and feline scabies and canine flea allergy are notable exceptions.

Seasonality or Pattern (Predictability). Atopy and flea allergy are seasonal diseases in many areas of the world. Food allergy is continuous unless the diet is changed.

Response to Previous Therapy. Food allergy is less responsive to corticosteroids than atopy or flea allergy.

Original chapter written by Peter J. Ihrke

Ectoparasitic diseases, pyoderma, and seborrhea are among the more common pruritic skin diseases in which primary skin lesions are identified. Conversely, primary lesions are uncommon in atopy and food allergy.

DIAGNOSTIC PLAN

Skin Scrapings.   Multiple skin scrapings should be performed on all pruritic animals.

Smears and Tape Preparations.   The contents of pustules and exudates should be smeared, stained with a rapid stain such as Diff-Quik, and examined microscopically.

Feces.   Fecal examination may document worm burdens.

Skin Biopsy.   Biopsy of primary lesions free of self-trauma is most rewarding.

Fungal Culture.   Most animals with dermatophytosis are not pruritic.

Elimination Diets.   Such foods as mutton, whitefish, rabbit, cottage cheese, and tofu mixed with either rice or potatoes are commonly tried in the dog. Cats are given mutton, rabbit, or pork, frequently without an additional food source.

Intradermal Skin Testing.   Substantial training is required.

Trial Therapy.   Trial therapy with parasiticidal agents is used in suspected cases of canine scabies or flea allergy. Since canine superficial pyoderma may be pleomorphic, trial use of antibiotics frequently is indicated in undiagnosed pruritic crusted papular dermatoses.

GOALS OF THERAPY (p. 219)

The successful management of a pruritic animal usually requires a definitive diagnosis.

CHAPTER 49

LUMPS, BUMPS, MASSES, AND LYMPHADENOPATHY
(pages 219–223)

Neoplasms, abscesses, cysts, hematomas, granulomas, and excessive fibrous scar tissue account for most of the masses in veterinary medicine. When dealing with masses, the information we would like to obtain is: How long has the mass been present? Has it changed in shape or color? Has it been painful to the animal? After a complete examination of the primary lesion, the possible spread of the mass to other areas should be assessed.

DIAGNOSTIC PLAN (pp. 221–223)

Radiographs are used to evaluate the primary mass and to detect metastasis if the mass is a malignant neoplasm. *Ultrasound examina-*

Original chapter written by Dudley McCaw

tions are useful for defining masses. They can help to determine whether the mass is cystic or solid. *Cytologic examination* should be performed on all masses because it is quick, inexpensive, and carries little risk. Basically, inflammation contains neutrophils, eosinophils, or macrophages. Carcinomas are round or polygonal cells that tend to be in clumps. Sarcomas are spindle-shaped and tend to be individual. Normal lymph nodes contain 75 to 90 per cent small lymphocytes. Lymphosarcoma is characterized by the smear composed of lymphoblasts.

Histopathologic examination of formalin-fixed tissue is needed for a definitive diagnosis. If the lump is small it can be removed in its entirety. If the specimen contains a large quantity of blood or exudate, it may be rinsed with fixative of physiologic saline. Tissues should never be rinsed with tap water, which is hypotonic and causes cell lysis. Biopsy of abdominal masses can be accomplished by the use of biopsy instruments or by removal of the entire mass. Laparoscopy, ultrasound guided biopsy, and laparotomy can all be used for obtaining biopsies of intra-abdominal masses. Each technique has its own advantages and disadvantages, with laparotomy being the only one that usually allows complete mass removal.

CHAPTER 50

CHROMOSOMAL AND GENETIC DISORDERS
(pages 223–226)

See the textbook for a brief discussion of the causes of congenital defects and inheritance patterns.

Susceptibility to injurious environmental or genetic agents varies with the stage of development and decreases with fetal age. Diagnosis of genetic defects is based on the rule that genetic diseases run in families in typical intergenerational and intragenerational patterns. Identification of these defects requires enumeration of normal and abnormal offspring as well as their familial relationships. Breeding trials may be necessary to confirm inheritance patterns, with many congenital diseases following simple mendelian inheritance, mostly simple autosomal recessive. Surgical correction of defects should not be performed on breeding animals.

It is recommended that practitioners do the following:

1. Take greater interest in perinatal puppy and kitten mortality.
2. Become familiar with the common gross findings in dead perinates.
3. Encourage clients to consult them concerning perinatal problems.
4. Monitor perinatal problems by routinely performing necropsy on dead puppies and kittens.
5. Take an interest in canine and feline teratology.
6. Become familiar with the common congenital defects in dogs and cats.

Original chapter written by Horst W. Leipold and Deryl Troyer

CHAPTER 51

NUTRITIONAL MANAGEMENT OF HEPATIC AND ENDOCRINE DISEASES
(pages 228–233)

NUTRITIONAL MANAGEMENT OF HEPATIC DISEASE
(pp. 228–231)

The objectives of nutritional therapy in dogs and cats with liver disease are to provide optimal conditions for hepatic repair and regeneration and to prevent or manage complications of hepatic failure, such as hepatic encephalopathy or ascites. Attention should be turned to nutritional considerations simultaneously with obtaining a diagnosis and restoration of fluid, electrolyte, and acid-base homeostasis.

CALORIES AND FEEDING FREQUENCY

If energy needs are not met, the patient will remain in a catabolic state. The quantity of food fed must be adjusted to achieve and maintain an optimal body weight. Small meals should be fed often (four to six times daily) to minimize HE and reduce fasting hypoglycemia.

PROTEIN

The amount of ammonia delivered to the liver is determined by the level of dietary protein, the activity of colonic bacteria, and the amount of nondietary nitrogen entering the colon (Chapter 106).

Protein Quantity. Animals with impaired hepatic function should be fed as much protein as they will tolerate; the dietary goal in hepatopathy patients is to control signs associated with encephalopathy. Dietary protein restriction can worsen already impaired hepatic protein synthetic functions—for example, causing serum albumin to decrease further when it is already low. The protein intake of patients with hepatic insufficiency is restricted only when signs of HE are unmanageable. In all other cases, the level of dietary protein should be at least a minimum for maintenance (18 per cent for adult dogs based on an energy density of 3.5 kilocalories [kcal] metabolizable energy [ME] per gram of food on a DM basis).

The diet should have high digestibility so that it is nearly completely absorbed in the small intestine. If signs of HE develop, nondietary strate-

---

Original chapter written by P. Jane Armstrong and Sherri L. Ihle

gies for managing HE should be attempted before imposing protein restriction (Chapter 106). Encephalopathic dogs should be fed a minimum of 0.95 gm of highly digestible protein per pound of body weight (BW) per day. Protein of high biologic value, such as milk or egg protein, is recommended. Examples of such diets include dry canine k/d Prescription Diet and dry NF-Formula Canine Veterinary Diet.

Protein restriction usually is not necessary in cats with acquired liver disease, as encephalopathy is an uncommon finding. Protein requirements of cats with liver disease are likely to be as high or higher than for healthy cats. In cats with hepatic lipidosis, diets such as Pulmocare, feline p/d Prescription Diet, and a/d Prescription Diet have been used with success. If there are clinical signs of encephalopathy, feed a diet with approximately 2 gm protein/lb BW—for example, dry feline k/d Prescription Diet.

Protein Source. The source of protein fed to dogs with PSS has proved to be important to survival and development of clinical signs. Equivalent feline studies have not been performed. Meat is not recommended as a protein source.

CARBOHYDRATE AND FAT

Most nonprotein calories should come from easily digested carbohydrates. Cooked white rice is an excellent carbohydrate source. Dietary fats are required as a source of essential fatty acids and for absorption of fat-soluble vitamins, and are useful to increase diet palatability and energy density. Moderate levels of dietary fat are usually well tolerated. However, with cholestatic liver disease and cirrhosis, reduced bile salt excretion may result in steatorrhea.

SALT

Avoidance of excess dietary sodium is indicated in the long-term management of ascites. For a dog with ascites, gradually modify the diet to reduce the dietary sodium content to 0.1 to 0.3 per cent. Diets formulated for canine renal disease typically have a sodium content lower than 0.3 per cent.

COPPER

Restricting dietary copper is one arm of the management strategy for Bedlington terriers, and potentially other breeds, with copper toxicosis (Chapter 106). Canine u/d Prescription Diet is one commercially available food that is low in copper. The protein content of canine u/d may be lower than desired and can be increased by combining one cup of dry diet with one-half cup cottage cheese or one hard-cooked egg. The absorption of copper is reduced by other dietary constituents such as zinc, ascorbic acid, and fiber.

VITAMINS

There is little indication that fat-soluble vitamins are a necessary adjunct therapy for liver disease unless lipid malabsorption is present. Deficiencies of water-soluble vitamins are unlikely in anorectic animals, but may develop when intake resumes.

NUTRITIONAL MANAGEMENT OF ENDOCRINE DISEASE (pp. 231–232)

DIABETES MELLITUS

In most cases dietary control cannot replace insulin therapy but works synergistically to improve glycemic control (Chapter 117).

Correct Obesity and Maintain an Optimal Body Weight. The insulin resistance of obesity resolves with weight loss. Some overweight diabetic cats may even have resolution of their diabetes mellitus following weight loss. Insulin requirements often decrease with weight reduction. If the diabetic patient is thin, caloric intake should be increased initially to allow the animal to replace lost body tissue.

Meal Timing. Feeding must be adjusted to the schedule of insulin injections. If the animal is receiving one insulin injection daily, three equal meals should be fed. If the animal is receiving two insulin injections daily, four equal meals are fed. However, adequate glycemic control can usually be achieved by feeding two equal meals.

Diet Composition. Complex carbohydrates should be fed. Semi-moist and soft dry foods, which contain a high proportion of simple sugars, should be avoided. Glycemic control is improved by consumption of a diet high in fiber. Increased dietary fiber results in less postprandial increase in blood glucose and promotes weight loss. It is recommended that diabetic dogs be fed a relatively high-carbohydrate, moderate-fiber diet (e.g., dry or canned canine w/d Prescription Diet, or dry Canine Science Diet Custom Care Light). This recommendation may be most important if the dog is overweight or glycemic control is poor. Data regarding optimal diet composition for diabetic cats are not available. Feeding diets with increased fiber (e.g., dry or canned feline r/d or w/d Prescription Diets) may improve glycemic control in some cats, especially those that are overweight. A high-fiber diet should not be used initially for a thin patient. A dog with pancreatitis may require an easily digested, low-fat diet such as cooked rice and cottage cheese.

INSULINOMA

Frequent feeding (four to six times daily) of meals moderately high in complex carbohydrates and protein will help to minimize clinical signs associated with large fluctuations in serum glucose concentrations. The owner should be instructed to feed the dog immediately if any sign of weakness is observed. If possible, avoid giving table sugar, corn syrup, honey, or dextrose solutions. Their use may avert one hypoglycemic episode, but predispose to another within 30 to 120 minutes. A diet high in complex carbohydrate and moderately high in protein is recommended.

CHAPTER 52

DIETARY MODIFICATIONS IN CARDIAC DISEASE
(pages 233–238)

IMPORTANT DIETARY CONSIDERATIONS (pp. 234–236)

Reduce Sodium Intake to Prevent Accumulation. The dietary level of sodium that can be tolerated without the appearance of clinical signs depends on the type and severity of the cardiac lesions, neurohumoral mechanisms, and the state of congestion present. Dietary sodium restriction as a clinical tool is divided into three levels: reduced salt, 7 to 13 mg/lb; moderate restriction, 5 to 7

Original chapter written by Mark L. Morris, Jr. and Stephen J. Ettinger mg/lb; and severe restriction, 2 to 6 mg/lb. Dogs in phase II/IV heart disease can be effectively maintained with minimal clinical signs only on moderately restricted sodium diets. Severely restricted sodium diets are required for all dogs exhibiting phases III/IV and IV/IV classification.

Maintain Total Body Potassium Balance. This is an important consideration due to the common use of diuretic agents. However, foods likely to be fed to dogs receiving higher dosages of these drugs already contain levels of potassium shown to be adequate for puppy growth. Of concern are recent reports of hyperkalemia in dogs being given certain ACE inhibitors. Therefore, potassium supplementation of restricted sodium dietary foods appears to be contraindicated.

Provide Taurine. All feline foods produced today should contain added taurine unless the food has been shown to maintain normal taurine blood levels.

Control Caloric Intake and Body Weight. Cardiac cachexia develops progressively in most animals with chronic cardiac disease. This occurs despite what appears to be adequate caloric intake.

Excessive weight increases the stress of cardiac function and exacerbates clinical heart failure. The best way to manage and control weight excess in the cardiac patient is to reduce the total intake of the sodium-restricted dietary food. Caution is advised, since progressive weight loss may continue to the point of cachexia.

SOURCES OF SODIUM INTAKE OTHER THAN DIET

Treats. If the owners feel they must give treats to the pet, the treat should be limited to pieces of the sodium-restricted diet, fruits, vegetables, or lower-sodium treats.

Fresh Water. A significant source of sodium intake occurs when the water has been softened by an ion exchange softener which uses salt. Distilled or nonsoftened water should be given if possible.

PRACTICAL CONSIDERATIONS

The therapeutic objective is to reduce the sodium intake by feeding a food with a lower sodium content. Table 52–1 eliminates the need to know the content of each specific brand of dog and cat food.

TABLE 52–1. CLASSIFICATION OF PREPARED PET FOODS BY SODIUM CONTENT

	AVERAGE SODIUM CONTENT (% DRY MATTER)
High (>0.5% DM)	
Popular Canine and Feline canned	0.9–1.0
Reduced-salt diets (0.35–0.5% DM)	
Popular Canine and Feline dry	0.40–0.44
Premium Canine and Feline canned and dry	0.35–0.42
Moderate salt restriction (0.1–0.35% DM)	
Canine Geriatric/Senior	0.12–0.17
Dietary-Canine and Feline renal	0.23–0.33
Dietary-Feline cardiac	0.23
Severe salt restriction (<0.1% DM)	
Dietary-Canine cardiac	0.08–0.12
Minimum Adult Requirement	
Canine	0.06
Feline	0.20

TABLE 52–2. RECIPES FOR LOW-SODIUM DIETS

Low-Sodium Diet for Dogs	Low-Sodium Diet for Cats
¼ lb lean ground beef	1 lb regular ground beef
2 c cooked rice without salt	¼ lb liver
1 tbsp vegetable oil	1 cup cooked rice without salt
2 Tums tablets, crushed	1 tsp vegetable oil
Braise meat, retaining fat.	1 tsp calcium carbonate or
Add other ingredients and mix.	10 Tums tablets, crushed
Yield: 1.1 lb (480 g)	Braise meat and liver, retaining fat.
Sodium content: 0.05% in dry matter	Add other ingredients and mix.
	Yield: 1.7 lb (750 g)
	Sodium content: 0.16% in dry matter

Changing the Diet. Many pets, especially dogs, readily accept a change to a restricted sodium diet by the third day. If a complete switch cannot be accomplished at one time, restriction should be initiated by selecting a lower-sodium diet (e.g., foods designed for renal failure). Another alternative is to change to a "senior" diet.

Homemade Diets. Some owners choose not to feed prepared foods to their pets or refuse to believe that their pet will consume a commercially prepared food. The owner must be advised that a home-made diet restricted in both salt and calories is a less than ideal alternative and that such a diet may not meet nutritional needs. Table 52–2 gives some recipes for low-sodium diets, and Table 52–3 shows the sodium and calorie content of foods. Anorexic pets brought home after a bout with heart failure may be a challenge. Never allow a dog or cat on high-dose diuretics to starve, as this will seriously aggravate hyponatremia, hypochloremia, and renal dysfunction.

Veterinary Instructions. Owners may find that commercial preparations appear unpalatable. Warming, chopping, or even pan frying such foods often changes the presentation to one that is more familiar to both the pet and the owner. Supplementing such food with garlic or onion powder, honey, maple syrup, oregano, or parsley is likely to make the product more familiar or tasty.

LOW-SALT DIETS IN HYPERTENSIVE CARDIAC DISEASE

Gradual introduction of "renal diets" is the recommended approach to these patients.

TABLE 52–3. SODIUM AND CALORIE CONTENT OF FOODS

FOOD	AMOUNT	SODIUM (MG)	CALORIES
Bread, cereals, and potatoes			
Recommended			
Potato	1 (small)	1	70
Polished rice	½ cup	1–10	360
Macaroni	1 cup	1–10	465
Puffed wheat	1 oz	1–10	100
Spaghetti	1 cup	1–10	355
Not recommended			
Bread	1 slice	200	60
Pretzel	1	275	58
Potato chips	1 oz	300	170
Cheese pizza	1 slice	650	245
Margarine and oil			
Recommended			
Unsalted margarine	1 tsp	0–1	50
Vegetable shortening	1 tbs	0–1	120
Not recommended			
Mayonnaise	1 tbs	60–90	110
Dairy products			
Not recommended			
Milk (regular)	1 cup	122	160
Milk (skim)	1 cup	122	90
Cream cheese	1½ oz	100–120	160
Cottage cheese	3 oz	200–300	90
American cheese	1 oz	200–300	105
Butter	1 tsp	50	50
Meats, poultry, fish			
Recommended			
Beef (fresh)	3½ oz	50	200
Pork (fresh)	3½ oz	62	275
Lamb (fresh)	3½ oz	84	175
Veal	3½ oz	67	300
Chicken (no skin)			
Light meat	3½ oz	64	180
Dark meat	3½ oz	86	180
Turkey (no skin)			
Light meat	3½ oz	82	230
Dark meat	3½ oz	98	230
Not recommended			
Egg	1	70	80
Bacon	2 slices	385	95
Ham (processed)	3 oz	940	225
Frankfurter	1	560	310
Vegetables (fresh or dietetic canned)			
Recommended			
Asparagus	½ cup	<5	20
Green beans	½ cup	<5	15
Peas	½ cup	<5	55
Green pepper	¼ cup	<5	10
Tomato	1	<5	30
Lettuce	¼ head	<5	15
Corn	½ cup	<5	70
Cucumber	½ cup	<5	<20
Fresh fruits			
Most are low in sodium and are permitted			
Desserts			
Recommended			
Sherbet	½ cup	15–25	120
Not recommended			
Gelatins	½ cup	60–85	50–80
Ice cream	½ cup	60–85	200
Puddings	½ cup	100–200	175

Modified from Ettinger SJ, Suter PF: Canine Cardiology. Philadelphia, WB Saunders, 1970.

CHAPTER 53

DIETARY CONSIDERATIONS FOR UROGENITAL PROBLEMS
(pages 238–243)

In this chapter, we address considerations related to the nutritional management of chronic renal failure in dogs and cats. With chronic renal failure, the goals of dietary management are to maximize the quality and quantity of life by ensuring adequate intake of energy, limiting the extent of uremia, and slowing the rate of progression of renal disease.

RESTRICTION OF NUTRIENTS: UREMIA (pp. 240–241)

In uremic animals, restriction of dietary protein intake has routinely been recommended to reduce the generation of a variety of toxins derived from protein metabolism. A recently completed clinical trial supports the use of dietary protein restriction for this purpose. Since marked restriction of dietary protein intake has been associated with protein malnutrition and increased mortality, unwarranted excessive restriction should be avoided. The degree of protein restriction should be individualized and based on the patient's clinical response.

Some pets will find special diets unpalatable. Modifications include warming the diet or supplementing it with a small amount of a substance to enhance palatability (e.g., turkey fat). Restriction of dietary intake of phosphorus reduces the extent of renal secondary hyperparathyroidism. The extent of dietary phosphorus restriction should parallel the degree of renal dysfunction. A diet with minimal phosphorus content usually must be supplemented with intestinal phosphate binders dosed to effect to achieve normophosphatemia. If dogs with renal failure and normophosphatemia exhibit manifestations attributable to renal secondary hyperparathyroidism, the oral administration of calcitriol may be used as adjunct therapy (Chapter 134).

Metabolic acidosis may also contribute to uremic complications. Dietary protein restriction may normalize acid-base status. Dietary alkalinization (e.g., calcium carbonate) will effectively control acidosis without the need for other dietary manipulations.

RESTRICTION OF NUTRIENTS: PROGRESSIVE NEPHROPATHY (pp. 241–242)

Progressive decrements of renal function may be observed in animals in which the primary disease has been eliminated. It has been proposed that once renal disease reaches a certain degree of severity, progression to end-stage renal disease is inevitable. Alterations in dietary intake can modify both the extent and nature of renal adaptations and can serve to restore homeostasis, theoretically limiting progressive renal injury.

RESTRICTION OF DIETARY PROTEIN INTAKE

Dietary protein restriction may limit the genesis of nitrogenous wastes and thus lessen the extent of uremic complications of chronic renal failure, such as lethargy and vomiting. However, most studies do not support the use of low-protein diets to slow the progression of renal

---

Original chapter written by Scott A. Brown, Delmar R. Finco, and Jeanne A. Barsanti failure in dogs. Many questions remain unanswered, and only general guidelines for dietary protein intake can be suggested. A moderate protein diet (15 to 25 per cent protein content) is appropriate for dogs with moderate azotemia that do not exhibit signs of uremia. Further restriction (9 to 15 per cent protein content) is warranted only if uremia is present. Dietary protein restriction in cats with azotemic renal failure should be attempted much more cautiously (28 to 32 per cent protein). Diets supplying less protein seem unwarranted.

RESTRICTION OF DIETARY PHOSPHORUS INTAKE

Dietary phosphorus restriction should be in proportion to the degree of renal dysfunction. In general, diets comprised of less than 0.5 per cent phosphorus should be employed initially. It is likely that further reductions in phosphorus intake will be necessary to achieve normophosphatemia in some affected animals. Intestinal phosphorus binders should be added in animals remaining hyperphosphatemic despite dietary phosphate restriction. Calcium-containing phosphorus binding agents may induce hypercalcemia and should not be employed in animals with hypercalcemia or in conjunction with vitamin D therapy.

RESTRICTION OF DIETARY SODIUM INTAKE

The rationale for dietary sodium restriction is to combat systemic hypertension. However, it has not been clearly established that moderate dietary sodium restriction will lower systemic arterial pressure in dogs and cats with spontaneous renal disease. In animals with renal failure in the presence of systemic hypertension, dietary sodium restriction is an appropriate therapeutic maneuver. It should be moderate, with a goal of approximately 7 to 18 mg/lb/day. Changes in sodium intake should be accomplished gradually, over 7 to 14 days. Effectiveness of sodium restriction should be assessed by blood pressure measurements.

MAINTENANCE OF DIETARY POTASSIUM INTAKE

In cats, hypokalemic renal failure has been associated with polymyopathy. It is hypothesized that renal failure leads to kaliuresis and hypokalemia, which reduce renal function. Reduced renal function further enhances kaliuresis. It is important to ensure adequate potassium intake for cats (and dogs) with renal failure. Dietary supplementation with potassium salts (Chapter 134) should be utilized, if needed, to maintain eukalemia.

DIETARY ALKALINIZATION

Metabolic acidosis in animals with renal failure can be ameliorated by dietary alkalinization, restriction of dietary protein intake, or changing from an animal protein to a vegetable-source protein. A reasonable goal is to achieve the lower limit of the normal range for plasma bicarbonate or total carbon dioxide content.

COMMERCIALLY AVAILABLE DIETS (pp. 242–243)

A commercially available preparation is likely to be most practical when dietary modification is instituted. Pet food companies are not required to demonstrate efficacy for claims they may make, and they may alter the content and nutrient profiles of foods without notice. Consequently, the veterinarian is left with considerable uncertainty about what food to use. Serial measurements of serum concentrations of creatinine, blood urea nitrogen, phosphate, calcium, bicarbonate, protein, and albumin and a complete blood count and urinalysis should be performed one month after a diet change and repeated every 3

TABLE 53-1. NUTRIENT INFORMATION FOR COMMERCIALLY AVAILABLE DIETS* FORMULATED FOR ANIMALS WITH RENAL FAILURE

DIET	NUTRIENT CONTENT† (% DRY WEIGHT)				NUTRIENT INTAKE‡			
	Protein	P	Na	K	Protein (gm/kg)	P (mg/kg)	Na	K
Canine Diets:								
Hill's K/D canned	16.1	0.26	0.22	0.30	2.1	34.4	29.1	39.7
Hill's K/D dry	14.6	0.28	0.23	0.38	2.1	40.7	33.4	55.2
Hill's U/D canned	11.5	0.14	0.25	0.39	1.5	18.6	33.1	51.7
Hill's U/D dry	9.3	0.15	0.26	0.62	1.3	21.6	37.4	89.1
Waltham canned	16.7	0.50	0.33	0.90	2.2	65.5	43.2	117.9
Purina NF canned	16.5	0.26	0.23	0.33	2.3	35.5	31.4	45.0
Purina NF dry	14.9	0.27	0.23	0.36	2.3	41.2	35.1	54.9
Rx148 canned	17.4	0.27	0.22	0.87	2.5	39.1	31.9	126.0
Rx148 dry	17.4	0.27	0.22	0.87	2.5	39.1	31.9	126.0
Renalcare canned	15.2	0.66	0.30	0.73	1.8	77.1	35.0	85.2
Feline Diets:								
Hill's K/D canned	29.3	0.48	0.28	0.93	3.8	62.7	36.6	121.5
Hill's K/D dry	28.1	0.57	0.25	0.89	4.2	86.0	37.7	134.3
Rx248 canned	28.4	0.44	0.27	0.82	4.4	67.4	41.4	125.6
Rx248 dry	28.4	0.44	0.27	0.82	4.4	67.4	41.4	125.6
Renalcare canned	30.5	0.66	0.36	0.76	4.2	90.9	49.6	104.7

*Prescription Diet Canine K/D, Prescription Diet Canine U/D, and Prescription Diet Feline K/D (Hill's Pet Products, Topeka, Kansas); Waltham Low Protein Canine Diet (KalKan Inc., Vernon California); Purina NF Diet (Ralston-Purina, St. Louis, Missouri); Rx148 and Rx248 (KenVet, Ashland, Ohio); and RenalCare Canine and Feline Liquid Diets (Pet-Ag, Inc., Elgin, Illinois).

†Average nutrient content of diet on a dry weight basis, as currently formulated (based on information supplied by producers).

‡Nutrient intake for a 44 lb dog consuming 1250 calories daily (canine diets) or an 8.8 lb cat consuming 280 kcal daily (feline diets). These calculations assume apparent digestibility of 80 per cent for protein, 90 per cent for fat, and 85 per cent for carbohydrate and represent approximations only. Factors such as digestibility, palatability, biologic value of protein, availability of phosphorus for absorption, and fatty acid profiles are likely to vary substantially between diets.

months throughout the life of an animal. This will allow the veterinarian to identify abnormalities and institute appropriate therapy.

Nutrient information on commercially available preparations demonstrates that while several of the commercially available preparations are similar, there are some important differences in protein, phosphorus, sodium, and potassium contents (see Table 53–1).

CHAPTER 54

ENTERAL AND PARENTERAL NUTRITIONAL SUPPORT
(pages 244–252)

PATIENT SELECTION (p. 244)

Table 54–1 contains clinical and laboratory findings that serve as general indicators of poor nutritional status. In studies of veterinary patients, history, physical examination, assessment of body condition, and serum proteins are most commonly used to select patients in need of assisted feeding.

TABLE 54–1. INDICATORS OF POOR NUTRITIONAL STATUS

Historical findings
    Poor food intake for >3 days (adults); >1 day (neonates)
    Unplanned weight loss of >10% (adults); >5% (neonates)
Physical findings
    General debilitation
    Poor haircoat quality
    Muscle wasting
    Loss of body fat stores
Laboratory findings
    Hypoproteinemia
    Hypoalbuminemia
    Lymphopenia
    Anemia
    Hypokalemia
Recognition of conditions causing increased nutrient demands
    Trauma
    Surgery
    Infection/fever
    Cancer
    Burns
Recognition of conditions causing increased nutrient losses
    Gastrointestinal losses
    Urinary losses
    Draining wounds/abscesses
    Burns

Original chapter written by Deborah J. Davenport

ENTERAL FEEDING METHODS (pp. 244–247)

Enteral feeding is the simplest, safest, least expensive, and most physiologic route; it should be used whenever possible, and it is best to use diets that are formulated for veterinary use.

Coax Feeding.   At times, hospitalized dogs and cats will eat more readily when they are out of their cage or fed by their owners. Warming food to body temperature will also enhance palatability.

Appetite Stimulation.   Appetite stimulants include diazepam and derivatives, anabolic steroids, vitamin B complex, and cyproheptadine. Appetite stimulation should be considered a "jumpstart" mechanism, at best.

Force Feeding.   Forcing food into an animal's pharynx should stimulate the swallowing reflex, leading to food ingestion. Force feeding should only be attempted for a short time (2 to 3 days).

Tube Feeding.

Orogastric.   Commonly used in the management of orphaned puppies and kittens, this technique is stressful to adult pets, particularly cats. There is a risk of aspiration if the feeding tube is inadvertently placed in the trachea.

Nasoesophageal.   Nasoesophageal (NE) catheters are useful for feeding anorexic patients. NE tubes are well tolerated by most animals, and pets are commonly discharged from the hospital with tubes in place. Serious complications are uncommon. The greatest drawback is their small diameter, which necessitates the use of commercial enteral diets rather than blenderized pet foods.

Pharyngostomy.   Because of the small diameter of NE tubes, some clinicians prefer pharyngostomy tubes. When properly placed, these are used for long-term feeding.

Esophagostomy.   Such tubes are reportedly well tolerated. The disadvantages include the need for sedation or general anesthesia and the small diameter of the tubes.

Gastrostomy.   Gastrostomy tubes can be placed at the time of abdominal surgery or through an endoscope. Most animals tolerate gastrostomy tubes extremely well, allowing these tubes to be left in place for weeks to months if necessary.

Duodenostomy/Jejunostomy.   In dogs or cats with serious disease of the proximal gastrointestinal tract, the use of jejunostomy tubes for nutritional support may be indicated. The use of these tubes is limited to hospitalized patients. The small size of the catheters demands the use of commercial enteral diets.

Diet Selection

Water.   It is crucial to postpone feeding anorexic animals until fluid, electrolyte, and acid-base balance have been reestablished. Only then should feeding be initiated.

Energy.   The equation for Resting Energy Requirement (RER) is:

$$\text{RER (kcal/day)} = 70 \, (BW_{kg})^{0.75}$$

It is necessary to factor a value to account for the increased energy needs of illness. I recommend the use of the term *Illness Energy Requirement (IER)*, which can be determined by the following formula:

$$\text{Canine IER (kcal/day)} = 1.25 \text{ to } 1.50 \times \text{RER}$$

$$\text{Feline IER (kcal/day)} = 1.10 \text{ to } 1.25 \times \text{RER}$$

This method calculates the energy needs of dogs and cats suffering from a variety of illnesses.

Protein.   It is assumed that hospitalized cats require at least maintenance amounts of protein in their diet and perhaps as much as two to

Parenteral Feeding Worksheet

1. Calculate Resting Energy Requirement (RER)

Animals between 2 kg and 45 kg body weight:*

$$30 \quad \boxed{} \quad + 70 = \boxed{}$$

body weight (kg)   RER (kcal/day)

*Animals < 2 kg or > 45 kg use 70 $(BW_{kg})^{0.75}$

2. Calculate Illness/Infection/Injury Energy Requirement (IER)

Illness Factor = 1.25 - 1.50 Canine
               1.10 - 1.25 Feline

$$\boxed{} \quad \times \quad \boxed{} \quad = \quad \boxed{}$$

factor chosen   RER (kcal/day)   IER (kcal/day)

3. Calculate Protein Requirement

	Canine	Feline
Standard requirement	4.0-8.0 g/100 kcal	6.0-9.0 g/100 kcal
Decreased reqt. (hepatic or renal failure)	≤ 4.0 g/100 kcal	≤ 6.0 g/100 kcal
Increased reqt. (protein losing conditions)	≥ 8.0 g/100 kcal	≥ 9.0 g/100 kcal

122

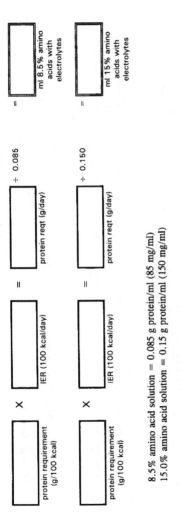

8.5% amino acid solution = 0.085 g protein/ml (85 mg/ml)
15.0% amino acid solution = 0.15 g protein/ml (150 mg/ml)

4. Calculate Non-Protein Calorie Requirement

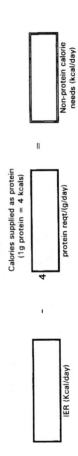

Figure 54-1. Representative parenteral worksheet.

Figure continued on next page

5. Calculate Fluid Quantities to Meet Non-Protein Calorie Requirement

Caloric densities

Dextrose solutions:
10% = 0.34 kcal/ml
20% = 0.68 kcal/ml
50% = 1.70 kcal/ml

Lipid solutions:
10% = 1.1 kcal/ml
20% = 2.0 kcal/ml

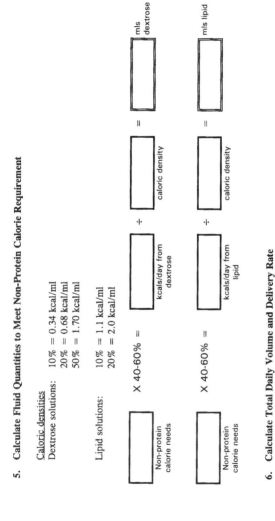

| Non-protein calorie needs | X 40-60% = | kcals/day from dextrose | ÷ | caloric density | = | mls dextrose |

| Non-protein calorie needs | X 40-60% = | kcals/day from lipid | ÷ | caloric density | = | mls lipid |

6. Calculate Total Daily Volume and Delivery Rate

Volume dextrose = ☐ ml

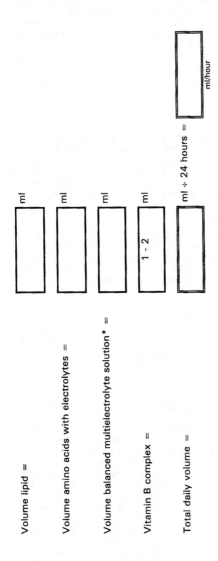

Volume lipid = ☐ ml

Volume amino acids with electrolytes = ☐ ml

Volume balanced multielectrolyte solution* = ☐ ml

Vitamin B complex = ☐ 1 - 2 ml

Total daily volume = ☐ ml ÷ 24 hours = ☐ ml/hour

*Calculate based on animal's fluid and electrolyte requirements.
Daily fluid reqt(ml) - TPN solution volume (ml) = required volume
of balanced multielectrolyte solution

Figure 54-1. *Continued*

125

three times that quantity. If a dog or cat is suffering from a protein-losing disorder, additional dietary protein may be necessary. Alternatively, in cases of uremia or hepatic encephalopathy, it may be necessary to reduce protein intake. One must also consider protein quality, in particular taurine and arginine.

Minerals and Vitamins.   It seems prudent to provide at least maintenance levels of these nutrients to hospitalized patients except in those situations (e.g., renal failure) in which they would be contraindicated. Vitamin B depletion is known to depress appetite, and repletion can serve as a stimulus for food consumption.

Food Dosage Calculations

Calculations are determined from an animal's energy requirement and the energy density of the selected diet.

Diet Types

Energy-dense, recuperative-type canned cat foods are commonly used. The consistency of such diets precludes their use in feeding tubes less than 8 F in diameter. Commercial enteral diets are available as ready-to-use liquids and gels or as powders that must be reconstituted with water. These products are easily digested, readily absorbed, and useful for feeding patients with severe gastrointestinal disease.

Diet Administration

It is extremely important to initiate feeding in the anorexic animal gradually. On the first day of feeding, no more than one-third of the calculated caloric requirement should be provided. Full feeding can often be provided by day 3. *Continuous infusion* of enteral diets is a useful technique in animals being fed via enterostomy.

RETURN TO VOLUNTARY FEEDING

This decision should be based on a number of factors: (1) improvement in the patient's condition, (2) demonstrated interest in food, (3) tube feeding complications, and (4) expected difficulty in replacing the feeding tube if necessary. In general, feeding tubes should be left in place until the patient is consuming at least 50 per cent of its caloric needs voluntarily.

PARENTERAL FEEDING METHODS (pp. 247–252)

Specific indications for the use of parenteral feeding include intolerance of enteral feeding as manifested by vomiting or diarrhea, severe malabsorption syndromes, and the risk of aspiration if the patient is fed via the gastrointestinal tract. The three basic components of parenteral feeding solutions are dextrose (50 to 70 per cent solutions), crystalline amino acids (8.5 or 15 per cent solutions), and lipid emulsions (20 per cent). Varying mixtures of these components can be prepared to meet the needs of the individual patient. In general, the animal's nonprotein caloric requirements are met using a 1 to 1 ratio of 50 per cent dextrose and 20 per cent lipids, while protein requirements are met via the administration of 8.5 per cent amino acids. The use of a parenteral feeding worksheet (Fig. 54–1) can facilitate such calculations.

Solutions must be administered through a central vein. Parenteral nutrition catheters must be placed aseptically to avoid the complication of sepsis. Parenteral support should be initiated gradually. When it is no longer necessary, fluid administration rates should be decreased incrementally over 2 to 3 days. Careful monitoring is necessary to avoid complications. Allow for close observation of the catheter site for any evidence of infection. Serial monitoring of serum potassium, triglycerides, and glucose is important for all patients. Urinary glucose determinations are also recommended. For animals with hepatic disease, plasma ammonia measurement is advised.

In veterinary patients, hypokalemia and hyperglycemia are the most common metabolic consequences of parenteral feeding. Sepsis is the most serious potential sequela of parenteral nutritional support.

CHAPTER 55

DEVELOPMENTAL ORTHOPEDICS: NUTRITIONAL INFLUENCES IN THE DOG
(pages 252–258)

Nutrition is one of the single most important factors influencing development of the musculoskeletal system. The vast majority of developmental skeletal disorders diagnosed in veterinary practice are in large and giant breeds and are associated with excess (inappropriate) intake of a commercial diet and/or supplementation.

NUTRIENTS AND SKELETAL DISEASE (pp. 253–254)

ENERGY (CALORIES)

Growing dogs require approximately two times as much energy per unit of body weight immediately after weaning as adult animals of the same breed. This is arbitrarily decreased to 1.6 times when the dog reaches 40 per cent of adult body weight. The link to skeletal disease appears to be when energy contributes to rapid growth rates and excessive body weight.

PROTEIN

Like excess energy, protein has been incriminated in the development of skeletal disease. If requirements for essential amino acids are met, there are no known benefits to feeding excess protein to healthy, young, growing dogs.

CALCIUM

There are three specific hormonal regulators of plasma calcium concentration: parathyroid hormone (PTH), calcitonin (CT), and 1,25 dihydroxycholecalciferol (1,25 vit D). Hormone release is influenced by plasma calcium concentration, which regulates calcium dynamics in the respective target organs.

Chronic high calcium intake in large-breed dogs has been associated with hypercalcemia, concomitant hypophosphatemia, rise in serum alkaline phosphatase, retarded bone maturation, higher percentage of total bone volume, retarded bone remodeling, decrease in osteoclasts, and retarded maturation of cartilage. The clinical diseases associated with these changes are osteochondrosis, retained cartilage cones, radius curvus syndrome, and stunted growth.

VITAMIN C

Excess vitamin C supplementation is generally considered to have little or no effect on the skeleton. The relationship between vitamin C and developmental disorders of the skeletal system in the dog has not been proved.

OTHER NUTRIENTS

Clinical cases of vitamin D deficiency (rickets) are extremely rare. In the growing dog, supplementation with vitamin D can result in marked disturbance of normal skeletal development. Copper deficiency in the dog has been associated with hyperextension of the distal phalanges. Long-term studies of dietary zinc levels showed no significant clinical influence on skeletal development.

PRIMARY DEVELOPMENTAL SKELETAL DISEASES (pp. 254–255)

CANINE HIP DYSPLASIA (CHD)

Canine hip dysplasia is the most frequently encountered orthopedic disease in the practice of veterinary medicine. It appears that the period from 3 to 8 months of age is important in the development of CHD, and the first 6 months are generally believed to be the most critical. Frequency and severity of CHD is influenced by weight gain in growing dogs, especially if sired by parents with CHD. Dogs with weight gains exceeding breed standards have a higher frequency of CHD as well as more severe CHD than dogs with weight gain below the standard curve.

PROTEIN AND CHD

High-protein intake does not appear important for the development of normal hip joints.

ENERGY AND CHD

Other than when overall food consumption is reduced by restricted intake, dietary energy has minimal to no influence on the production or prevention of CHD.

VITAMIN C AND CHD

No studies have adequately demonstrated a positive effect of oral supplementation of vitamin C in preventing CHD in growing dogs genetically at risk for the disease.

ELECTROLYTE BALANCE AND CHD

A role for dietary electrolytes has been proposed as a preventative for CHD. Studies suggesting an association did not prove a mechanism of action and were not definitive.

OSTEOCHONDROSIS (OCD) (pp. 255–256)

Osteochondrosis (OCD) is a focal area of disruption in endochondral ossification. In the dog, OCD risk factors are associated with age, gender, breed, rapid growth, and nutrient excesses (primarily calcium). All large and giant breeds are at increased risk for OCD. The highest risk is in the Great Dane, Labrador retriever, Newfoundland, and rottweiler breeds. Males have an increased risk of OCD in the proximal humerus, but gender relationships are not found for OCD involving other joints. While generalized nutrient excesses have been incriminated with OCD lesions, there is increasing evidence implicating specific nutrients (e.g., calcium and vitamin C).

NUTRITIONAL MANAGEMENT OF THE GROWING DOG (p. 256)

ENERGY

Energy alone is not a key factor, but energy as a component of the diet when fed in excess is likely to result in a more rapid rate of growth. Although energy is needed for normal development, there are differing needs based on breed, age, neuter status, and activity levels.

PROTEIN

Protein has not been demonstrated to have any negative consequences on calcium metabolism or skeletal development in the dog. A growth diet should contain >28 per cent protein of high biologic value supplying at least 16 per cent of the dietary energy.

CALCIUM

The absolute level of calcium, rather than an imbalance in the calcium/phosphorus ratio, is responsible for negatively influencing skeletal development. Calcium levels for a growth diet should be between 1 per cent and 1.6 per cent (dry matter basis). Feeding treats containing calcium and/or providing calcium supplements increases daily calcium intake.

FEEDING TECHNIQUES (pp. 256–257)

There are three basic methods of feeding the growing dog, free-choice (ad libitum), food-restricted, or time-restricted. In general, free-choice feeding is contraindicated in "at risk" dogs until they have reached at least 80 to 90 per cent of adult size and weight. Food-restricted feeding requires frequent calculations of MER and is used as the basis for food amount. Frequent body weights are needed.

Time-restricted feeding is the feeding method of choice for most large and giant breeds. Having food available for a set period of time, two to three times per day, not only controls intake but can help in discipline and house training of the young puppy. If fed based on energy requirements, activity level, and body condition, growth diets do not increase the risk of developmental bone disease in large- and giant-breed dogs. It is not only important to feed the appropriate diet, but to feed the diet appropriately!

CHAPTER 56

ADVERSE REACTIONS TO FOODS: ALLERGIES
(pages 258–262)

An *adverse reaction to food* is a clinically abnormal response to an ingested food or food additive. Adverse reactions to food have been blamed for a variety of clinical syndromes in the dog and cat, usually involving the skin and gastrointestinal tract.

TERMINOLOGY (p. 258)

Food allergy (food hypersensitivity) is an adverse reaction to a food or food additive with a proven immunologic basis. *Food intolerance* is a nonimmunologic adverse physiologic response to a food or food additive, which can be subcategorized as a food idiosyncrasy, food poisoning, or pharmacologic reaction to food. Adverse reactions due to gluttony, pica, or consumption of indigestible materials are called *dietary indiscretion*.

IMMUNOLOGIC REACTIONS TO FOOD (pp. 258–261)

Food allergens incriminated in North American dogs and cats include preservatives, dyes, and wheat, beef, egg, corn, fish, poultry, soy, and dairy products.

Mucosal Barrier and Oral Tolerance

See textbook.

Clinical Features in Dogs and Cats

Adverse food reactions are usually suspected when a client or veterinarian establishes a historical association between ingestion of certain foods and the appearance of certain clinical signs. Dogs and cats may develop food allergy after prolonged exposure to one brand, type, or form of food.

Dermatologic signs include severe, generalized pruritus without lesions; miliary dermatitis; pruritus with self-trauma centered around the head, neck, and ears; alopecia; and scaling dermatoses, self-inflicted alopecia, eosinophilic plaques, and indolent ulcers of the lip in some cats. Absolute peripheral eosinophilia occurs in 20 to 50 per cent of these cats.

Food allergy can mimic idiopathic miliary dermatitis, atopy, flea bite hypersensitivity, psychogenic alopecia, dermatophytosis, and parasitic infestation. As many as 20 per cent of cats with suspected food allergy may have concurrent flea allergy dermatitis or atopy.

In dogs, food allergy typically occurs as nonseasonal pruritic dermatitis that is occasionally accompanied by gastrointestinal signs. Pruritus is often indistinguishable from that seen with inhalant allergies—feet, face, axilla, perineal region, inguinal region, rump, and ears. Dogs with chronic or recurrent otitis externa should be closely evaluated for food allergy.

A variety of primary and secondary skin lesions occur in dogs with food allergy. These include papules, erythroderma, excoriations, hyper-

Original chapter written by Philip Roudebush

pigmentation, epidermal collarettes, pododermatitis, seborrhea sicca, and otitis externa. Gastrointestinal signs include intermittent vomiting and/or mild to severe diarrhea.

DIAGNOSIS

Dietary elimination trials are the main diagnostic method used in dogs and cats. It is useful for the client to keep the dog or cat on its usual food for 7 to 14 days. The patient is then placed on a controlled elimination diet for 4 to 12 weeks. The ideal elimination diet should include a novel, highly digestible protein source, avoid protein excesses, be free of additives, and be nutritionally adequate for the animal's life stage and condition. *No* other ingested substances should be offered. Observation of at least 50 per cent improvement in clinical signs is necessary to make a tentative diagnosis of food allergy.

Ingredients recommended most often for home-made feline diets include lamb baby food, lamb, rice, and rabbit. Ingredients for home-made canine diets include lamb, rice, potato, fish, rabbit, venison, and tofu. Home-made diets are often nutritionally inadequate for adult maintenance. These deficiencies are not considered worrisome if the elimination diet is to be used for only several weeks. Alternative nutritionally adequate home-made diet recipes are available and may be used.

A definitive diagnosis is made if the elimination diet resolves all clinical signs and if the former diet is subsequently offered as a challenge, with a return of clinical signs within a few minutes to a week. Elimination trials are difficult to interpret in some dogs and cats because of concurrent allergic skin disease. Flea-allergic dermatitis and atopy are the most common allergies and should be eliminated through other diagnostic testing.

TREATMENT

For most food allergies, avoiding the offending foods is the most effective treatment. How selective or meticulous an avoidance diet must be depends upon the individual animal's sensitivity. Concurrent allergies will influence the threshold level of clinical signs. Symptomatic therapy can include corticosteroids and antihistamines. It is important that any home-made recipe for long-term maintenance should ensure a nutritionally adequate ration. An attempt should always be made to find an acceptable commercial diet.

NONIMMUNOLOGIC REACTIONS TO FOOD
(pp. 261–262)

Nonimmunologic reactions to food include food intolerance and dietary indiscretion. Dietary indiscretions are easily diagnosed by a thorough environmental and dietary history. Food additives, preservatives, or dyes are frequently mentioned as dietary items that cause adverse food reactions in dogs and cats. Additives are found least often in canned pet foods and most commonly in soft-moist foods, treats, snacks, and dry foods. Reactions to food additives are best described as food intolerance because they cause clinical signs due to nonimmunologic mechanisms. Another cause of food intolerance is pharmacologic reactions to substances found in food—for example, vasoactive amines. What role histamine and other vasoactive amines play in food intolerance in animals is unknown. Vasoactive amines may not be present in levels high enough to cause clinical signs but could lower the threshold levels for allergens in individual dogs and cats.

CHAPTER 57

PHARMACOLOGIC PRINCIPLES
(pages 264–272)

PHARMACOLOGIC PRINCIPLES (pp. 264–265)

DRUG DISTRIBUTION

Most drugs easily distribute from the intravascular compartment to the extracellular fluid through the fenestrations in capillaries. Capillaries that are not fenestrated or have a continuous epithelial layer ordinarily prevent diffusion of water-soluble drugs into certain tissues. Examples of such tissues are the central nervous system, the cerebrospinal fluid (CSF), aqueous humor, joint fluid, and the prostate. Lipid-soluble drugs can diffuse across these barriers. Intracellular penetration is not necessary for the action of most drugs, which for many drugs is carried out simply by binding to cell surface receptors. A drug's *volume of distribution* can be a clue to its ability to diffuse across membranes.

DRUG DIFFUSION

The ability of a drug to diffuse from one body compartment to another is determined by the difference in drug concentration between compartments, the thickness of the barrier between the compartments, the lipid/water partition coefficient, and the surface area available for diffusion. Drugs may also be transported across membranes via active transport, which can occur against a concentration gradient.

DRUG PERMEABILITY

Drug permeability is a function of its molecular size and shape, protein binding, and ionization. Molecular size has little effect on drug permeability. Most drugs exist either in an ionized or un-ionized state. An ionized (polar) drug is poorly lipid-soluble, but an un-ionized (nonpolar) drug diffuses across a membrane more easily. The pH of the drug milieu and the drug's pKa determine whether a drug is primarily in an ionized or un-ionized form.

Original chapter written by Mark G. Papich

DRUG ABSORPTION (pp. 267–268)

The measure of a drug's absorption is called *bioavailability*, which is determined by both the *extent* and *rate* of drug absorption. A measure of the amount of drug that reaches the systemic circulation following a dose is called the *systemic availability*.

ORAL DRUG ADMINISTRATION

Drugs absorbed from the intestine must pass through the liver before reaching the systemic circulation. The metabolism or inactivation of a drug by the liver before it reaches the systemic circulation is called *presystemic metabolism*, and is responsible for a *first-pass* effect. Lidocaine, propranolol, and opiates are examples of drugs that undergo significant presystemic metabolism.

Factors That May Decrease Drug Absorption. The presence of food and other drugs also may affect oral absorption. Some drug interactions are listed in Table 57–1.

Drugs that are degraded in acid are absorbed better if the stomach is empty when they are administered—for example, the penicillin class of antibiotics. For other drugs, availability increases if the patient has been fed. Systemic availability of fat-soluble drugs such as griseofulvin and vitamin K also is increased if they are administered with a meal that contains fat.

The dose formulation often affects the absorption of oral drugs. Drugs that are in an oral liquid may be absorbed more easily because dissolution of a tablet does not have to occur. Enteric coating of some tablets that are intended for people may exhibit decreased absorption in dogs.

INTRAMUSCULAR DRUG ADMINISTRATION

Intramuscular (IM) drug administration is convenient for drugs that cannot be administered orally and when it is not possible to administer the drug intravenously. Injections in the muscle usually are absorbed rapidly and completely, but the absorption is perfusion-rate-limited. Therefore, conditions such as shock will decrease muscular blood flow and delay absorption.

Some drugs are formulated in a liquid suspension that is poorly soluble. These drugs are absorbed slowly but continuously into the circulation. Examples are methylprednisolone acetate, microcrystalline deoxycorticosterone pivalate, testosterone cypionate, and benzathine

TABLE 57–1. EXAMPLES OF INTERACTIONS AFFECTING DRUG BIOAVAILABILITY

	Drug Interactions
Tetracycline	Absorption is inhibited by concurrent administration of drugs that contain calcium, other divalent cations (e.g., iron or magnesium), or trivalent cations (e.g., aluminum).
Enrofloxacin	Absorption is inhibited by concurrent administration of sucralfate.
Ketoconazole	Absorption may be inhibited by drugs that decrease stomach acidity (e.g., antacids or H_2 blockers).
	Disease Interactions
Chloramphenicol	Hydrolysis of the palmitate is decreased in cats that have not been eating.
Mitotane (Lysodren)	Absorption is increased in dogs with hyper-adrenocorticism.

penicillin G. Important disadvantages of an IM injection are the pain and irritation produced.

OTHER ROUTES OF ADMINISTRATION

Water-soluble drugs injected subcutaneously (SC) are usually absorbed rapidly and completely. If an animal is volume depleted, drugs may not be absorbed readily from this site. One also should avoid the administration of a depot drug via the SC route. Rectal administration may be an alternative to an injection. Ketamine and diazepam have been administered via the rectal route, resulting in the desired sedative or anesthetic effect.

Intratracheal Administration.   For most drugs to obtain sufficient delivery to the lower respiratory tract, nebulization is necessary. Via nebulization, as much as 85 per cent of the drug may be deposited in the mouth and upper respiratory tract. The tracheal route has been used successfully to administer drugs such as epinephrine, but the systemic absorption is poor from most drugs.

DRUG METABOLISM AND EXCRETION (pp. 268–270)

The major organ of drug metabolism is the liver, although metabolism may occur at other sites, such as the kidneys and gastrointestinal epithelium.

RENAL DRUG CLEARANCE

Effects of Disease on Renal Clearance.   Renal disease can directly affect the clearance of a parent drug or active metabolites and may alter the distribution of drugs. Uremia may decrease drug tissue binding, decrease the drug's volume of distribution, and decrease the plasma drug protein binding, increasing the proportion of active drug in the blood.

Changes in Drug Dosage for a Patient with Renal Failure. For drugs with a moderate to high therapeutic index, a change in drug dose or interval probably is not necessary if the loss of renal function is not greater than two-thirds. If the extent of renal failure suggests that a dose should be adjusted, the dose can be reduced by first determining the fraction (F) of renal function remaining by estimating renal clearance. Renal clearance may be estimated by measuring creatinine clearance or may be estimated. The dose can be reduced by the fraction of renal nephron loss (F) while keeping a constant dose interval:

$$\text{Dose}_{(RENAL\ FAILURE)} = \text{Dose}_{(NORMAL)} \times F$$

Alternatively, the dose may be kept constant and the dose interval adjusted:

$$\text{Dose Interval}_{(RENAL\ FAILURE)} = (\text{Dose Interval}_{(NORMAL)}) \times \frac{1}{F}$$

However, a decrease in dose with a constant interval probably is best except for drugs such as the aminoglycoside antibiotics. Here, an adjustment in the dose interval while keeping a constant dose is better and less likely to produce toxicosis.

HEPATIC DRUG CLEARANCE

Lidocaine, propranolol, nitroglycerin, and diazepam are examples of drugs that have a high *first-pass effect*. The clearance of these drugs is significantly reduced by any condition (e.g., portal systemic shunt) that decreases hepatic blood perfusion.

Hepatic Drug Metabolism.   The process of biotransformation by the liver usually occurs in two phases. *Phase I* is one of a metabolic conversion involving oxidation, reduction, hydrolysis, and hydration. The responsible enzymes are often referred to as the *microsomal enzymes* of the liver. *Phase II* is one of conjugation, in which endogenous compounds are conjugated to the drug. Examples are glucuronidation, sulfation, acetylation, and conjugation to glutathione and amino acids. The result of biotransformation is a drug that is less active, more active, or more toxic in comparison to the parent drug.

Factors That Influence Hepatic Metabolism. Diseases such as hepatic cirrhosis decrease functional liver mass. Drug interactions decrease hepatic drug metabolism by inhibiting the activity of hepatic metabolic enzymes. Cimetidine, chloramphenicol, ketoconazole, and erythromycin are examples of enzyme inhibitors. Drug administration can increase the activity of hepatic microsomal enzymes. Phenobarbital, rifampin, estrogens, griseofulvin, and phenylbutazone are examples of hepatic enzyme inducers. The hormones of pregnancy also can induce microsomal enzymes.

CHAPTER 58

ANTIMICROBIAL DRUGS
(pages 272–284)

IMPORTANT TERMINOLOGY: MIC, MBC, MAC
(pp. 272–273)

The *minimum inhibitory concentration* (MIC) is the lowest concentration that inhibits visible bacterial growth. The MIC value represents the concentration necessary for an inhibitory effect in the plasma or tissues of the patient. The *minimum bactericidal concentration* (MBC) is the lowest concentration that kills 99.9 per cent of the bacteria. It represents the concentration in the patients' plasma or tissues that is bactericidal. The lowest concentration that produces an antibacterial effect is the *minimum antibacterial concentration* (MAC). This concentration interferes with normal bacterial proliferation but is not lethal or inhibitory.

BACTERICIDAL AND BACTERIOSTATIC ANTIBIOTICS

It has been common to classify antibiotics into those that are *bactericidal* and those that are *bacteriostatic*. This distinction is not exact, and it is possible for a drug to fall in both classes, depending on the concentration reached and the organism involved. For most drugs, the ratio of MBC to MIC must be less than 4 to 6 in order for a drug to be considered bactericidal.

ANTIMICROBIAL DRUG CLASSES: AN OVERVIEW
(pp. 273–283)

BETA-LACTAM ANTIBIOTICS

Penicillins, cephalosporins, and the carbacephems are β-lactam antibiotics.

Original chapter written by Mark G. Papich

Mechanism of Action

Beta-lactam antibiotics bind enzymes (penicillin-binding proteins [PBPs]) near the bacterial cell wall. Binding to PBPs decreases cell wall rigidity and strength, and affects cell division, growth, and septum formation.

Bacterial Resistance Mechanisms

Resistance mechanisms are (1) failure to penetrate the outer membrane of gram-negative bacteria, (2) penicillin-binding proteins that may have a decreased affinity for the antibiotic, and (3) synthesis of β-lactamase enzymes, which inactivates the drug. Bacteria that lack a cell wall are resistant to the effects of β-lactam antibiotics.

PENICILLINS

Benzylpenicillin (Penicillin G)

Penicillin G is effective primarily against gram-positive bacteria, but it is also effective against obligate gram-positive and gram-negative anaerobes that do not produce a β-lactamase. Staphylococci and gram-negative bacteria are the organisms that most often produce a β-lactamase that hydrolyzes penicillin G.

Formulations Available. Penicillin G may be injected intravenously, intramuscularly, or subcutaneously. Procaine penicillin G is slowly absorbed following IM or SC injection. Antibacterial effects persist for at least 24 hours after a single injection.

Pharmacokinetics. Penicillins reach concentrations in the interstitial fluid of most tissues that are similar to the concentrations in plasma. However, the diffusion into the central nervous system, prostate, and eye is poor. All penicillins rely on renal elimination and reach high drug concentrations in the urine.

Adverse Effects. Adverse effects are rare. The most common is an allergic reaction. There is also the chance of a *Clostridium* bacterial intestinal overgrowth.

Aminopenicillins (Amoxicillin, Ampicillin, Hetacillin)

These have a spectrum of activity that includes those listed for penicillin but also is extended to many of the gram-negative bacteria (e.g., many Enterobacteriaceae). The most important resistance mechanism is inactivation by bacterial β-lactamases.

Formulations Available. Ampicillin sodium can be injected IV, IM, or SC. Oral tablets, capsules, and suspensions are available. Oral hetacillin does not have any advantage over ampicillin.

Pharmacokinetics. The elimination of the aminopenicillins is slightly longer than what is reported for penicillin. Amoxicillin has twice the systemic bioavailability of ampicillin when administered orally in dogs. The bioavailability of both ampicillin and amoxicillin are reduced when they are administered with food.

Antipseudomonas Penicillins (Carbenicillin, Ticarcillin, Piperacillin, Azlocillin)

These are able to penetrate the outer wall of *Pseudomonas* and other gram-negative bacteria. They are susceptible to β-lactamase inactivation and have synergistic activity when administered with the aminoglycosides. These drugs are primarily used for resistant gram-negative infections, especially infections caused by *Pseudomonas aeruginosa*. Their pharmacokinetics are similar to those of other penicillins. There are no orally effective formulations in this class except indanyl carbenicillin, which should not be used for systemic infections.

Antistaphylococcal Penicillins

This group includes oxacillin, cloxacillin, dicloxacillin, methicillin, and nafcillin. Their value lies in their resistance to the β-lactamase of *Staphylococcus* spp. Their most common use is for treating skin and soft tissue infections. Staphylococcal resistance is possible, but fortunately it is rare.

Pharmacokinetics. Usually only the oral forms of oxacillin, cloxacillin, and dicloxacillin are used. The drug concentrations are sufficient to reach the MIC of susceptible bacteria. Methicillin and nafcillin are not absorbed orally.

Beta-Lactamase Inhibitors

These have little antibacterial activity of their own, but they inhibit the β-lactamase enzyme. An inactive enzyme complex is formed, and the co-administered antibiotic is allowed to exert its antibacterial effect. The primary drugs are *clavulanic acid*, which is combined with amoxicillin, and *sulbactam*, which is combined with ampicillin. These combinations have the same pharmacokinetic properties as other drugs in the β-lactam class.

CEPHALOSPORIN ANTIBIOTICS

These are used routinely in veterinary medicine for a variety of infections, including skin, urinary tract, soft tissue, and bone infections, as well as before and after a surgical procedure. The cephalosporins bind to PBPs and disrupt the cell wall. They have the advantage of antibacterial activity against β-lactamase-producing *Staphylococcus* spp., and many Enterobacteriaceae. There are tablets, capsules, and liquid suspensions available for most of the first-generation cephalosporins that are well absorbed after oral administration.

Classification

First-Generation Cephalosporins. These are effective against almost all gram-positive bacteria, including β-lactamase-positive staphylococci and streptococci. Resistance to gram-negative bacteria is common.

Second-Generation Cephalosporins. These have greater activity against resistant *E. coli, Klebsiella, Proteus, and Enterobacter* but are no more active against gram-positive bacteria than first-generation cephalosporins.

Third-Generation Cephalosporins. This group has more activity against gram-negative bacteria than first- or second-generation cephalosporins. They have less activity against staphylococci and streptococci.

Pharmacokinetics

Most cephalosporins rely primarily on renal mechanisms for elimination. They achieve effective concentrations in the synovial, pericardial, pleural, and peritoneal fluid, as well as in urine, bile, and skin. They have poor penetration into the central nervous system, prostate, or aqueous humor. The third-generation cephalosporins can achieve effective concentrations in the central nervous system.

Adverse Effects

There seems to be a lower incidence of allergic reactions. The most common reaction seen with the oral products is gastric irritation. A positive Coombs test reaction, not associated with hemolytic anemia, can occur with patients receiving cephalosporins.

NEW BETA-LACTAM ANTIBIOTICS

Carbapenems (Imipenem)

Imipenem has been used primarily for serious, resistant infections that would otherwise require multiple drugs. It has the broadest antibacterial action of any systemic antimicrobial and includes even some strains of enterococci. Imipenem is combined with cilastatin to avoid renal toxicity and achieve high urine concentrations of active drug.

AMINOGLYCOSIDE ANTIBIOTICS

The aminoglycosides include gentamicin, tobramycin, kanamycin, dihydrostreptomycin, netilmicin, amikacin, and neomycin. They are bacterial protein synthesis inhibitors and are rapidly *bactericidal*. The aminoglycosides are primarily used for gram-negative infections that are resistant to β-lactam drugs. They are particularly valuable for treating patients that have acute, overwhelming sepsis. There are topical preparations for superficial skin, eye, and external ear canal infections.

Spectrum of Activity and Resistance

Aminoglycosides are effective against most gram-negative bacteria, including Enterobacteriaceae and *Pseudomonas aeruginosa*. They are somewhat effective against staphylococci, although resistance can occur. Aminoglycosides have a synergistic effect with β-lactam antibiotics against streptococci, enterococci, *Pseudomonas aeruginosa*, and other gram-negative bacteria. Anaerobic bacteria are intrinsically resistant. Bacterial synthesis of enzymes is probably the most important resistance mechanism for organisms encountered in veterinary medicine.

Pharmacokinetics

Distribution into the respiratory fluids, eye, prostate, and the central nervous system is poor, but distribution to the pleural space, bone, joints, and peritoneal cavity is relatively good. None of these drugs is absorbed orally or from a topical application. Aminoglycosides rely almost exclusively on renal clearance for elimination.

Adverse Effects

Nephrotoxicosis. The most serious adverse effect is renal toxicosis. Animals that are dehydrated, have electrolyte losses, or have existing renal disease are at a higher risk for toxicity.

Ototoxicosis and Vestibulotoxicosis. Ototoxicosis may result from prolonged use. The incidence of these effects in animals is unknown.

Neuromuscular Blockade. This effect has been known to occur when certain anesthetic agents are administered concurrently with aminoglycosides.

TETRACYCLINES

The tetracyclines include chlortetracycline, oxytetracycline, doxycycline, and minocycline. They are bacterial protein synthesis inhibitors. Tetracyclines are bacteriostatic and are active against gram-negative and gram-positive bacteria, as well as *Chlamydia*, rickettsia, spirochetes, *Mycoplasma*, bacteria L-forms, and some protozoa (*Haemobartonella*). They have been used to treat urinary tract infections, respiratory infections, chlamydial infections, *Ehrlichia canis*, haemobartonellosis, and Lyme disease.

Pharmacokinetics

Absorption is best if administered on an empty stomach. Tetracyclines rely on glomerular filtration for elimination. Doxycycline is excreted in the intestine. Tetracyclines are distributed well to most tissues, except to those of the central nervous system. Minocycline and doxycycline are more lipid-soluble than others and more effective for infections in some tissues.

Adverse Effects and Interactions

Calcium-containing products or other di- or trivalent cations (Mg^{+2}, Fe^{+2}, Al^{-3}) will chelate with tetracyclines and interfere with oral absorption. Doxycycline is the least affected by this interaction. Tetracyclines will produce tooth discoloration and inhibit long bone growth in young animals.

The most serious toxic effect is renal injury, associated with high doses or the administration of outdated products. Tetracycline has been known to cause hepatic lipidosis, but this effect has been rare in animals. Hypersensitivity and drug fever have been seen. Cats appear to be more prone.

CHLORAMPHENICOL

Chloramphenicol is a protein synthesis inhibitor that is bacteriostatic. It is a broad-spectrum drug with activity against streptococci, *Haemophilus, Salmonella, Brucella*, staphylococci, *Pasteurella* spp., *Mycoplasma*, anaerobic bacteria (*Bacteroides*), *Rickettsia, Chlamydia*, and *Haemobartonella*. Chloramphenicol has been effective for infections in the central nervous system, pneumonia, enteritis caused by *Salmonella* spp. and *E. coli*, intracellular infections, anaerobic bacterial infections, and skin and soft tissue bacterial infections. It also is often used as a topical antibiotic for eye infections.

Pharmacokinetics

Chloramphenicol is well absorbed after oral administration, but sick cats may not absorb chloramphenicol from the ester well. It is metabolized by the liver and enters the central nervous system and the eye better than most other antibiotics.

Adverse Effects and Interactions

A dose-related, reversible bone marrow suppression has been reported in dogs and cats. Cats are most susceptible. An idiosyncratic (non-dose-related), irreversible form of pancytopenia has been described in people who have received chloramphenicol. There is no evidence that this reaction occurs in dogs or cats. Chloramphenicol is a hepatic microsomal enzyme inhibitor.

THE MACROLIDE ANTIBIOTICS, CLINDAMYCIN, AND LINCOMYCIN

Clindamycin is a derivative of lincomycin; this difference results in increased intestinal absorption, lower toxicity, and greater activity. The drug group interferes with the growth of a bacterial peptide chain. They are considered bacteriostatic for most bacteria. Susceptible bacteria include staphylococci, streptococci, *Campylobacter jejuni, Clostridium* spp., *Mycoplasma*, and *Chlamydia*. Lincomycin and clindamycin also are active for the bacteria listed for erythromycin. Clindamycin may be more active against anaerobes and has good activity against *Toxoplasma gondii*, although higher doses are needed. Clindamycin distributes to bones and joints, and it has been used to treat osteomyelitis caused by staphylococci. The routine use of erythromycin has been limited because of the development of resistance.

Pharmacokinetics

All drugs in this group are metabolized in the liver to some extent. They do not achieve high concentrations in the urine. Erythromycin and clindamycin can concentrate in leukocytes.

Adverse Effects and Interactions

This group of antibiotics is associated with very few adverse reactions. Intramuscular injections are very painful and should be avoided.

TRIMETHOPRIM-SULFONAMIDE COMBINATIONS

This combination is effective for osteomyelitis, prostatitis, pneumonia, tracheobronchitis, staphylococcal pyoderma, and urinary tract infections. Together, they may be bactericidal. Bacteria resistant to either drug alone may be susceptible against the combination.

Spectrum of Activity

The spectrum of activity is broad. *Streptococcus, Pasteurella* spp., *Proteus mirabilis, Salmonella* spp., *Toxoplasma*, and *Coccidia* usually are susceptible. A susceptibility test is advised to guide drug selection. Treatment of infections caused by *Nocardia asteroides* usually requires high doses.

Pharmacokinetics

Oral absorption is rapid, and good in small animals. Veterinarians continue to disagree regarding whether trimethoprim should be administered once or twice daily. Many of the dosage regimens for these drugs continue to be based on empiricism rather than pharmacokinetic data.

Adverse Effects and Toxicities

Anemia and leukopenia are rare but have been described. Allergic reactions have been described in dogs; they can be acute or can be seen as a type III hypersensitivity reaction. The serum sickness reaction was originally described in Doberman pinschers but is possible in other breeds. The lesions include glomerulopathy, polymyositis, polyarthritis, skin rash, fever, and anemia. The reaction appears to be caused by the sulfonamide component. When drug administration is stopped, improvement is seen within 24 hours. Drug-induced anemia, skin eruptions, and hepatitis are other possible reactions. Drug-induced keratoconjunctivitis sicca has been observed, most commonly after chronic treatment.

FLUOROQUINOLONE ANTIBIOTICS

The only drug in this class approved at the present time for veterinary use is *enrofloxacin*. The quinolones inhibit the enzyme DNA gyrase, which causes a decrease in transcription and translation of the genetic code and inhibits protein synthesis. The mammalian enzyme is resistant to the usual antibacterial concentrations achieved. Quinolones are rapidly bactericidal. They have been used for soft tissue infections, pneumonia, osteomyelitis, and urinary tract infections caused by gram-negative organisms and staphylococci. These drugs are valuable because of their activity against bacteria that have developed resistance to other drugs.

Spectrum of Activity

Enrofloxacin and ciprofloxacin have excellent activity against most bacteria, particularly the Enterobacteriaceae and *Pseudomonas aeruginosa*. Other susceptible bacteria include staphylococci, including methicillin-resistant staphylococci. The activity against anaerobic bacteria is poor. Enrofloxacin is effective against rickettsial infections in dogs. Organisms that may develop resistance include *Pseudomonas aeruginosa*, *E. coli*, enterococci, and staphylococci.

Pharmacokinetics

Enrofloxacin is absorbed orally. Oral absorption is inhibited by co-administration of magnesium, aluminum, or other divalent cations because of chelation. The concentrations achieved in lungs, kidneys, liver, muscle, prostate, heart, and intestine are likely effective. Concentrations in the bile and urine are many-fold higher. The concentrations in the cerebrospinal fluid or brain are probably not high enough for treating infections in these tissues. The elimination of fluoroquinolones is primarily renal. Enrofloxacin (Baytril), in tablet form and an injectable solution, is the only veterinary preparation at the present time. The injectable solution is intended for IM administration; some dogs have received this drug IV without any complications.

Adverse Effects and Toxicities

Reports have been rare. An increase in the incidence of seizures has been reported with enrofloxacin in dogs. Because of the risk of developmental arthropathy, avoid the administration to young animals less than 30 weeks old, especially rapidly growing breeds. Administration to pregnant animals also should be cautioned.

METRONIDAZOLE

Metronidazole is highly effective against anaerobic gram-negative bacteria (e.g., *Bacteroides* spp. or fusobacteria), but it is not effective against organisms that may be facultative anaerobes. It probably has acceptable activity against *Clostridium* spp. It has good activity against the protozoa *Giardia lamblia* and *Entamoeba*. Aerobic bacteria lack the reductive pathway necessary to produce cytotoxicity. Diseases that have been treated with metronidazole include oral infections (bacterial stomatitis), osteomyelitis, pneumonia (lung abscesses), and intra-abdominal infections. It is the drug of choice for giardiasis. Many patients with idiopathic colitis also respond to a trial. Metronidazole is distributed into all tissues, including eyes, central nervous system, bone, and abscess cavities.

Adverse Effects

Its use in pregnant animals should be cautioned, but is not contraindicated. Serious neurotoxicosis has been described in dogs. Signs included ataxia, lethargy, anorexia, vomiting, nystagmus, and seizures. Dogs have recovered, but the recovery requires 1 to 2 weeks.

CHAPTER 59

USE OF CORTICOSTEROIDS AND NONSTEROIDAL ANTI-INFLAMMATORY AGENTS
(pages 284–293)

GLUCOCORTICOIDS (p. 284)

Corticosteroids are hormones secreted principally by cells of the adrenal cortex. These hormones vary in their actions to inhibit the inflammatory response and promote gluconeogenesis (glucocorticoids) and promote sodium retention and potassium loss from the body (mineralocorticoids). Exogenous corticosteroids are perhaps the most widely used therapeutic agents in veterinary practice. They are most commonly used by clinicians to treat inflammatory, pruritic, and immunologically mediated diseases; therefore, the term *corticosteroids* is generally assumed to mean glucocorticoids.

PHYSIOLOGY OF GLUCOCORTICOIDS (pp. 284–285)

Structure and Mechanism of Action

All adrenocortical hormones are derivatives of the cyclopentanoperhydrophenanthrene nucleus. Corticosteroids bind to cytoplasmic receptors, which then migrate to the cell nucleus, where they attach to chromatin and activate the transcription process of DNA into messenger RNA formation. Messenger RNA codes for enzyme and protein production, which are responsible for the biologic effects.

PHYSIOPHARMACOLOGIC PROPERTIES (pp. 285–286)

Glucocorticoids raise blood glucose by increasing gluconeogenesis and insulin antagonism. They also promote gluconeogenesis and facilitate the breakdown of tryglycerides in adipose tissue. Glucocorticoids have mineralocorticoid effects that promote the retention of sodium, excretion of potassium, and expansion of extracellular fluid volume. They promote diuresis by increasing glomerular filtration rate, inhibiting the action of antidiuretic hormone on the renal tubules, and increasing ADH inactivation. They also cause increased gastric acid and pepsin secretion and stimulate pancreatic secretions, and may cause vacuolization of hepatocytes and the induction of an alkaline phosphatase isoenzyme in dogs. Glucocorticoid administration may cause muscle weakness and atrophy. Other hormone secretion—including thyroid stimulating hormone, growth hormone, follicle stimulating hormone, luteinizing hormone, and prolactin—may be adversely affected. Glucocorticoids stimulate red blood cell production and increase platelets in circulation, increase the number of circulating neutrophils, and decrease the number of lymphocytes, eosinophils, and basophils.

Anti-Inflammatory and Immunosuppressive Properties

The arachidonic acid cascade is affected by glucocorticoids. Lipomodulin, induced by steroid-receptor-nuclear interaction, inhibits phospholipase A_2, which normally converts membrane phospholipid into

Original chapter written by Robert K. McDonald and Vernon C. Langston

TABLE 59–1. COMPARISON OF THE POTENCY AND DURATION OF ACTION OF COMMON GLUCOCORTICOIDS

DRUG	ANTI-INFLAMMATORY POTENCY*	DURATION OF ACTION (hr)
Short-acting		
Hydrocortisone (Cortisol)	1	8–12
Intermediate-acting		
Prednisone	4	12–36
Prednisolone	4	12–36
Methylprednisolone	5	12–36
Triamcinolone	5	12–36
Long-acting		
Dexamethasone	30	>48
Betamethasone	35	>48

*Values compared by assigning cortisol a potency of 1.0.

arachidonic acid (AA). Arachidonic acid is the precursor of potent mediators of inflammation through both the cyclooxygenase and lipoxygenase pathways, i.e., prostaglandins, prostacyclin, thromboxane, and leukotrienes. Glucocorticoids are the only therapeutic agents that inhibit both AA inflammatory pathways.

COMPARISON OF COMMON GLUCOCORTICOID PREPARATIONS (pp. 286–289)

Glucocorticoids can be characterized into short-, intermediate-, and long-acting agents (Table 59–1). Oral dose forms of glucocorticoids are usually tablets containing the free steroid alcohol. A number of topical glucocorticoids are available as ointments, creams, lotions, foams, gels, and solutions. Some shampoos contain glucocorticoids for more generalized application. Glucocorticoid enemas are available to treat diseases such as ulcerative colitis. Chronic topical therapy with ointments or creams should be the lowest effective concentration of 0.25 to 2.5 per cent hydrocortisone. Parenteral glucocorticoid preparations are administered subcutaneously (SQ), intramuscularly (IM), or intravenously (IV), depending on the desired effect and the formulation used. Administration of some parenteral preparations is intralesional, sublesional, or intra-articular.

COMMON CLINICAL USES OF GLUCOCORTICOIDS

When treating with a glucocorticoid, there should be convincing evidence that the benefits of therapy outweigh the potential of adverse effects. Treatment with these drugs should not be used as a substitute for establishing a definitive diagnosis.

Endogenous Glucocorticoid Deficiency

Treatment of primary hypoadrenocorticism requires replacement of both mineralocorticoids and glucocorticoids. Many dogs require low doses, and some develop polyuria/polydipsia at recommended doses.

Anti-Inflammatory (Anti-Allergic) Applications

Inflammation in response to allergic conditions, such as dermatopathies or insect bites or stings, usually responds to glucocorticoid therapy. Induction doses of oral prednisone or prednisolone are given until the pruritus improves. Then the dose is tapered to the lowest alternate-day dose that will control the signs. In some animals, therapy can be extended to every third or fourth day.

Immunosuppression

Glucocorticoids are commonly used for the treatment of immune-mediated diseases (e.g., hemolytic anemia, thrombocytopenia, systemic lupus erythematosus, and pemphigus), and can be lifesaving. The induction dose should be continued for 7 to 10 days or as needed, depending on the patient's response, and gradually tapered. Some patients cannot be maintained on alternate-day therapy and may require adjunctive immunosuppressive therapy.

Cerebrospinal Trauma and Edema

Glucocorticoids have been used to decrease edema and inflammation associated with brain tumors, but are most commonly used in treating brain and spinal cord trauma. Available reports suggest that relatively high doses are necessary. Treatment beyond 5 to 7 days is not usually recommended.

Shock

Glucocorticoids have been advocated in a variety of shock states. Their role in these conditions has remained controversial. Septic (endotoxic) shock is perhaps most responsive to glucocorticoid treatment. Large doses of glucocorticoids are typically employed as early in the condition as possible. Glucocorticoids are not substitutes for aggressive fluid therapy and other supportive measures.

ADVERSE EFFECTS OF GLUCOCORTICOID ADMINISTRATION

Iatrogenic Hyperadrenocorticism

Iatrogenic hyperadrenocorticism may develop following therapy with any glucocorticoid preparation. This would include use of oral, topical, and ophthalmic preparations. Cats are relatively resistant to iatrogenic hyperadrenocorticism.

Iatrogenic Adrenocortical Insufficiency

Exogenous glucocorticoids cause a negative feedback and directly inhibit ACTH release from the anterior pituitary. Signs may develop when long-term glucocorticoid therapy is suddenly stopped or when patients are stressed by trauma, surgery, or infection. Clinical signs may manifest as depression, anorexia, and vomiting, or as acute shock. A diagnosis is confirmed by the ACTH stimulation test.

Precautions and Contraindications

Infectious Disease. Glucocorticoids are usually contraindicated in the treatment of bacterial or fungal infections. If an animal is on prolonged glucocorticoid therapy, host defenses are suppressed and frequent monitoring for infection is necessary (e.g., UTI).

Gastric and Intestinal Bleeding/Perforation. Glucocorticoids have been shown to impair mucosal blood flow, alter mucus production, stimulate gastrin secretion, and decrease gastrointestinal mucosal cell renewal.

Diabetes Mellitus. Glucocorticoids have anti-insulin actions that interfere with the control of diabetes mellitus.

Pancreatitis. Glucocorticoid therapy may contribute to the development of acute pancreatitis, but conflicting data exist in the literature.

Renal Disease. Glucocorticoids may exacerbate existing renal failure and azotemia.

Corneal Ulceration. Ophthalmic glucocorticoids are contraindicated in patients with corneal ulceration.

Interference with Pituitary Hormones. Baseline T_4 concentrations and response to TSH are blunted in dogs receiving glucocorticoids. Glucocorticoids have suppressive effects on growth hormone and somatomedin secretion. Glucocorticoid therapy may interfere with fertility and may cause abortion in pregnant animals, failure to cycle in the bitch, and testicular atrophy and oligospermia in the male.

OTHER ANTI-INFLAMMATORY AGENTS (pp. 289–293)

Cromolyn

Cromolyn stabilizes mast cells, thereby preventing degranulation and subsequent histamine release. Because topical application is required, cromolyn is seldom used in veterinary medicine.

Antihistamines

Antihistamines act to block the binding of histamine to the H_1 receptors of effector cells, thereby diminishing the well-known effects of histamine. Antihistamines have been used most commonly prophylactically when an allergic incident was expected or in the treatment of atopy in dogs and cats. When antihistamines are used, the following points should be kept in mind:

1. Antihistamines do not reverse the effects of histamine but only prevent its binding.

2. Antihistamines commonly possess anticholinergic properties and cause a drying effect on epithelial surfaces.

3. The majority of antihistamines used in veterinary medicine cross the blood-brain barrier and may cause sedation. Paradoxically, sudden high concentrations may cause agitation and excitement; therefore, rapid IV administration is ill-advised.

NONSTEROIDAL ANTI-INFLAMMATORY DRUGS (NSAIDs)

NSAIDs are cyclooxygenase inhibitors. These agents typically possess a triad of properties, namely, antipyretic, analgesic, and anti-inflammatory effects. They are most commonly used for fever reduction and pain control. Only the cyclooxygenase pathway of the arachidonic acid cascade is inhibited; the precursor mediators are free to enter the lipoxygenase pathway and still produce considerable inflammation.

Normal prostaglandin synthesis results in the production of the cytoprotective mucus of the GI tract. GI ulceration represents the most frequent adverse effect. Renal papillary necrosis is the second most commonly encountered toxic lesion seen. Cytoprotective drugs such as sucralfate or prostaglandin analogs are receiving increasing preference in both preventing and treating NSAID-induced GI ulceration.

Aspirin

It is administered orally to all species and can control fever, mild to moderate somatic pain, and some inflammatory conditions (e.g., degenerative joint disease). Higher plasma concentrations are generally required for an anti-inflammatory effect as opposed to antipyresis or analgesia. Buffered products (e.g., Ascriptin) may decrease local gastric irritation and can be used in animals; however, enteric-coated aspirin products are not recommended. Aspirin permanently inactivates platelet cyclooxygenase. Lower doses of aspirin are recommended for anticoagulant purposes. Cats excrete aspirin much more slowly than do dogs, but it can be safely used in cats provided appropriate dosage regimens are followed.

Phenylbutazone

Phenylbutazone possesses the typical triad of NSAID effects. It has gained a reputation for being effective in the control of mild to moderate visceral and somatic pain, particularly in musculoskeletal disorders. Phenylbutazone-induced bone marrow suppression (including aplastic anemia) is an infrequent side effect.

Dipyrone

It has an excellent reputation as an antipyretic and can control mild to moderate somatic and visceral pain. There have been questionable interactions between dipyrone and phenothiazine tranquilizers whereby animals apparently lost their ability to thermoregulate. Some authors have advised against its use in cats.

Flunixin

A distinguishing feature is its ability to control moderate to severe visceral and somatic pain. It is also often used to minimize the effects of endotoxemia. Repeated doses in dogs have resulted in severe GI ulceration and renal damage.

Piroxicam

The antineoplastic effects of piroxicam were evaluated. On the basis of this evidence and anecdotal clinical use, piroxicam may be considered an alternative NSAID in dogs that have failed to respond to traditional therapy.

Acetaminophen

It produces few GI side effects. It is limited to the treatment of fever and mild to moderate somatic pain. In cats, the use of acetaminophen is strictly contraindicated.

See textbook for naproxen, ibuprofen, and other NSAIDs.

AGENTS AFFECTING FREE RADICAL REMOVAL

Superoxide Dismutase

Superoxide dismutase is a naturally occurring enzyme that converts H_2O_2 into oxygen and water. The efficacy of the product in most inflammatory conditions is unclear.

Dimethyl Sulfoxide (DMSO)

DMSO is the best-known agent for scavenging free radicals. It may also potentiate endogenous glucocorticoid effects, decrease the influx of WBCs into an area, and limit fibrous tissue formation following injury. DMSO can be used to treat tendonitis or desmitis. It is also used extra-label to treat CNS edema and trauma. Besides the possible side effects of hemolysis and histamine release, DMSO is a potential teratogen. DMSO may potentiate the effects of organophosphate insecticides or phenothiazine tranquilizers.

CHRYSOTHERAPY

Gold therapy is indicated for the treatment of certain immune-mediated diseases, such as rheumatoid arthritis or pemphigus, that have failed to respond to conventional glucocorticoid or NSAID therapy. Daily oral therapy with auranofin is preferred by some. Response is not usually seen for 6 to 12 weeks after initiation of therapy. The most common toxicity is the development of dermatitis. Stomatitis also is common. Gold salt therapy can also produce nephrosis, hepatitis, diarrhea, and interstitial pneumonitis. Chelation therapy with penicillamine or dimercaprol may speed the recovery from toxicosis.

CHAPTER 60

FLUID THERAPY, ELECTROLYTES, AND ACID-BASE CONTROL
(pages 294–312)

GENERAL GUIDELINES FOR FLUID THERAPY
(pp. 295–297)

The goal of fluid therapy is to restore the volume and composition of body fluids to normal and, once this is achieved, to maintain external fluid and electrolyte balance so that input by treatment matches fluid losses. The history should include information on food and water intake, gastrointestinal losses, urine output, recent exercise, exposure to heat, trauma, hemorrhage, excessive panting, fever, and diuretic use.

Careful physical examination can determine hydration status. Regular reassessment during fluid therapy is important. In monitoring treatment, the most frequently performed tests are packed cell volume, total plasma protein, urine specific gravity, blood urea nitrogen (BUN), blood glucose, and electrocardiogram (ECG). Other tests indicated include serum and urine creatinine; serum and urine Na^+; serum potassium, chloride, and bicarbonate (or total CO_2); serum calcium and inorganic phosphorus; blood gas values; and serum and urine osmolality. From these values the anion gap, osmolar gap, and fractional excretion of sodium (FE_{Na}^+) can be calculated.

An indwelling urinary catheter allows an accurate measurement of urine output to aid in the calculation of fluid requirements, determine renal function, and assess the response to diuretics. Central venous pressure is useful in determining excessive plasma volume expansion.

Intravenous fluid administration is preferred. Intraperitoneal and subcutaneous routes also can be used, but absorption can be unreliable and too slow in severe dehydration. The major parenteral fluids can be divided into colloidal solutions, electrolyte solutions, and 5 per cent dextrose in water (Table 60–1). A number of supplements can be added to the basic electrolyte solutions to provide more precise treatment tailored to the special needs of individual patients (Table 60–2).

DISORDERS OF TOTAL BODY SODIUM (pp. 297–300)

VOLUME CONTRACTION

Reduced fluid intake or nonrenal and renal Na^+ and water loss can cause volume contraction (Table 60–3).

Original chapter written by David F. Senior

TABLE 60-1. SOLUTIONS FOR FLUID THERAPY

	ELECTROLYTE CONCENTRATION mEq/L					BUFFER mEq/L	pH	OSMOLALITY mOsm/L	CALORIC VALUE kcal/L
	Na+	K+	Ca²⁺	Mg²⁺	Cl⁻				
Colloidal Solutions									
Hetasta ch 6% in 0.9% saline	154	—	—	—	154		5.5	300–303	
Dextrar 70 6% w/v in 0.9% saline	154	—	—	—	154		4.5–7		
Plasma (average values, dog)	145	4.2	5	2.5	108	20	7.4	290	
Electrolyte Solutions									
REPLACEMENT SOLUTIONS:									
Lactated Ringer's	130	4	3	—	109	Lactate 25	6.5	273	9
Ringer's solution	147	4	5	—	156	—	5.8	310	—
Formal saline	154	—	—	—	154	—	5.4	308	—
Normosol R	140	5	—	3	98	Acetate 27 Gluconate 23	6.2	295	18
MAINTENANCE SOLUTIONS:									
2½% dex/0.45% saline	77	—	—	—	77	—	4.8	280	85
2½% dex/½ str lactated Ringer's	65	2	1	—	54	Lactate 14	5.0	263	89
Normosol M	40	13	—	3	40	Acetate 16	6.0	112	0
Normosol M in 5% dextrose	40	13	—	3	40	Acetate 16	5.2	363	175
Other Solutions									
5% dextrose in water	—	—	—	—	—	—	5.0	252	170

TABLE 60–2. SPECIAL SOLUTIONS FOR SUPPLEMENTATION OF PARENTERAL FLUIDS

	CONCENTRATION/ml
Potassium chloride	2 mEq K^+
Calcium gluconate 10%	0.465 mEq Ca^{2+}
Calcium chloride 10%	1.36 mEq Ca^{2+}
Sodium bicarbonate 5%	0.59 mEq HCO_3^-
Sodium bicarbonate 8.4%	1 mEq HCO_3^-

Clinical Signs

Clinical signs of dehydration become evident when body weight is reduced by 5 to 8 per cent. The signs are obvious at 10 per cent, and animals with 15 per cent loss show all the signs of hypovolemic shock (Table 60–4). When gastroenteritis causes fluid loss equal to 5 per cent of body weight, signs of plasma volume depletion are marked. When reduced water intake and insensible water loss cause a 5 per cent reduction in body weight, hypovolemia is barely perceptible.

Treatment

Volume. Fluid therapy for volume contraction must replace deficits, provide maintenance requirements equivalent to normal insensible losses, and take into account ongoing losses such as those incurred by continued vomiting and diarrhea or through burns. The general formula for calculation of fluid requirements is:

Fluid required (ml) = deficit:
    BW (kg) × per cent dehydration × 1000
    + maintenance (40 to 60 ml/kg/day)
    + extraordinary losses

A precise calculation of volume contraction can be determined from the body weight, packed cell volume (PCV), and total plasma protein if prevolume contracted values are known. The reduction in body weight in kilograms equals the volume of fluid lost in liters. Maintenance fluid requirements are the sum of urinary and insensible fluid losses, which include pulmonary, cutaneous, and fecal losses. Combined urinary, fecal, and insensible losses usually amount to about 20 ml/lb/day. Most clinicians calculate daily maintenance fluid requirements as 20 to 30 ml/lb/day, using the lower value for large dogs and the higher value for small dogs and cats.

TABLE 60–3. CAUSES OF VOLUME CONTRACTION

NONRENAL	RENAL
Vomiting	Osmotic diuresis
Diarrhea	Diabetes mellitus
Small bowel obstruction	Mannitol
Pancreatitis	Radiographic contrast
Peritonitis	Diuretics
Burns	Hypoadrenocorticoidism
Hemorrhage	Polyuric phase of acute renal failure
Paracentesis	Postobstructive diuresis
Thoracentesis	
Insensible water loss in water deprivation	

TABLE 60–4. CLINICAL SIGNS OF ECF VOLUME DEPLETION AND OVERLOAD

DEPLETION	OVERLOAD
Increased temperature	Restlessness, coughing
Weak rapid pulse	Increased respiration rate
Pale, dry mucous membranes	Subcutaneous edema
Slow capillary refill time	Ascites
Poor skin elasticity	Chemosis
Cool distal extremities	Exophthalmos
Sunken orbits	Vomiting
Reduced urine output	Serous nasal discharge
Microcardia on thoracic radiographs	Increased urine output (assumes normal kidney function)

In dogs and cats with normal renal function, excessive fluid administration is of little consequence. However, in animals with acute renal failure and those with heart failure, continued rapid fluid administration can result in overhydration and pulmonary edema.

Rate. Animals suffering from sudden severe blood loss and hypovolemic shock require immediate rapid intravenous fluid treatment. In the absence of cardiopulmonary disease, intravenous fluids can be safely administered to dogs and cats at 45 ml/lb/day. Patients with mild volume depletion require much less aggressive treatment. Fluid deficits can be corrected over a 4- to 6-hour period.

Composition. The choice of fluids should be based on the degree of volume depletion and the nature of the fluid loss. For an animal in shock, replacement fluids are preferred. When plasma volume depletion is secondary to hemorrhage, the best replacement fluid is immunologically compatible whole blood. Isotonic electrolyte solutions should be used as initial treatment for shock only until plasma or another colloidal solution is available. Hypertonic saline may be superior to isotonic saline. Colloidal solutions may benefit animals with hypoalbuminemia secondary to ongoing losses due to nephrotic syndrome or protein-losing enteropathy.

Intravenous administration of colloidal solutions can prevent and treat hypotension, whereas replacement with electrolyte solutions is often inadequate. In animals that do not require colloidal solutions, replacement solutions should be used to replace deficits caused by balanced ECF losses, maintenance solutions can be used to replace normal urinary and insensible fluid losses, and sodium-free solutions should be used to replace deficits in patients suffering from insensible or pure water losses.

Supplementation of replacement fluids may be required to correct acid-base imbalance and K^+ deficits. Vomiting due to pyloric outflow obstruction causes metabolic alkalosis and renal K^+ wasting. Replacement solutions, such as Ringer's solution and 0.9 per cent NaCl, should be used and K^+ supplementation may be required. However, most causes of vomiting other than pyloric outflow obstruction induce a mild metabolic acidosis. Thus Ringer's lactate or Normosol R can be used. Fluid losses due to diarrhea may need to be supplemented with K^+ and HCO_3^-.

Maintenance electrolyte solutions with reduced Na^+, such as 2.5 per cent dextrose in half-strength lactated Ringer's solution or 2.5 per cent dextrose in 0.45 per cent NaCl, are recommended. Animals that dehydrate owing to insensible fluid losses and failure to drink water have a pure water loss and should receive 5 per cent dextrose in water as the main replacement fluid.

VOLUME EXPANSION

Excessive fluid administration to patients with acute renal failure and chronic renal failure patients supplemented with too much dietary Na^+ results in excessive volume expansion. Cardiac failure, hepatic disease, and hypoalbuminemia also cause ECF volume expansion.

Clinical Signs and Diagnosis

Signs of overhydration due to excessive fluid administration are shown in Table 60–4. Once the mechanism of edema formation has been identified, an appropriate list of differential diagnoses is apparent.

Treatment

Treatment should include an attempt to correct the primary cause. Judicious use of diuretics may alleviate the problem sooner. Treatment of edema due to sodium retention consists of a low-sodium diet combined with diuretics.

DISORDERS OF WATER METABOLISM (pp. 300–302)

HYPONATREMIA

Isotonic hyponatremia (pseudohyponatremia) occurs with extreme hyperlipidemia and hyperglobulinemia. Estimations using more recently available ion-specific electrode methodology avoid this error. Hypertonic hyponatremia occurs with hyperglycemia in uncontrolled diabetes mellitus and mannitol after intravenous infusion. Hypotonic hyponatremia is seen in congestive heart failure, severe liver disease, the nephrotic syndrome, hypoadrenocorticoidism, during postobstructive diuresis, and during vigorous long-term diuretic treatment in animals fed a low-sodium diet. Hypotonic hyponatremia also occurs in the syndrome of inappropriate secretion of ADH (SIADH).

Major signs are usually those of the underlying condition rather than those due to hyponatremia per se. Hyponatremia causes weakness, depression, vomiting, muscle fasciculations, seizures, and coma, and the CNS signs are due to enlargement of the ICF with cerebral swelling.

Treatment

Access to water may need to be restricted and use of drugs with an antidiuretic effect withdrawn. Replacement electrolyte solutions should be given if the serum Na^+ concentration is above 120 mEq/L. Hypertonic saline solutions and potent diuretics may be necessary when the serum Na^+ concentration is less than 120 mEq/L. Extremely rapid correction may cause dangerous brain shrinkage because "ideogenic osmoles" cannot be rapidly regenerated. Gradual restoration over a 24 to 48 hour period is preferable.

HYPERNATREMIA

Etiology

Hypernatremia is often iatrogenic. The most common causes are shown in Table 60–5.

Clinical Signs

The signs of hypernatremia include anorexia, vomiting, weakness, thirst, muscle fasciculations, disorientation, depression, seizures, and coma. Clinical signs are likely to become apparent when plasma osmolality exceeds 350 mOsm/kg H_2O. Rapidly increasing osmolality is more likely to induce CNS signs because brain cells are unable to develop "ideogenic osmoles" sufficiently fast to prevent severe brain cell shrinkage.

TABLE 60–5. CAUSES OF HYPONATREMIA AND HYPERNATREMIA

HYPONATREMIA	HYPERNATREMIA
Isotonic (pseudohyponatremia)	Pure water loss
Hyperlipidemia	Diabetes insipidus
Hyperglobulinemia	Dementia
Hypertonic	Hypertonic $NaHCO_3$ administration
Diabetes mellitus	Cardiac arrest
Mannitol treatment	Feline urethral obstruction
Hypotonic	Inappropriate Na^+ administration
Hypoadrenocorticoidism	Acute renal failure
Postobstructive diuresis	Hypodipsia
Diuretic treatment	Miniature schnauzers
Postoperative	
SIADH	
Congestive heart failure	
Severe liver disease	
Nephrotic syndrome	

Treatment

The primary underlying cause of hypernatremia must be addressed. Hypernatremia due to pure water loss is treated either with oral water replacement or intravenous 5 per cent dextrose in water. Hypernatremia due to excessive administration of hypertonic saline and $NaHCO_3$ may be treated the same way. More rapid reduction can be achieved by simultaneous treatment with furosemide.

In chronic hypernatremia, plasma osmolality should not be reduced too rapidly. If ECF osmolality is decreased too fast, cerebral edema can occur. Serum osmolality should not be reduced faster than 2 mOsm/kg H_2O/hour over the first 48 hours. Complete correction should be extended over 2 to 3 days.

Hypernatremia caused by excessive Na^+ administration in patients with oliguric renal failure often fails to respond to diuretic treatment. If ECF volume expansion is life-threatening, excess sodium can be removed by peritoneal dialysis.

POTASSIUM IMBALANCE (pp. 302–305)

HYPOKALEMIA

Etiology

Hypokalemia usually arises from reduced intake or excessive losses via renal or extrarenal routes. On occasion, hypokalemia is the result of ECF to ICF translocation of K^+. The most common causes of hypokalemia in dogs and cats are shown in Table 60–6.

Clinical Signs

Signs begin to develop once serum K^+ levels drop below 3.0 mEq/L and include impaired gastrointestinal motility with ileus and constipation, generalized skeletal muscle weakness, and ECG abnormalities. In cats, rear limb weakness and ventroflexion of the neck may be observed. ECG abnormalities in dogs are variable and include prolonged Q-T interval, sagging S-T segment, depressed T wave amplitude, and atrial and ventricular premature contractions.

Treatment

Correction of K^+ deficits involves treating the underlying disease and providing K^+ supplementation. Several precautions should be

TABLE 60–6. CAUSES OF HYPOKALEMIA AND HYPERKALEMIA

HYPOKALEMIA	HYPERKALEMIA
Reduced K+ intake	*Increased intake*
Anorexia	Rapid infusion of K+ salts
Potassium-poor fluid infusion	High doses of potassium penicillin G
Nonrenal K+ losses	*Decreased renal elimination*
Diarrhea	Oliguric acute renal failure
Enemas	Terminal stages of chronic renal failure
Renal K+ losses	Urethral obstruction
Diuretic use	Lower urinary tract rupture
Polyuric phase of acute renal failure	Hypoadrenocorticoidism
Postobstructive diuresis	*Translocation*
Vomiting with metabolic alkalosis	Metabolic acidosis
Renal tubular reabsorption defects	*Pseudohyperkalemia*
Glucosuria	Thrombocytosis
Amphotericin B treatment	Stored blood or hemolysis (Akitas)
Chronic renal failure in cats	
Acidified diet with marginal K+ (cats)	
Hyperadrenocorticoidism	
Translocation	
Metabolic alkalosis—any cause	
Insulin treatment	

taken to prevent fatal hyperkalemia during treatment. These include making sure there is adequate renal function, giving K+ slowly and in dilute concentrations, and using the oral rather than the parenteral route of administration whenever possible. During K+ supplementation, plasma K+ concentration should be checked routinely and deficits re-estimated to monitor progress toward normokalemia.

Several different K+ salts are available. If only one salt is to be stocked, potassium chloride should be chosen because it is adequate for most disorders. The oral route of administration is best if this is clinically feasible, and the wax matrix tablet and microencapsulated forms are preferred. If the subcutaneous route is used, the concentration of K+ should not exceed 30 mEq/L. Intravenous fluids should never exceed 80 mEq/L. In severe K+ depletion, the rate can be increased to as high as 0.25 mEq/lb/hour (0.5 mEq/kg/hour), but this rate should never be exceeded.

Optimal management of K+ depletion requires recognition of clinical situations in which hypokalemia may develop so that preventive K+ supplementation can be provided on a maintenance basis. The main complication of K+ supplementation is hyperkalemia, and care should be taken to prevent cardiotoxicity, particularly with intravenous treatment.

HYPERKALEMIA

Etiology

The most common causes of hyperkalemia in dogs and cats are shown in Table 60–6.

Clinical Signs

Pseudohyperkalemia can be differentiated from true hyperkalemia by remeasurement of K+ levels in plasma rather than serum. There are no clinical signs. The signs of hyperkalemia usually develop once plasma K+ exceeds 6.5 mEq/L and include weakness and cardiac conduction abnormalities usually associated with bradycardia.

Treatment

The urgency to counteract hyperkalemia should match the severity of ECG abnormalities as well as the degree of hyperkalemia. With severe abnormalities, the ECG should be monitored while calcium, insulin combined with dextrose, and bicarbonate are given intravenously.

A 10 per cent solution of calcium gluconate should be given by slow intravenous infusion to provide 0.25 ml/lb. The effect begins within minutes and lasts about 30 minutes. Regular insulin combined with glucose may be given intravenously to dogs at 2.5 U/lb/hour and to cats at 0.25 U/lb. Insulin should be combined with glucose at 2 gm/unit of insulin. The onset of action is immediate and can last several hours. Sodium bicarbonate given at 0.5 to 1 mEq/lb also induces transfer of K^+ to the ICF, and the effect lasts as long as the effect of insulin combined with glucose.

The foregoing measures are only transient. Volume contraction should be corrected, and ECF expansion will both dilute ECF K^+ levels and increase renal perfusion, possibly leading to better K^+ excretion. The cation exchange resin, sodium polystyrene sulfonate, can be given orally or by retention enema. If hyperkalemia persists, dialysis represents the only alternative to further reduce ECF K^+ levels.

ACID-BASE IMBALANCE (pp. 305–307)

The normal values of arterial and venous blood gas values for dogs and cats are shown in Table 60–7.

Definitions

Acidemia refers to reduced plasma pH, and animals in this condition are said to be *acidotic*. *Alkalemia* refers to increased plasma pH, and animals in this condition are said to be *alkalotic*.

Metabolic acidosis means a primary decrease in plasma HCO_3^-.
Metabolic alkalosis means a primary increase in plasma HCO_3^-.
Respiratory acidosis means a primary increase in plasma $PaCO_2$.
Respiratory alkalosis means a primary decrease in plasma $PaCO_2$.

The term *primary* denotes that the disturbance referred to is the initiating event and the pH is shifted, at least initially, in the same direction. Thus, *primary metabolic acidosis* refers to decreased plasma HCO_3^- as an initiating event that tends to cause acidemia or reduced pH. There is always a secondary or compensatory response that tends to return plasma pH toward, but not completely back to, normal. Therefore, a primary metabolic acidosis leads to a compensatory respiratory alkalosis. The expected compensatory responses to primary disturbances of acid-base balance in dogs are shown in Table 60–8. The expected responses in cats have not been defined.

TABLE 60–7. NORMAL ARTERIAL AND VENOUS BLOOD GAS VALUES IN DOGS AND CATS

| | CANINE | | FELINE | |
	Arterial	Venous	Arterial	Venous
pH	7.407 ± 0.028	7.405 ± 0.0097	7.386 ± 0.038	7.300 ± 0.087
P_{CO_2} (mmHg)	36.8 ± 3.0	36.6 ± 1.21	31.0 ± 2.9	41.8 ± 9.12
P_{O_2} (mmHg)	92.1 ± 5.6	52.1 ± 2.11	106.8 ± 5.7	38.6 ± 11.44
HCO_3^- (mEq/L)	22.2 ± 1.7	22.3 ± 0.43	18.0 ± 1.8	19.4 ± 4.0

TABLE 60–8. RELATIONSHIP BETWEEN HCO_3^- AND $PaCO_2$ IN SIMPLE ACID-BASE DISTURBANCES

PRIMARY DISTURBANCE	EXPECTED COMPENSATORY RESPONSES
Metabolic acidosis	$\Delta PaCO_2$ mmHg = $0.7 \times \Delta HCO_3^-$ mEq/L
Metabolic alkalosis	$\Delta PaCO_2$ mmHg = $0.7 \times \Delta HCO_3^-$ mEq/L
Respiratory acidosis	
Acute ;	ΔHCO_3^- mEq/L = $0.15 \times \Delta PaCO_2$ mmHg
Chronic	ΔHCO_3^- mEq/L = $0.35 \times \Delta PaCO_2$ mmHg
Respiratory alkalosis	
Acute	ΔHCO_3^- mEq/L = $0.25 \times \Delta PaCO_2$ mmHg
Chronic	ΔHCO_3^- mEq/L = $0.53 \times \Delta PaCO_2$ mmHg

METABOLIC ACIDOSIS (pp. 307–309)

Etiology

Metabolic acidosis can be due to the addition of a strong acid to ECF, loss of HCO_3^- from ECF, or ECF expansion with a bicarbonate-poor solution. The more common causes of metabolic acidosis are shown in Table 60–9.

Clinical Signs

In most conditions the clinical signs are those of the initiating disease. However, the signs of severe metabolic acidosis may include hypotension and deep, rapid respiration (Kussmaul breathing). Laboratory findings include reduced plasma pH, reduced plasma HCO_3^- and pH, with reduced $PaCO_2$ as compensation. Plasma K^+ may be normal or increased even if total body K^+ is depleted because of an ICF to ECF shift. Serum electrolyte values allow calculation of the anion gap:

$$\text{Anion gap} = [Na^+] - ([Cl^-] + [HCO_3^-])$$

The anion gap allows differentiation of some causes of metabolic acidosis (Table 60–9). Production of organic acids causes depletion of HCO_3^- stores with subsequent increase in anion gap, whereas loss of HCO_3^- in diarrhea or renal tubular acidosis is matched by an equivalent renal retention of Cl^-, and the anion gap remains unchanged.

TABLE 60–9. CAUSES OF METABOLIC ACIDOSIS

NORMAL ANION GAP	INCREASED ANION GAP
Diarrhea	Azotemia
Renal tubular acidosis	Acute renal failure
Proximal: Fanconi syndrome	Chronic renal failure
Distal: amphotericin B	Diabetic ketoacidosis
Drugs	Lactic acidosis
Acetazolamide	Cardiac arrest
NH_4Cl administration	Shock
	Hypoxemia
	Toxins
	Ethylene glycol
	Metaldehyde

Treatment

The first priority is accurate identification and treatment of the primary cause. No further treatment is usually required. Intravenous alkali treatment usually should be considered only if plasma pH is less than pH 7.1 to 7.2.

The organic acidoses rarely require HCO_3^- treatment except for a small initial dose to raise the plasma pH to 7.1 if the patient is extremely acidemic. Once the primary cause is corrected, both ketoacids and lactate are rapidly converted to bicarbonate, and metabolic acidosis corrects itself. The deficit of HCO_3^- is extremely difficult to calculate. In those few cases in which the plasma pH is less than 7.1, it is best to empirically treat with 0.5 mEq/lb intravenously and then recheck the acid-base status. If too much HCO_3^- is given, rapid metabolism of ketoacids or lactate can lead to metabolic alkalosis and severe overshoot alkalemia. When metabolic acidosis is caused by a process other than an excess of organic acids—as in diarrhea, renal tubular acidosis, and ammonium chloride intoxication—bicarbonate needs can be crudely calculated:

$$\text{Bicarbonate deficit} = BW \text{ (kg)} \times 0.3 \times (\text{desired} - \text{observed plasma } HCO_3^-)$$

In severe acidemia (pH less than 7.1), 25 per cent of the calculated dose may be given by bolus over 10 to 15 minutes so that plasma pH rises above 7.1. Then the balance can be given over the following 12 to 18 hours. In less urgent circumstances, the deficit should be corrected gradually over 12 to 24 hours. If accurate blood-gas or total HCO_3^- estimations are unavailable, a total dose of 0.5 to 1 mEq/lb HCO_3^- may be given empirically.

Several precautions must be taken. Careless use of hypertonic $NaHCO_3$ solutions can easily cause excessive hyperosmolality. Rapid HCO_3^- infusion can lead to hypocalcemic tetany, paradoxical CSF acidosis with seizures, hypokalemia, and a shift of the oxygen-hemoglobin dissociation curve to the left so that O_2 release from hemoglobin is reduced.

METABOLIC ALKALOSIS (pp. 309–310)

Metabolic alkalosis is due to an increase in plasma HCO_3^- above 24 mEq/L.

Etiology

Vomiting, diuretic use, and excessive alkali administration are the most common causes of metabolic alkalosis.

Clinical Signs and Diagnosis

The signs are nonspecific, and patients usually manifest signs of the disease process causing metabolic alkalosis. In severe cases muscle twitches and tetany may occur, and affected animals are much more likely to have ventricular arrhythmias. The usual laboratory findings include elevated plasma pH, elevated plasma HCO_3^-, elevated $PaCO_2$, reduced plasma Cl^-, and, often, reduced plasma K^+. The diagnosis is confirmed by the presence of an elevated plasma HCO_3^- level.

Treatment

When kidney function is normal, metabolic alkalosis rapidly responds to ECF fluid expansion by the administration of normal saline. With concurrent hypokalemia, intravenous fluids may need to be supplemented with K^+.

RESPIRATORY ACIDOSIS (p. 310)

Respiratory acidosis occurs when $PaCO_2$ rises above the normal level of 40 mmHg. Hypercapnia results from decreased effective alveolar ventilation so that CO_2 production transiently exceeds CO_2 excretion.

Clinical Signs

The signs are those of the primary respiratory disease, and these may include dyspnea, tachypnea, restlessness, and stupor ultimately leading to coma. Typical laboratory findings include decreased plasma pH, elevated $PaCO_2$, slightly elevated plasma HCO_3^-, and reduced PaO_2. The causes of respiratory acidosis are discussed in Chapters 87 through 90 (Table 60–10).

Treatment

Treatment of acute respiratory acidosis should be aimed at restoring effective ventilation. Mechanical ventilation may be necessary. If correction of the pulmonary disturbance is to be delayed, sufficient HCO_3^- to increase pH above 7.2 may be given, but further HCO_3^- treatment should be avoided. Treatment of chronic respiratory acidosis also involves treatment of the primary cause; however, this is frequently impossible because chronic pulmonary diseases are often irreversible. Oxygen supplementation without ventilation may induce life-threatening respiratory acidosis.

RESPIRATORY ALKALOSIS (pp. 310–311)

Respiratory alkalosis refers to the reduced $PaCO_2$ below the normal level that occurs when CO_2 excretion by the lungs exceeds tissue production. The signs of respiratory alkalosis are usually those of the underlying condition causing hyperventilation. If alkalemia is severe, tetany, seizures, and cardiac arrhythmias may be seen. Laboratory evaluation reveals elevated plasma pH, reduced $PaCO_2$, reduced plasma HCO_3^-, and slightly elevated plasma Cl^-. Causes of respiratory alkalosis are shown in Table 60–10. Treatment requires correction of hyperventilation.

TABLE 60–10. CAUSES OF RESPIRATORY ACIDOSIS AND ALKALOSIS

RESPIRATORY ACIDOSIS	RESPIRATORY ALKALOSIS
Neuromuscular Disturbances	*Central Stimulation*
Tick paralysis	Anxiety
Polyradiculoneuritis	CNS disease
Narcotic, sedative, or tranquilizer overdose	Fever
Myasthenia gravis	Pain
Organophosphate intoxication	
Severe hypothyroidism	*Peripheral Stimulation*
	Pneumonia
Respiratory Disorders	Interstitial lung disease
Airway obstruction	
Pneumothorax	*Other*
Pleural effusion	Gram-negative septicemia
Severe pneumonia	Mechanical hyperventilation
Severe pulmonary edema	
Diffuse metastatic disease	
Massive pulmonary embolism	
Cardiopulmonary arrest	

MIXED ACID-BASE DISORDERS (p. 311)

Mixed acid-base disturbances result when two conditions that affect acid-base balance occur concurrently in the same patient. Mixed disturbances can be diagnosed when the expected compensation for a suspected primary disturbance fails to develop (Table 60–8). When the compensatory changes fail to fall within the expected range, the patient must be evaluated for possible causes of the second acid-base disturbance. Even if the $PaCO_2$ or HCO_3^- values fall within the normal range, they still may represent an acid-base disturbance if the expected compensation means the value should be a lot higher or lower. When mixed disturbances alter pH in the same direction (e.g., metabolic acidosis combined with respiratory acidosis), extremely dangerous plasma pH values may develop. However, when disturbances alter pH in different directions (e.g., metabolic alkalosis combined with respiratory acidosis), the plasma pH may be nearly normal.

Mixed acid-base disturbances often require that both conditions be treated at once. When the disturbances have a concurrent effect on lowering or raising plasma pH, dangerous values inconsistent with survival often develop, and immediate treatment is required. When the disturbances have a disparate effect, treatment of one condition without the other will cause plasma pH values to move away from normal; that is, the second disturbance will be unmasked.

CHAPTER 61

TOXICOLOGY
(pages 312–326)

THE EMERGENCY CASE (pp. 312–313)

IMMEDIATE MEASURES

Life-threatening toxic conditions must be dealt with immediately by ensuring a patent airway, assisting respiration, providing oxygen, and dealing with cardiovascular insufficiencies as indicated during physical examination. Only after life-threatening situations have been dealt with can further evaluation of the case be considered. The axiom, "treat the patient and not the poison" has more than a grain of truth. Table 61–1 lists steps for preventing further absorption of ingested toxicants.

INSECTICIDES (pp. 313–314)

ORGANOPHOSPHORUS AND CARBAMATE INSECTICIDES

Toxicity and Clinical Signs. These are anticholinesterase insecticides. Onset of signs generally occurs within minutes of exposure. Dermal contact may have a longer period to onset of poisoning. Salivation, lacrimation, urination, and defecation (SLUD) can occur in acutely poisoned animals. Muscle fasciculations are prominent, and the pupils are constricted unless the animal is in shock. Convulsions may be present in severe cases. Bronchoconstriction, pulmonary conges-

---

Original chapter written by Steven S. Nicholson

TABLE 61–1. PREVENTING FURTHER ABSORPTION AND HASTENING ELIMINATION OF TOXICANTS*

A. Induction of emesis
  i. Make sure stomach contains food material or liquid before inducing vomiting. Don't induce if animal is already vomiting, is severely depressed, does not have gag reflex, is known to have ingested caustic or petroleum products, has convulsed, or may convulse.
  ii. Apomorphine (0.02 mg/lb or 0.04 mg/kg IV, 0.04 mg/lb or 0.08 mg/kg IM, SQ) is most effective in the dog. Respiratory depression and protracted vomiting are adverse effects. For cats, xylazine is given at a dose of 0.25 mg/lb (0.5 mg/kg) IV or 0.5 mg/lb (1.0 mg/kg) IM.
  iii. Antagonists to apomorphine
    a. Naloxone hydrochloride (Narcan), 0.02 mg/lb (0.04 mg/kg) IV, IM, SQ.
    b. Levallorphan tartrate (Lorfan), 0.01 to 0.1 mg/lb (0.02 to 0.2 mg/kg) IV, IM, SQ.
    c. Nalorphan hydrochloride (Nalline), 0.05 mg/lb (0.10 mg/kg) IV, IM, SQ.
B. Gastric lavage—most effective if performed within 2 hours of ingestion.
  i. Animal should be unconscious or under light anesthesia.
  ii. Cuffed endotracheal tube placed in trachea; tube tip should extend 2 inches (5 cm) beyond incisor teeth to prevent laryngotracheal aspiration.
  iii. Use large-bore stomach tube, at least as large as endotracheal tube.
  iv. Lower head and thorax slightly below rest of the body.
  v. Pass lubricated stomach tube after premeasurement to xiphoid cartilage.
  vi. Use 3 to 5 ml/lb (6 to 10 mg/kg) of water or saline or part saline to lavage. Aspirate, repeat lavage 10 to 15 times. Activated charcoal in saline can be used as the lavage solution.
C. Gastrointestinal absorbents
  i. Activated charcoal—several commercial types are available. Activated charcoal tablets are easiest to handle.
  ii. Add one gram charcoal per 5 to 10 ml to make slurry.
  iii. Dose at 5 ml slurry/lb body weight (10 ml/kg).
  iv. Follow in 30 minutes with 40% saline cathartic–sodium sulfate, 0.5 gm/lb (1 gm/kg) orally. Lower doses of activated charcoal (0.25 gm/lb or 0.5 gm/kg) given at 3-hour intervals for 72 hours are recommended for slowly excreted substances. A cathartic should follow the first and second doses only.
D. Enemas. Use tepid water.
E. Hasten elimination in urine.
  i. Maintain renal function. Correct dehydration.
  ii. Diuretics—once animal is well hydrated.
    a. 10% dextrose in water, 10 ml/lb (20 ml/kg) alternated with 10 ml/lb (20 ml/kg) normal saline solution or lactated Ringer's IV over 6 to 8 hours.
    b. 20% mannitol, 2.5–5 ml/lb (5–10 mg/kg) IV over 30 minutes as single dose.
    c. Furosemide—initial dose 1–2 mg/lb (2–4 mg/kg) IV. If no response, give second and third doses of 2–4 mg/lb (4–8 mg/kg).
  iii. Ion trapping—ionized compounds are poorly reabsorbed by renal tubules.
    a. Alkaline urine facilitates ionization of acid compounds, i.e., aspirin, barbiturates.
    b. Acidic urine tends to ionize basic compounds, i.e., amphetamines, strychnine.
  iv. Peritoneal dialysis

*Modified from Hoskins JD, Nicholson SS: Toxicology. In Hoskins JD: Veterinary Pediatrics. Philadelphia: WB Saunders Co, 1990, p 499.

tion, and edema contribute to respiratory distress. Death results from paralysis of respiration and pulmonary edema.

Diagnosis. Laboratory confirmation of a very low red blood cell cholinesterase level confirms exposure. Stomach contents, liver, urine, and hair/skin are sampled for chemical analysis.

Treatment. A response to atropine supports the diagnosis. Severely poisoned cyanotic animals may require additional oxygen prior to atropinization. Repeated administration of atropine, as needed to control signs, can be given. Carbamate poisoning usually responds promptly. Recovery from OP poisoning is not as dramatic.

Activated carbon in the gastrointestinal tract may trap additional pesticide. Continued absorption from contaminated skin and hair should be prevented. Prolonged muscle weakness is seen in dogs and cats in some cases. Diphenhydramine has antinicotinic activity and may be useful in dogs and cats. Pralidoxime chloride (2-PAM, Protopam chloride) should be administered. Treatment should begin within 24 to 48 hours.

ORGANOCHLORINE INSECTICIDES

Endosulfan (Thiodan) remains in use for gardens and agricultural application.

Toxicity and Clinical Signs. Convulsions sometimes occur as myoclonic jerking, but often as violent seizures. Muscle twitching is common. Excitement or handling causes the signs to increase.

Diagnosis. Diagnosis depends on history and classic signs. Serum, vomitus, liver, fat, and brain may be submitted for analysis.

Treatment. Control seizures with pentobarbital or diazepam, and apply detoxification procedures to remove the poison.

PYRETHRIN AND PYRETHROID INSECTICIDES

This class of chemical is relatively safer than the others.

Toxicity and Clinical Signs. Signs include tremors, increased salivation, ataxia, vomiting, depression, hyperexcitability or hyperactivity, seizures, dyspnea, and death.

Diagnosis. Based on history, clinical signs, and chemical analysis for residues in vomitus, skin, and hair.

Treatment. Control seizures or hyperactivity. Remove pesticide from skin and digestive tract and provide supportive care.

RODENTICIDES (pp. 314–316)

ANTICOAGULANT TOXICANTS

Long-acting anticoagulants have largely replaced the much safer (for pets) warfarin-based coumarins because of resistance. Brodifacoum is the most commonly used and is the most toxic. Secondary or relay poisoning may occur.

Toxicity and Clinical Signs. These toxins depress the hepatic vitamin K–dependent synthesis of prothrombin (factor II) and factors VII, IX, and X. Lethargy, respiratory distress, dyspnea, and ventral hematomas are prominent initial signs. Internal bleeding constitutes a diagnostic challenge.

Diagnosis. History of exposure, compatible signs and lesions, extended prothrombin time, and response to vitamin K_1 therapy provide for a presumptive diagnosis.

Treatment. Blood or plasma transfusions, combating shock, oxygen therapy, and drugs for pulmonary edema must be considered. Vitamin K_1 should be administered SQ in multiple sites using a small-gauge needle. Administer orally for at least 14 days unless the anticoagulant was known to be a short-acting coumarin. Prothrombin time should be checked 2 to 3 days after cessation of therapy.

HYPERCALCEMIA-INDUCING TOXICANT

Toxicity and Clinical Signs. Poisoning results in hypercalcemia (>11.5 mg/dl) which, if not successfully treated, leads to calcification of soft tissues and nephrosis. Signs and lesions attributed to cardiac, pulmonary, renal, gastrointestinal, and nervous system effects may be seen.

Diagnosis. Suspicion may come from a routine serum chemistry panel indicating a serum calcium concentration above 12 mg/dl. History and clinical findings provide the basis for presumptive diagnosis. Elevation in serum 25-OH has been suggested for diagnosing vitamin D_3 poisoning in the dog.

Treatment. Prompt evacuation of the stomach and instillation of activated charcoal/cathartic mixture is indicated. Normal saline and furosemide are administered. Prednisolone is given. Salmon calcitonin can be used. A low-calcium diet should be fed.

BROMETHALIN

Bromethalin is an acute, single-feeding rodenticide in Vengeance, Assault, and Trounce.

Toxicity and Clinical Signs. A large dose causes a convulsant syndrome, generally within 24 hours, characterized by tremors, hyperthermia, extreme hyperexcitability, and focal motor and generalized seizures. A lower dose induces signs of hindlimb ataxia and/or paresis and/or central nervous system depression.

Diagnosis. Signs may mimic other convulsive syndromes, spinal cord injuries, and cerebral edema from other causes. Detection of bromethalin in tissues may be offered by some laboratories.

Treatment. Removal of the poison from the digestive tract may successfully prevent poisoning. Treatment administered once clinical signs have become apparent has not proved effective.

STRYCHNINE AND (1080/1081)

Strychnine has presented veterinarians with emergency situations for many years. Use of 1080/1081 is restricted, and it is seldom, if ever, used in the United States anymore.

Toxicity and Clinical Signs. Strychnine symptoms include nervousness and apprehension, which precede tetanic seizures. Seizures are triggered by noise, bright light, and touch. Death is the result of respiratory paralysis. Signs for 1080/1081 poisoning develop within 40 minutes to 2 hours. Dogs may become apprehensive, vomit, urinate, defecate, and suddenly commence running and howling or barking. Tetanic convulsions may occur and are not inducible. Cardiac abnormalities may be detected, especially in the cat.

Diagnosis. Vomitus or stomach contents may be colored green or pink by the dye marker in the bait. Alkaloid can be identified in stomach contents, liver, and urine.

Treatment. Pentobarbital given IV to effect is effective for control of the tetanic seizures. Gastric lavage followed by instillation of actived charcoal is recommended. Acidification of the urine may enhance urinary excretion.

The prognosis for 1080/1081 poisoning is grave. Glycerol monoacetate has been used as a competitive antagonist.

ZINC PHOSPHIDE

Toxicity and Clinical Signs. These include severe gastrointestinal inflammation, pulmonary congestion and edema, and cardiovascular insufficency.

Diagnosis. Promptly frozen stomach contents should be submitted for analysis. Zinc content in blood, liver, kidney, and stomach contents will be elevated.

Treatment. Control seizures, treat acidosis and shock, perform gastric lavage, and provide supportive care.

METALDEHYDE

Toxicity and Clinical Signs. Vomiting may occur due to stomach irritation. Hypersalivation, abdominal pain, tremors, hyperesthesia, nystagmus, and incoordination are seen. Significant elevation of body temperature is common. Opisthotonos and continuous tonic convulsions are noted in moderate to severe intoxications. Cholinergic signs may be present if a carbamate is included. Severe acidosis develops.

Diagnosis.　Tests for metaldehyde or acetaldehyde in stomach contents or suspect bait are offered by some laboratories.

Treatment.　Treatment consists of the usual detoxification procedures, control of seizures with diazepam or methocarbamol, correction of acidosis with sodium lactate in fluids, and supportive care.

ETHYLENE GLYCOL (pp. 317–318)

Toxicity and Clinical Signs.　Signs of intoxication become apparent within an hour. Vomiting, ataxia, knuckling, polydipsia, polyuria, dehydration, and depression may be noted. If the dog or cat survives the initial phase of intoxication, the first 12 hours after ingestion, the second clinical phase of poisoning, 24 to 96 hours later, is associated with renal failure and severe metabolic acidosis.

Diagnosis.　Ethylene glycol can be detected in serum and urine for up to 48 hours after ingestion. This common toxicosis may not be suspected if the history does not provide a clue. Calcium oxalate crystals may be seen in urine 5 hours after ingestion in dogs and 3 hours after ingestion in cats. Increases in serum osmolality correlate with increases in ethylene glycol concentrations. The osmolar gap remains markedly wide for the first 6 hours, then gradually decreases. If there is a high anion gap, metabolic acidosis is present. Isosthenuria is a constant finding.

In the second phase, hypocalcemia and elevated BUN and creatinine occur. Renal biopsy or cytologic examination of renal cortex scrapings at necropsy for crystals is diagnostic.

Treatment.　Therapy can be successful if begun in the early stages prior to renal damage. Emesis can be induced if the gag reflex is functional. Activated carbon and sodium sulfate should be given by stomach tube during the first 3 hours after ingestion. Dehydration and acidosis must be corrected and fluid therapy maintained. Peritoneal dialysis may be a lifesaving procedure when oliguria/anuria is present. Ethanol or 4-methylpyrazole (4-MP) will inhibit ethylene glycol metabolism and prevent or reduce the effects of the renal phase. Ethanol requires a longer hospital stay and frequent patient monitoring.

METALS (pp. 318–320)

LEAD

Toxicity and Clinical Signs.　Gastrointestinal and neurologic signs are commonly observed. Anorexia, vomiting, abdominal pain, diarrhea, constipation, and megaesophagus are seen. Hysteria characterized by increased irritability, whining or barking, continuous running, and snapping may occur. Opisthotonos, apparent blindness, dullness, or unusual behavior may be noticed.

Diagnosis.　Presentation of a young animal with GI signs should raise suspicions. Nucleated red blood cells accompanied by a packed cell volume of not less than 30 per cent, also supports toxicosis. Blood lead and tissue levels combined with the history and signs of lead poisoning confirm the diagnosis. Whole blood is the preferred sample. If blood lead levels are not conclusive, the urinary CaEDTA post-cheation test is recommended

Treatment.　Removal of lead from the digestive tract with magnesium or sodium sulfate cathartic may be indicated. Surgical removal might be necessary. Favorable response to chelation therapy can be expected in many cases. Thiamine is beneficial in alleviating signs. Chelation therapy using calcium EDTA is recommended. D-penicillamine is also effective.

THALLIUM

Clinical Signs. Intense congestion of the oral mucous membranes produces a brick red color. Neurologic signs such as muscle fasciculations, ataxia, convulsions, hyperesthesia, and coma are seen. Subacute poisoning is characterized by moderate gastroenteritis, brick red gingiva, reddened skin, and pustule formation. Weight loss, lethargy, dehydration, vomiting, alopecia, and hyperkeratosis are typical of the chronic form.

Diagnosis. The presence of thallium in urine is confirmatory.

Treatment. Emesis and/or activated charcoal is suggested acutely. Oral administration of potassium ferric-cyanoferrate has been recommended. Potassium chloride is suggested unless azotemia is present. Diphenylthiocarbazone has been recommended, but not for cats.

MERCURY

Clinical Signs. Methylmercury and elemental mercury vapor produce CNS damage. Inorganic salts and aryl forms of mercury cause gastrointestinal and renal tubular damage.

Diagnosis. Blood, urine, kidney, and stomach content samples may be analyzed.

Treatment. Milk and eggs, given orally, may be beneficial in acute poisonings; 2,3-dimercaptosuccinic acid has been used successfully in human cases.

ZINC

Toxicity and Clinical Signs. Zinc is eroded from pennies or metal nuts, retained in the stomach. Hemolytic anemia is a consistent finding. Signs of depression, abdominal discomfort, vomiting, diarrhea, and anorexia may precede the appearance of red urine and icterus. Pancreatic necrosis in the dog has been reported.

Diagnosis. Abdominal survey radiographs may reveal a retained metal object. Elevated serum zinc levels confirm exposure. Special blood tubes (metal-free) should be used.

Treatment. Treatment includes general supportive measures and removal of the metal object. Blood transfusion may be indicated. Chelation therapy with calcium EDTA should be administered.

IRON

Clinical Signs. Gastroenteritis, often hemorrhagic, with nausea and vomiting may be accompanied by shock and lethargy in moderate to severe poisoning. There may be remission of signs followed by liver or renal failure.

Diagnosis. Diagnosis is dependent on history, clinical signs, and serum iron concentrations.

Treatment. Early treatment measures include oral milk of magnesia and induction of emesis. Gastric lavage with normal saline can be preceded by instillation of 100 ml of 1 per cent bicarbonate solution. Deferoxamine mesylate is the antidote, but is hazardous to patients in renal failure.

COPPER

Clinical Signs. Copper is corrosive to mucous membranes of the GI tract and causes hepatic necrosis, methemoglobinemia, and hemolysis.

Diagnosis. Diagnosis is based on history, clinical signs, and high copper concentration in stomach contents and serum.

Treatment. Initial treatment consists of water or milk and removal by gastric lavage. Induction of emesis is not recommended. D-penicillamine can be used as a chelating agent.

ARSENIC

Clinical Signs. Arsenic damages gastric submucosal vasculature. Signs and lesions vary from mild to severe gastroenteritis. Severe diarrhea leads to dehydration, shock, metabolic acidosis, and anuria. Hepatic necrosis and renal tubular necrosis are additional findings. Death may occur.

Diagnosis. History and clinical signs merit a tentative diagnosis. Urine and kidney are submitted for toxicologic analysis.

Treatment. Intensive fluid and electrolyte therapy is needed. Activated charcoal is beneficial. British antilewisite (BAL) is the antidote for inorganic arsenic poisoning. Penicillamine has been used in human medicine either with BAL or to continue chelation after BAL.

HERBICIDES (pp. 320–321)

PARAQUAT AND DIQUAT

Clinical Signs. Corrosive effects may be seen on the oral membranes, eyes, and skin. Gastroenteritis and hepatic and renal damage is evident. Paraquat is concentrated in the lung. Pulmonary edema develops, followed by fibrosis and death.

Diagnosis. Serum, urine, stomach contents, hair, and the suspect substances should be saved for confirmation.

Treatment. Prompt removal of paraquat from skin and hair is imperative. Reduce GI tract absorption by gastric lavage with Fuller's earth or bentonite. A saline cathartic containing Fuller's earth is recommended. Oxygen therapy is contraindicated.

CHLOROPHENOXY COMPOUNDS

Clinical Signs. Poisoned dogs show vomiting, diarrhea, ataxia, posterior weakness, and myotonia.

Diagnosis. Urine is the specimen of choice to confirm exposure.

Treatment. Apply detoxification methods, treat metabolic acidosis, provide supportive care, and promote renal excretion with fluid therapy.

GLYPHOSATE

Transient irritation to the eyes and skin, vomiting, staggering, and hindlimb weakness have been seen.

Diagnosis. Diagnosis is based on history and clinical signs.

Treatment. Signs disappear when the animal is removed from the source and bathed.

BIOTOXINS (pp. 321–323)

SNAKEBITE

Toxicity and Clinical Signs. Pit viper toxins cause local tissue damage, blood vessel injury, red blood cell changes, coagulation defects, and shock. Severity of a pit viper bite depends on the location and amount of venom injected, the size of the animal, and the type of snake. Pit viper envenomation causes swelling within 20 to 30 minutes, and pain is usually present. In evaluation of crotalid bites, mild cases have minimal local reaction; moderate cases have intense local reaction; and in severe cases, both local and systemic effects are severe.

Signs of neurotoxic elapid venom poisoning are manifested as cranial motor nerve paralysis involving the eyelids, extrinsic musculature of the eyeball, and paralysis of respiration. Hemolysis, hemoglobinuria, and excessive salivation may occur.

Diagnosis. Identification of the snake and evidence of envenomation are needed for positive diagnosis. One or more fang marks are seen. Without the history or a fang mark, it may be difficult to differentiate coral snake envenomation from polyradiculoneuritis, tick paralysis, botulism, and myasthenia gravis.

Treatment. Crotalid antivenin, tetanus antitoxin, broad-spectrum antibiotics, and anti-inflammatories are utilized in the treatment of pit viper envenomation. Prenisolone sodium succinate should be given IV or IM. Antivenin is recommended in the treatment of moderate to severe envenomations. It is administered IV. Supportive treatment and antibiotics may be required for several days in severe cases.

Coral snakebites require antivenin within the first 4 hours. Broad-spectrum antibiotics and tetanus antitoxin are included in the treatment. Ventilatory assistance must be available.

TOAD POISONING

The Colorado river toad *(Bufo alvarius)* and the marine toad *(Bufo marinus)* are the most toxic.

Clinical Signs. Hypersalivation, vomiting, and pawing at the mouth are signs commonly seen when dogs or cats have mouthed a toad. Bufo toxins induce cyanosis, weakness, pulmonary edema, collapse, and convulsions. Death may occur.

Diagnosis. A history is helpful.

Treatment. The mouth should be flushed with copious amounts of water. Atropine will reduce salivation and the risk of aspirating saliva contaminated with toxin. Immediate administration of propranolol has been recommended in dogs.

ARTHROPOD BITES AND STINGS

Toxicity and Clinical Signs. Each species of Hymenoptera has unique venom. Local erythema and pain accompanied by swelling are seen. A pustule forms within 24 hours at the site of the fire ant sting. Large numbers of stings may result in death caused by pain and vascular effects. Anaphylaxis has occurred in hypersensitive animals.

Diagnosis. Depends on a clinician's ability to differentiate stings from mechanical punctures, snakebite, and angioneurotic edema.

Treatment. No treatment may be required. Alternatively, antihistamines and/or corticosteroids may be deemed necessary when moderate to severe local reactions or systemic signs are present. Epinephrine is indicated if anaphylaxis is evident. Methocarbamol, in conjunction with calcium gluconate, is recommended in black widow spider envenomizations. An antivenin is available for black widow bites. Corticosteroids are recommended for treatment following the bite of the brown recluse spider. If ulceration occurs, the lesion should be treated as an open wound.

MUSHROOM POISONING

Toxicity and Clinical Signs. *Amanita* spp. and *Galerina* spp. cause gastroenteritis, followed by rising hepatic enzymes and hepatic failure. Delayed gastroenteritis followed by renal failure is caused by *Cortinarius* spp. Hallucinations occur in *Psilocybe*. Several common lawn mushrooms contain the cholinergic toxicant muscarine. The anticholinergic agents in certain *Amanita* spp. and *Gyromitra* spp. cause gastroenteritis. Persistent abdominal pain, pyrexia, hepatotoxic effects, and icterus can occur.

Diagnosis. History, mushroom fragments in stomach contents, and identification of the mushroom are useful.

Treatment. Removal of toxins by emesis, lavage, and activated charcoal/laxative is essential. Vitamin B_6 leads to a faster recovery in Gyromitra poisoning. Supportive treatment should be given as required.

POISONOUS PLANTS

Table 61–2 lists plants that may cause poisoning that is more serious than mild gastroenteritis.

TABLE 61–2. PLANTS HAZARDOUS TO PETS BASED ON TOXICITY AND LOCATION

SCIENTIFIC NAME	COMMON NAME	TOXICANT/EFFECTS	REMARKS/TREATMENT
Allium spp (Liliaceae)	Onions	n-Methyl sulfide/Heinz body anemia, hemolysis	Blood transfusion if indicated, supportive
Aesculus spp (Hippocastanaceae)	Buckeye, horse chestnut	Nuts/gastroenteritis, narcosis	Emesis, lavage, control seizures
Aleurites fordii (Euphorbiaceae)	Tung-oil tree	Toxic protein, nuts/severe gastroenteritis	Lavage, activated charcoal, fluids
Brunfelsia spp (Solanaceae)	Yesterday, today and tomorrow	Alkaloids, leaves, seeds/convulsions, coma	Emesis, lavage, activated charcoal, control seizures, symptomatic
Caladium spp (Araceae)	Caladium	Calcium oxalate crystals, toxic protein/pain, erythema, edema of oral mucus membranes	Flush mouth with lime juice, water, milk; control pain
Calycanthus spp (Calycanthaceae)	Carolina allspice bubby-bush	Alkaloids, seeds/tremors, convulsions	Emesis, lavage, activated charcoal, cathartic
Cycas revoluta (Cycadaceae)	False sago palm	Cycasin, seeds/hepatic necrosis, icterus, bleeding	Emesis, lavage, activated carbon, vitamin K_1
Dieffenbachia (Araceae)	Dumbcane	Crystals, protein/stems, stalk most toxic	Same as caladium
Kalanchoe spp	Kalanchoe	Glycosides, others/seizures, paralysis	Emesis, lavage, activated charcoal, monitor heart
Cotyledon spp (Crassulaceae)	Pigs ears		
Hoya carnosa (Asclepiadaceae)	Wax plant	Unknown/tremors, convulsions	Lavage, activated charcoal, cathartic, control seizures
Hyacinthus spp and others (Liliaceae)	Hyacinth	Alkaloid, bulbs/gastroenteritis	Activated charcoal
Narcissus spp (Amaryllidaceae)	Daffodils	Alkaloids?/gastroenteritis	Same as hyacinth
Nerium spp	Oleander	Cardioactive glycosides/severe gastroenteritis	Emesis, lavage, activated charcoal, monitor heart, treat same as for digitalis poisoning
Thevetia (Oleaceae)	Yellow oleander		
Persea americana (Lauraceae)	Avocado	All parts, fruit poisons budgerigars/edema, chemical mastitis in lactating mammals	Emesis, lavage, activated carbon cathartic
Philodendron spp (Araceae)	Ivy, philodendron	See caladium: CNS signs, ataxia reported in cats	See caladium; cat—control CNS signs
Rhododendron spp (Ericaceae)	Azaleas, rhododendrons	Gray anatoxins, all parts/salivation, central vomiting, hypotension, weakness	Lavage, activated charcoal, supportive
Sanseveria spp (Agavaceae)	Snake plant, mother-in-laws tongue	Unknown/gastroenteritis	Activated charcoal, fluids
Taxus cuspidata (Taxaceae)	Japanese yew	Alkaloids/cardiotoxic	Emesis, lavage, activated charcoal, atropine

FEED- AND FOOD-RELATED TOXICOSES

Toxicity and Clinical Signs.   Corn, grain by-products, peanut meal, and soybean meal used in production of pet foods are potential sources of aflatoxins, ochratoxin, zearalenone, fumonisins, and other mycotoxins. Aflatoxins have caused acute and chronic hepatotoxicity in dogs. Simple stomached animals are susceptible to tubular necrosis and fibrosis caused by ochratoxins. Tremorgens produced by *Penicillium* spp. in cream cheese and walnuts have induced tremors and convulsions in dogs. Garbage poisoning in dogs may cause brief, mild gastroenteritis or a more serious intoxication with weakness, incoordination, dyspnea, abdominal pain, shock, coma, and death. Botulism may result from ingestion of carrion or other spoiled material. Onion powder added in excess to homemade diets for the dog has caused hemolysis and hemoglobinuria.

Diagnosis.   Is dependent on history. Radiographs may reveal bones or other objects in the stomach and intestines in cases of garbage poisoning. Consult your state veterinary medical laboratory to report suspicion of toxicant in a commercial pet food and request microscopic and toxicologic analysis.

Treatment.   Apply principles listed in Table 61–1.

MISCELLANEOUS TOXICOSES (pp. 323–325)

ACETAMINOPHEN

Cats are more susceptible than dogs to this medication. Methemoglobinemia, hemolysis, icterus, anemia, and hemoglobinuria develop. Cyanosis and subcutaneous edema of the face and extremities are characteristic findings. Heinz-body anemia is present. Diagnosis is based on history and confirmation by analysis of urine or serum. Dogs require a much larger dose, and the major response is hepatotoxicosis. Treatment in cats includes osmotic cathartic if vomiting has already occurred and administration of N-acetylcysteine. Activated charcoal is not recommended. Vitamin C can be given to cats to reverse methemoglobinemia. Methylene blue has been recommended.

ASPIRIN

Anorexia, abdominal discomfort, hyperpnea, pyrexia, and depression are seen in dogs. Signs may progress to coma and death. Metabolic acidosis and hypokalemia require correction. Activated charcoal and a saline cathartic are indicated. Alkalinization of the urine increases excretion of salicylate.

CHOCOLATE

Theobromine causes gastrointestinal, nervous, and cardiovascular symptoms. Cardiac effects can cause sudden death. Vomiting, thirst, diarrhea, restlessness, nervousness, agitation, urinary incontinence, muscle twitches, seizures, and death have been reported. Treatment includes administering a saline cathartic and activated charcoal. Monitoring for cardiac dysrhythmias is recommended (see textbook).

CHAPTER 62

ADVERSE DRUG REACTIONS
(pages 326–335)

An adverse drug reaction is defined as any noxious and unintended response to a drug that occurs at appropriate doses of a given drug used for prophylaxis, diagnosis, or therapy and that occurs within a reasonable time frame of administration of the drug.

FACTORS RELATED TO THE DEVELOPMENT OF ADVERSE DRUG REACTIONS (pp. 327–328)

Adverse reactions in animals may occur in response to components of the dosage form other than the active drug. Adverse reactions related to dose, variations in bioavailability, incorrect route of administration, or oral dosage forms given intravenously may occur. The incidence of adverse drug reactions is greater in the very young and the very old animal, and the very obese as well as the asthenic animal. Sensitivity to drugs and drug disposition may vary during pregnancy and parturition.

The presence of dysfunctions of various organ systems is an important factor in the occurrence of adverse drug reactions. Atopic individuals are at much greater risk than the general population of suffering adverse reactions to drugs. A number of congenital disorders that may predispose affected individuals to adverse drug effects occur in various breeds of dogs and other species (see textbook).

The incidence of adverse drug reactions increases dramatically with the number of drugs given simultaneously to the patient. Crowding of animals in high-confinement situations may result in unusual responses. Altitude and extremes of ambient temperature could provoke adverse reactions to drugs. Adverse drug reactions can occur at any time during therapy.

ALLERGIC DRUG REACTIONS (pp. 328–331)

Allergic reactions generally cannot be anticipated by the veterinarian unless the animal has a prior history of allergy to some drug. Atopic individuals have a greater tendency to develop an allergy to therapeutic agents.

CHARACTERISTICS OF ALLERGIC RESPONSE TO A DRUG

1. Generally allergic responses are not dose-related.
2. The presence of antibodies may be demonstrated in the patient.
3. The same or greater reaction occurs when a test dose of the drug is given.
4. Eosinophilia is a common concomitant finding.
5. The clinical picture conforms to a known allergic pattern (e.g., anaphylaxis, hemolytic anemia, systemic lupus erythematosus).
6. The reaction does not resemble any known pharmacologic action of the drug.
7. There is a delay in the development of the allergic state following initial exposure.

nal chapter written by Lloyd E. Davis

CLINICAL MANIFESTATIONS OF ALLERGIC DRUG REACTIONS

Immediate Hypersensitivity. Anaphylaxis is an acute, systemic, life-threatening, allergic reaction characterized by hypotension, bronchospasm, angioedema, urticaria, erythema, pruritus, pharyngeal and/or laryngeal edema, cardiac dysrhythmias, vomiting, colic, and hyperperistalsis. Anaphylactic manifestations most commonly follow parenteral administration of drugs. If the reaction is not fatal, the manifestations subside over a period of hours.

Treatment. The clinician can reduce the release of mediators by administering epinephrine, beta-adrenoceptor agonists, or phosphodiesterase (or adenosine) inhibitors such as theophylline. Corticosteroids modify the effects of the mediators on target tissues but do not modify the initial secretory response.

Typical Reactions. Dogs have a high density of mast cells present in their liver. Anaphylaxis is generally manifested by vomiting and diarrhea followed by profound shock due to obstruction of the hepatic circulation, although cutaneous manifestations may appear. Cats seem to react most commonly with acute respiratory distress due to bronchospasm.

Serum Sickness. Serum sickness is a systemic allergic reaction that occurs in response to some drugs and to biologics, and is manifested by lymphadenopathy, neuropathy, vasculitis, nephritis, arthritis, urticaria, and fever. The pathogenesis appears to be associated with the formation of immune complexes of antigen with IgG antibody. Generally, the onset is delayed until 10 to 20 days after the beginning of therapy. An accelerated form of the reaction may occur in individuals that have been previously sensitized. Antimicrobial drugs that have been incriminated most frequently include the sulfonamides, penicillins, para-aminosalicyclic acid, and streptomycin.

Hematologic Manifestations. The adverse drug reactions of hemolytic anemia, thrombocytopenia, and agranulocytosis may in some cases be immune-mediated. Drugs associated with immune-mediated thrombocytopenia include stibophen, sulfonamides, isoniazid, and rifampin. Drugs that most frequently cause immune-mediated hemolytic anemia in humans are penicillin, alpha-methyldopa, dipyrone, quinine, quinidine, stibophen, p-aminosalicylic acid, phenacetin, and rifampin.

Drugs most frequently associated are phenylbutazone, amidopyrine, oxyphenbutazone, sulfonamides, cephalothin, semi-synthetic penicillins, chloramphenicol, p-aminosalicylic acid, phenothiazines, gold compounds, anticonvulsants, propylthiouracil, indomethacin, dipyrone, tolbutamide, barbiturates, antihistamines, and arsenicals.

Autoimmune Reactions Induced by Drugs. Certain drugs may induce the formation of antibodies directed against the recipient's own tissues. Drugs have been implicated in the development of systemic lupus erythematosus (SLE), polymyositis, hepatitis, tubular nephropathy, and inhibition of coagulation factor VIII. Drug-induced SLE has been observed in patients treated with isoniazid, griseofulvin, tetracycline, and antimalarial drugs.

Cutaneous Manifestations. A fairly common allergic drug reaction seen in animal patients as well as in veterinarians who handle drugs is contact dermatitis.

DIAGNOSIS OF DRUG ALLERGY

Patch testing is useful for the diagnosis of contact sensitivity due to a delayed hypersensitivity reaction to a suspected drug or chemical. Intradermal tests for immediate hypersensitivity may be misleading. Serologic tests have limited value for the prediction of allergic drug reactions.

ACUTE ADVERSE DRUG REACTIONS RESEMBLING ALLERGY (pp. 331–332)

These reactions may be due to nonspecific release of mediators of hypersensitivity or due to direct effects of the drug on responding tissues.

CARDIOVASCULAR REACTIONS

Cardiovascular effects of chloramphenicol, aminoglycosides, tetracyclines, polymyxins, propylene glycol, and several other drugs can produce sudden ataxia, shivering, dyspnea, and collapse following intravenous administration. These clinical signs are associated with various cardiac arrhythmias, hypotension, brief cardiac standstill, and decreased pulmonary and renal blood flow. Rapid IV administration of drugs that are contained in propylene glycol vehicles may produce acute collapse through cardiovascular effects of the solvent.

HEMATOLOGIC REACTIONS

Administration of drugs contained in hypotonic solutions or in some organic vehicles can cause rapid lysis of circulating erythrocytes. Oxidant drugs and chemicals can cause hemolytic anemia accompanied by methemoglobinemia and Heinz-body formation. Heinz-body anemia in response to oxidant drugs is encountered most frequently in cats and in neonates. Suspect drugs include sulfonamides, quinacrine, nitrofurans, neoarsphenamine, and nalidixic acid.

DRUG FEVER

Drug fever may be produced as a result of drug allergy or by mechanisms that are not immune-mediated. Drug fevers may result in body

TABLE 62–1. DRUGS PRODUCING NEPHROTOXICITY

Antimicrobial Drugs	Analgesics
Ampicillin, I	Ibuprofen, I
Amphotericin B, T	Naproxen, I
Bacitracin, T	Phenacetin, T
Cephaloridine, T	Phenylbutazone, T, V
Colistin, T	Salicylates, T
Gentamicin, T	Antineoplastic Drugs
Kanamycin, T	Adriamycin, N
Methicillin, I	Cis-Platin, T
Neomycin, T	Cyclophosphamide, T, V
Oxacillin, I	Daunorubicin, N
Penicillin, I, V	Methotrexate, O
Polymyxin B, T	Mithramycin, T
Sulfonamides, O, I	Diuretics
Tetracyclines, T, V	Furosemide, I
Tobramycin, T	Mannitol, T
Heavy Metals	Thiazides, I, V
Arsenicals, T, N	Miscellaneous
Bismuth, T	Captopril, N
Cadmium, T	Dextrans, V
Copper, T	EDTA, T
Gold salts, T, N	Lithium, N
Mercurials, T, N	Penicillamine, N
Uranium, T	Phenazopyridine, T
	Phenindione, I
	Probenecid, N

Mechanisms are indicated by I = interstitial, N = nephrotic syndrome, O = obstructive, T = tubular and V = vasculitis.

temperatures that exceed those commonly seen with infections. Commonly, one encounters sustained fever of 103 to 104°F during the course of drug therapy. If the patient is bright, alert, eating, and active, it is likely that the fever is caused by the therapy rather than a disease. Penicillins and cephalosporins are the most common cause of drug fever in dogs, and tetracycline the most common cause in cats.

TOXIC DRUG REACTIONS (pp. 332–334)

Often the mechanisms for these effects are complex and obscure.

NEPHROTOXICITY

Nephrotoxicity may be manifested as nephrotoxic renal failure, acute glomerulonephritis, interstitial nephritis, lower nephron nephrosis, and nephrotic syndrome. Drugs that are nephrotoxic are listed in Table 62–1.

HEPATOTOXICITY

Hepatotoxic reactions should be suspected in any patient developing icterus, abnormal serum concentrations of transaminases or alkaline phosphatase, or hepatomegaly while receiving a drug. Hepatotoxicity is more commonly associated with chronic administration of medication or gross overdoses of certain drugs than with short courses of therapy. Drugs causing hepatotoxicity are listed in Table 62–2.

APLASTIC ANEMIA

Aplastic pancytopenia is an uncommon adverse drug reaction. The mechanism is not understood. Drugs that have been implicated as

TABLE 62–2. DRUGS CAUSING HEPATOTOXICITY

Anesthetics	Cardiovascular Agents
Chloroform	Procainamide
Halothane	Quinidine
Methoxyflurane	Warfarin
Anticonvulsants	Antineoplastics
Carbamazepine	Busulfan
Phenobarbital	Cyclophosphamide
Primidone	L-Asparginase
Valproic acid	6-Mercaptopurine
Antimicrobials	Methotrexate
Ampicillin	Mithramycin
Carbenicillin	Urethane
Erythromycin estolate	Endocrine Agents
5-Fluorocytosine	Anabolic steroids (C-17
Griseofulvin	alkylated)
Isoniazid	Corticosteroids
Nitrofurantoin	Methimazole
Quinacrine	Propylthiouracil
Tetracyclines	Tranquilizers
Thiabendazole	Diazepam
Analgesics	Haloperidol
Acetaminophen	Phenothiazines
Ibuprofen	Other Drugs
Indomethacin	Cimetidine
Naproxen	Danthron
Phenylbutazone	Dapsone
Salicylates	Iodochlorhydroxyquin
	Nicotinamide
	Stibophen
	Vitamin A

TABLE 62–3. DRUGS CAUSING APLASTIC ANEMIA

Antineoplastic	Endocrine Agents
Busulfan	Estrogens
Cyclophosphamide	Thiouracil
Cytosine arabinoside	Thiocyanate
Methotrexate	Methimazole
Mustargen	Tolbutamide
Vinblastine	Tranquilizers
Vincristine	Meprobamate
Antimicrobials	Phenothiazines
Amphotericin B	Antihistaminics
Chloramphenicol	Chlorpheniramine
Methicillin	Tripelennamine
Pyrimethamine	Miscellaneous
Quinacrine	Benzene
Sulfonamides	Carbamazepine
Tetracyclines	Carbon tetrachloride
Analgesics	Chlordane
Phenylbutazone	DDT
Phenacetin	Disophenol
Indomethacin	Gamma-Benzene hexachloride
Heavy Metals	
Organic arsenicals	
Gold salts	
Colloidal silver	

causes of aplastic anemia in humans are listed in Table 62–3. Chloramphenicol-induced aplastic anemia is probably rare among animals. Probably the most commonly encountered cause of pancytopenia in the dog is estrogen toxicity.

MEDICATION ERRORS

Errors encountered in a veterinary hospital may consist of omission of a dose, miscalculation of dosage, administration of a wrong drug, or improper administration of a drug.

MANAGEMENT OF ADVERSE DRUG REACTIONS
(pp. 334–335)

The main objectives to pursue in any animal that develops an adverse reaction to a drug are (1) provide life support; (2) stop administration of the drug; (3) enhance elimination of the drug; (4) if continued therapy is required, modify the dosage regimen or change to another drug; and (5) if available, administer drug antagonists or antidotes.

Cardiopulmonary resuscitation should be undertaken if there are signs of cardiac arrest present. Acute hypersensitivity reactions can have a rapid onset and must be treated immediately. In less urgent situations, stop therapy and allow time for the processes of biotransformation and excretion to remove the drug from the body. In some cases, active efforts should be made to enhance elimination of the drug following an overdose (e.g., increase the renal clearance of salicylate by maintaining a brisk alkaline diuresis). If acute renal failure has occurred, the only way of enhancing removal of the drug may be by peritoneal dialysis. In a small number of circumstances, antagonists may be available to prevent or mitigate the adverse effects. The most discouraging adverse drug reaction to manage is aplastic anemia. A high percentage of these patients eventually succumb to hemorrhage or overwhelming sepsis.

CHAPTER 63

ACUPUNCTURE THERAPY IN SMALL ANIMAL PRACTICE
(pages 336–347)

PRECAUTIONS (p. 336)

The most important contraindication for acupuncture is treating before an adequate diagnosis has been made, or before at least an honest and diligent attempt has been made to determine the etiology of the condition being treated. This is contraindicated because acupuncture may mask or alter clinical signs so that later accurate diagnosis is more difficult (e.g., pain and neurologic syndromes) or more advanced.

If possible, acupuncture should be avoided under the following conditions: immediately after a heavy meal; after exertion or on a fatigued animal; on a subject that is extremely frightened, enraged, or emotional; on pregnant animals, especially if points caudal to the umbilicus are to be used; if the subject has just been bathed; if injections of atropine, narcotics, narcotic antagonists, or corticosteroids have been used; or if the animal cannot be comfortably restrained. The practitioner should always be aware of the anatomy to avoid traumatizing underlying internal structures. In addition, it is inadvisable to insert needles in animals with severe blood dyscrasias or clotting deficiencies or into areas where local malignancies or skin infections are present.

SEQUELAE (p. 336)

The most common is exacerbation of the problem being treated, especially pain. The worsening of pain is usually short-lived (less than 24 to 48 hours) and usually is not a poor prognostic sign. Some other sequelae are broken needles; needles caught in tissue; injury to vital organs such as the heart, liver, kidneys, and spleen; hematomas; pneumothorax; infections; nausea; vomiting; and in one instance, syncope.

TECHNIQUES (pp. 336–346)

See textbook.

Original chapter written by Sheldon Altman

CHAPTER 64

BLOOD BANKING AND TRANSFUSION MEDICINE
(pages 347–360)

GENERAL CONSIDERATIONS (p. 347)

Blood transfusion is a simple form of transplantation. Blood (the organ), with its oxygen-carrying red cells and clotting proteins and platelets, is transferred from donor to patient to temporarily correct a deficiency or dysfunction. The organ and patient must be tested to ensure compatibility. A transfusion can be rejected and can cause profound complications in the recipient.

CANINE BLOOD GROUPS (p. 348)

The dog has eight different blood groups identified as dog erythrocyte antigens (DEA; Table 64–1). Transfusion reactions usually do not occur unless the canine patient has been previously transfused with incompatible blood. The use of blood negative for DEA 1.1, 1.2, and 7, so-called universal blood, prevents the formation of antibodies against these determinants in the transfused recipient. Many patients can realistically receive incompatible products if crossmatch compatibility is established.

FELINE BLOOD GROUPS (p. 348)

Cats have naturally occurring antibodies in their plasma against the other blood group. All type B cats have strong titers of anti-A alloantibodies. In contrast, type A cats have low anti-B alloantibody titers, and the extremely rare AB cat has no alloantibodies. In the United States, nearly all domestic long- and shorthaired cats (99.7 per cent) have type A blood. Type B cats have been found among domestic cat breeds and Abyssinian, Birman, British shorthair, Devon Rex, Himalayan, Persian, Scottish fold ear, and Somali cats.

TABLE 64–1. CANINE BLOOD GROUPS

CURRENT NAME	COMMON NAME	POPULATION INCIDENCE (%)
DEA 1.1	A1	40
DEA 1.2	A2	20
DEA 3	B	5
DEA 4	C	98
DEA 5	D	25
DEA 6	F	98
DEA 7	Tr	45
DEA 8	He	4

Data from Paradis MR: Neonatal transfusion medicine. Adv Vet Sci Comp Med 36:225, 1991.

Original chapter written by Annemarie T. Kristensen and Bernard F. Feldman

FELINE NEONATAL ISOERYTHROLYSIS

All of the cases studied exhibited queens with type B blood and may have been primiparous, while males and NI kittens had type A blood. With intake of colostrum containing high titers of maternal alloantibodies, these kittens may stop nursing, fail to thrive, and develop pigmenturia, icterus, and anemia, or they may die without showing any specific signs during the first few days of life. Upon first recognition, affected type A kittens should be removed from their mother for the next 3 days and can be successfully foster-nursed. Neonatal isoerythrolysis can be avoided by breeding type B queens to blood compatible mates.

INDICATIONS FOR TRANSFUSION AND CHOICE OF COMPONENT (pp. 352–355)

The major indications, dosages, and administration rates for different components are listed in Table 64–2; the general guidelines for dogs and cats are listed in Table 64–3. A crossmatch should be performed in both dogs and cats prior to any red cell administration. In dogs in which there is no time for crossmatching, universal donor blood (DEA 1.1, 1.2, and 7 negative) should be administered. Intravenous administration is preferable, but in kittens and puppies, intraperitoneal or intramedullary access may be more practical. An in-line filter should always be used.

SPECIFIC CONSIDERATIONS FOR BLOOD COMPONENT THERAPY

Need for Oxygen-Carrying Capacity

In general 5 ml/lb of PRBCs or 10 ml/lb of whole blood will increase the PCV 10 per cent. A more accurate estimation can be calculated using the formula in Table 64–2. All of these estimations assume that the patient has normal blood volume. In patients with cardiac disease or circulatory overload, administration should take 4 hours.

Replacement in Acute Blood Loss. Red cell replacement is necessary if: (1) PCV drops rapidly to less than 20 per cent in the dog, or less than 12 to 15 per cent in the cat; (2) more than 30 per cent of blood volume is lost; (3) blood loss is associated with collapse; (4) ongoing hemorrhage is present; and (5) there is poor response to conventional shock therapy. Whole blood has no advantage over PRBCs.

Replacement in Chronic Blood Loss. Administration of blood should be based on clinical signs, but all patients need a transfusion if the PCV is less than 10 per cent.

Replacement in Immune-mediated Hemolytic Anemia (IHA). Patients with IHA with clinical signs of life-threatening anemia should always be transfused. Crossmatching may be difficult. Hypoxic injury to vital organs could be the result of withholding therapy.

Replacement in Feline Neonatal Isoerythrolysis. Washed red cells from the queen or from a known type B cat should be given if transfusion support is necessary during the first 3 days of life, or transfusion of type A blood thereafter.

Replacement Using Autologous Transfusions. *Autotransfusion* is considered when a patient is bleeding or has bled into one of the major body cavities. Autotransfusion is contraindicated if bleeding is due to an infectious process or neoplasia. *Autologous donation* is the donation of blood from a patient prior to elective surgery and return during surgery if needed. Good candidates include patients undergoing elective amputation, rhinotomy, or thoracotomy.

Need for Restoration of Hemostatic Function

Replacement of Dysfunctional or Decreased Coagulation Proteins. The most common clinical situations are DIC, coumarin

TABLE 64-2. BLOOD COMPONENT STORAGE, DOSE, AND ADMINISTRATION RATES

COMPONENT	STORAGE	INDICATION	DOSE & ADMINISTRATION RATE†
Fresh whole blood	<12 hours (CPDA1)	Hemostatic dysfunction with severe bleeding (1) Coagulopathy (DIC, coumarin toxicity, von Willebrand's disease [VWD], hemophilia) (2) Thrombocytopenia/thrombocytopathia Anemia	10 ml/lb will ↑ PCV 10%‡ 30 (cat)
Stored whole blood	37 days (ADSOL), 4°C 21 days (CPDA1), 4°C	Anemia	10 ml/lb will ↑ PCV 10%‡
Packed red cells	37 days (ADSOL), 4°C 20 days (CPDA1), 4°C	Anemia	5 ml/lb will ↑ PCV 10%‡
Platelet rich plasma	1–3 days (CPDA1), 22°C	Thrombocytopenia (1) Associated with life-threatening bleeding (2) Prior to surgery Thrombocytopathia (1) Congenital (2) Acquired (nonsteroidal anti-inflammatory drugs)	0.5 unit/10 lbs (1 unit/10 kg)

Product	Storage	Indications	Dosage
Fresh frozen plasma	1 year, minus 30°C; 3 months, minus 18°C	Coagulopathy associated with acute blood loss (1) Congenital (VWD), hemophilia controlled (2) Acquired (DIC, coumarin toxicity) Prior to (during) surgery in patient with coagulopathy Dilutional coagulopathy after massive transfusion Hypoproteinemia Acute volume expansion	5 ml/lb (10 ml/kg) repeat until bleeding controlled
Cryoprecipitate	1 year, minus 30°C; 3 months, minus 18°C	Coagulopathy associated with acute blood loss (1) Congenital (VWD, hemophilia) (2) Acquired (DIC, coumarin toxicity) Prior to (during) surgery in patient with coagulopathy	0.5 unit/10 lbs, repeat until bleeding controlled
Plasma/Cryopoor plasma	5 years, minus 30°C	Hypoproteinemia Colostrum replacement Coagulopathy with loss of factor II, VII, IX, X (coumarin toxicity) Hypofibrinogenemia Hemophilia B (IX deficiency)	5 ml/lb (10 ml/kg) repeat until bleeding controlled

†All blood products should be administered within 4 hours according to standards set by the American Association of Blood Banks. Within this guideline should be administered according to amount to be administered, size, and clinical status of the patient.

‡Or calculated more accurately as weight (lbs) $\times \dfrac{40 \text{ (dog)}}{30 \text{ (cat)}} \times \dfrac{\text{Desired PCV} - \text{Patient PCV}}{\text{PCV of donor blood}}$

CPDA1 = citrate-phosphate-dextrose-adenine; ADSOL = commercial additive which prolongs red cell viability; DIC = disseminated intravascular coagulation.

TABLE 64–3. GENERAL GUIDELINES FOR USE OF BLOOD COMPONENT THERAPY

Anemia	PCV <10%
	PCV drops rapidly to less than 20% in the dog, or less than 12–15% in the cat
	More than 30% of the blood volume is lost (30 ml/kg for the dog; 20 ml/kg for the cat)
	Blood loss is associated with collapse
	Acute hemorrhage with poor response to conventional shock therapy
Coagulopathy	Associated with life-threatening bleeding or surgery is needed†
Thrombocytopenia/ thrombocytopathia	Associated with life-threatening bleeding or surgery is needed†
Hypoproteinemia	Albumin concentrations <1.5 gm/ml (TPP <3.5 gm/ml) and compromise due to hypoproteinemia or surgery is needed
Hypovolemia	No other means of fluid therapy is adequate

†Coagulation tests or absolute platelet counts are not necessarily helpful; need for component therapy should be established based on clinical condition of the patient.
PCV = packed cell volume.

toxicity, von Willebrand's disease, and hemophilia. Fresh frozen plasma or cryoprecipitate are the blood products of choice in these processes.

Replacement of Dysfunctional or Decreased Platelets. The most common clinical situation is in dogs with IMT.

Need for Restoring Plasma Volume

This should preferentially be accomplished with crystalloids or with plasma expanders. Stored plasma can be used as well.

Need for Restoring Oncotic Pressure

Plasma products can be used as acute therapy in hypoproteinemic patients. The necessary calculations for albumin replacements are given in Table 64–4.

COMPLICATIONS OF TRANSFUSION (pp. 355–357)

An approach to prevention of transfusion reactions is outlined in Table 64–5.

TABLE 64–4. CALCULATION OF AMOUNT OF PLASMA NEEDED TO REPLACE ALBUMIN DEFICIT

Normal albumin (40% intravascular + 60% extravascular) = 3.5 gm/dl

Step 1: Normal plasma volume = A = 4.5% of body weight (kg)

Step 2: Normal plasma albumin (g) = 3.5 (gm/dl) $\times$ A (dl)

Step 3: Patient plasma albumin (g) = patient albumin (gm/dl) $\times$ A (dl)

Step 4: Plasma deficit = B = normal plasma albumin (gm) - patient plasma albumin (gm)

Step 5: Total albumin deficit = T = (B/40) $\times$ 100 (gm)

Step 6: Plasma units needed = T (gm)/5 gm* = _____

*Approximately 5 gm albumin/unit canine plasma.

TABLE 64–5. MEASURES TO PREVENT
TRANSFUSION REACTIONS

Proper handling of the blood before, during, and after collection
Crossmatch if red cell preparations are administered, or
Use universal donor blood
Proper handling of the blood prior to and during administration
Proper prophylaxis
Proper monitoring during administration (Table 64–5 in textbook)

Disease Transmission.   It is imperative that potential blood donors be screened for certain potentially infectious diseases. The extent of screening is determined by geographic area.

Hypothermia.   Cold blood components can lead to hypothermia in severely debilitated animals, in neonates, in young puppies or kittens, and in small-breed dogs.

Metabolic Abnormalities.   Citrate toxicity is occasionally observed if large amounts of components, especially plasma, are administered rapidly. The result is hypocalcemia. Storage of red cell components leads to accumulation of ammonia. This may be a cause for concern in patients with renal or hepatic disease.

Febrile Reactions.   Fever may be caused by a multitude of factors—infectious, immunologic, and hemolytic. The febrile response may be the first clinical sign of a more severe reaction.

Allergic Reactions.   Allergic reactions are usually immediate, and typical clinical signs include facial edema, pruritus, and urticaria. Most allergic reactions will resolve after administration of antihistamines and glucocorticoids. The transfusion should not be resumed until the patient is stable and only if it is necessary.

Hemolytic Reactions.   These can be due to mishandling of the blood product prior to transfusion or may be immune-mediated. Clinical signs vary, but signs of hypotension and shock predominate, followed by hemoglobinemia, hemoglobinuria, DIC, and acute oliguric renal failure.

BLOOD BANKING FOR THE SMALL ANIMAL PRACTITIONER (pp. 357–360)

See textbook.

CHAPTER 65

SMALL ANIMAL ZOONOSES
(pages 362–367)

PARASITIC DISEASES (pp. 362–364)

VISCERAL LARVA MIGRANS

Visceral larva migrans may occur following human ingestion of the infective ova of the roundworm *Toxocara canis*. Migration of larvae occasionally can cause significant eosinophilic granulomatous reactions in the myocardium and central nervous system. Larval migration in the eye (ocular larva migrans) may lead to blindness. Most clinical cases occur in young children (1 to 4 years old). Prompt disposal of fecal material before ova can become infective is important in the prevention of human disease.

CUTANEOUS LARVA MIGRANS

Cutaneous larva migrans occurs following the penetration of the infective larvae of *Ancylostoma caninum* (dogs) or *A. braziliense* (dogs, cats, other carnivores) through the intact skin of human beings. The parasite causes intense pruritus as it migrates through the dermal tissue before being destroyed by the immune system. Preventive measures described for control of roundworms should be used.

DIPYLIDIASIS

Human beings may become infested with the adult tapeworm *Dipylidium caninum* following ingestion of the intermediate host, the flea. Human infestation usually shows no clinical signs.
Prevention. Is through flea control.

ECHINOCOCCOSIS

Human ingestion of the ova of *Echinococcus granulosus* leads to cyst formation in the liver, lungs, and other organs. It is a potentially fatal disease in man. Sheep act as the primary intermediate host for the parasite, and most dogs are infested through the ingestion of sheep entrails.

Both the dog and the cat may be definitive hosts for *Echinococcus multilocularis*. The cysts grow by exogenous budding and lead to a serious and potentially fatal disease in human beings.

Original chapter written by James B. Miller

Prevention. If *E. granulosus* is diagnosed in a dog, the animal should be treated appropriately and the owner should be informed of the public health significance.

DIROFILARIASIS

The transmission of the parasite to human beings can occur via the mosquito. Human dirofilariasis is caused by emboli of dead larvae of the parasite in the lung. The disease is frequently asymptomatic.

Prevention. Is dependent on decreasing the incidence of canine dirofilariasis.

TOXOPLASMOSIS

Human infection occurs with ingestion of trophozoites in raw or undercooked meat, ingestion of oocyst from cat feces, and by transplacental route. The disease rarely causes clinical manifestations in adult humans unless they are immunocompromised. Congenital infection presents the greatest threat to human beings.

Prevention. Pregnant women should not clean cat litter boxes; they should be cautious when working in gardens and clean all garden vegetables well before eating.

GIARDIASIS

Transmission to man has not been established.

CRYPTOSPORIDIOSIS

Cryptosporidia have been the cause of diarrhea in man. Infection in humans is often asymptomatic or self-limiting except in immunosuppressed patients, in whom the disease may be fatal.

ROCKY MOUNTAIN SPOTTED FEVER

RMSF is a rickettsial disease caused by *Rickettsia rickettsi*. Although the disease may be subclinical, signs of vasculitis occur in humans.

Prevention. Dogs should be checked daily for the presence of ticks during times of the year when ticks are abundant.

EHRLICHIOSIS

Recent evidence suggests that human beings may become infected with *Ehrlichia canis* or a similar organism. The human disease causes fever, nausea, vomiting, rash, and weight loss.

Prevention. Tick control similar to RMSF would be appropriate.

PLAGUE

Infection with the bacterium *Yersinia pestis* causes plague in human beings, dogs, and cats. Wild rodents serve as the primary reservoir. Transmission occurs when the animal is bitten by a flea from an infected rodent or by ingestion of an infected rodent.

Prevention. Prevention is best accomplished by not allowing pet exposure to wild rodents in endemic areas.

TULAREMIA

The bacterium *Francisella tularensis* causes tularemia in humans, dogs, and cats. Rabbits and rodents appear to be the primary reservoir for the disease. The disease is transmitted by blood-sucking arthropods. Symptoms include pulmonary signs and lymphadenopathy.

Prevention. Prevention is dependent primarily on prevention of pet exposure to the wild reservoir.

LYME DISEASE

Lyme disease is caused by the spirochete *Borrelia burgdorferi*. It is still unclear whether there should be concern for zoonotic potential from dog to man.

LEISHMANIASIS

Visceral leishmaniasis is a chronic protozoal disease of human beings transmitted by the sandfly and caused by *Leishmania donovani*.

Prevention.   There appears to be little means by which the veterinarian can help in the prevention of animal-to-human transmission other than destroying an infected animal.

BACTERIAL/RICKETTSIAL INFECTIONS (pp. 365–366)

BRUCELLOSIS

Human infection with *Brucella canis* is by direct transmission from genitourinary secretions of infected dogs. Human illness is characterized by fever, headache, and myalgia.

Prevention.   It is reasonable to recommend that all positive testing dogs be neutered.

LEPTOSPIROSIS

Human infection may occur following exposure to urine, blood, or tissues from infected dogs.

Prevention.   Prevention is primarily through vaccinating dogs against the disease.

Q FEVER

Q fever is a rickettsial disease caused by the organism *Coxiella burnetii*. The domestic cat may be a source for transmission to human beings. The human disease is characterized by fever, respiratory signs, and cardiac signs.

Prevention.   Gloves and masks should be worn for the handling of fetal and placental tissues from aborting cats.

CAMPYLOBACTERIOSIS AND SALMONELLOSIS

Both dogs and cats may harbor *Campylobacter jejuni* and a variety of nontyphoidal *Salmonella* species. Bacteria have been isolated from the feces of healthy animals. Most cases of human enteric disease are not associated with pet exposure.

CAT SCRATCH DISEASE

Cat scratch disease occurs in human beings following cat scratches or the handling of cats. The disease is characterized by a primary papule or pustule, followed in several weeks by regional lymphadenopathy.

Prevention.   Prevention is best accomplished by advising cat owners of ways to avoid exposure.

GROUP A STREPTOCOCCAL INFECTIONS

Group A streptococcal infections in human beings can lead to asymptomatic carrier states, sore throat, otitis externa, systemic bacteremia, rheumatic fever, or poststreptococcal glomerulonephritis. Humans are the natural reservoir for the bacteria, but dogs and, occasionally, cats can harbor the bacteria in the oral pharynx.

MYCOTIC DISEASES (p. 366)

DERMATOMYCOSIS

Direct transmission of *Microsporum canis* from dogs and cats does occur. Owners should wash their hands well following the handling of an infected dog or cat.

SPOROTRICHOSIS

Recent reports indicate that infected cats can transmit the infection directly to human beings.

MISCELLANEOUS DISEASES (pp. 366–367)

RABIES

Despite the low incidence of human rabies in this country, the near 100 per cent mortality rate in human beings makes the prevention of this zoonosis of particular importance.

Prevention. Many effective vaccines are available for use to protect both dogs and cats from rabies. It is important to have owners understand that there is still a large reservoir of endemic rabies, especially in skunks and bats.

FLEAS AND MITES

Canine and feline scabies (*Sarcoptes scabiei* var. *canis* and *Notoedres cati*), cheyletiellosis (*Cheyletiella* spp.), and fleas (*Ctenocephalides* spp. and *Pulex* spp.) can all have zoonotic potential.

CHAPTER 66

BACTERIAL DISEASES
(pages 367–376)

SALMONELLOSIS (pp. 367–368)

Source of Infection. The most common source of infection, which occurs through the gastrointestinal route, is contact with contaminated food, water, or fomites.

Clinical Signs. Clinical findings in salmonellosis vary (see textbook). The syndromes can be artificially divided into gastroenteritis, bacteremia/endotoxemia, organ localization, and persistence of an asymptomatic carrier state.

Diagnosis. Diagnosis is based on clinical suspicion. Isolation of *Salmonella* organisms is the most definitive means. However, mere isolation from the gastrointestinal tract does not indicate that the organisms are causing clinical disease. Finding organisms in samples of normally sterile secretions or body fluids or tissues allows for the most definitive diagnosis of systemic salmonellosis.

Original chapter written by Craig E. Greene

Treatment. Acute *Salmonella* gastroenteritis, without systemic signs, is best treated with parenteral polyionic isotonic fluids. Routine antimicrobial treatment may not be indicated because *Salmonella* gastroenteritis is usually self-limiting (see textbook).

Prevention. Prevention involves hygiene and strict isolation of infected animals.

CAMPYLOBACTERIOSIS (pp. 368–369)

Source of Infection. Fecal contamination can serve as sources of infection.

Clinical Signs. In general, animals are asymptomatic carriers. When clinical illness develops, it is usually in animals less than 6 months of age. *Campylobacter*-associated diarrhea has a wide clinical spectrum.

Diagnosis. Fresh fecal samples are examined microscopically for *C. jejuni*. Culture the organism from feces on specific *Campylobacter* media. Gross and microscopic lesions are an acute to chronic ileocecocolitis.

Treatment. Erythromycin is the drug of choice for *Campylobacter*-induced diarrhea.

TYZZER'S DISEASE (p. 369)

Sources of Infection. Dogs and cats presumably acquire infection by contact with or ingestion of rodent feces.

Clinical Signs. Include lethargy, depression, anorexia, abdominal discomfort, hepatomegaly, abdominal distention, hypothermia, obtundation, and death within 24 to 48 hours. Scant amounts of pasty feces are characteristic. Icterus in cats has been apparent.

Diagnosis. Diagnosis is usually limited to necropsy because of the rapid progress of this disease.

Treatment. Treatment has not been successful.

L-FORM INFECTIONS (p. 369)

Cell wall–deficient or L-form bacteria have been isolated from cats with a syndrome of fever and persistently draining, spreading cellulitis and synovitis. The condition usually involves the extremities. Infection may result in polyarthritis or distant abscess formation. Tetracycline is the treatment of choice.

MYCOBACTERIOSIS (pp. 369–370)

Dogs and cats are susceptible to infections by *M. tuberculosis* and *M. bovis* but are relatively resistant to infection by *M. avium*. Tubercle bacilli induce granuloma formation at the site of inoculation, usually the respiratory or gastrointestinal tracts or the local lymph nodes. Host immunity determines whether the infection is contained or spreads from these sites. The *nontuberculous* forms include feline leprosy, caused by *M. lepraemurium*. Transmission is thought to occur from contact with infected rats.

Clinical Signs. Tubercular mycobacterial infections: bronchopneumonia, pulmonary nodule formation, hilar lymphadenopathy, fever, weight loss, anorexia, and harsh, nonproductive coughing. Cats develop primary intestinal localization more commonly than dogs, and exhibit weight loss, anemia, vomiting, and diarrhea. With dissemination, the clinical signs reflect the organ system of involvement.

The lesions associated with feline leprosy are usually soft, fleshy, focal nodules in the skin and subcutis, and occur most often on the head and extremities of healthy-appearing cats. Atypical mycobacteriosis in cats most commonly occurs with multiple fistulous draining tracts associated with purulent drainage into the caudal abdominal, inguinal, and lumbar subcutaneous tissues.

Diagnosis. Radiographically visible masses may be seen in the chest, abdomen, or skeleton. Culture is the definitive means of identifying the specific mycobacterial agent; however, these pathogens are slow-growing, requiring special media and several weeks to establish visible colonies. Definitive diagnoses can be made by demonstrating organisms within a lesion via biopsy and histologic examination of the lesion or via direct smears of exudates or fluids. Lepromatous infections in cats demonstrate large numbers of acid-fast bacilli. Confirming atypical mycobacteriosis is not always easy. Bacterial culture is essential for definitive diagnosis.

Treatment. The zoonotic aspect of a pet harboring *M. tuberculosis* must be considered. Dogs and cats usually are euthanized. Surgical removal of lepromatous granulomas is the desired treatment. Atypical mycobacteria respond variably to aminoglycosides, tetracyclines, and quinolones.

BRUCELLOSIS (pp. 370–371)

Brucella canis causes an insidious bacteremia and reproductive disturbances.

Clinical Signs. The main features seen in male dogs are epididymitis and scrotal enlargement or dermatitis. Pregnant bitches usually abort dead pups following 40 to 60 days of gestation, but show no other clinical signs. Conception failures can also occur. Nonreproductive abnormalities may include spinal hyperesthesia, paresis, or paralysis. Recurrent anterior uveitis has been described.

Diagnosis. Serologic testing is the most frequently used method for detecting canine brucellosis. The tube agglutination test (TAT) is used by some laboratories following a positive RSAT to confirm and quantitate a titer. Hemoculture is the only definitive diagnostic method.

Treatment. Therapy of *B. canis* is difficult because of the intracellular persistence, and relapses are common once antimicrobial therapy is discontinued. It is recommended that brucella-positive pets be neutered. Combination therapy with tetracyclines and aminoglycosides offers the best chance for eliminating infection. Gentamicin with doxycycline or minocycline is suggested.

ACTINOMYCOSIS AND NOCARDIOSIS (pp. 371–372)

Actinomyces infection follows puncture wounds or tissue trauma. *Nocardia* enters the body through contamination of wounds or by respiratory inhalation.

Clinical Signs. Actinomycosis produces localized pyogranulomatous infections, including localized abscesses, chronic draining fistulas, bony infections, and infections of body cavities. The drainage often contains small yellow granules. Paraspinal or appendicular osteomyelitis may occur. *Nocardia* may cause clinical syndromes similar to those of actinomycosis. A disseminated form has been seen, primarily in young dogs.

Diagnosis. Cytologic examination of lesion exudate is most helpful, particularly if granules are present. Preparations consist of colonies of gram-positive branching, filamentous rods and cocci. Definitive diagnosis is obtained through culture.

Treatment. For both diseases, this involves surgical drainage and debridement of affected areas except in disseminated cases. For *Actinomyces*, treatment with anaerobic antimicrobials such as penicillin, chloramphenicol, or clindamycin is indicated. For *Nocardia* infections, trimethoprim-sulfonamide is the first choice, followed by aminoglycosides or tetracyclines. Treatment is usually for a 6-week period.

STREPTOCOCCOSIS (p. 372)

Group A streptococci are primarily commensal and pathogenic in people. *S. pneumoniae* has been isolated in only one case—from a cat. *Group B streptococci* have been reported to cause endometritis, with birth of pups that develop bacteremia, pyelonephritis, and necrotizing pneumonia. *Group C streptococci* have been described only in dogs with hemorrhagic and purulent pneumonia. *Group G streptococci* in neonatal animals cause cervical lymphadenitis, which may spread to joints in surviving juveniles. As with other streptococci, those in group G are sensitive to penicillin.

RHODOCOCCOSIS (p. 372)

R. equi has been isolated from abscesses in cats. Diagnosis is made by culture, and treatment involves surgical drainage and antimicrobial therapy.

BORRELIOSIS (pp. 372–373)

This is a complex multiorgan disorder caused by the spirochete *Borrelia burgdorferi.*
Clinical Signs.   In dogs these include fever, inappetence, lethargy, lymphadenopathy, and episodic lameness related to polyarthritis. Renal glomerular lesions may develop.
Laboratory Findings.   Findings on synovial fluid analysis may reveal a suppurative polyarthritis, with leukocyte counts ranging from 2000 to 100,000 nucleated cells/μl. IgM titers usually increase within the first weeks of infection, and then the response is mainly that of IgG. Antibody titers between clinically ill and asymptomatic dogs often overlap in endemic areas, making titer information difficult to interpret. Identification or isolation of *B. burgdorferi* from tissues or body fluids is definitive but extremely difficult.
Treatment.   The antibiotics that are most effective for treating borreliosis are tetracycline, ampicillin, and erythromycin and its derivatives. Doxycycline is usually the drug of first choice for treatment of dogs with acute infections.

LEPTOSPIROSIS (pp. 373–374)

Leptospirosis is caused by infection with the motile spirochetal bacterium *Leptospira interrogans. L. icterohaemorrhagiae, L. canicola,* and *L. grippotyphosa* are the most common serovars isolated from dogs. Clinical reports in cats are rare.
Clinical Signs.   Peracute infections are manifested by massive leptospiremia, shock, and death. Less severe infections are manifested by fever, anorexia, vomiting, dehydration, increased thirst, and reluctance to move. Progressive deterioration in renal function is manifested by oliguria or anuria. Icterus is common in some cases.
Hematologic findings include leukocytosis and thrombocytopenia. Serum urea nitrogen and creatinine concentration increases are found with varying severity of renal failure. Liver damage is demonstrated by high serum hepatic transaminase activity and bilirubinuria. Demonstration of a fourfold rise in a titer is often required for serologic confirmation of disease. The urine is the best fluid for darkfield examination and culture purposes.
Treatment.   Fluids must be given to overcome shock and dehy-

dration, and chemical diuresis with osmotic agents or tubular diuretics is needed for oliguric patients. Penicillin is the antibiotic of choice for terminating leptospiremia. Following recovery, tetracyclines should be given to eradicate the carrier state.

TETANUS (p. 374)

Tetanus is caused by the action of a potent neurotoxin formed in the body by *Clostridium tetani*. Environmentally resistant spores enter the body when wounds become contaminated. Dogs and cats are relatively resistant to the effects of the toxin.

Clinical Signs. Signs usually occur within 5 days to 3 weeks of injury. Localized tetanus is manifested by increased stiffness of a muscle or entire limb. The stiffness usually spreads gradually from there and may involve the entire nervous system. The animal with tetanus holds its ears erect and has its ears and facial muscles drawn back with protrusion of the third eyelid. Other signs include trismus, increased salivation, altered heart and respiratory rates, laryngeal spasm, and dysphagia. Mild stimulation may precipitate tonic contraction of all muscles or grand mal convulsions. Death results from respiratory dysfunction.

Diagnosis. The history of a recent wound and the clinical signs are the primary means of making a diagnosis of tetanus.

Treatment. Mildly diseased animals will recover with wound management alone. Antitoxin is administered IV. Precautions must be taken to reduce anaphylaxis. Local and parenteral antibiotic therapy should be instituted in an attempt to kill any vegetative *C. tetani* organisms present in the wound. Penicillin G is the drug of choice. Sedation with phenothiazines may be needed for excitable animals, even though they are contraindicated in most seizure disorders. Supportive measures are imperative. Fluids and tracheostomy, esophagostomy, or gastrostomy tubes may be needed.

BOTULISM (pp. 374–375)

Clostridium botulinum produces a neurotoxin that causes neuromuscular paralysis. Most cases are caused by ingestion of the preformed toxin in food. There are no reports of the naturally occurring disease in cats.

Clinical Signs. Signs consist of a symmetric, ascending weakness from the rear to the forelimbs. Limb reflexes are depressed and cranial nerve motor responses are affected, causing mydriasis, decreased jaw tone, decreased gag reflexes, and excess salivation. Megaesophagus may be present. Pain perception is intact. Death may result from respiratory paralysis.

Diagnosis. The diagnosis is confirmed by finding the toxin in serum, feces, vomitus, or samples of ingested food.

Treatment. Supportive treatment is most important, since spontaneous recovery will occur in moderately affected animals if the respiratory and urinary tract infections can be avoided. Penicillin or metronidazole has been recommended to reduce any potential intestinal population of *Clostridia*.

FELINE ABSCESSES (p. 375)

Abscesses usually result from bites and scratches. The most common organisms found within them are resident oral microflora, and anaerobes predominate.

Clinical Signs. Abscesses are usually located around the cat's legs, face, back, and base of the tail. Some cats develop mild swellings with few other signs of illness; others have fever, anorexia, depression, hyperesthesia, and regional lymphadenopathy. In complicated cases, the abscess can migrate in tissues or infection can disseminate hematogenously.

Treatment.   Deeper or more extensive abscesses require surgical drainage. Antibiotics alone are ineffective. Penicillin derivatives are the antibiotics of choice. Drugs such as metronidazole can be used if discharges suggest a predominance of anaerobic infection.

CHAPTER 67
THE RICKETTSIOSES
(pages 376–383)

ROCKY MOUNTAIN SPOTTED FEVER (pp. 376–378)

The causative agent, *Rickettsia rickettsii*, induces direct cytopathic vascular endothelial injury. Distribution of the disease is related to the distribution of the vector ticks *Dermacentor variabilis*, found in the eastern United States, and *Dermacentor andersoni*, the principal vector in the western United States. Rickettsiae cause direct damage to endothelial cells, resulting in vascular inflammation, necrosis, and, subsequently, increased vascular permeability. Central nervous system edema may contribute to the development of neurologic signs. Myocardial inflammation can induce potentially life-threatening arrhythmias. Pulmonary edema may cause tachypnea, dyspnea, or coughing. Ocular abnormalities, including subconjunctival hemorrhage, retinal petechiae, and focal areas of retinal edema, and perivascular inflammatory cell infiltrate may occur. Gangrene may affect the distal extremities, scrotum, mammary glands, nose, or lips. In severe cases, decreased renal perfusion can predispose to acute renal failure.

Other clinical abnormalities include fever, anorexia, depression, mucopurulent ocular discharge, scleral injection, tachypnea, coughing, vomiting, diarrhea, muscle pain, neutrophilic polyarthritis, hyperesthesia, ataxia, vestibular signs, stupor, seizures, and coma. Retinal hemorrhages are a consistent finding. Epistaxis, melena, hematuria, and petechial to ecchymotic hemorrhages occur in some dogs. Scrotal edema, hyperemia, hemorrhage, and epididymal pain are frequently observed in male dogs.

DIAGNOSIS

Seasonal occurrence, history of tick infestation, fever, and the clinical findings should suggest RMSF. Thrombocytopenia is the most consistent hematologic finding. Leukopenia is followed by progressive leukocytosis. Anemia may occur. Hypoproteinemia, hypoalbuminemia, azotemia, hyponatremia, hypocalcemia, and increased liver enzymes may occur. Synovial and cerebrospinal fluid analyses generally reflect a mild increase in protein and neutrophils.

Confirmation of a diagnosis requires direct immunofluorescent testing for *R. rickettsii* antigen in tissue biopsy and necropsy specimens, serologic testing, or rickettsial culture. Documentation of a fourfold or greater increase in antibody titer between acute and convalescent sera confirms a diagnosis.

Original chapter written by Edward B. Breitschwerdt

TREATMENT

Tetracyline is the treatment of choice. Chloramphenicol and enrofloxacin are equally effective. Due to severe vascular damage, fluid therapy should be utilized with caution.

CANINE MONOCYTIC EHRLICHIOSIS (pp. 378–380)

The distribution of ehrlichiosis is related to the distribution of the vector tick, *Rhipicephalus sanguineus*. Clinical signs during the acute phase of disease will vary from depression, anorexia, and fever to severe loss of stamina, weight loss, ocular and nasal discharges, dyspnea, lymphadenopathy, and edema of the limbs or scrotum. Despite moderate to severe thrombocytopenia, hemorrhages are rarely observed. A variety of central nervous system signs, including hyperesthesia, muscle twitching, and cranial nerve deficits, may occur. Clinical findings in the acute phase can be identical to those of canine RMSF.

Clinical signs associated with the chronic phase would be characterized as mild to asymptomatic in some dogs but severe in other dogs. A combination of bleeding tendencies, pallor due to anemia, severe weight loss, debilitation, abdominal tenderness, anterior uveitis, retinal hemorrhages, and neurologic signs consistent with meningoencephalitis typify dogs that are affected chronically. Epistaxis, once considered a hallmark of the disease, occurs infrequently.

Hematologic abnormalities including pancytopenia, aplastic anemia, and thrombocytopenia would be consistent with *E. canis* infection. Finding *E. canis* morulae in peripheral blood smears or buffy-coat smears is diagnostic. Morulae are generally found only during the first 2 weeks following infection and usually in low numbers.

Anemia will vary in degree of severity. Positive Coombs' tests suggest that autoimmune damage can contribute to an acute hemolytic crisis in some dogs. However, a nonregenerative anemia is most frequently documented in chronically infected dogs. Bone marrow examination usually reveals a hypocellular marrow. Plasmacytosis is a frequently reported bone marrow finding in ehrlichiosis.

Hyperglobulinemia is characterized by increased beta and/or gamma globulins. Serum protein electrophoresis may reveal a polyclonal or monoclonal gammopathy. Hypoalbuminemia occurs. In the chronic disease phase, *E. canis* can induce a severe protein-losing nephropathy. Serologic diagnosis of ehrlichiosis is currently the only widely available procedure for confirming a diagnosis. A positive titer is considered indicative of infection. Infection with *E. canis* does not confer protective immunity; therefore, subsequent exposure to infected ticks after treatment will result in disease.

Tetracycline or doxycycline represents the treatment of choice for ehrlichiosis. Chloramphenicol and enrofloxacin may be effective. Although imidocarb dipropionate has gained clinical acceptance, lack of efficacy has been demonstrated in some dogs. The prognosis for canine ehrlichiosis is generally good.

CANINE GRANULOCYTIC EHRLICHIOSIS (p. 380)

E. equi has a broad host range, including dogs. *E. ewingii* has been most frequently described in dogs in Missouri, Oklahoma, and Tennessee. Clinical signs include lameness, muscular stiffness, a stilted gait, reluctance to rise, and joint swelling and pain. Polyarthritis is the most frequently reported abnormality. Detection of morulae in granulocytic cells in conjunction with *E. canis* seropositivity can be used to confirm a clinical diagnosis. Tetracycline or doxycycline elicits rapid improvement in clinical status.

CANINE CYCLIC THROMBOCYTOPENIA (pp. 380–381)

Canine cyclic thrombocytopenia is caused by *E. platys*, a rickettsial organism that replicates only in platelets. The mode of transmission is presumed to be by tick vector. The organism is considered to be minimally pathogenic and is generally recognized as an incidental observation during blood smear examination. It causes thrombocytopenia at approximately 10- to 14-day intervals. At its nadir, thrombocytopenia can be severe (20,000 to 50,000 platelets/µl). Diagnosis requires visualization of rickettsiae in platelets or detection of antibodies by indirect immunofluorescence in a serum sample. Treatment with oral tetracycline or presumably doxycycline should eliminate the organism.

FELINE EHRLICHIOSIS (p. 381)

Although the precise clinical significance of this disease awaits the results of future studies, it seems probable that cats can be infected by one or more rickettsia of the genus *Ehrlichia*. Serologic evidence of ehrlichiosis was detected in 12 sick cats with clinical and laboratory abnormalities including fever, malaise, weight loss, anorexia, lymphadenopathy, nonseptic suppurative polyarthritis, anemia, thrombocytopenia, neutropenia, and polyclonal or monoclonal gammopathy. Each of these cats responded favorably to doxycycline.

SALMON POISONING DISEASE (p. 381)

Salmon poisoning disease is caused by two rickettsiae, *Neorickettsia helminthoeca* and the Elokomin fluke fever agent. It is limited geographically to the coastal areas of Washington, Oregon, and California, and is characterized by a sudden onset of fever (higher than 40°C), depression, and anorexia. Vomiting and diarrhea, accompanied by weight loss, contribute to dehydration and hypokalemia. There is progressive lymph node enlargement and splenomegaly. In untreated dogs, death usually occurs 7 to 10 days after the onset of clinical signs. The diagnosis can be implied by the discovery of operculated trematode eggs in dog feces. Identification of rickettsial inclusion bodies on a lymph node aspirate confirms the disease. Tetracycline is the drug of choice.

HEMOBARTONELLOSIS (pp. 381–382)

Haemobartonella are differentiated on the basis of their host range and include *H. felis*, infecting cats, and *H. canis*, infecting dogs. It is probable that transmission of *H. felis* occurs by bloodsucking arthropods and potentially by cat-bite wounds.

Feline hemobartonellosis is characterized by acute or chronic anemia, pallor, weight loss, anorexia, and occasionally splenomegaly or icterus. Many infected cats become Coombs' test–positive, indicating the presence of infection-induced antierythrocyte antibodies. Without therapy, approximately one-third of cats with acute hemobartonellosis die as a result of severe anemia. Cats that recover without treatment develop recurrent episodes of rickettsemia and remain chronically infected for months to years, if not indefinitely. Chronically infected carrier cats appear clinically normal, but may have a mild regenerative anemia. Failure to visualize *H. felis* organisms on a blood smear does not eliminate the possibility that hemobartonellosis is responsible for anemia.

Risk factors include anemia, FeLV-positive status, lack of vaccinations, a history of cat-bite abscesses, age under 4 years, and outdoor roaming status. Immunosuppression potentiates visualization of rickettsia on blood smears and may influence disease susceptibility and severity.

It is generally accepted that *H. canis* is an incidental finding during blood smear examination, that the rickettsia is of minimal pathogenic significance, and that concurrent infectious or noninfectious disease should be sought in a rickettsemic dog. Tetracycline appears to be the treatment of choice.

COXIELLA BURNETII (p. 382)

The extent to which *C. burnetii* causes illness in cats or dogs remains unclear.

ROCHALIMAEA HENSELAE (pp. 382–383)

Recent evidence indicates that cat scratch disease in people is most frequently caused by *Rochalimaea henselae*, and less frequently by *Afipia felis*. Exposure to *R. henselae* is prevalent in the healthy cat population. Until the zoonotic potential of *R. henselae* infection in cats has been determined, the potential risk of cat ownership for immunocompromised humans should not be underestimated.

CHAPTER 68

PROTOZOAL AND MISCELLANEOUS INFECTIONS
(pages 384–397)

ENTERIC PROTOZOAL DISEASES (pp. 384–386)

TRICHOMONIASIS

Trichomoniasis is caused by *Pentatrichomonas hominis*. Whether the trichomonads are actually pathogenic and cause the diarrhea has not been established.

AMEBIASIS

Amebiasis is caused by *Entamoeba histolytica*. Transmission is by the direct fecal-oral route. Infections may be inapparent or may cause large intestinal disease ranging from mild catarrhal inflammation to severe ulcerative colitis. Anorexia and weight loss may also be seen. Diagnosis is made by identification of trophozoites on examination of direct fecal smears or biopsy specimens of colonic mucosa. Metronidazole is the treatment of choice.

BALANTIDIASIS

Balantidiasis is caused by *Balantidium coli*. Most canine infections are probably inapparent, but severe large intestinal diarrhea can occur. Diagnosis is made by demonstrating ciliated trophozoites on direct fecal smears or spherical cysts using zinc sulfate flotation. Metronidazole or tetracycline should prove effective in dogs.

Original chapter written by Joseph Taboada and Sandra R. Merchant

ENTERIC COCCIDIOSIS

Most coccidial infections in dogs and cats are subclinical. Puppies, kittens, immunosuppressed animals, and animals stressed by concurrent illness are more likely to have diarrhea. Diagnosis is based on demonstration of oocysts in the feces.

Cystoisospora

Oocysts are often found in association with diarrheic stools, especially in puppies and kittens. Whether the coccidia are the cause of the diarrhea or just incidentally present is difficult to determine. Sulfonamides are efficacious, but most small animals are believed capable of spontaneously eliminating *Cystoisospora* spp. infections.

Cryptosporidium

Cryptosporidium parvum infects the microvilli of host small intestinal epithelial cells and has been associated with severe gastroenteritis in animals and humans. Infection is most likely in neonates and immunocompromised animals. Diagnosis is made by demonstrating *Cryptosporidium* in intestinal biopsy specimens, gastroduodenal aspirates, and feces. An accurate enzyme-linked immunosorbent assay (ELISA) procedure to detect cryptosporidial antigen in feces has also been developed. No drug has shown efficacy against cryptosporidiosis in the dog and cat, but infections in immunocompetent animals are self-limiting.

Hammondia, Besnoitia, and Sarcocystis

Clinical disease has not been attributed to *Hammondia* or *Besnoitia*.

Sarcocystis. *Sarcocystis* species are generally not considered pathogenic for dogs and cats, but fatal, possibly *Sarcocystis*-induced, encephalitis, dermatitis, and myocarditis has been reported in rottweilers. Disseminated sarcocystosis has been reported in a cat with lymphosarcoma.

GIARDIASIS

Giardiasis is caused by *Giardia intestinalis*, a flagellate protozoan parasite of the intestinal tract of many host species.

Clinical Features. When signs are noted, acute or chronic malabsorptive diarrhea is characteristic. The feces are usually pale, malodorous, and soft. The affected animal may have weight loss, poor weight gain, or anorexia. Occasionally, animals are presented with signs indicative of large intestinal disease.

Diagnosis. Diagnosis is made by demonstration of *Giardia* or *Giardia* antigen in feces or aspirates of intestinal contents. The simplest way of demonstrating trophozoites is by direct fecal smear. Concentration techniques such as zinc sulfate flotation increase the likelihood of finding cysts. At least three samples should be examined. ELISA kits for the detection of *Giardia* antigen in feces are available.

Treatment. Metronidazole and quinacrine are the drugs used most often to treat dogs and cats with giardiasis. Neither drug is 100 per cent effective. Albendazole has recently proved safe and effective for treating *Giardia* infections in dogs.

NONENTERIC COCCIDIAN PROTOZOAL DISEASE
(pp. 386–390)

TOXOPLASMOSIS

Toxoplasmosis is caused by *Toxoplasma gondii*, an obligate intracellular coccidian parasite with a world-wide distribution. The domestic cat and other Felidae are the definitive hosts, and many species of animals can serve as intermediate hosts.

Clinical Features.

Clinical Features in the Cat. *Toxoplasma* can affect any organ system in the cat. Clinical manifestations may include anorexia, lethargy, fever, weight loss, diarrhea, vomiting, icterus, respiratory disease, muscle hyperesthesia, lameness, pancreatitis, abdominal effusion, central nervous system disease, ocular dysfunction, myocardial disorders, and sudden death. Disease varies from mild and self-limiting to fatal. The organs most commonly affected are the eyes and the lungs. Approximately 75 per cent of cats with anterior uveitis are seropositive for *Toxoplasma*. Transplacentally infected kittens may be stillborn or die shortly after birth. Cats infected with (FIV) are more likely to become infected with *Toxoplasma* and are more likely to have severe clinical disease.

Clinical Features in the Dog. Clinical illness is rare in dogs. Two forms of disease are primarily observed: (1) severe, often fatal multisystemic disease and (2) disease localized to the central and peripheral nervous systems. Generalized infections and infections localized to the respiratory and gastrointestinal systems are usually rapidly fatal and seen most commonly in dogs less than 1 year of age. Most reported cases have been in dogs concurrently infected with distemper. Dogs with nervous system involvement usually lack other signs. Lower motor neuron disease with spastic rigidity in the hind limbs is most commonly reported, especially in puppies. Neurologic signs in adult dogs may include hyperexcitability, depression, tremor, paresis, paralysis, and seizures. Concurrent distemper virus infection is common.

Diagnosis. Creatinine kinase is often increased owing to muscle cell damage. Thoracic radiographs reveal a diffuse interstitial to alveolar pattern that may have a patchy lobar distribution. Mild pleural effusion is occasionally seen. CSF is characterized by increased protein and a lymphocytic pleocytosis, with neutrophils occasionally seen. Rarely, tachyzoites may be noted.

Definitive antemortem diagnosis can be difficult. Because *Toxoplasma* organisms are rarely detected, serologic examination becomes the primary means of diagnosis. Paired titers revealing a fourfold increase can document recent infection. However, many cats are not evaluated until after their IgG titer has reached its maximum. A positive IgM titer should always be interpreted in light of the total clinical picture. Criteria for an antemortem diagnosis of clinical feline toxoplasmosis have been proposed (Table 68–1).

Treatment. Clindamycin is the drug of choice for treating clinical toxoplasmosis in dogs and cats. Cats with anterior uveitis may require the addition of topical or parenteral corticosteroids. The combination of rapid-acting sulfonamides and pyrimethamine is synergistic in the treatment of toxoplasmosis. However, there is a high incidence of side effects, making this regimen less suitable than clindamycin.

NEOSPOROSIS

N. caninum is a recently recognized protozoan parasite of dogs and other animals that has previously been confused with *T. gondii*. The

TABLE 68–1. ANTEMORTEM DIAGNOSIS OF CLINICAL FELINE TOXOPLASMOSIS

Demonstration of serologic evidence of recent or active infection
    IgM titer >1:256
    Increasing IgG titer
    Circulating antigens without antibodies
Clinical signs of disease referable to toxoplasmosis
Exclusion of other common etiologies
Response to appropriate treatment

clinical signs vary with the organ system involved and are indistinguishable from toxoplasmosis. The most severe disease occurs in transplacentally infected puppies. Signs begin after 4 weeks of age and consist of stiffness, ataxia, and muscle atrophy that progress to rigid contracture of the hind limbs. The retina, choroid, and extraocular muscles are also commonly involved. Adult dogs may have localized or generalized disease. Central nervous system involvement as well as polymyositis, myocarditis, hepatitis, dermatitis, and multifocal dissemination has been reported.

Definitive diagnosis of neosporosis is dependent on demonstration of *Neospora* tachyzoites or tissue cysts in infected nervous tissues. Tachyzoites may be found in cerebrospinal fluid or in tissue from many organs. Clindamycin, sulfadiazine, trimethoprim, and pyrimethamine have been used to treat dogs with neosporosis, but successful treatment has not been reported.

HEPATOZOONOSIS

Hepatozoon canis is the causative agent. In the United States it is limited to the area around the Gulf Coast. Transmission is primarily via ingestion of the vector tick, *Rhipicephalus sanguineus*.

Clinical Features.   Concurrent infection with other protozoal parasites *(Babesia canis, Ehrlichia canis)* transmitted by the same tick, may be important to the clinical picture. The typical presentation is chronic intermittent fever, weight loss, stiffness, oculonasal discharge, and pain that is often localized to the rear limbs or lumbar spine. Other reported clinical signs include diarrhea, cough, oral lesions, and polyuria/polydipsia.

Diagnosis.   A complete blood count usually reveals anemia of chronic disease. A marked leukocytosis and lymphocytosis is common. The most consistent chemistry panel abnormalities are increased serum alkaline phosphatase and hypoglycemia. Proteinuria may be noted in dogs with glomerular lesions. Radiographs characteristically reveal periosteal bone proliferation at origins and insertions of skeletal muscles on the vertebrae, pelvis, radius, ulna, humerus, femur, fibula, tibia, and mandible. Definitive diagnosis is dependent on demonstration of the parasite on cytology or histopathology. The most consistent means of demonstrating the parasite is histopathology of muscle tissue.

Treatment.   No effective treatment for hepatozoonosis has been reported. Primaquine may be most effective. Palliative treatment with nonsteroidal anti-inflammatory drugs seems to be the most important aspect of therapy at this time.

MISCELLANEOUS COCCIDIAN INFECTIONS

See textbook for discussions of cutaneous coccidiosis, biliary coccidiosis, and pulmonary coccidiosis.

NONENTERIC MISCELLANEOUS PROTOZOAL DISEASES (pp. 390–394)

BABESIOSIS

Babesia gibsoni and *B. canis* affect the dog; *B. felis, B. cati, B. herpailuri,* and *B. pantherae* affect wild and domestic cats. *Babesia* are introduced into the host by the bite of infected ixodid ticks.

Clinical Features.   Two syndromes, one characterized by hypotensive shock (hyperacute disease) and the other by hemolytic anemia (acute disease), account for most of the clinical signs observed in dogs. Hyperacute disease is characterized by hypotensive shock, hypoxia, extensive tissue damage, and vascular stasis. It may occasionally occur in infected puppies. Acute disease is characterized by hemolytic anemia, thrombocytopenia, and splenomegaly. Anorexia, lethargy, and vomiting are commonly observed. Hematuria, icterus, and generalized lymphadenopathy and periorbital edema can be seen. Immune-mediated hemolytic anemia is the primary disease that must be differentiated from babesiosis.

A wide variety of atypical signs have been reported, including upper respiratory signs, gastrointestinal signs, vascular manifestations, musculoskeletal manifestations, and neurologic manifestations. Dual infections with *Babesia* spp. and *E. canis* probably contribute to the diversity of clinical signs. Cats with babesiosis may be presented for lethargy, anorexia, weakness, rough hair coat, or diarrhea. Chronic anemia can be severe.

Diagnosis. A mild, normocytic, normochromic anemia is generally noted in the first few days after infection. The anemia becomes macrocytic, hypochromic, and regenerative as the disease progresses. Serum chemistry values are usually normal. Hyperbilirubinemia is a consistent finding during acute disease caused by *B. canis*, but not by *B. gibsoni*. Liver enzyme activities may be increased during severe disease. Diagnosis of babesiosis is made by demonstrating the presence of *Babesia* organisms within infected erythrocytes. While the organisms are sometimes easy to find in acutely infected animals, they are rarely evident in chronically infected or asymptomatic carriers. An indirect fluorescent antibody test is useful in the diagnosis.

Treatment. The most effective drugs, diminazene aceturate and imidocarb dipropionate, are not available and are not approved for use. There are anecdotal clinical reports of successful treatment with clindamycin. Immunosuppressive therapy directed at the immune response would seem warranted. Intravenous fluids should be administered to animals that are dehydrated or in shock. Whole blood or packed erythrocytes should be transfused if necessary. Treatment of concurrent stressors, especially gastrointestinal parasitism, is important.

CYTAUXZOONOSIS

Feline cytauxzoonosis is an often fatal blood protozoal disease caused by the piroplasm *Cytauxzoon felis*. Clinical signs are initially nonspecific, with high fever and dyspnea. Most cats die 2 to 3 days after the body temperature peaks. Anemia, thrombocytopenia, icterus, and splenomegaly develop at the time of parasitemia. Increased BUN and serum liver enzymes may be noted in the terminal stage of disease.

Cytauxzoonosis is diagnosed by demonstrating single round-to-oval "signet ring"–shaped organisms within erythrocytes. Care must be taken, as *Haemobartonella felis* has a similar appearance. Successful treatment has not been reliably reported. Anecdotal reports of success using paravaquone or thiacetarsamide exist, however.

LEISHMANIASIS

Leishmania donovani causes visceral and cutaneous disease in both the Old and New Worlds, while *L. mexicana* and *L. braziliensis* cause cutaneous and mucocutaneous disease in only the New World. Sandflies of the genus *Phlebotomus* in the Old World and *Lutzomyia* in the New World are the primary vectors.

Clinical Features. Leishmanial lesions occur in the skin and visceral organs. Symptoms of immune complex disease are prominent. Exfoliative dermatitis with alopecia; ulcerations; onychogryposis; sterile pustule and nodule formation; paronychia; muzzle and foot pad hyperkeratosis and depigmentation; focal pinnal, muzzle, and periocular scaling and alopecia; erythematous plaques; diffuse erythema; and a dull, brittle, poor-quality haircoat are potential dermatologic patterns.

Localized or generalized lymphadenopathy is seen. The most common signs associated with visceral involvement are weight loss and decreased activity. Complex-induced renal failure is the major cause of death. Immune complex disease is probably also involved in the pathogenesis of polyarthritis, vasculitis, and thrombocytopenia. Splenomegaly is obvious in many cases. Epistaxis may occur. Ocular involvement can include conjunctivitis and, less commonly, keratitis, anterior uveitis, and panophthalmitis.

Diagnosis. In the vast majority of cases, a polyclonal hyperglobulinemia and a hypoalbuminemia are seen. Complete blood count abnormalities include anemia, thrombocytopenia, leukocytosis with a left shift, or leukopenia. Increased BUN and creatinine with proteinuria and hematuria are usually noted in dogs with renal involvement. Liver enzymes may be increased.

The most reliable diagnostic test for leishmaniasis is identification of the organism either free or in macrophages. Lymph node aspirate, bone marrow or splenic aspirates, or skin or liver biopsies may reveal organisms. A definitive diagnosis may be established by culturing the organism from tissue and serologic tests can also be useful in establishing a diagnosis.

Treatment. At present, the pentavalent antimonial compound meglumine antimonate is considered the most effective drug for treatment of canine leishmaniasis. Unfortunately, the majority of patients relapse within a few months to 1 year of treatment. Clinical signs usually resolve with retreatment.

AMERICAN TRYPANOSOMIASIS

Chagas' disease is caused by the hemoflagellate protozoan parasite *Trypanosoma cruzi*. Dogs become infected when a kissing bug defecates trypomastigote-containing feces into a wound created while feeding. Acute disease is characterized by anorexia, generalized lymphadenopathy, diarrhea, and myocarditis. Chronic disease occurs 8 to 36 months after initial infection and is characterized by ventricular arrhythmias and dilated cardiomyopathy.

Diagnosis during the acute phase is based on demonstration of trypomastigotes in the blood. Lymph node aspirates may also reveal organisms. In chronic cases, serologic tests can be used. There is no approved treatment available in the United States.

ENCEPHALITOZOONOSIS

Encephalitozoonosis is caused by the microsporidian protozoan, *Encephalitozoon cuniculi*. Clinical disease is most common in young puppies. The most common clinical signs are stunted growth and general unthriftiness. Other signs are related to renal failure and central nervous system involvement. A positive antibody test for antibody against *E. cuniculi* is considered indicative of active infection. No specific treatment exists.

PNEUMOCYSTOSIS

Pneumocystosis is caused by *Pneumocystis carinii*. The parasite is an opportunistic invader, causing disease almost exclusively in animals that are immunosuppressed. In these, severe pneumonia may occur. Diagnosis is made by demonstrating organisms in bronchial lavage, transtracheal wash, or transthoracic aspirates. Glucocorticoids should be given for the first 5 to 10 days of therapy at anti-inflammatory doses. Trimethoprim-sulfamethoxazole is the preferred therapy.

ALGAL AND PROTISTAN DISEASE (pp. 394–395)

PROTOTHECOSIS

Protothecosis is caused by *Prototheca wickerhami* and *Prototheca zopfii*. Most infected animals have defective cell-mediated immunity or neutrophil function. Females and collies appear to be predisposed. The most common signs are diarrhea and weight loss. Ocular and CNS involvement is occasionally seen. Less commonly, the kidneys, skin, lymph nodes, lungs, and heart may be affected. Feline prototohecosis is characterized by firm cutaneous nodules occurring on the limbs, feet, nose, head, pinna, or base of the tail. Diagnosis is based on culture or cytologic demonstration of the organism. Most attempts to treat dogs and cats with prototohecosis have failed.

PYTHIOSIS

Pythiosis is caused by *Pythium insidiosum*.

Clinical Features. The gastrointestinal form of the disease predominates in the dog. Vomiting, weight loss, and a palpable abdominal mass are typical clinical findings. The cutaneous form of the disease is less common. The German shepherd may be predisposed. Lesions may occur as slightly pruritic, poorly defined nodules that soon become ulcerated. Cutaneous, nasal, and retrobulbar pythiosis has been reported in the cat.

Diagnosis. Diagnosis is based on demonstration of *Pythium* organisms in lesions from affected patients. An ELISA test has been developed and tested. Definitive diagnosis is dependent on culture.

Treatment. Wide surgical excision is the treatment of choice. Unless the lesions are completely resectable, the prognosis is poor. Long-term itraconazole may be useful.

CHAPTER 69

CANINE VIRAL DISEASES
(pages 398–409)

RABIES (pp. 398–400)

Because of its fatal nature, rabies is a most important zoonotic disease. The virus is classified in the Rhabdoviridae family and is a member of the genus *Lyssavirus*. Sunlight, warm temperatures, drying, heat, and common disinfectants all destroy its infectivity. All species of warm-blooded animals are susceptible, although there are differences in susceptibility. Rabies virus must contact nerve endings and enter nerve fibers before infection occurs, primarily by contact of infected saliva from a rabid animal with nerve endings or damaged nerve fibers as a result of a bite wound. Contact with the conjunctivum or olfactory mucosa can also result in transmission. Bites that occur on the face, head, and neck result in shorter incubation periods. The virus migrates centripetally in peripheral nerve fibers to the central nervous system. After it reaches the brain and multiplies, it migrates centrifugally in nerve fibers to the salivary glands, allowing for shedding of virus in the saliva.

CLINICAL SIGNS

Three clinical stages of rabies have been defined: the prodromal, excitative, and paralytic stages of the disease. The prodromal stage of

---

Original chapter written by Larry J. Swango

the disease is characterized by change in behavior. Wild animals may lose their fear of humans, and friendly, affectionate pets may become apprehensive and may hide out of fear. The prodromal stage may last for 1 to 3 days and is followed by the excitative or hyperreactive stage. Animals may attempt to bite anything. It is this stage that typifies the association of rabies with a "mad dog." If manifestations of hyperreactivity are prominent, the animal is regarded as having "furious" rabies. Some animals may be oblivious to their surroundings and appear to be in a state of stupor. Such animals are regarded as having "dumb" rabies. Viral-induced damage to motor neurons results in paralysis, which is usually an ascending ataxia of the back legs. Paralysis of muscles of deglutition is responsible for drooling of saliva and inability to swallow. The paralytic stage may last for 1 to 2 days and is followed by death due to respiratory arrest. Death usually occurs within 2 to 7 days after the onset of clinical signs.

DIAGNOSIS

Rabies should be suspected on the basis of clinical signs. Confirmation of the diagnosis depends on postmortem examination for rabies virus in portions of the brain. The fluorescent antibody test is more than 99 per cent accurate. If there has been possible human or animal exposure from an animal with clinical signs suggestive of rabies, mouse inoculation is usually done to verify negative fluorescent antibody results. Intracytoplasmic inclusion bodies in neurons are pathognomonic for rabies in dogs but are not always present.

TREATMENT AND PREVENTION

Treatment is not recommended for animals with rabies because of the risk of human exposure. Rabies is preventable by immunization of dogs and cats and by control of stray animals. It is recommended that dogs and cats be vaccinated at 3 to 4 months of age, again one year later, and either annually or triennially thereafter, depending upon the vaccine.

Management of Dogs and Cats That Have Bitten a Human

A dog showing signs of neurologic disease at the time it bites a human and an unwanted or stray dog or cat that has bitten a person should be euthanized immediately and its brain examined for rabies virus. Healthy dogs or cats that are owned pets should be confined for 10 days after the bite and observed for signs of rabies. This is based on the knowledge that dogs and cats do not shed rabies virus in their saliva for more than a few days before the onset of rabies. There are no provisions for confinement and observation of other species. As a result, all "biters" except owned, healthy dogs and cats should be euthanized immediately after the bite and examined for rabies virus.

Management of Dogs and Cats Exposed to Rabies

Dogs or cats that are currently immunized against rabies according to recommendations and are bitten by a proven rabid animal or by a wild animal in a rabies endemic area should be revaccinated immediately. Unvaccinated dogs or cats should undergo euthanasia or be confined in strict isolation for 6 months. The dog or cat should be vaccinated at the fifth month of isolation and, if healthy by 6 months, may be released to the owner.

CANINE DISTEMPER (pp. 400–402)

Canine distemper is the most prevalent viral disease of dogs and causes more morbidity and mortality than any other virus that infects dogs. The incidence of disease is greatest in young dogs 3 to 6 months of age, after maternally derived passive immunity has waned. Paramyxoviridae are relatively labile viruses, destroyed by heat, drying, detergents, and routine cleaning and disinfection procedures.

EPIZOOTIOLOGY

The virus is transmitted primarily by aerosol and infective droplets from body secretions of infected animals. Immunosuppression is an important factor in determining the outcome of infection. Secondary bacterial and other infections are often responsible for many of the clinical signs, and they contribute to increased mortality.

CLINICAL SIGNS

Seven to fourteen days postinfection, there is a rise in body temperature accompanied by conjunctivitis and rhinitis. Coughing, diarrhea, vomiting, anorexia, dehydration, and weight loss with debilitation are commonly observed in dogs with acute distemper. Mucopurulent oculonasal discharges and pneumonia often result. A skin rash progressing to pustules may occur on the abdomen. Signs of acute encephalitis may develop. Myoclonus or involuntary twitching of muscles, "chewing gum" seizures, ataxia, incoordination, circling, hyperesthesia, muscle rigidity, vocalization, fear responses, and blindness are commonly observed signs. The magnitude of neurologic involvement has a major influence on the prognosis.

Neurologic signs may occur with delayed onset weeks or months after recovery. The clinical signs observed are similar to those in acute distemper; the most characteristic sign is myoclonus or flexor spasm. Dogs that survive may have permanent neurologic deficits. CDV has also been associated etiologically with two different forms of chronic encephalitis. Multifocal encephalitis and "old dog encephalitis" both show progressive neurologic deterioration.

DIAGNOSIS

The diagnosis is usually based on history and clinical signs. Ophthalmoscopic examination may detect chorioretinitis or "gold medallion" lesions in dogs that have chronic infection. Hypoplasia of enamel may occur. Lymphopenia and thrombocytopenia may be present early. A definitive diagnosis can be made by fluorescent antibody examination or by isolation of the virus. The fluorescent antibody test is usually done on epithelial cells collected from the conjunctivum or buffy coat cells. Success is good during the first few days of acute signs. The test is usually negative in cases of subacute, delayed-onset, or chronic distemper.

TREATMENT AND PREVENTION

Broad-spectrum antibiotics are indicated to control secondary bacterial infections, and fluids, electrolytes, B vitamins, and nutritional supplements are indicated for supportive therapy. Dexamethasone has been reported to be of some value in treating dogs with postdistemper neurologic signs.

A single dose of MLV distemper vaccine usually immunizes dogs that are free of antibody and are susceptible to distemper. Approximately 95 per cent of puppies are immunizable to distemper by 13 weeks of age. See Table 69–1 in the textbook for vaccination schedules.

INFECTIOUS CANINE HEPATITIS (pp. 402–404)

Most infections with ICH virus in dogs are inapparent, but occasionally it causes acute, fatal disease that clinically resembles distemper and canine parvovirus disease. Infectious canine hepatitis virus is classified as canine adenovirus type-1 (CAV-1).

CLINICAL SIGNS

Clinical signs are most frequently observed in young dogs. Fever with rectal temperature from 103°F to 106°F occurs at the onset of the clinical signs, which may be accompanied by depression and lethargy. In dogs with moderate disease, tonsillitis, pharyngitis, and cervical lymphadenopathy are common findings. Dogs with uncomplicated cases usually recover after an illness lasting 3 to 5 days. Corneal opacity due to immune-mediated corneal edema may occur during convalescence. In more severely affected dogs, hemorrhagic diathesis with petechial and ecchymotic hemorrhages may occur. Coughing may develop. Bloody diarrhea may occur with or without vomiting. Neurologic signs related to vascular damage may occur. Hepatomegaly occurs in some cases Dogs may develop hepatic coma and die, or they may die suddenly of shock. Peracute disease with sudden death may occur.

DIAGNOSIS

Combined neutropenia and lymphopenia occur early. Thrombocytopenia usually occurs. Prolonged bleeding time and coagulation abnormalities occur in the more severe cases. Serum alanine aminotransferase may become elevated in moderate to severe cases. Demonstration of rising titer of antibody in paired serums confirms the diagnosis.

TREATMENT AND PREVENTION

Therapy for ICH is symptomatic. Most dogs recover without supportive therapy. Prevention is afforded by immunization with vaccines containing either attenuated CAV-1 or CAV-2. Vaccines containing MLV CAV-2 provide effective immunity and are essentially free of postvaccinal reactions or complications.

INFECTIOUS TRACHEOBRONCHITIS (KENNEL COUGH) (pp. 404–405)

Viruses involved in kennel cough include CDV, CAV-1, CAV-2, and canine parainfluenza virus. Canine parainfluenza virus and CAV-2 are considered together. Canine parainfluenza (CPI) virus is in the *Paramyxovirus* genus. Canine adenovirus type 2 is classified in the Adenoviridae family.

CLINICAL SIGNS

The primary manifestation is paroxysmal coughing of varying frequency and intensity. Fever is variable. Dogs usually recover within 3 to 7 days after the onset of clinical signs.

DIAGNOSIS

An etiologic diagnosis cannot be made on the basis of clinical signs. Practically speaking, it is not necessary to establish the etiology.

TREATMENT AND PREVENTION

There are no specific antiviral drugs or chemotherapeutic agents for treatment of either CAV-2 or CPI virus infections. Most animals recover spontaneously without complications or sequelae. Treatment with broad-spectrum antibiotics is indicated when there is evidence of secondary bacterial infection. Attenuated virus vaccines are available for both CAV-2 and CPI virus. Recovery from an infection confers immunity of long duration.

VIRAL GASTROENTERITIS (pp. 405–408)

CANINE PARVOVIRUS

Etiology. It is classified in the Parvoviridae family, and it is closely related antigenically to feline panleukopenia and mink enteritis viruses. Sodium hypochlorite (common household bleach) is the only disinfecting agent that is effective against CPV.

Clinical Signs. Most infections with CPV are clinically inapparent. In dogs that develop clinical disease, vomiting and diarrhea are the first signs observed. Fever is variable, but leukopenia is a consistent finding. Lymphopenia is more pronounced than neutropenia. More severely affected dogs may require symptomatic and supportive therapy, but most recover after 3 to 5 days of illness. If the vomiting is protracted and if severe hemorrhagic diarrhea occurs, the prognosis is less favorable. The acute fatal disease is more common in young pups, some of which may have myocarditis if infected when younger than 8 weeks of age.

Diagnosis. A definitive diagnosis is made on detection of viral antigen in feces or by demonstrating a rising titer of antibody to CPV. Commercially available diagnostic test kits are available for office use. All are based on detection of CPV in fecal samples. Positive results are confirmatory; negative results may or may not rule out CPV.

Treatment and Prevention. Treatment for gastroenteritis caused by CPV is symptomatic and supportive. Fluids and electrolytes are indicated based on evaluation of the clinical condition. Broad-spectrum antibiotics may be indicated to guard against secondary bacterial infections. High dosages of penicillin derivatives and aminoglycosides administered IV together are indicated when there is evidence of septicemia. Antiemetics are indicated in dogs with persistent vomiting. Antidiarrheal drugs should be used with caution. Transfusion with plasma or whole blood may be indicated in dogs with hypovolemia due to severe intestinal loss of serum proteins. Plasma or serum with high titer of antibody to CAV has therapeutic benefits.

The currently available vaccines for CPV are safe and effective. The primary cause of failure of CPV vaccines is interfering levels of maternally derived antibody to CPV (see textbook). It is recommended that pups of unknown immune status be vaccinated at 6, 9, 12, 15, and 18 weeks of age, followed by revaccination annually.

CANINE CORONAVIRUS

Etiology. It is classified in the Coronaviridae family and is antigenically related to transmissible gastroenteritis virus of swine and feline infectious peritonitis virus.

Clinical Signs. Sudden onset of diarrhea with or without vomiting is most commonly reported. Vomiting usually subsides within 24 to 36 hours. The diarrhea may vary from a soft or loose stool to a frothy orange-colored semisolid material to projectile watery diarrhea with mucus and blood. Fever is variable. Dogs generally recover spontaneously, although treatment may be necessary in the more severe cases. The mortality rate is low.

Diagnosis. The clinical signs are similar to signs of gastroenteritis caused by other viruses. A definitive diagnosis is not essential when therapy is needed, because treatment is nonspecific and supportive.

Treatment and Prevention. Treatment is symptomatic and supportive. The approach to therapy is the same as for parvovirus disease. Inactivated virus vaccines are currently marketed for use in preventing CCV infection. They provide incomplete protection against infection.

CANINE HERPESVIRUS INFECTION (p. 408)

Its primary role as a pathogen of dogs is in causing a generalized, fatal, hemorrhagic disease in newborn puppies less than two weeks of age. Affected puppies cease sucking, cry persistently, become weakened and depressed, often pass soft, yellow-green feces, and develop a nasal exudate. Petechial hemorrhages often occur in mucous membranes. Mortality is high in pups less than 3 weeks of age. Pups that survive may develop signs of neurologic disease characterized by ataxia and blindness. Multifocal petechial and ecchymotic hemorrhages are consistent findings in fatal cases.

Treatment is usually unrewarding. Intraperitoneal injection of serum containing antibody to CHV lessens the mortality in a litter of affected pups. There is no specific antiviral therapy of practical value, and there are no vaccines for use in prevention of infections.

Infection of the genital tract is the most important problem of CHV in adult dogs. Most infections are inapparent with occasional mild vaginitis or balanoposthitis. Lesions regress with apparent recovery, but the virus persists as a latent infection. Recrudescence of lesions can occur during stress.

PSEUDORABIES (p. 408)

Dogs have sudden onset of clinical signs usually characterized by sudden change in behavior and intense pruritus of the head. The disease progresses rapidly, and death usually occurs within 48 hours. Intense scratching results in self-mutilation. Generalized convulsions often follow an episode of frantic scratching. Definitive diagnosis is dependent upon histopathologic examination of the brain and/or by virus isolation.

CHAPTER 70
FELINE VIRAL DISEASES
(pages 409–439)

FELINE RETROVIRUS INFECTIONS (pp. 411–421)

FELINE IMMUNODEFICIENCY VIRUS

Feline immunodeficiency virus (FIV) is a lentivirus associated with an immunodeficiency disease in domestic cats.

Epizootiology and Transmission of FIV

Male cats are approximately three times as likely to be infected as female cats. Free-roaming cats are much more likely to be infected than cats housed strictly indoors; very few purebred cats housed in catteries are infected. The prevalence of FIV infection increases with age, with a mean age of about 5 years at the time of diagnosis. Feline immunodeficiency virus has been demonstrated to be efficiently transmitted through bite wounds, with virus being shed in the saliva of infected cats. Transmission through casual contact is at best inefficient under natural conditions. Transmission from a queen to her offspring occurs infrequently. Fetuses or kittens exposed to FIV prior to antibody development in the queen appear to be at highest risk of infection.

Original chapter written by Margaret C. Barr, Christopher W. Olsen, and Fred W. Scott

Immunopathogenesis of FIV Infection

FIV infects both feline CD4+ (helper) and feline CD8+ (cytotoxic) T lymphocytes. FIV appears to selectively and progressively decrease feline CD4+ cells *in vivo*.

Clinical Presentation of FIV-Associated Diseases

The clinical signs are diverse due to the immunosuppressive nature of the disease. The acute phase begins about 4 weeks after infection and lasts for up to 4 months. Some cats experience lymphadenopathy, neutropenia, fever, and diarrhea. Many cats exhibit no clinical signs during acute infection. The asymptomatic carrier (AC) stage, during which clinical evidence of disease is absent, may last several months to years. A short period (2 to 4 months or less) of persistent generalized lymphadenopathy (PGL) follows the AC stage. Cats with AIDS-related complex (ARC) usually suffer from chronic respiratory, gastrointestinal, and skin disorders, accompanied by PGL. The development of opportunistic infections, severe emaciation, and lymphoid depletion signals a progression to AIDS. Many FIV-positive cats have histories of recurrent illnesses with periods of relative health between episodes; however, the general trend seems to be progressive. In general, the life expectancy of cats in the ARC or AIDS stage of disease is less than 1 year.

Among the most common clinical findings in FIV-infected cats are gingivitis, stomatitis, and periodontitis. Oral lesions, reported in 25 to 50 per cent of positive cats, may be ulcerative, proliferative, or a combination of both types. Both ulcerative and proliferative lesions frequently consist of lymphocytic and plasmacytic infiltrates. Chronic, nonresponsive, or recurrent infections of the external ear and skin are commonly seen. *Otodectes cyanotis* and *Demodex cati* infestations may be responsible for purulent otitis externa. Generalized notoedric and demodectic mange have been reported in FIV-positive cats. Dermatophytosis may be particularly aggressive and difficult to treat.

Chronic upper respiratory tract disease occurs in about 30 per cent of FIV-positive cats, and persistent diarrhea due to chronic enteritis occurs in 10 to 20 per cent of infected cats. Pyrexia is a frequent finding in the later stages of disease. Severe wasting occurs in some cats. Abortion, infertility, and other reproductive failures have been reported in infected queens. Some FIV-infected cats have experienced seizures, behavioral abnormalities, and other neurologic disorders, usually in the terminal stages of disease.

Anemia, lymphopenia, neutropenia, and hypergammaglobulinemia are the most frequent laboratory findings. Thrombocytopenia is often seen in FeLV-infected cats but is uncommonly found in FIV-infected cats. Bone marrow abnormalities may include increased cellularity due to elevated numbers of lymphocytes, plasma cells, or eosinophils; myeloproliferative disease; dysmorphic syndromes; and neoplasia. Cats infected with FIV may be more susceptible to *Haemobartonella felis*–induced anemia and related disease. Three types of ophthalmic disease common in FIV-positive cats are anterior uveitis, pars planitis, and glaucoma. Opportunistic infections, such as cytomegalovirus and *Toxoplasma gondii* infections, may be involved in FIV-associated intraocular disease. Lentiviruses are not considered to be directly oncogenic; however, several types of neoplasia have been reported in FIV-positive cats. Lymphomas associated with FIV infection frequently are extranodal in origin. Other neoplastic diseases that have been reported in FIV-positive cats include fibrosarcoma, mastocytoma, squamous cell carcinoma, and myeloproliferative disease.

Co-infection of cats with FIV and FeLV occurs under natural conditions, although infection with one virus does not appear to predispose the cat to infection with the second virus. Researchers have demonstrated that preexisting FeLV infection acts as a potentiator for FIV-related disease. Cats with naturally acquired dual infections also suffer from severe disease. Cats co-infected with FIV and FeLV have an extremely poor prognosis.

Prevention and Control of FIV Infection

Prevention of exposure to FIV-infected cats is the only available method of control.

FELINE LEUKEMIA VIRUS

FeLV is believed to have originated more than 1 million years ago when an endogenous rat retrovirus somehow infected an ancestor of the domestic cat and became an exogenous cat virus. The virus is classified as an oncovirus and is associated with both neoplastic and non-neoplastic (immunosuppressive) diseases.

Epizootiology and Transmission of FeLV

The highest concentration of FeLV infection is found in multiple-cat households in which FeLV is enzootic. The male-to-female ratio of FeLV antigen-positive cats is 1.7:1. The prevalence of FeLV infection is highest for cats between 1 and 6 years of age, with a mean age of about 3 years.

Persistently viremic cats shed large amounts of FeLV in their saliva; virus is shed also in urine, tears, and milk. Cat-to-cat transmission occurs through exposure to any of these fluids by fighting, grooming, or contact with contaminated food, water, or litter pans. Infection results in fetal and neonatal death of kittens from 80 per cent of affected queens. Transplacental and transmammary transmission of FeLV occur in at least 20 per cent of surviving kittens from infected queens.

Pathogenesis of FeLV Infection

Susceptibility to persistent FeLV viremia is strongly influenced by the age of cats at exposure. Most neonatal kittens become persistently viremic when exposed to FeLV, whereas only 30 to 50 per cent of kittens older than 8 weeks and less than 30 per cent of adolescent and adult cats develop persistent viremia.

The initial pathogenesis of FeLV infection can be divided into five partially overlapping stages: (1) viral replication in the tonsils and pharyngeal lymph nodes or in regional lymph nodes (2) infection of small numbers of circulating lymphocytes and macrophages, which serve to disseminate the virus throughout the cat's body; (3) replication of FeLV in the spleen, gut-associated lymphoid tissues, lymph nodes, intestinal crypt epithelial cells, and bone marrow precursor cells; (4) release of infected neutrophils and platelets from the bone marrow into the circulatory system; and (5) infection of multiple epithelial and glandular tissues, with subsequent shedding of large quantities of virus into the saliva and urine. An adequate immune response curtails the progression of infection at stage 2 or 3 and forces the virus into latency. Cats that become persistently viremic progress through all five stages; persistent viremia (stages 4 and 5) frequently develops beginning 4 to 6 weeks after infection. Persistently viremic cats usually succumb within 2 to 3 years of infection.

Clinical Presentation of FeLV-Associated Diseases

The diseases associated with FeLV infection can be categorized as neoplastic or non-neoplastic in nature. Most of the non-neoplastic or degenerative diseases are the result of immunosuppression. Immune complex diseases, including thrombocytopenia, immune-mediated hemolytic anemia, and glomerulonephritis, appear to be more common in FeLV-infected cats than in FIV-positive cats. Thymic atrophy is observed in young kittens infected with FeLV. Erythroblastopenia (non-regenerative anemia) is a common clinical finding in FeLV-infected cats. True aplastic anemia may be induced by FeLV-C infection.

Lymphoma is the most common FeLV-associated neoplastic disease. Lymphomas can be classified as thymic, multicentric, alimentary, or miscellaneous according to their location or distribution in the affected cat. Thymic and multicentric lymphomas are highly associated with FeLV infection in cats. Clinical signs depend on the organs affected. Alimentary lymphomas are associated with FeLV infection in only about 50 per cent of affected cats and may cause intestinal blockages or malabsorption syndromes. Miscellaneous lymphomas are found in nonlymphoid tissues and most frequently involve the eye and nervous system of FeLV-positive cats. Lymphoid and nonlymphoid leukemias are less common than solid tumors. Fibrosarcomas may develop in cats that are co-infected with FeLV and FeSV. They occur most frequently in young cats.

Prevention and Control of FeLV Infection

The ideal method of FeLV control is to prevent contact between infected and uninfected cats. Test and removal programs have been effective in controlling FeLV-related disease in many catteries and multiple-cat households. A typical program is described on page 418 of the textbook.

Vaccination can be used to control the spread of FeLV; it is most effective when it is considered as an adjunct to appropriate husbandry practices. The general consensus is that the efficacy of most FeLV vaccines is somewhat less than 100 per cent. However, vaccination against FeLV infection is recommended for all cats that are at risk of exposure to FeLV.

DIAGNOSIS OF FELINE RETROVIRUS INFECTIONS

Feline immunodeficiency virus and FeLV infections can be differentiated only by appropriate laboratory tests. In most circumstances, concurrent testing for both viruses is indicated.

Diagnostic Tests for FIV

The diagnosis usually depends on the detection of FIV-specific antibodies in serum, plasma, or whole blood. The presence of FIV antibodies correlates well with persistent FIV infection. Positive ELISA tests for FIV antibody should be confirmed by IFA or immunoblot, especially when the cat is asymptomatic or at low risk for infection, or when euthanasia may be considered. The presence of maternally derived FIV antibody in kittens less than 4 to 5 months of age results in false-positive tests with any of the antibody assays. Cats with indeterminate or discordant results should be retested in 6 to 8 weeks; most cats have a clearly positive or negative result on retesting.

Diagnostic Tests for FeLV

An IFA test is available. It identifies p27 in leukocytes and platelets in fixed smears of whole blood or buffy coat preparations; a positive result indicates a productive FeLV infection in the bone marrow cells. Most (97 per cent) IFA-positive cats remain persistently infected and viremic for life. False-negative results may be obtained early in infections before FeLV has reached the bone marrow. When testing leukopenic cats, buffy coat smears provide a much better substrate for the IFA than whole blood smears.

Several commercial manufacturers produce ELISA tests for detection of FeLV antigen in whole blood, serum, plasma, saliva, or tears.

These tests are more sensitive than the IFA at detecting early or transient FeLV infections; however, a single positive ELISA test cannot predict which cats will be persistently viremic. Most of the FeLV ELISAs provide an excellent method of screening for FeLV-positive cats. To identify persistently viremic cats, a positive ELISA should be confirmed by a positive IFA. Cats with discordant test results should be retested in 12 weeks. Cats with persistently discordant tests may have sequestered areas of FeLV replication in lymphoid tissues, salivary glands, or other tissues; these cats are considered to be aviremic and are unlikely to shed infectious virus. Previous vaccination does not interfere with the ability to detect FeLV infection.

TREATMENT OF FELINE RETROVIRAL INFECTIONS AND ASSOCIATED DISEASES

Antiviral Therapeutic Agents

Safe and consistently effective antiviral agents are not available for use in FIV- and FeLV-infected cats. Two primary approaches to antiretroviral therapy have been used in cats: (1) reverse transcriptase inhibitors have been administered to suppress viral replication, and (2) immunomodulatory drugs have been given to potentiate the cat's immune response against the retrovirus. General clinical improvement of FIV-associated stomatitis, gingivitis, and diarrhea was observed after PMEA or AZT treatment in a small field trial. However, the risks of toxicity often outweigh the therapeutic benefits.

Low-dose, orally administered human recombinant alpha interferon has been successful in increasing survival rates and improving clinical status of FeLV-infected cats. Oral IFN treatment is believed to act by stimulating the release of soluble cytokines, such as IL-1. Additional drugs that have shown some promise in the treatment of feline retroviral diseases include acemannan, *Propionibacterium acnes* and staphylococcal protein A. All of these drugs induce the release of endogenous interferons and IL1.

Treatment of Diseases Associated with FeLV and FIV Infections

Management of secondary and opportunistic infections is a primary consideration in the treatment of cats immunosuppressed by FeLV or FIV. Supportive therapy, such as parenteral fluids and nutritional supplements, may be required. Yearly vaccination for respiratory and enteric viruses with inactivated vaccines is recommended. However, the ability of some FIV- and FeLV-infected cats to respond appropriately to vaccination is questionable. Retrovirus-related gingivitis tends to be refractory to treatment. Antibacterial or antimycotic drugs using prolonged therapy or increased dosages may be required. Metronidazole or clindamycin may be useful in treating anaerobic bacterial infections. Judicious but aggressive use of corticosteroids or gold salts may be helpful in controlling immune-mediated inflammation.

The underlying cause of anemia should be determined before treatment is attempted. *Haemobartonella* should be suspected in all cats with regenerative hemolytic anemias; treatment consists of oxytetracycline with short-term glucocorticoids in severe cases. Blood transfusions can provide emergency support. Management of weight loss and cachexia associated with FIV and FeLV infections is critical. Anorexic cats may benefit from diazepam or oxazepam. Anabolic steroids may be useful for more prolonged stimulation of appetite and reversal of cachexia. Treatment for anterior uveitis consists of application of topical corticosteroids. Systemic corticosteroids should be used with caution. Many cases of lymphosarcoma in FeLV-positive cats have been managed successfully with combination chemotherapy. Regimens using vincristine, cyclophosphamide, and prednisone are most commonly used. Myeloproliferative disease and leukemias are more refractory to treatment.

PUBLIC HEALTH SIGNIFICANCE OF FELINE RETROVIRUS INFECTIONS

FIV infection in domestic cats poses little or no public health hazard. Most of the recent studies have found no evidence of FeLV infection in nonfeline species.

FELINE CORONAVIRUS INFECTIONS (pp. 421–425)

There is no conclusive method of diagnosis that can differentiate between a cat's exposure to a feline infectious peritonitis virus (FIPV) and a feline enteric coronavirus (FECV). Multiple strains of both FIPV and FECV exist, which vary greatly in virulence, and antigenic differentiation between the FIPV and FECV groups of viruses remains difficult. Because of this, there is no serologic test that can distinguish between these viruses.

Pathogenesis of FIPV and FECV Infections

Following oronasal infection, FCoV first replicate in pharyngeal, respiratory, or intestinal epithelial cells. Thereafter, FECV and FIPV differ in their target cells for replication. Infection with FECV occurs primarily at the level of intestinal epithelial cells. In contrast, following epithelial cell replication of FIPVs, a cell-associated viremia occurs and monocytes distribute the virus systematically.

One of the most interesting aspects of the pathogenesis of FIP is the frequent development of an accelerated, more fulminant form of FIP upon experimental infection of cats with preexisting FCoV antibodies (seropositive) compared to seronegative cats. One explanation for this phenomenon is the fact that immune-complex deposition incites the pathologic lesions in FIP. Once this pathogenetic cascade is initiated, the prognosis for recovery is extremely poor.

Not all cats that are exposed to FIPV develop clinically apparent FIP. The incidence of FIP peaks in young cats (6 to 24 months of age) and then to a lesser degree in elderly cats. Cats that are infected with FeLV are clearly at a higher risk for developing FIP following FIPV exposure, but this does not appear to be the case with concurrent FIV infection. Nonspecific stress factors are also important. Certain breeds of cats (Siamese, Burmese, Persian) seem to be over-represented among FIP victims.

Clinical Signs

The spectrum of clinical signs is broad. The two major forms of FIP are the effusive or "wet" form and the noneffusive, granulomatous or "dry" form. Although these are presented as separate entities, they probably represent two ends of a continuum of disease progression.

In effusive FIP, increased vascular permeability secondary to perivasculitis leads to the accumulation of protein-rich fluid in the peritoneal and pleural spaces, as well as in potential spaces such as the pericardial cavity. Fluid accumulation is often palpable. Extension of the inflammatory process to other organs in the abdomen can produce signs of hepatic disease and exocrine or endocrine pancreatic insufficiency. Clinical signs such as anorexia, weight loss, listlessness, and dehydration are characteristic.

The clinical presentation in cases of noneffusive FIP is often vague. Fever is a hallmark clinical sign in both forms of FIP. Signs of central nervous system and ocular disease can either accompany or be the sole evidence of FIP, particularly noneffusive FIP. Clinical signs may include ataxia, seizures, behavioral changes, vestibular signs, cranial nerve dysfunctions, paresis, hyperesthesia, and urinary incontinence. Obstruction of cerebrospinal fluid flow has also produced hydrocephalus. Lesions in the eye occur most commonly in the uveal tract, producing hypopyon, vascular engorgement, hyphema, and hypotony, as well as secondary corneal edema, keratic precipitates, and retinal hemorrhage and detachments.

Diagnosis

Histopathologic examination of affected tissues is the *only* definitive method for diagnosing FIP. Without histopathologic evidence, a clinician is forced to assemble information from a variety of parameters "in support of" a diagnosis of FIP. In cases of effusive FIP, the fluid is generally straw-colored and viscous with visible strands of fibrin. The fluid should have a high specific gravity with variable numbers of inflammatory cells Likewise, CSF analysis may reveal elevated protein levels and cellularity when FIP affects the CNS. Demonstration of a polyclonal gammopathy pattern by serum protein electrophoresis is also consistent with, but not pathognomonic for, FIP. Analysis of serum proteins rather than effusion may yield a lower sensitivity. Serologic testing *must* be approached with great care because available tests cannot differentiate between FIPV and FECV. Arbitrary cut-off values such as "less than 100" or "greater than 400" are unacceptable. An added complication is that cats can produce Ab to bovine serum components (which may be present in routine vaccine preparations), which cross-react in tests for FCoV Ab.

Treatment

Treatment is largely palliative (fluid therapy and nutritional support). Aspiration of effusion fluids may result in relief from dyspnea and may temporarily improve a cat's appetite and attitude. Immunosuppressive doses of corticosteroids should be prescribed, along with broad-spectrum antibiotics. Immunosuppressive drugs such as cyclophosphamide or melphalan have also been used. At this time, there is no antiviral agent that is useful clinically.

Control and Prevention of FCoV Infection

FCoV transmission is believed to occur via ingestion or inhalation of the virus, which is shed from infected cats in their feces and oronasal secretions. In most cases, cats will not be shedding the virus at the time of clinical illness. Activation of clinical disease on subsequent infection with FeLV or corticosteroid treatment indicates the existence of FIPV latent carrier cats. In cattery populations, basic management practices, such as avoiding overcrowding stress, limiting movement into and out of the cattery, isolation of cats coming into or returning to the cattery, sound genetic breeding decisions, control of FeLV, and regular use of disinfectants should be used.

Vaccination. The development of Primucell FIP vaccine marks the first time that a significant level of protection against experimental FIPV infections has been attained with a commercially available vaccine. This vaccine strain is a temperature-sensitive mutant of FIPV that is administered intranasally; thus it is able to replicate at the relatively cooler temperatures of a cat's nasal passages, but not at systemic body temperatures. The mean vaccine efficacy for 11 experimental studies was 78 per cent. However, some cats may develop accelerated FIP.

FELINE VIRAL RESPIRATORY DISEASES (pp. 425–433)

FELINE VIRAL RHINOTRACHEITIS

Feline viral rhinotracheitis (FVR), also known as feline herpesvirus infection, is an acute viral infection of the upper respiratory tract and conjunctiva of domestic and exotic cats. FVR is caused by feline herpesvirus 1 (FHV-1), classified in the family Herpesviridae.

Epizootiology

The mortality is usually low, but may approach 30 per cent in young kittens. Most infections occur at 5 to 8 weeks of age before kittens are routinely vaccinated. The more closely cats are housed, the greater the chances of an enzootic.

Transmission.   Aerosol and direct cat-to-cat transmission during the acute disease plus vertical transmission from carrier queens to their susceptible kittens ensure survival of the virus in nature. During the acute disease large quantities of virus are shed in the oral, nasal, and ocular discharges. Cats normally will shed virus for a period of 7 to 21 days after infection; then recovered cats will shed virus intermittently in low titers for long periods of time. This chronic viral carrier status is a true latent infection with no shed of virus from these cats during the latent infection between the actively shedding periods. Stress plays a role in the stimulation of herpesvirus shed from carrier cats.

Pathogenesis and Host Response

See textbook.

Clinical Signs

In the typical case, an acute attack of sneezing is the first clinical sign observed. This is followed shortly by conjunctivitis with ocular discharge and rhinitis with nasal discharge. Fever, anorexia, and depression are present in varying degrees. Conjunctivitis may begin unilaterally, but bilateral involvement within hours is typical. The ocular discharge usually changes from serous to mucoid or mucopurulent, and in many cases it becomes purulent. The eyelids may become stuck together.

Concurrent with the development of conjunctivitis, rhinitis usually develops with a serous nasal discharge, which later becomes mucoid or mucopurulent. Involvement of the trachea and bronchi results in inflammatory exudate, rales, and coughing. Excessive salivation may occur in those rare cases of ulcerative stomatitis.

Viral infection of the cornea and the resulting ulcerative keratitis are serious manifestations of FVR. FVR produces either numerous, small, punctate epithelial ulcers or the linear and zigzagging dendritic ulcers. The small ulcers may coalesce to form larger ulcers and subsequent descemetocele formation.

If FVR occurs in a pregnant queen, infection of the fetuses and/or abortion may occur shortly after the acute disease. Fetuses may be born with a generalized infection, or they may be born without evidence of clinical illness but develop clinical signs shortly after birth. Complications of FVR include a chronic bacterial sinusitis, scarring and occlusion of the nasolacrimal duct, and keratoconjunctivitis sicca.

Diagnosis

Feline respiratory disease is easily diagnosed by clinical signs, but the exact etiologic agent involved is often difficult to accurately identify without laboratory back-up. The diagnosis of "viral respiratory disease" is often sufficient, since treatment and management of the infectious respiratory diseases of the cat are similar in most cases regardless of the cause. If ulcerative keratitis occurs, chances are excellent that the causative agent is FHV-1.

Laboratory confirmation of a diagnosis of FVR can be done by viral isolation, by identification of specific viral antigens in cells of nasal or conjunctival smears by immunofluorescence, or by finding typical herpesviral intranuclear inclusions in cells from conjunctival or nasal scrapings.

Differential Diagnosis. FVR must be differentiated from calicivirus infection and chlamydiosis (pneumonitis). Bacterial infections with *Bordetella bronchiseptica* and *Pasteurella* should be considered.

Treatment

The treatment of cats with FVR involves supportive and good nursing care, broad-spectrum antibiotics for secondary bacterial infections, and specific antiviral therapy if severe ocular disease is present. Decongestants, antihistamines, and vaporization may be indicated to relieve the nasal congestion. Parenteral fluids and oxygen may be needed in severe cases. Insertion of a feeding tube can be beneficial. Antibiotic ophthalmic ointment is usually indicated for prevention or treatment of secondary bacterial infections.

Corticosteroids should not be used in FVR for routine treatment of conjunctivitis or for treatment of epithelial ulceration of the cornea. However, their use in the treatment of stromal keratitis may be beneficial. Antiviral therapy is limited to topical treatment of ocular infections. Idoxuridine, adenine arabinoside, or trifluridine may be considered.

Prevention and Control

Inactivated or modified-live-virus (MLV) vaccines are available. These FVR vaccines produce significant protection following vaccination and should be part of the routine vaccination program. Intranasal vaccines may produce mild sneezing and slight ocular and nasal discharge 4 to 7 days after vaccination.

FELINE CALICIVIRUS INFECTION

Feline calicivirus (FCV) is characterized by upper respiratory disease, pneumonia, ulcerative stomatitis, and occasionally enteritis or arthritis.

Epizootiology

FCV is a common infection in unvaccinated cats world-wide. Routine vaccination has greatly reduced clinical disease. Transmission occurs primarily by direct contact with acutely infected cats, but the virus is maintained by persistently infected carrier cats. Large quantities of virus are shed in the secretions of the mouth, nose, and feces.

Clinical Signs

The clinical signs vary greatly depending on the strain of virus, the age of the cat, and any coexisting infections. The types of disease may be listed as: (1) upper respiratory infection (URI), (2) pneumonia, (3) ulcerative stomatitis, (4) enteritis, (5) acute arthritis, and (6) chronic stomatitis.

Fever is a consistent finding. In the upper respiratory form there is mild serous ocular and nasal discharge for one to a few days. The discharge usually remains serous or possibly mucoid or mucopurulent. The conjunctivae may be mildly hyperemic.

Many strains will produce some degree of pneumonia. FCV is the most common cause of interstitial pneumonia in the cat. In the initial stages, abnormal respiratory sounds are not prominent on auscultation. Cats may mask the lung involvement for the first 1 or 2 days of illness, then suddenly exhibit severe respiratory distress. Radiographs of the chest will reveal a generalized increased density of the lungs.

In the ulcerative form, ulcers may occur on the tongue, the hard palate, at the angle of the jaws, on the tip of the nose, and rarely on the skin or around the claws. The most characteristic ulcers occur on the dorsum of the tongue either as discrete, circular shallow ulcers or as a large horseshoe-shaped necrotic ulcer on the anterior-dorsal surface of the tongue. These ulcers last for 7 to 10 days and heal without complications. In rare instances, ulcerations occur around the claws, to produce the condition referred to as "paw-and-mouth disease."

Certain strains may produce an acute arthritis as part of the "limping kitten syndrome." Cats exhibit acute swelling and pain of the joints of the distal limbs. Affected cats are reluctant to move, and they cry out in pain if these joints are manipulated. This form of FCV infection usually occurs in young kittens. Clinical enteritis has been associated with natural infections with FCV. Nothing is known about the disease-producing capabilities of the enteric caliciviruses of the cat.

Diagnosis

A presumptive diagnosis can be made in some cases based on history and clinical signs, especially if these include ulceration of the tongue. If severe pneumonia is present, a tentative diagnosis of FCV is warranted. Laboratory confirmation can be done by viral isolation or by demonstration of seroconversion to FCV.

Differential Diagnosis. FCV infection must be differentiated from FVR and pneumonitis. Eosinophilic granuloma produces ulcerations on the lips, which tends to be chronic without the respiratory signs of FCV. The acute severe respiratory distress could be mistaken for acute congestive cardiomyopathy, feline leukemia, or feline infectious peritonitis.

Treatment

Treatment involves supportive and good nursing care, broad-spectrum antibiotics for secondary bacterial infections, and specific therapy to relieve the respiratory distress from the interstitial pneumonia. Most cases subside satisfactorily without treatment. The ulcerations of the tongue and mouth do not require specific therapy.

Treatment of the pneumonia should receive prompt and careful attention. Supportive therapy, especially oxygen, can make the difference between death and survival. Antibiotics that are effective against respiratory bacteria should be given until the pneumonia has resolved.

Prevention and Control

Inactivated or MLV vaccines are available. These FCV vaccines produce significant protection following vaccination and should be part of the routine vaccination program. Intranasal FVR-FCV vaccines may produce mild sneezing and slight ocular and nasal discharge 4 to 7 days after vaccination. Most vaccination programs start when the kittens are about 8 weeks old, with a second dose 3 to 4 weeks later.

FELINE VIRAL INTESTINAL INFECTIONS (pp. 433–434)

FELINE PANLEUKOPENIA

Feline panleukopenia (FP) is characterized by sudden onset, fever, leukopenia, vomiting, diarrhea, dehydration, depression, and a high mortality rate. It is caused by a virus classified in the family Parvoviridae.

Epizootiology

Routine vaccination programs have almost completely eliminated FP from the pet cat population. Younger cats are more susceptible than adult cats. Transmission is usually by direct contact of infected and susceptible cats. Large amounts of virus are shed from all secretions and excretions during the acute disease, and this resistant virus may remain infectious in a contaminated environment for years.

Clinical Disease

Peracute FP is characterized by acute, severe disease with severe depression, subclinical temperature, and death within 24 hours.

Typical or acute FP is the usual form of disease. There is sudden onset of fever, anorexia, and depression. Vomiting and a severe fetid diarrhea often follows within a day or two. Cats often adopt a typical attitude characterized by a crouched position with the head between the front paws. The haircoat becomes dull and rough, and there is severe dehydration. Temperature may become subnormal, with coma and death following shortly. Mortality may vary from 25 to 90 per cent. The affected cat that survives about 5 days of illness, in most cases, will have a rapid recovery.

Subacute or mild FP presents as a mild disease. Illness lasts for 1 to 3 days without mortality and with rapid, uncomplicated recovery.

Subclinical FPV infection is a common occurrence, especially in adult cats. There is a mild leukopenia and mild fever, but no outward signs of illness are evident. Cats develop a rapid, lifelong immunity without complications.

In utero FPV infection can result in fetal death or in teratologic effects due to cerebellar or retinal dysplasia.

Diagnosis

Clinical diagnosis is based on history, clinical signs, hematologic findings, and identification of FPV antigen in feces. Hematologic findings include a moderate to severe panleukopenia.

Laboratory Diagnosis.   The antigen can be detected in the feces by the CITE canine parvovirus test.

Treatment

This involves extensive supportive therapy to overcome the severe dehydration and electrolyte imbalances. If the cat can be supported for a few days with fluids and electrolytes, and nutritional supplements as indicated, serum neutralizing antibodies will shut off the infection and result in an uncomplicated recovery. The use of broad-spectrum antibiotics is indicated, since there is a severe depletion of leukocytes and severe damage to the small intestinal mucosa.

Prevention

This involves routine vaccination with either inactivated or attenuated vaccines. FP vaccines are safe and extremely effective, and all cats should be routinely vaccinated as kittens, with periodic boosters. Recommendations usually include vaccinations at 8 to 10 weeks of age with a second dose of vaccine given at 12 to 14 weeks. The last vaccination must be given when kittens are at least 12 weeks of age.

FELINE ROTAVIRUS INFECTION

The importance of this pathogen in the cat is yet to be established. Infection produces cytolysis, which results in a shortening of the villi and a repopulation of immature enterocytes. Osmotic diarrhea results. Studies to date indicate that feline rotavirus by itself probably produces only a mild or subclinical infection.

FELINE RABIES (pp. 434–435)

Since 1981 the number of cases of rabies in cats in the United States has exceeded the number of cases in dogs. Rabies is caused by rabies virus, a member of the Rhabdoviridae family. The main sources of feline rabies in the United States are the raccoon and skunk strains of virus. Contact of cats with a rabid bat can also occur. Transmission is almost exclusively from contact with infected wildlife, primarily through bite wounds.

Clinical Disease

Clinical signs in cats usually parallel those seen in dogs and other animals. During the *prodromal phase* (1 or 2 days), cats show erratic or unusual behavior. Cats may hide or withdraw, or they may become unusually friendly. Other signs may include a slight fever, slight dilation of pupils, or pruritus at the bite site. The second phase, either *furious phase* or *dumb phase*, lasts for 1 to 4 days. Unpredictable, vicious behavior often is the main clinical sign of the furious form. Neuromuscular signs include generalized muscle twitching, incoordination, and weakness. Some cats may exhibit the dumb form of rabies. The *paralytic phase* quickly follows the furious or dumb phase and lasts for 1 to 4 days. This is characterized by posterior paresis with an ascending paralysis, followed by coma, respiratory arrest, and death.

Diagnosis

Rabies should be suspected anytime an attitude or behavioral change occurs in a cat or when an unidentifiable neurologic disease occurs. The diagnosis generally is confirmed only by tests performed on postmortem tissues.

Therapy

Treatment for rabies in cats is not recommended. Suspected cases should be quarantined and observed as recommended (see Compendium on Animal Rabies Control, 1993). Routine vaccination is the main method of controlling rabies in the cat population. Restriction of contact with wildlife in endemic rabies areas also is an effective preventive measure.

CHAPTER 71
DEEP MYCOTIC DISEASES
(pages 439–463)

BLASTOMYCOSIS (pp. 439–444)

ETIOLOGY AND EPIZOOTIOLOGY

Blastomyces dermatitidis is a thermal dimorphic fungus and the etiologic agent of blastomycosis in dogs and cats. The yeast form of *B. dermatitidis* is found in tissues; the mycelial phase exists in soil. The organism is endemic world-wide and particularly in certain regions of the United States, which include most of the eastern seaboard, southern Canada, the Great Lakes region, and the Mississippi, Ohio, and St. Lawrence river valleys. Several reports suggest a seasonal occurrence of canine blastomycosis from June through September and in the

---

Original chapter written by Alice M. Wolf and Gregory C. Troy

autumn months. Routes of infection include inhalation of windborne or soilborne spores and direct inoculation of spores into the skin.

CLINICAL MANIFESTATIONS

The clinical signs depend on whether or not the disease remains localized to the pulmonary tissue or becomes disseminated. The localized pulmonary form in the dog may go unrecognized, with only patients with the disseminated form of the disease being presented for veterinary care.

Young large-breed, male dogs have the greatest risk of infection. Dogs with localized pulmonary disease usually exhibit anorexia, depression, exercise intolerance, weight loss, fever, cough, and/or dyspnea. The skin, lymphatic system, ocular, skeletal, male genital, and the central nervous systems may be affected with disseminated blastomycosis. Respiratory signs noted in affected dogs include cough, dyspnea, and ocular and nasal discharges. The cough is usually nonproductive. Cutaneous signs may be observed and include small and slightly raised lesions with central ulcers and fistulous tracts. Exudates from skin lesions may be serosanguineous to purulent. Generalized lymphadenopathy is commonly present.

Ocular disease is a frequent finding and includes uveitis, glaucoma, subretinal granuloma formation, and retinal detachment. Blindness can result from optic neuritis, panophthalmitis, retinal detachment, chronic uveitis, and glaucoma.

Osseous involvement occasionally occurs. Lesions usually involve the long bones of the appendicular skeleton. The lesions are characterized by periosteal reactions and osteolysis and are suggestive of neoplastic diseases.

Urogenital tract involvement is common in males. Clinical signs include hematuria, dysuria, nocturia, and tenesmus, which may result from urinary bladder or prostatic involvement. Lesions can also be found in the testicles.

Involvement of the central nervous system is uncommon. Most reports of blastomycosis in the cat have described disseminated lesions.

DIAGNOSIS

Hematologic and Biochemical Findings.   Nonregenerative anemia attributed to chronic inflammatory disease is frequently observed. Leukocytosis with a left shift, monocytosis, and lymphopenia are usually present. Serum proteins may reveal decreased albumin levels plus increased inflammatory proteins and immunoglobulins. Seven of 114 confirmed cases of blastomycosis have demonstrated hypercalcemia.

Cytologic Findings.   Cytologic evaluation of specimens obtained by aspiration or impression smears yields a definitive diagnosis in the majority of animals. Suitable specimens include lymph node, tracheobronchial secretions, bone, fine-needle lung and ocular aspirates, and impression smears of cutaneous lesions, bronchoscopic brushings, urine specimens, bone biopsies, pleural fluids, bronchoalveolar lavage, transtracheal washings, and cerebrospinal fluid.

Radiographic Findings.   The most common pulmonary change is a generalized, diffuse, miliary nodular interstitial pattern. Mediastinal and tracheobronchial lymphadenopathy may be observed. Mixed interstitial alveolar or peribronchial patterns can also be observed. Osseous lesions usually affect the epiphyseal region of long bones below the stifle and elbow.

Serology.   The AGID test has an accuracy greater than 90 per cent and is the serologic test used most frequently.

TREATMENT

All animals infected with *Blastomyces* and demonstrating clinical signs warrant medical therapy. The notable exception is the rare case of primary cutaneous or isolated ocular blastomycosis that may be amenable to surgical excision. The discussion of antifungal therapy below will focus on the systemic mycotic infections in general, and specific dosages and recommendations will be made as appropriate, depending on the etiologic agent.

Amphotericin B is effective against, in decreasing order of susceptibility, *Blastomyces, Histoplasma, Cryptococcus, Candida, Sporothrix*, and *Coccidioides*. Common routes of administration are intravenous and subconjunctival. Penetration of amphotericin B across the blood-brain barrier, joint spaces, and ocular tissues is poor.

The clinical use of amphotericin B is not without potential complications. Anorexia, nausea, vomiting, chills, seizures, fever, thrombophlebitis, hypokalemia, anemia, cardiac arrest or arrhythmias, and renal impairment or dysfunction are common side effects. The encapsulated liposomal product has significantly reduced the occurrence of side effects. Nephrotoxicity is the major reason for interruption or cessation of therapy. Toxicity may become evident as early as one hour after administration. Renal dysfunction may persist for long periods after cessation or termination of therapy.

Mannitol, sodium bicarbonate, saralasin, dopamine, furosemide, and salt loading have been used to decrease the frequency and severity of the nephrotoxicity. Two intravenous methods of amphotericin B administration are used frequently. A slow drip method is recommended for use in debilitated animals. A rapid bolus technique is used in animals that are treated on an outpatient basis or do not require additional supportive care.

When amphotericin B nephrotoxicity occurs, ketoconazole or itraconazole should be considered as the alternate drug of choice. Blood urea nitrogen (BUN) and creatinine determination should be performed prior to each dose. If BUN concentrations are greater than 50 mg/dl, therapy should be discontinued until there is improvement in renal function.

Ketoconazole is a substituted imidazole that has been used in the treatment of blastomycosis, cryptococcosis, histoplasmosis, coccidioidomycosis, sporotrichosis, and aspergillosis in dogs and cats. Combination therapy with amphotericin B and ketoconazole resulted in cure rates comparable to those of amphotericin B given alone in dogs with blastomycosis. With ketoconazole, clinical response is slower than with amphotericin B. Anorexia, vomiting, fever, diarrhea, reversible elevation in liver enzymes, reversible alopecia, lightening of the haircoat, and teratogenesis have resulted from its use. Ketoconazole should be administered with food.

Itraconazole has a lower toxicity than ketoconazole and has been used to treat blastomycosis, coccidioidomycoses, cryptococcosis, and histoplasmosis in the dog and cat. The major advantage of fluconazole over ketoconazole and itraconazole is that it penetrates into the CSF. It would appear that this drug may be warranted when central nervous involvement is present with the systemic mycotic infections, such as with cryptococcus in cats.

PROGNOSIS

Animals with more severe lung lesions and higher absolute nonsegmented neutrophil numbers have the worst prognosis. Females have higher survival rates but are more likely to suffer relapses. One study in dogs treated with amphotericin B showed an 88 per cent survival rate over a period of 6 years.

COCCIDIOIDOMYCOSIS (pp. 444–448)

Coccidioides immitis is a geophilic, dimorphic fungus. The free-living mycelial phase in the soil produces the source of infection for mammals. Animals are infected following inhalation of the small arthroconidia, although direct inoculation through the skin has caused infection. Once inside the mammalian host, the arthroconidia are transformed to the parasitic spherular phase. Environmental distribution of *C. immitis* in the United States is restricted to parts of California, Nevada, Utah, Arizona, New Mexico, and Texas.

CLINICAL MANIFESTATIONS

Acute, primary pulmonary coccidioidomycosis usually occurs within one to three weeks following infection. Early clinical signs may be absent or include a mild nonproductive cough, low-grade fever, partial anorexia, and weight loss. This form of disease is often self-limiting but may progress to disseminated infection. Primary cutaneous coccidioidomycosis usually results in a regional lymphadenitis and lymphangitis. Disseminated pulmonary coccidioidomycosis causes a more severe productive cough. Systemic signs include an antibiotic-unresponsive fluctuating fever, depression, weakness, anorexia, and weight loss. Significant respiratory tract signs may not be observed prior to the development of other systemic involvement. Bone is a common site for *C. immitis* dissemination. Most lesions occur in the metaphyseal regions of long bones, and most dogs have multiple bone involvement.

Variable findings include fever, regional lymphadenopathy, and superficial draining tracts. Infection of the heart and pericardium results in granulomatous myocarditis and effusive or constrictive pericarditis. Lesions associated with ocular involvement include granulomatous retinitis, uveitis, and keratitis. Skin lesions include superficial nodules and chronic draining tracts. Infection of the reproductive tract has caused prostatitis, epididymitis, and orchitis. Central nervous system infection is associated with encephalitis and meningitis, causing ataxia, seizures, or coma.

DIAGNOSIS

Mild, nonregenerative anemia, mild to moderate neutrophilic leukocytosis with or without a left shift, and an increased erythrocyte sedimentation rate are common. Hypoalbuminemia and hyperglobulinemia are consistent changes. Direct observation of the *C. immitis* organism is the most definitive method of diagnosis. Unfortunately, there are usually few organisms present in affected tissues. Exfoliative cytology is useful to evaluate tracheal and bronchoalveolar wash specimens, exudate from draining tracts or skin lesions, and lung, lymph node, or tissue aspirates. Bone specimens should be taken from several sites. Thoracic radiographs reveal a wide spectrum of pulmonary parenchymal changes. Interstitial or mixed interstitial/bronchovascular distribution is most common. Hilar lymphadenopathy is a prominent feature of all forms of pulmonary coccidioidomycosis. Bone lesions are usually more productive than destructive. Serologic testing is a useful adjunct in diagnosis and an aid in monitoring the response to therapy (see textbook).

TREATMENT

Systemic antifungal chemotherapy is recommended for all forms of coccidioidomycosis except primary cutaneous disease. Ketoconazole and itraconazole are the two agents currently recommended. Amphotericin B can be used for patients that cannot tolerate oral imidazole therapy. Liposome-encapsulated amphotericin B is the preferred formulation. Treatment with azole antifungals should continue for at least

2 months following the resolution of clinical signs in localized pulmonary disease and for a total of 6 to 12 months in animals with disseminated disease. Amphotericin B may be used concurrently with azole therapy. Primary pulmonary coccidiodomycosis usually responds well to antifungal chemotherapy; disseminated canine coccidioidomycosis carries a guarded prognosis. Most dogs respond well initially but relapse when treatment is discontinued. Caution should be used in handling animals with draining cutaneous wounds.

HISTOPLASMOSIS (pp. 448–450)

ETIOLOGY AND EPIZOOTIOLOGY

American histoplasmosis is a systemic mycotic infection caused by the soil-borne, dimorphic fungus *Histoplasma capsulatum*. The mycelial stage in soil produces the source of infection for mammals. The majority of cases occur in the region comprising the drainage and tributary system of the Ohio, Missouri, and Mississippi rivers. Pulmonary histoplasmosis is acquired by inhalation of microaleuriospores. *Histoplasma* aleuriospores convert to the yeast phase in the lung and are engulfed by cells of the mononuclear phagocyte system. Systemic hematogenous dissemination results.

CLINICAL MANIFESTATIONS

Cats show more evidence of pulmonary involvement and generalized disseminated disease, whereas dogs frequently develop severe gastrointestinal involvement.

Feline Histoplasmosis. Histoplasmosis in the cat is usually an insidious disease characterized by nonspecific signs, including depression, weight loss, fever, anorexia, and pale mucous membranes. Dyspnea and abnormal lung sounds are identified in about one-half of these cats, but coughing is uncommon. Other findings include hepatomegaly and visceral or peripheral lymphadenopathy. Ocular lesions can include conjunctivitis, anterior uveitis, granulomatous chorioretinitis, retinal detachment, and optic neuritis. Several cats have had osseous involvement. Skin lesions have been seen.

Canine Histoplasmosis. Clinical signs referable to gastrointestinal dysfunction (weight loss and diarrhea) are most common. Diarrhea is often "large bowel" in character, with mucus, tenesmus, and fresh blood. More extensive intestinal infiltration can produce a profuse, watery stool with an accompanying protein-losing enteropathy. Pulmonary involvement is a fairly common finding and may cause dyspnea, coughing, abnormal lung sounds, pale mucous membranes, and a low-grade fever. Hepatomegaly, splenomegaly, icterus, and ascites have been reported. Unusual signs include peripheral lymphadenopathy, pleural effusion, ocular lesions, skin lesions, lameness, and neurologic dysfunction.

DIAGNOSIS

Normocytic, normochromic, nonregenerative anemia is the most common hematologic abnormality. Leukocyte counts are variable. *Histoplasma* organisms may occasionally be seen in monocytes or neutrophils. Buffy coat examination increases the chance of finding infected cells. Some cats have had hyperproteinemia, hyperglobulinemia, or hypoalbuminemia. Dogs may have hypoproteinemia and profound hypoalbuminemia associated with a protein-losing enteropathy. Liver dysfunction may be evident biochemically.

Histoplasma organisms are usually numerous in affected tissues. In the cat, organisms are most likely to be found in the bone marrow, lung, and lymph node. Rectal scrapings, imprints of colonic biopsies, and aspirates of liver, lung, and bone marrow are most productive in the dog. Bronchoalveolar lavage may be a useful method of diagnosis in some patients.

The most common radiographic finding in active pulmonary histoplasmosis is a diffuse or linear pulmonary interstitial pattern. Hilar lymphadenopathy is a prominent finding in some dogs but is not common in cats. Calcified pulmonary nodules, indicative of inactive pulmonary histoplasmosis, have been found in dogs but not cats. Plain film abdominal examinations may demonstrate hepatomegaly, splenomegaly, and ascites. Osseous lesions are rare.

TREATMENT

Pulmonary histoplasmosis in the dog can be self-limiting and may resolve without treatment. However, antifungal therapy is recommended. Early or mild cases may respond to ketoconazole or itraconazole alone. Combination therapy with amphotericin B and ketoconazole or itraconazole is preferred in patients with severe or fulminating disease. In most cases, treatment with oral azole antifungals should be continued for at least 6 months.

Dogs with intestinal involvement and most cats have extensive fungal dissemination by the time their disease is recognized. Aggressive antifungal therapy with oral azole drugs alone or in combination with amphotericin B is suggested.

CRYPTOCOCCOSIS (pp. 450–453)

ETIOLOGY AND EPIZOOTIOLOGY

Cryptococcus neoformans is a saprophytic, budding yeast with world-wide distribution. Growth of *C. neoformans* is enhanced in avian excreta, particularly pigeon droppings. The primary portal of entry for *C. neoformans* is the respiratory tract. Extension of infection from the respiratory tract occurs by local invasion and hematogenous or lymphatic dissemination. Concurrent feline leukemia virus or feline immunodeficiency virus infection have been found in some cats with cryptococcosis. In most cases in companion animals, an underlying immunosuppressive disorder has not been identified.

CLINICAL MANIFESTATIONS

Feline Cryptococcosis. *Cryptococcus neoformans* most commonly affects the nasal cavity and sinuses of cats. Clinical signs include sneezing, stertorous breathing, and chronic nasal discharge. The nasal discharge may be unilateral or bilateral and serous to mucopurulent to hemorrhagic. Granulomatous lesions may protrude from the external nares or cause swelling over the facial bones. Local extension of infection may cause regional lymphadenopathy. Signs of CNS involvement may result from direct invasion through the cribriform plate into the brain.

Skin lesions are fairly common in cats. These lesions occur as single or multiple rapidly enlarging nodules that may ulcerate and exude a slimy serous material. Most of these skin lesions are the result of disseminated disease.

Cryptococcal infection of the CNS occurs. Diffuse meningoencephalitis occurs most commonly; granulomatous mass lesions of the brain and spinal cord have also been reported. *Cryptococcus neoformans* occasionally affects the eye. Clinical signs include ocular discharge, optic neuritis, granulomatous chorioretinitis, retinal detachment, and anterior uveitis. Signs of systemic illness are uncommon.

Canine Cryptococcosis. The disease appears in large breeds more commonly than in small breeds. The CNS is the most common site for infection. Neurologic derangements are usually caused by granulomatous meningoencephalitis, and ocular lesions are common. In dogs, signs of vestibular system dysfunction are especially prominent. Skin lesions are found in dogs. Other sites of involvement are less frequent.

DIAGNOSIS

Erythrocyte and leukocyte counts are often normal. Biochemistry profiles are generally unremarkable. Radiographs of the nasal cavity and frontal sinuses usually reveal increased soft tissue density on one or both sides; however, bone destruction is uncommon. Examination of the CSF of animals with CNS involvement often reveals *Cryptococcus* organisms, increased cellularity, neutrophilia, eosinophilia, and elevated protein concentrations.

Cryptococcus organisms are usually numerous in aspirates from impression smears prepared from affected tissues or body fluids. Cryptococcal antigen titers parallel the severity of infection, and sequential samples may be used to monitor the patient's response to therapy.

TREATMENT

Even with solitary cutaneous cryptococcal lesions, antifungal chemotherapy is recommended. Ketoconazole, itraconazole, or fluconazole may be used to treat nasal and cutaneous cryptococcosis. The duration of treatment should be based on the response of the patient, negative follow-up cytology or culture results, and changes in the serum titer.

SPOROTRICHOSIS (pp. 453–455)

Sporotrichosis is a chronic pyogranulomatous infectious disease of dogs and cats caused by the dimorphic fungus *Sporothrix schenckii*, a ubiquitous saprophyte with a world-wide distribution. Infection is usually the result of accidental or traumatic inoculation of the fungus into the skin by thorns or plant materials. Inhalation, ingestion, and mechanical vectors (animal bites) are also means by which infection can be established. Once infection is established, it is usually localized to the cutaneous tissues; however, involvement of the lymphatics draining the area may occur. Dissemination can occur but is considered rare in the dog and cat.

CLINICAL MANIFESTATIONS

The cutaneous and cutaneous-lymphatic forms of sporotrichosis are the most common. Lesions are usually confined to the dorsal aspects of the head and trunk. Multiple, raised, circular lesions characterized by alopecia, crusts, and central ulceration are typical. These papular or nodular lesions may be linear in nature, which is usually indicative of a concurrent lymphangitis. Involved areas are usually nonpainful and nonpruritic. Ocular, central nervous, osseous, and lymphatic abnormalities may be present with disseminated disease.

DIAGNOSIS

The diagnosis can be made by demonstrating the organism in exudates or tissue specimens, by isolation of the organism by culture techniques, or by laboratory animal inoculation with infected material. Culture of exudates, tissues, or aspirates from unopened lesions provides the most reliable method of sporotrichosis diagnosis. Serologic tests are not currently available for use in animals.

TREATMENT

The drugs of choice for the treatment of cutaneous or cutaneous-lymphatic sporotrichosis are the inorganic iodides, ketoconazole and itraconazole. Because of the marked sensitivity of the feline species to iodide preparations, cats should be monitored closely for evidence of toxicity. Amphotericin B, alone or in combination with iodides keto-conazole or itraconazole, should be used in the treatment of animals with disseminated disease. Care should be exercised in the handling of infected animals, exudates, or contaminated materials.

ASPERGILLOSIS (pp. 455–458)

ETIOLOGY AND EPIZOOTIOLOGY

Aspergillus fumigatus is the most common species found in animals with primary respiratory tract involvement. *Aspergillus terreus, A. deflectus*, and *A. flavipes* have been isolated from dogs with disseminated aspergillosis. The respiratory tract is the primary portal of entry for *Aspergillus* spores. Although immune system defects have been demonstrated in some dogs with localized or nasal aspergillosis, there is not a consistent association with a specific immunodeficient state. An apparent defect in IgA production has been demonstrated in some German shepherd dogs.

CLINICAL MANIFESTATIONS

Canine Nasal Aspergillosis. Most affected dogs are young to middle-aged. Males predominate. There does not appear to be a specific breed predisposition for nasal aspergillosis. Dolichocephalic breeds are affected more frequently. The nasal discharge is usually serous initially and later becomes purulent and is often hemorrhagic. Sneezing, stertorous breathing, and facial pain are occasional associated clinical findings. Most infections are initially unilateral. Signs of systemic illness are not usually present. In rare cases the infection may erode through the cribriform plate and produce signs of central nervous system involvement.

Canine Disseminated Aspergillosis. German shepherd dogs are predisposed to develop disseminated aspergillosis. Common clinical signs are weight loss, anorexia, depression or lethargy, weakness, fever, lameness, back pain, and paresis or paralysis. Ocular signs include anterior uveitis, enophthalmitis, or chorioretinitis.

Focal Aspergillus: Osteomyelitis and Pulmonary Disease. Three German shepherd dogs have been identified with unifocal *Aspergillus* osteomyelitis or discospondylitis not associated with disseminated disease. *Aspergillus* bronchopneumonia was reported in another young German shepherd dog.

Feline Aspergillosis. Two cases of nasal aspergillosis have been reported in cats; concurrent feline leukemia virus infection was present in one of them. Systemic aspergillosis has been reported in 22 cats, primarily affecting the lung, intestinal tract, liver, spleen, and/or kidneys. Clinical signs were often vague and nonspecific, and mycosis was not suspected prior to postmortem examination. Feline leukemia virus or feline infectious peritonitis virus infections were identified as underlying disorders in some cats.

DIAGNOSIS

Nasal Aspergillosis. Characteristic findings on radiographs of the nasal cavity include nasal turbinate loss, causing increased lucency rostrally and a mixed density pattern in the caudal portion of the nasal cavity. Fifty per cent of cases demonstrate changes in both nasal cavities. Biopsy is most likely to provide a definitive diagnosis. *Aspergillus* infection produces white or yellow-green to gray-black fungal plaques on the nasal mucosa and in the sinuses. Material may be collected for cytologic examination. Branching, septate fungal hyphae can be seen.

Aspergillus spp. grow well on most fungal culture media. Isolation of *Aspergillus* should be interpreted with caution because it is a normal contaminant in the upper respiratory tract. Failure to culture this organism does not rule out a diagnosis of aspergillosis. Serology is used to detect the presence of systemic antibody directed against *A. fumigatus*. A positive result strongly supports the presence of active infection.

Canine Extranasal Aspergillosis. Leukocytosis with a mature neutrophilia and elevations of blood urea nitrogen, serum alkaline phosphatase, and total serum protein levels are common findings. *Aspergillus* can be seen in the urine sediment or cultured from the urine in many patients. Radiographs are useful in demonstrating fungal osteomyelitis and discospondylitis. Osseous lesions are primarily lytic. Thoracic radiographs in dogs with lung involvement may reveal a generalized granulomatous interstitial pattern.

Feline Aspergillosis. Anemia was present in a number of cats; leukocyte counts were extremely variable. The approach to diagnosis of aspergillosis in the cat should be the same as for the dog.

TREATMENT

Treatment of canine nasal aspergillosis has been difficult. Topical clotrimazole has been used successfully. This solution is either instilled twice daily into indwelling nasal cavity catheters or applied in continuous contact with the nasal cavity for one hour during surgical exploration. Ketoconazole has been used alone or following surgery, with complete resolution of the fungal infection in about half the reported cases. Itraconazole has produced similar results. Enilconazole is another effective compound against fungal rhinitis which is instilled into the nasal cavities and sinuses via indwelling catheters for 7 to 14 days. Follow-up therapy with oral ketoconazole or itraconazole is recommended. Treatment of disseminated aspergillosis in dogs has generally been unsuccessful. Itraconazole has produced remission in some dogs.

RHINOSPORIDIOSIS (pp. 458–460)

Rhinosporidiosis is a rare, chronic infection involving the mucous membranes of the nasal cavity. The etiologic agent is *Rhinosporidium seeberi*. The infection mainly involves the anterior nares and is unilateral. Sneezing, epistaxis, and stertorous breathing are the major clinical signs. The mass is usually single, polypoid, and located at the anterior naris. Masses may be pedunculated or sessile. The diagnosis is established by demonstration of the organism in nasal exudates or tissue specimens. Treatment is usually surgical. The mass can be removed through the external nasal orifice or by rhinotomy. Regrowth may occur. One canine case treated with dapsone had a favorable response.

PROTOTHECOSIS (pp. 460–462)

Two species, *Prototheca wickerhamii* and *P. zopfii* are pathogenic for mammals. The route of infection is uncertain. Percutaneous inoculation via trauma or wound contamination is the most likely route for localized cutaneous infections. In the cat, several cases of the cutaneous form of protothecosis have been reported. The disease produced solitary, soft or firm, mass lesions most commonly found on the limbs or head. Canine protothecosis is usually a disseminated disease that produces a variable spectrum of clinical signs. The collie predominates in reported cases. Colonic involvement occurs in many dogs, causing a chronic, intermittent, bloody diarrhea. Ocular lesions are frequently present, including chorioretinitis, exudative retinitis with retinal detachment, anterior uveitis, and panophthalmitis. Central nervous system and kidney involvement may produce characteristic signs.

Hematologic and biochemical parameters are often normal. Proctoscopic examination may reveal diffuse thickening, reddening, and hemorrhage in the colonic and rectal mucosa. The diagnosis is made most readily by identification of the organism on cytologic or histopathologic examination. *Prototheca* have been recovered from rectal scrapings and biopsies, aspirates of cutaneous masses, CSF, the vitreous or aqueous humor of the eye, and biopsies of other affected tissues. Definitive diagnosis and speciation can be determined by fluorescent antibody techniques.

The treatment of choice for cutaneous prototheriosis is surgical removal of affected tissues. Several cats have apparently responded to excision of well-circumscribed cutaneous lesions. To date, amphotericin B, ketoconazole, oral nystatin with tetracycline, and simazine have not been effective in the treatment of disseminated prototheriosis in dogs. One dog was apparently successfully treated with liposomal amphotericin B.

CHAPTER 72

TUMOR BIOLOGY
(pages 466–473)

CELLULAR BIOLOGY OF CANCER (pp. 466–468)

SIGNAL TRANSDUCTION

Genes called oncogenes represent the driving force behind the uncontrolled growth of many cancer cells. Present in the normal cell as proto-oncogenes, these growth regulatory genes become inappropriately activated and result in the conversion of the normal founder cell into a cancer cell.

CANCER INITIATION

The genetic mechanisms that initiate cancer do not seem to be necessarily involved in the progression of cancer. Therefore, the key element of the current tumor progression model is that a genetic event initiates the cancer process via activation of an oncogene and alters the operation of the regulatory network (i.e., epigenetic event), thereby channeling it into an evolutionary pathway not consistent with the program of the genome. The drift of the network out of control is attributed to the presence of the oncogene product, which is part of the network, but is either present in cells in which it is normally absent or present at a time in the growth cycle in which it should be absent.

IMPLICATIONS FOR THE WHOLE ANIMAL (pp. 468–469)

By locally invading at the primary site and impinging on the function of that tissue, cancer may disrupt important body functions. Tumors may also cause paraneoplastic syndromes. Even though tumors usually follow relatively reproducible metastatic patterns, the cause of organ-specific metastasis is poorly understood, and atypical metastatic patterns are frequently seen in clinical practice.

BIOLOGY OF METASTASIS (pp. 469–470)

Metastasis is a selective process, not a random event. The competent metastatic cell must complete a series of linked, sequential complex interactions between tumor cells and normal cells and tissues. After transformation of normal cells, angiogenesis occurs to nourish the

---

Original chapter written by Ralph C. Richardson, Kevin A. Hahn, and Deborah W. Knapp

growing tumor. Tumor cells detach from the primary tumor and travel through the extracellular matrix. Tumor cells then penetrate and enter a blood vessel (intravasation). Once in the circulation, tumor cells must survive in this environment, avoid immune attack, and settle at a new site. Arrested tumor cells penetrate the vessel wall, leave the circulation (extravasation), proliferate in the new organ, undergo angiogenesis, and continue growing. Once metastases are established, secondary metastasis (the metastasis of metastases) can occur.

PRINCIPLES OF CANCER THERAPY (p. 470)

Specific treatment methods for cancer are described in the next few chapters, but the practicing veterinarian must diligently maintain an overall view of the patient and its therapy if care is to be optimum. Treatment choices begin with an accurate diagnosis and clinical staging of the patient. A diagnosis is best confirmed through cytologic and histopathologic methods. It is the clinician's responsibility to determine that the microscopic diagnosis is consistent with the patient's clinical presentation. Localized tumors and tumors demonstrating limited regional invasion are best treated by a localized form of therapy.

IMPROVEMENTS IN CANCER THERAPY (pp. 470–471)

Areas of possible advancement in the quest to improve treatment for metastatic neoplasia include intensification of existing therapy, improvement in drug screening methods to maximize use of existing and new drugs, and development or discovery of new drugs that target different sites in the cancer cell or its environment.

INTENSIFICATION OF THERAPY

One way to improve chemotherapy efficacy is to increase intensity (increasing the dosage or decreasing the treatment interval) of therapy in patients with susceptible tumors. In veterinary medicine, investigations of potential ways to offset chemotherapy toxicity include stimulation of bone marrow progenitor cells with colony-stimulating factors during chemotherapy, use of renal protective protocols during nephrotoxic chemotherapy, and vigorous use of antiemetics.

Another way to intensify therapy is to use combination chemotherapy. These principles include (1) using only drugs that are at least partially effective when used alone, (2) attempting to prevent overlapping toxicity, (3) using each drug at its optimal dose and schedule, and (4) developing a consistent treatment protocol with the shortest possible treatment-free interval between doses.

Intensification of therapy has also been applied to the primary tumor site by exposing the localized tumor to high chemotherapy concentrations. The same principles used in selection of combination chemotherapy should be applied when one is developing multimodality therapy.

DRUG SCREENING METHODS

Expanding knowledge of biochemical mechanisms associated with tumor growth or differentiation provides many new pharmacologic targets for novel anticancer agents.

NEW TARGETS FOR ANTICANCER DRUGS (pp. 471–472)

One drug discovery group is screening for agents that inhibit multiple drug resistance (MDR), protein kinase C (PKC), and protein tyrosine kinase. Other potential targets for antitumor agents are proteins in signal transduction pathways. Growth factors and their receptors, the first messengers in signal transduction, are also potential targets for anticancer drugs. Other new targets for cancer therapy include the host's immune system, the metastatic process (if instituted before metastasis occurs), dietary factors, and the cancer cell genome (gene therapy). Goals of effective immunotherapy include making the tumor more antigenic so that it is recognized as foreign, and improving the host response to these foreign cells.

CHAPTER 73

CHEMOTHERAPY
(pages 473–484)

Chemotherapy may help to control generalized, rapidly progressive disease that is not amenable to surgery or radiotherapy or may help to increase the disease-free interval after other initial treatment. It may help to prevent spread of a neoplasm by controlling early metastases that are proliferating at a high rate and have a relatively small likelihood of containing resistant cells. Chemotherapy may also benefit patients by providing symptomatic relief of related problems and temporary restoration of deteriorated function.

A prudent handler of anticancer drugs takes a conservative but reasonable approach to all aspects of storing, preparing, administering, and disposing of these agents.

BIOLOGIC BASIS (pp. 474–475)

See Chapter 72. In both normal and neoplastic cell populations, there are relatively more dividing cells in a small population and relatively fewer dividing cells in a large population. It is evident that the cytoreductive effects of surgery or radiation therapy can induce a renewed level of proliferative activity within a tumor and render the tumor more susceptible to chemotherapeutic attack.

PHARMACOLOGIC FACTORS (p. 475)

To affect a tumor, the chemotherapeutic agent must reach the site of action. The blood-brain barrier represents such a problem in distribution. Drug resistance, interactions, and toxicities all may affect the usefulness of a theraputic agent. Direct chemical or physical interactions, interference with absorption or receptor binding, or altered metabolism or excretion each might have an impact on a drug's net effect. The amount of drug given or the dosage interval may need to be adjusted to compensate for impaired excretion, but for the most part, strict guidelines have not been established in veterinary medicine.

DRUG RESISTANCE (pp. 475–476)

Acquired resistance may occur with decreased activation or increased deactivation of the drug by neoplastic cells. Resistance may

Original chapter written by Robert C. Rosenthal

also be related to impermeability of the tumor cell to the drug, increased rates of removal of drugs from tumor cells, shifts in enzyme specificity, increased repair of cytologic lesions, or bypassing of inhibited reactions with alternate biochemical pathways.

TOXICOSES (p. 476)

The most commonly encountered problems relate to gastrointestinal toxicity, bone marrow suppression, and immunosuppression. Generally, chemotherapy can be reinstituted in 1 to 2 weeks based on a return to normal white blood cell parameters. When resuming chemotherapy, it may be advisable to decrease the dosage of the offending drug by 25 per cent. The kidneys are subject to damage from methotrexate, streptozotocin, L-asparaginase, and other chemotherapeutic agents. Skin reactions and alopecia are less frequent in animals than in humans, but they do occur. Clipped hair may not regrow or may regrow a different color.

DRUGS USED IN CHEMOTHERAPY (pp. 476–480)

Comments on selected drugs (see Table 73–1 in the textbook) aid in effective, rational chemotherapy. Tables 73–1 and 73–2 in this pocket companion list conversions for dogs and cats.

ALKYLATING AGENTS

The alkylating agents are not specific for the cell cycle phase. Cyclophosphamide is the most widely used alkylating agent in veteri-

TABLE 73–1. CONVERSION OF BODY WEIGHT IN KILOGRAMS TO BODY SURFACE AREA IN METERS SQUARED FOR DOGS

KG	M²	KG	M²
0.50	0.06	26.00	0.88
1.00	0.10	27.00	0.90
2.00	0.15	28.00	0.92
3.00	0.20	29.00	0.94
4.00	0.25	30.00	0.96
5.00	0.29	31.00	0.99
6.00	0.33	32.00	1.01
7.00	0.36	33.00	1.03
8.00	0.40	34.00	1.05
9.00	0.43	35.00	1.07
10.00	0.46	36.00	1.09
11.00	0.49	37.00	1.11
12.00	0.52	38.00	1.13
13.00	0.55	39.00	1.15
14.00	0.58	40.00	1.17
15.00	0.60	41.00	1.19
16.00	0.63	42.00	1.21
17.00	0.66	43.00	1.23
18.00	0.69	44.00	1.25
19.00	0.71	45.00	1.26
20.00	0.74	46.00	1.28
21.00	0.76	47.00	1.30
22.00	0.78	48.00	1.32
23.00	0.81	49.00	1.34
24.00	0.83	50.00	1.36
25.00	0.85		

**TABLE 73–2. CONVERSION OF BODY WEIGHT
IN KILOGRAMS TO BODY SURFACE AREA
IN METERS SQUARED FOR CATS**

KG	M²	KG	M²
0.50	0.06	5.50	0.29
1.00	0.10	6.00	0.31
1.50	0.12	6.50	0.33
2.00	0.15	7.00	0.34
2.50	0.17	7.50	0.36
3.00	0.20	8.00	0.38
3.50	0.22	8.50	0.39
4.00	0.24	9.00	0.41
4.50	0.26	9.50	0.42
5.00	0.28	10.00	0.44

nary medicine. It has been administered for lymphoreticular neoplasia, various sarcomas and carcinomas, mast cell tumors, and transmissible venereal tumors as a single agent and with other drugs. Hematologic and gastrointestinal toxicoses are dose limiting. Leukopenia is most severe within a week or two of administration.

A unique and important problem associated with the administration of cyclophosphamide is sterile hemorrhagic cystitis. Early recognition of signs, diuresis, and cessation of cyclophosphamide administration help to limit the problem. Chlorambucil is often used in chemotherapy of canine lymphoma as a replacement for cyclophosphamide. Melphalan is most useful in multiple myeloma but has also been used in lymphoreticular neoplasia, mammary and lung carcinomas, and osteogenic sarcoma. Dacarbazine may be useful in lymphoma in dogs but is not widely employed. Nitrogen mustard is rarely used systemically, but topical application is helpful in cutaneous lymphoma.

ANTIMETABOLITES

The antimetabolites are S-phase-specific drugs. They are highly schedule dependent, and questions regarding their best use remain unanswered. Methotrexate is used in the treatment of lymphoreticular neoplasms and myeloproliferative disorders as well as metastatic transitional cell tumor, transmissible venereal tumor, Sertoli cell tumor, and osteogenic sarcoma. Damage to the bone marrow and gastrointestinal tract can be severe. The purine analog 6-mercaptopurine interferes with purine synthesis and interconversion and is used for lymphocytic and granulocytic leukemias. 5-Fluorouracil is used in the treatment of various carcinomas. Hematologic and gastrointestinal toxicoses are important. 5-Fluorouracil should not be used in cats because of severe neurotoxicosis. The use of cytosine arabinoside in various hematologic and lymphoid malignancies has been suggested, but its true role in the management of these diseases is not known.

ANTIBIOTICS

They are cytotoxic, nonspecific for cell-cycle phase, and damage DNA by binding DNA and inhibiting DNA or RNA synthesis. Hematologic, gastrointestinal, and cardiac toxicoses are important. Renal disease may be significant in cats.

Doxorubicin is administered slowly through a free-flowing intravenous line. Extravasation causes serious sloughing and is treated promptly with saline dilution through the same (unremoved) needle used to administer the drug after attempts to aspirate extravasated drug.

Restlessness, facial swelling, or head shaking may signal excessively rapid administration. Doxorubicin has had wide application in the treatment of canine lymphosarcoma as both a first- and second-line drug and for various carcinomas and sarcomas with limited success. Unlike doxorubicin, *mitoxantrone* does not seem to have significant potential for cardiotoxicity; however, gastrointestinal upset and myelosuppression are potential problems. To date, mitoxantrone has been used with limited success in a variety of tumor types including carcinomas, sarcomas, and lymphoid malignancies. The best results were noted with squamous cell carcinoma and lymphoma. *Bleomycin* has had limited use in squamous cell carcinoma in animals. Pulmonary fibrosis may be a lethal complication.

PLANT ALKALOIDS

Although vincristine and vinblastine have a common mechanism of action, M-phase activity, resistance to one does not imply resistance to the other. Vincristine affects the peripheral nervous system. Vinblastine toxicity is primarily hematologic. Both are used to treat lymphoreticular neoplasms. Vincristine is the treatment of choice for transmissible venereal tumor and is used for sarcomas and carcinomas. Vinblastine is used to treat carcinomas and mast cell tumors.

HORMONES

Adrenal corticosteroids have important uses in therapy of lymphoma and mast cell tumors and may be of benefit in central nervous system neoplasms because of their ability to cross the blood-brain barrier. The major effects of these drugs in brain tumors relates to the reduction of peritumor inflammation and edema. Sex hormones have been used in the treatment of hormone-dependent tumors of mammary, prostatic, or perianal gland origin.

MISCELLANEOUS AGENTS

L-Asparaginase acts against cells in G1. It is effective in canine lymphoreticular neoplasms. Anaphylaxis has been the most dangerous side effect. The cell cycle–nonspecific drug o,p′-DDD directly suppresses both normal and neoplastic adrenocortical cells. Streptozocin has been suggested for islet cell carcinoma but has generally been considered too toxic for use in dogs. Cisdichlorodiammineplatinum (CDDP) causes nausea and vomiting, which may be severe and prolonged. Renal insufficiency is usually the dose-limiting toxicosis, but myelosuppression may also occur. Brisk saline diuresis before and after administration and use of antiemetics help to limit renal damage and gastrointestinal disturbances. CDDP, as administered to dogs, should not be given to cats because of dose-related primary pulmonary toxicosis. The most clearly defined indication for CDDP is adjunctive treatment of osteosarcoma in dogs. Carboplatin is a platinum compound that is less nephrotoxic than CDDP and may be useful in the management of osteosarcoma, melanoma, and various carcinomas in dogs.

MULTIMODALITY THERAPY (pp. 480–481)

Present practice includes adjuvant chemotherapy as part of the initial treatment plan when appropriate. When applied to the much smaller tumor burdens that remain after surgery, chemotherapy may have a better chance of being effective. Another means of combining modalities is neoadjuvant chemotherapy, the use of drugs before the definitive treatment (surgery or radiation) for the primary tumor. By moving chemotherapy "up front," it may be possible to reduce the size of the surgical or radiation field even if the chemotherapy is not itself cura-

TABLE 73–3. PROTOCOL FOR LYMPHOMA IN DOGS: INITIAL EIGHT-TREATMENT CYCLE

Week 1:	Asparaginase 10,000 IU/m^2 IM
	Vincristine 0.6 mg/m^2 IV
	Prednisone 2.0 mg/kg PO q24h
Week 2:	Cyclophosphamide 200 mg/m^2 IV
	Prednisone 1.5 mg/kg PO q24h
Week 3:	Vincristine 0.6 mg/m^2 IV
	Prednisone 1.0 mg/kg PO q24h
Week 4:	Doxorubicin 30 mg/m^2 IV
	Prednisone 0.5 mg/kg PO q24h
Week 6:	Vincristine 0.6 mg/m^2 IV
Week 7:	Cyclophosphamide 200 mg/m^2 IV
Week 8:	Vincristine 0.6 mg/m^2 IV
Week 9:	Doxorubicin 30 mg/m^2 IV

tive. Also, early chemotherapy may have an effect on undetected micrometastatic disease, which theoretically is kept somewhat in check by a suppressive effect from the primary tumor. In general, in combined modality treatments, chemotherapy and biologic therapy can be considered useful to combat micrometastatic disease, radiation to sterilize local or regional disease, and surgery to remove the gross tumor. In any case, adjuvant chemotherapy should not be undertaken unless there is some evidence that the tumor being treated is at least somewhat responsive to the drug or drugs used.

SELECTED PROTOCOLS (pp. 481–482)

Lymphoma in dogs is very responsive to medical management. Response rates are high, and survival times are significant compared to the outcome in untreated animals (see Table 73–3 for protocol). Second and subsequent cycles are similar to the first with a few exceptions. Treatments are administered at 2-week intervals in the second eight-treatment cycle, 3-week intervals in the third cycle, and approximately monthly thereafter. Asparaginase and prednisone are used only in the first cycle. In the second and third cycles, the fourth treatment is methotrexate (0.65 mg/kg or 20 mg/m^2 IV); in cycles after the third, doxorubicin is replaced entirely by methotrexate. In the second and all subsequent cycles, Leukeran (1.4 mg/kg PO) replaces cyclophosphamide. Therapy is planned for 3 years. Cats may not as easily enter

TABLE 73–4. PROTOCOL FOR LYMPHOMA IN CATS: INITIAL EIGHT-TREATMENT CYCLE*

Week 1:	Asparaginase 10,000 IU/m^2 IM
	Vincristine 0.7 mg/m^2 IV
	Prednisone 2.0 mg/kg PO q24h (continues throughout protocol)
Week 2:	Cyclophosphamide 200 mg/m^2 IV
Week 3:	Vincristine 0.7 mg/m^2 IV
Week 4:	Doxorubicin 20 mg/m^2 IV
Week 6:	Vincristine 0.7 mg/m^2 IV
Week 7:	Cyclophosphamide 200 mg/m^2 IV
Week 8:	Vincristine 0.7 mg/m^2 IV
Week 9:	Methotrexate 10–15 mg/m^2 IV

*In the second and third cycles, starting at week 11, asparaginase is not given. Treatments are administered at two week intervals in the second cycle and at three week intervals in the third cycle.

or remain in remission. Feline leukemia virus–positive cats have a worse prognosis (see Table 73–4).

Multiple myeloma is responsive to drug therapy, and good responses may be expected in dogs without negative prognostic factors such as hypercalcemia and Bence Jones proteinuria. Treatment with melphalan and prednisone is very likely to result in a good response.

Transmissible venereal tumors are highly responsive to chemotherapy. Vincristine (0.5 mg/m² IV) can be administered intravenously weekly until complete remission is attained and then for an additional two treatments with excellent results.

Mast cell tumors have traditionally been difficult to manage with drugs. Prednisone will induce remission in some dogs with systemic disease that are not candidates for surgery or radiotherapy, currently the most effective approach for localized disease. Occasionally, other carcinomas and sarcomas will respond to chemotherapeutic management. The sarcoma best demonstrated to be responsive to adjunctive chemotherapy is *hemangiosarcoma.* A protocol including vincristine, doxorubicin, and cyclophosphamide (VAC) has been shown to increase median survival from approximately 60 days (with surgery alone) to 172 days. A 3-week cycle of therapy is recommended. Neutropenia is marked, and the prophylactic use of antibiotics for the first 14 days of each cycle seems to be helpful.

CHAPTER 74

IMMUNOTHERAPY OF CANCER
(pages 484–493)

TUMOR IMMUNOLOGY OVERVIEW (pp. 484–485)

T LYMPHOCYTES

T cells play a central role in delayed-type hypersensitivity reaction, resistance to certain bacteria, viruses, and tumors, and rejection of organ transplants. T cells have important regulatory functions because of their ability to produce cytokines that act on other T cells, B cells, and macrophages, and their ability to directly interact with other lymphocytes. See Table 74–2 in the textbook.

CURRENT APPROACHES TO IMMUNOTHERAPY
(pp. 485–491)

NONSPECIFIC IMMUNOMODULATORS

Nonspecific host immunostimulators fall into several categories and are listed in Table 74–3 in the textbook.

Nonspecific Bacterial Agents

The principles of therapy using nonspecific bacterial vaccines are as follows:

1. The tumor burden should be small. Ideally, these agents would be

---

Original chapter written by E. Gregory MacEwen

more effective when used in conjunction with cytoreductive surgery or following radiation or chemotherapy.

2. An immunocompetent host is most desirable or, at least, a host capable of immunorestoration. Patients who have been heavily pretreated with chemotherapy are unlikely to respond.

3. Immunosuppressive therapy such as corticosteroids must be avoided.

4. Therapy may be timed to be given following chemotherapy after the rebound from immunosuppression.

5. The effectiveness of the vaccine may be improved if administered in close proximity to the tumor via intratumor, intracavity, or regional lymph node injection.

Galactomannans

Acemannan has been shown to enhance macrophage release of IL-1_β, TNF_α, IL-2, IL-6, IFN_γ, and GM-CSF, and has been found to enhance T-cell function. It also has been shown to delay the development of clinical signs in cats infected with the feline leukemia virus. Acemannan is currently available commercially for use in animals with fibrosarcoma. Studies in our clinic show that tumors that are less than 1 to 2 cm in size are more likely to respond to acemannan.

Systemic Activation of Macrophages by Liposome-Muramyl Tripeptide

Encapsulation of MDP into multilamellar phospholipid vesicles or liposomes results in effective delivery of the MDP to monocytes and macrophages, resulting in activation and in situ antitumor activity. Two studies clearly indicate that L-MTP-PE is an effective agent for the treatment of micrometastases in dogs with osteosarcoma. With the addition of the chemotherapy, we can greatly enhance the survival time of dogs with osteosarcoma.

Currently, we are conducting a trial in canine oral melanoma combined with surgery: in dogs with splenic hemangiosarcoma combined with splenectomy and chemotherapy, and in cats with mammary adenocarcinoma combined with a radical mastectomy. In all these studies, we are utilizing the L-MTP-PE in an adjuvant setting, that is, treating the minimal residual tumor or microscopic metastatic disease.

Levamisole

Levamisole has been shown to increase both T-cell numbers and proliferative responses, if depressed. Levamisole also enhances phagocytic and chemotactic activities of polymorphonuclear leukocytes and monocytes. Clinical use is still under investigation.

Prostaglandin Antagonists

PGE_2 inhibits several lymphocyte functions: proliferation, lymphokine production, cytotoxic activity, and suppressor activity. PGE_2 has also been shown to down-regulate gene expression of TNF_α in activated monocytes. Cyclo-oxygenase inhibitors inhibit the production of PGE_2 and have been shown to have immunomodulating activity, as well as inhibition of tumor growth in a number of experimental tumors. The nonsteroidal anti-inflammatory drug (NSAID) piroxicam (Feldene), a PGE_2 antagonist, has been shown to have antitumor activity in canine bladder carcinoma.

Cimetidine

Cimetidine may modulate T suppressor activity. However, its use as a therapeutic immunomodulator is still unproven.

LYMPHOKINES/MONOKINES

Interleukin-2 (IL-2)

In man, the major drawback for this therapy is toxicity (e.g., fever, hypotension, pulmonary edema secondary to capillary leakage, liver damage, and renal insufficiency). IL-2 administration produces a hemodynamic pattern similar to that of septic shock, with decreased vascular resistance leading to hypotension and oliguria. Overall, the toxicity in dogs was minimal and mainly confined to gastrointestinal signs. In one study, objective antitumor responses were seen in dogs with oral melanoma and mast cell tumors when IL-2 was combined with TNF.

Tumor Necrosis Factor (TNF$_\alpha$)

When TNF$_\alpha$ is produced acutely and released in large quantities into the circulation during a serious septic condition, it triggers a state of shock and tissue injury (septic shock syndrome) that has a high mortality rate. When produced during chronic disease states, TNF$_\alpha$ produces a syndrome characterized by accelerated catabolism, weight loss, anemia, and loss of lean body mass, as well as lipid stores.

The tumoricidal effects of TNF$_\alpha$ are not clearly understood. However, it is known that TNF$_\alpha$ can induce changes on the cell membrane, especially those having a strong effect on lipids, leading to lysosomal damage. TNF$_\alpha$ will also cause the formation of pores to develop within the cell membrane, thus leading to cytopathic effects.

Results of clinical trials using hrTNF$_\alpha$ have been disappointing. Little antitumor activity has been documented and excessive toxicity has been noted. It is likely that recombinant TNF$_\alpha$ will be effective when used in combination with other treatments.

Interferons: α, β, γ

Gamma (γ) IFN is a more potent immune system modulator than is alpha (α) or beta (β) IFN. IFN-α is a more powerful antitumor agent. IFN-γ plays an extremely important role in the function of CD4 (T_H1) cells, NK cells, B cells, and macrophages. The recombinantly synthesized IFNs (human, mouse, bovine, feline) are generally species-specific for γ and β and not for α.

Clinically, IFN-α has been studied in cats infected with FeLV. The mean survival time for cats given HuIFN-α was significantly longer than those given no treatment (control). We recommend 30 U/cat given orally once daily for 7 days, on a week-off schedule. The clinical responses reported with IFN-β and IFN-γ in human cancers have been minimal.

MONOCLONAL ANTIBODIES

A number of factors will influence the effectiveness of MAb therapy. These include number of antigen molecules per cell surface, number of cells expressing the antigen, size of the tumor mass, degree of tumor vascularization, presence and reactivity of circulating antigen in the blood, presence of antigen on non-neoplastic (normal) tissues, clearance of MAb from blood, dose and route of administration, and development of an immune response—antimonoclonal antibodies.

Antibodies against cancer can be used both for their cytotoxic effects or through conjugation of radioactive materials. A monoclonal antibody has been developed that has been reported to mediate ADCC against a canine lymphoma cell line. This antibody has been reported to prolong remission duration when used following chemotherapy in dogs with lymphoma.

HEMATOPOIETIC GROWTH FACTORS

The CSFs and the target cells are presented in Table 74–5 in the textbook. G-CSF (rcG-CSF) has potential therapeutic value to reduce the duration of neutropenia following chemotherapy and total body radiation therapy. In one study, it was determined that serum from dogs taken during the neutropenia period contained antibody to human recombinant G-CSF (rhG-CSF), which neutralized the stimulatory effects of both rhG-CSF and endogenous cG-CSF.

GM-CSF supports the growth of multipotential hematopoietic progenitor cells, as well as cells already committed to myeloid, erythroid, or megakaryocytic lineages. GM-CSF also enhances multiple functions of mature cells, including oxidative metabolism, phagocytosis, lysozyme secretion, and ADCC. We have studied rhGM-CSF in normal dogs. We suspect that antibodies to rhGM-CSF developed and resulted in inactivation of the rhGM-CSF.

M-CSF has been shown to increase circulatory peripheral blood monocytes, promonocytes, and large vacuolated macrophage-like cells, although platelet counts decline with M-CSF. M-CSF has been shown to induce secretion of IL-1 and TNF_α and to increase ADCC in selected *in vitro* tumor systems. It appears that rhM-CSF has no activity in canines.

Gene Therapy

A major goal of gene therapy may be to inhibit the expression of endogenous genes using antisense oligonucleotides. These can be introduced into cells using viral vectors, liposomes, and cationic lipid complexes. Only liposomes can be used to package anionic and nonionic oligonucleotides.

Gene therapy is being used to introduce cytokine-expressing genes into tumor-infiltrating lymphocytes (TILs). Another exciting area of research is the incorporation of the gene that induces multidrug resistance (mdr) into bone marrow cells to increase the therapeutic index of chemotherapy. To date, no trials using gene therapy have been reported in clinical veterinary oncology.

It is unlikely that biotherapy will be a "stand alone" treatment for cancer. Just as surgery, radiation, and chemotherapy are used in combination, biotherapy is most likely to be used in combination with other modalities.

CHAPTER 75

RADIATION THERAPY: PRINCIPLES AND CLINICAL APPLICATIONS
(pages 493–506)

RADIATION BIOLOGY (pp. 493–499)

Injury to the DNA is believed to be the primary mechanism by which radiation kills cells. In general, tissues with the highest percentage of regularly dividing cells are the most sensitive to the acute effects of radiation. For example, tissues such as the skin, bone marrow, and gastrointenstinal mucosa require continued cellular prolifera-

Original chapter written by G. Neal Mauldin and Karri A. Meleo

tion for normal function. Furthermore, in general the radiosensitivity of tumor cells parallels the sensitivity of the cells of the tissue of origin. Consequently, tumors of the hematopoietic system are the most sensitive to the effects of radiation, followed by epithelial tumors (carcinomas) and, finally, mesenchymal tumors (sarcomas).

In clinical practice, radiation is delivered in multiple fractions. As cells within the sensitive phases of the cell cycle are killed by one fraction, cells in the less sensitive phases progress along the cycle and may be killed by subsequent fractions. Oxygen enhances the effects of ionizing radiation by inhibiting the repair of DNA damage. Cells that are separated from the capillary beds by more than 100 μm are hypoxic and may be protected from the effects of radiation. Cells that are more than 150 μm from the capillaries are anoxic and often necrotic.

CELL RESISTANCE

Tumor tissues may also increase the overall rate of cell division in response to radiation therapy. This tumor regeneration has important clinical implications in planning radiation therapy: interruptions in therapy should be avoided; if an interruption in treatment is necessary because of acute toxicity, it should be kept as short as possible; postponements in therapy for nonmedical reasons (machine breakdown, holidays) may sometimes warrant "catch-up" treatments, provided the patient can tolerate the potential increase in acute toxicity.

Radiation Therapy and Surgery

The general rationale for combining surgery and radiation therapy is that the mechanism of failure for the two techniques is quite different. Radiation rarely fails at the periphery of tumors, where cells are small in number and well vascularized. If surgery fails under these circumstances, it is usually due to the presence of residual microscopic tumor cells at the periphery of the surgical field.

Since radiation therapy kills a constant percentage of tumor cells with each fraction, cytoreduction via surgery prior to radiotherapy may increase the probability of a cure. In addition, decreasing the tumor size with surgery often encourages recruitment of tumor cells from the nonproliferating population into the growth fraction, thus increasing the percentage of cells within the tumor that are sensitive to radiation. If surgery can significantly decrease the size of the tumor, the number and percentage of hypoxic cells within the tumor may also be decreased. In general, a delay of 1½ to 3 weeks before beginning radiotherapy is recommended.

Preoperative radiotherapy also has certain advantages. By decreasing the tumor size prior to surgery, radiation therapy may improve the ease of resection. Radiation may also eradicate subclinical disease beyond the margins of surgical resection. Ionizing radiation may also influence the viability of tumor cells and decrease the chance of tumor implantation or dissemination that could occur as a result of surgical manipulation. Intraoperative radiation therapy has been used successfully to treat dogs with nonmetastatic prostatic adenocarcinoma.

Radiosensitizers and Protectors

Agents that enhance the damage to hypoxic cells have been intensively studied as radiosensitizers, since tumors often contain a percentage of hypoxic cells while normal tissues do not. We have treated two cats with oral squamous cell carcinoma with misonidazole and radiation therapy. Both cats developed severe neurologic signs that were reversible when the radiosensitizer was discontinued. Other nitroimidazoles are currently being studied in both clinical and laboratory trials.

The perfluorochemicals increase the local concentration of oxygen within tumor tissue, and thus may potentiate the radiosensitivity of tumor cells. Diethylmaleate (DEM) and buthionine sulphoxamine (BSO) are both effective radiosensitizers, and clinical trials are under way in both veterinary and human oncology to determine their safety and efficacy.

Combined treatment using standard chemotherapeutic agents may also enhance the effects of radiation. Both actinomycin D (Dactinomycin) and doxorubicin (Adriamycin) decrease the shoulder of the radiation survival curve, and thus enhance the effects of radiation, especially at low dosages. Chemicals may also interact with radiation by preferentially killing cells that are more resistant to radiation.

Radiation Therapy and Hyperthermia

Hyperthermia is an ideal radiosensitizer in that it preferentially increases the toxicity of radiation to tumor tissue without significantly enhancing the toxicity to normal tissue. In veterinary medicine, radiation and hyperthermia have been combined to treat patients with oral squamous cell carcinoma, soft tissue sarcomas, mast cell tumor, malignant melanoma, and mammary carcinoma. Improved complete and long-term control rates have been reported in some patients when compared to the results of radiation therapy alone.

Radiation therapy is a local treatment. Therefore, complete staging of every patient is necessary prior to therapy in order to ensure that local therapy is indicated.

Radiation Simulation

See textbook.

Dosimetry

See textbook.

CLINICAL RADIATION THERAPY (pp. 501–505)

HEMOLYMPHATIC NEOPLASIA OF DOGS AND CATS

Tumors that arise from hemolymphatic tissues are among the most responsive to radiation therapy.

Lymphoma

Because of the systemic nature of this cancer in both species, chemotherapy remains the cornerstone of treatment (Chapter 73). Radiotherapy may be used to alleviate any physical problems caused by a lymphomatous mass, such as breathing difficulty caused by a large thymic mass, pelvic canal obstruction due to intrapelvic lymph nodes, or central nervous system (CNS) signs secondary to brain or spinal LSA. Radiation therapy may also play a role in the treatment of animals that have developed a drug-resistant form of LSA, or in those less frequent cases that present as LSA confined to a single site, such as solitary cutaneous lesions in the dog or nasal lymphoma in the cat. Other diseases of malignant lymphoid cells—such as multiple myeloma, solitary plasmacytomas, and mycosis fungoides—may benefit from RT.

Mast Cell Tumor

The use of RT for the treatment of MCT is limited to animals with local or regional disease. Dogs with grade II or III MCT and unclean margins have a high risk of recurrence and are good candidates for adjunct therapy with RT.

Thymoma

Dogs and cats with thymomas of predominantly lymphoid origin may be treated with RT, especially if surgical excision is incomplete or impossible.

Reticulosis

The reticuloses that involve lymphoid cell lines may respond to radiotherapy in much the same way as CNS lymphoma and may in fact be the same disease.

EPITHELIAL NEOPLASIA OF DOGS AND CATS

Very little structured work has been done with treatment of the epithelial tumors, and much of the information is currently anecdotal. Table 75–1 in the textbook summarizes many carcinomas that may be treated with RT and lists their relative radiosensitivities and metastatic potentials.

Nasal Carcinoma. In dogs, a distinction must be made between nasal adenocarcinoma (AdCa) and a more aggressive and anaplastic tumor that is variably known as nasal squamous cell carcinoma (SCCa) or nasal solid carcinoma. More aggressive radiotherapy protocols utilizing a higher cumulative dose may improve the survival times for dogs with both nasal adenocarcinoma and nasal sarcomas. Combination chemotherapy and radiotherapy protocols may be necessary to significantly increase the survival of dogs with nasal SCCa.

Oral Squamous Cell Carcinoma. Aggressive radiation therapy and radiation-hyperthermia protocols have not significantly improved survival times over those of untreated animals. One promising new protocol combines radiation therapy and chemotherapy using mitoxantrone (Novantrone). Squamous cell carcinomas of the nasal planum and ear tips are solar radiation–induced tumors in the cat. They usually respond well to radiation therapy alone, and the prognosis is good. Nasal planum SCCa in the dog is an aggressive tumor that frequently fails to respond to radiotherapy.

Thyroid Carcinomas. Functional thyroid tumors in both dogs and cats are best treated with radionuclide therapy, such as ^{131}I. Radiation resistance combined with aggressive biologic behavior require innovative treatments to achieve adequate tumor control in dogs with nonfunctional thyroid malignancies.

Epithelial Tumors of the Central Nervous System

Primary carcinomas of the CNS are rare with the exception of pituitary tumors. Most other epithelial tumors of the CNS will be metastatic from some other site, and animals with a diagnosis of CNS carcinoma must be carefully screened for systemic cancer.

Animals that do not tolerate or respond to medical treatment for pituitary dependent hyperadrenocorticism (PDH) might benefit from radiotherapy. At the present time, radiotherapy may be the only therapy that can be offered cats with pituitary tumors.

Carcinomas of the Skin

As a general rule, carcinomas arising from the skin and adnexal structures are radioresponsive.

Cutaneous Squamous Cell and Basal Cell Carcinoma. Radiation therapy can induce remissions in animals with incompletely resected or unresected lesions, leading to disease-free survival times exceeding 1 year in many cases.

Perianal Gland Tumors. Complete and durable remissions

have been attained after RT in dogs with perianal adenomas and adenocarcinomas in which surgery was either not attempted or impossible. Irradiation of most or all of the anal sphincter increases the risk of rectal stricture as a possible late complication.

Urogenital Carcinomas

Transitional Cell Carcinoma of the Urinary Bladder. Surgical removal is the treatment of choice but is often impossible because of involvement of the trigone of the bladder. A protocol incorporating RT and cisplatinum chemotherapy in dogs has shown the most promise of increasing survival with a reasonable quality of life.

Mammary Gland Carcinoma. Aggressive surgical resection is the recommended treatment in both species. Treatment of recurrent or inoperable thoracic or abdominal wall mammary gland tumors with radiotherapy can result in remissions.

MESENCHYMAL TUMORS OF THE DOG AND CAT

Biologic characteristics make the sarcomas the most radioresistant of all the classes of tumors. This does not mean, however, that RT cannot be used to effectively treat many mesenchymal tumors, especially as an adjunct to surgical resection. Table 75–2 in the textbook summarizes the soft tissue sarcomas most commonly treated with RT.

Soft Tissue Sarcomas

This group includes fibrosarcomas, hemangiopericytomas, neurofibrosarcomas, and malignant fibrous histiocytomas. The combination of local aggression and infrequent metastasis make combination radiation and surgery ideal for the treatment of these tumors.

Central Nervous System Sarcomas

Complete surgical resection or combination surgery and RT may be especially appropriate for the treatment of meningiomas, which tend to be superficial and resectable.

Osteosarcoma

Amputation alone is frequently curative in the cat and is well tolerated. Osteosarcoma in the dog is a rapidly progressive tumor that is best treated with amputation and a chemotherapy protocol incorporating cisplatinum. In dogs that are unable to undergo amputation, radiation may play a role in the palliation of the pain associated with this tumor.

CLINICAL RADIATION TOXICITY

The normal tissue response is always the dose-limiting toxicity for radiotherapy.

Cutaneous Toxicity

Cutaneous reactions are the most common form of toxicity seen with radiation therapy. Although frequently uncomfortable and requiring treatment, these skin reactions rarely result in the discontinuation of therapy. As a general rule, the acute skin reactions are worse in protocols that have a high dose per fraction delivered over a short period of time. Cobalt or other megavoltage radiation tends to be skin-sparing, since it must pass through a few millimeters of absorbing tissue before maximal radiation dose is achieved. Another property of orthovoltage radiation is that bone absorbs relatively more radiation than does soft tissue, and this may result in bone necrosis and sequestrum formation.

Ocular Complications

Toxicity to the eye frequently results from treatment of tumors of the head and neck, especially nasal carcinomas. All parts of the eye can be affected and can exhibit damage in different ways.

Radiation Sickness

Radiation-induced nausea and vomiting are usually seen only in animals that undergo abdominal irradiation. However, many animals may become anorexic during their tumor response.

CHAPTER 76
SURGICAL ONCOLOGY
(pages 506–513)

APPLICATIONS OF SURGICAL ONCOLOGY (pp. 506–511)

Surgery in cancer therapy initially involves the establishment of a diagnosis, usually best determined by biopsy and histologic evaluation of the tissue. Cytology is a useful preliminary study of cells that precedes the tissue biopsy for histopathologic diagnosis. Standard methods of obtaining tissue for a histopathologic diagnosis include needle core biopsy, incisional biopsy, and excisional biopsy (Chapter 49). Excisional biopsy is the preferred method if the mass can be removed completely and the results of the biopsy will not alter the treatment recommendation. Preoperative biopsy is indicated for determining the grade of a tumor, staging the extent of tumor, and determining whether aggressive surgery is required, such as limb amputation versus local excision of the tumor, or whether alternative therapy is indicated.

Serious complications such as tumor dissemination, hemorrhage, and infection may result from improper biopsy techniques. The external edges of an excisional biopsy should be marked so that the pathologist can determine whether neoplastic cells are at the surgical margins.

SURGERY FOR TREATMENT

One of the most important roles surgery plays in cancer therapy is that of primary treatment. Tumor behavior and extent of tumor (stage) are important predictors of a tumor's response to surgical excision. Concurrent conditions in a patient may influence the type of surgical procedure that can be performed, so thorough preoperative patient evaluation and tumor staging are recommended.

Principles of Oncologic Surgery

There are four classifications for surgical resection of a tumor (see Table 76–1 in the textbook). Generally one should be at least one tissue plane away from the malignant tumor. Tumors should be removed in one piece and should include a surrounding layer of normal tissue as well as any previous biopsy tract or surgical incision. Tumor manipula-

---

Original chapter written by Maura G. O'Brien and Stephen J. Withrow

tion should be minimized to prevent rupture of the mass and limit local tumor dissemination. When possible the vascular drainage (veins) of a tumor should be ligated early in the procedure, in an attempt to prevent embolization of large aggregates of tumor cells into the bloodstream. Excessive undermining of normal tissue should be avoided because it leads to potential contamination of previously uninvolved tissue planes and may promote seroma formation.

To avoid dissemination of malignant cells to other sites, contaminated instruments, gloves, and drapes should be changed frequently, especially between excisions of different masses or when beginning new procedures. "Clean," non-oncologic procedures should be performed before the primary surgery.

The removal of a tumor-bearing lymph node is practical if the lymphatic vessels draining the primary tumor can also be removed (e.g., *en bloc* excision). Enlarged, tumor-bearing lymph nodes that are fixed to surrounding tissues are generally not removed because complete excision is impossible and their removal may cause excessive morbidity. Palliative removal or cytoreductive surgery is warranted when nodes become enlarged and cause clinical signs. The wound should be closed using the patient's own tissues, provided they have an adequate blood supply and there is minimal tension on the suture line. If an extensive tumor resection is planned and it is believed that primary wound closure may be difficult, it is better to leave the wound open than to perform a marginal resection, close the wound, and leave tumor *in situ*. The open wound should heal by second intention or can be closed with reconstructive procedures such as free flaps or axial pattern grafts.

Postoperative Care

Surgical oncology procedures are frequently associated with intraoperative blood loss, extensive soft tissue resection, and pain. Animals should be monitored closely to prevent self-trauma to incisions, grafts, and bandages. Provision of an adequate nutritional plane is important to place the animal in a positive energy balance and speed the healing process (Chapter 54).

Complications that may occur in surgical oncology patients are infection, wound dehiscence, immunosuppression, local tumor recurrence, and metastatic disease.

ADDITIONAL USES FOR SURGERY IN ONCOLOGY
(pp. 511–512)

SURGERY FOR COMPLICATIONS OF CANCER THERAPY

If extensive damage due to extravasation of a chemotherapeutic agent occurs, the damage may require debridement and skin grafting procedures. Radiation therapy may result in soft tissue and bone necrosis that may not appear until months after therapy. Bone necrosis may result in chronic deep-seated infections and osteomyelitis, which often requires surgery to remove avascular tissue and reconstruct the region with skin and muscle flaps to restore blood supply, function, and cosmesis.

SURGERY FOR PALLIATION

In some oncology patients there is no valid, curative treatment because of the type or extent of disease. Surgery can sometimes be offered to palliate symptoms and improve the quality of the patient's life, even if only for a brief period. The surgeon should always remember that the palliative procedure must never induce more morbidity than the disease itself or worsen the patient's quality of life.

RECENT ADVANCES IN ONCOLOGIC SURGERY

New operative procedures are available to treat forms of cancer previously believed unresectable. Limb-sparing techniques now substitute for amputation in dogs affected with osteosarcoma and other bone tumors. Procedures such as maxillectomy, mandibulectomy, and orbitectomy are now used successfully to excise many tumors of the head with minimal morbidity and surprisingly good functional and cosmetic results. Recently, hemipelvectomy has been described for the excision of pelvic bone tumors.

CHAPTER 77
PARANEOPLASTIC SYNDROMES
(pages 513–521)

Remote effects of malignancy are known as paraneoplastic syndromes. The best known and characterized paraneoplastic syndromes are those produced by tumors that secrete a hormone such as parathormone or insulin. In veterinary medicine, the etiology of most paraneoplastic syndromes is unknown.

CANCER CACHEXIA (pp. 513–515)

Cancer causes profound alterations in carbohydrate, protein, and lipid metabolism which result in the syndrome known as cancer cachexia. Cancer cachexia causes weight loss in spite of adequate nutritional intake.

CANCER AND CARBOHYDRATE METABOLISM

In tumor cells, glucose is the preferred substrate for energy production. Relative insulin resistance has been reported in both human cancer patients and dogs with cancer. Alterations in carbohydrate metabolism result partially because tumors preferentially metabolize glucose, use anaerobic glycolysis for energy, and form lactate as an end product. The host must convert the majority of the lactate back to glucose, which results in a net energy gain by the tumor and an energy loss by the host.

CANCER AND PROTEIN METABOLISM

In cancer cachexia, protein degradation often exceeds protein synthesis, which results in a negative nitrogen balance. Because all protein is functional, net protein loss in cancer cachexia results in decreased cell-mediated and humoral immunity, gastrointestinal function, and wound healing. Loss of body protein is manifested clinically as atrophy of skeletal muscle and hypoalbuminemia. Because fatty acids cannot serve as gluconeogenic precursors in these animals, amino acids are the primary substrate for gluconeogenesis in cancer cachexia.

Original chapter written by Gregory K. Ogilvie

CANCER AND FAT METABOLISM

Patients with cancer cachexia have increased fat breakdown, which correlates with increased levels of free fatty acids and certain plasma lipoprotein. Knowledge that tumor cells have difficulty utilizing lipids as a fuel may be of value clinically, especially since host tissues can continue to oxidize lipids for energy. Experimentally, specific types of triglycerides and fatty acids have minimized cancer cachexia and, in some circumstances, had anticancer effects. Medium-chain triglycerides, 3-hydroxybutyrate, and diets that are high in fish oils and rich in omega-3-type polyunsaturated fatty acids EPA (20:5, omega-3) and DHA (C22:6, omega-3) are effective for promoting weight gain and have an anticancer effect.

TREATMENT: ENTERAL AND PARENTERAL THERAPY FOR THE CANCER PATIENT

Nutrient profiles that contain 30 to 50 per cent of nonprotein calories as fat instead of carbohydrate decrease glucose intolerance, fat loss, and tumor growth while host weight, nitrogen, and energy balance increase. The addition of medium-chain fatty acids and omega-3 fatty acids may be beneficial in treating dogs with cancer. Diets based on shark cartilage may also be therapeutic. As an example, to calculate the number of calories needed for the dog with cancer, the basal energy requirement (Kcal/day) is determined by multiplying 70 times the animal's weight in kg and then multiplying by 1.2 to 2. The protein requirements for dogs without renal disease are approximately 4 to 6 gm/kg/day. Lactate- and glucose-containing parenteral fluids should be avoided for critically ill animals with cancer that require acute, intensive fluid therapy.

HYPERCALCEMIA (pp. 515–516)

Cancer is the most common cause of hypercalcemia in the dog and cat. Any neoplastic process has the potential to cause elevated calcium. In the veterinary patient, alterations in renal function are the most common clinical manifestations of hypercalcemia caused by malignant disease. The algorithm (see Fig. 77–1). reviews laboratory findings of common causes of hypercalcemia.

TREATMENT OF HYPERCALCEMIA OF MALIGNANCY

The most important therapy for hypercalcemia of malignancy is identification and elimination of the tumor. Premature and inappropriate administration of symptomatic therapy may interfere with identification of the source of the electrolyte abnormality. The decision to specifically treat hypercalcemia depends on its severity and the severity of related clinical signs. For mild elevations (e.g., 12.5 mg/dl) in animals with minimal clinical signs, the situation is often controlled by adequate hydration. In cases of moderate hypercalcemia with concurrent clinical signs, more aggressive management is indicated, which often entails the use of intravenous saline in volumes that exceed daily maintenance (290 ml/lb$^{0.75}$ [132 mls/kg$^{0.75}$]). Furosemide is often administered concurrently to well hydrated hypercalcemic patients; the drug inhibits calcium resorption at the level of the ascending loop of Henle. Prednisone is effective in treating hypercalcemia because it inhibits osteoclast activating factor, prostaglandins, vitamin D, and the absorption of calcium across the intestinal tract. Other treatments that can be considered in unusual cases include calcitonin, mithramycin, prostaglandin synthetase inhibitors, bisphosphonates, gallium nitrate, and oral phosphate.

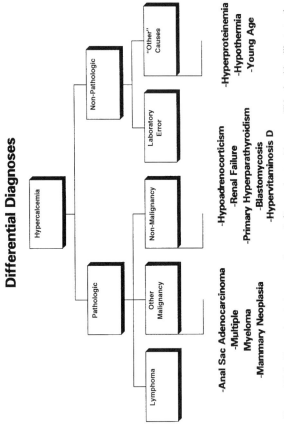

Differential Diagnoses

Figure 77–1. Hypercalcemia is commonly seen in dogs and cats with cancer. This algorithm illustrates the most common differential diagnoses of this electrolyte disorder in the veterinary patient.

HYPOCALCEMIA (pp. 516–517)

Hypocalcemia is a rare complication in veterinary and human cancer. Hypocalcemia of magnesium deficiency can occur from prolonged intestinal drainage procedures, parenteral hyperalimentation without magnesium supplementation, cisplatin therapy, and severe liver disease. The tumor lysis syndrome also may be associated with hypocalcemia secondary to elevated phosphate levels.

TREATMENT OF HYPOCALCEMIA OF MALIGNANCY

The underlying cause should be identified and treated as soon as possible. When hypocalcemia is associated with clinical signs, intravenous administration of calcium should be initiated followed by oral calcium supplements, and vitamin D if needed.

HYPOGLYCEMIA (p. 517)

Insulinoma is the most common malignancy associated with hypoglycemia (blood glucose <70 mg/dl) in the dog. In contrast to insulinomas that produce excessive quantities of insulin, hypoglycemia of extrapancreatic tumors in the dog has been associated with low to low-normal insulin levels. The most common differential diagnoses of non-malignant causes of hypoglycemia include hyperinsulinism, hepatic dysfunction, adrenocortical insufficiency, hypopituitarism, extrapancreatic tumors, starvation, sepsis, and laboratory error.

Animals with hypoglycemia secondary to malignancy are often presented to a veterinarian with neurologic signs. These include weakness, disorientation, and seizures that may progress to convulsions, coma, and death. The identification of malignancy-associated hypoglycemia is made when the blood glucose is dramatically reduced, but insulin levels are elevated.

TREATMENT OF MALIGNANCY-ASSOCIATED HYPOGLYCEMIA

Surgical extirpation may be the treatment of choice for tumors that produce hypoglycemia. Surgery often is not curative. Prednisone is often effective in elevating blood glucose levels by inducing hepatic gluconeogensis and decreasing peripheral utilization of glucose. Diazoxide may be effective in elevating blood glucose levels by directly inhibiting pancreatic insulin secretion and glucose uptake by tissues, enhancing epinephrine-induced glycogenolysis, and increasing the rate of mobilization of free fatty acids. Diazoxide's hyperglycemic effects can be potentiated by concurrent administration of hydrochlorothiazide. Propranolol, a β-adrenergic blocking agent, may also be effective in increasing blood glucose levels.

ERYTHROCYTOSIS (p. 517)

Erythrocytosis secondary to malignancy results from increased production of erythropoietin or occurs secondarily as a result of tumor-induced hypoxia, which subsequently triggers the production of erythropoietin. Tumors that infrequently induce a pathologic increase in the red blood cell mass by direct or indirect means include renal cell tumors, lymphoma, and hepatic tumors. Other causes of erythrocytosis include dehydration, pulmonary and cardiac disorders, venoarterial shunts, Cushing's disease, the chronic administration of adrenocortical steroids, and polycythemia vera. Erythrocytosis of paraneoplastic origin can be distinguished from polycythemia vera by the absence of pancytosis or splenomegaly, and from secondary polycythemia by the absence of decreased arterial oxygen saturation.

TREATMENT OF TUMOR-INDUCED ERYTHROCYTOSIS

Surgical removal of the tumor that induces regional or systemic hypoxia is the treatment of choice. Phlebotomies may temporarily reduce the red blood cell load. The chemotherapeutic agent hydroxyurea can be used to induce reversible bone marrow suppression.

OTHER SYNDROMES OF ECTOPIC HORMONE PRODUCTION (pp. 517–518)

Diagnostic criteria for the syndrome of inappropriate secretion of antidiuretic hormone include hypo-osmolality and hyponatremia of extracellular fluids, urine that is less than maximally dilute, absence of volume depletion, sustained renal excretion of sodium, and normal renal and adrenal function. The clinical signs result from excess retention of water with clinical manifestations of weakness and lethargy that may progress to seizures, coma, and death.

The ectopic production of adrenocorticotropic hormone (ACTH) or related polypeptides has been described for a variety of cancers in man. This condition was reported in a primary lung tumor in a dog. Clinical signs are similar to those of Cushing's disease.

HYPERTROPHIC OSTEOPATHY (p. 518)

Hypertrophic osteopathy is a disorder that occurs primarily in bones of the extremities in dogs, and rarely in cats. This paraneoplastic syndrome, often associated with primary and metastatic lung tumors, may cause lameness and painful swellings of affected bones. Other neoplastic and non-neoplastic conditions associated with hypertrophic osteopathy include esophageal sarcoma, rhabdomyosarcoma of the urinary bladder, pneumonia, heartworm disease, congenital and acquired heart disease, and focal lung atelectasis.

TREATMENT OF HYPERTROPHIC OSTEOPATHY

Glucocorticoid therapy offers temporary improvement in clinical signs and may reduce the extent of swelling. Removal of the tumor can result in resolution of clinical signs and regression of the bony changes. Other treatments such as unilateral vagotomy on the side of the lung lesion, incision through the parietal pleura, subperiosteal rib resection, bilateral cervical vagotomy, and the use of analgesics have been suggested.

ANEMIA (pp. 518–519)

This paraneoplastic syndrome may be caused by anemia of chronic disease, bone marrow invasion by tumor cells, blood loss, marrow suppression by chemotherapy, hypersplenism, immune-mediated disease, megaloblastic anemia, vitamin and iron deficiency, microangiopathic hemolytic anemia, and pure red cell aplasia. Clinically, anemia of chronic disease is recognized as normocytic, normochromic, normal bone marrow cellularity, depressed iron metabolism, and reticuloendothelial iron sequestration. Treatment is directed at elimination of the neoplastic condition.

Blood loss anemia is recognized clinically when the red blood cells are microcytic and hypochromic due to decreased hemoglobin synthesis. Poikilocytosis, microleptocytosis, inadequate reticulocytosis, increased total iron binding capacity, decreased serum iron concentrations, and elevated platelet counts may also be seen in this condition. The marked decrease in serum iron concentration may be treated with ferrous sulfate along with appropriate steps to eliminate the tumor.

Hemolysis and schistocytosis is the hallmark of microangiopathic hemolytic anemia. Although hemangiosarcoma is the most common cause of this type of anemia, it can be seen with a variety of neoplastic diseases. Removal of the tumor and appropriate supportive care (e.g., intravenous fluids) may be beneficial in this type of anemia.

Diagnosis of immune-related hemolytic anemia is based on finding antibody or complement on the surface of the patient's red blood cells through a Coomb's test or slide agglutination test, spherocytosis, and a regenerative anemia. Medical management with prednisone and azathioprine may be indicated if rapid resolution of the underlying neoplastic condition is not possible. The degree of anemia associated with the administration of chemotherapeutic agents is generally mild and without clinical signs.

LEUKOCYTOSIS (p. 519)

An elevation in white blood cell count has been seen in a variety of canine tumors including lymphoma and hemangiosarcoma. Generally, the condition is not clinically significant.

THROMBOCYTOPENIA (pp. 519–520)

Platelet consumption is the most significant hemostatic abnormality in tumor-bearing dogs. If DIC is suspected, prolongation of clotting times (ACT, OSPT, APTT) and an elevated fibrinogen may be identified along with the thrombocytopenia. In these cases, elimination of the neoplastic condition, intravenous fluids, and heparin may be of therapeutic value.

Immune-mediated thrombocytopenia is also a significant cause of decreased platelet numbers in dogs with cancer. Immune-mediated thrombocytopenia has been successfully resolved in the dog by elimination of the tumor and treatment with immunosuppressive drugs such as prednisone and azathioprine. Vincristine can be used to temporarily increase platelet numbers.

HYPERGAMMAGLOBULINEMIA (p. 520)

These diseases result from excessive secretion of a monoclonal line of immunoglobulin-producing cells. IgG, IgA, IgM, and light-chain protein classes are produced in large quantities and may be identified by performing a protein immunoelectrophoresis on serum. In addition, Bence Jones proteins (light chains) may be identified in the urine. Approximately 75 per cent of plasma cell tumors in dogs have M-component disorders. Other tumors associated with this syndrome include lymphoma, lymphocytic leukemia, and primary macroglobulinemia.

Bleeding disorders, commonly noted clinically as epistaxis, are the result of elevated proteins interfering with normal platelet function. A hyperviscosity syndrome becomes clinically apparent as elevated protein decreases fluidity of the blood, which results in central nervous system signs, retinopathies, visual disturbances, congestive heart failure, and renal decompensation.

TREATMENT OF M-COMPONENT DISORDERS

The treatment of M-component disorders revolves around appropriate antitumor and supportive therapy. The hyperviscosity syndrome may require immediate therapy directed toward reduction of protein levels in the blood such as plasmapheresis. Antibiotics often are indicated because myeloma cells secrete an immunosuppressive substance that suppresses macrophage and lymphocyte function.

FEVER (p. 520)

Tumor-associated fever usually is defined as unexplained fever that coincides with the growth or elimination of a tumor.

TREATMENT OF TUMOR-INDUCED FEVER

Fever that is directly related to malignant disease can be treated symptomatically with antipyretics or nonsteroidal anti-inflammatory agents.

NEUROLOGIC ABNORMALITIES (p. 520)

There are several reports in the veterinary literature of cancer-induced peripheral neuropathies, including a case of trigeminal nerve paralysis and Horner's syndrome in the dog. Animals also exhibit neurologic signs secondary to endocrine, fluid, and electrolyte disturbances caused by neoplasia. Hypercalcemia, hyperviscosity syndrome, and hepatoencephalopathy are common examples. The neurologic syndromes of myasthenia gravis secondary to thymoma are well described in the literature.

CHAPTER 78

OCULAR MANIFESTATIONS OF SYSTEMIC DISEASES
(pages 524–533)

This chapter outlines specific ocular abnormalities. See other chapters for details on systemic signs, diagnosis, and treatment of these diseases.

PARASITIC AND INFECTIOUS DISEASES (pp. 524–527)

PARASITIC DISEASES

Toxoplasmosis. The most common ocular lesion is multifocal posterior chorioretinitis, which may result in retinal detachment. Ocular disease is more common in cats than in dogs (see Chapters 82 and 83). Anterior uveitis can be exudative or granulomatous in the cat; generally granulomatous inflammation is seen in the dog.

Leishmaniasis. Ocular signs can be associated with general disease or may be isolated. Chronic keratoconjunctivitis and keratouveitis are the prominent signs. "Spectacle blepharitis" with skin surface desquamation and loss of hair is characteristic. Granulomatous and nongranulomatous uveitis are observed; anterior uveitis is the most frequent.

Ehrlichiosis. Ehrlichiosis (tropical canine pancytopenia) is associated with ocular signs that include conjunctivitis, corneal opacities, conjunctival hemorrhage, and hyphema. Horseshoe-shaped, gray, perivascular lesions characteristic of nongranulomatous chorioretinitis develop and later regress, resulting in focal or diffuse retinal atrophy.

Ophthalmomyiasis. Ophthalmomyiasis interna may be anterior when the larvae are found in the anterior segment and posterior when larvae are found posterior to the lens. Clinical abnormalities included uveitis, multiple curvilinear tracks involving both tapetal and nontapetal fundi, and low-grade chorioretinitis.

Other Diseases. *Rocky Mountain spotted fever* is a rickettsial infection inducing scleral vascular congestion, conjunctivitis, chemosis, and mucopurulent ocular discharge. Petechial retinal hemorrhages, anterior uveitis with deep corneal vascularization, corneal edema, aqueous flare, and miosis have been described. *Visceral larva migrans,* caused by the migratory stages of *Toxocara canis,* may result in ocular

---

Original chapter written by Bernard Clerc and Hervé LaForge

granulomatous inflammation. Chronic, low-grade anterior uveitis may be associated with *D. immitis* larvae and/or a toxic effect of its metabolic products.

BACTERIAL AND MYCOBACTERIAL DISEASES

Endophthalmitis, intraretinal hemorrhage, and toxic anterior uveitis have been reported in dogs with endocarditis and pyometra. Systemic infection with *Brucella canis* may cause chronic anterior uveitis or endophthalmitis, and *Leptospira icterohaemorrhagiae* has been associated with episcleral injection, yellowing of the sclera, conjunctival petechiae, and anterior uveitis. *Tuberculosis* has been reported to cause ocular granulomatous inflammation in the cat.

FUNGAL AND ALGAL DISEASES

Cryptococcosis can produce subretinal granulomas, retinal detachments, hyphema, anisocoria, papilledema, papillitis, and orbital cellulitis. Systemic *blastomycosis* can be associated with severe granulomatous chorioretinitis with retinal detachment, optic neuritis, anterior uveitis, and secondary glaucoma. Ocular manifestations of *coccidioidomycosis* include granulomatous panuveitis with infiltration of inflammatory cells into the cornea and iridocorneal angle. A severe interstitial keratitis may accompany the anterior uveitis.

Focal granulomatous anterior and posterior uveitis occur infrequently with disseminated *histoplasmosis*. *Geotrichosis*, a rare mycosis, can generate panuveitis with focal inflammatory infiltration of uveal tissue and exudative retinal detachment. Granulomatous necrotizing chorioretinitis with retinal detachment and hemorrhagic gastroenteritis characterize the pathology of *Prototheca*.

VIRAL DISEASES

Infectious Canine Hepatitis. The typical ocular lesion of infectious canine hepatitis is unilateral or bilateral anterior uveitis called "blue eye" or "blue keratitis."

Canine Distemper. Ocular manifestations of canine distemper are, by decreasing frequency, conjunctivitis, chorioretinitis, keratoconjunctivitis sicca (KCS), and optic nerve lesions. Conjunctivitis is always present in an acute form. Acute distemper retinal lesions are characterized by hazy areas of retinitis and perivascular infiltration. After several weeks, this area is marked by bright, hyperreflective lesions in the tapetal retina. In the nontapetal area, depigmented patches and areas of light-gray color appear.

Feline chlamydiosis **(Chlamydia psittaci).** Purulent discharge is often seen even in early cases. Chronic cases exhibit thickened conjunctiva, minimal exudate, and occasionally follicles.

Mycoplasma felis and M. gatae. There is usually a monocular purulent ocular discharge with a mildly hyperemic conjunctival surface.

Feline Herpesvirus. It can produce three different forms of ocular troubles, which appear to be age-dependent. Intense chemosis, conjunctival vascular injection, partial prolapse of the nictitans, and mucopurulent ocular discharge characterize the fulminant viral disease in kittens 2 to 4 weeks old. A more benign conjunctivitis that is usually self-limiting in 10 to 14 days is seen in kittens 4 weeks to 6 months old. Older cats develop a keratoconjunctivitis with mild, short-lived respiratory signs. Ulcerative keratitis is remarkable for early punctate or dendritic (branching) superficial corneal ulcers, although geographically deeper ulcers and interstitial keratitis can occur. Topical trifluridine is the most effective viricidal agent for feline herpes.

Feline Infectious Peritonitis. A typical ocular lesion is severe pyogranulomatous anterior uveitis, although both anterior and posterior segments may be involved. When the fundus is visible, focal retinal hemorrhages, perivascular edema, chorioretinitis, and sometimes retinal detachment can be noted.

METABOLIC AND NUTRITIONAL DISORDERS
(pp. 528–530)

METABOLIC DISORDERS

Diabetes Mellitus.   Diabetes mellitus is associated with a high incidence of bilateral cataracts. Diabetic cataracts exhibit three distinguishing clinical features: (1) the most prominent is its rapid development, within a few days in some cases; (2) as in all the cataracts of adult animals, subepithelial cortical vacuoles appear during cataract formation, but they are numerous in this case; and (3) lens intumescence is common in diabetic cataracts.

Disorders of Lipid Metabolism.   Hyperlipidemia and hyperlipoproteinemia may be associated with corneal lipodystrophies, lipid-laden aqueous humor, and lipemia retinalis. Lipid deposits in the canine cornea must be differentiated from calcium keratopathies, which can occur secondary to hypercalcemia or chronic severe inflammation. The clinical aspect of the lipid deposit is usually suggested by bilateral deposits localized at the periphery of the cornea. Inherited corneal dystrophies (Siberian husky, pinscher) are bilateral but usually central.

Inborn Errors of Metabolism.   See Table 78–7 in the textbook.

Neuronal Ceroid Lipofuscinosis.   Clinical signs begin at one year of age with a decrease in visual acuity, followed by behavioral abnormalities. Nervous symptoms appear with depression, ataxia, muscular pain, and masseter muscle hypersensitivity; convulsions are then observed and animals die approximately one year after the onset of clinical signs.

Gangliosidosis GM_1.   This disease is found in the Siamese cat. Visual deficits, multiple opacities in the cornea, and small, gray, multifocal retinal lesions may be observed.

NUTRITIONAL DISORDERS

Taurine Deficiency.   This is an important diagnostic consideration in cats with central retinal or panretinal degeneration.

Thiamine Deficiency.   The pupils of an affected animal become dilated and fixed, although vision is retained. Papilledema and retinal neovascularization have been observed.

Vitamin A Deficiency.   An entire spectrum of disease is seen, including retinopathy, conjunctival and corneal xerosis, corneal ulceration and melting, and less obvious changes in the epithelial structure of a number of organs.

Vitamin E Deficiency.   This condition in the dog has been accompanied by the development of ocular lesions similar to central retinal atrophy.

Other Deficiencies.   Replacements for bitch's milk may be associated with the development of cataracts, which usually occur in the posterior cortical area and do not cause blindness.

VASCULAR DISEASES (p. 530)

These diseases (hyperviscosity, polycythemia, and systemic hypertension) have in common vascular engorgement and perivascular hemorrhage, differing by size and location. They are frequently complicated by retinal detachment.

Clotting Disorders.   Signs include hyphema and uveal and retinal hemorrhages. Retinal hemorrhage is the hallmark of ocular hypertensive disease. Other ocular signs include nongranulomatous chorioretinitis, exudative retinal detachment, "cotton wool spots" (areas of retinal hemorrhage in the nerve fiber layer), sclerosis of retinal vasculature, vitreous hemorrhage, secondary uveitis, and glaucoma.

ALLERGIC AND IMMUNE-MEDIATED DISEASES
(pp. 530–531)

CONJUNCTIVA AND EYELIDS

The immediate-type lesion (histamine and IgE-mediated disease) is seen after food absorption, insect bites, and drug administration. Swelling of eyelid and conjunctival tissue is rapid and impressive.

Delayed Reactions. Eyelids and conjunctiva may appear red and swollen in dogs with atopic disease. Chronic blepharoconjunctivitis may be complicated by infection.

Blepharitis. Blepharitis may be part of a generalized or an extensive immunologic disease with pemphigus-like lesions, discoid lupus lesions, and lupus erythematosus disseminated (LED) lesions.

CORNEA

Keratoconjunctivitis Sicca (KCS). A breed predilection for the miniature schnauzer, cocker spaniel, and West Highland white terrier has been reported with the immune-mediated form. Oral sulfonamides can be responsible for KCS, and we have observed other cases associated with pheneturide, or phenytoin, administration. Cyclosporin A, an immunosuppressive drug, applied topically to dogs with KCS gives dramatic improvement. In the few cases of complete gland destruction, the only possibility of improvement is the use of tear substitutes or parotid duct transposition.

UVEA

Some of the generalized infectious diseases that cause a local reaction of uveitis are listed in Table 78–4 in the textbook. A uveodermatologic syndrome characterized by chronic or recurrent uveitis and dermal depigmentation has been described in several breeds of dogs, including the Akita, Samoyed, Irish setter, Siberian husky, Shetland sheep dog, Ainu dog, and Shiba dog. Retinal detachment, secondary glaucoma, and cataracts are seen in a high percentage of both canine and human patients.

CANINE OCULAR TUMORS (pp. 531–533)

OCULAR TUMORS

Primary Neoplasms with Possible Extension. *Primary ocular melanomas*, the most common ocular tumors in dogs, seldom metastasize. *Adenocarcinomas*, the most common nonpigmented anterior uveal tumors, are invasive as well as proliferative, and are known for their pulmonary and liver metastases.

Metastatic Ocular Neoplasms. *Malignant lymphoma*, the most common secondary intraocular tumor in the dog, may involve ocular or periocular structures, although the uvea is the most frequently affected intraocular tissue. Conjunctivitis is common, and corneal infiltration with cells and vessels occurs. Anterior uveal infiltration results in mild uveitis, flare, and hypopyon with keratic precipitates. Choroidal involvement is less frequent and occurs primarily adjacent to the optic disc. Retinal involvement is characterized by increased vascular tortuosity, papilledema, intraretinal hemorrhage, and localized or complete retinal detachment. As in all cases of uveitis, complications such as synechia, glaucoma, hyphema, and complete retinal detachment may occur.

The uvea is the major site of involvement of ocular metastatic carcinoma; common clinical signs include intraocular hemorrhage, iridocyclitis, nonpigmented uveal nodules, and secondary glaucoma. The intraocular extension from optic nerve tumors is seen with meningiomas, astrocytomas, gliomas, gangliogliomas, and reticulosis. These cases may appear clinically as optic neuritis.

FELINE OCULAR TUMORS

Primary Intraocular Tumors. Intraocular malignant melanoma, the most common primary ocular tumor of cats, tends to metastasize. Primary ocular sarcomas other than malignant melanomas are uncommon.

Metastatic Ocular Tumors of the Cat. Secondary intraocular tumors of the eye of the cat include the feline lymphosarcoma leukemia complex (FeLV), reticulosis, plasma cell myeloma, and intraocular extension of tumors of the orbit, optic nerve, and adjacent tissues. Carcinoma metastases to the anterior and posterior uvea from primary sites in the lung, uterus, and mammary gland have been known to occur. Intraocular tumors may present with a variety of signs and should be suspected in all cases of otherwise inexplicable inflammation, uveitis, hyphema, and/or glaucoma.

BLINDNESS (p. 533)

Blindness is often the result of ocular lesions but may be related to a general disease. Practitioners should be aware of the main causes of blindness: intraocular inflammation, glaucoma, and retinal dystrophy.

CHAPTER 79
DISEASES OF THE EAR
(pages 533–550)

DISEASES OF THE PINNA (pp. 534–538)

CLINICAL MANIFESTATIONS, DIAGNOSIS, AND THERAPY OF SPECIFIC DISEASES OF THE PINNA

Nonpruritic Alopecia

Acquired Pattern Alopecia (Pattern Baldness). A progressive, symmetric alopecia of the pinna is seen primarily in dachshunds, but also occurs in Boston terriers, Chihuahuas, whippets, Manchester terriers, and Italian greyhounds. The alopecia seldom develops before 1 year of age and is slowly progressive. Diagnosis is based on the process of elimination and on skin biopsy. There is anecdotal suggestion that thyroid hormone, sex hormones, or etretinate may produce some regrowth in affected cases.

Periodic Pinnal Alopecia of Miniature Poodles. Mature miniature poodles are known to undergo a sudden loss of hair over one

---

Original chapter written by Rod A.W. Rosychuk and Patricia Luttgen or both ears. Over several months there is progression to complete bilateral pinnal alopecia. Spontaneous hair regrowth is noted within several months.

Idiopathic Pinnal Alopecia of Siamese Cats. Spontaneous, symmetric pinnal alopecia is noted to gradually develop in affected cats. In some, the alopecia will be periodic, with spontaneous regrowth after several months.

Ear Margin Dermatoses

Sarcoptic and Notoedric Mange. *Sarcoptes scabiei* produces an intensely pruritic dermatitis primarily directed at the head, convex (outer) aspect of the pinna, lateral elbows, stifles, and ventrum of the dog. Pinna lesions consist of patchy alopecia, erythema, scaling, and crusting. Diagnosis is made by skin scrapings or response to trial therapy. Therapy involves oral ivermectin once weekly for 4 to 6 weeks or until lesions and pruritus have completely resolved. To hasten resolution and reduce the potential for contagion, topical therapy with 2 per cent lime sulfur dips administered once weekly, or amitraz (Mitaban), 0.025 per cent administered once weekly, may be considered. *Notoedres cati* primarily affects cats but may be found on foxes, dogs, and rabbits. Signs, diagnosis, and treatment are similar those for sarcoptic mange.

Fly Strike Dermatitis. Lesions consist of small erythematous papules or ulcers with hemorrhagic crusts. Resolution can be facilitated by restricting outdoor exposure and/or using commercial or homemade fly protectants or repellents at least twice daily.

Canine Ear Margin Seborrhea. Oily/waxy or scaly accumulations are noted on both the lateral and medial margins of the pinna, most commonly in the dachshund. Diagnosis is by rule-out and skin biopsy. Ceruminolytics (e.g., propylene glycol 50:50 with water) can be applied daily, followed in several hours by antiseborrheic shampoos (sulfur–salicylic acid, benzoyl, peroxide, or coal tar), which are allowed to remain on the ear for 10 to 15 minutes and then thoroughly rinsed off. Boston terriers appear to be predisposed to a similar keratinizing disorder, which affects the margins of the ears, concave surface of the pinna, and bridge of the nose. Good responses have been achieved with etretinate.

Actinic Dermatitis and Squamous Cell Carcinoma (SCC). Nonpigmented areas of the margins and apex of the ears are involved initially. Affected areas are erythematous, with variable degrees of alopecia and scaling. More advanced cases may ulcerate and crust. Diagnosis is based on history, physical examination, and skin biopsy.

Therapy for precancerous actinic dermatitis includes sun restriction, topical sunscreens (SPF of 15 or greater), topical glucocorticoids, and possibly a short course of oral prednisone at anti-inflammatory dosages. Etretinate may benefit both cats and dogs with actinic dermatitis (see Table 79–5 in the textbook). Hyperthermia, cryosurgery, or photochemotherapy can be used to successfully treat small, focal solar lesions or early SCC. Radiation therapy and surgical excision can be effective for treating established SCC.

Frostbite. After thawing, affected tissues become erythematous, scaly, alopecic, and variably painful. Subsequently the ear tips may curl, necrose, and slough. Frozen tissue should be rapidly thawed with warm water. Erythematous, scaly skin can be lightly covered with a bland ointment such as petrolatum. In severe cases, amputation of the affected tissue should be performed, but only after enough time has elapsed to more accurately determine the amount of nonviable tissue.

Inflammation/Ulceration/Necrosis of the Ear Apex

Vasculitis. Lesions of vasculitis often affect the apex of the ears, with variable patchy involvement of the concave surface of the pinna.

Lesions are erythematous, crusty, eroded, and occasionally ulcerated. A diagnosis of vasculitis is confirmed by skin biopsy. Potential causes of vasculitis include systemic lupus erythematosus, discoid lupus erythematosus, rickettsial disease, infectious disease (deep staphylococcal pyoderma), polyarteritis nodosa, and drug reactions. Many cases are idiopathic. Therapy involves resolving underlying disease when possible. Idiopathic, suspected immune-mediated vasculitis is treated with immunosuppressive dosages of glucocorticoids, with or without other immunosuppressive drugs.

Proliferative Thrombovascular Necrosis. This disease has been recognized in the Chihuahua, terrier crosses, Labrador retriever, dachshund, and Rhodesian ridgeback. The treatment of choice is surgical removal of the affected portion of the pinna.

Ear Fissures. Ear fissures often originate from the trauma of severe head shaking or scratching. Lesions begin as small lacerations which may bleed profusely. With chronicity and further trauma, the lesions may become full-thickness wedge-shaped defects. Therapy is directed at relieving the underlying disease. Medical failure usually warrants surgical amputation of the affected portion of the pinna.

Relapsing Polychondritis. A polychondritis affecting the ear margin apex has been described in cats. The distal margins of the ears are curled, erythematous, and thickened. Diagnosis is based on pinna biopsy, and treatment consists of immunosuppressive dosages of glucocorticoids.

Diffuse Erythema

Atopy and Food Sensitivities. Fifty to 80 per cent of both atopic and food-sensitive dogs are subject to inflammatory ear disease. Three to 5 per cent of atopics will have their disease restricted to the ears, but it is estimated that up to 20 per cent of food-sensitive dogs will have ear disease as the only manifestation of their food sensitivity. Affected dogs usually manifest aural pruritus (scratching, rubbing) and head shaking.

Diffuse inflammation is primarily noted in the more proximal portion of the concave pinna and in the proximal portion of the vertical canal. With chronicity, affected skin becomes thickened, cobblestone in appearance, and variably hyperpigmented and waxy/oily. Thickening may eventually result in almost complete occlusion of the entrance to the canals. Secondary *Malassezia* and bacterial infections are common. Allergic reactions less commonly are manifested as acute, diffuse erythema and swelling of the entire concave surface of the pinna.

Topical otic combination products that contain a glucocorticoid, antibiotic, and antifungal (see Otitis Externa) are usually used to treat "flares" of otitis. For severe cases, attempts should also be made to control the underlying allergy (e.g., systemic glucocorticoids, antihistamines, fatty acids, hyposensitization for atopy, and an appropriate diet for food-sensitive individuals).

Contact Hypersensitivities, Irritant Dermatitis, and Reactions to Systemic Drug Administration. Contact hypersensitivities are uncommonly noted to affect the ear in both dogs and cats. The neomycin in topical otic preparations is most commonly incriminated. Similar reactions may be seen to propylene glycol. Reactions to systemically administered drugs commonly affect the ears, causing diffuse pinnal erythema with variable degrees of swelling and exudation. Therapy involves discontinuation of the offending drug. Oral glucocorticoids may be of benefit.

Idiopathic Pinnal Erythema. An acute diffuse inflammation and swelling sometimes affect the pinna of dogs. Pruritus is usually present and may be severe. Affected patients initially require aggressive glucocorticoid therapy.

Crusting/Inflammation

Lichenoid-Psoriaform Dermatitis of the Springer Spaniel. This is a rare skin disease that begins in young English springer spaniels under 2 years of age. Affected dogs develop erythematous to yellow, waxy, crusty papules and plaques over the medial aspect of the pinna, ear canals, periocular and periorbital skin, lips, prepuce, and ventral abdomen. Therapy with etretinate should be considered.

Cellulitis

Juvenile Cellulitis (Juvenile Sterile Granulomatous Dermatitis and Lymphadenitis). Juvenile cellulitis is an uncommon acute dermatitis of mainly young dogs 3 weeks to 6 months of age. Characteristic features include a marked submandibular and prescapular lymphadenopathy, severe edema, exudation, pustules, and inflammatory nodules affecting the concave aspect of the pinna, muzzle, and periocular region. Treatment consists of immunosuppressive dosages of oral glucocorticoids for 1 to 2 weeks, which are then tapered over 2 to 4 weeks. Systemic antibiotics are given for suspected secondary pyoderma.

Pustules/Vesicles/Bulla

The most common causes are autoimmune diseases of the pemphigus complex and bullous pemphigoid. Bacterial infections, drug eruptions, and contact hypersensitivities may produce similar lesions.

Papules/Nodules

Auricular tumors are found more commonly in cats than in dogs. In cats, they also have a greater tendency to be malignant. The most common pinnal neoplasms in dogs are histiocytomas and papillomas; in cats, squamous cell carcinomas (see Actinic Dermatitis).

Aural Hematoma

The hematoma arises within the cartilage of the ear but is most evident on the concave surface of the pinna. Affected patients almost always have some underlying ear disease or disorder (e.g., atopy, food sensitivity, foreign body). Therapeutic options include needle aspiration (rarely successful), drainage with a self-retaining disposable teat cannula, and surgical incision with postoperative maintenance of surgical apposition (e.g., mattress sutures). In addition, regardless of the mode of therapy selected, it is of paramount importance to remove or control the underlying irritative disease if rapid resolution of the hematoma is to be achieved.

DISEASES OF THE EXTERNAL EAR CANAL (pp. 538–543)

OTITIS EXTERNA

The clinical signs associated with otitis externa include variable degrees of head shaking, pruritus, pain, odor, and exudation. Table 79–2 in the textbook presents the pathogenesis of the condition. The bacteria that proliferate in association with otitis externa are usually opportunists but contribute significantly to pathologic changes. The most common bacterial isolate associated with otitis externa is *Staphylococcus intermedius*. As the otitis externa becomes more chronic, or if there is a history of chronic topical antibiotic therapy, the incidence of gram-negative infections increases, with *Pseudomonas aeruginosa* predominating. *Malassezia* is considered an opportunist that proliferates in otherwise inflamed ears.

Diagnostic Principles

When excessive amounts of waxy debris or inflammatory exudate are encountered within the canals, a cytologic examination should be performed and repeated at each follow-up visit.

Culture and sensitivity testing are recommended only if resistant strains of bacteria are suspected. Resistance is suggested if there has been a history of chronic topical therapy or if bacteria persist in spite of appropriate therapy. In all cases of chronic or recurrent otitis externa in which the tympanic membrane is perforated, is abnormal, or cannot be seen because of canal swelling or proliferation, the tympanic bulla should be radiographed.

General Principles of Management

The general goals of therapy of otitis externa are to control or remove primary factors, reduce inflammation, resolve bacterial or yeast infections, and clean and dry the ears. Ear cleaning is generally accomplished through the use of a topical ceruminolytic and/or a flushing system. Examples of ceruminolytics include dioctyl sodium sulfosuccinate (DSS), carbamide peroxide, squalene, propylene glycol, glycerin, and oil. If a ruptured tympanum is noted or suspected, only water or saline should be used for cleansing and flushing purposes.

Flushing solutions include dilute chlorhexidine, povidone-iodine (see Table 79–5 in the textbook), or water/saline.

Topical Therapy. Eighty to 85 per cent of acute otitis externa cases can be managed with topical therapy alone. Most topical medications indicated for the treatment of otitis externa contain an antibiotic, a glucocorticoid, and an antifungal agent. DMSO may significantly potentiate the anti-inflammatory effects of glucocorticoids. The long-term, frequent use of especially more potent topical products can cause iatrogenic hyperadrenocorticism.

First-line products generally contain neomycin or chloramphenicol and are used to treat acute or infrequently recurrent otitis externa (e.g., Tresaderm). Second-line products generally contain gentamicin and are used when resistance is suspected. The drugs most commonly found in otic preparations for treatment of *Malassezia* include thiabendazole, nystatin, clotrimazole, and cuprimyxin. Rechecks should be scheduled every 10 to 14 days until the problem is resolved.

Systemic Therapy. Oral antibiotics appear to be beneficial when there is moderate to severe thickening of the canals/proximal pinna, significant periaural skin dermatitis, ulcerative changes in the ear, or large numbers of inflammatory cells seen cytologically. Systemic antibiotics are indicated in all cases that involve a concurrent otitis media.

CLINICAL MANIFESTATIONS, DIAGNOSIS, AND THERAPY OF SPECIFIC DISEASES OF THE EAR CANAL

Ear Mites. Infestations are generally encountered in dogs and cats less than one year of age. The development of a hypersensitivity to the mite may explain the variable degrees of inflammation associated with infestations. Diagnosis is generally made by direct otoscopic or cytologic examination.

Carbaryl (Mitox) and pyrethrins (Cerumite), among others, are commonly used to kill adult and immature mites. A thiabendazole-containing product (Tresaderm) is favored because thiabendazole is believed to kill all stages of the mite. It is recommended that topical otic therapy be combined with a total body miticide treatment (e.g., flea powder, spray, or dip) for 3 to 4 weeks. All dogs and cats in contact should be treated. Ivermectin, given PO once weekly for 4 weeks or SQ every 10 to 14 days for two or three treatments, has been effective. The ears are generally not affected in dogs with fleabite hypersensitivities, unless the problem is severe.

Swimmer's Ear. In many instances, patients prone to otitis who are frequent swimmers have underlying low-grade inflammatory disease (e.g., atopy) that makes maceration more likely to exacerbate problems. Drying agents primarily contain alcohol or astringents and have mild antibacterial and antifungal activity. The aforementioned products are generally used on the day of swimming and for 2 to 5 days thereafter.

Ceruminous Otitis Externa (Seborrheic Otitis). Ceruminous otitis externa is most commonly associated with endocrinopathies (e.g., hypothyroidism, sex hormone imbalances, and the idiopathic seborrheas seen in the spaniel breeds). Management of ceruminous accumulations and the mild to moderate inflammation that accompanies this syndrome is best achieved by initially using a first-line topical preparation to resolve secondary bacterial and yeast infections. Longer-term maintenance therapy can be achieved by ear flushes with a combination cleansing/drying agent one to three times a week and application of a glucocorticoid/astringent every 2 to 3 days.

Idiopathic Inflammatory/Hyperplastic Otitis in the Cocker Spaniel. Cocker spaniels, and occasionally individuals of other spaniel and non-spaniel breeds, may develop a gradually progressive inflammatory, proliferative otitis externa that eventually results in calcification of the auricular cartilages. Proliferative otitis is best treated with a combination of anti-inflammatory dosages of oral glucocorticoids, a potent topical glucocorticoid/antibiotic/antifungal preparation, and possibly oral antibiotics.

***Pseudomonas* Otitis.** *Pseudomonas* infections are most commonly encountered in chronic otitis externa or after prolonged or intermittent topical antibiotic therapy. Suspected *Pseudomonas* infections are usually first treated with topical gentamicin therapy. When resistance is encountered, therapy is based on culture and sensitivity testing. When *Pseudomonas* spp. are resistant to all routinely tested antibiotics, therapies to consider include silver sulfadiazine, polyhydroxidine iodine complex (Xenodyne), tris-EDTA (increases *Pseudomonas* sensitivity to several antibiotics, including gentamicin), and 1.5 per cent chlorhexidine in propylene glycol (see Drug Appendix in the textbook for specifics). White vinegar (5 per cent), diluted 1:1 to 1:3 with water, is the ear flush of choice for *Pseudomonas*-infected ears.

Refractory *Malassezia* Infections. When *Malassezia* appears to be refractory to therapy, extensive efforts must be directed toward recognizing and controlling underlying inflammatory primary factors. Topical alternative therapies include imidazoles, clotrimazole (Otomax), or 1 per cent miconazole lotion (Conofite). A 2- to 4-week course of oral ketoconazole is effective.

Neoplasia. The neoplasms encountered within the ear canals of dogs include ceruminous gland adenomas and carcinomas, papillomas, basal cell carcinomas, squamous cell carcinomas, and sebaceous adenocarcinomas. In cats, ceruminous gland adenomas and carcinomas, sebaceous gland adenomas and carcinomas, squamous cell carcinomas, and papillomas have been reported.

Ceruminous gland tumors are the most common tumor found in the canine and feline external ear canal. Metastasis is usually to regional lymph nodes, lungs, and distant viscera. The therapy of choice is surgical excision. Squamous cell carcinomas are generally amenable to surgical excision and radiation therapy.

ROLE OF SURGERY IN THE MANAGEMENT OF OTITIS EXTERNA

Lateral ear resections are primarily indicated as adjunctive therapies to improve drainage and aeration and to facilitate medication administration in patients with chronic otitis externa. They are of most value when disease is restricted to the vertical canal. Intractable disease associated with severe proliferation of the horizontal canal and calcification of the auricular cartilages is usually not amenable to successful medical management. Ablation of the entire ear canal combined with bulla osteotomy and curettage has proved extremely beneficial in such cases.

DISEASES OF THE MIDDLE AND INNER EAR
(pp. 543–550)

OTITIS MEDIA

Bacterial infections are most commonly incriminated as the cause of otitis media. These are commonly associated with perforating foreign bodies (e.g., grass awns), or they occur as a sequela to chronic, usually proliferative or severe otitis externa. Other etiologies of otitis media include fungal infections (*Malassezia, Aspergillus,* candidiasis), foreign bodies, neoplasia, inflammatory polyps, trauma, primary bone tumors, and aural cholesteatoma.

Patients with otitis media generally have signs of otitis externa (e.g., head shaking, rubbing or scratching at ears, discharge, odor). Signs more suggestive of the presence of otitis media include otic pain, swelling or stenosis of the ear canal, purulent otitis externa, or facial nerve palsy and/or Horner's syndrome. Signs of abnormal peripheral vestibular function suggest the presence of otitis interna. The lack of visible perforation of the tympanic membrane does not preclude middle ear involvement. It may be difficult to ascertain if the tympanum is intact. Radiographic studies of the bulla are indicated whenever otitis media is suspected, but the tympanum or a tympanic rupture cannot be visualized. Increased tissue opacity within the bulla may signify acute or chronic otitis media, neoplasia, or hemorrhage. Sclerosis and thickening of the bulla wall are considered to be normal changes in aged animals (primarily cats), chronic otitis media, and nasopharyngeal polyps. Lysis of the tympanic bulla and/or petrous temporal bone is seen with malignant neoplasia, chronic otitis media, and osteomyelitis. Unfortunately, the absence of radiographic changes does not preclude a diagnosis of otitis media.

When otitis externa is suspected, but the tympanum is visualized and intact, myringotomy may be performed to harvest samples for cytologic examination and culture and sensitivity testing. Surgical exploration remains the most accurate and cost- effective means of diagnosing otitis media in questionable cases. Medical management is usually unsuccessful unless, at some time, the middle ear can be thoroughly cleaned out. Appropriate systemic antibiotic therapy should be continued for at least 4 to 6 weeks. Topical therapy should be continued until evidence of infection has resolved. If the tympanum fails to heal, regular flushing, possibly combined with a lateral ear resection to facilitate drainage, may offer control. Otherwise, a surgical resolution of the problem should be considered (ear ablation and bulla osteotomy or ventral bulla osteotomy).

Neoplasia of the Middle Ear

It is more common to see extension from the canals into the middle ear. Major clinical signs include otic discharge and discomfort. Although the therapy of choice is surgical excision, other alternatives are possible. The prognosis is poor.

Inflammatory Polyps of the Middle Ear in Cats

Clinical signs are dependent on the site of origin and extent of mass development. They include respiratory stridor, dyspnea, dysphagia, and signs of external or middle/inner ear disease. Diagnosis is based on careful oropharyngeal evaluation and otoscopic and radiographic examination of the middle ear and nasal cavity. Treatment is surgical excision. The prognosis is generally good.

OTITIS INTERNA

Otitis interna most commonly arises as a progression from infection or neoplastic disease related to otitis media. The clinical signs of otitis interna include asymmetric ataxia (falls or drifts to side of lesion), head tilt, usually toward the side of the lesion, circling to the side of the lesion, and horizontal or rotatory nystagmus with the quick phase away from the side of the lesion. Facial nerve paralysis or Horner's syndrome may be present. Signs of paresis or proprioceptive deficits associated with a head tilt usually indicate central vestibular disease.

The diagnosis of otitis interna is generally established on the basis of neurologic examination and work-up as for otitis media. Therapy is the same as for otitis media. Aggressive medical or surgical management is indicated to prevent the spread of infectious disease into the brain stem.

The prognosis for the medical management of infectious otitis media/interna is poor if the ear canals remain stenotic, if the middle ear cannot be thoroughly cleaned and kept clean, if there is osteomyelitis or significant bony proliferation/lysis, or if resistant organisms are encountered. Dogs and cats learn to compensate for vestibular disorders. Facial paralysis and keratoconjunctivitis sicca, when encountered, are usually permanent.

OTOTOXICITY

Potential ototoxic drugs are listed in Table 79–3 of the textbook. Vestibular signs generally improve once the offending drugs are discontinued, but deafness is often permanent.

IDIOPATHIC VESTIBULAR/FACIAL NERVE DISEASES

Canine and Feline Idiopathic Vestibular Disease. An acute, nonprogressive, unilateral or occasionally bilateral vestibular disease is noted in cats and older dogs. Dogs and cats with unilateral involvement develop severe peracute or acute head tilt, disorientation, falling, rolling, and nystagmus. Ear canals and bulla are normal, and the animals are otherwise healthy. Spontaneous improvement is usually noted within 72 hours and recovery within 1 to 3 weeks. Residual mild ataxia and head tilt may persist for as long as several months.

DEAFNESS

Inherited deafness has been reported in dogs (see Table 79–4 in the textbook) and cats.

Behavioral Evaluation. An animal suspected of being deaf should be challenged with sounds of varying intensity and frequency from different directions and observed for a response. Care should be taken to avoid making sounds that could alert the animal through "feel" (i.e., slamming a door) or visual cuing (i.e., clapping hands in front of the animal). Other animals and people should not be present during the evaluation to avoid visual cuing.

Electrodiagnostic Evaluation of Hearing Loss

Impedance audiometry and audiometry evoked response testing provide a quantitative way to determine the type (conduction versus sensorineural) and degree (partial versus complete) of deafness present, and the symmetry (unilateral versus bilateral) of dysfunction. Brain stem auditory evoked response (BAER) provides a fairly good evaluation of brain stem integrity in general and can be used in cases of head trauma, inflammatory disease, and other conditions in which an animal is comatose and cranial nerve reflexes cannot be evaluated.

Senile or age-related deafness can be entirely sensorineural in nature or a combination of sensorineural and conduction if chronic otitis and/or otosclerosis are also a component of the dysfunction. It should be pointed out that very few animals learn to tolerate the presence of a hearing aid in the ear canal.

CHAPTER 80
DISEASES OF THE NOSE
(pages 551–567)

Given the limitations of anterior and posterior rhinoscopy, radiography remains the one important noninvasive diagnostic procedure for routine application.

CONDITIONS OF THE RHINARIUM (pp. 555–557)

CLEFT OF THE PRIMARY PALATE

The primary palate consists of the lip and premaxillae, and the term *harelip* is used to describe the unilateral or bilateral congenital clefts that are occasionally seen in the dog, but rarely in the cat. Suckling is almost impossible because any communication with the rhinarial airway interferes with the creation of negative pressure within the mouth. Full depth closure of the cleft is easily accomplished even when the tissue deficiency is considerable.

CONGENITAL STENOSIS OF THE EXTERNAL NARES

At rest the airway through the external naris is extremely narrow but patent. During inspiration the naris does not dilate, but the wing of the nostril is sucked medially against the philtrum, thus closing down the air space. The relief of dyspnea caused by stenotic nares is simply obtained by abducting the wing of the nostril surgically or removing part of its structure.

TRAUMA AND FOREIGN BODIES

Wounds of the rhinarium usually heal without complication, but when there is damage to the dorsolateral nasal cartilages, stenosis and collapse of the nares may occur.

DISCOID LUPUS ERYTHEMATOSUS

The condition is similar clinically to pemphigus erythematosus, being characterized by hypopigmentation, depigmentation, erythema, scaling, crusting, erosion, and ulceration of the rhinarium. The two conditions are usually limited to the face and pinnae but, unlike pemphigus vulgaris, do not involve the oral cavity, and patients are not ill systemically. The initial lesions often involve the planum nasale, the alar folds, or the

Original chapter written by Peter G. C. Bedford

lips, and the margo-intermarginales of the eyelids can be affected. The clinical picture is often complicated by bacterial contamination.

Diagnosis requires biopsy of a non-ulcerated erythematous or depigmented diseased area and the demonstration of autoantibodies by direct immunofluorescence. Treatment is always difficult. In early disease sunscreens may be helpful, and topical fluorinated steroids should be used q24h for the first 14 days. Systemic corticosteroid therapy usually proves effective. Azathioprine given at 1 to 2 mg/lb q24h can be prescribed as a replacement for systemic corticosteroids and may be used with corticosteroids on occasion.

NEOPLASIA

Squamous cell carcinoma of the rhinarium is seen with equal frequency in the dog and cat. Although the tumor is slow to metastasize, excision is followed by rapid recurrence, and early radiotherapy or cryotherapy is the treatment of choice. Fibrosarcomas or malignant melanomas can involve the rhinarium. Recurrence usually follows excision.

CONDITIONS OF THE NASAL CAVITY (pp. 557–564)

TRAUMA

Simple measures such as cage rest and possibly ice packs are often sufficient to control minor hemorrhage, but pressure packing of both the rhinarial airway and the internal nares with gauze sponges under general anesthesia can prove essential when severe epistaxis is present. Obstruction of the nasal cavity following trauma is due to the presence of blood clots and edema, and mouth breathing may persist for several days. The displacement of fractured maxillary and nasal bone should be repaired or the bone fragments removed. Splitting of the hard palate along the maxillary and palatine symphyses can occur during the jumping cat's five-point landing.

FOREIGN BODY RHINITIS

The entry of foreign body material into the nasal cavity is invariably of sudden onset and accompanied by violent and persistent sneezing, together with head shaking and nose-pawing. Sneezing and discharge persist when the foreign body is retained. With time, these initial features give way to a clinical picture characterized by chronic nasal discharge with secondary bacterial and possible fungal infections complicating the situation. Gagging and retching due to the nasopharyngeal drainage of discharge may be a feature. Anterior rhinoscopy may allow identification and removal of foreign body material. Rhinotomy may prove necessary in the treatment of foreign body rhinitis.

RHINITIS DUE TO PALATINE DEFECTS

See Chapter 100.

RHINITIS DUE TO DENTAL DISEASE

Periapical abscess together with caries and dental fractures is seldom involved in rhinitis. Treatment consists of removal of the diseased tooth and curettage of the alveolus. Oronasal fistula formation following this surgery and the loss of canine teeth in older animals may result in low-grade nasal discharge. Such defects can be sealed with pedicle flaps of buccal mucosa.

VIRAL RHINITIS

Most viral-induced rhinitis in the dog is seen as acute, but transient, relatively low-grade disease that may predispose the patient to secondary, often chronic, bacterial infection. A specific rhinitis immuno-deficiency syndrome attributed to primary herpes virus infection with secondary *Bordetella bronchiseptica* and *Pasteurella multocida* involvement has been described in Irish wolfhound pups.

In cats, feline rhinotracheitis virus (FVR), a herpes virus, is extemely contagious, and the disease produced is more severe than that caused by FCD. Mild to severe rhinitis occurs, and although the picture can be complicated by bacterial and mycoplasmal infections, turbinate osteolysis can be produced by the virus acting alone. A 2- to 3-week course of ampicillin (15 mg/lb q12h) or a potentiated sulfonamide (10 mg/lb q12h) can be accompanied by multivitamin therapy. Hydration states and nutritional concerns should also be addressed.

Failure of the rhinitis to respond to systemic antibiotics may be corrected by administering antibiotic through the frontal sinuses. Unfortunately, the acute disease situation often gives way to a chronic rhinitis.

BACTERIAL RHINITIS

A number of bacteria can be isolated from rhinitis patients, and while some are of contaminant significance only, others exert a pathogenic effect. It is likely that most require predisposing inflammation or damage to create an environment in which they can multiply in order to exert their pathogenic effect as secondary invaders. Hyperplastic changes within the mucosa can result from uncontrolled infection. Antibiotics will have some effect, but dyspnea, inadequate drainage, and recurrence of infection will be prevented only by turbinectomy. Unlike cats, dogs tolerate this procedure well.

FUNGAL RHINITIS

Nasal mycosis is a relatively common cause of rhinitis and sinusitis in the dog, but occurs much less frequently in the cat. In the cat it is *Cryptococcus neoformans* that is the most common fungal pathogen, with both *Aspergillus* and Penicillium species being isolated rarely.

Aspergillosis is primarily a disease of the young to middle-aged dolicocephalic dog. An intermittent serosanguineous nasal discharge is indicative of endonasal neoplasia as a rule, whereas the profuse production of a purulent discharge characterizes aspergillosis. Sneezing is commonplace, and severe epistaxis may accompany these episodes. Pain and discomfort are usually present. The positive identification of *Aspergillus* in nasal discharge does not always mean a diagnosis of rhinomycosis. An agar gel double-diffusion test can confirm the presence of *Aspergillus* antibodies in the serum, but false positives are possible. Radiographs will reveal loss of turbinate pattern as the result of the destruction caused by the fungus. It is likely, though, that most rhinomycoses follow tissue damage caused by trauma, bacterial or viral infection, and neoplasia.

Itraconazole is offering an improved cure rate of about 70 per cent in preliminary trials and may prove to be the most effective therapeutic approach in the future. Currently, however, it is the use of topical enilconazole through frontal sinus irrigation that offers the best chance of success.

A noninvasive type of aspergillosis, which occurs infrequently in the dog, is characterized by compact masses of mycelia ("fungal balls") filling the larger conchal air spaces without damaging the surrounding tissue. Anterior rhinoscopy or rhinotomy is necessary, and treatment calls for turbinate dissection with routine postoperative antibiotics.

Cryptococcus in cats causes a severe chronic rhinitis with persistent sneezing and discharge is accompanied by the destruction of facial bone, and radiographs demonstrate osteolysis of the maxillae and the nasal and frontal bones. See Chapter 71 for a more complete discussion of the diagnosis and treatment of this condition.

PARASITIC RHINITIS

Disease due to the tongue worm of the dog, *Linguatula serrata,* may be characterized by a severe rhinitis in which coughing and violent sneezing occur and a blood-stained discharge is seen. Eggs may be present in the nasal discharge. Rhinotomy may thus prove necessary, and the parasite's physical removal is the only certain method of treatment.

NEOPLASIA

Benign fibrous polyps that originate within the anterior nasal cavity are an occasional finding in both the dog and cat. Enlargement causes airway obstruction, and pressure-induced destruction of the anterior ethmoidal conchae can cause hemorrhage and a blood-stained nasal discharge. The presence of a polyp is confirmed by anterior rhinoscopy and radiography, and anterior rhinotomy is necessary to effect removal.

The adenocarcinoma is the most common neoplasm in the dog's nasal cavity, but fibrosarcoma, chondrosarcoma, osteosarcoma, and squamous cell carcinoma have all been recorded. The discharge may be blood-stained, and bouts of epistaxis can occur spontaneously or during violent sneezing. The radiographic features are those of bone destruction or proliferation and the replacement of air space with soft tissue shadow.

Curettage is not an effective treatment for endonasal neoplasia, and no matter how complete the turbinectomy, recurrence should be expected, usually within three months. The prognosis is therefore grave.

Lymphosarcoma as part of a multicentric tumor problem is the most common endonasal neoplasm in the cat, but other carcinomas are seen occasionally. Dyspnea, purulent nasal discharge, epistaxis, and facial distortion are the expected clinical features, and treatment is not advisable, given the nature of these two tumor types.

CONDITIONS OF THE PARANASAL SINUSES
(pp. 564–567)

Primary conditions of the paranasal sinuses in both the dog and cat are rare occurrences. Sinusitis, when it occurs, is thus an extension of a rhinitis, and both bacterial and fungal infections as well as neoplasia may be present. Disease based within the ethmoidal conchae can interfere with the normal drainage of the frontal sinus, and resultant retention mucocoele formation may eventually disrupt the continuity of the frontal bones. The canine maxillary sinus or recess, an outpouching of the nasal cavity at the level of the carnassial tooth, which is in open communication with the middle and ventral nasal meati, can be involved occasionally in cyst formation and periapical carnassial tooth abscessation.

CHAPTER 81

DISEASES OF THE THROAT
(pages 567–575)

DISEASES OF THE PHARYNX (pp. 568–572)

Diseases of the pharynx are usually associated with abnormal deglutition. However, dyspnea or inspiratory stridor may be the sole sign of disease. The history in cases of dysphagia can be confusing, because a variety of signs such as coughing, vomiting, regurgitation, and nasal discharge may accompany the "swallowing disorder." Clinical signs in acute pharyngeal disease may be dominated by pain. The animal usually refuses to eat or drink. The neck is extended, there is often drooling of saliva and there are weak swallowing movements independent of intake. In chronic pharyngitis the predominant signs are gagging, regurgitation, and often sudden episodes of pica.

Pharyngeal disease is a component of many systemic diseases, but at the same time it can be complicated by such things as abscesses following foreign body trauma, by pneumonia associated with dysphagia, or by metastasis in the case of pharyngeal tumors. Since a thorough inspection of the pharyngeal cavities cannot be performed without anesthesia, plans should be made for electromyography and radiography while the dog is sedated. The inspection of the nasopharynx can be facilitated by use of a Mathieu retractor and a dentist's mirror or a flexible endoscope, which can be turned through 180 degrees. The laryngeal pharynx can best be inspected with a laryngoscope. Abnormal radiographic findings in the pharyngeal area always should be confirmed by pharyngeal inspection before diagnostic conclusions are made.

Computed tomography is extremely helpful in the diagnosis of lesions in the rostral part of the nasopharynx and at the base of the skull. Contrast videofluorography is almost indispensable in diagnostic studies of dysphagia. Electromyography of the pharyngeal muscles is useful when no abnormalities are found during inspection. Biopsies for histologic examination are helpful for diagnosis. Samples for bacteriologic culture from the pharyngeal cavity seldom lead to a diagnosis.

DYSPHAGIA

Neurogenic dysphagia can be caused by interruption of the peripheral innervation or by processes in the brain. Neuromuscular dysphagia is represented by myasthenia gravis. Dysphagia in these cases is usually associated with a megaesophagus. Myogenic dysphagia is a rare sign in polymyopathies of various causes, but was the main sign in the muscular dystrophy described in 24 Bouviers.

CONGENITAL MALFORMATION

Hypoplasia usually results in an opening between the oropharynx and the nasopharynx. Depending on the size of the defect, clinical signs may be negligible or considerable, including swallowing problems and misdirection of milk and, later, food in the pup or kitten. Surgical repair has the best prognosis when the cleft involves only the soft palate and there is still a substantial muscular layer.

Hyperplasia of the soft palate is associated with brachycephaly and a relative narrow pharynx. Clinical signs associated with an overlong

Original chapter written by Anjop J. Venker-van Haagen

soft palate consist of snoring, regurgitation, and dyspnea, usually increasing in severity during the second and third years of the dog's life. In some dogs the pharyngeal mucosa and soft palate are very thick and the musculature is insufficient, resulting in snoring during closed-mouth breathing. When at a later age these dogs develop dyspnea, little can be done. This is in contrast to the overlong soft palate, which can be reduced in length so that it no longer covers the laryngeal inlet.

PHARYNGITIS

Acute pharyngitis, a typical symptom of viral infections, is characterized by pain, fever, and extreme discomfort. The dog or cat does not attempt to eat, often salivates, and makes inefficient swallowing movements. Symptomatic treatment of acute pharyngitis consists of parenteral broad-spectrum antibiotics, fluids, or parenteral nutrition as needed. The painful period of 3 to 5 days is followed by a week of convalescence during which liquid food may be given in small portions several times a day. Antibiotic therapy is given to prevent secondary bacterial infections and pneumonia.

Chronic pharyngitis is characterized by retching independent of the intake of food, normal swallowing, and sudden periods of pica. In most cases in dogs and cats the cause is obscure. In cats there may be focal eosinophilic granulomas, which respond to corticosteroid therapy. All symptomatic treatment is directed at diminishing the irritation to the pharyngeal mucosa.

TONSILLITIS

When the tonsils are both indurated and enlarged, they may be painful during swallowing even though the pharyngitis has long since resolved. Only in such cases of chronic tonsillitis should the tonsils be removed. In all other cases, the tonsils should be recognized as being lymph nodes reacting to inflammation in the pharyngeal area, and they should be left *in situ*. The tonsils are enlarged in inflammatory diseases affecting the pharynx and in feline leukemia and lymphoma.

PHARYNGEAL MUCOCELE

The pharyngeal mucocele is a rather common anomaly in dogs and a rare finding in cats. The clinical signs are related to its location and consist of dyspnea and, to a lesser extent, dysphagia. Therapy consists of removal of the thick mucus and excision of the bulging and obstructing tissue. Care should be taken to suture the pharyngeal mucosa after removing the tissue.

NASOPHARYNGEAL POLYPS

See Chapter 79.

PHARYNGEAL TRAUMA AND FOREIGN BODIES

The animal's initial response to penetration of a fish hook or needle is to try to remove it by movements of the tongue, by gagging and chewing, and, in cats, by use of the front paws. These efforts are accompanied by excessive salivation. With obvious signs, the animal should be anesthetized as soon as possible so that the search for the foreign body can be started before deeper foreign body penetration occurs. Trauma in the pharyngeal area caused by bite wounds may include fracture of the hyoid bone, large hematomas, and lacerations caused by the canine teeth of the attacker. A tracheostomy, suturing of the pharyngeal mucosa, and placement of drains are the principal steps in treatment. Removal of the fractured hyoid parts may be needed if painful swelling persists.

NEOPLASMS

In dogs and cats, most tumors of the pharyngeal area are malignant. The most common tumors are squamous cell carcinomas in dogs and lymphomas in cats. The tonsillar carcinoma in the dog is remarkable because of its misleading presentation as a painful process rather than an obvious mass in the oropharyngeal area. The tonsil may not be significantly enlarged, but it is often yellowish-pink, and the surrounding tissue is retracted and indurated owing to infiltration by the tumor. The pain caused by this tumor gradually becomes severe, and together with anorexia and emaciation, it provides adequate justification for euthanasia.

REVERSE SNEEZING

This consists of short periods (1 to 2 minutes) of severe inspiratory dyspnea characterized by extension of the neck, bulging of the eyes, and abduction of the elbows. Swallowing causes the attack to stop. The owner should be instructed to induce the dog's swallowing reflex by massaging the pharyngeal area or briefly closing the nares.

DISEASES OF THE LARYNX (pp. 572–575)

HISTORY AND CLINICAL SIGNS

The history and clinical signs in laryngeal disease are often dyspnea, exertional stridor, dysphonia, and coughing.

PHYSICAL EXAMINATION

If the patient is in a state of severe dyspnea or is in rapidly increasing distress, emergency laryngotracheal intubation precedes clinical examination.

DIAGNOSTIC PROCEDURES

A lateral radiograph can be helpful in detecting ossification and neoplasia. Laryngoscopy, the direct inspection of the larynx via the oropharyngeal cavity, is most informative. When the appropriate anesthesia is used, the respiratory movements of the arytenoid cartilages and the vocal folds can be assessed. Electromyography of the intrinsic laryngeal muscles is indicated when the clinical signs and the insufficient glottic movements revealed by laryngoscopy both indicate laryngeal paralysis.

LARYNGEAL PARALYSIS

See textbook.

CONGENITAL MALFORMATION

Hypoplasia of the laryngeal structures, causing laryngeal collapse, is a common finding in brachycephalic breeds. The dogs are dyspneic, and a laryngeal stridor is present. Inspection reveals the larynx to be remarkably small for the dog's size, and a small rima glottidis is visible when the collapsed epiglottis is unfolded. There is no satisfactory treatment as yet.

In dogs and cats congenital malformations are found occasionally and usually cause laryngeal dysfunction, indicated by stridorous breathing and dyspnea at an early age. Many variations are found, and the possibility of surgical enlargement of the laryngeal opening dictates the prognosis.

LARYNGITIS

Laryngotracheitis caused by viral or bacterial infection is characterized initially by a persistent, rough, dry cough and no further signs of illness. Bronchitis or bronchopneumonia may complicate the infection. Acute laryngitis is therefore treated with house rest and cough syrups to limit irritation of the laryngeal mucosa. In cats, tracheobronchitis also causes acute inflammation of the larynx, but the symptoms are dominated by fever and distress, salivation, conjunctivitis, and sometimes dyspnea caused by edema of the laryngeal mucosa. Antibiotic treatment and fluid therapy are indicated.

Acute laryngeal edema can be caused by insect poison or other allergens. Corticosteroids are indicated, and when necessary, a tracheostomy should be performed without hesitation. Chronic laryngitis, common in dogs and cats, results from continuous barking, panting, and straining on the leash during training. Severe chronic laryngitis may result in recurrent coughing and a hoarse voice. Chronic irritation of the larynx may cause laryngeal spasm, which causes severe dyspnea, a heavy stridor, and cyanosis. The spasm usually occurs during special exercises in the training program. It becomes a permanent hazard for the dog and can be avoided only by stopping the training.

TRAUMA

Laryngeal trauma is often life threatening because the passage of air through the larynx is obstructed. When the larynx is partially lacerated, emphysema develops in the cervical area. Surgical examination of the larynx and suturing of the laceration are necessary. In most cases of severe trauma, a tracheostomy is indicated. One of the most feared complications of laryngeal, vocal fold, or arytenoid surgery is webbing, the forming of scar tissue in the laryngeal lumen. In cats almost every intervention in the larynx causes edema, so corticosteroids are indicated when the first signs of laryngeal obstruction are observed.

NEOPLASMS

In dogs, leiomyomas, rhabdomyosarcomas, and squamous cell carcinomas, as well as other types of tumors, have been reported. In cats, lymphosarcoma and squamous cell carcinoma are the most frequent tumors. Squamous cell carcinomas and lymphosarcomas invade the laryngeal structures rapidly and are inoperable by the time they are diagnosed.

SECTION VII
THE NERVOUS SYSTEM

CHAPTER 82

DISEASES OF THE BRAIN
(pages 578–629)

DIAGNOSTIC APPROACH (pp. 578–580)

Historical Review and Client Complaints. The history may suggest a dysfunction of the nervous system, such as epilepsy, narcolepsy, or myasthenia gravis, whereas the neurologic examination may be normal. The patient's signalment, use, age, breed, gender, environment, diet, history of prior illness, or injury should be reviewed. Onset, progression, and aggravating factors should be discussed.

THE NEUROLOGIC EXAMINATION (pp. 582–599)

The examination should consist of observing an animal, watching its gait, carefully palpating it for abnormal muscle tone and mass, and performing tests of reflexes and reaction. Leave painful portion for the last. An abnormality may suggest a lesion in either the sensory or motor side of the arc. If all the signs cannot be explained with a single lesion, the patient probably has a disseminated disorder, such as an inflammation or degeneration.

GENERAL OBSERVATIONS

Head Posture. In patients with vestibular disorders, the head is often tilted (usually toward the side of the lesion). These patients may also have torticollis (a twisted neck). Patients with cervical spinal injuries may also have torticollis, but without the associated head tilt. Inability to raise the head has been seen with feline hypokalemic polymyopathy, occipital dysplasia in the dog, botulism, cervical vertebral malformations, and feline thiamine deficiency.

Head Coordination. Disturbances of head coordination typically appear as head tremor, which implies a cerebellar lesion (or a cerebellar peduncle lesion). Such tremor is often exaggerated when the animal attempts purposeful movement, such as eating or drinking (intention tremor).

Circling. Patients with vestibular system injuries usually have concomitant head tilts and also are more likely to circle in only one direction. Patients with cerebral injuries rarely have head tilts, and may circle in both directions (wander aimlessly).

Original chapter written by William R. Fenner

STANCE AND GAIT

Animals with lesions of the conscious proprioceptive system (PNS, spinal cord, brain stem, or cerebrum) often stand "knuckled over." Animals with special proprioceptive (vestibulocerebellar) dysfunction tend to have a broad-based stance. Ataxia (an unconscious proprioceptive sign) may appear as swaying, veering, crossing over of the limbs, scuffing of the toes, and the like. Ataxia may be seen with cerebellar, brain stem, spinal cord, or PNS injuries (of spinal nerves or cranial nerve VIII). Weakness is characterized by stumbling, falling, tripping, or inability to initiate or sustain an activity. Weakness may be caused by injury to the cerebrum, brain stem, spinal cord, or peripheral spinal nerves. Spasticity (an increase in muscle tone) may be seen with injuries to the cerebrum, brain stem, or spinal cord. Dysmetria may be seen with injury to the cerebellum, spinal cord, brain stem, peripheral spinal nerves, and cranial nerve VIII.

ATTITUDINAL AND POSTURAL REACTIONS

Cerebral injuries depress the A&P reactions in both thoracic and pelvic limbs on the opposite side of the body from the damaged hemisphere (contralateral). With brain stem injuries, the reactions are also depressed or absent, and the clinical signs are usually bilateral, but more severe on the same side of the body as the side of the brain stem injury (ipsilateral). With cerebellar injuries, the A&P reactions are usually still present, but ataxic. With peripheral vestibular injuries, the A&P reactions are preserved, but the patient tends to lean, fall, and roll to the affected side when the maneuvers are performed. With lesions in the spinal cord and peripheral spinal nerves, the A&P reactions tend to be depressed or absent on the side of the NS injury.

True A&P prescriptions include proprioceptive positioning, hemihopping/hemistanding/hemiwalking, wheelbarrowing, and hopping. Additional A&P reactions include the extensor postural thrust reaction, righting reaction, visual placing reactions, tactile placing reactions, and tonic neck reaction.

CRANIAL NERVE EXAMINATION

Normally, except for Horner's syndrome, a cranial nerve deficit indicates a lesion above the foramen magnum.

Anatomic Review

Unlike spinal nerves, some cranial nerves are purely sensory and others purely motor; thus, testing a cranial nerve reflex usually tests two peripheral cranial nerves, one motor and one sensory; a central connection (usually in the brain stem); and a higher regulatory center (usually in the cerebrum).

Tests of Cranial Nerve Function

See Table 82–4 in the textbook.

The Pupillary Light Reflex (PLR). Non-neurologic causes of an abnormal PLR include posterior synechia, iris atrophy, glaucoma, other ophthalmic diseases, excessive sympathetic tone (excitement), a weak light source, and prior administration of cycloplegic drugs.

Pupil Size. Abnormally large pupils may be seen with excitement (sympathetic stimulation), bilateral CN II injury, CN III injury, and/or ophthalmic disease. Abnormally small pupils may be seen with loss of sympathetic tone (Horner's syndrome), excess parasympathetic tone, and ophthalmic disease.

Ocular Position. A lesion of CN III or CN VIII may result in a ventrolateral strabismus. A lesion of CN IV will produce intorsion (rotation) of the eye, which can only be detected on retinal examination in the dog. A lesion of CN VI will produce a medial strabismus. Animals with retrobulbar masses may show a strabismus.

Ocular Motility (Voluntary and Involuntary). With cerebral lesions, both eyes are involved and there is a tendency for the eyes to look toward the side of the diseased cerebral hemisphere (conjugate gaze deviation). With a cranial nerve lesion, one eye tends to have a strabismus at rest and lacks the ability to move.

Pathologic Nystagmus. This usually results from an imbalance in the special proprioceptive system, which includes the inner ear, CN VIII, the brain stem, and the cerebellum. Horizontal nystagmus is most commonly seen in patients with peripheral vestibular injuries. The fast component of the nystagmus is typically away from the diseased side. Vertical nystagmus is most commonly seen in patients with central vestibular disease. Rotatory nystagmus has components of both horizontal and vertical movement and is not localizing; it may be seen with a lesion anywhere in the special proprioceptive system. *Resting* nystagmus is most characteristic of peripheral vestibular disease. Positional nystagmus is most characteristic of central vestibular dysfunction, e.g., brain stem and cerebellar lesions, but is also seen during the compensation phase of peripheral vestibular diseases.

Most pathologic nystagmus resulting from an injury to the peripheral vestibular system spontaneously resolves during the 10 to 14 days following the initial injury. Few patients can compensate for brain stem or progressive cerebellar injuries, in which case the pathologic nystagmus persists over time.

Cranial Muscle Symmetry. The muscles of facial expression are innervated by CN VII and include the muscles of the eyelid and lip. Facial muscle paralysis may result from injury to the contralateral cerebrum, ipsilateral brain stem, or ipsilateral CN VII. Clinically, drooping of the lip, deviation of the nasal philtrum, an increase in palpebral fissure width (pseudoptosis), and, in some animals, true ptosis (drooping of the eyelid) are seen. The muscles of mastication are innervated by CN V and include the temporal and masseter muscles. Masticatory muscle paralysis may result from ipsilateral injury to the brain stem or peripheral CN V. The clinical appearance is loss of muscle mass and weakness of the jaw, often manifested as a dropped jaw and inability to close the mouth.

Facial Reflexes

Facial Sensory Examination. By lightly stimulating the nasal mucosa, which should produce an avoidance response such as head turning, CN V and its cerebral connections can be tested.

Summary

If the cerebrum is damaged, abnormalities of learning, behavior, and vision are seen in addition to cranial nerve deficits. If the midbrain is abnormal, there is abnormal eyeball function. If the pons is abnormal, the face does not function properly. If the medulla is abnormal, the mouth, tongue, and throat do not function normally. With brain stem diseases, there may also be disturbances of vegetative functions (e.g., consciousness, heart rate, and respiration) as well as limb signs. If the cerebellum is diseased, dysregulation of voluntary motor coordination occurs, with associated tremors of head and body and with limb ataxia (see Table 82–2 in the textbook).

SPINAL SEGMENTAL REFLEXES

Discovering a diminished reflex precisely localizes a lesion to the reflex arc tested (lower motor neuron, or LMN). Loss of upper motor neuron (UMN) regulation results in reflex exaggeration.

Thoracic Limb Reflexes. The *triceps reflex* tests the radial nerve, which arises from spinal cord segments C7-T1 (T2). The *extensor carpi radialis reflex* tests the radial nerve, and thus also tests spinal cord segments C7-T1 (T2). The *biceps reflex* evaluates the musculocutaneous nerve, which arises from spinal cord segments C6-C8.

Pelvic Limb Reflexes. The *patellar reflex* tests the femoral nerve, which arises from spinal cord segments L4-L6. In patients with sciatic nerve paralysis, the functional loss of the antagonist muscles of the quadriceps may result in an excessively brisk patellar reflex, which falsely resembles an UMN reflex change. The *anterior tibialis reflex* tests the peroneal branch of the sciatic nerve, which originates from spinal cord segment L6-S1 (S2). The *gastrocnemius reflex* tests the tibial branch of the sciatic nerve, which originates from spinal cord segment L6-S1 (S2). The expected normal response is extension of the tarsus; however, in my experience, many patients have had tarsal flexion instead.

Nociceptive Reflexes

These reflexes only test the spinal reflex arc integrity.

Flexor Reflexes. The thoracic limb flexor response uses all peripheral nerves of the thoracic limb and tests spinal cord segment C6-T2. The pelvic limb flexor reflex tests primarily the sciatic nerve and its branches and L6-S2 nerve roots.

Perineal Reflexes. These reflexes test the perineal and pudendal nerves, spinal cord segments S1-S3, and the cauda equina.

Panniculus Reflex (Cutaneous Trunci Reflex). The stimulus is carried to the CNS by the dorsal root that supplies the dermatome being stimulated and travels cranially in the CNS to synapse on the lateral thoracic nerve's LMNs (C8-T1 spinal cord segments). This reflex helps to localize transverse spinal cord lesions when there is a clear demarcation between an area of absent reflex and a zone of normal reflex activity. The reflex also helps to distinguish between injuries to the brachial plexus (reflex should be present) and injuries to the thoracic limb nerve roots (reflex often absent).

Special (Released) Reflexes

The ability to elicit these reflexes in an adult animal indicates loss of UMN inhibition to a reflex arc and the presence of a CNS lesion.

Babinski Reflex. This reflex, only elicited in the pelvic limbs, is seen when the plantar metatarsus is lightly stroked.

Crossed Extensor Reflex. In the face of an UMN injury, when the stimulated limb flexes, avoiding the flexor reflex evaluation, the contralateral paired limb involuntarily extends.

Nociceptive Evaluation

Diminished Pain Perception. To test for diminished pain perception, enough pain must be produced by compressing the digits vigorously; the expected response is turning of the head and/or vocalization. Peripheral nerve lesions usually cause focal sensory loss, confined to the distribution of the involved nerve(s). Spinal cord lesions cause a bilateral, symmetric sensory loss that is apparent caudal to the injury level. Brain stem lesions rarely produce detectable analgesia, since a brain stem lesion severe enough to affect nociception would result in the patient's death. Cerebral lesions produce only hypalgesia, usually unilateral and contralateral to the diseased hemisphere.

Exaggerated Responsiveness to Pain. This is tested by digital manipulation of the paraspinal region with a hemostat or safety pin. An exaggerated response normally indicates a nerve root or meningeal lesion.

DIAGNOSTIC TESTING (pp. 599–603)

CEREBROSPINAL FLUID EVALUATION

Many nervous system diseases, especially inflammations and neoplasms, will affect CSF composition. A disease must involve either the ventricular system or the subarachnoid space for cells to be shed into CSF. CNS disorders involving deeper parenchyma may disrupt the blood-brain barrier (BBB), allowing protein leakage, without shedding cells into CSF.

Spinal Fluid Collection

Complications of CSF collection include anesthetic misadventures, CNS damage from the spinal needle, and/or brain herniation (uncommon, but fatal). If the pressure appears to be elevated or if a patient appears to be in danger of herniation, hyperventilation with oxygen may decrease the intracranial pressure (ICP) sufficiently to avoid problems. Overflexing the neck and occluding the jugular veins will artifactually elevate the ICP and increase the potential for brain herniation. If the fluid appears bloody at the onset of collection, the stylet should be replaced and the needle left in place for 30 to 60 seconds.

CSF Analysis

Cerebrospinal fluid from the cerebellomedullary cistern tends to have slightly more cells and lower protein than the fluid from the lumbar space.

Pressure. The normal pressures in dogs ranged from 50 to 140 mm H_2O, depending on body size. Typically, patients with meningitis have moderate to severe elevations of CSF pressure above the normal. Patients with tumors are more likely to have massive elevations of CSF pressure.

Gross Evaluation. Free hemoglobin suggests previous subarachnoid hemorrhage. Yellow-orange (xanthochromic) CSF generally indicates breakdown of hemoglobin from previous hemorrhage or severe elevations of CSF protein, and is seen in some cases of protracted icterus.

Cytologic Evaluation. There should be fewer than 5 WBC/μl in normal CSF. Cell numbers may increase with inflammations, tumors, necrosis, trauma, and vascular injuries to the CNS. Cytology is most changed with inflammations. CSF cytology is most reliable in acute, untreated CNS infections.

Some inflammatory diseases and many neoplasms are associated with normal CSF cytology. Suppurative meningitis is a pathologic response to bacterial infection; to acute, severe viral encephalitis; to presumed immune vasculitis/meningitis of young dogs; following myelography; and with some tumors, especially meningiomas.

Mixed inflammatory cytology is generally the result of a granulomatous inflammation, such as occurs with fungal, protozoal, and some idiopathic diseases, in inadequately treated chronic bacterial infections, and in response to foreign bodies. Nonsuppurative inflammation is most characteristic of viral and rickettsial infections, but is also seen with neoplasms and uncommonly with an acute bacterial infection of the nervous system. In any inflammatory process, but especially one with visible organisms, CSF should be cultured.

Biochemical Evaluation. In dogs and cats, protein from a cerebellomedullary cisternal tap is generally less than 25 mg/dl, whereas that from a lumbar puncture may be as high as 45 mg/dl. CSF protein is elevated in many diseases of the nervous system, including encephalitis, meningitis, neoplasms, trauma, and infarcts.

Total protein quantitation and protein electrophoresis should be performed on all CSF samples. Over 75 per cent of CSF protein should be albumin. If the elevated protein is predominantly globulin, this is most consistent with an inflammatory process of the CNS (encephalitis). With a combination of elevated albumin and globulin in CSF, an inflammatory process that affects both CNS and meninges (e.g., FIP) should be suspected. Normal CSF glucose is about 60 to 80 per cent of blood levels. A meningitic patient that was also bacteremic would be expected to have a concomitant drop in CSF glucose.

The presence of intrathecal antibodies serves as evidence that the organism against which the antibodies are found is the cause of the encephalitis. Increased albumin on CSF electrophoresis would support a false-positive diagnosis, as it indicates an increased BBB permeability. If both serum and CSF titers are elevated, there is a greater possibility that the CSF titer is the result of leakage. If only CSF titers are elevated, it is most likely intrathecal production.

ELECTRODIAGNOSTIC EVALUATIONS

Electroencephalography (EEG). EEG does not allow a clinician to establish a precise etiologic diagnosis. EEG changes are most likely to be seen with metabolic diseases, inflammatory diseases, and mass lesions.

Brain Stem Auditory Evoked Response (BAER, BER). The BAER has proved to be highly useful in the evaluation of deafness. The BAER will also be altered by brain stem and some cerebral lesions, so it is a useful tool in confirming the presence of a central lesion in patients with vestibular dysfunction.

RADIOGRAPHIC AND ALTERNATE IMAGING EVALUATION

Routine Radiographic Procedures

In general, plain skull films are of limited value in patients with brain disease. Calcified brain tumors or A-U malformations, foramen and magnum deformities (open mouth frontal view), fractures, hydrocephalus, and middle/inner ear problems may be identified.

Contrast Radiography

This requires an experienced interpreter and a rapid film changer for arterial studies.

Ultrasonography. In patients with an open fontanelle, ultrasonography has been of great value in the diagnosis of hydrocephalus.

Computerized Tomography (CT Scans). CT scanning has become routine in veterinary neurology, allowing for antemortem localization of mass lesions, granulomas, and inflammatory disorders.

Magnetic Resonance Imaging (MRI). The ability of MRI to detect subtle differences in tissues makes it ideal for early neoplasm detection. MRI also recognizes inflammatory diseases with greater reliability than CT scans.

BRAIN BIOPSY

Brain biopsies have been beneficial in the antemortem diagnosis of brain tumors and in inflammatory diseases that may mimic neoplasms, especially granulomatous meningoencephalitis (GME).

PRINCIPLES OF THERAPY (pp. 603–604)

Treatment of Edema/Elevated Intracranial Pressure. As CO_2 levels decline, intracranial volume decreases, lowering ICP. *Hyperventilation* is a simple and effective means of lowering a patient's CO_2 level.

Diuretics lower ICP, by both removing edema and decreasing intracranial volume. *Corticosteroids* have been successfully used to treat the edema associated with brain tumors and may also alleviate the edema following CNS injury, provided it is administered in high doses and within 8 hours of trauma.

Anti-Inflammatory Therapy. The most effective therapy for inflammations is the judicious use of corticosteroids.

Anticonvulsant Therapy. The choice of a drug should be based on the ability to achieve and maintain therapeutic levels, with minimal side effects. In general, if the epilepsy is idiopathic, about 80 per cent of patients may be treated effectively.

Antineoplastic Therapy. Brain tumor therapy may consist of surgical removal, chemotherapy, radiation therapy, or a combination of two or more methods. Concomitant with the tumor treatment is treatment of secondary effects, such as edema.

DISEASES OF THE BRAIN (pp. 604–627)

FOCAL DISEASES

Cerebral disorders, associated with a guarded prognosis, tend to cause changes in mental status and vision, as well as seizures. Many patients with cerebral diseases will circle. Most patients with cerebral diseases have weakness of limbs, with increased spinal reflexes and decreased postural reactions.

Cerebellar disorders, associated with a fair prognosis, tend to cause ataxia of head and limbs. These patients may have tremor of the head, as well as postural tremor of the trunk when the patient is standing. Many patients with cerebellar diseases have head tilts and pathologic nystagmus. If the lesion involves the cerebellar peduncles, the patient may also have torticollis.

Brain stem disorders, associated with a poor prognosis, tend to cause cranial nerve deficits and weakness of limbs. Most brain stem disorders cause vestibular signs. Rostral brain stem lesions often depress consciousness. Caudal brain stem lesions often result in an abnormal heart rate and rhythm or respiratory distress.

FOCAL BRAIN DISEASES OF RAPID ONSET

These diseases tend to be caused by one of four major disease categories; head trauma, vascular injuries, idiopathic disorders, or neoplasms. Of these, neoplasms tend to be rapid in onset as a result of secondary changes, such as obstruction of CSF movement, with secondary hydrocephalus.

Head Trauma

Traumatic nervous system injuries not only produce immediate and direct injury to nervous tissues (primary events); secondary events (related to sympathetic nervous system activation) such as increased ICP, systemic hypertension, myocardial necrosis, cardiac arrhythmias, pulmonary edema, and increased nutritional requirements can occur after CCT.

Pressure Changes. ICP rises in most patients with CNS trauma. Elevated ICP should be treated with diuretics, osmotic agents, and steroids. Intracranial blood volume is decreased by hyperventilation and elevation of the head.

Edema. Cytotoxic edema accumulates in cells, particularly neurons and astrocytes, and usually arises from cellular hypoxia. Vasogenic edema is extracellular, primarily affects white matter, and is more amenable to therapy than cytotoxic edema.

Seizures. Many patients with CCT experience seizures, either immediately or as a delayed sequela to the trauma.

Diagnostic Approach. Patients with PNS injury usually survive without serious sequelae. In contrast, patients with CNS injury may not survive, and those that do survive may have serious sequelae including epilepsy, personality changes, and severe paralysis of limbs.

Therapeutic Approach

Medical Therapy. Intubation and *hyperventilation* constitute the quickest way to reverse both hypercarbia and hypoxia in a stuporous or comatose patient. *Steroids* reduce edema, stabilize cell membranes, stabilize the BBB, and decrease the inflammatory response that results from tissue necrosis, decreasing the secondary demyelination that occurs 1 to 5 days following CCT.

Surgical Therapy. Surgery is rarely needed following CCT unless the patient has depressed skull fractures compressing neural tissue or an open wound that may introduce an infection.

Vascular Disorders

In most cases the initial CNS injury is focal. Nervous system vascular injury may result from a variety of causes, including neoplasms, CNS infection, aneurysms, atherosclerosis, arteriovenous malformations, cardiogenic emboli, vasospasm, atrial fibrillation, mitral stenosis, hematologic disorders, vasculitis, polycythemia, hyperviscosity syndromes (plasma cell myeloma, macroglobulinemia), bleeding disorders, immune disease, uremia, sepsis, disseminated intravascular coagulation (DIC), vascular tumors, and cardiomyopathy.

Clinical Presentation

In most patients, clinical signs of vascular injury are acute, focal, asymmetric, and nonprogressive. In ischemic injuries, the signs develop over a fixed period (usually less than a day), then stabilize and begin to improve within several days. In patients with hemorrhage into the nervous system, the course is less predictable. Many patients with brain stem or cerebellar peduncular injuries have significant torticollis. Some patients with vascular injuries, especially to the brain stem, have brain-heart syndrome.

Diagnostic Approach.

The initial laboratory screening should include an evaluation for extracranial disorders (thyroid assay, retroviral testing in cats, hemostasis screen, serum protein levels, electrocardiogram, echocardiogram, and ophthalmic examination). With subarachnoid or intraventricular hemorrhage, there is free blood in the early stages, then *erythrophagocytosis* occurs, followed by xanthochromia. In patients with severe necrosis and malacia, there may be mononuclear cells, both lymphocytes and macrophages. The lack of organisms and the presence of predominantly albumin on CSF electrophoresis will distinguish this inflammatory response from that seen in patients with CNS infections.

Enhanced Imaging. CT scan, MRI, and/or scintigraphy may demonstrate the vascular lesion.

Therapy.

Unless the patient is shocky, moderate fluid restriction is indicated to prevent worsening of the brain edema. Supportive therapy and monitoring for systemic problems such as cardiac arrhythmias, nutritional changes, albumin levels, electrolyte levels, and seizures should be instituted. Corticosteroids decrease CNS inflammation and edema. If the MRI or CT scan identifies both extracellular and intracellular edema, furosemide is added to the therapy. Mild hypoglycemia during the postischemic interval might reduce the degree of necrosis in the brain.

Prognosis.

Brain stem injuries carry a poor prognosis, regardless of cause. However, patients with cerebral and cerebellar vascular injuries often recover. Some patients with cerebral injuries have permanent behavioral changes, especially patients with feline ischemic encephalopathy (FIE).

Aberrant Parasite Migration

The parasites most commonly found in the CNS are *Dirofilaria immitis* and *Cuterebrae.* Others include *Toxascaris, Ancylostoma, Taenia,* and

Angiostrongylus. The signs are referable to the portion of the CNS involved. On CSF evaluation, eosinophils are seen. A definitive diagnosis rests on necropsy. There is no effective therapy.

Idiopathic Disorders

Idiopathic Vestibular Disease. This disorder is seen in both cats and dogs. The signs are usually acute to peracute in onset, often peaking in less than 24 hours. The clinical signs include loss of balance, severe (often incapacitating) disorientation, ataxia, nystagmus, and head tilt. Nausea may be seen initially. Clinical signs stabilize rapidly, the nystagmus disappears over several days, and the ataxia gradually resolves over 3 to 6 weeks. Supportive therapy to prevent self-injury and maintain good nutrition is important. There is rarely any sequela (occasionally a mild head tilt), and recovery occurs in all patients.

Idiopathic Trigeminal Neuropathy (Canine Dropped Jaw Syndrome). The patient appears unable to close its mouth, and the owner may complain that the patient appears dysphagic. Clinical signs are acute to peracute in onset. Sensory abnormalities, muscle atrophy, and other motor cranial nerve changes are rarely seen. Most patients recover rapidly and completely (4 to 8 weeks). Teach the owner to feed the dog with the head elevated.

Idiopathic Facial Paralysis. Affected animals have an acute onset of facial paralysis (unilateral or bilateral), including loss of eye blink, drooping of the lip, and sagging of the ear. If the lacrimal gland is denervated, the eye on the affected side will be dry, as will the nostril on the same side.

Clinically, this condition has been associated with endocrine dysfunction (hypothyroidism and Cushing's disease primarily) and toxins such as lead poisoning. If neoplasia or middle ear infection are serious differentials, skull films should be obtained. There is no agreement in the veterinary literature on the benefits of steroids. With idiopathic facial paralysis, some degree of functional recovery over a 1- to 2-month time period is common.

FOCAL DISEASES OF INTERMEDIATE ONSET

Focal Inflammations

Brain Abscesses. There is often a prior history of inner ear, respiratory, or oral infection. Brain abscesses usually progress steadily unless they are being treated.

CSF analysis and enhanced imaging are the tests of choice for the diagnosis of brain abscesses. If the abscess is extradural, the CSF is normal. Abscesses of hematogenous origin are frequently multiple and occur in any part of the brain. Most brain stem abscesses are cerebellopontine in location and arise from otogenic infections. Necrosis of tissue adjacent to an abscess is common. Cerebellar herniation is often seen as a terminal event in patients with unsuccessfully treated brain abscesses.

Therapy. Antimicrobials are the basis of therapy. In most cases of brain abscess, the prognosis appears to be grave.

FOCAL DISEASES OF SLOW ONSET

The major example of focal brain disorders that are chronic in their progression are brain tumors.

Neoplastic Disorders

These result in a gradual progression of *focal* neurologic impairment that is clinically *progressive.* Secondary vascular injury may present acutely. Other common secondary changes include edema and inflammation around the tumor site, and ventricular obstruction with secondary hydrocephalus. In patients with *metastatic* neoplasms, the signs may be multifocal. Primary brain tumors are typically solitary. The major exception to this rule is the occurrence of meningiomas in cats, in which multiple tumors are noted in one-third of the cases.

Clinical Presentation. Seizures are among the most commonly reported first sign in patients with cerebral neoplasms. Animals with brain tumors may have endocrine signs such as polydipsia or polyuria, gonadal atrophy, unexplained obesity, or an abnormal haircoat, especially with pituitary neoplasms.

The most common early signs in patients with brain stem neoplasms are vestibular signs, which are usually acute in onset. With extramedullary neoplasms, cranial nerve deficits are often the principal early clinical sign. With mass lesions at the cerebellopontine angle, you may see *paradoxical vestibular syndrome.* Tremor, ataxia, and vestibular signs are the hallmark of cerebellar neoplasms.

Diagnostic Approach. All patients suspected of having a brain tumor should be thoroughly screened for primary tumors in other organs.

CSF Tap. The classically described CSF changes in patients with brain tumors are an elevation in pressure and albumin, with normal WBC count (occurs in <50% of patients). A significant number of tumor patients have some form of inflammatory CSF response, characterized by mild to severe elevations of WBCs. Elevated CSF pressure is seen in most patients with intramedullary tumors. Elevated CSF protein is generally seen with intramedullary tumors, especially in choroid plexus tumors and CNS lymphoma.

Electroencephalography (EEG). The EEG is helpful in confirming the presence of a localized process in about two-thirds of patients with brain tumors.

Ophthalmic Examination. Some patients with elevated intracranial pressure have optic nerve edema visualized on ocular fundus examination. Computerized axial tomography (CT scan) and magnetic resonance imaging (MRI), especially when combined with contrast enhancement, have proved to be the diagnostic tools of choice in CNS mass lesions.

Therapeutic Approach. Palliative therapy usually consists of administering glucocorticosteroids and anticonvulsants if needed. Primary therapy of the neoplasm itself may consist of surgical removal, radiation therapy, chemotherapy, or a combination of one or more of these modes of therapy. If the tumor is superficial, a biopsy should be performed. Megavoltage or orthovoltage radiation without surgery has increased both survival and quality of life in several reports. If the patient appears to have metastatic disease or a primary CNS lymphoma, chemotherapy may be rewarding.

DISSEMINATED DISEASES OF RAPID ONSET

These conditions tend to be toxic, metabolic, and nutritional in etiology. Congenital anomalies and inflammatory disorders may also present in this manner. Metabolic abnormalities are usually manifest as cerebral dysfunction.

Manifestations of Metabolic Encephalopathies

Altered Consciousness. Altered consciousness, confusion, delirium, obtundation, stupor, or coma may occur.

Oculomotor Responses. The pupillary light reflex is usually preserved in metabolic diseases, the exceptions being thiamine deficiency, hypothermia, anoxia, and anticholinergic intoxication. These four conditions all produce mid-position or dilated nonresponsive pupils. The corneal reflexes and oculovestibular reflexes (OVRs) should remain intact in most patients with metabolic encephalopathies.

Abnormal Motor Responses. Many patients with metabolic abnormalities have nonspecific motor abnormalities, which center around abnormal tone, including spasms of rigidity, tremors, paratonia, flaccidity, and seizures. Focal myoclonus and focal seizure are less common and are usually seen in patients suffering from hypoxia, hypoglycemia, lead poisoning, and uremia. Generalized myoclonus occurs in alkalotic and hypocalcemic patients.

Abnormal Respiration. Many patients with metabolic encephalopathies have ataxic respiration. Among the ventilatory disturbances reported in metabolic encephalopathies are hyperventilation with hepatic encephalopathy, diabetic ketoacidosis, and uremia.

Classification of Acquired Metabolic Encephalopathies

Thiamine Deficiency (Feline and Canine). Thiamine must be provided in the diet. In addition, certain fish (e.g., tuna and salmon) contain the enzyme thiaminase. Clinical signs of thiamine deficiency are usually acute in onset and rapidly progressive. Affected patients have vestibular "seizures," fixed and dilated pupils, loss of physiologic nystagmus, plus stupor or coma. Routine laboratory tests are normal, although serum can be tested for vitamin B_1 metabolite levels to confirm a deficiency state. The response to therapy is dramatic and the treatment innocuous, so clinicians often treat whenever the diagnosis is suspected. The first step is to reverse the immediate disease with injectable thiamine hydrochloride at a dose of 4.5 mg/lb (10 mg/kg). This should be followed by dietary evaluation and supplementation if necessary.

Hypoglycemia. Reported causes of hypoglycemia are identified in Chapters 116 and 117. The most commonly seen signs include clouding of consciousness, shifting focal deficits (may mimic stroke), collapse, and/or seizures. Blindness, weakness, and ataxia are other frequent signs of hypoglycemia. Hypoglycemia should be one of the first disease processes considered in young puppies and toy breeds, hunting dogs that show signs only when working, middle-aged and older dogs with seizures of recent onset, and diabetics with acute onset of neurologic signs. Many animals with hypoglycemia may also be thiamine-deficient, and if they receive glucose before thiamine, it could worsen their signs.

Hepatoencephalopathy (HE). This neurologic condition is associated with the liver's failure to remove toxins and digestive by-products from the systemic circulation. HE may result from the shunting of portal blood directly into the systemic circulation, from structural liver disease, or from a deficiency of urea cycle enzymes.

Animals with HE generally have waxing and waning alterations of consciousness and dementia as the primary signs. Other neural signs include seizures, visual deficits, circling, ataxia, and weakness. The client may connect the onset of signs with eating. Systemic signs such as abdominal pain, icterus, cachexia, ascites, polydyssia, polyuria, and diarrhea may be present. In cats, gagging and increased salivation are frequently reported signs associated with HE. See Chapter 106 regarding therapy.

Hypocalcemia. Generally hypocalcemia is seen in postpartum toy breed dogs. The condition may also occur in association with hypoparathyroidism (any age or breed) and other causes of hypocalcemia including hypoalbuminemia, renal failure, pancreatitis, GI malabsorption of either Ca^{++} or vitamin D, ethylene glycol poisoning, and following blood transfusions. The principal signs include restlessness and apprehension, muscle tremors and fasciculations, hyperthermia, weakness, generalized seizures, tachycardia, and behavior changes.

The diagnostic approach consists of measuring serum calcium levels. Hypoalbuminemia may falsely lower the plasma calcium level, as will alkalosis. Immediate therapy consists of administering intravenous calcium gluconate (slow infusion of 10% solution) for seizures or severe tremors.

Hypoxia and Anoxia.   Hypoxia may be associated with primary hypoventilation, pulmonary disease, or decreased O_2 transport. Ischemia may be seen with shock, with decreased cardiac output (arrhythmias, pump disturbances), or with cerebrovascular accidents. The chief clinical feature of hypoxia is clouding of consciousness or confusion. Causes of hypoxia include cardiac diseases, pulmonary disease, anemia, polycythemia, and hyperviscosity syndromes. Anesthetic arrest and resuscitation produce a characteristic syndrome. With mild anoxia, the animal may be transiently demented and later become epileptic, but is otherwise normal. With severe anoxia, the patient is severely demented, has cortical blindness (with normal pupillary reflexes), and may not be able to stand and walk.

Therapy for an acute hypoxic or anoxic episode includes mannitol, 0.45 gm/lb (1 gm/kg) as a slow intravenous bolus, and dexamethasone, given intravenously at 0.1 mg/lb every 6 hours for 24 hours. In addition, the underlying cause must be corrected.

Renal Failure.   Uremic encephalopathy usually presents as an acute confusional state with nonfixed focal deficits. Many patients display what is known as the "twitch-convulsive state," in which there is a combination of tremor, myoclonus, and seizures all in the same patient. There may be severe electrolyte, osmolality, and acid-base disturbances associated with the renal failure. The principal therapy is treatment of the underlying condition. Acute renal failure patients are more likely to have seizures; chronic renal failure patients are more likely to have dementia.

Hyperthyroidism.   Although the hallmarks of hyperthyroidism are systemic signs, including weight loss, polyphagia, polydipsia, polyuria, hyperactivity, and cardiac dysfunction, a recent report described CNS manifestations in a group of cats. Affected cats displayed both CNS and neuromuscular signs. They are restless, hyperexcitable, and aggressive, and may have generalized or focal seizures. The diagnosis rests on diagnosing the hyperthyroidism. Treatment is directed toward returning the cat to the euthyroid state (Chapter 114).

Metronidazole Intoxication.   Both cats and dogs are reported to develop CNS signs as a result of metronidazole intoxication. The clinical signs included ataxia, weakness, disorientation, diminished postural reactions, seizures, and apparent blindness. In all cases, the signs were acute in onset. The diagnosis rests primarily on a history of metronidazole being administered in excessive doses and the clinical response to cessation of therapy.

 Lead Poisoning.   Intoxication with lead causes primarily a cerebral disturbance with seizures and behavioral changes, although megaesophagus has been seen. Gastrointestinal signs such as diarrhea are common. Approximately half of affected cases will have nucleated RBCs on the complete blood count and 25 per cent will have basophilic stippling. Blood lead levels above 40 µg/ml are abnormal in patients with clinical signs.

Therapy consists of administering chelating agents (e.g., calcium disodium edetate) and eliminating lead exposure.

DEVELOPMENTAL DEFECTS

Hydrocephalus.   This may be a primary or a secondary condition, and does not always result in clinical signs. It may be seen in both dogs and cats. The highest incidence is in toy breeds (Chihuahua, Yorkshire terrier, Manchester terrier, Pomeranian, toy poodle) and in brachycephalic breeds (e.g., English bulldog, Boston terrier, Pekingese, Lhasa apso).

The most common clinical findings in patients with hydrocephalus include seizures, visual deficits, slowed learning, and dementia. Some affected patients have a bilateral divergent strabismus, referred to as a "setting sun sign." Although the clinical course in congenital hydrocephalus is usually slowly progressive, the condition appears to stabilize in some patients. A small number of patients with hydrocephalus have a sudden, catastrophic worsening of their condition. Secondary hydrocephalus is often rapidly progressive and is associated with massive elevations of ICP.

In primary hydrocephalus, skull radiographs may demonstrate a thin calvarium and loss of the radiographic, bony gyral pattern. Enhanced imaging techniques, such as MRI or CT scanning, confirm the presence of hydrocephalus (whether primary or secondary) and may reveal the underlying cause in secondary hydrocephalus.

Steroids may be used in either primary or secondary hydrocephalus to increase CSF absorption. Diuretics, such as furosemide, diminish CSF production.

Cerebellar Hypoplasia. Cerebellar hypoplasia results from a failure of cerebellar development in utero. The condition is most common in cats. The condition may be heritable, may result from in-utero viral or toxic injury, or may not have a known cause. In most patients the signs are static, as this is not a progressive condition. The principal clinical sign seen in this condition is cerebellar tremor. The tremors worsen with excitement or stress and abate during rest.

Cerebellar hypoplasia is a diagnosis of exclusion. Some canine patients with cerebellar hypoplasia may also have *occipital dysplasia,* and plain skull radiographs will demonstrate the associated bony malformation. The lack of clinical progression of a pure cerebellar disorder is often the basis for diagnosis. Currently no therapy is available.

Lissencephaly. The gyri and sulci fail to form, and the brain surface is nearly smooth. This rare condition is most widely reported in the dog, especially Lhasa apsos, wirehaired fox terriers, and Irish setters. The disease is characterized by dementia, seizures, blindness, and severe behavior changes. The diagnosis is established at necropsy, and there is no effective therapy.

Hypomyelinogenesis/Dysmyelinogenesis.

Since the pathology affects primarily proprioceptive fibers, the clinical signs of affected patients closely resemble those of patients with cerebellar disease. Tremors (myoclonus) of limbs and head, a base wide stance, ataxia without weakness, and tremors that are enhanced with excitement and movement, but usually abate with rest and sleep are the typical signs.

This disease usually affects multiple animals in a given litter. The signs are not usually progressive. Rather, many patients improve over several weeks to months, even becoming normal in some cases. Known causes of hypomyelinogenesis/dysmyelinogenesis include inheritance and in-utero infections.

Scotty Cramp.

This hyperkinetic syndrome is associated with episodes of spasticity and alternating hyperflexion/hyperextension of the limbs in Scottish terriers. All available evidence suggests that there is a deficiency in the amount of serotonin available in these patients.

Clinical signs first appear at 6 weeks to 18 months of age. Typically the signs are induced by exercise or excitement and will disappear with rest. The signs last 1 to 30 minutes and are primarily characterized by a goose-stepping gait. The methysergide challenge is a provocative test for the condition.

Diazepam, a centrally acting muscle relaxant, may reduce the severity of the signs. Vitamin E has been shown to decrease the frequency of the events. Avoid antiprostaglandins (e.g., aspirin), indomethacin, phenylbutazone, banamine, and penicillin—all of which will exacerbate the disease.

IDIOPATHIC DISORDERS

Diffuse Diseases of Slow Onset. These processes, which include degenerations and most inflammations, affect multiple CNS areas at the same time and are almost always progressive. Degenerations tend to be more symmetric than inflammations and are less likely to be associated with a febrile response.

DEGENERATIVE DISORDERS

Lysosomal Storage Diseases (LSD). The cell's metabolic function is compromised because of lysosomal hypertrophy, which crowds out normal organelles and impairs cellular respiration. The waste product build-up injures the cell. All these disorders are rare. All known disorders are inherited by an autosomal recessive pattern. Generally, affected patients are normal at birth. Most of them fail to thrive and do not develop concomitantly with the rest of the litter. These are always progressive fatal disorders, which usually result in death of affected animals within 4 to 6 months after the onset of clinical signs. There is no therapy for these conditions, and the definitive diagnosis requires necropsy confirmation.

Cerebellar Abiotrophy. This group of generally inherited, slowly progressive, degenerative diseases of the cerebellum has been reported in many species and breeds. In most animals signs begin at 2 months of age or older. Affected animals show only cerebellar signs. Clinical signs are slowly progressive, eventually incapacitating the animal.

The history is the tool used to establish this diagnosis. This condition is generally easy to separate from hypoplasia at necropsy, since cerebellar abiotrophies reflect cell dysfunction and death in a previously normal tissue.

Neuroaxonal Dystrophies (NAD). Neuroaxonal dystrophies are inherited CNS degenerations of both dogs and cats. In most patients, clinical signs begin at an early age and progress steadily. The predominant signs are cerebellar, including tremor and ataxia. Progression in rottweilers is slow (up to 6 years); in all other species it is more rapid. Confirmation requires histopathology.

Bull Mastiff Cerebellar Degeneration and Hydrocephalus. Clinical signs begin at 1 to 2 months of age and include ataxia and tremor initially. Cerebral signs include visual deficits, behavior changes, and depression. No treatment is successful, and the prognosis is poor.

Rottweiler Leukoencephalomyelopathy. This disease is a progressive, heritable, white matter degeneration of rottweilers. Affected patients have symmetric limb ataxia and weakness without cranial nerve deficits. Signs typically begin at 1.5 to 3.5 years of age, then slowly progress. All diagnostic tests are normal and no therapy has been reported effective.

INFLAMMATORY DISORDERS

Nervous system inflammations usually produce subacute, multifocal symptoms. They are most common in the young animal. The random progression is often one of the best clues that a patient has an inflammatory process. CNS inflammations are characterized by increased blood flow, exudation of fluids, leukocyte migration into the affected area, and altered CNS function. In addition to infections, other causes of CNS inflammation include trauma, some neoplasms, and immune and idiopathic disorders.

The most common focal inflammation is an abscess, a local region of necrosis and suppuration, usually in response to bacterial infection. Another form of localized inflammation is the granuloma. Granulomas tend to develop more slowly than abscesses and are generally progressive. Disseminated inflammations are usually subacute in onset. Some disseminated inflammations, especially some viral infections, may be acute in onset.

The most common infection routes include hematogenous spread, via the systemic circulation; direct invasion; contiguous or parameningeal spread; and entry along a nerve root. The principal barrier to hematogenous entry is the BBB, which provides both an anatomic and a physiologic barrier between the systemic circulation and the parenchyma of the CNS. In the dog and cat, transneuronal spread of organisms appears rarely. Organisms that may use this route are rabies, herpes suis, and *Listeria monocytogenes*. The organism itself may play a role in the production of clinical signs by producing toxins, vasculitis, or neural destruction. The local host defenses in the nervous system itself are generally inadequate to reverse most infections unassisted.

Clinical Features of CNS Inflammation. Many patients with CNS infections will also be systemically ill. Fever, tremors, ophthalmic signs, cardiac abnormalities, and respiratory insufficiency may be seen. There are large differences in clinical appearance between the patient with meningitis (pain and fever), meningoencephalitis (pain, fever, and CNS dysfunction), and encephalitis alone (CNS dysfunction).

Encephalitis and/or meningitis should be suspected in any patient who presents with progressive CNS dysfunction without localizing signs.

Supportive Therapy. Supportive therapy is directed toward treating or preventing brain edema by fluid restriction and diuretics. If steroids are used, it appears that dexamethasone is more effective than prednisone in relieving the secondary effects of meningitis. Antipyretics, anticonvulsants, and good nursing care may be necessary.

The most common (or significant) causes of encephalitis in cats include rabies, feline infectious peritonitis, toxoplasmosis, neosporosis, feline immunodeficiency virus, and systemic fungal diseases. The most common (or significant) causes of encephalitis in dogs include rabies, granulomatous meningoencephalitis (GME), canine distemper, toxoplasmosis, neosporosis, and systemic fungal diseases.

Diagnostic Tests. CSF analysis remains the diagnostic test of choice in CNS inflammations. Generally, the WBC numbers will be elevated, the highest counts being seen with granulomatous diseases (e.g., FIP and GME) and bacterial meningitis. With systemic fungal, protozoal, and parasitic infections, eosinophils may also be present in the CSF. CSF protein levels should be increased with globulin elevations. In some viral diseases, such as canine distemper and rabies, the protein elevation may be minimal.

Listeriosis (Circling Disease). The disease is usually seen in ruminants but may occur in cats and dogs. The clinical signs center around the nerve traveled following oral abrasion entry; usually cranial nerves V, VII, IX, and X are involved. The neurologic signs, generally confined to the brain stem, include asymmetric cranial nerve deficits, limb weakness, depression, and vestibular dysfunction. Torticollis, circling, head tilts, ataxia, and weakness are other common signs.

The CSF pressure is normal to increased, and the CSF WBC count is increased, with a predominately monocellular pleocytosis. Usually there is an elevated protein as well. Vigorous therapy with chlortetracycline or high doses of penicillin is indicated. If the disease is treated early and vigorously, the prognosis is good. Residual signs, including head tilts, may be seen for several weeks following treatment but usually resolve.

Rabies Encephalitis. See Chapters 69 and 70.

Postvaccinal Rabies. There are no reports of this condition occurring following vaccination with killed virus vaccines. All affected animals developed a progressive caudal paresis beginning 12 to 17 days after vaccination with a modified live virus (MLV) rabies vaccine. Over time, the signs progress to involve the brain stem. The disease starts in the LMN and then progresses up to the UMN. The signs are rapidly progressive.

Aujesky's Disease (Pseudorabies). The reservoir for this herpesvirus disease is pigs, but it may occur in dogs and cats. Dogs and cats usually acquire the infection by ingesting infected tissue. The viral infection of the ganglion and spinal cord segment initiate the localized or generalized pruritus so characteristic of this disease. The disease is rapidly lethal in carnivores. If found alive, the affected patients show a profound dementia, pain, seizures, and self-mutilation that progresses quickly to death. At autopsy, the disease is diagnosed by serology, mouse inoculation, and histopathology. There is no effective therapy, and the prognosis is poor.

Infectious Canine Distemper Viral Encephalitis (CDVE). It is apparent that dogs with CDVE infection may have direct virus-induced damage to the CNS as well as later indirect damage as a result of developing immunity. Very young puppies are more likely to have gray matter infection, severe neuronal necrosis, minimal inflammation, and a high mortality rate. Older animals are more likely to develop an inflammatory white matter disease. Young dogs (6 to 12 weeks of age) typically have a neuronal disease. This is also the form usually seen in postvaccinal distemper. Clinical signs include seizures, dementia, severe personality changes, weakness, and ataxia. The postvaccinal disease occurs 7 to 10 days after vaccination and is seen only in immature dogs. This form of the disease is most likely to produce distemper myoclonus.

A chronic progressive multifocal CNS disease may occur in adult animals, regardless of age. This is primarily a white matter disease which often has predominantly cerebellar vestibular signs. These patients often show spinal cord signs as well as brain involvement. Old dog encephalitis (ODE) may occur at any age. The most prominent clinical sign is dementia with ataxia and central blindness. Patients with ODE rarely have seizures.

In multisystemic distemper, there are generally no diagnostic challenges. Affected patients have respiratory signs, chorioretinitis, and CNS disease. In mature patients, however, the diagnosis is often less certain. CSF is often normal in affected patients, although there may be an increase in mononuclear cells or protein. CSF serology may be helpful, but is not conclusive in vaccinated patients. Testing the cells in CSF for CDVE antigen will allow for a specific diagnosis if the results are positive.

Epithelial inclusions from vagina, prepuce, and conjunctiva are rarely present in the CNS form of CDV. There is no therapy known to be effective in the treatment of CDVE. A small percentage of patients do recover, but these animals are generally left with sequelae such as myoclonus or seizures.

Herpes Canis Encephalitis. This virus encephalitis is occasionally seen in nursing puppies and is often fatal. Clinically, the patients have predominantly brain stem and cerebellar signs; some patients have a trigeminal ganglioneuritis. If patients survive the initial systemic illness, the neurologic disease appears self-limiting.

Parvovirus Encephalitis. This has been seen in puppies. Unlike the disease in the cat, the pathology and clinical signs are not confined to the cerebellum. In many patients, the disease is rapidly progressive and fatal.

Feline Infectious Peritonitis (FIP). FIP is a coronavirus disorder of cats that causes polyserositis with peritoneal and pleural effusions. The virus also produces a nonsuppurative meningoencephalitis in about 63 per cent of cases, with resultant clinical signs in about 29 per cent of cases. Signs begin acutely to subacutely and are multifocal and slowly progressive. Patients display fever, choriorctinitis, keratic precipitates, and/or anterior uveitis. Cats with FIP encephalitis rarely have pleural or peritoneal effusions; however, many have renal involvement with irregular kidney size. Affected patients are often anemic and hyperglobulinemic. The CSF is consistent with a granulomatous inflammation; usually there is an increase in lymphocytes or neutrophils and in protein. Serology is less helpful. There is no effective therapy for FIP encephalitis, and the prognosis is poor.

Protozoal Encephalitis. The most widely reported are *Toxoplasma gondii* and *Neosporum caninum;* however, a new protozoa has recently been identified in cats. In patients with clinical neurologic signs, there are two different illnesses based on age. In adults, there is typically a multifocal histiocytic inflammation and CNS malacia. In animals under 6 months of age, a generalized inflammatory muscle disease (polymyositis) and widespread nerve root inflammation (polyradiculoneuritis) are more likely to result. Respiratory illness and radiographic pneumonia may be seen with toxoplasmosis. Icterus from liver involvement may also be seen. Muscle pain will be seen with myositis in protozoal infections. Serologic confirmation for the appropriate protozoan is the definitive antemortem diagnostic tool. Cats are the only species known to shed *T. gondii* oocysts in the feces; accurate identification requires a parasitologist.

Mycotic Encephalitis. Fungal organisms which have been reported in the CNS include *Cryptococcus neoformans* (the most frequent), *Coccidioides immitis, Histoplasma capsulatum, Blastomyces dermatitides, Aspergillus* spp., and *Mucor* spp. Prototheca, an achlorophyllous alga, and phaeohyphomycosis may also cause a disseminated CNS infection. All fungal organisms can cause encephalitis and chorioretinitis. Chronic rhinitis is common with cryptococcal infection. With CNS histoplasmosis, there may be an antecedent history of colitis or vague weight loss. Neurologic signs include depression, dementia, ataxia, weakness, cranial nerve deficits, and LMN paralysis.

When CSF is examined, the organism may be seen on cytologic examination, especially with cryptococcal infections. There are increased numbers of WBCs and increased CSF protein, including elevated globulins. Serologic assays are available to test for both antigen of organism and antibody against organism. Ketaconazole and itraconazole are more expensive, but safer for the patient. Therapy should continue for at least 6 weeks after remission of clinical signs.

Meningitis. The primary complaints are usually hyperesthesia, neck pain, depression, and fever. CSF should show normal to increased pressure, normal to increased cell number (the cell type will reflect the cause of meningitis), and increased protein. Depending on the etiology, organisms may be found. In the sterile suppurative meningitis of young dogs, the predominant cell type will be mature, healthy-appearing neutrophils without organisms. In bacterial meningitis, the neutrophils are often toxic and organisms are seen.

If bacterial meningitis is confirmed, 4 to 6 weeks of appropriate antibiotic therapy, as determined by CSF culture and sensitivity, is essential. There is some evidence that treatment with steroids for the first 24 hours of treatment with antibiotics will both hasten and improve the degree of recovery. If the meningitis is immune or sterile, the use of immunosuppressive doses of corticosteroids is indicated.

Granulomatous Meningoencephalitis (GME, Inflammatory Reticulosis). GME is a nonsuppurative inflammatory disease of the CNS of dogs and, less commonly, cats and is associated with a marked perivascular proliferation of reticuloendothelial (RE) cells. Although lesions may occur in any portion of the CNS, there appears to be a predilection for the cerebrum and the cerebellopontine angle. The disease, which tends to occur more commonly in female toy-breed dogs, is primarily a disease of the young or middle-aged (1 to 8 yr), but may occur at any age. The onset is usually rapid, although indolent cases have been reported. Without treatment, the disease usually progresses to death within several months.

Ocular Form. The ocular form is relatively uncommon. It is characterized by acute visual loss in the affected eye(s) with loss of the pupillary light reflex if the affected eye is illuminated (optic neuritis). This disease is the slowest to progress, often remaining static for months.

Focal Form. The focal form mimics an expanding mass, with the signs reflecting the site of the granuloma. This form is intermediate in progression, with signs partially responsive to therapy.

Disseminated Form. This is the most rapidly progressive form of the disease. Because this is a multifocal disease, any neurologic sign can be seen.

Diagnosis. The diagnosis can be confirmed only at necropsy or by brain biopsy; however, with improved diagnostic techniques, a reliable tentative diagnosis can be made without histopathology. The principal diagnostic aid is CSF analysis. There should be an elevated WBC consisting of about 10 to 20 per cent PMNs in the CSF, 10 to 20 per cent monocytes and macrophages, and 60 to 80 per cent lymphocytes and plasma cells. In some cases, large anaplastic-looking mononuclear cells may be seen, and these cells are considered to be diagnostic of this condition. The protein generally is elevated (40 to 1000 mg/dl), with significant elevation of IgG on electrophoresis. CSF normalizes rapidly with steroid therapy, so treatment with steroids should not be given before CSF is collected.

Treatment. The drug most often used is prednisolone; however, other drugs such as cytoxan and azathioprine are being considered as well. Radiation therapy is showing promising results. In spite of current advances, therapy is limited to remission rather than a cure in most cases.

Pug Encephalitis. This chronic granulomatous meningoencephalitis that affects adult pugs bears many similarities to GME histologically, except that there is more malacia and eosinophils may be found in the lesions. The onset of CNS signs is 9 months to 4 years. The disease is multifocal; however, cerebral signs, including seizures and dementia, are often the earliest complaint. Circling, head tilts, nystagmus and other brain stem signs are common in the later stages of the disease. The diagnosis is based on abnormal CSF, with a mixed inflammatory picture. Corticosteroids may alleviate the clinical signs for short periods. This appears to be an invariably fatal disease.

Feline Polioencephalomyelitis. This slowly progressive chronic disease of cats does not appear to have an age predilection. The signs are spinal cord and cerebellar, rarely brain stem or cerebral. Many affected animals have nonregenerative anemias.

Rickettsial Diseases. Several rickettsial diseases, including Rocky Mountain spotted fever and ehrlichiosis, can produce meningoencephalitis in dogs. The most common neurologic signs are vestibular, but any portion of the neuraxis may be affected clinically or pathologically.

OTHER DIFFUSE DISORDERS

Idiopathic Tremor Syndrome (White Dog Shaker Syndrome). It may be a diffuse demyelinating disorder or possibly a generalized neurotransmitter deficiency, on the order of Parkinson's disease or Huntington's chorea in humans. The signs are usually acute in onset, and for unknown reasons the condition is seen primarily in young to middle-aged dogs with white hair coats, especially the Maltese, West Highland white terrier, Bichon Frisc, and poodle. The principal clinical sign is diffuse tremor of the entire body. Chaotic, random eye movements (opsoclonus) are a characteristic feature of this condition on neurologic examination. All diagnostic tests are normal in these patients. Steroids are generally effective in reversing the clinical disease. Diazepam appears to abort the tremors, allowing the nervous system to recover.

Feline Spongioform Encephalopathy. A progressive neurologic disease has been identified in five cats in Great Britain. Affected cats had ataxia of limbs, especially the pelvic limbs, behavior changes, hyperesthesia, head tremor, muscle fasciculations, and hypersalivation. The signs and lesions appeared identical to those of scrapie and bovine spongioform encephalopathy (BSE).

Feline Immunodeficiency Virus (FIV). It appears that as many as 30 per cent of cats infected with FIV may develop neurologic signs unrelated to secondary infections. The principal changes reflect cerebral injury and include depression, behavior changes, dementia, loss of toilet training, and aggression. At present, the attribution of CNS signs to FIV infection requires proof that FIV is present in the affected patient and that there are no other well-established causes of neurologic disease present in the patient concurrently. The presence of FIV antibodies is considered diagnostic of CNS infection, provided there was no blood contamination of the CSF. Currently the prognosis for FIV encephalopathy is poor.

CHAPTER 83

DISEASES OF THE SPINAL CORD
(pages 629–696)

DIAGNOSTIC APPROACH TO A SPINAL CORD PROBLEM

Minimum Data Base

Initial clinicopathologic tests include a complete blood count, blood chemistry profile, and urinalysis. Thoracic or abdominal radiographs may be obtained as part of the minimum data base in dogs or cats with a spinal cord disorder.

Ancillary Diagnostic Investigations

The recommended essential procedures for diagnosis of a myelopathy in advised order of completion are noncontrast vertebral radiography, cerebrospinal fluid (CSF) analysis, and myelography.

Noncontrast Vertebral Radiography. Correct technique, exact positioning, and use of appropriate projections are essential considerations for the production of noncontrast vertebral radiographs that are of diagnostic quality.

Cerebrospinal Fluid Analysis. It should be noted that normal values differ in CSF collected from lumbar and cisternal collection sites.

Myelography. Myelography should only be considered if positive findings are essential for diagnosis and prognosis, or to determine a precise site for surgery.

Original chapter written by Richard A. LeCouteur and Georgina Child

Electrophysiology. Abnormal EMG results associated with spinal cord disease are seen only when the lower motor neurons (LMNs) in the ventral horn of the spinal cord or their axons in the ventral root are affected by a pathologic process. Electromyographic examination may be used to define the extent of a lesion affecting the brachial or lumbar enlargement of the spinal cord.

Sensory or motor nerve conduction velocities may also aid in identification of nerve roots affected by a spinal cord disorder. Spinal cord potentials (cord dorsum potentials) evoked by stimulation of a peripheral sensory nerve may be used in combination with sensory nerve conduction velocity determinations to determine involvement of sensory nerve roots proximal to the dorsal root ganglia. Cystometry, urethral closure pressure profile recording, electromyography of urethral sphincter, uroflowmetry, and evoked spinal cord potential measurements following pudendal nerve stimulation may provide information regarding the functional status of spinal cord segments involved in micturition.

Additional Diagnostic Techniques. The lumbosacral junction, with overlying bodies of the ileum, and the thoracic vertebral column, with overlying ribs, are regions of the spine in which linear tomography has particular application in vertebral radiography. X-ray computed tomography (CT) and magnetic resonance imaging (MRI) are being used with increasing frequency in the diagnosis of spinal cord disorders of dogs and cats.

CLINICAL SIGNS OF SPINAL CORD DISEASES
(pp. 633–635)

A complete neurologic examination is described in Chapter 82. Diseases of the spinal cord may also result in dysfunction of bladder, urethral sphincter, and anal sphincter, and in loss of voluntary control of urination and defecation. This may be due to interruption of spinal cord pathways connecting brain stem and cerebrum to bladder and rectum that are important in normal detrusor reflex function and voluntary control of micturition and defecation, or it may be due to interruption of the parasympathetic nerve supply to the bladder and urinary and anal sphincters (L7 to S3 spinal cord segments and spinal nerves).

Voluntary Movement. Ataxia (incoordination) is seen in association with paresis and probably occurs due to interference with both ascending and descending spinal cord pathways.

Spinal Reflexes. Depression of a spinal reflex in association with spinal cord disease most frequently occurs as a result of involvement by a pathologic process of spinal cord segments mediating the reflex. Exaggeration of a spinal reflex in association with spinal cord disease occurs when a lesion affects the spinal cord cranial to segments that mediate a reflex. It is important to remember that reflex exaggeration may result from a brain lesion as well as from a spinal cord lesion.

Muscle Tone. Alterations of muscle tone are interpreted in a similar fashion to that for alterations in spinal reflexes.

Muscle Atrophy. Denervation atrophy is seen when α motor neurons (LMNs) that innervate a muscle are damaged by a lesion affecting their spinal cord segment(s) of origin. Denervation atrophy is evident within a week of injury, usually is severe, and is associated with EMG abnormalities. Disuse atrophy may be seen in muscles innervated by LMNs caudal to a spinal cord lesion. Disuse atrophy usually is slower in onset and progression than denervation atrophy, most often is less severe in character, and is not associated with EMG alterations.

Sensory Dysfunction. Conscious proprioception is a sensitive indicator of spinal cord function, and depression or loss of conscious proprioception frequently is the sign first produced by a myelopathy. Areas of decreased or absent cutaneous pain perception may aid in identification of specific nerves, nerve roots, and spinal cord segments involved in a pathologic process. Deep pain perception appears to be the sensory function that is most resistant to a spinal cord disease and is the last spinal cord function to disappear in myelopathies of any type. Therefore, loss of deep pain perception is a very grave prognostic sign. Hyperesthesia in association with a spinal cord disease may indicate nerve root or spinal nerve involvement, or may be consistent with meningeal irritation.

ALPHABETICAL LISTING OF DISEASES (pp. 638–693)

ATLANTOAXIAL SUBLUXATION (ATLANTOAXIAL INSTABILITY) AND MALFORMATIONS OF THE ODONTOID PROCESS

Subluxation, instability, or malformation of the atlantoaxial joint that permits excessive flexion of the joint may result in compression of the spinal cord due to dorsal displacement of the cranial portion of the body of the axis into the vertebral canal. These conditions may result from congenital or developmental abnormalities, trauma, or a combination. Agenesis or hypoplasia of the dens, non-union of the dens with the axis (odontoid process dysplasia), absence of the transverse ligament of the atlas, and dorsal angulation of the odontoid process with compression of the spinal cord have been associated with atlantoaxial instability in dogs. Traumatic atlantoaxial luxation occurs in all breeds of dog or cat and usually results from rupture of the atlantoaxial ligaments or fracture of the dens at its junction with the axis. Onset of signs is usually acute and coincides with the trauma.

Clinical Findings. Congenital or developmental malformations occur most frequently in toy or miniature breeds of dog. Animals with congenital or developmental abnormalities of the atlantoaxial joint usually develop clinical signs during the first year of life, although clinical signs may occur at any age. Clinical signs associated with congenital atlantoaxial instability may have an acute onset, may be slowly progressive, or may be intermittent. Signs are indicative of a transverse myelopathy between C1 and C5. Clinical signs associated with traumatic atlantoaxial instability vary from reluctance to be patted on the head and cervical pain to tetraparesis or tetraplegia. Severe spinal cord trauma as a result of atlantoaxial luxation may result in death due to respiratory paralysis.

Diagnosis. Atlantoaxial instability is best demonstrated by means of a lateral radiographic projection of the cervical spine with the neck in slight ventroflexion. Extreme care must be taken when manipulating an animal suspected of having atlantoaxial instability under anesthesia or during radiography, as flexion of the animal's neck may result in further spinal cord compression. Abnormalities of the dens may be seen on ventrodorsal views or slightly oblique lateral views.

Treatment. Animals with an acute onset of neurologic deficits resulting from atlantoaxial instability or traumatic atlanto-occipital luxation should be treated medically, as described for other forms of spinal cord trauma. In addition, the head and neck should be splinted in extension. Animals with mild luxations and cervical pain only or with minimal neurologic deficits, or animals with multiple vertebral abnormalities such as atlantoaxial instability and shortening of the body of C1, may respond to splinting of the head and neck in extension and strict cage rest for at least 6 weeks.

Surgical stabilization and/or decompression is indicated in animals with moderate to severe neurologic deficits or recurrent episodes of neck pain unresponsive to medical therapy or splinting, and in animals in which angulation of the dens results in spinal cord compression. Prognosis is fair to good for those with mild to moderate neurologic deficits and guarded for those with an acute onset of tetraplegia.

BACTERIAL, FUNGAL, RICKETTSIAL, OR PROTOTHECAL MENINGOMYELITIS

Etiology and Pathogenesis. Bacterial or fungal meningitis and/or myelitis occur infrequently in dogs and cats. Meningitis and/or myelitis may be focal, multifocal, or disseminated in distribution and are frequently accompanied by meningoencephalitis. Bacteria that have been isolated from cats or dogs with meningitis and myelitis include *Staphylococcus aureus, S. epidermidis, S. albus, Pasteurella* spp., *Actinomyces,* and *Nocardia.* Fungal infections have been caused by *Cryptococcus neoformans, Blastomyces dermatitidis, Histoplasma capsulatum,* and *Coccidioides immitis.* Cryptococcosis is more common in cats than dogs, and infection may result from extension of nasal infection through the cribriform plate. Focal epidural infections have been reported to occur, generally as a result of migrating grass awns or penetrating wounds. Ehrlichiosis (*Ehrlichia canis* infection) and Rocky Mountain spotted fever (RMSF, caused by *Rickettsia rickettsii*) may cause meningoencephalitis or meningomyelitis in dogs. Acutely, both diseases may induce immune-mediated vasculitis in a variety of tissues including the CNS. Protothecosis rarely occurs.

Clinical Findings

Bacterial or Fungal Infections. Clinical signs of meningitis include apparent spinal pain, hyperesthesia, and cervical or thoracolumbar rigidity, occasionally manifest as a "sawhorse" posture. Fever is intermittent and is more likely to occur in association with concurrent bacteremia or disseminated fungal infection. Neurologic deficits are indicative of associated myelitis or radiculitis, and abnormalities depend on the location and extent of infection. Paraparesis and pelvic limb ataxia are common presenting signs in animals with cryptococcal meningitis and/or myelitis. Progressive paralysis of a single pelvic limb has been reported in two cats with cryptococcal infection of the lumbar spinal cord.

Rickettsial Infections. Central depression is the most consistent clinical finding in dogs with rickettsial infection. Other abnormalities indicative of spinal cord and/or meningeal involvement include paraparesis, tetraparesis, ataxia, and generalized or localized hyperesthesia. Intermittent neck pain was the predominant clinical sign in two dogs with positive *E. canis* titers seen by these authors. Neurologic abnormalities indicative of cerebral involvement include vestibular disturbances, seizures, cerebellar abnormalities, and coma.

Prototothecal Infections. Clinical signs reported in dogs have included ataxia, circling, and paresis or paralysis. Only the cutaneous form of this disease has been reported in cats.

Diagnosis. A diagnosis of bacterial or fungal meningitis and/or myelitis is made on the basis of results of CSF analysis and isolation of a causative organism by culture of CSF. See Chapter 82 for CSF characteristics.

Bacterial or Fungal Infections. A diagnosis of bacterial or fungal meningitis and/or myelitis is made on the basis of results of CSF analysis, and isolation of a causative organism by culture of CSF. See Chapter 82 for CSF characteristics. Focal epidural inflammatory lesions may appear as an extradural mass on myelography.

Rickettsial Infections. Diagnosis of RMSF or erlichosis is based on serology. A single positive serum titer for *E. canis* using an indirect immunofluorescent antibody technique is considered diagnostic for ehrlichiosis. A fourfold increase in serum antibody titer in samples collected 2 to 3 weeks apart is considered diagnostic for RMSF.

Treatment. See Chapter 82.

Bacterial Infections. The blood-brain, blood–spinal cord, and blood-CSF barriers are most permeable to antimicrobials with high lipid solubility, low ionization potential, and low protein binding affinity. See Table 82–11 in the textbook. Corticosteroids may decrease inflammation and thereby decrease the resulting spinal cord and nerve root damage; however, such treatment may also decrease host defense mechanisms, which may result in worsening of clinical signs and in a higher incidence of relapse.

Fungal Infections.   Fungal infection of the CNS of dogs or cats is extremely difficult to eliminate.

Rickettsial Infections.   Rickettsial organisms appear to be extremely sensitive to tetracyclines (10 mg/lb orally three times a day for 14 days). Doxycycline has better CNS penetration than that seen with oxytetracycline or tetracycline.

CALCINOSIS CIRCUMSCRIPTA

Etiology and Pathogenesis.   Calcinosis circumscripta is usually idiopathic and presents in the form of circumscribed single or multiple calcium deposits, often in periarticular connective tissue. The condition occurs mainly in young dogs of large breeds, with an apparently high incidence in German shepherd dogs.

Clinical Signs.   Masses in the cervical region result in a progressive tetraparesis and generalized ataxia, whereas thoracic lesions result in a progressive pelvic limb paresis and ataxia. Affected dogs are apparently free of spinal pain.

Diagnosis.   Radiography and myelography usually reveal a solitary, rounded, mineralized mass dorsal to the spinal cord, resulting in severe extradural spinal cord compression.

Treatment.   Complete surgical removal of the mass provides long-term resolution of clinical signs in affected dogs.

CALCIUM PHOSPHATE DEPOSITION DISEASE IN GREAT DANE DOGS

Etiology and Pathogenesis.   A disease characterized by progressive incoordination and paralysis has been described in Great Dane puppies (1 to 2 months old). Bones are shorter than normal and have a thin cortex and increased medullary trabeculae and curvature. Caudal cervical vertebral canal stenosis results from dorsal displacement of C7, and deformation of the vertebral articular processes results in spinal cord compression.

Treatment.   Treatment for this condition has not been described.

CERVICAL SPONDYLOMYELOPATHY

Etiology and Pathogenesis.   Several terms have been used to describe a disease of the cervical vertebral column of Great Dane dogs, Doberman pinscher dogs, and other large breeds of dog. Vertebral instability, either alone or in combination with vertebral malformation and/or soft tissue stenosis, has been suggested as an initiating cause of spinal cord compression and associated neurologic abnormalities. Chronic progressive compression of the spinal cord results from stenosis of the vertebral canal that is caused by a combination of these factors. Cervical spondylomyelopathy occurs most frequently in young (less than 2 years of age) Great Dane dogs, and middle-aged or older (3 to 9 years of age) Doberman pinscher dogs. The C5-6 and C6-7 interspaces appear to be affected most commonly.

Clinical Findings.   Clinical signs are most often insidious in onset and are gradually progressive over several months or years. A mild pelvic limb ataxia progresses in severity until a wide-based, crouching stance and dragging or knuckling of the toes of the pelvic limbs may be seen. Neurologic abnormalities that may be noted in the pelvic limbs include depression or loss of conscious proprioception and exaggerated spinal reflexes. Thoracic limb abnormalities most often occur after the development of neurologic deficits in pelvic limbs, and thoracic limb deficits seldom progress to the level of severity of pelvic limb abnormalities. Neurogenic atrophy of supraspinatus or infraspinatus muscles may be detected; however, widespread lower motor neuron involvement in thoracic limbs rarely is seen. Although affected dogs may resist extension of the neck, apparent neck pain, as seen frequently with an acute cervical disk protrusion, is seldom elicitable.

Diagnosis. Diagnosis of cervical vertebral canal stenosis has been made on the basis of noncontrast lateral radiographs of the cervical spine; however, numerous studies have emphasized that noncontrast radiographs of the cervical spine may be normal in affected dogs. Myelography is essential to determine the location or locations, and nature and extent, of spinal cord compression present. The importance of ventrodorsal projections in defining lateral spinal cord compression, and dynamic or "stressed" radiographs in outlining dorsal spinal cord compression, in combination with myelography, has been emphasized by several authors.

Dynamic or "stress" radiography, following myelography, is of particular value in demonstration of instability, ventral spinal cord compression as a result of dorsally protruding intervertebral disks, or dorsal spinal cord compression as a result of ventrally protruding interarcuate ligament or joint capsule, but should be performed with caution. "Traction" views are recommended following myelography, as they do not appear to increase spinal cord compression and do provide information that is useful in the selection of an appropriate surgical technique.

Treatment. Medical therapy consists of use of anti-inflammatory medications and management procedures that reduce neck movement, such as close confinement or use of a neck brace. Some affected dogs may be maintained at an acceptable level of neurologic function for months to years by means of corticosteroid administration. Adverse effects of long-term corticosteroid therapy must be considered, and it must be remembered that this approach does not address the underlying sustained spinal cord compression in most cases. Use of a neck brace or cage confinement is likely to be useful only in those dogs in which there is a dynamic component to the spinal cord compression.

The primary objective of all surgical procedures is decompression of the spinal cord, stabilization of the vertebral column, or both. Prognosis for dogs with cervical spondylomyelopathy is difficult to determine. Dogs with acute onset of signs, mildly affected dogs, and dogs with a single level of compression appear to have a better prognosis.

CONGENITAL VERTEBRAL ANOMALIES

Etiology and Pathogenesis. If a vertebral anomaly causes instability or deformity of the vertebral canal, spinal cord compression and associated clinical signs may result. The most frequently recognized vertebral anomalies are alteration in location of the anticlinal vertebra, anomalies of articular processes, variations in numbers of vertebrae, transitional vertebrae, butterfly vertebrae, block vertebrae, nonfusion of sacral vertebrae, or hemivertebrae. Of these anomalies, hemivertebrae are the most significant as a cause of neurologic abnormalities.

Hemivertebrae. Hemivertebrae are wedge-shaped, and the apex may be directed dorsally, ventrally, or medially across the midline. Hemivertebrae may be associated with moderate to severe angulation of the spine (kyphosis, scoliosis, or lordosis), and may be displaced dorsally during growth by pressure from adjacent vertebrae. They occur most commonly in the thoracic spine of "screw-tailed" brachycephalic breeds (French and English bulldogs, pugs, and Boston terriers) but may occur at any location in any breed of dog. Thoracic hemivertebrae are inherited (autosomal recessive).

Block Vertebrae. Block vertebrae involve the vertebral bodies, vertebral arches, dorsal spinous processes, or entire vertebrae. The sacrum is considered a "normal" block vertebra, with remnants of disk material or intervertebral disk spaces frequently seen radiographically. Block vertebrae may be the same length as the number of involved vertebrae, or may be shorter, and can result in abnormal angulation of the spine.

Butterfly Vertebrae. Butterfly vertebrae result from persistence of the notochord. On a dorsoventral radiograph of the vertebral column, such vertebrae resemble a butterfly with wings spread. Butterfly vertebrae are most common in brachycephalic "screw-tailed" breeds.

Transitional Vertebrae. Dogs may have variations in the number or shape of cervical, thoracic, lumbar, or sacral vertebrae. Vertebrae that have the characteristics of two major divisions of the vertebral column are referred to as transitional vertebrae. Alterations may be unilateral or bilateral, and most commonly involve vertebral arches and transverse processes and less frequently the vertebral bodies.

Clinical Findings. Hemivertebrae may result in vertebral instability and/or narrowing of the spinal canal, especially in the dorsoventral plane, owing to moderate to severe angulation of the spine, which can result in spinal cord compression or intermittent trauma to the spinal cord. Clinical signs produced depend on the location of the anomaly and usually reflect a progressive or intermittent transverse myelopathy. Acute onset of neurologic deficits may occur following trauma to an already unstable spine, or clinical signs may become evident as a dog grows, owing to spinal cord compression that results from progressive spinal deformity. Clinical signs usually occur in dogs less than one year of age.

Diagnosis. Diagnosis of a vertebral anomaly is made by means of radiographs of the vertebral column. Hemivertebrae should be differentiated from vertebral compression due to a traumatic fracture, pathologic fracture due to vertebral neoplasia, or osteomyelitis.

Treatment. Vertebral anomalies resulting in spinal cord compression and instability of the vertebral column may be treated by means of surgical decompression and stabilization. It is important to determine that a congenital anomaly is the cause of an animal's myelopathy by ensuring that the clinical signs are consistent with the observed abnormality. Animals may have more than one spinal abnormality, and vertebral anomalies may be associated with congenital spinal cord anomalies that are not amenable to surgical treatment.

CORTICOSTEROID-RESPONSIVE MENINGITIS (ASEPTIC MENINGITIS)

Etiology and Pathogenesis. Corticosteroid-responsive meningitis occurs in young dogs of medium to large breeds and may be the most frequently occurring form of meningitis in dogs.

Clinical Findings. Clinical signs include reluctance to move, arched back, stiff gait, apparent cervical and/or thoracolumbar pain, fever, muscle rigidity or spasms, apparent pain on opening the mouth, and, less commonly, neurologic deficits such as decreased conscious proprioception, paraparesis, or tetraparesis. Clinical signs are indistinguishable from those of meningitis and myelitis due to other causes (bacterial, fungal, viral) and necrotizing vasculitis of spinal meningeal arteries. Clinical signs may be acute in onset and progressive or may have a waxing and waning course over a period of weeks or months.

Diagnosis. Diagnosis is made on the basis of increased white blood cells in CSF, failure to isolate an infectious agent from CSF, and response to therapy with corticosteroids.

Treatment. Initially, a corticosteroid is given at a dose sufficient to produce a remission of clinical signs, then the dose is slowly tapered. Therapy for up to 6 months may be necessary to prevent recurrence of clinical signs.

DEGENERATIVE MYELOPATHY OF DOGS

Etiology and Pathogenesis.   Degenerative myelopathy (also called chronic degenerative radiculomyelopathy) is characterized by slowly progressive ataxia and paresis of the pelvic limbs. Dural ossification (osseous metaplasia or "ossifying pachymeningitis"), spondylosis deformans, chronic intervertebral disk protrusion, or infectious or vascular disorders may occur concurrently.

Clinical Findings.   Degenerative myelopathy generally occurs in dogs 6 years of age or older. It has been reported most commonly in German shepherd dogs and German shepherd mixed-breed dogs, although it does occur in other large and medium breeds of dog. Neurologic deficits often are more noticeable when the dog walks on smooth surfaces. Paraparesis and ataxia progressively worsen so that most affected dogs become nonambulatory within several months to one year after neurologic deficits are first detected. Apparent pain or discomfort is not evident. Voluntary control of urination and defecation is retained, although affected dogs may not be able to urinate or defecate in an appropriate place owing to severe paraparesis or inability to assume a voiding posture. Muscle atrophy is not severe in the initial stages of the disease but may become noticeable in later stages. Cutaneous and deep pain perception remains intact throughout the course of the disease.

Neurologic examination findings usually are indicative of a transverse myelopathy between T3 and L3. It is important to note that patellar reflexes may be decreased or absent unilaterally or bilaterally in some cases.

Diagnosis.   Diagnosis of degenerative myelopathy is based on clinical findings, age and breed of the dog, and the ruling out of all other causes of a transverse myelopathy in the T3 to L3 region. Diseases to be considered in the differential diagnosis include diskospondylitis, myelitis, spinal cord compression due to type II intervertebral disk protrusion, or spinal neoplasia. Significant myelographic abnormalities are not found.

Treatment.   Effective treatment has not been reported.

DEGENERATIVE MYELOPATHY OF CATS

Clinical Findings.   In the single report of degenerative myelopathy, the affected cat showed progressive symmetric paraparesis over a period of several months. Neurologic deficits were consistent with a transverse myelopathy between T3 and L3 spinal cord segments. Clinical improvement was not apparent after treatment with corticosteroids.

DEMYELINATING MYELOPATHY OF MINIATURE POODLES

Etiology and Pathogenesis.   Demyelination of the brain stem and spinal cord has been reported in young miniature poodles.

Clinical Findings.   Affected dogs are between 2 and 5 months of age. Initially, progressive paraparesis is seen, followed by tetraparesis, paraplegia, and tetraplegia over a period of 2 weeks. Withdrawal reflexes are normal, and extensor thrust reflexes are present. Muscle tone in all limbs is increased, and tetraplegic dogs may lie in lateral recumbency with forelimbs held in extension. Pain perception remains normal. Cranial nerve deficits are not present, and affected animals are alert and responsive. Affected animals are not in apparent pain.

Treatment.   Effective treatment for this disorder has not been described and prognosis is hopeless.

DISKOSPONDYLITIS (SPONDYLITIS, VERTEBRAL OSTEOMYELITIS)

Etiology and Pathogenesis.   Diskospondylitis and spondylitis result from implantation of bacteria or fungi introduced by migrating plant awns (grass seeds, foxtails), hematogenous spread, extension of a paravertebral infection, a penetrating wound, or previous disk or vertebral surgery.

Organisms most commonly isolated are coagulase-positive *Staphylococcus* spp. *(aureus, intermedius).* Other organisms that have been isolated include *Bacteroides capillosus, Brucella canis, Nocardia* spp., *Streptococcus canis, Corynebacterium* sp., *Escherichia coli, Proteus* spp., *Pasteurella* spp., *Paecilomyces* spp., *Aspergillus* spp., and *Mycobacterium* spp. *Coccidioides immitis* may cause vertebral body osteomyelitis. *Hepatozoon canis* infection has been associated with periosteal bone proliferation of the vertebrae as well as other bones of the body. *Spirocerca lupi* infection may cause productive bony changes on the ventral aspect of thoracic vertebrae where the aorta and the esophagus run in parallel course. Diskospondylitis has been reported to occur in cats.

Clinical Findings. Diskospondylitis is most commonly seen in giant and large breeds of dog. The most common clinical signs are weight loss, anorexia, depression, fever, reluctance to run or jump, and apparent spinal pain (which may be severe).

Diagnosis. Diskospondylitis should always be considered in an animal with fever of unknown origin. Neurologic deficits associated with a transverse myelopathy (T3-L3) occur most commonly and include paraparesis, decreased conscious proprioception, exaggerated spinal reflexes, and much less commonly, paraplegia. Cervical lesions most commonly cause only apparent cervical pain, and lumbosacral lesions may cause neurologic deficits due to compression of nerves of the cauda equina. Affected animals may have a normal or elevated peripheral white blood cell count. Infection may be difficult to distinguish from a healing fracture, unstable fracture, congenital malformation, or postoperative changes. Diskospondylitis usually can be distinguished from a neoplastic lesion, as neoplasms rarely cross intervertebral disk spaces.

Occasionally, clinical signs may occur before characteristic radiographic changes are evident. Well-positioned, good-quality radiographs, usually with the animal under general anesthesia, are required for diagnosis of early cases. Cerebrospinal fluid may be normal or may have an increased protein content or increased WBC count in cases in which diskospondylitis lesions cause extradural compression of spinal cord or result in meningitis and/or myelitis. Myelography is indicated in animals with neurologic deficits indicative of spinal cord compression and is mandatory in cases in which decompressive surgery is considered.

Efforts should be made to diagnose *B. canis* infection in all dogs with diskospondylitis. Surgical biopsy may be indicated in affected dogs in which a causative organism is not isolated from blood or urine, and/or animals that are unresponsive to treatment with broad-spectrum antibiotics.

Treatment. Treatment of diskospondylitis in animals without neurologic deficits, or with mild neurologic deficits, consists of long-term use of an antimicrobial that is effective against the causative organism(s) determined by results of blood and/or urine cultures. Antibiotics that are most effective for this purpose are cephalosporins, or β-lactamase resistant penicillins such as oxacillin and cloxacillin. Treatment is continued for at least 6 weeks, and vertebral radiographs are done every 2 to 3 weeks to monitor progression/regression of a lesion. Antibiotic administration may be necessary for up to 6 months before radiographic evidence of resolution of lesions is seen.

Lesions resulting from *B. canis* infection appear to be less severe and more slowly progressive than those caused by other bacterial diskospondylitides. A combination of minocycline or tetracycline and streptomycin is recommended for treatment of *B. canis* infections. Recrudescence of infection after cessation of antibiotic therapy occurs commonly although periodic antibiotic therapy may keep affected dogs free of clinical signs. Infected dogs should be neutered to eliminate risk of transmission. *B. canis* infections have public health significance, as people may become infected. Clinical improvement in animals with diskospondylitis should be seen within 2 weeks of starting antibiotic therapy.

Surgical exploration of a lesion should be considered in animals that are unresponsive to treatment or have persistent draining tracts suggestive of grass seed migration. Decompressive surgery is indicated if evidence of spinal cord compression is found on myelography and if animals show severe or progressive neurologic deficits.

DISTEMPER MYELITIS AND MYOCLONUS

Etiology and Pathogenesis.   See Chapter 82.

Clinical Findings.   Canine distemper myelitis may occur as a focal or a diffuse disease at any location in the spinal cord. The T3-L3 spinal cord segments are affected most often, and clinical signs indicative of a transverse myelopathy in this region are seen. Neurologic deficits are progressive and are bilateral; however, they may be asymmetric. Neurologic deficits commonly seen in dogs with CD infection are vestibular and/or cerebellar abnormalities and visual deficits. Chorioretinitis with retinal hyperreflectivity and "medallion" lesions may be present on ophthalmoscopic examination. Self-mutilation (limbs and tail) occasionally is seen in dogs with CD infection.

Diagnosis and Treatment.   See Chapter 82.

Distemper Myoclonus.   See Chapter 82.

DURAL OSSIFICATION

Etiology and Pathogenesis.   Dural ossification is the formation of bony plaques on the inner surface of the dura mater. Bony plaques are found most commonly in the cervical and lumbar spine and may occur laterally, ventrally, or dorsally. Dural ossification is found in over 40 per cent of large and small breeds of dog over 2 years of age, and in over 60 per cent of dogs 5 years of age or older.

Clinical Findings.   Dural ossification rarely results in neurologic deficits or apparent spinal pain in dogs.

Diagnosis.   Radiographically, bony plaques appear as thin radiopaque lines (linear shadows), which are most easily viewed at the site of intervertebral foramina.

Treatment.   There is no specific treatment for dural ossification; however, surgical removal of a bony plaque from the vicinity of a nerve root rarely may be necessary to alleviate apparent pain due to nerve root compression.

FELINE INFECTIOUS PERITONITIS, MENINGITIS, AND MYELITIS

Etiology and Pathogenesis.   See Chapter 82.

Clinical Findings.   With spinal cord involvement, the most commonly recognized neurologic signs are pelvic limb ataxia, hyperesthesia (especially over the back), and generalized ataxia.

Diagnosis and Treatment.   See Chapter 82.

FELINE POLIOENCEPHALOMYELITIS (FELINE NONSUPPURATIVE MENINGOENCEPHALOMYELITIS)

Etiology and Pathogenesis.   The chronic clinical course, distribution of lesions, and lack of inclusions distinguish this disease from rabies, pseudorabies, and FIP.

Clinical Findings.   Clinical signs include ataxia, paraparesis, tetraparesis, hypermetria, head tremors, and localized hyperesthesia. Spinal reflexes, pupillary light reflexes, and postural reactions may be normal or depressed. Clinical signs are slowly progressive over several months.

GLOBOID CELL LEUKODYSTROPHY (KRABBE TYPE LEUKODYSTROPHY)

Clinical Findings. See Table 82-10 in the textbook. Affected cats usually show abnormalities by 6 weeks of age. Progressive paraparesis and paraplegia predominate in some affected animals. Spinal reflexes in the pelvic limbs may be normal, exaggerated, or decreased. Clinical signs in cats with globoid cell leukodystrophy are generally more indicative of cerebellar disease and are more rapidly progressive than in dogs.

Diagnosis. Cerebrospinal fluid may contain phagocytic cells containing PAS-positive material (globoid cells), and CSF protein content may be increased. Brain and/or peripheral nerve biopsy may show characteristic demyelination and globoid cell accumulation.

GRANULOMATOUS MENINGOENCEPHALOMYELITIS (GME)

Etiology and Pathogenesis. See Chapter 82.

Clinical Findings. Granulomatous meningoencephalomyelitis may involve the spinal cord at any level; however, lesions appear to be most severe in the cervical spinal cord, and clinical findings are often indicative of cervical spinal cord disease. Findings include apparent cervical pain, rigidity, reluctance to move, hyperesthesia, cervical paraspinal muscle spasms, exaggerated spinal reflexes, decreased conscious proprioception, paraparesis, tetraparesis, or paraplegia.

Diagnosis. Noncontrast radiography and myelography may confirm an intramedullary space-occupying lesion of the spinal cord (Fig. 83–14 in textbook).

Treatment. See Chapter 82.

HEMORRHAGE

Etiology and Pathogenesis. Intramedullary, intrameningeal, or epidural hemorrhage may be due to coagulopathies including thrombocytopenia, clotting factor deficiencies, disseminated intravascular coagulation, and anticoagulant poisonings (warfarin and the like). Acute hemorrhage may also occur in association with tumors, vascular malformations, acute intervertebral disk protrusion, trauma, parasitic migration, or meningitis. Spontaneous intramedullary hemorrhage with hematoma formation has been reported in the cervical spinal cord of a dog. Spontaneous subperiosteal vertebral hemorrhage and hematoma formation associated with spinal cord compression and transverse myelopathy have been reported in dogs.

Clinical Findings. Observed neurologic deficits depend on the location of the hemorrhage and usually indicate a focal or multifocal myelopathy. Clinical signs most often are acute in onset and neurologic deficits may be severe. Epidural hemorrhage may result in spinal cord compression and transverse (focal) myelopathy. Subarachnoid hemorrhage may result in clinical signs suggestive of meningitis, including cervical rigidity, hyperesthesia, and increased body temperature.

Diagnosis. Diagnostic tests for coagulopathy include determination of prothrombin time, partial thromboplastin time, platelet count, activated clotting time, fibrinogen levels, and evaluation of specific clotting factor activity. Subarachnoid CSF puncture may be contraindicated in animals with a coagulopathy because of the high probability of inducing further hemorrhage. Red blood cells may be present in CSF for a short time following subarachnoid hemorrhage, and CSF supernatant may be red or pink in color. Xanthochromia may be present in CSF 48 hours or more after the hemorrhage has occurred. Epidural hemorrhage is not distinguishable from other extradural space-occupying lesions on myelography.

HEREDITARY ATAXIA (ATAXIA IN SMOOTH-HAIRED FOX TERRIERS AND JACK RUSSELL TERRIERS)

Etiology and Pathogenesis. An inherited, progressive, generalized ataxia has been reported to occur in young smooth-haired fox terriers in Sweden and Jack Russell terriers in England.

Clinical Findings. Neurologic abnormalities are first seen between 2 and 6 months of age and include pelvic limb ataxia and "swinging" of the hindquarters. Ataxia becomes progressively worse over 6 months to 2 years and involves all four limbs. Affected animals often have a "prancing" pelvic limb gait. Dysmetria may be severe, and affected dogs fall to the ground with slight change in position.

Diagnosis. Diagnosis is made on the basis of age, breed, and clinical findings.

Treatment. Treatment is not effective. Affected animals are eventually unable to walk.

HEREDITARY MYELOPATHY OF AFGHAN HOUNDS (NECROTIZING MYELOPATHY OR MYELOMALACIA OF AFGHAN HOUNDS)

Etiology and Pathogenesis. Hereditary myelopathy is a disease characterized by extensive spongiform degeneration of myelin with micro- and macrocavitation within the spinal cord white matter of young Afghan hounds. Typically, paresis and ataxia in pelvic limbs that progress to paraplegia within 10 to 14 days occur in affected dogs.

Clinical Findings. Clinical signs most commonly occur between 3 and 8 months of age. Pain perception initially is normal but, with progression of the disease, becomes impaired caudal to the cranial thoracic region. Neurologic deficits are indicative of a caudal cervical or cranial thoracic myelopathy.

Diagnosis. Diagnosis is made on the basis of age, breed of dog, and clinical signs and by ruling out other causes of rapidly progressive caudal cervical or cranial thoracic myelopathy in young dogs, including canine distemper myelitis and necrotizing vasculitis of the spinal meningeal arteries.

Treatment. Treatment has not been described; prognosis for affected animals is hopeless.

HOUND ATAXIA

Clinical Findings. Affected animals (male and female) were between 2 and 7 years of age. The clinical findings are indicative of a transverse myelopathy between T3 and L3 spinal cord segments. A gradual onset of ataxia in the pelvic limbs, paraparesis, and a "stilted" gait in the pelvic limbs (without evidence of pain) characterize this disease. In most affected animals, the panniculus reflex is absent bilaterally caudal to the midthoracic or cranial lumbar spinal cord segments. Affected hounds are usually severely debilitated within 6 to 18 months of the onset of clinical signs.

Diagnosis. Diagnosis is made on the basis of a compatible dietary history, age, breed of dog, and clinical findings and by ruling out other causes of progressive T3 to L3 myelopathy, including compressive lesions of the spinal cord (type II intervertebral disk protrusion, diskospondylitis, neoplasia) and intramedullary lesions such as neoplasia.

Treatment. Therapy has not been described.

HYPERVITAMINOSIS A OF CATS

Etiology and Pathogenesis. Hypervitaminosis A in cats is characterized by extensive confluent exostosis that is most prominent in the cervical and thoracic spine. It is caused by a chronic excess of dietary vitamin A and is usually a result of feeding a diet consisting largely of liver. Exostosis may extend to involve the entire spine, ribs, and pelvic and thoracic limbs with complete fusion of the spine and joints. Compression of spinal nerve roots or nerves may occur if new bone formation extends into intervertebral foramina.

Clinical Findings. Clinical signs in affected cats include apparent cervical pain and rigidity, thoracic limb lameness, ataxia, reluctance to move, paralysis, and hyperesthesia or anesthesia of the skin of the neck and forelimbs. The three most proximal diarthrodial joints of the cervical spine are almost always first affected. Osseous lesions develop insidiously, and clinical disease usually is advanced in cats older than 2 years of age before significant clinical features are recognized.

Diagnosis. Radiographic evidence of extensive exostosis of the cervical vertebral column and a history of excessive dietary intake of vitamin A or liver are necessary for diagnosis.

Treatment. Reduction of dietary intake of vitamin A prevents the development of further exostosis.

INTERVERTEBRAL DISK DISEASE

Etiology and Pathogenesis. Degeneration of intervertebral disks may result in protrusion or extrusion of disk material into the spinal canal, causing spinal cord compression and clinical signs ranging from apparent pain to complete transverse myelopathy. Degenerative changes may occur in any of the intervertebral disks (C2-3 to L7-S1); however, disk protrusion or extrusion occurs most commonly in the cervical, caudal thoracic, and lumbar spine. Type I disk herniation occurs with degeneration and rupture of the dorsal anulus fibrosus and extrusion of nucleus pulposus into the spinal canal. Type II disk protrusion is characterized by bulging of the intervertebral disk without complete rupture of the anulus fibrosus.

Chondroid metaplasia of the nucleus pulposus and type I disk extrusion occur most commonly in chondrodystrophoid breeds including dachshund, beagle, Pekingese, Lhasa apso, Shih Tzu, and breeds with chondrodystrophoid tendencies including miniature poodle and cocker spaniel. Fibroid disk degeneration (type II) occurs in older dogs of all breeds but is most often recognized as a clinical problem in older, large-breed, nonchondrodystrophoid dogs and is characterized by fibrous metaplasia of the nucleus pulposus.

Intervertebral disk protrusion or extrusion may occur in a ventral, dorsal, or lateral direction. In most instances, only dorsal protrusions or extrusions are of clinical significance as meningeal irritation and nerve root and/or spinal cord compression may occur. Occasionally a lateral disk protrusion or extrusion may result in nerve root or spinal nerve compression with associated clinical signs.

Type I disk extrusion often results in more severe clinical signs than type II protrusion, although the mechanical distortion and compression of the spinal cord caused by type II protrusion may be greater. Hemorrhage, edema, and necrosis of spinal cord gray and white matter are characteristic of acute spinal cord injury associated with acute type I disk extrusion. Degenerative disk disease also occurs in cats, although the incidence of clinical signs associated with disk protrusion is low. Degenerative changes and distribution of disk protrusions are similar to type II disk protrusions in nonchondrodystrophoid dogs.

Clinical Findings. Chondroid degeneration and type I disk extrusion most commonly occur in dogs 3 years of age and older. Fibroid degeneration and type II disk protrusion most commonly occur in dogs older than 5 years of age. Clinical signs seen in association with type I disk extrusion include apparent pain and/or motor and/or sensory deficits. These clinical signs usually develop rapidly, within minutes or hours of disk extrusion. Clinical signs associated with type I disk extrusion in the cervical spine usually are less severe than those associated with extrusions in the thoracolumbar region. Apparent neck pain is the most common clinical finding in dogs with cervical disk extrusion. Neurologic deficits indicative of a cervical myelopathy such as proprioceptive deficits, tetraparesis, or tetraplegia are seen less commonly. Thoracic limb lameness may also be seen in caudal cervical disk extrusions as a result of nerve root compression.

Clinical findings in animals with thoracolumbar type I disk extrusion depend on the severity of spinal cord injury and range from apparent back or abdominal pain to complete paraplegia and loss of deep pain perception. Neurologic deficits usually are indicative of a transverse myelopathy between T3 and L3, as most disk extrusions in this region occur between T11 and L3. Lower motor neuron signs may be seen in the pelvic limbs if disk extrusion occurs caudal to L3 as a result of compression of the lumbosacral spinal cord or nerves of the cauda equina. Lower motor neuron signs also may be seen in paraplegic animals with progressive hemorrhagic myelomalacia (PHM).

Clinical signs associated with type II disk protrusion generally are slowly progressive over a period of months. Paraparesis or tetraparesis, depending on the site of the lesion, is the most common clinical finding, and deficits may be asymmetric. Apparent neck or back pain may or may not be a feature of type II disk protrusion.

Diagnosis. Spinal radiographs and, in almost all cases, CSF analysis and myelography are necessary to confirm a diagnosis of disk extrusion or protrusion. Calcified material within the nucleus pulposus is indicative of disk degeneration, but alone is not of clinical significance.

The disk space of an extruded disk may be narrower than adjacent disk spaces and may be wedge-shaped with a decrease in the width of the disk space dorsally. However, positioning is important in evaluating some disk spaces (C7-T1, T9-10 or T10-11, and L7-S1). Calcified material may be present within the vertebral canal or in the area of the intervertebral foramina.

Type II disk protrusion may be associated with narrowing of the disk space, osteophyte production, and end-plate sclerosis. Calcification of disk material rarely is seen in association with type II disk protrusion. In some animals with type I or type II disk herniation obvious abnormalities are not seen on noncontrast vertebral radiographs.

Myelography is most important in determining the site (or sites) of disk herniation and in lateralization of disk material within the spinal canal prior to surgical decompression and is necessary for diagnosis in most cases of type II disk protrusion as a means of distinguishing disk protrusion from other causes of slowly progressive transverse myelopathy such as spinal neoplasia and degenerative myelopathy.

The characteristic myelographic findings in both type I and type II disk herniation into the spinal canal are extradural compression of the spinal cord with displacement of the spinal cord and narrowing of the subarachnoid space on lateral and/or ventrodorsal views, depending on the location of the compressive mass. With spinal cord edema and swelling, the spinal cord may be widened over several spinal cord segments and the myelographic appearance is similar to that of an intramedullary mass, making precise determination of the site of disk extrusion difficult. Rarely, in the cervical region, type I disk extrusion may occur laterally or intraforaminally, resulting in neck pain or thoracic limb pain due to nerve root compression. In such cases myelograms may be normal.

Treatment

Type I Disk Extrusion. Medical treatment directed at decreasing spinal cord edema by means of corticosteroids is indicated in all animals with an acute onset of neurologic deficits. Nonsurgical (medical or conservative) treatment is recommended for animals with apparent pain only or animals that have mild neurologic deficits but are ambulatory and have not had previous clinical signs associated with disk disease. These animals should be strictly confined to a small area such as a hospital cage or a quiet place away from other pets for at least 2 weeks and walked (on a leash or harness) only to urinate and defecate.

Use of analgesics, muscle relaxants, and anti-inflammatory drugs such as corticosteroids is not recommended in most cases as it is believed that their use encourages animals to exercise and risk further disk extrusion. Owners should also be warned that an animal's neurologic status may deteriorate owing to extrusion of further disk material despite this treatment and to observe the animal very carefully.

Animals with severe cervical pain frequently do not respond to cage rest. Dogs that do not show improvement after 7 to 10 days of confinement should be evaluated further by means of radiographs and possibly myelography, and ventral cervical decompression should be considered.

Fenestration does not prevent recurrence of disk extrusion in all animals. The effectiveness of fenestration depends largely on the amount of nucleus pulposus removed.

Animals with neurologic deficits such as paresis or paralysis with deep pain perception intact, animals with recurrent bouts of apparent back or neck pain, and animals with apparent back or neck pain (or mild neurologic deficits) that are unresponsive to strict confinement should be evaluated by means of spinal radiographs, CSF analysis, and myelography. Surgical decompression of the spinal cord and removal of disk material from the spinal canal should be considered. If the owner opts for surgery, surgical decompression should be done as soon as possible to prevent further spinal cord damage incurred as a result of sustained compression or further extrusion of disk material.

Prognosis for neurologic recovery in animals that retain deep pain perception postsurgically is fair to very good. Animals that have severe neurologic signs, a rapid onset of clinical signs (hours), and a long period of time before surgery generally have a prolonged recovery period and may have varying degrees of permanent neurologic deficit.

In animals with clinical signs of a complete transverse myelopathy, without deep pain perception for a period of more than 24 hours, the prognosis for return of spinal cord function is poor despite medical or surgical treatment. In cases in which deep pain perception has been absent for less than 24 hours, the prognosis for return of spinal cord function is guarded to poor; however, surgical treatment may increase the likelihood of neurologic improvement in this group.

Neurologic improvement may take weeks or months, and this requires owner cooperation and enthusiasm regarding care and physical therapy. Physical therapy should not be attempted in animals treated medically for at least the first 2 weeks following onset of signs, as further extrusion of disk material may occur.

Type II Disk Protrusion. Treatment with corticosteroids may result in neurologic improvement for variable periods of time in animals with type II disk protrusion. In the thoracolumbar spine, surgical removal of protruded disk material is generally impossible without causing further spinal cord damage. Surgical decompression without removal of protruded disk material may result in improvement; however, the neurologic status of some dogs is worsened permanently despite careful surgical technique. Ventral decompression in the cervical spine allows removal of protruded type II disk material and neurologic improvement may occur; however, some dogs, especially those with moderate to severe neurologic deficits prior to surgery, may manifest temporary or permanent worsening of clinical signs postoperatively.

Acupuncture. Acupuncture is an excellent adjunctive therapy in nonsurgical management of affected dogs. However, the use of acupuncture as an alternative to surgery for dogs that have severe spinal cord compression resulting from disk extrusion is not recommended at this time.

Chemonucleolysis.   This is not indicated in cases of type I disk extrusion, as the enzyme is unable to reach sequestered nucleus pulposus within the spinal canal. Chemonucleolysis has been used in the treatment of type II disk protrusion in the cervical spine of large breeds of dog. The majority of dogs in one study improved clinically despite persistence, or only slight decrease, in the degree of spinal cord compression on myelography.

ISCHEMIC MYELOPATHY DUE TO FIBROCARTILAGINOUS EMBOLISM

Etiology and Pathogenesis.   Ischemic myelopathy results from ischemic necrosis of spinal cord gray and white matter associated with fibrocartilaginous emboli that occlude arteries and/or veins of the leptomeninges and spinal cord parenchyma. This disease is characterized by an acute onset of neurologic deficits and is generally nonprogressive after several hours.

Clinical Findings.   Ischemic myelopathy most commonly occurs in large and giant breeds of dog, generally between 1 and 9 years of age. Apparent pain usually is not present at the time of examination or during the course of the disease, although dogs are often reported to "cry out" at the onset of clinical signs.

Neurologic deficits usually are bilateral and are often (but not always) asymmetric. Clinical signs seen depend on the location and extent of the spinal cord lesion. Many spinal cord segments may be involved (see Table 82–4 in the textbook). A Horner's syndrome may also be seen in severe lesions in the cervical spinal cord.

Diagnosis is made by ruling out other causes of myelopathy.

Treatment.   Corticosteroids (as recommended for spinal trauma) may be given initially to reduce any secondary spinal cord edema. Good nursing care is essential in recumbent animals to prevent pressure sores, urinary tract infections, and contracture of denervated muscles. Animals that retain pain perception in affected limbs and tail usually regain neurologic function, although recovery may take several weeks to months and LMN signs may persist (muscle atrophy and/or paresis). Many animals show improvement within 2 weeks of onset of signs, unless extensive gray matter destruction has occurred.

LEUKOENCEPHALOMYELOPATHY OF ROTTWEILER DOGS

See Chapter 82.

LUMBOSACRAL VERTEBRAL CANAL STENOSIS

Etiology and Pathogenesis.   Lumbosacral vertebral canal stenosis is a term that encompasses a spectrum of disorders that result in narrowing of the lumbosacral vertebral canal with resulting compression of the cauda equina. The term *cauda equina syndrome* describes a group of neurologic signs that result from compression, destruction, or displacement of those nerve roots and spinal nerves that form the cauda equina. We use the term *lumbosacral vertebral canal stenosis* to describe an acquired disorder of large breeds of dog that results from several or all of the following: type II disk protrusion (dorsal bulging of the anulus fibrosus), hypertrophy/hyperplasia of the interarcuate ligament, thickening of vertebral arches or articular facets, and (infrequently) subluxation/instability of the lumbosacral junction. Cauda equina syndrome may result from numerous causes other than lumbosacral vertebral canal stenosis.

Clinical Findings.   Acquired degenerative lumbosacral vertebral canal stenosis occurs most commonly in large-breed male (especially German shepherd) dogs. Dogs with the congenital ("idiopathic") form appear to be of the smaller breeds. Affected dogs in both categories are usually between 3 and 7 years of age. Signs of cauda equina compression seen frequently in affected dogs include the following: apparent pain on palpation of the lumbosacral region, on caudal extension of the pelvic limbs, or on elevation of the tail; difficulty rising; pelvic limb lameness (often unilateral); pelvic limb muscle atrophy; paresis of the tail; scuffing of the toes; urinary and/or fecal incontinence, or "inappropriate" voiding due to an inability to assume a voiding posture; self-mutilation of the perineum, tail, or pelvic limbs; and rarely, paraphimosis. These signs most often are insidious in onset and progress gradually over months, and they are easily confused with those of hip dysplasia or degenerative myelopathy.

Abnormalities detected on neurologic examination include gait deficits related to sciatic nerve paresis (e.g., dragging of toes). In addition, depression or loss of conscious proprioception, normal or slightly exaggerated patellar reflexes, depressed or absent flexion reflexes in pelvic limbs, decreased anal tone and anal sphincter reflexes, atonic bladder, hypesthesia of the perineum and tail, and muscle atrophy may be seen. These abnormalities relate to deficits of the sciatic, pudendal, caudal, and pelvic nerves, whose nerve roots comprise the cauda equina.

Diagnosis. Rarely can this condition be diagnosed on the basis of plain radiographic findings alone. Plain radiographic findings include spondylosis deformans ventral and lateral to the lumbosacral articulation, sclerosis of vertebral end-plates, "wedging" or narrowing of the L7-S1 disk space, secondary degenerative joint disease in the region of L7-S1 articular facets, ventral displacement of the sacrum with respect to L7 ("retrolisthesis"), and diminished dorsoventral dimensions of the lumbosacral spinal canal.

"Stressed" plain radiographic projections (flexed and extended views), completed with careful attention to avoid rotation, often assist in determining the presence of instability or "retrolisthesis." Electromyography may complement information available from a neurologic examination and from plain spinal radiographs by confirming denervation in muscles innervated by the nerves of the cauda equina. Contrast radiographic techniques are necessary for demonstration of soft tissue vertebral canal stenosis.

Treatment. Some affected dogs in which clinical signs are mild or in which apparent lumbosacral pain is the sole problem improve temporarily after strict confinement and restricted leash exercise for a period of 4 to 6 weeks. Use of analgesic drugs or corticosteroids has been recommended; however, their use must be accompanied by strict confinement.

Dogs with recurrence of signs, or dogs that are moderately to severely affected at the time of initial presentation (especially those with urinary/fecal incontinence), should be considered candidates for surgical therapy. Dorsal decompressive laminectomy of L7 and S1 vertebrae is recommended. Attention to bladder emptying may be necessary in dogs with bladder atony prior to surgery. Prognosis for affected dogs is dependent on the severity of signs prior to surgery. Dogs with bladder atony or a flaccid anal sphincter prior to surgery have the poorest prognosis.

MUCOPOLYSACCHARIDOSIS

Etiology and Pathogenesis. Mucopolysaccharidosis VI is the result of a deficiency of the lysosomal enzyme arylsulfatase B and, in addition to causing characteristic physical deformities, can result in skeletal changes, including fusion of the cervical vertebrae, variable fusion of thoracic and lumbar vertebrae, bony proliferation and bony protrusion into the vertebral canal in the thoracic and lumbar spine causing compression of the spinal cord, and bony proliferation in the intervertebral foramina causing nerve root compression. Mucopolysaccharidosis VI is an inherited abnormality of siamese cats and has an autosomal recessive mode of inheritance.

Mucopolysaccharidosis I due to a deficiency in α-L-iduronidase has been reported in a domestic shorthaired cat. The clinical features were similar to MPS VI, but bony proliferative changes and associated spinal cord compression were not found.

Clinical Findings.   The characteristic physical findings in cases of MPS VI are small head, flat broad face, widely spaced eyes, corneal clouding, small ears, depressed bridge of the nose, large forepaws, and concave deformity of the sternum. Neurologic deficits due to skeletal changes and spinal cord compression are seen between 4 and 7 months of age and progress over 2 to 4 weeks. Neurologic findings are indicative of a transverse myelopathy between T3 and L3. The thoracic limb gait may be normal or affected cats may have a crouching posture.

Diagnosis.   Radiographs of the spine show vertebral fusion and bony protrusions into the spinal canal and intervertebral foramina of the thoracolumbar spine. Myelography is necessary to demonstrate spinal cord compression. MPS VI can be confirmed by measurement of arylsulfatase B activity in leukocytes.

Treatment.   As skeletal changes are nonprogressive after about 9 months of age, decompressive surgery may result in improvement in neurologic signs.

MYELODYSPLASIA

Etiology and Pathogenesis.   Myelodysplasia is considered to be an inherited condition in the Weimaraner dog, transmitted by a mutant gene with some degree of dominance but reduced penetrance and variable expressivity. Myelodysplasia has been described in other breeds of dogs or cats, including a Dalmatian, a rottweiler, a West Highland white terrier, an English bulldog, mixed-breed dogs, and Manx cats.

Clinical Findings.   Clinical abnormalities usually are evident at 4 to 6 weeks of age, when puppies become ambulatory. The major clinical finding in affected dogs is a symmetric "bunny-hopping" pelvic limb gait. Other clinical findings are crouching stance, abduction or overextension of one or both pelvic limbs, decreased conscious proprioception in the pelvic limbs, scoliosis, and in one case, torticollis. In Weimaraner dogs, other findings include abnormal hair "streams" in the dorsal neck region, koilosternia (gutter-like depression in the chest), and occasionally, a head tilt. Myelodysplasia of Weimaraner dogs is a nonprogressive condition.

Diagnosis.   Diagnosis is made on the basis of history, signalment, clinical signs, plain radiography, CSF analysis, and myelography. Advanced imaging techniques such as CT have also been used.

Treatment.   There is no effective treatment.

NECROTIZING VASCULITIS

Etiology and Pathogenesis.   Necrotizing vasculitis of the extradural and intradural spinal meningeal arteries has been reported to occur in young dogs of several breeds, including Bernese mountain dogs, German shorthaired pointers, and beagle dogs.

Clinical Findings.   Affected dogs usually are 4 to 12 months of age. Clinical signs include fever, anorexia, cervical rigidity, hunched posture, apparent spinal pain, shifting lameness, apparent pain on opening the mouth, and, in some animals, neurologic deficits, including paraparesis, tetraparesis, and paraplegia.

Diagnosis.   Cerebrospinal fluid generally has a marked pleocytosis (may be greater than 10,000 WBC/μl) with predominantly mature nontoxic neutrophils present. Cerebrospinal fluid protein concentration also is elevated. This disease often cannot be distinguished from other meningitides (including viral, bacterial, or fungal meningitis; GME; or corticosteroid responsive meningitis) on the basis of clinical and CSF findings.

Treatment.   Treatment with corticosteroids usually results in a rapid improvement in clinical signs. However, relapses commonly occur when treatment is discontinued. Treatment for longer than 6 months may result in permanent resolution of clinical signs.

NEOPLASIA

Etiology and Pathogenesis.   Retrospective studies have shown the most commonly occurring spinal tumors in dogs to be primary and secondary bone tumors, and tumors of spinal nerves and nerve roots. Primary intramedullary tumors occur less commonly than extradural or intradural-extramedullary tumors. Spinal tumors of all types occur more frequently in large breeds of dog. Epidural lymphosarcoma is the most commonly occurring spinal tumor in cats. Although tumors more commonly occur in animals more than 5 years of age, spinal cord blastoma (nephroblastoma) in dogs and lymphosarcoma in cats are found most commonly in young animals.

Clinical Findings.   See Table 82–5 in the textbook. Clinical signs depend on the location of the tumor. Most animals present with clinical signs referable to a transverse myelopathy, and progressive neurologic deficits usually result. Tumors of nerves of the brachial plexus initially cause progressive LMN signs in the ipsilateral thoracic limb, including muscle atrophy and paresis. The affected limb is often painful on palpation or movement; cutaneous sensation generally remains intact. Apparent pain is a common finding associated with extradural and intradural tumors, and was the predominant clinical sign in a study of dogs with vertebral tumors. Intramedullary tumors are reported to cause a more rapid progression of clinical signs and are much less likely to be painful than extradural or intradural-extramedullary tumors.

Diagnosis.   A tentative diagnosis of spinal tumor can be made on the basis of radiographic, CSF, and myelographic findings. Definitive diagnosis can only be made after biopsy of a suspected lesion.

Radiography.   Bone lysis with a cortical "break" is the most common radiographic finding in animals with vertebral tumors. Other radiographic findings include destruction of vertebral end-plates, collapse of an adjacent disk space, collapse and shortening of a vertebral body, pathologic fracture, bone sclerosis and bony production, cyst-like expansile lesions, or adjacent soft tissue masses. Bone tumors most commonly occur in the vertebral body but may also be found in the dorsal spinous processes, transverse processes, and articular facets. Primary bone tumors usually involve one vertebra but may involve multiple vertebrae. Rarely, metastatic tumors (e.g., carcinoma) may arise within a disk space. Metastases from intrapelvic soft tissue tumors often produce periosteal new bone on the ventral aspect of multiple lumbar vertebral bodies in association with paravertebral soft tissue mass formation. Vertebral lesions of multiple myeloma are characterized by "punched out" lytic lesions. Expanding tumors may result in widening of the vertebral canal or widening of intervertebral foramina.

Cerebrospinal Fluid Analysis.   Cerebrospinal fluid may be normal or may have an increased protein concentration and/or white blood cell count. Tumor cells rarely are found in CSF, except in CSF from animals with lymphosarcoma.

Myelography.   It is important to obtain survey radiographs of the entire vertebral column prior to and after injection of contrast, as more than one tumor may be present and the neurologic deficits of one tumor may "mask" those produced by another. Tumors may have a mixed myelographic appearance, with extradural, intradural, and/or intramedullary components (e.g., nerve root tumors, meningioma, and spinal cord blastoma). Other mass lesions resulting in spinal cord compression, intramedullary swelling, and intradural lesions must be considered in the differential diagnosis of spinal tumors. Such mass lesions include intervertebral disk protrusion, epidural abscess or granuloma formation, spinal cord edema associated with spinal cord trauma, vascular malformation, or subarachnoid cyst.

Other Diagnostic Tests. As many spinal tumors are secondary tumors and primary vertebral tumors commonly metastasize, careful attention should be directed toward eliminating the presence of other tumors by performing a thorough physical examination, survey thoracic and abdominal radiographic examinations, rectal examination, complete blood count, and other diagnostic tests as necessary. Both CT and MRI aid in exact determination of location and extent of spinal tumors.

Treatment. The majority of vertebral tumors are not surgically resectable, owing to the malignant characteristics of the tumor and the decreased stability of the vertebral column that may result from extensive surgery. Surgical decompression of the spinal cord and debulking of tumor mass may be palliative in some cases. Some tumors within the spinal canal are surgically resectable, including some tumors that appear intramedullary on myelography, such as spinal cord blastoma.

Corticosteroids may decrease spinal cord edema associated with spinal cord tumors and result in clinical improvement for a variable period of time. Radiation therapy and chemotherapy may be helpful in animals with spinal lymphosarcoma. Several chemotherapeutic agents, including methotrexate and cytosine arabinoside, may be given intrathecally and have been used in the treatment of meningeal lymphosarcoma and leukemic meningitis. Chemotherapy may be helpful in the treatment of plasma cell myeloma. In general, the prognosis for animals with nonresectable spinal tumors is poor.

NEUROAXONAL DYSTROPHY OF ROTTWEILER DOGS

See Chapter 82.

OSTEOCHONDROMATOSIS (MULTIPLE CARTILAGINOUS EXOSTOSES)

Etiology and Pathogenesis. Feline osteochondromatosis is characterized by an initial appearance of lesions in the skeleton of mature cats (2 to 4 years of age). Growth of the lesions is progressive. Malignant transformation to osteosarcoma has been reported to occur in an osteochondroma of a cervical vertebra in a cat.

The disease is frequently demonstrated in the skeleton of dogs radiographed for unrelated reasons. Onset of clinical disease is usually in dogs less than 18 months of age. Continued growth or reactivation of growth of exostoses in dogs is suggestive of neoplastic transformation.

Clinical Signs. Osteochondromatosis may occur anywhere in the vertebral column but most commonly is found in the thoracic and lumbar spine. The disease may result in spinal cord compression and clinical signs indicative of a progressive transverse myelopathy between T3 and L3.

Diagnosis. Radiographically, vertebral lesions tend to be circular and smooth, with sclerotic borders. Lesions are usually multiple and may be cystic or proliferative, with an increased radiodensity. Myelography is necessary to demonstrate associated spinal cord compression. Surgical biopsy is necessary to differentiate osteochondromatosis from benign bone tumors (osteomas), neoplastic lesions, or infectious processes.

Treatment. Treatment of canine osteochondromatosis affecting the vertebral column is unnecessary unless a lesion results in clinical sequelae or impinges on the spinal cord, or if malignant transformation is suspected. The prognosis for dogs that have stopped growing is good; however, the prognosis for animals that are still growing is guarded, as lesions may continue to expand and subsequently result in spinal cord compression.

Treatment of feline osteochondromatosis is complicated by the association with FeLV and the progressive nature of lesions in cats. It seems that at best the surgical removal of a lesion may provide only temporary relief to a cat because of the tendency for excised lesions to recur and for new lesions to develop.

PILONIDAL SINUS, EPIDERMOID CYST, AND DERMOID CYST (DERMOID SINUS, PILONIDAL CYST)

Etiology and Pathogenesis. A pilonidal sinus is an invagination of the skin dorsal to the spine, extending below the skin to variable depths and in some cases as far as the dura mater, where it may communicate with the subarachnoid space. Pilonidal sinuses may occur anywhere along the dorsal midline from cervical to sacrocaudal regions and may be single or multiple. Dermoid cysts have been reported to occur in the brain and spinal cord of dogs or cats. Epidermoid cysts have been reported to occur rarely in the brain and spinal cord of dogs.

Clinical Signs. Clinical signs of meningitis and myelitis may be seen in animals as a result of extension of infection from a pilonidal sinus to the subarachnoid space. Neurologic signs resulting from a spinal dermoid or epidermoid cyst depend on its location.

Diagnosis. A pilonidal sinus may be palpable as a cord of fibrous tissue under the skin of the dorsal midline. Fistulography performed by injecting a radiographic contrast material such as metrizamide, which is not an irritant to nervous tissue, into the sinus demonstrates whether pilonidal sinuses are continuous with the subarachnoid space. Typically an epidermoid cyst should be suspected in the presence of an intramedullary, expansile lesion on myelography in a young dog with progressive neurologic deficits. Diagnosis is confirmed by means of an open surgical biopsy, which may provide the only means to rule out spinal neoplasia (e.g., spinal cord blastoma).

Treatment. Animals with meningitis and/or myelitis associated with a pilonidal sinus should be treated in the same way as an animal with meningitis and myelitis due to another cause. Complete surgical excision of the pilonidal sinus is essential. Treatment of spinal dermoid or epidermoid cysts of dogs has not been reported.

PROGRESSIVE HEMORRHAGIC MYELOMALACIA

Etiology and Pathogenesis. Acute, severe spinal cord injury may result in progressive ascending and descending infarction and hemorrhagic necrosis of the spinal cord parenchyma. Progressive hemorrhagic myelomalacia (PHM) occurs infrequently; it usually follows peracute explosive extrusion of a thoracolumbar disk but may also be seen in animals after spinal cord trauma.

Clinical Signs. Clinical signs depend on the location of the lesion; however, most affected animals initially have clinical signs indicative of a transverse myelopathy between T3 and L3, with UMN signs in the pelvic limbs. Clinical signs indicating a diffuse myelopathy progress over a period of hours to 1 to 2 days. Affected animals often are in extreme pain, are anxious, and show an increased body temperature.

Treatment. Progressive hemorrhagic myelomalacia is in most cases fatal within 24 to 48 hours due to respiratory paralysis. Effective medical or surgical treatments do not exist, and euthanasia is recommended.

PROTOZOAL MYELITIS

See textbook.

Clinical Findings. In dogs less than one year of age, a syndrome of progressive paralysis and rigid extension of one or both pelvic limbs may be seen in association with *Toxoplasma gondii* infection. Muscle atrophy and contracture of affected limbs is seen, and limbs cannot be flexed. Neosporosis causes severe disease in young, congenitally infected pups. Young dogs develop an ascending paralysis, with pelvic limbs affected more severely than thoracic limbs. Other signs of dysfunction include difficulty in swallowing, paralysis of the jaw, muscle flaccidity, and muscle atrophy.

Diagnosis. Antemortem confirmation of CNS toxoplasmosis in dogs or cats is extremely difficult. Cerebrospinal fluid may be normal, or it may have an elevated white blood cell count with a mixed mononuclear pleocytosis and an elevated protein concentration. *Toxoplasma* organisms may be identified in cytologic preparations of thoracic or peritoneal effusions, in biopsies of lymph node or muscle examined by conventional histopathologic techniques, or by other methods such as immunoperoxidase staining.

Serologic testing for antibody (immunoglobulin G or IgG) is of limited use for determining active infection, unless paired titers done 2 to 3 weeks apart demonstrate a fourfold increase. Currently it is recommended that for serologic diagnosis of toxoplasmosis in dogs or cats a single serum sample should be submitted for immunoglobulins G and M (IgG and IgM) determinations, and for calculation of levels of circulating antigen for *T. gondii.* Smears of CSF, bronchial lavage fluid, or dermal lesions may be examined for *Neospora tachyzoites.* The detection of antibodies to *Neospora caninum* in serum may aid in diagnosis.

Treatment. Available drugs are effective in CNS tissues only against actively proliferating forms of the organism and are not active against encysted forms, which are dependent on host humoral and cell-mediated immune responses for eradication. The effectiveness of clindamycin in penetrating CNS tissues of dogs or cats has not been determined, and it is therefore recommended that sulfadiazine or triple-sulfas be given orally at a daily dosage of 50 mg/lb divided q12h for CNS toxoplasmosis. Addition of pyrimethamine permits reduction of the sulfadiazine dosage by half. The public health risk posed by a cat with active *T. gondii* infection must be considered.

PYOGRANULOMATOUS MENINGOENCEPHALOMYELITIS

Etiology and Pathogenesis. Pyogranulomatous meningoencephalomyelitis is an acute, rapidly progressive disease that has been described in mature pointers. Pathologic changes are most severe in the cranial cervical spinal cord and caudal brain stem.

Clinical Findings. Clinical signs are indicative of meningitis and cervical myelopathy, and include cervical rigidity, kyphosis, nose held to the ground, reluctance to move, incoordinated hypermetric gait, and atrophy of cervical muscles. Other reported abnormalities are bradycardia, vomiting, trigeminal and facial nerve paralysis, and Horner's syndrome. Clinical signs are rapidly progressive over 2 to 3 weeks.

Diagnosis. There is an increased CSF white blood cell count (500 to 1000 cells/μl) with predominance of polymorphonuclear cells. Protein concentration is also increased in CSF, and may be greater than 700 mg/ml.

Treatment. Temporary remission of clinical signs may occur with antibiotic therapy; however, prognosis for recovery is poor.

SACROCAUDAL DYSGENESIS IN MANX CATS

Etiology and Pathogenesis. Sacrocaudal dysgenesis and associated malformations have been recognized in most breeds of cats.

Clinical Findings. Clinical signs are variable, depending on the degree of spinal cord and cauda equina malformation, and include paraparesis, paraplegia, megacolon, atonic bladder, absent anal and urinary bladder sphincter tone, absent anal reflex, urinary and fecal incontinence, and perineal analgesia. Affected cats often walk plantigrade in the pelvic limbs with a "bunny-hopping" gait. Vertebral abnormalities may be palpable in the lumbosacral region, and in some cats a meningocele, congenital or the result of necrosis of the overlying skin, may exit through the skin and drain CSF.

Clinical signs usually are evident soon after birth and may remain static or may be progressive. Worsening of neurologic deficits may be due to progressive syringomyelia in the lumbar and sacral spinal cord.

Diagnosis. Diagnosis is made on the basis of clinical findings and radiographic findings indicative of dysgenesis or agenesis of the sacral and caudal vertebrae. Clinical findings are the most important factors to consider in determining prognosis.

Treatment. Prognosis for severely affected cats is hopeless, and treatment is not available. Many tailless cats do not have neurologic deficits, and sacral and caudal deformities often are an incidental radiographic finding.

SPINA BIFIDA

Etiology and Pathogenesis. *Spina bifida* is a term used to describe a group of developmental defects characterized by failure of fusion of the vertebral arches with or without protrusion or dysplasia of the spinal cord, meninges, or both. It has been described in both dogs and cats. Myelodysplasia consisting of hydromyelia, syringomyelia, anomalies of the dorsal septum, anomalies of the central gray matter, abnormal position of the central gray matter, anomalies of the dorsal and ventral horns, and myeloschisis (cleft in the dorsal part of the spinal cord) may occur in association with spina bifida. The most severe defects involve myelorachischisis with superficial location of the neuroectoderm that is continuous with the skin.

Clinical Findings. Spina bifida is usually an incidental radiographic finding; however, if associated with spinal cord malformations, it may result in clinical signs of spinal cord or cauda equina dysfunction. Spina bifida may occur anywhere in the spinal column but occurs most commonly in the caudal lumbar spine, where clinical signs are indicative of a transverse myelopathy from L4 to S3 spinal cord segments. Clinical signs usually become evident when affected animals start to walk.

Diagnosis. Absence of the vertebral arch or failure of fusion of the dorsal spinous processes in one or more vertebrae may be evident on plain radiographs.

Treatment. Treatment is not effective for affected animals with clinical signs of spinal cord malformation. Meningocele may be amenable to surgery if neurologic abnormalities are not evident. Treatment is not necessary for animals with vertebral defects in the absence of spinal cord dysfunction (spina bifida occulta).

SPINAL ARACHNOID CYSTS (MENINGEAL, LEPTOMENINGEAL CYSTS)

Clinical Findings. In reported cases a single arachnoid cyst was found in either the cranial cervical or caudal thoracic spinal canal, and neurologic deficits were indicative of a progressive transverse myelopathy in either the C1-C5 or T3-L3 spinal cord region.

Diagnosis. Plain radiographs of the spine may be normal or may show enlargement of the vertebral canal with smooth cortical margins, presumably as a result of pressure atrophy of bone overlying the cyst. Pooling of contrast material within the subarachnoid space, resulting in widening of the subarachnoid space and spinal cord compression, is seen on myelography. In all reported cases, lesions have been intradural-extramedullary and located on the dorsal midline.

Treatment. Surgical exploration is necessary to confirm a diagnosis of subarachnoid cyst and to decompress the spinal cord.

SPINAL NEMATODIASIS

Clinical Findings. Clinical signs depend on location of the lesions. Lesions may be focal or multifocal. Spinal nematodiasis usually is seen in immature animals, with the exception of *Dirofilaria immitis*. Clinical signs often have an acute onset and usually are progressive.

Diagnosis. Definite diagnosis is difficult antemortem, as it requires isolation or demonstration of the parasite within the CNS. An increase in white blood cell count, especially eosinophils, and/or protein may be present in the CSF. Lesions may be located by means of myelography.

Treatment. Medical therapy often is ineffective in eliminating parasites in the CNS.

SPINAL CORD TRAUMA

Etiology and Pathogenesis. Acute spinal cord injuries of dogs or cats result most commonly from direct physical trauma such as missile injury or vertebral fracture or luxation. Also, spinal cord trauma is the underlying cause of neurologic signs in numerous myelopathies (e.g., intervertebral disk protrusion or extrusion). Chronic spinal cord compression usually is seen in association with chronic progressive diseases such as neoplasia or type II disk protrusion.

The severity of a spinal cord injury, as determined by the eventual degree and quality of recovery, is related to three factors: the velocity with which the compressive force is applied, the degree of compression (transverse deformation), and the duration of the compression. An understanding of differences between acute and chronic spinal cord injury is essential for effective management and determination of prognosis in cats or dogs with spinal trauma.

Chronic Spinal Cord Compression. In contrast to acute spinal cord injury, chronic compression affects white matter more severely than it affects gray matter. Hemorrhage and edema, the major findings of acute trauma, are not significant in chronic compression.

Clinical Findings

Acute Spinal Cord Injury. Dogs or cats with a spinal injury frequently have serious injuries to other organ systems. A neurologic examination should be done with care to prevent further injury resulting from excessive movement of a vertebral instability.

Recognition of the Schiff-Sherrington sign is important. Following trauma, this sign must be differentiated from other postures associated with cranial injury (e.g., decerebrate rigidity or decerebellate posture). Both deep and cutaneous pain perception should be assessed, as results of these tests are important in determining prognosis.

Chronic Spinal Cord Compression. Clinical signs of chronic spinal cord compression may progress over weeks or months, or may be seen to occur acutely. Acute onset of neurologic signs with chronic spinal cord compression frequently is seen in association with such disorders as spinal neoplasia or type II disk protrusion. Sudden onset of signs may accompany pathologic fracture of a vertebra and spinal cord hemorrhage or infarction.

Diagnosis

Acute Spinal Cord Injury. The objectives of radiographic examination of an animal following acute spinal trauma are the following: precise determination of location and extent of a lesion, demonstration of multiple lesions that may not be apparent on the basis of a neurologic examination, and assessment of the need for surgical therapy and determination of the most appropriate surgical procedure to be used. We recommend that a myelogram be completed in animals that have sustained spinal trauma (and likewise for *chronic spinal cord compression.*)

Treatment.

Acute Spinal Cord Injury. Treatment of acute spinal cord trauma should always be instituted as soon as possible following injury. The specific objectives of therapy are the following: relief of edema, control of intra- or extramedullary hemorrhage, relief of spinal cord compression, and, in cases of vertebral fracture/luxation, removal of bone fragments from the spinal canal and stabilization of the vertebral column. Treatment of acute spinal cord trauma may be medical, surgical, or a combination of both. The use of low or high doses of corticosteroids in the treatment of spinal trauma has yielded conflicting results.

Indications for surgery following spinal cord injury are the following: moderate to severe paresis, or paralysis, associated with myelographic evidence of spinal cord compression; progressive worsening of neurologic signs despite adequate medical therapy; and luxation or fracture of the vertebral column, in association with distraction, malalignment, instability, or myelographic evidence of spinal cord compression. Any animal with sustained compression of the spinal cord following injury, regardless of the cause, must be considered a candidate for surgical decompression of the spinal cord.

Prognosis for an animal with an acute spinal cord injury depends on numerous factors; however, results of a neurologic examination should be the main determinant. Following a severe spinal injury, an animal may require many months to recover, and residual neurologic deficits may persist.

Chronic Spinal Cord Compression. Occasionally, animals may be maintained for months or years by means of corticosteroid therapy alone. Surgical decompression of the spinal cord should be approached with caution in animals with chronic spinal cord compression. Pathologic alterations within the spinal cord may be irreversible, in which case the most that may be achieved is to arrest progression of neurologic deficits. Neurologic status may be worsened by surgical decompression, even with meticulous surgical technique. However, surgical decompression should be considered in most animals that have neurologic deficits associated with chronic spinal cord compression.

SPINAL STENOSIS

Etiology and Pathogenesis. *Spinal stenosis* is a term indicating a narrowed vertebral canal, which may produce a variety of neurologic syndromes. Stenosis may be focal, segmental (affecting several adjacent vertebrae), or generalized (throughout the vertebral column). Spinal stenosis may result either from bony impingement on neural elements or from compression of neural tissue by nonosseous components of the walls of the vertebral canal.

Congenital Spinal Stenosis. Congenital stenosis may occur as a primary lesion or may be seen in association with other congenital anomalies of the spinal cord or vertebral column (such as block vertebrae, hemivertebrae, or transitional vertebrae). Despite the congenital origin of this stenosis, initial manifestation of clinical signs may not be seen until after an animal reaches skeletal maturity.

Thoracic Vertebral Canal Stenosis of Doberman Pinscher Dogs. Vertebrae T3 through T7 are affected most frequently. A decrease in the dorsoventral diameter of the vertebral canal (as compared with adjacent vertebrae) is seen, although spinal cord compression is seen infrequently.

Developmental Stenosis Resulting from Inborn Errors in Skeletal Growth. These conditions result in generalized spinal stenosis, which is more pronounced in the lumbar vertebral column. As with congenital stenosis, clinical signs may not develop until later in life and may be related to only a single level of the stenotic vertebral canal.

Idiopathic Developmental Stenosis. Clinical signs of spinal stenosis may result should some additional factor (e.g., disk protrusion) compromise the available diameter of the spinal canal in adult life.

Hypertrophy of the Nonosseous Components of the Vertebral Canal.

Spinal stenosis resulting from ligamentous proliferation at C2-C3 has been reported in young rottweiler dogs.

Clinical Findings.   Clinical signs of spinal stenosis reflect the location of the lesion, regardless of the precise cause.

Diagnosis.   Myelography is essential for precise localization.

Treatment.   This may be either medical or surgical.

SPONDYLOSIS DEFORMANS

Etiology and Pathogenesis.   Spondylosis deformans is characterized by the formation of osteophytes (bony spurs) around the margins of vertebral end-plates. Osteophytes may form at one or multiple intervertebral disk spaces and may appear to bridge or almost bridge intervertebral disk spaces. Osteophyte production in spondylosis deformans is the noninflammatory bony response to degenerative changes in the intervertebral disks. The incidence and size of vertebral osteophytes increases with age. All breeds of dog are affected. The caudal thoracic, lumbar, and lumbosacral spinal segments are affected most frequently.

Clinical Findings.   In most affected animals, spondylosis deformans is not of clinical significance. Rarely, bony spurs may project into the spinal canal or intervertebral foramina, resulting in compression of spinal cord or spinal nerves. Localized pain or lameness is reported to occur in animals with fracture of vertebral osteophytes.

Diagnosis.   A diagnosis of spondylosis deformans is based on results of radiographs of the spine. Myelography is necessary to determine whether disk protrusion or dorsal vertebral osteophyte formation is causing spinal cord compression.

Treatment.   If spinal cord compression or nerve root entrapment is indicated on a myelogram of an animal with neurologic deficits, surgical decompression may result in clinical improvement. Removal of dorsally projecting osteophytes should not be attempted. In most animals, spondylosis deformans is not of clinical significance and treatment is not necessary.

SYRINGOMYELIA AND HYDROMYELIA

Etiology and Pathogenesis.   A distinction cannot be made clinically between syringomyelia (cavitation of the spinal cord) and hydromyelia (dilation of the central canal). Syringomyelia may be associated with spinal cord tumors, myelitis, meningitis, and spinal cord trauma. Hydromyelia with or without syringomyelia may be associated with congenital malformations such as myelodysplasia; meningomyelocele or hydrocephalus; or lesions resulting in obstruction of CSF flow into the spinal subarachnoid space at the foramen magnum such as chronic arachnoiditis, trauma, congenital malformations, and vascular malformations; or it may be idiopathic.

Clinical Findings.   Clinical signs depend on the location of the lesion and whether or not other spinal cord lesions are present. Clinical findings include progressive spinal deformity (scoliosis, torticollis) LMN or UMN signs, depending on location, and apparent spinal pain. Clinical signs may be acute or may be progressive over weeks to several years.

Diagnosis.   Cisternal puncture for the collection of CSF is contraindicated in these animals owing to likely inadvertent puncture of the spinal cord. Computed tomography of the spinal cord may be useful in the diagnosis of cavitary lesions of the spinal cord.

Treatment.   Treatment in dogs has not been reported.

VASCULAR MALFORMATIONS AND BENIGN VASCULAR TUMORS

Clinical Findings.   Arteriovenous malformations and vascular tumors may occur anywhere in the spinal canal, and clinical signs usually reflect a progressive transverse myelopathy. An acute onset or sudden worsening of clinical signs may occur as a result of hemorrhage or thrombosis associated with abnormal vasculature of the malformation or tumor.

Diagnosis. Cerebrospinal fluid may be normal or may have an elevated protein concentration. Cerebrospinal fluid may be xanthochromic, and the white blood cell count may be mildly elevated if subarachnoid hemorrhage has occurred or a meningeal inflammatory response is associated with tumor growth. Myelography may show evidence of an intradural or intramedullary mass. Surgical biopsy is necessary to identify these lesions.

Treatment. Surgical removal of a vascular malformation or vascular tumor may be possible.

CHAPTER 84

NEURO-OPHTHALMOLOGY
(pages 696–701)

One of the most reliable indicators of a cerebral lesion is a loss of vision with preservation of pupillary light responses. While watching the dog walk, without and then with obstacles, a visual deficit may be apparent.

MENACE RESPONSE (pp. 696–697)

The menace response is elicited by making a threatening gesture with the hand at each eye while the other hand covers the opposite eye. If the other eye is not covered, an alert animal may be blind in the eye being tested but pick up the threat with its normal eye and respond by blinking bilaterally. It is crucial to the validity of this test that the threatening hand not touch the patient or create enough air currents to be felt by the patient. This response may not become fully developed until 10 to 12 weeks of age in some small animals.

A loss of menace response on one side is a reliable indicator of a lesion in the opposite central visual pathway even though there are still intact optic nerve axons projecting ipsilaterally. Serious cerebellar lesions prevent the menace response but do not interfere with visual perception. Animals with such lesions always have significant signs of cerebellar ataxia. A unilateral cerebellar lesion causes an ipsilateral menace deficit.

If the menace response does not occur, the clinician should first check the facial nerve innervation of the orbicularis oculi by touching the eyelids to see that they close the fissure normally. If a facial paralysis exists, then observe for head or eyeball retraction when that eye is threatened. If there is no facial paralysis and no menace response occurs, lightly strike the animal two to three times with the threatening hand and then repeat the threat without touching the patient. With all young animals who may not yet have learned this response and occasionally with stoic, older animals, the clinician can assess their vision

---

Original chapter written by Alexander de Lahunta

by rolling a roll of tape by them on the floor from different directions or dropping cotton balls in front of them. The visual placing postural reaction test also tests their vision.

PUPILLARY LIGHT REFLEX (pp. 697–698)

The size and response of pupils to light should be assessed following the menace test. It is important to evaluate the size of the pupils in normal room light before stimulating the retina with a strong accessory light source. Animals with extensive retinal or optic nerve disease (optic neuritis, progressive retinal degeneration) can be functionally blind, and yet the pupils may still respond to a bright light. The clinician who is unaware of this fact may direct a strong light source into the fundus of a blind dog, observe a pupillary response, and erroneously diagnose a lesion in the central visual pathway in the brain. Although blind with pupils that respond to a bright light source, these animals have pupils that are dilated more than normal in room light.

Remember that it takes a serious lesion of the afferent side of this reflex to cause an abnormality. It would be rare for this reflex to be abnormal in an animal with an afferent lesion that was not blind in that eye. As a rule, afferent lesions that interrupt this reflex occur in the eyeball, optic nerve, or optic chiasm.

Animals with unilateral lesions in the retina or optic nerve have no menace response in that eye. Frequently there is no asymmetry of pupil size, or the pupil in that eye is slightly larger. Light directed into the affected eye causes no response in either eye. Light directed into the unaffected eye elicits a bilateral response. Further confirmation of a unilateral lesion is made by covering the normal eye and observing further dilation of the pupil in the affected eye.

A lesion of the efferent pathway in the parasympathetic component of the oculomotor nerve causes a widely dilated pupil in the ipsilateral eye at rest. The menace response is normal in each eye. Light directed into either eye only causes constriction of the pupil in the eye on the side opposite the lesion.

A retrobulbar or intracranial lesion that affects both the optic nerve and the parasympathetic part of the oculomotor nerve on the same side causes a widely dilated pupil in the ipsilateral eye at rest. There is no menace response from this affected eye. Light directed into the affected eye elicits no response in either eye. Light directed into the unaffected eye causes pupillary constriction only in that eye.

PUPIL SIZE (pp. 698–699)

The influence of lesions in the eyeball, optic nerve, and oculomotor nerve has been considered. The one remaining neurologic component that can influence the size of the pupil is the sympathetic innervation of the iris smooth muscle that dilates the pupil. A defect in the sympathetic innervation of the structures of the head is referred to as Horner's syndrome; anisocoria results from the loss of innervation of the dilator of the pupil, producing miosis on the affected side. Due to loss of tone in smooth muscle normally maintained by sympathetic innervation, there is also a protrusion of the third eyelid and slight narrowing of the palpebral fissure (ptosis). Enophthalmos results from loss of tone in the periorbital smooth muscle, but distinguishing this feature from the other eyelid changes is both difficult and unimportant.

Lesions involving the LMN are the most common causes of Horner's syndrome. Severe cervical spinal cord lesions that interrupt the upper motor neuron can also cause Horner's syndrome. Such a bilateral lesion is life threatening due to its simultaneous interference with the upper motor neuron that controls respiration. Acute unilateral lesions such as an intervertebral disc extrusion on one side or infarction from fibrocartilaginous emboli cause hemiplegia and an ipsilateral Horner's syndrome. There are many lesions that can interfere with the lower motor neuron sympathetic innervation of the head. Examples are given in Table 84–1. A rare observation is a mildly dilated, slowly responsive pupil that occurs in animals with severe cerebellar disease that affects the cerebellar nuclei.

Evaluation of the size of the pupils is important in assessing the location and extent of brain damage from intracranial injury and following the response to therapy. Brain stem contusion interrupts the parenchymal components of the oculomotor neurons, causing bilateral, widely dilated, unresponsive pupils, which is a grave sign. Injuries that predominantly involve the prosencephalon often result in extremely miotic pupils, a condition that is assumed to represent a release of the parasympathetic oculomotor neurons from upper motor neuron inhibition. These can change rapidly to dilated, unresponsive pupils if there is progressive brain stem edema or hemorrhage. They can just as readily return to normal size if the cerebral edema resolves. Frequently, there is remarkable anisocoria with one mydriatic and one miotic pupil. Usually each shows a slight response to light. These should be carefully observed and utilized as indicators of whether to treat the patient more vigorously. Severe caudal brain stem lesions that are life threatening often result in partly dilated, fixed, unresponsive pupils.

Anisocoria can also result from specific diseases of the eye. Keratitis or uveitis may cause miosis in the affected eye, and glaucoma causes mydriasis. Iris atrophy is a common cause of dilated, unresponsive pupils in older animals and usually is bilateral. Animals consumption of drugs containing atropine. plants with belladonna alkaloids, or administration of a mydratic drug can cause dilated, nonresponsive pupils.

PHARMACOLOGIC TESTING

Further localization of autonomic lesions is based on the phenomenon of denervation hypersensitivity that occurs with second neuron lesions and uses low concentrations of the drug. In the parasympathetic system, lesions of the second neuron that denervate the pupil constrictor make it hypersensitive to low concentrations of the direct-acting drug pilocarpine. A 0.1 per cent solution causes constriction of the pupil of the denervated iris but not a normal iris or an iris in which the lesion involves the first neuron. With first neuron lesions, indirect-acting drugs cause pupil constriction by way of the intact second neuron. These drugs include physostigmine and phospholine iodine. These do not produce pupillary constriction with second neuron lesions.

The same concept applies to the sympathetic system innervation of the dilator of the pupil. For the direct-acting drug, a 1/10,000 dilution of epinephrine can be used. This should only cause dilation of a denervated pupil. Alternatively, 0.1 ml of a 0.001 per cent epinephrine solution causes dilation in 20 minutes if the pupil is denervated and 30 to 40 minutes if the lesion is in the preganglionic neurons. Cocaine (10 per cent solution) or hydroxyamphetamine (1 per cent solution) can be used as the indirect-acting drugs.

PALPEBRAL FISSURE (pp. 699–700)

A small palpebral fissure or ptosis results from a lesion in the oculomotor or sympathetic neurons that supply the eye. With a complete oculomotor paralysis, the ipsilateral pupil is dilated and unresponsive to light directed into either eye. There is also a lateral and slightly ventral strabismus, with decreased ability to adduct the eye normally, and an elevated third eyelid and miosis.

A small palpebral fissure occurs indirectly when extensive atrophy of

TABLE 84–1. LESION LOCATION AND ASSOCIATED NEUROLOGIC SIGNS

LOCATION	LESION	ASSOCIATED NEUROLOGIC SIGNS
T1–T3 spinal cord	Injury Neoplasia Embolic myelopathy	Tetraparesis to tetraplegia with LMN forelimb signs and UMN hindlimb signs
T1–T3 ventral roots proximal spinal nerves	Avulsion	Diffuse LMN paralysis of ipsilateral thoracic limb
Cranial thoracic sympathetic trunk	Lymphosarcoma, other neoplasms	None
Cervical sympathetic trunk	Neoplasia Injury-surgical; drug injection; dog bites	None or laryngeal hemiplegia
Postganglionic axons in middle ear	Otitis media	Peripheral vestibular ataxia, facial paralysis
Retrobulbar	Injury Neoplasia	Optic and oculomotor nerve defects

the muscles of mastication occurs and the eyeball retracts into the orbit. A narrowed palpebral fissure occurs with spasm of the facial muscles on one side. Similarly, the ear on the affected side is elevated slightly and the lips are retracted. This disease rarely occurs bilaterally. Tetanus regularly produces a bilateral narrowing of the palpebral fissures due to the uninhibited facial neuron activity. Occasionally animals with serious cerebellar disease that involves the cerebellar nuclei have one palpebral fissure that is slightly wider or a mildly elevated third eyelid.

THIRD EYELID (p. 700)

Lesions of the sympathetic neurons cause a constant protrusion of the third eyelid that is a feature of Horner's syndrome. The third eyelid also passively protrudes if the eyeball is actively retracted (as in tetanus) or the eyeball sinks in the orbit from severe weight loss or atrophy of the muscles of mastication (trigeminal nerve paralysis).

STRABISMUS (p. 700)

Strabismus is an abnormal position of the eyeball resulting from lesions of the cranial nerves that innervate the striated extraocular muscles (cranial nerves III, IV, and VI), in some head positions with lesions in the vestibular system, or as a result of orbital malformation. Oculomotor nerve lesions cause a lateral and slightly ventral strabismus, and eyeball adduction is deficient. As the head is moved in a dorsal plane, side to side, the eyeballs normally develop a jerk nystagmus with the quick phase in the direction of the head movement. The jerk-like movement toward the nose is adduction from the action of the medial rectus innervated by the oculomotor nerve (III). The same abrupt movement away from the nose, abduction, is a function of the lateral rectus innervated by the abducent nerve (VI). The latter is deficient in lesions of the abducent neurons, and a medial strabismus is observed. Trochlear nerve (IV) lesions are rare or unrecognized. Strabismus is often seen in hydrocephalic animals that have an enlarged cranial cavity. Both eyes often deviate ventrolaterally. Strabismus can also be observed in some positions of the head when animals have lesions in the vestibular system. This involves the eye on the same side as the vestibular abnormality, is usually a ventrolateral strabismus, and is present only in some positions of the head.

NYSTAGMUS (pp. 700–701)

Abnormal nystagmus most commonly occurs with disturbances of the vestibular system. In acute or progressive lesions, it may be spontaneous or resting, which means it is constant regardless of the position of the head. In more prolonged, less progressive lesions, it may be positional. With all disturbances of the peripheral components of the vestibular system, the quick phase of the abnormal nystagmus is opposite to the side of the head tilt and balance loss, which are on the same side as the lesion. This nystagmus can be horizontal or rotatory. With lesions of the central components of the vestibular system, the quick phase can be away from the lesion, be toward the lesion, change directions with different positions of the head, or be vertical. Congenital nystagmus is rare and usually is rapid and pendular (the speed is equal in both directions of the movement).

PALPEBRAL REFLEX (p. 701)

The sensory innervation occurs through branches of the ophthalmic and maxillary nerves from the trigeminal nerve (cranial nerve V). Sensory deficits are uncommon compared to facial paralysis and can be mistaken for the latter. Animals with only a trigeminal nerve lesion blink spontaneously and when the eye is menaced, provided they are visual. Loss of ophthalmic nerve innervation to the cornea via ciliary nerves may result in a neurotrophic keratitis.

CHAPTER 85

PERIPHERAL NERVE DISORDERS
(pages 701–726)

BIRMAN CAT DISTAL POLYNEUROPATHY (p. 702)

A degenerative polyneuropathy has recently been reported in several litters of Birman cats bred from the same parents. Clinical signs were first noted in cats 8 to 10 weeks of age. Affected cats fell frequently and had a tendency to stand and walk on their hocks, which were held in adduction. The gait was characterized by slight hypermetria in all limbs, and there was progressive pelvic limb ataxia. Analysis of blood and cerebrospinal fluid was normal. Nerve conduction velocity studies were normal; however, electromyography revealed the presence of fibrillation potentials and positive sharp waves in pelvic limbs. Prognosis is poor. Presently, there is no treatment.

BOTULISM (p. 702)

Clinical signs may occur within hours to several days following ingestion of toxin and reflect a progressive, symmetric disorder, ranging from mild weakness to severe flaccid tetraplegia with absent spinal reflexes and evidence of weakness in muscles of the face, jaw, pharynx, and esophagus resulting in dysphonia, dysphagia, facial paralysis, and megaesophagus. Electrodiagnostic studies may reveal a reduction in amplitude of evoked potentials and motor unit potentials, normal or decreased nerve conduction velocities, and sometimes fibrillation potentials and positive sharp waves, especially in distal limb muscles. Diagnosis is confirmed by identification of the toxin in the material ingested or in serum, feces, or vomitus of an affected animal with type-specific antitoxin using the neutralization test in mice. The prognosis is usually favorable in dogs.

BRACHIAL PLEXUS AVULSION (pp. 702–704)

Signs may vary from weakness of single muscle groups, without sensory loss, to paralysis of all thoracic limb muscle groups with accompanying sensory loss. Loss of ipsilateral panniculus or partial Horner's syndrome may be seen. Conscious pain presentation is usually impaired to a variable degree in all dogs with brachial plexus avulsion. Diagnosis is most commonly based on historical and clinical data. Electrodiagnostic testing is useful for detecting muscle denervation, especially minor degrees that cannot be uncovered by routine neurologic examination. The prognosis is guarded to poor. An electro-diagnostic evaluation of the radial nerve may provide early prognostic information, prognosis being poor in animals with initial, decreased radial nerve conduction velocity. Amputation of the affected limb or carpal fusion may be necessary.

BRACHIAL PLEXUS NEUROPATHY (p. 704)

This is a rare, bilaterally symmetric, neurologic condition in dogs and cats. Clinical signs may be characterized by acute onset of thoracic limb paresis with depressed or absent reflexes and hypotonia, facial paresis, and neurogenic atrophy in all thoracic limb muscles. Affected animals may show allergic episodes with facial edema and generalized urticaria a few days prior to development of neurologic signs. A milder form of brachial plexus neuropathy has been reported in several dogs presented with shifting thoracic limb lameness and diffuse electromyographic changes typical of denervation. Some of these dogs were steroid-responsive.

CHRONIC RELAPSING POLYNEUROPATHY (p. 704)

A 9-month-old female domestic short-haired cat was presented for slowly progressive tetraparesis of one month's duration. The cat was recumbent but alert, with generalized loss of muscle mass. Cranial nerve function was normal. Segmental spinal reflexes were depressed in all limbs, and postural reactions were clumsy. Proprioceptive deficits were noted in all limbs. Sensation was normal. The cat recovered spontaneously after 1 week, but relapsed 10 days later. Clinical signs abated gradually after 1 week of corticosteroid therapy, and no recurrence occurred during therapy. The cat remained neurologically normal, and corticosteroid therapy was terminated after 6 months.

In the Scott-Ritchey Neuromuscular Laboratory over the past several years, we have seen similar clinical and pathologic findings (in which paranodal demyelination is the dominant abnormality) in three other mature cats and nine mature dogs, many of which have been steroid-responsive.

DANCING DOBERMAN DISEASE (p. 704)

Doberman pinschers of either sex, from 6 months to 7 years of age, initially manifest flexion of one pelvic limb when standing. Similar signs may be noted in the opposite pelvic limb several months later, and affected dogs begin to alternately flex and extend each pelvic limb in a dancing motion and prefer to sit rather than stand. The condition progresses insidiously over several years, with pelvic limb weakness, proprioceptive deficits, and gradual atrophy of pelvic limb musculature, especially the gastrocnemius. Pelvic reflexes are reportedly normal or hyperactive. Affected dogs do not appear to be in pain. At present, there is no treatment. The long-term prognosis for a pain-free, acceptable pet is good.

DEAFNESS (pp. 705–706)

Neurogenic deafness or hearing impairment may be *central*, resulting from damage to central nervous system auditory pathways, or *peripheral*, resulting from cochlear abnormalities. Conductive deafness stems from problems within the external or middle ear cavities—external ear canal occlusion, rigidity or rupture of the tympanic membrane, damage to the ossicular chain (stapes, malleus, and incus), or fluid within the middle ear. The most common cause of conductive deafness is chronic otitis externa/media, sometimes in association with cholesteatomas.

Neural deafness resulting from cochlear abnormalities may be congenital or hereditary, associated with ototoxic drugs, or associated with normal aging. Congenital deafness is frequently associated with pigmentation disorders such as a white coat color and blue eyes. Deafness can also result from various ototoxic agents.

While all aminoglycoside antibiotics can damage auditory and vestibular receptors, streptomycin and gentomycin have their greatest effects on the vestibular system, whereas neomycin, kanamycin, tobramycin, and amikacin sulfate produce more damage to the auditory peripheral receptors. Other ototoxic antibiotics include topical polymixin B, chloramphenicol, antiseptic solutions (ethanol, iodine, iodophors, chlorhexidine, benzalkonium chloride, benzethonium chloride, and cetrimide), diuretics (ethacrynic acid, bumetanide, and furosemide), antineoplastic agents (cisplastin), propylene glycol, ceruminolytic agents, and detergents. While hearing is difficult to assess accurately by testing response to sounds such as clapping, electrodiagnostic testing using the brain stem auditory evoked response (BAER) method can provide early diagnosis of deafness. There is no treatment.

Deafness also has been reported in young dogs and cats accompanied by signs of peripheral vestibular disease. It has been seen in beagles, Akita and Doberman pinscher puppies, and Siamese kittens. Clinical signs, which usually begin at 3 to 12 weeks of age, include head tilt, circling, and ataxia. Nystagmus is not a feature of this disorder, but there is a deficit in normal eye movements. The vestibular signs are generally not progressive, and improvement is usually seen over a period of weeks or months, probably due to compensation. Deafness is usually permanent.

DIABETIC NEUROPATHY (p. 706)

Clinical signs are extremely variable, ranging from an insidious subclinical condition to one with an acute onset of progressive paraparesis, proprioceptive deficits, muscle atrophy, and depressed spinal reflexes. Cats often assume a plantigrade posture in pelvic limbs. Electrodiagnostic testing has revealed fibrillation potentials, positive sharp waves and fasciculation potentials in muscles, slow nerve conduction velocities, and decreased amplitudes of evoked muscle action potentials.

Diagnosis is based on laboratory evidence of diabetes mellitus and clinical, neurologic, electrophysiologic, and nerve biopsy data. Prognosis is guarded.

DISTAL DENERVATING DISEASE (pp. 706–707)

This degenerative neuropathy is reportedly the most common canine polyneuropathy in the United Kingdom, but has not been reported elsewhere. The condition is clinically similar to coonhound paralysis (see Polyradiculoneuritis).

DISTAL SYMMETRIC POLYNEUROPATHY (p. 707)

We have seen a distal symmetric sensorimotor polyneuropathy in several breeds of large dogs. Clinical signs include chronic pelvic limb paresis, which progresses to involve thoracic limbs, and bilateral atrophy of head (masticatory) and distal limb muscles. A reduced response to painful stimuli has been observed. Electrodiagnostic studies reveal fibrillation potentials, positive sharp waves in distal limb muscles (below stifle and elbow), and absence of evoked muscle action potentials. Diagnosis is based on clinical, electrodiagnostic, and nerve biopsy data. Prognosis is poor.

DYSAUTONOMIA (p. 707)

This disease has been reported frequently in cats but only rarely in dogs. Clinical signs suggest involvement of the parasympathetic nervous system. In the majority of cases, clinical signs develop in less than 48 hours, but may take up to 7 days. Historically, cats begin vomiting/retching and become depressed and anorexic. The third eyelid protrudes, pupils are dilated and poorly responsive to light stimulation, and lacrimation is reduced. Cats may be febrile, emaciated, constipated, and dehydrated. Urinary and fecal incontinence may develop. Sneezing may occur, and the nose is often dry. Occasionally, mild posterior ataxia or more generalized paresis, depressed proprioception, and absent anal reflex have been detected. Megaesophagus is often present and is usualy associated with regurgitation. Many cats have bradycardia of less than 120 beats/minute. Pharmacologic testing may confirm sympathetic and parasympathetic dysfunction.

In dogs, signs may be nonspecific—lethargy, depression, anorexia, retching, regurgitation, vomiting, constipation, or, more commonly, diarrhea. Other signs include dry, crusty nose, dry oral mucous membranes, subnormal Schirmer tear tests, dilated or anisocoric pupils (poorly responsive to light), prolapsed nictitating membranes, megaesophagus, and distended incontinent urinary bladder. Heart rate is often less than 120 beats/minute (even after exercise). No specific treatment is available, but supportive therapy is indicated. Prognosis in dogs and cats is guarded to poor, especially in animals that suffer from persistent regurgitation/vomiting. Clinical recovery may take as long as 12 months.

FACIAL PARALYSIS (pp. 707–708)

Idiopathic facial nerve paralysis of acute onset has been reported in mature (e.g., >5 years) dogs and cats. There is an apparent predisposition for cocker spaniels, Pembroke Welsh corgis, boxers, English setters, and domestic long-haired cats. Clinical signs are characterized by ear drooping, lip commissural paralysis, sialosis, deviation of the nose away from the affected side, and collection of food on the paralyzed side of the mouth. Menace response testing and palpebral reflexes are absent. Bilateral facial paralysis may be observed in some animals.

Electrodiagnostic testing may reveal spontaneous denervation potentials in superficial facial muscles. Stimulation of the facial nerve external to the stylomastoid foramen may fail to evoke muscle action potentials. Prognosis is guarded. Improvement may take place in a few weeks or months, or may never occur. Treatment is empiric. Artificial tears may assist with corneal dryness.

Unilateral or bilateral facial paresis or paralysis in animals has also been seen in association with polyradiculoneuritis (e.g., coonhound paralysis), insulinomas, laryngeal paralysis-polyneuropathy complex, myasthenia gravis, botulism, brain stem inflammation or neoplasia, middle ear infection, trauma external to the stylomastoid foramen, or in conjunction with petrosal bone fracture. It may occur secondary to surgical ablation of the external ear canal or bulla osteotomy for chronic otitis.

GANGLIOSIDOSIS (p. 708)

See Table 82–10 in the textbook. Peripheral neuropathies are not typically associated with gangliosidoses in animals; however, axonal degeneration and demyelination, along with lamellar inclusion bodies in Schwann cells, fibroblasts, macrophages, and endoneurial cells have been observed in peripheral nerves from cats with GM_2 gangliosidosis.

GIANT AXONAL NEUROPATHY (p. 708)

Giant axonal neuropathy, a rare neurologic disease of German shepherd dogs, is inherited as an autosomal recessive trait. Clinical neurologic signs are noted around 14 to 16 months of age, are more obvious in pelvic limbs, and are progressive. They are characterized by paresis, proprioceptive loss, diminished patellar reflexes, and pelvic limb hypotonia with atrophy of muscles below the stifles. Conscious perception of pain is gradually reduced in pelvic limbs. Bark may be lost or diminished, and there may be fecal incontinence. Megaesophagus develops around 18 months. By 18 to 24 months of age, tetraparesis is pronounced. Electrophysiologically, amplitudes of evoked compound muscle action potentials are decreased, then denervation potentials are demonstrable in the limbs. Prognosis is poor. There is no treatment.

GLOBOID LEUKODYSTROPHY (p. 708)

See Table 82–10 in the textbook and Chapter 83.

GLYCOGENOSIS (p. 708)

Glycogen storage diseases or glycogenoses are rare inborn errors of metabolism due to deficient activity of one of the enzymes involved in glycogen degradation or synthesis. Young Norwegian forest cats may develop fever, generalized muscle tremors, bunny-hopping gait, and weakness at 5 to 6 months of age, which may progress to tetraplegia. Seizures may be seen as well as severe generalized muscle atrophy with contracture of the limb muscles. Prognosis is poor. There is no treatment.

HYPERADRENOCORTICAL (CUSHING'S) NEUROPATHY (p. 709)

We have found evidence of a peripheral neuropathy in several dogs with hyperadrenocorticism. Changes have been observed in dogs with and without histopathologic evidence of hyperadrenocortical myopathy. Reversibility and long-term prognosis are unknown.

HYPERCHYLOMICRONEMIA (p. 709)

Hyperchylomicronemia or hyperlipoproteinemia is a familial condition in cats with a world-wide distribution. Peripheral neuropathies may include (1) Horner's syndrome (ptosis, miosis, enophthalmos, and prolapse of the third eyelid), (2) facial nerve paralysis (absence of corneal and palpebral reflexes), (3) tibial nerve paralysis (overflexion of the tarsus), (4) femoral nerve paralysis (atrophy of quadriceps muscles and absence of patellar reflex), (5) trigeminal nerve paralysis (temporal muscle atrophy, inability to prehend and chew food), (6) radial nerve paralysis (inability to extend digits), and (7) recurrent laryngeal nerve paralysis (dyspnea and cyanosis due to impaired abduction of vocal cords). Neuropathic signs are usually not seen until cats are at least 8 months of age. Peripheral neuropathies in affected cats resolve after 2 to 3 months on a low-fat diet.

HYPEROXALURIA (p. 709)

Primary hyperoxaluria is considered to be an autosomal recessive disorder associated with renal failure and neurologic signs in young domestic shorthaired cats of either sex, resulting in death before 1 year of age. Signs include anorexia, dehydration, weakness, and depression.

Kidneys are often enlarged and seem to be painful when palpated. Affected cats develop a crouching, cow-hocked stance and are reluctant to stand or walk. Neurologic examination reveals deficiencies in postural reaction testing, depressed patellar and withdrawal reflexes, and a reduced response to pain. Diagnosis may be made in affected cats before they develop clinical signs by identifying L-glycerate in urine. Prognosis is grave. There is no treatment.

HYPERTROPHIC NEUROPATHY (pp. 709–710)

Hypertrophic neuropathy is an autosomal recessive neurologic disease that has been reported in Tibetan mastiff dogs. Clinical signs appear in animals from 7 to 10 weeks of age and consist of rapidly developing generalized weakness, hyporeflexia, muscle hypotonia, and dysphonia. Severely affected puppies may become totally recumbent within 3 weeks of onset with subsequent development of sternal compression and limb contractures. Electrodiagnostic studies reveal moderate to severe reduction in nerve conduction velocities. Diagnosis is based on signalment and clinical, electrodiagnostic, and nerve biopsy data. Prognosis is guarded. There is no treatment.

HYPOGLYCEMIA (p. 710)

See Chapters 82 and 116. Clinical signs of polyneuropathy range from paraparesis to tetraplegia, facial paresis/paralysis, hyporeflexia, hypotonia, and muscle atrophy, usually in conjunction with seizures.

HYPOMYELINATION NEUROPATHY (p. 710)

In contrast with CNS hypomyelination, hypomyelination of the peripheral nerves is rare, but has been recently reported in two golden retriever littermates. Both dogs were presented for pelvic limb ataxia at 7 weeks of age. Both had a crouched stance, mild pelvic limb atrophy, and weakness. Circumduction was evident in pelvic limbs when they walked, and a bunny-hop gait was present when they ran. Segmental spinal reflexes were depressed or absent in all limbs. Motor nerve conduction velocities were markedly reduced in sciatic-tibial and ulnar nerves. The defect appears to be reversible, since both dogs have clinically improved.

HYPOTHYROID NEUROPATHY (p. 710)

A hypothyroid-associated neuropathy does appear to exist in mature to middle-aged dogs, usually of the large-breed variety. Clinical signs may include progressive weakness, muscle atrophy (mainly appendicular), and depressed spinal reflexes. Facial nerve paresis/paralysis may also be present. Electrodiagnostic studies have revealed multifocal patterns of fibrillation potentials, positive sharp waves, and decreased motor nerve conduction velocities.

In four other dogs with hypothyroidism, a spectrum of neurologic signs referable to the cranial nerves was seen, ranging in duration from 2 weeks to 6 months. Clinical signs improved or returned to normal in all dogs within 3 to 4 months of thyroid hormone supplementation. However, we have seen a number of dogs in which there is less dramatic or no clinical response to long-term thyroid hormone supplementation.

ISCHEMIC NEUROMYOPATHY (pp. 710–711)

This disorder occurs in cats with cardiomyopathy and thromboemboli (Chapter 96). Clinical signs are acute in onset and usually include pelvic limb pain during the first 24 hours, plantigrade stance, and paraparesis or paralysis. Femoral pulse may be weak or absent, the gastrocnemius muscle is firm and often painful, and the limbs are cool. The nail beds of pelvic limbs are cyanotic. Although the collateral circulation does return in the majority of cases, return of function to varying degrees may take 6 weeks to 6 months, and the long-term prognosis is guarded to poor. At present there are no results that show that any treatment of the aortic thromboembolism produces a significantly better recovery than no therapy.

LARYNGEAL PARALYSIS (p. 711)

The idiopathic form has been reported mostly in middle-aged and older large- and giant-breed dogs, such as Saint Bernard, Chesapeake Bay retriever, and Irish setter, but medium and small/toy breeds also may be affected. Acquired laryngeal paralysis may result from lymphomatous infiltration of the vagus nerve, foreign bodies penetrating the wall of the esophagus, a complication of lead poisoning, or rabies, and is sporadically observed in animals with idiopathic polyradiculoneuritis.

Onset of clinical signs in the hereditary form in dogs is from 4 to 6 months of age. The acquired form may develop in animals from 1.5 to 13 years of age. Clinical signs reflect respiratory, primarily inspiratory, distress and are characterized by increasing loss of endurance, progressive laryngeal stridor, voice changes, dyspnea, cyanosis during episodes of severe dyspnea, and collapse with complete airway obstruction. Clinical signs are usually of several months' duration. In cats, excessive head shaking and abnormal purring may be noted. Laryngeal paralysis has also been noted in dogs with clinical, electrodiagnostic, and pathologic evidence of a more generalized polyneuropathy.

Diagnosis of laryngeal abductor dysfunction is made by laryngoscopy. Recurrent laryngeal nerve paralysis is confirmed by electromyographic detection of denervation potentials in individual intrinsic laryngeal muscles and by evidence of neurogenic atrophy in biopsy specimens of laryngeal muscles (e.g., the cricoarytenoid muscle).

Prognosis in animals with idiopathic paralysis is usually favorable with surgical management, such as arytenoidectomy and vocal fold removal, arytenoid lateralization, and castellated laryngofissure. However, prognosis is more guarded in animals with hereditary laryngeal paralysis. Based on our studies, prognosis is guarded to poor in affected Dalmatians.

MEGAESOPHAGUS (pp. 711–712)

The congenital form is common in Great Danes, German shepherds, Irish setters, Newfoundlands, Shar Peis, and greyhounds. The condition occurs as an inherited disease in wirehaired fox terriers and miniature schnauzers. Acquired megaesophagus may occur in dogs or cats at any age. In many cases, the cause is unknown; however, the condition has been observed in association with certain systemic neuromuscular disorders such as myasthenia gravis, botulism, hypothyroidism, hypoadrenocorticism, polymyositis, dermatomyositis, myotonic myopathy, polyradiculoneuritis, distemper, giant axonal neuropathy in German shepherds, tick paralysis, lead toxicosis, thallium toxicosis, canine and feline muscular dystrophy–like conditions, laryngeal paralysis–polyneuropathy complex, glycogen storage disorders, sensory ganglioradiculitis, and spinal muscular atrophy. In acquired myasthenia gravis in dogs, megaesophagus may be the only clinical sign. It has also been reported sporadically in dogs with tetanus and in cats with mannosidosis. Megaesophagus may also occur with brain stem lesions such as neoplasia, distemper encephalitis, granulomatous meningoen-cephalomyelitis, or trauma.

Clinical features are postprandial regurgitation of undigested food, with radiographic evidence of megaesophagus to the level of the diaphragm. In some dogs, respiratory signs such as cough, dyspnea, and/or abnormal secretions may be the only signs observed.

Prognosis of congenital megaesophagus in young dogs is guarded. Some animals appear normal by the time they mature. Acquired, idio-pathic megaesophagus has a poor prognosis for recovery, although transient megaesophagus followed by spontaneous recovery is seen occasionally in dogs. Cachexia becomes an important complication, and death is a common consequence of inhalation pneumonia. Clinical improvement has been noted in dogs with acquired megaesophagus following treatment of the primary disease process (e.g., myasthenia gravis, tetanus). Recommended management includes elevated feeding and/or gastrostomy tube feeding of high-caloric diets.

MYASTHENIA GRAVIS (pp. 712–713)

Acquired myasthenia gravis (MG) in dogs and cats has been seen in association with thymomas or other thymic abnormalities such as thymic cysts. In dogs, acquired MG has also been reported in associa-tion with other tumors, including cholangiocellular carcinoma and osteogenic sarcoma. Acquired MG has been observed in adult dogs of all sizes, but more commonly in medium-to-large breeds. A bimodal age of onset (<5 years and >7 years) has also been noted in affected dogs. In cats with MG, Abyssinians and a close relative, Somalis, seem to be over-represented.

Signs in dogs are often characterized by muscle weakness that is exacerbated by exercise. Additional signs may be lameness, collapse, regurgitation, drooling, ventroflexion of the head, and tremors. Megae-sophagus is common. In one study, 26 per cent of dogs with idiopathic megaesophagus, pharyngeal paralysis, and/or decreased palpebral reflexes had positive serum antibody titers against acetylcholine recep-tors. In cats, signs often include progressive lameness, weakness, drooling, and ventroflexion of the head. Other signs include head and body trembling, crouching posture, dysphagia, regurgitation, weight loss, and voice change. Many cats have facial weakness and are unable to close their eyelids (lack of menace and absent palpebral reflex). Megaesophagus has also been reported in cats.

Diagnosis is based on clinical signs, electrodiagnostic evidence of decremental response of muscle action potentials after repeated nerve stimulation, serologic testing for acetylcholine receptor antibodies (definitive), and amelioration of signs following administration of the short-acting anticholinesterase edrophonium chloride (Tensilon). How-ever, some dogs with myasthenia gravis may not respond, whereas dogs with other neuromuscular disorders may be responsive.

Prognosis is guarded. One potential complication is inhalation pneu-monia. Medical treatment usually entails a trial and error approach to the drug(s) used, dosage, frequency, or combination. In some dogs and cats, combination of corticosteroids and anticholinesterases may be necessary for effective treatment.

Congenital MG may occur as a postsynaptic and a presynaptic disor-der. Clinical signs and electrophysiologic findings in animals with postsynaptic congenital MG are similar to those described for acquired MG; however, signs of episodic weakness are often relentlessly pro-gressive, ultimately leading to generalized weakness, muscle wasting, and inability to ambulate, in spite of treatment. Clinical response to mestinon is often erratic, and prognosis is guarded to poor.

Presynaptic congenital MG has been reported in 12- to 16-week-old Gammel Dansk Honsehund dogs with autosomal recessive inheritance.

Signs are characterized by exercise-induced weakness, short strides with flexed limbs, head drooping, occasional falling, and crawling movements. Muscle tone and reflexes are normal during attacks; there is no facial weakness, no swallowing defect, no megaesophagus, and no change in voice. The condition is not progressive. Anti-cholinesterase treatment has no effect. The underlying defect may be due to a defect in the synthesis of acetylcholine, impaired release of acetylcholine, abnormality of acetylcholine-induced ion channels, or deficiency of end-plate acetylcholinesterase.

OPTIC NERVE HYPOPLASIA (pp. 713–714)

Optic nerve hypoplasia is an uncommon congenital abnormality of the posterior segment that may be unilateral or bilateral and may be accompanied by microphthalmia or other congenital ocular defects, such as retinal dysplasia, retinal detachment, and sometimes hydrocephalus. Diagnosis is suggested by a history of visual impairment (mydriasis, menace deficit, absent direct PLR) from birth. Ophthalmoscopic examination reveals variable reduction in the size of the optic disc with normal-appearing retinal vessels. Prognosis is poor. There is no treatment. Optic nerve aplasia is a rare congenital anomaly characterized by absence of optic nerve, optic disc, and retinal vessels.

OPTIC NEURITIS (p. 714)

Optic neuritis may be associated with primary ocular disease or can occur secondary to systemic inflammatory disease. In dogs, diagnostic considerations include canine distemper, the ocular form of granulomatous meningoencephalomyelitis, systemic mycosis (e.g., cryptococcosis), toxoplasmosis, neoplasia, trauma, and acute toxicity (e.g., lead or chlorinated hydrocarbon toxicity).

An apparently healthy animal may present with a history of unilateral or bilateral blindness of sudden onset. Pupils usually are unilaterally or bilaterally dilated and unresponsive to light stimulation. Ophthalmoscopic examination typically reveals an edematous, elevated optic disc and engorged retinal vessels. Focal hemorrhage may be present. Active or inactive chorioretinitis may accompany the optic neuritis. Optic neuritis is distinguished from papilledema in that vision is preserved in the latter condition.

If the cause is undetermined, the animal may be treated symptomatically with retrobulbar corticosteroids in conjunction with oral corticosteroid administration (gradual reduction to maintenance therapy every other day for as long as one year). Prognosis is guarded. Clinical response to treatment can be difficult to assess, and the course is unpredictable.

PARANEOPLASTIC NEUROPATHY (pp. 714–715)

Clinical neuropathies have been seen in dogs with bronchogenic carcinoma, insulinoma, leiomyosarcoma, hemangiosarcoma, undifferentiated sarcomas, synovial cell sarcoma, and adrenal adenocarcinoma.

PARANEOPLASTIC DISORDERS OF THE NEUROMUSCULAR JUNCTION

Acquired MG has been seen in association with mediastinal tumors, such as thymomas.

PERIPHERAL NERVE TUMORS (p. 715)

Tumors of cranial and spinal nerves and nerve roots commonly involve middle to low cervical nerve roots and the brachial plexus, resulting in slow, progressive unilateral thoracic limb lameness and muscle atrophy. Horner's syndrome is often present. These tumors may also involve other nerves, such as the trigeminal nerve, thoracic nerves, and lumbosacral plexus. The neoplasms commonly extend along peripheral nerves, resulting in intradural-extramedullary spinal cord compression. Various tumors of the ear canal may involve the facial nerve or one of its branches.

Diagnosis is confirmed by surgical biopsy. Peripheral nerve and nerve root tumors can be resected, but it is sometimes necessary to remove the affected nerve and nerve root. Complete amputation of the limb may be required if more than one root is involved or if atrophy of all muscle groups is extreme (as may occur with a tumor of the brachial plexus). Corticosteroids may ameliorate signs by reducing edema around the tumor and may produce temporary regression of lymphoid and reticulohistiocytic tumors.

POLYRADICULONEURITIS (pp. 715–717)

It is becoming evident that a number of nerve root disorders exist and are clinically characterized by sudden onset of paresis, paralysis, or tetraplegia. There may be increased levels of cerebrospinal fluid (CSF) protein without pleocytosis (albuminocytologic dissociation), and nerve root biopsy may show evidence of inflammatory cell infiltration.

COONHOUND PARALYSIS

The disease affects dogs of any breed, both sexes, and usually of adult age. Clinical signs frequently appear 7 to 11 days after an encounter with a raccoon. Onset is marked by weakness and pelvic limb hyporeflexia, although thoracic limb involvement may sometimes be the initial and dominant clinical sign. Paralysis progresses rapidly, resulting in a flaccid symmetric tetraplegia; however, milder forms without paralysis can occur. The duration of paralysis varies from several weeks to 2 or 3 months. Motor impairment is more pronounced than sensory changes, although many dogs appear to be hyperesthetic to sensory stimuli. Bladder or rectal paralysis usually is not observed. In severely affected animals, there may be complete absence of spinal reflexes, facial weakness, loss of voice, inability to lift the head, and labored respiration. Motor nerve conduction velocities may be markedly reduced, and electromyographic studies reveal widespread denervation 6 to 7 days after the onset. Prognosis is usually favorable, but dogs with severe axonal degeneration may die from respiratory paralysis or may have protracted, incomplete recoveries. Good nursing care is essential.

IDIOPATHIC POLYRADICULONEURITIS

A condition that appears to be identical to coonhound paralysis with respect to onset, clinical signs, clinical course, and pathology occurs in dogs that have had no possible exposure to raccoons. A similar, idiopathic polyradiculoneuritis occurs much less frequently in cats.

CAUDA EQUINA POLYRADICULONEURITIS

In rare instances, polyradiculoneuritis occurs in dogs with signs of a lumbosacral syndrome (pelvic limb paraparesis, muscle hypotonia and atrophy, loss of patellar reflexes, and proprioceptive loss). Pain sensation, bladder function, and anal reflex are intact. Motor nerve conduction velocity is decreased in the sciatic-tibial nerves.

CHRONIC RELAPSING POLYRADICULONEURITIS

This is a rare, chronic neurologic disorder seen in dogs and cats. Clinical and laboratory findings include tetraparesis, diminished or absent reflexes, muscle wasting, albuminocytologic dissociation (in CSF), muscle denervation potentials, and delayed peripheral nerve conduction velocities. The progressive course is interrupted by partial remission of signs.

INFECTIOUS POLYRADICULONEURITIS

See Chapter 83.

ROTTWEILER DISTAL SENSORIMOTOR POLYNEUROPATHY (p. 717)

A polyneuropathy has been recently reported in mature rottweiler dogs in the United States. Clinical signs are characterized by paraparesis that progresses to tetraparesis, spinal hyporeflexia and hypotonia, and appendicular muscle atrophy. Although signs may appear acutely, the course tends to be gradually progressive (up to 12 months or longer in some dogs) and may be relapsing. Numerous positive sharp waves and fibrillation potentials were detected in appendicular muscles by electromyographic testing, especially in muscles distal to the elbow and stifle. Motor nerve conduction velocities were reduced in some dogs. Hematology, blood chemistries, and spinal radiography/myelography were normal. Prognosis appears guarded to poor despite the fact that some dogs showed a temporary response to corticosteroid therapy.

SENSORY NEUROPATHIES (pp. 717–719)

Sensory neuropathies in dogs may be characterized by self-mutilation, loss of pain reflexes, or conscious proprioception. In general, paresis and muscle atrophy are not present, and no abnormal spontaneous potentials are detected on electromyographic testing. Nerve conduction studies may demonstrate slowed velocities in sensory but not motor nerves.

SENSORY GANGLIORADICULITIS

The clinical course is usually insidiously progressive over several months or years. Clinical signs are variable and include proprioceptive deficits, generalized ataxia with preservation of muscle strength, depression or absence of tendon reflexes, such as the patellar reflex, facial hypalgesia/paresthesia, megaesophagus, head tilt, loss of voice, hearing loss, anisocoria, dysphagia, stiff gait (often with hypermetria), and occasionally self-mutilation. Muscle atrophy is usually not a feature.

Hematologic values, cerebrospinal fluid (CSF) analysis, and radiographic studies are within normal limits; however, a mild increase in CSF cellularity and total protein may be present. Electromyographic findings are usually normal. Prognosis is guarded to poor. To date, corticosteroids have been ineffective.

SENSORY NEUROPATHY IN BOXERS

Sensory neuropathies have been reported in boxers, long-haired dachshunds, Jack Russell terriers, and English pointers.

SENSORY TRIGEMINAL NEUROPATHY

Clinical signs include acute onset of excessive salivation, coughing, and dysphagia. Prognosis is guarded.

IDIOPATHIC SELF-MUTILATION

Idiopathic self-mutilation or behavioral self-mutilation has been seen in both dogs and cats. Affected animals are often of nervous or high-strung breeds. In dogs, this self-mutilation may manifest itself as continued licking, biting, or scratching of one or more areas usually near the carpus or hock. In one blind clinical trial, the tricyclic antidepressant drug clomipramine resulted in significant improvement in the dogs' licking behavior.

SPHINGOMYELINOSIS (p. 719)

Signs in affected animals include absent conscious proprioception, severely depressed to absent spinal reflexes, hypotonia, fine generalized muscle tremors (especially in pelvic limbs), a palmigrade/plantigrade stance, and moderate hepatosplenomegaly. Pain perception and cranial nerve function are normal. Motor nerve conduction velocities are markedly depressed. All cats tested showed severe reduction in CNS and visceral lysosomal sphingomyelinase activity. Prognosis is poor. There is no treatment.

SPINAL MUSCULAR ATROPHY (pp. 719–721)

Clinical signs usually are progressive and tend to be dominated by neuropathies in pelvic and thoracic limbs that occur secondary to motor neuron involvement. Prognosis is guarded to poor, and there is no treatment. Spinal muscular atrophy with a distinct clinical picture has been seen in Swedish Lapland dogs, Brittany spaniels, English pointers, giant breed crosses, German shepherd dogs and rottweilers.

NEURONOPATHY IN CAIRN TERRIERS

Affected animals, of either sex, may show onset of signs at about 5 months of age. These signs are pelvic limb weakness that progresses to tetraparesis, depressed spinal reflexes and diminished proprioception, incoordination, hypermetria, and head tremor. A range of clinical and pathologic variations may occur in this condition.

TICK PARALYSIS (p. 721)

The common wood tick, *Dermacentor variabilis,* and the Rocky Mountain wood tick, *Dermacentor andersoni,* are incriminated most often. Onset of clinical signs is gradual, paralysis first becoming evident as an incoordination in the pelvic limbs, resulting in an unsteady gait. Altered voice, cough, and dysphagia can be early signs. Dogs become recumbent in 24 to 72 hours. Reflexes are lost, but sensation is preserved. Jaw muscle weakness and facial paresis may be present. Death may occur within several days from respiratory paralysis.

Electromyographic studies reveal absence of spontaneous potentials and lack of motor unit action potentials. No muscle response follows direct nerve stimulation. Motor and sensory nerve conduction velocity may be slower than normal.

Prognosis is usually good, with recovery occurring in 1 to 3 days following tick removal or dipping of the animal in an insecticide solution.

TOXIC NEUROPATHIES (pp. 721–722)

Vincristine, thallium poisoning, and lead poisoning have rarely induced peripheral neuropathies. A delayed neurotoxicity may occur in cats days or weeks after minimal exposure to organophosphates. Iatrogenic peripheral vestibular disease and/or deafness may result from use of various antibiotics and chemical agents that cause degeneration of vestibular and auditory peripheral receptors (see Deafness and Vestibular Disease).

TRAUMATIC NEUROPATHY (p. 722)

Nerve injuries may result from mechanical blows, gunshot wounds, fractures, pressure, and stretching (see Brachial Plexus Avulsion). Iatrogenic causes include crushing, cutting, or spearing the nerve with an intramedullary pin; compression by casts or splints; and injection of agents into or adjacent to the nerve.

Nerve integrity may be easily assessed by nerve stimulation proximal and distal to the site of the lesion. The closer the nerve injury is to the muscle it must reinnervate, the better the prognosis. Self-mutilation that results from abnormal sensation in an affected area produced by regeneration of sensory nerves can be a major complication.

Treatment may involve surgical anastomosis or neurolysis (i.e., freeing of a nerve from inflammatory adhesions). In those instances in which nerve damage is chronic, high, or severe, muscle relocation and muscle tendon transfer procedures can be considered.

TRIGEMINAL NEURITIS (pp. 722–723)

See Chapter 82.

VESTIBULAR DISEASE (pp. 723–724)

PERIPHERAL VESTIBULAR DISEASE

Labyrinthitis.   Signs may range from ipsilateral head tilt, nystagmus (frequently rotatory), and ataxia to torticollis, circling, falling, and rolling. Attendant middle ear inflammation may disturb function of the facial and sympathetic nerves, which course through the middle ear, resulting in ipsilateral facial paresis/paralysis and Horner's syndrome, respectively. Animals with labyrinthitis may have decreased tear production and develop ipsilateral keratitis sicca. Another structure commonly involved in labyrinthitis is the cochlear nerve, dysfunction of which results in deafness. Signs such as head shaking, pawing/rubbing of the ear, and discharge from the external ear canal may accompany the neurologic signs.

Otoscopy may reveal an otitis externa and evidence of erosion or rupture. Fluid in the middle ear produces bulging of the tympanic membrane, which may appear opaque and hyperemic. Prognosis is usually favorable with prolonged oral and topical antibiotics chosen from positive culture and sensitivity studies. In more chronic cases, surgical debridement and drainage of the middle ear may be required.

Idiopathic Vestibular Disease.   See Chapter 82.

Congenital Vestibular Disease.   Signs of peripheral vestibular disease without deafness have been observed in several breeds of puppies including English cocker spaniels, German shepherds, Tibetan terriers, and in Burmese kittens. Nystagmus is not a feature in these young animals. Prognosis is guarded, since clinical signs may regress completely, recur, or remain static.

Miscellaneous Causes of Peripheral Vestibular Disease. Osteosarcoma, fibrosarcoma, or chondrosarcoma may involve the osseous bulla or bony labyrinth, whereas squamous cell carcinoma and ceruminous gland adenocarcinoma may involve adjacent soft tissues. Inflammatory polyps are observed sporadically within the ear canal of cats.

Iatrogenic Peripheral Vestibular Disease.   This disease may result from the use of aminoglycoside antibiotics, fractures in the petrous temporal bone, or rupture of the tympanic bulla.

WALKER HOUND MONONEUROPATHY (p. 724)

An idiopathic neuropathy, usually involving one pelvic limb, has been reported in a kennel of Walker hounds in eastern North Carolina. Signs of pelvic limb monoparesis, areflexia, muscle atrophy, and deficient postural reactions were first seen in 2-week-old puppies. Signs progressed to severe paresis and self-mutilation.

CHAPTER 86

DISORDERS OF THE SKELETAL MUSCLES
(pages 727–736)

Myopathies affecting dogs and cats can be categorized as inflammatory or degenerative in nature (Table 86–1).

INFLAMMATORY MYOPATHIES (pp. 729–731)

INFECTIOUS MYOPATHIES

Bacterial Myositis

Infections in dogs and cats typically follow trauma, bite wounds, or contamination of a surgical wound. Antibiotic therapy should be based on culture and sensitivity. Surgical drainage may be indicated.

Protozoal Myositis

See Chapter 82.

IMMUNE-MEDIATED MYOPATHIES

Polymyositis

Polymyositis has been described rarely in dogs with systemic lupus erythematosus and neoplasia. Clinical signs compatible with polymyositis were noted in Doberman pinschers treated with trimethoprim-sulfadiazine. A syndrome in which dermatitis and myositis (dermatomyositis) occur together has been well characterized in collies, Shetland sheepdogs, and their crosses.

Clinical Findings. Polymyositis may affect dogs of any age and breed, although middle-aged larger dogs are most commonly affected. Hyperesthesia on muscle palpation is a common feature. Many affected dogs also have systemic signs, principally pyrexia and depression. Megaesophagus and associated regurgitation can be present. Muscle atrophy occurs chronically. The temporal muscles and face are particularly affected in dermatomyositis.

Diagnosis. Serum creatine kinase is variably elevated in affected dogs. Multiple muscles should ideally be biopsied to reach the diagnosis.

Treatment. Dogs with polymyositis generally improve on initia-

Original chapter written by Joe N. Kornegay

TABLE 86–1. CLASSIFICATION OF CANINE MYOPATHIES

I. Inflammatory
   A. Infectious
      1. Toxoplasmosis and neosporosis
      2. Bacterial
      3. Leptospirosis
      4. Parasitic
   B. Immune-mediated
      1. Polymyositis
      2. Masticatory muscle myositis
      3. Dermatomyositis
II. Degenerative
   A. Acquired
      1. Endocrine
         a. Hyperadrenocorticism
         b. Hypothyroidism
         c. Miscellaneous
      2. Fibrotic/ossifying
         a. Infraspinatus contracture
         b. Quadriceps contracture
      3. Ischemic
      4. Nutritional
      5. Neoplastic
   B. Inherited
      1. Muscular dystrophy
         a. X-linked muscular dystrophy
         b. Labrador retriever myopathy
      2. Myotonia
      3. Metabolic
         a. Glycogen storage diseases
         b. Miscellaneous

tion of glucocorticoid therapy. Glucocorticoids can be withdrawn after several weeks in certain dogs without recurrence of signs, whereas others require more lengthy therapy. In dogs that do not respond to glucocorticoids, chemotherapeutic agents may be beneficial.

Masticatory Muscle Myositis

Clinical Findings. Masticatory muscle myositis typically affects large dogs. In acute cases, the masticatory muscles may be swollen. Pain is noted when the jaw is opened. Chronically affected dogs have marked, generally symmetric atrophy of the temporalis and masseter muscles.

Diagnosis. On specialized histochemical evaluation, type 2M fibers are selectively affected.

Treatment. Many affected dogs improve after initiation of glucocorticoids at dosages similar to those described for polymyositis. Even dogs with advanced atrophy and trismus may improve. Long-term therapy is necessary in some dogs.

DEGENERATIVE MYOPATHIES (pp. 731–735)

Endocrine Myopathies

A myopathy has been described in dogs with both spontaneous and iatrogenic hyperadrenocorticism (Chapter 118). Affected dogs have characteristic signs of hyperadrenocorticism in addition to generalized muscle atrophy and weakness. Unilateral pelvic limb stiffness often is the initial sign, with the other pelvic limb and, to a lesser extent, the thoracic limbs becoming involved later. Type 2 myofiber atrophy, without evidence of clinical neuromuscular disease, was noted in two adult dogs with hypothyroidism. Hyperthyroidism may cause weakness and ventral neck flexion in cats.

Feline Polymyopathy

Clinical Findings. Cervical ventroflexion, episodic weakness, and myalgia occur frequently.

Diagnosis. In addition to the characteristic clinical syndrome, most affected cats have elevated serum creatine kinase and decreased serum potassium.

Treatment. Most affected cats improve when the diet is changed to one with a greater potassium content or after dietary supplementation with potassium.

Fibrotic and Ossifying Myopathies

In myositis ossificans and related disorders, focal calcified masses typically occur within or adjacent to muscles. Separate syndromes associated with fibrosis of the quadriceps femoris and infraspinatus muscles have been described in dogs. Quadriceps fibrosis results in rigid extension of the stifle joint and is noted most commonly in young dogs with fracture disease. Dogs with infraspinatus fibrosis typically have elbow adduction and outward rotation of the antebrachium. Surgical relief of adhesions may be helpful.

INHERITED MYOPATHIES

X-Linked Muscular Dystrophy

Etiology and Pathogenesis. Both conditions principally cause clinical diseases in males, with females serving as carriers. Affected dog breeds include golden retrievers, Irish terriers, Samoyeds, rottweilers, Belgian shepherds, and a miniature schnauzer.

Clinical Findings. Clinical signs often progress rapidly between 3 and 6 months of age and then stabilize. Stilted gait, atrophy of particularly the truncal and temporalis muscles, a plantigrade stance, excessive drooling, lumbar kyphosis and later lordosis, and exercise intolerance are noted. Aspiration pneumonia and cardiac failure may develop.

Diagnosis. All affected animals thus far examined have had dramatic elevation of serum creatine kinase. On electromyographic evaluation, there are prominent complex repetitive discharges. Dystrophin deficiency, demonstrated either immunocytochemically or by Western blot analysis, substantiates the diagnosis of X-linked muscular dystrophy.

Treatment. There is currently no proven treatment.

Labrador Retriever Myopathy

Clinical Findings. Both yellow and black Labrador retrievers have been affected. The age of onset of clinical signs varies from 6 weeks to up to 7 months. Affected dogs characteristically have a stilted gait and advance their pelvic limbs simultaneously. There may be significant ventral neck flexion. The temporalis muscles often are atrophied. Signs do not progress significantly beyond 6 to 8 months of age.

Diagnosis. Clinical signs are fairly characteristic. Serum creatine kinase is only mildly elevated, if at all.

Treatment. There is no specific treatment, although use of diazepam may be beneficial.

Myotonia

Clinical Findings. Prominent stiffness at gait is noted in dogs when they first become ambulatory and lessens with further exercise. The pelvic limbs are more severely affected and are often advanced simultaneously. Most muscles are hypertrophied. Joints are stiff and cannot be flexed when there is severe involvement.

Diagnosis.   A diagnosis of myotonia is based on characteristic clinical signs and electromyographic evidence of high-frequency discharges that wax and wane ("dive bomber" sound). Muscle percussion results in a characteristic dimple.

Treatment.   Use of procainamide has been somewhat effective in affected chow chows.

Metabolic Myopathies

Disordered energy metabolism in affected individuals typically causes weakness and cramping with minimal exercise. Inherited enzymatic defects within the mitochondrial electron-transport (respiratory) chain generally are responsible. Typical histopathologic changes include bizarre mitochondria on ultrastructural evaluation and histochemical evidence of "ragged red" fibers.

Glycogen storage disease type II with associated myopathy has been reported in Lapland dogs. Affected dogs had progressive weakness, vomiting, regurgitation, and dysphonia. Dyserythropoiesis, cardiomegaly, and polymyopathy characterized by gross muscle atrophy and histologic evidence of myofiber size variation and poorly defined inclusions have been reported in English springer spaniels. Episodic weakness with associated exertional lactic acidosis was noted in two male Old English sheepdog littermates. Lipid storage has been noted in muscle in dogs with assorted myopathies, particularly with carnitine deficiency.

Nemaline Myopathy

Five related cats were first noted to be weak between 6 and 18 months of age and later developed a characteristic rapid, choppy, hypermetric gait. The skin twitched vigorously when two of the cats were examined. General deterioration necessitated euthanasia in each cat. Characteristic nemaline rods were common.

NEUROMUSCULAR CONDITIONS CAUSING HYPERTONICITY OR MYOCLONUS (p. 735)

See textbook.

SECTION VIII
THE RESPIRATORY SYSTEM

CHAPTER 87
CLINICAL PULMONARY FUNCTION TESTS
(pages 738–754)

Pulmonary function testing determines whether the respiratory system is performing its tasks of oxygenation and elimination of carbon dioxide.

PHYSICAL EXAMINATION (pp. 738–739)

The respiratory rate is an objective measure that can be obtained in all animals by minimally trained observers. The respiratory rate, posture, and mental attitude should be assessed together, as a severely compromised animal usually stands or sits with the head and neck extended, elbows abducted, mouth open, and a glazed expression.

When respiratory drive is increased (owing to chemical, mechanical, or central neural inputs), additional muscles are recruited: upper airway nasal and pharyngeal dilators and additional accessory chest-wall muscles during inspiration, and abdominal muscles during expiration. The flare of nostrils or contraction of the abdominal muscles may be visible or palpable during physical examination.

Mechanical factors that can increase work include airway obstruction, stiff lungs, or abnormalities of the pleural space (e.g., pleural effusions, masses, or diaphragmatic hernia). The resulting movements are termed *paradoxical* because they oppose the natural, normal expansion of the thorax.

Very small tidal volumes and a high frequency are compatible with stiff lungs or restricted expansion due to space-occupying pleural or thoracic wall diseases. Prolonged, deep breaths may be taken when airway narrowing is present.

LUNG MECHANICS (pp. 739–745)

LUNG MECHANICS IN THE AWAKE PATIENT: TIDAL BREATHING FLOW-VOLUME LOOPS (TBFVL)

TBFVL in Respiratory Disease

TBFVL analysis has been used to quantitate a variety of airway disorders of dogs. Airway obstructions can be of two types: fixed or nonfixed. Fixed obstructions may include those caused by masses, strictures, or

Original chapter written by Lesley G. King and Joan C. Hendricks external compression of the airway. Such obstructions affect both inspiratory and expiratory phases of the TBFVL, with decreases in both inspiratory and expiratory flow rates. Fixed obstructions of both intrathoracic and extrathoracic airways cause similar changes in the TBFVL.

Nonfixed upper airway (extrathoracic) obstructions are mobile and therefore primarily affect inspiration. Examples of nonfixed upper airway obstructions might include laryngeal paralysis and brachycephalic airway syndrome. TBFVL analysis in nonfixed upper airway obstructions demonstrates decreased inspiratory flow rates and a flattened inspiratory loop, but generally normal expiratory function.

Nonfixed obstruction of the lower airways (intrathoracic) produces primarily a flattening or concavity of the expiratory curve, with decreased flow rates late in expiration. Disorders such as chronic bronchitis or feline asthma may lead to thickening of the bronchial wall or mucosa, edema, mucus accumulation, and/or bronchoconstriction, narrowing the lumen and obstructing expiratory flow.

LUNG MECHANICS IN THE ANESTHETIZED PATIENT: LUNG COMPLIANCE AND RESISTANCE

Lung Resistance

The term *lung resistance* describes the *nonelastic* component of the lungs and chest wall, which acts to resist changes in volume.

Lung Compliance

Dynamic compliance and static compliance assess the function of the *elastic* component of the lung-chest system that resists change in lung volume. Compliance may appear to be affected by disorders that decrease lung volume (for example, pneumonectomy), whereas in fact there is normal elasticity of the remaining lung, but simply a smaller volume. Any disease process that causes stiffening of the parenchyma (e.g., inflammatory or infiltrative disorders) may lead to decreases in compliance. Similar decreases in elasticity are expected when there is atelectasis or a decrease in pulmonary surfactant.

Disorders that increase compliance, such as emphysema, are unusual in veterinary patients. Decreases in dynamic compliance at higher respiration rates are used to indicate disease of the small airways (<2 mm diameter). Since parenchymal disease processes will also decrease dynamic compliance, the use of the frequency dependence of dynamic compliance as a test of small airway disease is only appropriate if static compliance (assessing parenchymal function) and lung resistance (assessing function of the larger airways) are normal.

NONINVASIVE MEASURES OF VENTILATION IN THE UNANESTHETIZED PATIENT (p. 745)

VENTILATION-PERFUSION SCINTIGRAPHY

Although lung perfusion is affected by pulmonary thromboemboli, it can also be affected by hypoxic pulmonary vasoconstriction in areas of lung disease or by capillary bed destruction in such conditions as emphysema. Areas that are poorly ventilated represent areas of lung or airway disease.

DIRECT MEASUREMENT OF GAS EXCHANGE (pp. 745–748)

ARTERIAL BLOOD GAS TENSIONS

The most definitive measure of lung function remains the analysis of PO_2 and PCO_2 in arterial blood. These tests accurately characterize gas transfer from the alveoli to the blood. Exposure to room air, excess dilution of sample with heparin, storage of blood, and failure to obtain the animal's body temperature can introduce significant error into PO_2 and PCO_2 measurement.

Interpretation of Arterial Blood Gas Analysis

Animals with normal lung function, breathing room air, should be expected to have PaO_2 values greater than 85 mm Hg. However, hyperventilation can result in PaO_2 values as high as 120 mm Hg. A useful clinical rule of thumb is that the PaO_2 should increase by about five times the inspired oxygen concentration: an animal receiving 100 per cent oxygen (anesthetized and intubated) should have a PaO_2 of 500 mm Hg or more, and an animal receiving 40 per cent oxygen (nasopharyngeal oxygen or oxygen cage) should have a PaO_2 of 200 mm.

Decreases in PaO_2 result from one of the following: (1) decreased partial pressure of oxygen in inspired air, such as might occur with decreased barometric pressure at high altitudes; (2) hypoventilation, with decreased movement of air into the lungs, leading to less availability of oxygen for gas transfer (see below); and (3) venous admixture, resulting from shunting, ventilation/perfusion mismatch, or diffusion impairment.

Venous admixture is the cause of decreased PaO_2 in the great majority of clinical patients. Shunting can occur either by venous-arterial shunts that deliver venous blood directly to the arterial circulation (e.g., reverse PDA, bronchial anastomoses) or by blood flow to completely nonfunctional areas of lung, such as severely atelectatic areas or neoplastic masses. If shunting occurs, there is absolutely no possibility of oxygenation of the venous blood, no matter how much the inspired oxygen concentration is increased.

Disease processes such as airway or alveolar disease can change the pattern of ventilation. Similarly, vascular disorders such as thromboembolic disease can change the pattern of perfusion. Thus, significant mismatch of ventilation and perfusion can result, causing hypoxemia. In such cases, increasing inspired oxygen concentration may increase PaO_2.

Diffusion of oxygen across the alveolar-capillary membrane may be impaired by any process that leads to thickening of that membrane. Since CO_2 is about 20 times more soluble than O_2, diffusion almost never limits CO_2 transfer in the lungs. Thus, $PaCO_2$ primarily depends on the extent of ventilation. Hyperventilation such as might occur with acidosis, fear, pain, or pulmonary parenchymal disease results in low $PaCO_2$. Hypoventilation leads to increases in $PaCO_2$ and is commonly seen with disorders that affect the mechanical ability to move air into the lungs. Examples of such disorders include neurologic disease affecting central medullary respiratory drive, and spinal cord, phrenic nerve, chest wall, or respiratory muscle dysfunction. Increased $PaCO_2$ in hypoventilation is accompanied by decreased PaO_2. In a hypoventilating patient, oxygen supplementation will increase the PaO_2 but will result in no change in $PaCO_2$ values.

Oxygen Tension Based Indices

Calculation of the alveolar-arterial oxygen gradient ($P(A-a)O_2$) gives an estimate of the effectiveness of gas transfer while removing the variable contribution of the extent of ventilation. At sea level, in room air, and assuming RQ for the dog to be about 0.9 on typical diets, the alveolar gas equation can be simplified as:

$$PAO_2 = 150 - (PaCO_2)1.1$$

$$P(A-a)O_2 = PAO_2 - PaO_2$$

Normal values for the $P(A-a)O_2$ are less than 15 mm Hg. Increased gradients are seen in patients with pulmonary parenchymal disease.

Factors Influencing Normal Arterial Blood Gases in Dogs

Studies of normal dogs give a mean pH for the dog of 7.407 ± 0.028, $PaCO_2$ of 36.8 ± 3.0 mm Hg, and PaO_2 of 92.1 ± 5.6 mm Hg.

Normal Arterial Blood Gases in Cats

All reported studies have been performed in cats with surgically placed indwelling catheters in the femoral artery, descending aorta, or carotid artery. Most studies agree that the normal range for PaO_2 in the cat is close to 106.8 ± 5.7 mm Hg. Normal pH is 7.38 ± 0.038, and normal $PaCO_2$ is 31.0 ± 2.9 mm Hg. A recent study suggests additionally that significant errors may occur in analysis of arterial blood samples that are obtained from indwelling catheters, resulting in an average reduction of $PaCO_2$ induced by their sampling procedures of 6 per cent, independent of tubing length.

COMPARISONS OF VENOUS OR CAPILLARY SAMPLES WITH ARTERIAL SAMPLES

In animals with normal circulatory status, jugular or mixed venous samples could be substituted for arterial to assess ventilatory and acid/base status. It is important to remember that such substitution may be invalidated by factors such as induction of venous stasis for sample collection.

The presence of hypovolemia significantly widens the difference between arterial and central venous PCO_2 values and pH. In the dog, toenail blood pH, PCO_2, and HCO_3 correlated well with arterial samples, but there was poor correlation of PO_2. In the cat, good correlation was obtained for all parameters including PO_2. In the feline study, various techniques were used to ensure that the blood was arterialized, including heating the paw to increase arterial flow and elevating the paw to decrease venous back flow.

Lingual venous PO_2 may be useful as a screening test, since acceptable PO_2 values in the lingual vein indicate that acceptable oxygen tensions exist in arterial blood. The finding of a low PO_2 in the lingual vein should prompt evaluation of PaO_2 to confirm hypoxemia.

INDIRECT MEASUREMENT OF GAS EXCHANGE
(pp. 748–751)

PULSE OXIMETRY

Although oxyhemoglobin saturation (SaO_2) is not linearly related to arterial PO_2, the SaO_2 provides information about tissue delivery of oxygen that is clinically important and is complementary to PO_2.

Respiratory wave-forms and movement have been noted to interfere with pulse oximetry in animals. Among the factors that interfere with accurate SPO_2 measurements in man, variation in skin color, decreased perfusion, hypothermia, increased serum bilirubin concentration, and anemia might be expected to be present in some small animal patients.

In general, the end-tidal CO_2 monitor should be used to provide complementary, additional information between arterial blood gas analyses. Appropriate uses include (1) identifying hypoventilation in nonpanting patients, (2) continuous monitoring between arterial blood samples, (3) reducing the frequency of arterial blood samples, (4) verifying continuity of the patient's airway, (5) serving as an apnea monitor, especially during weaning from mechanical ventilation, and (6) providing some information about CO_2 in patients in whom arterial samples absolutely cannot be obtained.

TRANSCUTANEOUS OXYGEN AND CARBON DIOXIDE MONITORING

In the presence of hypovolemia, hypothermia, vasculitis, or edema, significant differences may occur between measured transcutaneous and arterial O_2 values.

DYNAMIC IMAGING TECHNIQUES (pp. 751–753)

LARYNGOSCOPY

The vocal folds of the normally innervated larynx abduct to widen the airway during inspiration. As the plane of anesthesia lightens, the animal may begin vocalizing (whining), and this adduction narrows the airway during expiration. The depth of anesthesia at which these normal movements occur varies among animals; thus, some animals will not show obvious movement until they are nearly awake so that jaw tone and the gag reflex have returned.

FLUOROSCOPY

Fluoroscopy is perhaps most commonly used to evaluate the degree of airway collapse during expiration in dogs with suspected collapsing tracheas. We have also found it useful in documenting bronchial collapse, a common feature during expiration in chronic bronchitis. With disease that increases airway compliance, the intrathoracic airways dilate during inspiration and narrow during expiration. The pattern is reversed in the cervical trachea. Although the common conditions that lead to tracheobronchial collapse are those that increase airway compliance, changes in mechanics (such as increased force of inspiratory muscle action in the face of a more cranial obstruction) can also lead to changes in airway diameter. Diaphragmatic paralysis can also be appreciated with fluoroscopy.

CHAPTER 88

DISEASES OF THE TRACHEA
(pages 754–766)

HISTORY AND PHYSICAL EXAMINATION (p. 755)

The most commonly recognized clinical signs of tracheal disease are coughing; stertorous, noisy inspiratory sounds; stridulous or wheezing expiratory sounds; pulmonary edema; and occasionally cyanosis. The entire neck should be palpated for evidence of surrounding disease such as subcutaneous emphysema, lymphadenectomies, abscess, cyst, neoplasia, thyroid gland enlargement, or any other mass that may involve the trachea. Auscultation of the thorax and lung sounds, as well as respiratory sounds directly over the trachea, larynx, and nose, should be compared to help localize the lesion.

DIAGNOSTIC TESTS (pp. 755–756)

RADIOGRAPHY

The lateral radiographic examination must be performed with careful positioning of the patient to avoid artifactual deviations of the trachea, especially in the caudal cervical and cranial mediastinal regions. Dorsal deviation of the intrathoracic trachea can be due to cardiac enlargement (especially right heart enlargement), pleural effusion, cra-

Original chapter written by Kyle A. Brayley and Stephen J. Ettinger

nial mediastinal masses, and excessive ventroflexion of the neck. Ventral deviation of the thoracic trachea can be seen with a dilated, fluid-filled esophagus or with diseases of the dorsal cranial mediastinum.

Tracheal radiographs should be surveyed for continuity of the mucosal lining, diameter, and placement within the cervical and thoracic regions. The normal ventrodorsal diameter of the trachea at the third rib should be approximately three times the width of the third rib at the level of the trachea. Contrast studies of the tracheal lumen (bronchography) are indicated in cases showing signs of tracheal rupture or fracture, when suspected radiolucent foreign bodies may not be evident on noncontrast survey radiographs, and when a more detailed examination of the luminal surface is required. Contrast materials should not be introduced into the respiratory system when acute pulmonary disease is accompanied by fever or recent hemoptysis, when there is hypersensitivity to the contrast material, in chronic nephritis when iodine materials are being used, when vital lung capacity is depressed, in acute bronchitis, or with severe emphysema. Fluoroscopy is extremely valuable, if not indispensable, for the study of the collapsed trachea and other coughing syndromes.

TRACHEOSCOPY/BRONCHOSCOPY

Endoscopy can be used for direct visualization of the tracheal mucosa and identifying evidence of inflammation, ulceration, and edema; for visualizing and obtaining biopsy specimens of tumors and masses; for brush cytology, fluid aspiration, and cultures; for removal of foreign bodies; for demonstration of collapsed, hypoplastic, stenotic, disrupted, or compressed areas; and for evaluation of disease progression or response to therapy.

TRACHEOBRONCHIAL CULTURE AND CYTOLOGY

The tracheal cytologic specimen from a normal animal should include a few to a moderate number of neutrophils, epithelial cells, and goblet cells; a few macrophages; and a few to rare lymphocytes and eosinophils. Neutrophilic inflammation most often results from bacterial infections, which can be secondary to a number of other problems including, but not limited to, collapsed trachea, chronic bronchitis, neoplasia, allergic disease, and viral, mycotic, or parasitic infections. Major differential diagnoses of eosinophilic inflammation include allergic bronchitis, pulmonary parasites, heartworm disease, and hypersensitivity responses secondary to bacterial, protozoal, fungal, or neoplastic diseases. Chronic inflammation is indicated by a mixed inflammatory cell population with a predominant number of activated macrophages.

SPECIFIC TRACHEAL DISEASES (pp. 756–766)

NONINFECTIOUS TRACHEITIS

Noninfectious tracheitis is usually a secondary problem to prolonged barking, collapsing trachea, chronic cardiac disease, and diseases of the oropharynx. Tracheitis may be primary (inhalation of smoke or other noxious gases). Most patients with tracheitis are asymptomatic except for a cough, which is usually characterized as resonant, harsh, paroxysmal, and often terminated by nonproductive or slightly productive gagging.

Therapy should be directed at the primary underlying disease process. Tracheal coughing is often treated with antitussive and bronchodilating preparations. Many of these preparations also contain expectorants. Occasionally, short-term therapy with corticosteroids may be warranted. It is important to emphasize that this provides symptomatic relief only, and it may exacerbate the primary condition.

INFECTIOUS CANINE TRACHEOBRONCHITIS

Infectious canine tracheobronchitis is highly contagious and most commonly occurs where groups of dogs of different ages and susceptibilities are congregated. Clinical signs usually develop 3 to 5 days after initial exposure. The clinical signs are generally mild and self-limiting. A dry, hacking, and often paroxysmal cough is the most consistent sign.

Uncomplicated cases of tracheobronchitis probably do not require antimicrobials. Glucocorticoids, administered at anti-inflammatory doses, can be effective in suppressing the cough of uncomplicated infectious tracheobronchitis. However, glucocorticoids do not appear to shorten the clinical course of the disease. Antitussives, either alone or in combination with bronchodilators, may also be of benefit in suppressing the cough through their ability to prevent bronchospasm.

FILAROIDES OSLERI (Lungworm)

Filaroides osleri infection is a world-wide parasitic disease seen most often in dogs under 2 years of age. It can be seen in individual situations but is more often seen as a kennel-related problem (especially in greyhounds). Dogs usually present with chronic, mild to severe inspiratory wheezing sounds, dyspnea, coughing, and/or debilitation.

The radiographic examination is helpful if the disease process is extensive and the nodules are large. Direct bronchoscopic examination is safe and more specific. Cream-colored nodules, 1 to 5 mm high and wide, are usually diagnostic. The larvae are often seen peeking into the luminal edge of the growth. Brushings and biopsies of the nodules provide a definitive diagnosis. Larvae are occasionally detected in the feces.

Many drugs have been reported to be effective in treating lungworms, such as thiacetarsamide sodium, thiabendazole, diethylcarbamazine, levamisole, fenbendazole, and albendazole. Because of the lack of success with the previously mentioned drugs, one of the authors (SJE) has treated several dogs with oral ivermectin at 1000 µg/lb once weekly for 2 months. The nodules were reduced in size but did not resolve entirely. All of these dogs became asymptomatic and continued to thrive.

TRACHEAL HYPOPLASIA

This disease is recognized primarily in young, brachycephalic animals. Common clinical signs include dyspnea, stridor, and coughing. Occasionally, dogs present with a moist, productive cough, moist rales on auscultation, and a fever associated with bronchopneumonia.

The radiographic features are the most important and usually provide the definitive diagnosis. Many patients with slight to moderate hypoplastic tracheas can live normal, satisfactory lives with only an occasional need for bronchodilator therapy and antibiotics. We have also seen young dogs with this diagnosis apparently outgrow the condition.

SEGMENTAL TRACHEAL STENOSIS

Segmental tracheal stenosis may occur as a congenital lesion, or it may result from trauma to the trachea. The syndrome produces stridorous respiratory distress and subsequent cyanosis. Radiographic studies usually establish the diagnosis. The mainstay of treatment is surgical resection of the stenotic region.

COLLAPSED TRACHEA

The lateral form is unusual and occurs most commonly after central chondrotomy has been used as a method of treating the dorsoventral from of collapse. Dorsoventral flattening (narrowing of the trachea) is a commonly described lesion that is often associated with a pendulous, redundant dorsal tracheal membrane. The collapsed trachea may involve the cervical region only, but more commonly both the cervical and thoracic areas of the trachea are involved, and the collapse frequently extends into the bronchi.

Tracheal collapse sometimes produces a "respiratory distress syndrome." The disease is usually paroxysmal in nature, often with a long history of chronic coughing. With rare exception, the disease is recognized in toy and miniature breeds, most often Chihuahuas, Pomeranians, toy poodles, Shih Tzus, Lhasa apsos, and Yorkshire terriers. The characteristic cough is elicited by excitement, tracheal pressure (such as that caused by pulling on a leash), and drinking water or eating food. Perhaps the most significant finding during the physical examination is the elicitation of a "goose honk" cough when the trachea is palpated in the region of the thoracic inlet.

Radiographic examination of patients with collapsed tracheas requires both still and motion studies. Lateral radiographs made during both the maximum inspiratory phase and expiratory phase of the respiratory cycle are needed to demonstrate a dynamic collapsing trachea. The list of causes of coughing that could be confused with collapsed trachea is extensive (Chapter 12).

The majority of cases can be successfully treated symptomatically. Bronchodilator preparations containing expectorants and sedatives usually suffice to control this disease (see Table 88–1 in the textbook). In some cases, hospitalization with sedation for a period of several days, associated with corticosteroid therapy and nebulization, helps to reduce the degree of associated tracheitis. Occasionally, when other therapy fails, we have found that digitalization, for some unexplained reason, can be of assistance in controlling this cough. It is important to recognize that other disease states may be present. Variable results have been reported on the surgical correction of this condition.

OBSTRUCTIVE TRACHEAL MASSES

The lesion may be intraluminal, as in the case of primary tracheal neoplasia, or an extraluminal compressive mass. In dogs and cats, squamous cell carcinoma, histiocytic lymphosarcoma, lymphoblastic lymphosarcoma, osteosarcoma, adenocarcinoma, osteoma, chondroma, osteochondroma, chondrosarcoma, and leiomyoma have been described. Other types of intraluminal masses include nodular amyloidosis, eosinophilic granulomas, abscesses, chronic granulomas, and tracheal foreign bodies.

Clinical signs depend on the degree of obstruction present. Most animals present with stridor and loud ronchi (rattling in the throat). Overzealous examination and performance of diagnostic studies may disturb the patient, thereby worsening the condition.

Lateral and dorsoventral radiographic views should be obtained if the patient can tolerate them. Tracheal masses may decrease luminal size in a nonlinear manner, resulting in a mass protruding into the lumen. This is in contradistinction to the silhouette produced by masses that may be extraluminal, in which the line produced by the luminal air-mucosa interface is seen to pass uninterrupted through the mass. Concomitant narrowing of the trachea and esophagus in the cranial mediastinum is highly suggestive of an extraluminal mass. Bronchoscopy can also help in reaching a definitive diagnosis by allowing the retrieval of cytologic specimens of masses or even the obtainment of biopsies.

Some foreign bodies can be removed endoscopically, and some smaller tracheal masses may be removed by means of a suction biopsy device attached to the bronchoscope. For those that can't, the mainstay of therapy is surgical removal or resection. In the treatment of obstructive tracheal disease, the use of endotracheal intubation or tracheostomy, or both, is paramount.

TRACHEAL TRAUMA

Some relatively common causes of this condition include bite wounds to the neck incurred during a dog or cat fight, transtracheal wash procedure, and inadvertent laceration of the trachea during jugular venous puncture. In some cases, the subcutaneous emphysema involves only the peritracheal region, although it may become considerably more extensive and involve the entire subcutaneous area of the body. Such tears may also be responsible for the development of pneumomediastinum in both the dog and the cat.

Positive contrast studies, using water-soluble organic iodide solution instead of a barium suspension, are indicated when the location of the lesion is not obvious from the noncontrast radiographic examination. Bronchoscopy can also be used to visualize the point of tracheal mucosal interruption.

If the subcutaneous air collection is regressing and there are no signs of pulmonary distress, it is usually recommended that the patient be cage rested, allowing the emphysema to regress by slow absorption. If the condition is becoming further aggravated by continued air leakage, then closure of the laceration site with surgery is essential. Perhaps of greater importance is the effort to detect other pathologic conditions such as pneumothorax or hemothorax.

CHAPTER 89

DISEASES OF THE LOWER RESPIRATORY SYSTEM
(pages 767–812)

BRONCHIAL DISEASES (pp. 767–778)

Patients with bronchial disease commonly are presented with coughing as the major complaint. Other signs of lower respiratory tract disease are exercise intolerance, increased respiratory efforts, and cyanosis. Systemic signs such as weight loss, anorexia, and depression occur in severely affected animals.

Canine Infectious Tracheobronchitis

The organisms commonly associated with the disease are canine adenovirus 2 (CAV2), canine parainfluenza virus (CPV), and *Bordetella bronchiseptica*.

Presentation. Dogs are presented with an acute onset of bronchial signs. A honking cough is often worse with exercise and may be productive or nonproductive. Gagging, retching, or nasal discharge can occur. A careful history will frequently reveal exposure to a new puppy or to dogs during kenneling, hospitalization, or showing. Coughing can be induced by tracheal palpation.

Diagnostic Evaluation. The CBC is typically unremarkable. Thoracic radiographs are generally normal, although a mild bronchial

---

Original chapter written by Eleanor C. Hawkins

pattern can occur. Tracheal wash fluid analysis reveals increased neutrophils. Bacteria may be apparent. Virus isolation can be performed.

Treatment. Most cases resolve without treatment within 7 to 10 days, although some untreated dogs continue to cough for several weeks. *Cough suppressants* are indicated only if the cough is nonproductive and is persistent. Dextromethorphan hydrobromide is a mild suppressant. Hydrocodone bitartrate is a potent narcotic cough suppressant. Butorphanol is also a potent cough suppressant. Antibiotics are indicated when there are complications or signs of systemic involvement. Chloramphenicol, tetracycline, and quinolones have been found to be effective against *Bordetella* isolates *in vitro*. The high end of the recommended dosage range generally should be used. Clinical improvement should be noted within 3 to 5 days, but the drug should be continued for a minimum of 14 days. Unresponsive infections may benefit from nebulized antibiotics (e.g., gentocin).

Prevention and Control. Prevention in pet animals is best achieved through avoidance of exposure. Parenteral vaccines against CAV2 and CPV are readily available in combination with canine distemper virus vaccines. Vaccines against *Bordetella* are available for parenteral and intranasal administration. Vaccination against *Bordetella* is recommended only for high-risk patients or kennel situations, and intranasal vaccines are preferred.

Feline Bronchitis (Feline Asthma)

Moise and associates have suggested the following classification for feline bronchial disease based on nomenclature for bronchial disease in man.

Bronchial Asthma. Bronchial asthma refers to reversible lower airway obstruction resulting primarily from bronchoconstriction. Smooth muscle hypertrophy, increased mucus, and eosinophilic inflammation contribute to clinical signs. A type I hypersensitivity response is generally blamed. Often an inciting cause cannot be identified.

Acute Bronchitis. Acute bronchitis describes reversible airway inflammation of relatively short duration. Acute bronchitis may occur as a result of viral, bacterial, mycoplasmal, or parasitic infection.

Chronic Bronchitis. Chronic bronchitis refers to prolonged airway inflammation, usually for more than 2 to 3 months. Irreversible damage, such as fibrosis, occurs as a result of the chronic inflammation. Cats with chronic bronchitis may have concurrent bronchial asthma.

Emphysema. Emphysema refers to the enlargement of peripheral airspaces with destruction of bronchiolar and alveolar walls. Grossly visible cavitary lesions, bullae, can occur. Emphysema may be the result of, or occur concurrently with, chronic bronchitis.

Presentation. Most common presenting signs are cough and respiratory distress. Episodic respiratory distress, usually with cough, is suggestive of bronchial asthma. Such cats are often asymptomatic between episodes. Cough of sudden onset that resolves within several weeks is consistent with acute bronchitis. Long-standing cough, often with increased respiratory effort, is consistent with chronic bronchitis.

Physical examination findings vary. A cat presented between episodes may show no obvious abnormalities. Expiratory wheezes and crackles may be ausculted with more advanced disease. With severe involvement, the cat may be presented in severe respiratory distress with open mouth breathing, cyanosis, and a pronounced abdominal component to expiration. Occasionally, decreased sounds are ausculted due to air trapping.

Diagnostic Evaluation. Thoracic radiographs classically reveal a bronchial pattern. Interstitial patterns and patchy alveolar densities can occur. Cats with bronchial asthma may exhibit no radiographic changes. During severe asthmatic attacks or with chronic disease, hyperinflation of the lungs may result in increased radiolucency and flattening of the diaphragm. Circulating eosinophilia may be present in some cats with bronchial asthma. It is not a consistent finding.

Tracheal or bronchial wash fluid may consist primarily of eosinophils, nondegenerative neutrophils, or activated macrophages. Careful examination should always be performed for evidence of bacteria and parasitic ova *(Capillaria, Paragonimus)* or larvae *(Aelurostrongylus)*. Examination is also performed for protozoa *(Toxoplasma)*, fungal agents, and criteria of malignancy. Some clinically normal cats have high numbers of eosinophils in bronchoalveolar lavage specimens. Their significance must be determined in conjunction with other clinical information.

Bacterial and mycoplasmal cultures should be performed routinely. Cultured organisms can represent normal flora, the primary cause of signs, or secondary invaders of a diseased lung. Special fecal concentration techniques should be performed to investigate for underlying parasitic disease, particularly if eosinophilic inflammation is present. Heartworm testing should also be considered.

Treatment. A cat presenting in severe respiratory distress should be treated symptomatically until its condition will permit specific diagnostic evaluation. A rapid-acting corticosteroid should be administered intravenously or intramuscularly. Oxygen should be administered, preferably in a cage. Glucocorticoids, oxygen, and rest nearly always results in stabilization. In rare cases, more aggressive therapy with epinephrine is necessary.

In the stable cat, management of bronchitis consists of elimination of any identifiable underlying etiology, anti-inflammatory therapy, and bronchodilators. Environmental sources of antigen are rarely discovered.

Any infectious agents are treated directly. In most bacterial infections, routine administration of appropriate antibiotics is sufficient. Treatment of bacterial infection is ideally based on results of sensitivity testing. Chloramphenicol or a tetracycline should be administered if mycoplasmal infection is suspected. Parasitic organisms are treated as indicated.

If an infectious etiology is not identified, anti-inflammatory therapy with corticosteroids is rapidly effective in controlling signs in the majority of cases. Prednisone or prednisolone is preferred. Once signs are controlled, the amount of drug is rapidly tapered to alternate-evening therapy at the lowest effective dosage. The amount of steroids required to control signs is extremely variable. The duration of therapy necessary is also variable, with some cats requiring lifelong treatment and some cats requiring only a single or occasional course of therapy.

Bronchodilators can be helpful in controlling signs and may decrease the dosage of corticosteroids required. Methylxanthines, sympathomimetic drugs, and anticholinergic drugs can be used for their bronchodilating properties. In cases that do not respond to bronchodilator therapy or if toxicity is suspected, the dosage should be assessed by measurement of plasma concentrations. Sympathomimetic drugs cause bronchodilation through beta$_2$ adrenergic effects. The two most clinically useful sympathomimetic drugs for use in cats are epinephrine and terbutaline.

Cats that do not respond to therapy and those that experience sudden worsening of signs during constant levels of therapy should be reevaluated for inciting or complicating disease. Cats with severe chronic bronchitis may benefit from nebulization.

Canine Bronchitis

Acute bronchitis refers to inflammation of relatively short duration with reversible airway changes. Inflammation that persists longer than 2 months and results in permanent airway damage is referred to as chronic bronchitis. Underlying etiologies may be present. Considerations include viral, bacterial, or mycoplasmal infections, pulmonary parasites, heartworm disease, allergic disease, inhaled irritants, and foreign bodies. Many cases are idiopathic in origin.

Allergic bronchitis in the dog is not a well-defined clinical entity. The term is used to describe bronchitis with eosinophilic inflammation that responds to elimination of offending allergens or corticosteroid therapy. Dogs with signs of allergic bronchitis can have coexisting problems, such as chronic bronchitis, bacterial infection, and tracheal collapse.

Chronic bronchitis is defined as a persistent cough occurring for at least 2 consecutive months in the past year in the absence of a specific pulmonary disease. Factors initiating the pathologic changes are not known. Signs occur as a result of inflammation, increased secretions, and chronic obstructive pulmonary disease. As the chronic bronchitis progresses, bullous emphysema and bronchiectasis may further aggravate signs.

Presentation. Coughing is the classic presenting sign in dogs with bronchitis. The cough may or may not be productive and is often exacerbated by exercise or excitement. The attitude and appetite are usually normal. Small to medium-sized, middle-aged to older adult dogs are most commonly affected with chronic bronchitis. On physical examination the patients are often overweight. Auscultation may reveal normal airway sounds, increased breath sounds, crackles from excessive mucus or exudate, or expiratory wheezes from airway obstruction. A pronounced or split second heart sound may be heard due to secondary pulmonary hypertension. Tracheal collapse, tracheitis, or mitral insufficiency may be detected as a concurrent problem. Remember that dogs presenting with cough and a cardiac murmur are not always in heart failure, and treating them as such can be harmful.

Diagnostic Evaluation. Thoracic radiography classically reveals a bronchial pattern. Patchy peripheral alveolar densities can occur owing to decreased clearance of mucus, secondary bronchopneumonia, or, in cases with eosinophilic inflammation, a more generalized hypersensitivity reaction. Air trapping can sometimes be appreciated as hyperinflated lungs with flattening of the diaphragm.

Complete blood counts are generally unremarkable. Possible abnormalities include mature neutrophilia, polycythemia, neutrophilic leukocytosis and left shift, or eosinophilia. Tracheal wash fluid should be collected for cytologic and microbiologic analysis. Epithelial cells may demonstrate hyperplastic changes. Eosinophilic inflammation is consistent with allergic bronchitis. Septic inflammation suggests bacterial infection. Fluid from dogs with uncomplicated chronic bronchitis may have minimal inflammatory cell infiltrates. Bacteria may be isolated by culture, and sensitivity testing can be valuable. Ancillary tests include multiple fecal examinations for lungworms and heartworm testing.

Treatment. The treatment of choice for allergic bronchitis is the elimination of the offending antigen. If the antigen is infectious, the appropriate antimicrobial drug is given. If an underlying cause is not identifiable, corticosteroids are administered. There is no single treatment that will effectively control signs of chronic bronchitis in all patients. Intense management is often required.

Initial treatment should be aimed at eliminating factors contributing to the sudden worsening of signs. Such factors may include inhalation of irritants, excitement, and infection. Thereafter, a trial with *bronchodilator* therapy is instituted. The most useful bronchodilators are the theophyllines and beta$_2$ agonists. Systemic dehydration should be avoided and diuretics are contraindicated. Nebulization of saline increases the moisture content of airway secretions and has additional mucolytic properties. Nebulization is performed for 10 to 30 minutes at a time, one or more times daily, and should be followed by coupage or mild activity.

Weight loss should be aggressively pursued in all overweight patients. Cough suppressants are indicated to control continuous or fatiguing nonproductive coughs. Corticosteroids often improve clinical signs and may slow the airway changes associated with chronic inflammation, but the added insult to pulmonary defenses in an already compromised patient makes such therapy potentially harmful. If a beneficial effect is seen, the dosage is quickly tapered to the least effective amount.

Prognosis. The prognosis for controlling clinical signs of allergic bronchitis is good. However, intermittent therapy is often required.

Bronchiectasis

Bronchiectasis refers to dilation of bronchi, and it is generally an irreversible change. The dilation greatly interferes with normal airway clearance, and mucus and exudate tend to accumulate distal to the abnormality. Secondary infection is common. Diffuse bronchiectasis is most common, although the dependent lung lobes are often most severely involved. In small animals, bronchiectasis appears to occur as a complication of inflammatory pulmonary disease, such as infection, allergic bronchitis, or pulmonary infiltrates with eosinophils.

Presentation. Patients are presented with signs of chronic airway disease, primarily cough, and the cough is usually productive. Bacterial pneumonia may be present. The diagnosis is generally based on thoracic radiographs. The airway walls do not appear parallel and lose their normal gentle taper. The diameter of the airway lumina is greater than expected away from the central lung. Additional studies are rarely indicated solely to document bronchiectasis. Collection of airway specimens, through tracheal wash or bronchoscopy, is indicated for cytologic and microbiologic analysis.

Therapeutic recommendations are generally the same as for chronic bronchitis. These cases are especially prone to recurrent infections, and corticosteroid therapy should be avoided unless indicated for primary treatment. Surgical resection should be considered only if changes are localized and there is poor response to medical management. Bronchiectasis tends to be a permanent change, and chronic management is generally required.

Primary Ciliary Dyskinesia (Immotile Cilia Syndrome)

The respiratory system is extremely dependent on functioning cilia for effective clearance of respiratory secretions, inhaled particles, and infectious agents. Ciliary dyskinesia is a result of one or more defects of ciliary microtubules identifiable by electron microscopy. Many different clinical features are possible. Ciliary dysfunction can result in otitis media, hearing loss, hydrocephalus, dilated renal tubules, and male infertility. The majority of cases have been identified in puppies or young dogs. Persistent bilateral nasal discharge is a frequent presenting sign. A productive cough is common. Other organs can be affected.

In many cases routine diagnostic evaluation reveals evidence of respiratory infection. Radiographs may reveal bronchitis, bronchiectasis, or bronchopneumonia. Situs inversus in conjunction with respiratory infection or infertility is an extremely suggestive finding. Cytologic and microbiologic analysis of tracheal wash fluid is critical for successful management. Septic inflammation is often apparent cytologically. Bacterial and mycoplasmal cultures and sensitivity tests should be performed.

The definitive diagnosis is made by electron microscopy of nasal mucosa or tracheal mucosa or spermatozoa. Ciliary dyskinesia cannot be directly treated. Bacterial infections are treated with appropriate antibiotics as they occur. Cough suppressants and corticosteroids are contraindicated. Prognosis in canine cases is guarded. Some animals have been maintained for as long as 12 years.

Bronchial Foreign Bodies

Hunting breeds are prone to grass foreign bodies. Puppies may aspirate foreign bodies during play. Patients are often presented with an acute onset of severe, paroxysmal, nonproductive coughing or respiratory distress. Signs may be more consistent with chronic pneumonia. Presentation of dogs may be delayed for as long as 3 years following the initial development of signs. Radiographically, a soft tissue or mineral density may be apparent in the airways, although this finding is uncommon. With time, localized bronchial, interstitial, or alveolar densities may be visible owing to secondary infection.

The definitive diagnosis is generally made with bronchoscopy. Plant foreign bodies may be completely hidden with mucopurulent exudate. Careful suctioning of the airways is necessary. For animals with recurring pneumonia, thoracic radiographs should be evaluated soon after initiation of antibiotics and within 1 week of discontinuation of antibiotics in an attempt to identify a focal source of persistent infection or inflammation. Such a focus may represent a foreign body, and bronchoscopy or surgical exploration is indicated.

Treatment consists of removal of the foreign body, generally through bronchoscopy or lobectomy. Secondary bacterial infections are treated with appropriate antibiotic therapy. When a foreign body is identified and can be removed, the prognosis is excellent. Some foreign bodies, especially grass awns, may escape detection and result in chronic pulmonary disease. They may also migrate through the body to cause pneumothorax, pyothorax, discospondylitis, or signs of invasion of other organs. Delay in diagnosis and treatment of grass awn foreign bodies until after the development of diffuse pleuropneumonia is associated with a grave prognosis.

Bronchial Compression

Compression can be the result of hilar lymphadenopathy, left atrial enlargement, or pulmonary neoplasia. Compression generally involves the mainstem bronchi, identifiable radiographically.

Bronchoesophageal Fistulas

These occur most frequently as a result of esophageal foreign bodies, which penetrate the wall of the esophagus and involve an adjacent airway. Congenital fistulas or fistulas resulting from trauma or neoplasia also can occur. Recurrent aspiration pneumonia and sometimes pleuritis may be sequelae. The diagnosis is made through contrast radiography or bronchoscopy. The problem is corrected surgically.

PULMONARY DISEASES (pp. 778–809)

SUPPORT OF THE COMPROMISED PATIENT

Oxygen Supplementation

Hypoxemia can result from hypoventilation or from ventilation: perfusion abnormalities. Causes of hypoventilation include upper airway obstruction; diseases affecting pulmonary or thoracic wall compliance, such as pleural effusion, pneumothorax, and extreme abdominal distention; and decreased function of respiratory muscles. Most pulmonary parenchymal diseases cause ventilation : perfusion mismatching.

Degree of hypoxia is readily assessed by measurement of the partial pressure of oxygen in arterial blood (PaO_2). Therapeutic intervention is recommended when the PaO_2 falls below 60 mm Hg or the $PaCO_2$ rises above 60 to 75 mm Hg. In the absence of blood gas analysis, such signs as cyanosis, "muddy" mucous membranes, deterioration in mental status, or cardiac arrhythmias in conjunction with increased respiratory efforts are clear indications for treatment of hypoxemia. Cyanosis is generally observed at oxygen tensions less than 50 mm Hg.

Hypoxemia resulting from ventilation:perfusion abnormalities generally responds readily to increased alveolar oxygen concentration. An exception exists with complete arteriovenous shunts.

Some pulmonary parenchymal diseases are so severe that blood oxygen tensions cannot be adequately maintained without prolonged administration of 100 per cent oxygen, or are associated with collapse of alveoli and decreased compliance. In these situations positive pressure ventilatory support, as well as oxygen supplementation, is necessary. Humidification is essential if oxygen administration is necessary for more than a few hours to avoid severe airway drying. Oxygen supplementation can be provided through masks, transtracheal catheters, nasal catheters, oxygen cages, and tracheal tubes.

Patients that are sedated, unconscious, or otherwise limited in mobility are at increased risk for the development of atelectasis of the dependent lung lobes and pneumonia. Recumbent animals should be turned frequently. Coupage of conscious animals with limited mobility may encourage coughing and mobilization of airway secretions.

Airway Humidification

Maintaining airway hydration should be a consideration in all patients with lower respiratory disease. The most important method of maintaining airway hydration is maintaining the systemic hydration of the patient. The addition of water to inspired gases is indicated in patients receiving oxygen supplementation for more than a few hours. Nebulizers can be used to administer saline droplets to the airways. When oxygen therapy is being used, nebulization is recommended for 10 to 30 minutes every 4 to 8 hours.

Ventilation

Ventilatory support can be provided on an emergency basis with an anesthetic machine or ambu bag. The prolonged maintenance of a patient requires a ventilator. Four types of ventilatory support are intermittent positive pressure ventilation (IPPV), positive end-expiratory pressure (PEEP), continuous positive airway pressure (CPAP), and high-frequency ventilation (HF). Generally, patients are initially given IPPV, which is comparable to "bagging" the patient by hand. Pressures of 15 to 20 cm of water are generally adequate. Higher pressures may be necessary to overcome decreased compliance of diseased lungs.

Success of ventilation is judged by blood gas analysis. If there is inadequate response, PEEP can be initiated. The patient must exhale against the mild positive expiratory pressure, and early airway closure is countered. However, the increased pressure can severely compromise venous return. Continuous positive airway pressure is similar to PEEP except that increased pressure is maintained within the airways throughout expiration and inspiration. High-frequency ventilation has not gained widespread use in clinical veterinary medicine.

Patients who have been maintained with ventilatory support must be gradually weaned from the ventilator, since the maintenance of normal or low $PaCO_2$ will interfere with the normal respiratory drive. Support is discontinued slowly to allow the $PaCO_2$ to increase. If the patient does not begin normal, spontaneous ventilation, the support is resumed and discontinuation attempted later.

VIRAL DISEASES

Canine Distemper (see Chapter 69)

Other Canine Viral Pneumonias (see Chapter 69)

Feline Calicivirus Infection (see Chapter 70)

Feline Infectious Peritonitis (see Chapter 70)

Feline Retroviral Infections

Feline leukemia or feline immunodeficiency virus may result in other diseases with pulmonary involvement, such as malignant lymphoma, toxoplasmosis, and FIP.

RICKETTSIAL DISEASES

Rickettsia rickettsii and *Ehrlichia canis* may result in signs of pneumonitis, dyspnea, or cough.

BACTERIAL DISEASES

Bacterial Pneumonia

Primary bacterial infection in dogs can occur as a result of *Bordetella bronchiseptica* and possibly *Streptococcus zooepidemicus*. Other bacteria can also result in pneumonia, presumably as opportunistic invaders. Bacterial infection may complicate nearly any other pulmonary disease process. Possible primary etiologies include aspiration due to megaesophagus or bronchoesophageal fistulas, foreign bodies, viral infections, bronchial disease, neoplasia, contusions, lung parasites, mycotic infections, and others.

Presentation. Animals are often presented with localizing signs such as cough, exercise intolerance, respiratory distress, and nasal discharge. Mucopurulent nasal discharge and an increased respiratory effort may be apparent. Mucous membranes may be cyanotic with severe disease or following exertion. Lung sounds are usually increased, with crackles audible over all or part of the lung fields. Fever is inconsistently present.

Diagnostic Evaluation. Thoracic radiographs may show only an interstitial pattern early in the disease. An alveolar pattern develops as the disease progresses. Focal lesions may be associated with foreign bodies. Involvement primarily of the dependent lung lobes is supportive of concurrent airway disease or aspiration. Hematogenously borne infections may have a caudodorsal distribution.

Radiographs are examined for hilar lymphadenopathy, pulmonary artery enlargement, or mass lesions, which are characteristic of other diseases. It is common to find only a stress response or a normal leukogram.

Tracheal wash fluid analysis should be obtained *prior* to the administration of antibiotics in order to confirm the diagnosis and to obtain antibiotic sensitivity information. Cytologic evaluation typically reveals septic inflammation. The specimen always should be cultured for identification of bacteria and sensitivity testing. *Mycoplasma* cultures are considered, especially for evaluation of pneumonia in young dogs and pulmonary abscesses in cats. Cultures for anaerobic organisms should also be performed.

Bronchoscopy or lung aspiration may be necessary if the tracheal wash specimen is nondiagnostic. This situation may occur with localized disease. Further considerations include feline immunodeficiency and leukemia virus tests, tests for endocrinopathies, barium swallow for decreased esophageal motility, and biopsies or motility tests for ciliary dyskinesia.

Treatment. Antibiotic selection should be based on the results of sensitivity testing. Multiple organisms with different antibiotic resistance patterns may complicate the selection of effective antibiotics.

Reasonable initial antibiotic selection can be made based on microscopic examination of the specimen and tentative organism identification pending results of sensitivity testing. If marked respiratory compromise is present, combination therapy with ampicillin and an aminoglycoside is an appropriate first choice. In cases of persistent bronchial infections due to *Bordetella*, aerosol administration of antibiotics can be used. This route of therapy should be used in addition to, but not replace, systemic therapy.

General therapeutic measures should always be applied in addition to antibiotic therapy. Adequate oxygenation and maintaining airway hydration cannot be overemphasized. Mobilization of airway secretions may be facilitated by mild activity in sufficiently stable patients. *Coupage* may also be helpful. The use of bronchodilators is controversial. Corticosteroids and cough suppressants are avoided.

If improvement is observed, treatment should continue a minimum of one week beyond the total resolution of signs (including active radiographic changes). Usually a course of 3 to 6 weeks is required. Radiographs should be reevaluated approximately one week after discontinuation of therapy.

Pulmonary Abscessation

Pulmonary abscesses, though rare, can occur as a complication of bacterial pneumonia, foreign bodies, trauma, parasitic or fungal infections, and neoplasia.

Mycobacterial Infections

Dogs and cats are susceptible to infections caused by *Mycobacterium tuberculosis* and *M. bovis* ("true" tuberculosis) but are relatively resistant to infections by *M. avium*–complex organisms. Clinical signs in cats classically represent involvement of the intestinal tract, whereas signs in dogs are the result of pulmonary involvement.

Historic and physical findings in dogs with pulmonary involvement reflect lower respiratory tract disease and may mimic those of neoplasia, severe bacterial pneumonia, mycotic infection, or hypersensitivity/immune-mediated disease.

Thoracic radiographs often show hilar lymphadenopathy. Intersititial patterns, granulomas, lung lobe consolidation, mineralization of pulmonary lesions, and pleural or pericardial effusions may be apparent.

The diagnosis depends on the identification of organisms. Pleural fluid, lung aspirates, bronchoalveolar lavage, or lung biopsies may be required. Specimens should be cultured for *Mycobacterium* so that the organisms can be identified as saprophytic or nonsaprophytic.

PROTOZOAL DISEASES

Toxoplasmosis

Clinical disease can be acute or chronic. Historic and physical findings are typical of severe lower respiratory disease. Anorexia, weight loss, cough, exercise intolerance, and respiratory distress may be reported. Cough is uncommon in cats. Radiographs of the thorax reveal fluffy interstitial and alveolar densities throughout the lung fields. Other patterns can occur. Tracheal wash fluid analysis can show tachyzoites and could provide a definitive diagnosis. Lung biopsy may allow for the identification of organisms.

Pneumocystosis

Pneumocystis carinii is a protozoal organism that causes pulmonary disease in immunocompromised dogs. Dogs present with signs reflective of chronic pneumonia, including weight loss, exercise intolerance, respiratory distress, and sometimes a nonproductive cough. The majority of reported cases have involved young dachshunds. Trimethoprim and sulfamethoxazole combinations have been used to treat infections in man. Pentamidine isethionate can be administered.

FUNGAL DISEASES

Histoplasmosis

Lung involvement with histoplasmosis is common, and the signs are typical of chronic lower respiratory tract disease. Pleural effusion has been reported. Signs of involvement of other organs may occur concurrently with respiratory signs. The majority of dogs, however, are presented for signs of intestinal disease. Thoracic radiographs classically exhibit a diffuse interstitial pattern, which is often miliary. Hilar lymphadenopathy may be present in dogs. Calcification of pulmonary lesions can occur.

Cytologic identification of organisms is the preferred method of diagnosis. Organisms frequently cannot be identified in tracheal wash fluid. Pulmonary tissue can be sampled more deeply through transthoracic needle aspiration, bronchoalveolar lavage, or biopsy. The majority of cases are diagnosed following the development of overt clinical signs, often of disseminated disease. These patients require aggressive therapy as described in Chapter 71.

Blastomycosis

Client complaints relate to the organ systems involved. Lower respiratory signs were present in 43 per cent of 47 dogs. A diffuse, miliary interstitial pattern, as is seen with histoplasmosis, is typical. Hilar lymphadenopathy occurs, but probably less frequently than with other mycotic diseases. Pleural effusion may be apparent. Tracheal wash fluid should be examined carefully for organisms. Treatment, prognosis, and zoonotic potential are discussed in Chapter 71.

Coccidioidomycosis

Patients with pulmonary disease are presented with slowly progressive lower respiratory signs. Thoracic radiographs reveal changes similar to those seen with the other mycoses. Tracheal wash fluid should be carefully examined for organisms. If tracheal wash preparations are nondiagnostic, other specimens should be examined from organs suspected of being infected. Further diagnostic procedures, treatment, prognosis, and zoonotic potential are discussed in Chapter 71.

Cryptococcosis

Pulmonary lesions have been reported in 50 per cent of feline cases, but clinical signs relative to the lower respiratory tract are rare. Thoracic radiographs are normal in most cases in spite of pulmonary involvement.

PARASITIC DISEASES

Paragonimus kellicotti

Lung flukes cause pulmonary disease in dogs and cats in the states surrounding the Great Lakes, and in the midwestern and southern United States. Aquatic snails and crayfish are required intermediate hosts. When they occur, clinical signs may include coughing, hemoptysis, or wheezing. Crackles and wheezes may be ausculted with inflammatory disease, and decreased lung sounds with pneumothorax.

Thoracic radiographs demonstrate air-filled cysts or tissue density masses averaging 1 cm in diameter. The masses most commonly involve the caudal lung lobes. Pneumothorax may be present. Diffuse inflammatory signs may be apparent, resulting in bronchial, interstitial, or patchy alveolar patterns.

The disease is definitively diagnosed by the identification of eggs, which may be found in tracheal wash fluid or in feces. Sedimentation is the preferred fecal examination technique.

No treatment for *Paragonimus* has been well established. Praziquantel or fenbendazole may be considered. Radiographic lesions can take many weeks to resolve, and some abnormal density may persist.

Aelurostrongylus abstrusus

Aelurostrongylus abstrusus is a small (less than 1 cm) lungworm of cats. Adult worms reside primarily within the bronchioles. A mollusk intermediate host is required. Many infections are not associated with clinical signs, which can range from mild coughing to severe wheezing and respiratory distress. The clinical presentation mimics feline bronchitis.

Thoracic radiographs can show small, poorly defined, nodular densities throughout the lung fields, similar to metastatic neoplasia or mycotic disease. Inflammatory reactions can also result and can be confused with feline bronchitis. Tracheal wash fluid analysis may reveal eosinophilic inflammation, which can be reflected in the CBC.

The disease is definitively diagnosed by the identification of first-stage larvae in tracheal wash fluid or feces. Infection is usually self-limiting, and asymptomatic infections do not necessarily warrant treatment. Specific antiparasitic therapy can be attempted with fenbendazole. Ivermectin has been used successfully. Nonspecific treatment with corticosteroids and bronchodilators may be helpful in decreasing the severity of clinical signs.

Capillaria aerophila

Capillaria aerophila is a 2- to 4-cm lungworm that resides in the nasal cavity, trachea, and bronchi of dogs and cats. Infection is direct or through earthworm intermediate hosts. Occasionally a chronic cough is reported. Thoracic radiographs in symptomatic patients may reveal a bronchial or interstitial pattern. The diagnosis is made by the identification of eggs in tracheal wash fluid or in fecal specimens. Fenbendazole, levamisole, and ivermectin have been proposed for treatment, if necessary.

Filaroides osleri

Filaroides osleri is a lungworm that resides at the carina and in the major bronchi of dogs, forming inflammatory nodules. The initial presenting sign is generally an acute, nonproductive cough in an otherwise healthy, young dog. Over time, signs of chronic bronchitis develop. The diagnosis is based on the presence of larvae in tracheal wash fluid or on identification of the parasitic nodules by bronchoscopy.

Filaroides hirthi

Filaroides hirthi is a small lungworm (less than 2 mm) that resides in the terminal bronchioles and alveoli of dogs. Autoinfection can worsen the worm burden within the patient. Respiratory tract signs, including nonproductive cough, tachypnea, and respiratory distress, have been reported in small numbers of cases. Thoracic radiographs and tracheal wash specimens aid in the diagnosis. Albendazole and fenbendazole have been used to treat infections.

Crensoma vulpis

Crensoma vulpis is a worm that resides in the trachea, bronchi, and bronchioles of dogs. Mollusks serve as intermediate hosts. Infection is uncommon. Dogs are presented with signs of tracheobronchitis. The diagnosis is made by identification of larvae in tracheal wash fluid or in fecal specimens examined by the Baermann technique. Diethylcarbamazine, levamisole, and fenbendazole may be effective.

Intestinal Parasite Migration

Toxocara canis undergoes migration through the lungs of dogs following infection. In heavy infections pulmonary signs may result from damage and the inflammatory reaction to the migrating larvae. Coughing and tachypnea are usually noted in puppies less than 6 weeks of age. Larvae begin migrating prior to the shedding of eggs.

Signs are usually mild and resolve without treatment. Glucocorticoids can be administered in low dosages to control severe signs, but are rarely necessary. Routine anthelmintic therapy is not effective against the larvae, but should be initiated to prevent further propagation.

Other intestinal parasites with lung migration as part of their life cycle include *Ancylostoma caninum* and *Strongyloides stercoralis*. Transient signs, such as coughing, might be noted.

Dirofilaria immitis

See Chapter 98.

HYPERSENSITIVITY AND IMMUNE-MEDIATED DISEASES

Eosinophilic Diseases

For a discussion of bronchial eosinophilic diseases see Bronchial Diseases. Eosinophilic diseases predominantly involving the pulmonary parenchyma are also known as pulmonary infiltrates with eosinophils (PIE). Differential diagnoses for eosinophilic lung diseases include hypersensitivity reactions to pulmonary parasites, heartworms, drugs, or inhaled allergens. Occasionally, bacteria, fungus, or neoplasia can cause a hypersensitivity response.

Presentation. Signs of PIE are extremely variable. Coughing is often the primary complaint. Auscultation often reveals increased breath sounds or crackles.

Diagnostic Evaluation. The CBC classically reflects the eosinophilic response; however, peripheral eosinophilia may be absent. Radiographs can show a mild interstitial pattern, patchy alveolar densities, and even large masses that are indistinguishable from neoplasia or fungal granulomas. Hilar lymphadenopathy may be severe. Lymphomatoid granulomatosis has presenting and radiographic signs that are similar to those of eosinophilic pulmonary granulomatosis.

Cytologic evaluation is necessary for diagnosis. Tracheal wash fluid or deeper specimens may be required to obtain a diagnosis. Eosinophilic inflammation predominates, although other types of inflammatory cells are also present. Specimens should be critically evaluated for antigenic sources including parasites, bacteria, fungi, and neoplasia.

Treatment. When possible, an etiology should be identified and removed. If no allergen can be found, immunosuppression is required. Corticosteroids are frequently successful in controlling the inflammatory process, except in cases of eosinophilic pulmonary granulomatosis. With eosinophilic pulmonary granulomatosis cytotoxic drugs are often required.

Vasculitides/Lymphomatoid Granulomatosis

Reported cases in dogs have included lymphomatoid granulomatosis, granulomatosis associated with a positive LE cell test, and pneumonitis as a component of SLE. In other cases no etiology is found and resolution is achieved with immunosuppressant therapy.

Presentation. Lymphomatoid granulomatosis has only been described in the dog. Dogs are presented with any combination of respiratory signs, particularly cough and respiratory distress. Fever, anorexia, and weight loss may occur.

Diagnostic Evaluation. Thoracic radiographs reveal an interstitial pattern with multiple, ill-defined nodules of varying size. Hilar lymphadenopathy is frequently present. A peripheral basophilia, with or without eosinophilia, has been reported. Heartworm tests and fungal serology should be performed.

Cytologic evaluation of lung fluid reveals eosinophilic and neutrophilic inflammation with reactive macrophages. Lymphocytes and plasma cells may also be present. Histopathologic evaluation of a biopsy is required for a definitive diagnosis.

Treatment. Treatment consists of immunosuppression and should be withheld pending the elimination of infectious differential diagnoses. Combination therapy with prednisone and a cytotoxic agent is recommended.

PULMONARY NEOPLASIA

Primary Pulmonary Neoplasia

Fibrosarcomas, osteosarcomas, chondrosarcomas, hemangiosarcomas and benign adenomas occur infrequently. Metastatic disease resulting from primary lung tumors is common. The pulmonary metastatic lesions may be smaller than the original tumor. Another common site of metastasis is the bronchial lymph nodes. Extrathoracic metastatic lesions can occur.

Primary tumors and intrathoracic metastases can cause respiratory signs from compression or obstruction of airways, regional ventilation:perfusion abnormalities, or pleural effusion. Inflammatory reactions to the tumors, secondary infections, intrapulmonary hemorrhage, cavitary lesions, pneumothorax, and hemothorax also can contribute to respiratory signs.

Occasionally pulmonary tumors compress the major veins within the thorax and cause ascites, jugular distention, or edema of the head and neck. Esophageal compression can lead to dysphagia or regurgitation. Hypertrophic pulmonary osteopathy (HPO) is the most frequently reported paraneoplastic syndrome in dogs, with less frequent occurrence in cats.

Presentation. Client complaints can reflect respiratory signs, signs of metastases or HPO, or nonlocalizing signs, all of which are usually chronic. The lungs should be carefully auscultated for localized areas of increased or absent lung sounds, which can occur over regions of consolidation. Crackles or wheezes may be present. Pleural effusion or pneumothorax may result in a generalized decrease in lung sounds.

Diagnostic Evaluation. Thoracic radiographs are the most valuable diagnostic aid in the evaluation of patients with pulmonary neoplasia. Lung patterns are varied and include single circumscribed mass lesions, lobar consolidation, multiple circumscribed masses, and diffuse involvement. The last is common and can be demonstrated as reticular or nodular interstitial, alveolar, or peribronchial opacities.

Radiographs are insensitive to masses less than approximately 1 cm in diameter, and a definitive diagnosis of neoplasia cannot be made based upon radiographs alone. Radiographs of the bones should be evaluated in animals presenting with lameness, limb pain, or swelling for evidence of HPO or bone metastases.

A definitive diagnosis requires the cytologic or histologic evaluation of specimens. Pleural fluid, tracheal washings, bronchial brushings, and bronchoalveolar lavage fluid can be evaluated cytologically. Transthoracic or transbronchial biopsies can be obtained from lesions near the thoracic wall or involving the major airways, respectively. Thoracotomy is the most invasive method of obtaining lung tissue, but this approach has major advantages.

Treatment. Excision of tumor with wide surgical margins is the treatment of choice for primary pulmonary neoplasia. Lobectomy is usually required. Tumors that cannot be excised can be treated with systemic chemotherapeutic drugs, although promising results have not been published. Cyclophosphamide, doxorubicin, vindesine, vinblastine, and cisplatin have been used in man. Responses to cisplatin have been noted in dogs with pulmonary adenocarcinoma in ongoing studies, but final results have yet to be reported.

Prognosis.   Benign neoplasia carries an excellent prognosis, but is uncommon. The long-term prognosis for most primary pulmonary tumors is poor, although the time course may be slow.

Metastatic Pulmonary Neoplasia

The lungs are a common site of metastases, second only to lymph nodes draining the organ with the primary tumor. Tumor types with high incidences of pulmonary metastatic lesions include thyroid carcinomas and mammary carcinomas. Pulmonary metastases from osteosarcoma, hemangiosarcoma, transitional cell carcinoma, oral and digital melanoma, and squamous cell carcinoma also occur commonly.

Presentation.   Animals with pulmonary metastatic disease can be presented for signs caused by the primary tumor or for signs caused by the pulmonary involvement.

Diagnostic Evaluation.   A presumptive diagnosis of pulmonary metastatic disease frequently is made on the basis of a histopathologically diagnosed primary malignant tumor and suggestive thoracic radiographs. Radiographic patterns associated with metastatic tumors are the same as those described for pulmonary neoplasia.

Radiographic patterns that can be misinterpreted as metastatic disease can occur as a result of atypical bacterial infections, immune-mediated or hypersensitivity diseases, parasitic infections, fungal infections, and other non-neoplastic diseases. A definitive diagnosis of metastatic neoplasia is obtained through the cytologic or histologic evaluation of specimens as described for primary pulmonary tumors.

One study showed that conventional radiographs failed to detect 25 per cent of canine pulmonary metastases that were found at necropsy. Sensitivity can be improved by performing both right and left lateral recumbent views and by having multiple readers interpret the radiographs.

Treatment.   Surgical excision of metastatic lesions could potentially contribute to cure of disease. Unfortunately, metastatic disease is rarely identified prior to the development of diffuse, nonresectable, pulmonary lesions. Chemotherapeutic agents are recommended based on the sensitivity of the primary tumor. Other potential treatment modalities include immunotherapy and antimetastatic drugs.

Lymphoma

Lymphoma can involve the pulmonary parenchyma in the multicentric form of the disease in dogs and cats. Thoracic radiographs reveal an irregular reticular pattern, often with ill-defined nodular densities. Hilar, mediastinal, or sternal lymphadenopathy may be apparent. Rarely a single mass lesion or a peribronchial pattern occurs. Neoplastic cells within the lungs may be identifiable in bronchoalveolar lavage fluid, lung aspirates, or histologic specimens, but the disease is generally diagnosed through other more accessible systems, such as the peripheral lymph nodes.

Malignant Histiocytosis

Malignant histiocytosis is a malignant proliferative disorder of morphologically atypical histiocytes and their precursors. Signs of cough and respiratory distress rapidly progress. Radiographic abnormalities of the thorax include single or multiple mass lesions, hilar lymphadenopathy, and pleural effusion. Chemotherapy with doxorubicin, cyclophosphamide, and vincristine has been useful in the treatment of a few cases. The prognosis is poor.

PULMONARY THROMBOEMBOLIC DISEASE

Pulmonary thromboembolism is a relatively common disease, but is unrecognized by many clinicians. Lack of clinician awareness and the inability to readily make a definitive diagnosis interfere with the ante-mortem identification of these patients. Pulmonary thromboembolic disease is the result of the obstruction of pulmonary arteries and arterioles. Emboli can consist of bacteria, foreign bodies (e.g., intravenous catheters), air, fat, or parasites. The majority of emboli are fragments of thrombi (clots).

The principal result of interference in pulmonary blood flow is abnormal ventilation:perfusion relationships within the lung. Other effects of thromboembolism include decreased surfactant production, development of pulmonary edema due to overcirculation of unaffected regions of lung, pulmonary infarction, and the development of mild pleural effusion.

The most commonly recognized cause of pulmonary thromboembolism in small animal medicine is dirofilariasis. Other diseases include cardiac disease, nephrotic syndrome, immune-mediated hemolytic anemia, neoplasia, sepsis, pancreatitis, hyperadrenocorticism, and disseminated intravascular coagulation. Further conditions that can potentially result in thromboembolism include surgery, severe trauma, hyperlipidemia, and hyperviscosity syndromes.

Presentation. Patients generally experience a peracute onset of extremely severe respiratory distress and tachypnea. Less severely affected animals may demonstrate tachypnea only. Tachycardia is often present. A loud or split-second heart sound may occur as a result of pulmonary hypertension. Occasionally cough, hemoptysis, or crackles may be present.

Diagnostic Evaluation. Thoracic radiographs can be surprisingly normal. The predominant lung patterns include hyperlucent zones and alveolar pulmonary infiltrate secondary to edema or hemorrhage. Other potential abnormalities include interstitial pattern, mild pleural effusion, heart enlargement, and main pulmonary artery enlargement. Arterial blood gas analysis is particularly useful. Typical abnormalities are hypoxemia and hypocapnia.

A definitive diagnosis of pulmonary thromboembolic disease is obtained with contrast radiography. Nonselective angiography can be used and is a practical technique. Ventilation and perfusion scanning with radioisotopes can also be performed. If the perfusion scan is abnormal, ventilation scans are performed to determine whether hypoventilation could explain the decreased perfusion. It is normal for the lungs to shunt blood away from regions of the lung that have decreased ventilation (e.g., due to pneumonia or edema) in order to match ventilation and perfusion. Pulmonary thromboembolism typically results in abnormal perfusion in areas with normal ventilation.

Treatment. Animals with acute, severe embolism are treated for cardiovascular shock, administered oxygen, and given high doses of rapid-acting corticosteroids. Anticoagulant therapy with heparin, and possibly warfarin, is administered to prevent further clot formation. These drugs have no effect on the existing emboli. Hemorrhage is a potential complication. Treatment with heparin can be continued at home with subcutaneous injections. Animals that require prolonged treatment, usually because of a persistent predisposing problem that cannot be resolved, can be maintained with oral warfarin. Thrombolytic drugs, such as tissue plasminogen activator, have great potential for the treatment of pulmonary thromboembolism because existing clots can be dissolved, but these drugs have not gained widespread acceptance in veterinary medicine.

Prevention.   If prophylaxis is desired, heparin can be administered at low dosages. Treatment is discontinued once the predisposing factor has been controlled.

PULMONARY HYPERTENSION

Pulmonary hypertension is defined as increased pulmonary arterial pressure, and it is almost always a secondary problem. Causes can be classified as precapillary and postcapillary. Precapillary causes include lung disease, pulmonary thromboembolism, congenital heart disease, pulmonary vasculitis, high altitude disease, and pulmonary arteriovenous fistula. Postcapillary causes result in increased left atrial or pulmonary venous pressures and include left ventricular failure, mitral insufficiency or stenosis, left atrial masses (thrombus or neoplasia), and pulmonary venous obstruction. The right heart is secondarily affected by the pressure overload, and dilation and hypertrophy can develop. *Cor pulmonale* refers to these cardiac changes.

Presentation.   Exercise intolerance, respiratory distress, or cough may be present. Pronounced or split-second heart sounds may be auscultable, providing a valuable clue.

Diagnostic Evaluation.   Right heart enlargement, enlarged pulmonary arteries, or evidence of primary pulmonary disease may be observed. Echocardiography may be a more sensitive indicator of right heart involvement. Echocardiography with flow measurements can be used to estimate pulmonary pressure in some cases. A definitive diagnosis requires cardiac catheterization.

Treatment.   Treatment is aimed at eliminating the primary cause whenever possible. In animals in the acute setting (such as pulmonary thromboembolism), oxygen supplementation plays a major role in treatment. Use of vasodilator drugs is controversial.

PULMONARY EDEMA

Pulmonary edema is the accumulation of excess fluid within the lungs. Fluid homeostasis in the lungs is uniquely different from that in systemic capillary beds. Pulmonary edema is not a primary disease but occurs secondary to a disease process that upsets the balance of fluid accumulation and removal. Excess fluid within the lungs initially accumulates perivascularly and peribronchially in the interstitium. With increasing volumes, alveoli become flooded. Ventilation:perfusion mismatching and hypoxemia subsequently occur.

Causes of pulmonary edema can be grouped based on the major mechanisms resulting in edema formation: decreased plasma oncotic pressure, vascular overload, lymphatic obstruction, increased vascular permeability, and miscellaneous or unknown mechanisms.

Hypoalbuminemia alone is unlikely to cause pulmonary edema; however, it can be a contributing factor in conjunction with other predisposing problems. Albumin concentrations associated with edema formation are usually less than 1 gm/dl. Vascular overload can result from overcirculation (increased blood flow) or increased hydrostatic pressure. Cardiac disease and excessive fluid administration are the most common causes of vascular overload. Left heart failure, often due to mitral insufficiency or pump failure, is the most common cause of pulmonary edema. Lymphatic obstruction is an uncommon cause. It is usually the result of neoplasia.

Edema due to increased vascular permeability is described as the adult respiratory distress syndrome (ARDS) in man. The edema, by definition, is not cardiogenic and therefore is associated with normal pulmonary wedge pressures. Because the fluid results from vascular leakage, it is relatively proteinaceous fluid that does not readily resolve with diuretic therapy.

ARDS can occur secondary to pulmonary or systemic disease. Pulmonary diseases in which edema can result in significant signs include inhalation trauma (such as smoke inhalation, gastric acid aspiration, near-drowning, and oxygen toxicity) and direct trauma (pulmonary contusions). Systemic diseases that have been associated with ARDS include sepsis and endotoxemia, including parvovirus infection; pancreatitis; severe uremia; major trauma; drugs or toxins, such as cisplatinum in cats, snake venom, and paraquat; electrocution; and disseminated intravascular coagulation. Several other diseases have been associated with pulmonary edema, including thromboembolism, severe upper airway obstruction, neurogenic edema, and liver disease, unrelated to hypoalbuminemia.

Presentation. Animals with pulmonary edema show acute or subacute signs typical of lower respiratory tract disease. Crackles, and occasionally wheezes, are auscultated. They may be most pronounced in the central or caudodorsal regions. Cardiac auscultation and assessment of pulses are critical in the early identification of cardiogenic pulmonary edema.

Diagnostic Evaluation. Severely compromised animals are treated on the basis of presenting signs only. Following stabilization, thoracic radiography and complete systemic evaluation are performed.

Thoracic radiographs may be normal early in the development of edema. Interstitial densities appear, followed by an alveolar pattern demonstrating alveolar flooding. In dogs with cardiogenic edema, the lesions are usually most prominent in the perihilar regions. Cats with heart failure may have patchy areas of edema. Edema secondary to increased vascular permeability is often most pronounced in the caudodorsal regions.

Echocardiography is extremely valuable for evaluating the heart. Routine blood tests, areterial blood gases, and urinalysis are helpful in evaluating the systemic status of the patient.

Treatment. Oxygen supplementation, cage rest, and possibly sedation and bronchodilators are used initially to stabilize animals with pulmonary edema. Diuretics are indicated for treatment of some forms of edema, but in hypovolemic animals they can cause further deterioration of cardiac output. The concurrent administration of plasma to animals with hypoalbuminemia or positive inotropes to animals in heart failure may be warranted.

Animals with edema due to decreased oncotic pressure are treated with plasma infusions. Edema due to volume overload from excessive fluid administration will often resolve upon discontinuation of fluids. Furosemide is administered to treat marked edema. Edema due to increased vascular permeability is difficult to treat. Some mild cases respond to cage rest and oxygen supplementation alone. Unfortunately, most animals with ARDS do not respond adequately. Positive pressure ventilation, usually with PEEP, is needed. Diuretics can be administered to normovolemic animals, but they are minimally effective in most ARDS patients. The use of corticosteroids is controversial.

Cystic-Bullous Disease

Grossly visible circumscribed regions of air and fluid (cavitary lesions) can occur within the lung parenchyma owing to cysts, bullae, blebs, and pneumatoceles. Cysts are fluid-filled or air-filled lesions surrounded by a thin wall of respiratory epithelium. Bullae are gross air accumulations formed by the loss of alveolar walls. They are often multiple and can occur as a progression of emphysema (bullous emphysema). Pneumatoceles result from the entry of air into necrotic lesions. They may occur as a result of abscesses, granulomas, or neoplasia.

Patients generally are presented either with signs of a primary pulmonary disease or with signs of pneumothorax. Occasionally, lesions are incidental findings.

Most cavitary lesions are identified initially by thoracic radiography. Animals presented with pneumothorax and respiratory compromise are stabilized by thoracentesis prior to further diagnostic evaluation. Horizontal beam projections can be useful in enhancing the appearance of a fluid line. Cytologic evaluation may provide evidence of the cause of the cavitary lesion. For example, septic inflammation or *Paragonimus* ova might be found. Transthoracic lung aspiration is contraindicated because of increased risk of pneumothorax. A definitive diagnosis is obtained with thoracotomy, excision, and histopathologic examination.

Pneumothorax is managed as discussed in Chapter 90. Cavitary lesions may resolve with supportive care and treatment of primary disease. Surgical exploration and removal may be necessary.

TRAUMATIC LUNG DISEASE

Pulmonary Contusions

Pulmonary contusions refer to hemorrhage and edema within the lung and occur as a result of traumatic injury. The patient is presented with a history or physical findings that confirm a traumatic incident. The animal may be eupneic or in severe respiratory distress. Recent hemorrhage and edema result in crackles, whereas consolidated lobes cause absence or enhancement of sounds. Ribs should be carefully palpated for penetrating fractures. The overlying skin should be examined for penetrating wounds or subcutaneous emphysema. The patient should be carefully monitored; deterioration may occur for as long as 24 hours after the traumatic incident.

Pulmonary contusions are evidenced radiographically by localized areas of an interstitial pattern, alveolar pattern, or consolidation. Radiographic signs may be delayed for as long as 24 hours following trauma. With bite wounds, material should be submitted for bacterial culture and sensitivity testing.

The critical patient is stabilized according to the principles of shock-trauma management. Once the animal is stabilized, little therapy is generally required beyond cage rest. Antibiotics are indicated for puncture wounds. Improvement is usually seen within 24 to 48 hours of injury. Complications occasionally develop, and radiographic reevaluation is indicated for early detection.

Aspiration Pneumonia

Aspiration pneumonia occurs when foreign material is inspired into the lungs. Megaesophagus, cleft palate, bronchoesophageal fistula, therapeutic laryngoplasty, peripheral neuropathies, or abnormal consciousness due to sedation or severe debilitation are some underlying causes to consider. Aspiration can result in respiratory signs due to many mechanisms, including physical obstruction of airways; inflammation in response to gastric acid, food particles, mineral oil, or other reactive materials; bacterial infection; chemical damage to the respiratory epithelium; decreased pulmonary compliance; and bronchoconstriction.

Patients may be presented with acute respiratory signs following vomition or regurgitation, loss of consciousness, or forced oral administration of mineral oil, food, or drugs. Most cases demonstrate acute, severe respiratory distress, with signs apparent within hours of aspiration. Cardiovascular shock can occur. Physical examination reveals crackles, and sometimes wheezes, especially in the dependent (usually cranioventral) lung fields. A fever may be present.

Thoracic radiographs support a diagnosis of aspiration pneumonia in animals with a suggestive history. The characteristic change is a bronchoalveolar pattern involving primarily the dependent lung lobes. Radiographic changes may be inapparent initially, then progress for as long as 24 hours following aspiration. Tracheal wash fluid analysis shows acute or chronic inflammation, depending on the duration of injury. Bacterial culture and sensitivity testing should always be performed.

Bronchoscopy can be performed to remove large pieces of foreign material. Scoping is indicated only if large airway obstruction is suspected. Once the patient is stabilized, further diagnostic evaluation can be performed to identify underlying diseases.

Treatment. The severely distressed patient needs immediate oxygen supplementation. Positive pressure ventilation may also be necessary. Intravenous fluid therapy is indicated. High volumes are often required initially to treat shock. Nothing is administered orally until the patient is stabilized. If material is still present in the upper airways, airway suctioning or bronchoscopy and foreign body removal should be performed.

Bronchodilators can be beneficial in the immediate management of aspiration to overcome acute bronchoconstriction. The use of corticosteroids for treatment of acute aspiration is also controversial. In acute cases in which the patient is deteriorating, administration of short-acting corticosteroids is justified. Tracheal wash cytologic examination and culture are useful in determining the need for antibiotic therapy.

Near-Drowning

Aspiration occurs in most cases and results in severe pulmonary damage. In a small percentage of cases, laryngospasm prevents the aspiration of water. Dry-drowning results, and pulmonary disease is absent. Pulmonary damage occurs through a variety of mechanisms. Adult respiratory distress syndrome can occur secondary to near-drowning. Cerebral edema, herniation, and death can occur as a result of profound hypoxemia complicated by metabolic acidosis.

Presentation. History provides the diagnosis. Physical examination generally reveals loss of consciousness and either severe respiratory distress or respiratory arrest. Cardiovascular shock and hypothermia are common. Auscultation of the lungs reveals severe crackles and possibly wheezes.

Diagnostic Evaluation. Stabilization is the first priority. Radiographic changes may lag behind clinical signs during the initial 24 to 48 hours. A mixed bronchial, alveolar, and interstitial pattern is commonly seen. Radiographic evaluation should be continued during and following recovery for the detection of bacterial pneumonia, consolidation, or abscessation.

Treatment. Ventilation should be initiated as soon as possible. Mouth-to-muzzle resuscitation can be initiated on site, following clearing of any debris or obstruction from the oral cavity. Oxygen supplementation is provided when available. In the hospital, positive pressure ventilation is often required in addition to supplemental oxygen therapy. Shock is aggressively treated. Routine administration of corticosteroids or prophylactic antibiotics is not recommended.

Prognosis. Poor prognostic indicators are coma, severe acidosis, and the need for resuscitation or mechanical ventilation.

Smoke Inhalation

Pulmonary damage can occur during exposure to pollutants, poorly ventilated housing, exhaust from gasoline or diesel engines, improperly functioning heaters, and a variety of other sources. Smoke inhalation results in respiratory signs through several mechanisms.

Presentation. The presence of burns around the face, singed vibrissae, oral inflammation, and soot-stained nasal discharge or saliva are supportive of inhalation exposure. Mucous membranes may be bright red, due to carboxyhemoglobin, or cyanotic. Carbon monoxide intoxication may be significant in the absence of the characteristic reddening of mucous membranes. Stridor may be audible owing to laryngeal edema. Wheezes and crackles may be auscultated. Adult respiratory distress syndrome and secondary infections may occur days after exposure.

Diagnostic Evaluation.   Potential radiographic abnormalities include peribronchial infiltration, patchy consolidation, and hyperinflation. Lesions are often diffuse, with the caudodorsal lung fields most severely affected. Blood gas analyses must be evaluated with caution. The PaO_2 may be normal in spite of decreased oxygen content, since the carbon monoxide interferes with the oxygen saturation of hemoglobin. Carboxyhemoglobin concentrations in venous blood can be measured. The patient's cardiac and neurologic status should be carefully monitored. Deterioration in respiratory status can be a result of ARDS or bacterial infection.

Treatment.   A patent airway is essential, and animals with laryngeal obstruction may require tracheostomies. In compromised patients, oxygen supplementation should begin as soon as an airway is established. Oxygen therapy should be continued until carboxyhemoglobin concentrations are less than 10 per cent.

In the management of pulmonary injury, general principles of therapy should be applied: oxygenation, airway humidification, and physiotherapy. Positive pressure ventilation, bronchodilators, or antibiotic therapy may be indicated. Corticosteroids may be necessary for acute stabilization. Treatment of sequelae such as bronchitis, bronchopneumonia, abscesses, and consolidation are discussed in other sections.

MISCELLANEOUS CONDITIONS

Pulmonary Mineralization

Mineralized thoracic densities in the airways, pleura, parenchyma, or lymph nodes may be incidental radiographic findings. Chondrodystrophoid dogs may demonstrate airway mineralization at an early age. Diffuse nodular mineralization of unknown etiology involving the pulmonary parenchyma can be a nonprogressive lesion and can be misinterpreted as metastatic neoplasia. Mineralization can also occur in areas of inflammation or necrosis. Systemic diseases such as renal secondary hyperparathyroidism and hyperadrenocorticism can result in mineral deposition in the lungs.

Obesity (Pickwickian Syndrome)

The term *pickwickian syndrome* refers to a specific condition in man characterized by obesity, somnolence, hypoventilation, and erythrocytosis. A central neurologic abnormality may be involved. It should not be used indiscriminately to describe all obese patients with respiratory disease. The clinician should be careful not to use obesity as an excuse to avoid pursuing specific disease entities; however, the beneficial effects of weight reduction in patients with chronic bronchial or pulmonary disease can be dramatic.

Lobar Consolidation

Consolidation refers to the filling of alveoli and airways with cells or fluid and can occur with inflammatory, neoplastic, or hemorrhagic disease. Ventilation:perfusion abnormalities occur. Lobar consolidations are recognized radiographically as soft tissue densities with visible lung lobe borders.

Atelectasis

Atelectasis refers to the collapse (or incomplete expansion) of lung due to the loss of air from the alveoli. Atelectasis commonly results from pneumothorax and pleural effusion. Reexpansion almost always follows removal of the air or fluid from the pleural space. Atelectasis occasionally occurs as a complication of pulmonary disease due to total airway obstruction and the absorption of alveolar gases into the blood or by the loss of surfactant. Treatment is directed at the inciting cause. Prolonged atelectasis can potentially result in abscessation or fibrosis. Surgical intervention may be necessary if signs are persistent.

CHAPTER 90

MEDIASTINAL, PLEURAL, AND EXTRAPLEURAL DISEASES
(pages 812–842)

DISORDERS OF THE DIAPHRAGM (pp. 812–814)

DIAPHRAGMATIC DISPLACEMENT

Bilateral caudal displacement of the diaphragm is a characteristic of obstructive airway disorders. It is more profound in chronic disorders, causing air trapping and hyperinflation. Radiographically, the diaphragms are flattened; this may be more pronounced in the lateral radiograph. Pneumothorax displaces the diaphragm caudally. Cranial displacement may occur normally with obesity and pregnancy, whereas intra-abdominal disorders producing displacement include ascites, hepatomegaly, intra-abdominal masses, obstructive ileus, and acute gastric dilatation.

Unilateral caudal displacement of a hemidiaphragm may occur with unilateral pneumothorax, pulmonary cysts, or bullae. Pleural effusion or mass may produce displacement. Processes causing loss of lung volume, such as atelectasis or pulmonary resection, move a hemidiaphragm cranially.

EVENTRATION

Diaphragmatic eventration is a condition in which a hemidiaphragm is thinned and frequently is moved cranially. The etiology is unknown. The importance of this defect is that it masquerades as caudal or accessory lung lobe masses. Radiographic evaluation and ultrasonography are helpful in diagnosis.

PARALYSIS OF THE DIAPHRAGM

Diaphragmatic paralysis may be unilateral or bilateral and may be a permanent or transient phenomenon. Dysfunction arises from disruption of the phrenic pathway anywhere between its origin and the diaphragm. Unilateral paralysis may be caused by traumatic or surgical transection, infiltrative or mass lesions, and neuropathic disorders. Bilateral paralysis is most commonly a result of cervical spinal trauma but may be caused by the disorders previously mentioned. The diagnosis is made by fluoroscopic demonstration of diminished or absent diaphragmatic motion during normal inspiration.

Original chapter written by Timothy Bauer and Jerry A. Woodfield

DIAPHRAGMATIC HERNIA

The term *diaphragmatic hernia* loosely refers to all disorders in which abdominal viscera traverse the diaphragm and enter the thoracic cavity. The abdominal viscera may be contained within a hernial sac or may be free in the pleural space. Diaphragmatic rupture is most frequently associated with blunt trauma to the abdomen or lower chest. Radiographic and ultrasonographic evaluation remain the most important methods of confirming the diagnosis. Multiple positive or negative contrast studies may be helpful.

Frequently there is no known history of trauma. There may be a vague history of gastrointestinal distress that is episodic or consists of low-grade respiratory signs. Disorders may secondarily evolve, including gastric dilation, intrathoracic splenic torsion, intrathoracic bowel obstruction, and liver lobe incarceration. Late development of pleural effusion may complicate chronic herniation. Lung torsion may complicate pleural effusion.

Management. Diaphragmatic hernia is a surgical disorder; however, primary care in the acute patient is directed toward the management of concurrent injury if present. Treatment of hypotension, anemia, and acute ventilatory failure may be necessary prior to elective correction. Patients with long-standing herniation may present with pleural effusion of unknown etiology. Thoracocentesis is always indicated in such cases.

PERITONEAL PERICARDIAL DIAPHRAGMATIC HERNIA

This congenital condition is frequently an incidental finding in older patients who have been examined radiographically for other reasons. It is not known as an acquired anomaly. Radiographically the cardiac silhouette may appear to be a centrally located globular structure. There may be gas shadows present if bowel is involved, or there may be granular densities representing ingesta.

DISORDERS OF THE CHEST WALL (pp. 814–817)

BLUNT CHEST TRAUMA

A preponderance of these injuries result from motor vehicle trauma. Other causes include falls from heights, kicking, and sports-related injuries; pulmonary injuries such as contusion, laceration, or hematoma; chest wall disruption; fracture of the tracheobronchial tree; rupture of the diaphragm; and hemothorax, pneumothorax, or pneumomediastinum or potential sequelae.

The term *flail chest* refers to chest wall disruption with multiple linear rib fractures and associated paradoxical segmental motion of the fractured section. This phenomenon leads to hypoventilation. Radiographically, multiple rib fractures are evident; this may be accompanied by elevation of the affected hemidiaphragm and associated loss of lung volume.

Management is determined by the patient's respiratory status and concomitant chest injuries. Measures have been recommended to externally stabilize the flail segment. These appear to be of little use and may provoke further hypoventilation. Flail segments usually heal without surgical repair. Internal fixation of the rib fractures may be helpful in stabilizing extensive hemiflail segments.

Hemothorax or hemorrhage into the pleural space may be of intercostal or pulmonary origin. Signs and findings of pleural effusion, hypotension, and shock may be concurrent. Small hemothoraces may be treated conservatively and should resorb in 1 to 2 weeks. With large, trauma-related hemothoraces, tube thoracostomy is indicated to reduce hemothorax. Thoracotomy may be required for the rare case of persistent bleeding from systemic vessels. Chest wall bleeding in patients with coagulopathies should resolve with the appropriate therapy for the underlying disorder.

THORACIC WALL MASSES AND INFILTRATIVE DISORDERS

Chondrosarcoma. This is the most frequently encountered primary neoplasm of the chest wall. The tumors typically arise from the costochondral junction, the sternum, or the midportion of the first two ribs. Chondrosarcomas rarely metastasize; however, these tumors may be characterized as benign by pathologists only to return later and invade adjacent structures following resection.

Osteosarcomas. Osteosarcomas of the chest wall are typically nonpainful, rapidly growing tumors that most frequently arise at the costochondral junction. This tumor has a propensity for pulmonary metastasis. Surgical resection with chemotherapeutic follow-up with Platinol appears to increase survival time.

Soft Tissue Sarcomas. Hemangiosarcoma may occur anywhere in the chest wall. These tumors may not be as aggressive as the visceral forms and may not metastasize as rapidly.

Multiple Myeloma. Multiple "punch-out" lytic lesions may be present in the ribs and less frequently in the sternum. Systemic disease is usually concurrently present.

Osteochondromatosis. These are cartilage-covered bone tumors and are considered benign. They appear on ribs or vertebral segments and are frequently found in younger animals. Generally, lesions grow until skeletal maturation is complete. Some tumors may take on malignant characteristics. In dogs this condition may be heritable. C-type viral particles have been seen in feline tumors.

Metastatic Chest Wall Tumors. Osteosarcoma or mammary carcinoma in dogs may metastasize to ribs.

Infectious Chest Wall Disorders

Cellulitis, abscesses, or granuloma formation may be seen with *Actinomyces* species, *Nocardia* species, anaerobic organisms, aerobic organisms, and fungi, such as *Blastomyces, Aspergillus, Coccidioides,* and *Cryptococcus.* Some of these may be associated with migration of foreign bodies or bite wounds, others with systemic dissemination or local invasion.

PLEURA AND PLEURAL SPACE DISORDERS
(pp. 817–831)

CLINICAL MANIFESTATIONS OF PLEURAL EFFUSION

The most common sign associated with pleural effusion is shortness of breath. Some patients may have cough, fever, or the subjective finding of pleural pain (elicited by firm palpation of the intercostal spaces). Patients with large volumes of fluid may tolerate effusions with little dyspnea if they have accumulated chronically. Percussion over a normal lung produces a low-frequency vibration. When underlying structures are dense, such as over the cardiac region, consolidated lung, pleural fluid, or other thoracic masses, a characteristic dulling of the vibration is noted.

DIAGNOSIS

Diagnostic Thoracocentesis

Since all pleural fluids (blood, exudates, and transudates) are radiographically indistinguishable, thoracocentesis is essential for establishing a definitive diagnosis. In addition, removal of fluid improves radiographic visualization of lung and pleura and provides relief from associated dyspnea. However, patients with previously diagnosed disorders known to result in pleural effusion may not require initial diagnostic thoracocentesis.

A relative contraindication for thoracocentesis is the presence of a bleeding disorder. As with all diagnostic procedures, the risks of thoracocentesis versus its benefits must be evaluated for each patient's condition. In all but the most uncooperative patients, the procedure is accomplished without sedation. Samples are withdrawn for bacterial culture, cytologic evaluation, and biochemical or serologic analysis, when indicated. It is important to obtain both aerobic and anaerobic cultures from any fluid that suggests an infection.

Therapeutic Thoracocentesis

Thoracocentesis as a therapeutic procedure is frequently necessary when a large pleural effusion causes lung compression and hypoventilation. Wherever infected fluids are present, tube thoracostomy is mandatory and should be performed as the primary means of drainage. Likewise, when large sterile effusions are present in canine patients, a chest tube rather than needle aspiration should be used. The possible complications of needle drainage or tube thoracostomy include hemorrhage, pneumothorax, pulmonary edema, bradycardia, and laceration of abdominal or thoracic viscera.

Pleural Biopsy

Pleural biopsy is a particularly useful means of diagnosing pleural neoplasia and granulomatous disorders resulting in pleural effusion. Experience suggests that in veterinary patient populations, the two most frequent diagnoses obtained by closed pleural biopsy are mesothelioma and infiltrative chest wall neoplasia, such as hemangiosarcoma. Contraindications are bleeding disorders, significant pulmonary insufficiency, pyoderma or cellulitis over the biopsy site, and empyema. Possible complications include hemothorax, pneumothorax or subcuticular emphysema, empyema, and needle track implantation of neoplasms.

Thoracoscopy

See textbook.

Open Biopsy

Diagnostic thoracotomy should be used as a last resort. Such procedures should always include biopsy of pleura, mediastinum, tracheobronchial lymph node and, in most instances, lung. Open biopsy and exploration may not always identify the cause of the pleural effusion. Those patients subjected to open biopsy are those with the most elusive disorders.

DISEASES ASSOCIATED WITH PLEURAL EFFUSION

Congestive Heart Failure

Although pure right-sided heart failure or biventricular failure represents a major cause of pleural effusion, the clinician should remain vigilant for concurrent disorders masquerading as heart failure. Malignancy, parapneumonic effusion, and pulmonary embolism or thrombosis may all coexist with known heart disease, particularly in older patients.

In both canine and feline patients, biventricular failure may produce pleural effusion of significant magnitude (Chapter 91). The pleural effusion of congestive heart failure is a transudate and typically is straw-colored, although occasionally bloody or pseudochylous. Only initially is the specific gravity 1.013 or less with a protein below 3 gm/dl. Therapeutic pleural drainage is not unusual. Appropriate therapy for the underlying heart disease should result in medical management of the effusion.

Neoplastic Pleural Effusion

The majority of pleural tumors are metastatic in origin; primary pleural tumors are infrequent. Pleural spread of neoplasia is frequently accompanied by effusion, but this is not always the case. Neoplastic mediastinitis may limit the effusion to one hemithorax. Characteristically, the effusion rapidly returns after evacuation unless some intervention is instituted.

Cytopathologic examination of sediment is by no means invariably diagnostic. Definitive diagnosis is frequently not possible even for the most talented cytopathologists. Atypia, nuclear variation, high mitotic index, and acinar formation may be frequent findings with any process that irritates the pleura.

The treatment of neoplastic pleural effusion depends on multiple factors, e.g., type of neoplasia, anatomic involvement, anticipated prognosis, and clinical signs present. Systemic chemotherapy is suggested in patients with potentially responsive neoplasia, (e.g., lymphoma or mammary carcinoma). Pleurodesis is the most frequently used treatment for neoplastic effusions. The indication for pleurodesis is a patient whose signs of dyspnea are related solely to the presence of effusion and recur following thoracocentesis and re-accumulation. The long-term relief provided by pleurodesis is variable.

Pulmonary Infection/Parapneumonic Effusion

Patients with pneumonia may experience pleural effusions secondary to their infection in the absence of overt empyema. Parapneumonic effusions, although sterile inflammatory exudates, are grossly serous or hemorrhagic rather than purulent. The effusion resolves spontaneously with appropriate treatment of the pulmonary infection. Some have observed that *Klebsiella* and streptococcal infections appear to have the highest incidenceof parapneumonic effusions.

Empyema

Pyothorax, or empyema, is the accumulation of infected material and fluid within the pleural space. Causative agents may reach the pleural space by three routes: as a result of systemic sepsis (infection reaches the pleura by either lymphatics or blood); as a result of spread from an adjacent structure (pneumonia with bronchopleural communication and parapneumonic spread, rupture of the esophagus, mediastinitis, or subphrenic infection); or by direct introduction of organisms as a result of penetrating trauma, foreign bodies, thoracocentesis, or surgery.

Clinical Presentation. Fever, anorexia, weight loss, and shortness of breath are associated with empyema.

Radiographic Findings. In most cases, a moderate-to-large pleural effusion is present. Most effusions are bilateral; however, in a significant number, the exudate is unilateral because of pleural and mediastinal involvement. Pneumohydrothorax may be a finding in patients with anaerobic infections or necrotizing pneumonia.

Microbiology. The Gram stain is the most important tool for rapid assessment of microorganisms in pleural fluid. Both dogs and cats with empyema have a high incidence of anaerobic infection, either as a sole pathogen or in combination with aerobic organisms.

Therapy. Tube thoracostomy should be performed as soon as the diagnosis is made. Chest tube drainage is best accomplished by continuous water seal suction. Only a small number of patients require bilateral chest tube placement. Medical resolution cannot take place without complete drainage of the infected material. Restoration of blood pressure and intravascular volume prior to tube thoracostomy greatly reduces the incidence of hypotension or apnea during the procedure.

Cytologic examination of pleural fluid should be undertaken frequently to assess the effectiveness of antimicrobial therapy. An organism may be obtained on subsequent culture that was not isolated at the time of primary bacteriologic work-up. Therapy should be instituted with moderately high doses of parenteral synthetic penicillin. An oral agent may be substituted as the clinical condition improves. We arbitrarily use 3 months of oral therapy after complete tube drainage.

Ampicillin remains the drug of choice for most forms of anaerobic infection. *Bacteroides fragilis* has been shown to be penicillin-resistant. Either chloramphenicol or clindamycin is employed when it is isolated. All feline patients should initially be treated with a combination of ampicillin and clindamycin. Combination therapy should be discontinued if anaerobic cultures fail to demonstrate *B. fragilis*. Hospital-acquired infection is less predictable. Pending results of cultures, treatment with a combination of a cephalosporin and aminoglycoside is suggested.

Autoimmune Disorders

Many autoimmune disorders are associated with pleural effusion. The volumes tend to be small, often just large enough to be radiographically observable. Among the disorders producing effusion are systemic lupus erythematosus, rheumatoid arthritis, idiopathic thrombocytopenia, and autoimmune hemolytic anemia. Other diseases are angiitis, granulomatosis, and other poorly defined entities such as Wegener's granulomatosis. The effusions of these patients may be large. The effusion is usually an inflammatory exudate, although it may occasionally be a transudate. The cell population is variable but usually contains both lymphocytes and polymorphonuclear cells. There may be early detection of lupus erythematosus cells in SLE patients.

Hepatic Disorders

Pleural effusion may be seen with hepatic cirrhosis; almost invariably there is associated ascites. The effusions are described in Chapter 14.

Pancreatitis

Pleural effusion may be associated with acute fulminant pancreatitis and is described in Chapter 14.

Infrequent Causes of Pleural Effusion

Abdominal Surgery. The acute appearance of small postoperative pleural effusion usually is not clinically relevant.

Esophageal Rupture. The acute consequences may be a sterile pleural effusion. If the effusion is secondary to mediastinitis, esophageal secretions and bacteria are contained within the mediastinal pleura.

Glomerulonephritis. See Chapter 14.

Pyometra and Postpartum Status. These effusions are small, and the etiology is unknown. They resolve spontaneously and require no intervention. The exception is the syndrome of pulmonary eosinophilia, which is occasionally observed in the first few weeks postpartum.

Pulmonary Thrombosis or Embolism. The pleural effusions are usually small and may be exudative or transudative. Direct treatment of these effusions is unnecessary.

Hyperthyroidism. Feline patients with hyperthyroidism may develop effusion with or without documented cardiac failure, although the latter is by far more prevalent. The effusion is transudative and may be pseudochylous. Patients with overt congestive heart failure appear to be best managed with appropriate cardiac medication and surgical thyroidectomy.

Lung Torsion.   In some cases, it is questionable whether the pleural fluid was present prior to lung lobe torsion or was caused by the event. The effusion is typically an exudate and frankly hemorrhagic. Tube thoracostomy is advisable to remove the large volume of effusion and prevent recurrence prior to surgical intervention.

Trauma.   Most pleural effusions appearing immediately following major abdominal and/or thoracic trauma are hemothoraces. Most frequently, the effusions are self-limiting; however, tube thoracostomy may be necessary in nonresolving effusions to prevent pleural peel formation and fibrothorax.

Traumatic Diaphragmatic Hernia.   The effusion may be transudative or exudative and mildly hemorrhagic.

Central Venous Catheters.   Both large- and small-bore venous catheters may cause pleural effusion by thrombosis and venous obstruction. These effusions may be transudative and chylous or frank hemithoraces.

Coagulopathies.   Inherited coaguolapathies and warfarin toxicosis are the most common examples.

Pleural Effusion of Undetermined Etiology

Despite exhaustive evaluation, the causes of some pleural effusions will remain undetermined.

Pleural Effusion with Eosinophilia.   Pleural effusions with eosinophil counts higher than that of the peripheral blood appear to be encountered frequently. The significance of these mildly eosinophilic effusions and their relationships to the etiologic cause of the effusion is unknown. Although almost any disorder causing pleural effusion is capable of episodically being eosinophilic in veterinary patients, parasitic, immunologic, and hypersensitivity disorders appear to be the most frequent causes. The disorders that most frequently produce effusions with profound eosinophilia are those associated with angiitis and granulomatosis. Other disorders, such as heartworm disease, chronic eosinophilic pneumonia, and hypereosinophilic syndrome, may produce pleural effusions with significant eosinophilia.

CHYLOTHORAX AND PSEUDOCHYLOTHORAX

Chylothorax is the accumulation of chylous fluid in the pleural space. This fluid has a high triglyceride concentration and demonstrates a chylomicron band in lipoprotein electrophoresis. The fluid has the gross appearance of skim milk. The differentiation between chyle and pseudochyle may require the use of biochemical or dye tests. The differential diagnosis of chyle and pseudochyle may be made by adding diethyl ether and alkali to a sample of pleural fluid. When mixed, the milky nature of the fluid dissipates if it is due to chyle rather than pseudochyle. Pseudochylous effusions are invariably secondary to an underlying disorder, such as heart failure or malignancy, whereas true chylothorax more frequently exists as a primary entity (Table 90–1).

The etiology of chylothorax includes malignancy, trauma, congenital, pancreatic, parasitic, infectious, and idiopathic causes, as well as congestive heart failure. Conservative management should be considered for patients not having a neoplastic or infectious cause. This is achieved by decreasing fluid intake and feeding carbohydrate-rich diets that are free of fats. However, a recent study suggests that low-fat diets have little effect on the rate of chyle accumulation. Medium-chain triglycerides are substituted because they are taken up directly by the portal circulation. Chylothorax secondary to malignancy commonly does not resolve in the face of systemic chemotherapy except with lymphomas.

TABLE 90–1. MAJOR CHARACTERISTICS OF CHYLE AND PSEUDOCHYLE

Appearance	Milky	Milky
Stain with Sudan III	Positive	Negative
Clearing with ether	Positive	Negative
Triglycerides	High	Normal or slightly increased
Cholesterol	Low to normal	Normal to high
Cytology	Lymphocytes and fat globules	Few cells, may have PMNs and Lmphs

A recent study indicates that the long-term prognosis for chronic idiopathic chylous effusions in dogs and cats is poor despite frequent thoracocentesis and dietary changes. Many progress to severe fibrosing pleuritis. For patients in which conservative therapy fails, tube thoracostomy with water seal drainage is suggested. This is followed by pleurodesis. Attempts at thoracic duct ligation followed by pleurodesis do not appear to yield a higher rate of resolution then pleurodesis alone.

PNEUMOTHORAX

Pneumothorax may occur through one of four pathways. Air enters the pleural space via puncture of the pulmonary visceral pleura, chest wall disruption, entry of mediastinal air, and diaphragmatic rupture. Pneumothorax may occur under tension if the lung or pleura acts as a one-way valve, i.e., allowing air to pump into the pleural space by respiratory motions, but preventing its flow back toward the airway. In this case, the intrapleural pressures rise drastically and become supraatmospheric.

Traumatic Pneumothorax

This may be the most frequent cause of pneumothorax in veterinary patients. Findings other than pneumothorax may include rib fractures, subcuticular emphysema, pneumomediastinum, pulmonary contusions, and, in rare cases, rupture of the trachea or major bronchus.

Spontaneous Pneumothorax

We use this term to describe pneumothorax not associated with a known iatrogenic or traumatic case, and when no apparent pulmonary pathology is present. Spontaneous pneumothorax is seen most frequently in large, deep-chested dogs, particularly sight hounds. It is assumed that these cases represent rupture of a small subpleural bleb, the etiology of which appears to be unknown.

Pulmonary Cysts

The rupture of large pulmonary cysts or pneumatoceles may produce pneumothoraces with large volumes.

Lung Abscesses or Necrosis of Pulmonary Neoplasia Producing Pneumothorax

Frequently, these are under tension and are all life threatening when superimposed on the underlying illness.

Iatrogenic Pneumothorax

This may occur as a complication of a wide variety of both diagnostic and therapeutic maneuvers.

Diagnosis and Treatment of Pneumothorax

Radiographically, the dorsal ventral projection is most important, as it helps to identify both unilateral and tension pneumothoraces. The hallmark of pneumothorax is a lucent hemithorax with absence of vascular markings. Physical findings associated with a large pneumothorax include a resonant chest on percussion, but breath sounds are diminished or absent on auscultation. The degree of dyspnea is variable but usually significant.

A single-needle aspiration is the least effective treatment and usually will not resolve the problem; however, the course will probably not be complicated by such therapy. Tube thoracostomy and water seal drainage for 3 to 4 days allow prompt and complete re-expansion of the lung. Should recurrence be a problem in a patient without radiographic evidence of the cause, either pleurodesis or thoracotomy may be curative. Unlike spontaneous pneumothorax, traumatic or iatrogenic pneumothorax may reasonably respond to a single-needle aspiration. If dyspnea and radiographic evidence of pneumothorax return, tube thoracostomy and drainage should be instituted.

The radiographic presence of a pulmonary cyst, lung abscess, or lung torsion, or evidence of esophageal perforation is an indication for surgical intervention. Pneumothorax associated with necrotizing pneumonia in the absence of overt abscesses is not a surgical emergency. However, it necessitates chest tube insertion in all cases.

MEDIASTINAL DISORDERS (pp. 831–841)

The mediastinum is the central portion of the thoracic cavity, covered by the reflections of parietal pleura. In most dogs and cats, the mediastinum is incomplete; thus, a unilateral process causing effusion or pneumothorax affects the contralateral hemithorax. Inflammatory disorders may seal the mediastinal fenestrations, keeping a process unilateral.

HISTORY

A history of recent trauma or diagnostic or surgical procedures is critical to the diagnosis of hemomediastinum. A history of previous procedures or malignancy should be sought. Geographic location needs to be ascertained when contemplating exposure to specific fungal or parasitic disorders.

PHYSICAL FINDINGS

Extrathoracic abnormalities are frequently present in cases of lymphosarcoma, metastatic carcinoma, and systemic fungal dissemination. Large or infiltrative masses of the cranial segments of the ventral and central mediastinum may produce obstruction of the vena cava. Vena caval syndrome is characterized by edema and symmetric swelling of the head, neck, and frequently the front limbs.

Respiratory Signs. Signs are largely related to airway or pulmonary parenchymal compression. Mass lesions may compress the trachea or segmental bronchi, producing airway obstruction. Infiltrative processes may entrap peripheral nerves, causing laryngeal paralysis.

Dysphagia. Segmental esophageal dysfunction, megaesophagus, esophageal foreign bodies, tumors, or mediastinitis most frequently cause signs of dysphagia or regurgitation.

Ophthalmologic Changes. Infiltrative processes or mass lesions may produce Horner's syndrome.

DIAGNOSTIC STUDIES IN MEDIASTINAL DISEASE

Radiography

The cornerstone of recognition is the presence of a mediastinal abnormality on standard thoracic radiographs. The exact location of the lesion within the mediastinum is determined both to help select further diagnostic tests and to aid in establishing a differential diagnosis. See the textbook for other procedures.

DISEASES OF THE MEDIASTINUM

Disorders Causing Acute Widening of the Cranial Segments of the Ventral and Central Mediastinum

Factors such as obesity, variation in thymic size and rib cage conformation, and specific breed conformities make it difficult if not impossible to evaluate small or moderate degrees of mediastinal widening. In comparison, cats rarely have accumulations of mediastinal fat that mimic mediastinal widening. Their normal mediastinal width rarely exceeds that of the sternum.

Mediastinal Hemorrhage

Both dogs and cats may experience mediastinal hemorrhage secondary to trauma, thoracic surgery, or coagulopathies. It has been reported that young dogs may experience spontaneous and fatal hemorrhage related to thymic vascular disruption. Hemomediastinum virtually always represents a medical disorder, and surgical exploration is not warranted.

Mediastinitis

Acute Mediastinitis. Acute mediastinitis most frequently arises from perforation or rupture of the trachea or esophagus. These patients may have persistent radiographic findings suggesting the etiology, such as tracheal fracture or esophageal foreign body. Head and neck infection may extend via fascial planes and thoracic inlet into the mediastinum. Acute mediastinitis infrequently stems from sepsis, pneumonia, pericarditis, or empyema.

Chronic Mediastinitis. Granulomatous mediastinitis may result from infection by a number of agents. *Histoplasma, Cryptococcus, Coccidioides, Actinomyces,* and *Nocardia* species are the most frequently encountered organisms. *Actinomyces* species and *Corynebacterium* species have been reported as causes. Both mediastinal abscesses and granulomas may masquerade as neoplasia.

Treatment of Mediastinitis. Acute mediastinitis associated with esophageal perforation is a surgical emergency. If indicated, tube thoracostomy and pleural drainage should be instituted preoperatively and pleural fluid cultured both aerobically and anaerobically. Until culture results are available, antimicrobial therapy is started with both an aminoglycoside and penicillin. Whenever possible, chronic mediastinitis is treated surgically. Abscess drainage or granuloma removal may prove a formidable challenge. Chest tube drainage should persist for several days following surgical removal of infected material. Antifungal or antimicrobial therapy depends on the etiologic agent.

Pneumomediastinum

The presence of air within the mediastinum may occur seemingly spontaneously, secondary to trauma, as a result of mechanical ventilation, or related to both diagnostic and therapeutic maneuvers. Air may enter the mediastinum by several routes. Penetrating wounds of the head, neck, and cranial thorax may allow air to dissect into the mediastinum via the thoracic inlet. Air may move cranially from the abdomen and retroperitoneum; this may appear spontaneously following abdominal surgery or rupture of a gas-filled viscus, or on rare occasions may be associated with bowel obstruction without rupture. Most frequently, pneumomediastinum results from airway or alveolar rupture. It may occur as a sole event or in combination with pneumothorax. Radiographically, pneumomediastinum is characterized by ability to visualize mediastinal structures usually not seen (e.g., aorta, vena cava, azygous vein, and esophagus). In addition, there may be subcuticular emphysema present. On rare occasions, pneumocardium may be present.

Clinical Manifestation. Many patients are relatively asymptomatic. Markedly increased pressures within the mediastinum can produce acute catastrophic hypotension and ventilatory failure. Acute pneumothorax, which may be under tension, may produce profound dyspnea. Patients with esophageal rupture and mediastinitis may appear to be in pain and in extremis.

Treatment. Most uncomplicated cases require no treatment at all. However, it may take 10 to 20 days for all mediastinal and subcutaneous air to spontaneously resolve. Most patients who are significantly dyspneic have associated pneumothorax. Simple thoracocentesis may reduce dyspnea temporarily, but recurrence is frequent, requiring tube thoracostomy and water seal drainage. Patients in circulatory collapse should be volume expanded. Attempts to cannulate the mediastinum are ill-advised.

Benign Lymphadenopathy

Numerous infectious disorders produce thoracic lymph node enlargement. Bacterial infection causing empyema or mediastinitis produces adenopathy that may be radiographically recognizable. Frequently the primary process prevents recognition of node enlargement until pleural or mediastinal fluid is resolved.

Fungal Disorders

Mediastinal adenopathy may be the major radiographic finding in patients with systemic fungal disorders. Coccidioidomycosis, histoplasmosis, blastomycosis, and cryptococcosis may all produce mediastinal adenopathy in severe cases. Primary tuberculosis in dogs and cats may produce mediastinal node enlargement as a component of their complex. Mediastinal granulomas of identifiable or unknown etiology may cause mediastinal enlargement. *Actinomyces* and *Nocardia* species are the most frequently involved agents and may be responsible for both thoracic and extrathoracic spread. Adenopathy with pleural effusion is a frequent finding. These lesions may mimic neoplasia both clinically and radiographically.

Neoplastic Disorders

Neoplastic Lymphadenopathy. Lymphoma and lymphosarcoma frequently manifest their major clinical signs as those of mediastinal and pleura disease. Feline patients experience approximately 70 per cent of their tumor distribution in the mediastinum and alimentary tract; canine patients generally experience their disease as the multicentric form. Cats may have perihilar or sternal node involvement. In comparison, dogs infrequently have thymic lymphosarcoma.

Unlike thymoma, thoracic lymphosarcoma is frequently accompanied by pleural effusion. Dyspnea may be related to airway compression by large tumor masses or to pleural effusion. The presence of neoplastic cells in pleural fluid is variable but frequently diagnostically rewarding. Closed cutting needle biopsy is ill-advised. Infrequently, thoracotomy is necessary to confirm the diagnosis.

Metastatic Invasion of Mediastinal Lymph Nodes. Metastatic carcinoma and pulmonary carcinomas are the most common cause. In such cases there is usually a pulmonary mass or infiltrate that is a diagnostic aid. Pulmonary lymphosarcoma mimics this pattern. Mediastinal lymph node metastases may arise from tumors elsewhere in the body.

Thyroid Carcinoma. Extension of thyroid carcinoma into the cranial ventral mediastinum is more frequent in dogs than in cats but uncommon in both species.

Chemodectoma. Chemodectomas or heart-base, aortic body, or nonchromaffin paragangliomas are neoplasms of chemoreceptor cells of the aortic and carotid bodies. They may appear as discrete, well-encapsulated masses or infiltrative masses, intertwining themselves around the great vessels with direct cardiac extension. The recognition of such tumors often is related to intrapericardial invasion, with production of pericardial effusion and signs of right heart failure. Presumptive diagnosis may be established by aortography or echocardiographic evaluation.

Scirrhous Carcinoma. Carcinomas of the mediastinum are not frequently encountered and may pose a diagnostic challenge.

Thymoma

These tumors are solid and discrete when observed early in their course. Later they are expansile, making surgical removal impossible. Local invasion is common, but the metastatic potential of thymomas is apparently low. Surgical resection is a viable procedure that results in long-term survival in the majority of patients. The clinical signs are related to both tumor size and the presence or absence of paraneoplastic syndromes. Large pleural effusions are not typically present. If vomition is present, it is usually related to megaesophagus rather than obstruction. Cranial vena caval syndrome may be present. A number of associated disorders have been recognized: Cushing's syndrome, myasthenia gravis, hypogammaglobulinemia, and aplastic anemia. Surgical removal of the thymoma may palliate or resolve the signs of myasthenia gravis.

Cysts

Benign cysts of the ventral mediastinum are uncommon and arise from diverse cell lines. They typically are inadvertent findings on thoracic radiographs. Patients are typically asymptomatic, and these masses are not known to be pathologic.

CHAPTER 91

PATHOPHYSIOLOGY OF HEART FAILURE AND CLINICAL EVALUATION OF CARDIAC FUNCTION
(pages 844–867)

The syndrome of congestive heart failure represents a complex interaction of compensatory responses that attempt to preserve cardiac function and regional blood flow. Before rational decisions can be made regarding therapeutic options, it is essential that each patient be individually evaluated to determine what is causing the heart to fail and which compensatory responses are in greatest need of modification.

DETERMINANTS OF CARDIAC OUTPUT (pp. 845–851)

HEART RATE

Under normal circumstances, heart rate is the major determinant of transient changes in cardiac output.

PRELOAD

Blood volume expansion is an important determinant of preload and the adequacy of ventricular filling. Preload may be decreased in several clinical circumstances. Elevated intrathoracic pressure caused by pneumothorax or intermittent positive pressure respiration can have a major adverse effect on cardiac performance by impeding systemic venous return. Also, cardiac tamponade reduces the effective preload.

AFTERLOAD

The tension that develops in the wall of a contracting ventricle is designated the afterload. The systolic tension developed in muscle fibers is a powerful stimulus for hypertrophy. Myocardial hypertrophy compensates for chronic increases in afterload.

CONTRACTILITY

Chronic systolic mechanical overloading of any etiology requires the heart to perform more work at a given cardiac output. Unlike skele-

Original chapter written by David H. Knight

tal muscles, the heart is a functional syncytium and is therefore unable to recruit more motor units. Sustained systolic overloading of the heart usually leads to a decline in myocardial contractility.

COMPENSATORY MECHANISMS (pp. 851–855)

The integrity of cardiac function depends on three major compensatory mechanisms: (1) catecholamine release from cardiac adrenergic nerves and the adrenal medulla, (2) the Frank-Starling mechanism, implemented by blood volume expansion through the complex interplay of the renal-adrenal-pituitary axis, and (3) cardiac hypertrophy with or without chamber enlargement.

SYMPATHETIC NERVOUS SYSTEM

Vasoconstriction is a reflex response to falling cardiac output and blood pressure. Preservation of arterial blood pressure takes precedence over maintenance of cardiac output.

RENAL-ADRENAL-PITUITARY INTERACTIONS

Blood volume expansion is the result of renal conservation of sodium and water. The sequence of events begins with a fall in cardiac output and blood pressure.

CARDIORENAL INTERACTIONS (ATRIAL NATRIURETIC FACTOR)

The volume expansion induced by activation of the RAA system is helpful only to a point, after which deleterious side effects begin to develop. Although unable to normalize hemodynamics and natriuresis, ANF nonetheless appears to provide an important moderating effect on the pathogenesis of congestive heart failure.

CARDIAC HYPERTROPHY

One of two patterns of ventricular hypertrophy develops, depending on the nature of the stress. Pressure-overloaded ventricles adapt to increases in systolic wall tension by increasing wall thickness relative to the chamber volume (concentric hypertrophy). Volume-overloaded ventricles adapt to chronic, obligatory increases in stroke volume by undergoing extensive end-diastolic enlargement. Under these circumstances, wall thickness relative to chamber volume is normal at best and is usually reduced (*eccentric hypertrophy*).

CAUSES OF HEART FAILURE (pp. 855–859)

PRIMARY REDUCTION OF VENTRICULAR CONTRACTILITY

Dilated cardiomyopathy and chronic myocarditis of whatever etiology can produce profound depression of ventricular contractility and eventually lead to intractable heart failure. The clinical signs of heart failure develop over a relatively short period of time late in the clinical course.

SYSTOLIC MECHANICAL OVERLOAD

Pressure Overloading. Subaortic stenosis and pulmonary hypertension are two classic examples of pressure overloading. Chronic pressure-overloaded ventricles rely primarily on concentric hypertrophy to preserve stroke output. Once hypertrophy ceases to be an adequate response, the pressure-overloaded ventricle becomes increasingly dependent on preload. In this context, progressive ventricular dilatation is indicative of a decline in contractility.

Volume Overloading. In volume-overloaded conditions such as atrioventricular and semilunar valve regurgitation and left-to-right shunts, total stroke output exceeds the effective (forward) stroke output. As the ventricular chamber volume increases, eccentric hypertrophy normalizes systolic wall stress.

Aortic Versus Mitral Regurgitation. Left ventricular function is more seriously compromised by aortic regurgitation.

Ventricular Septal Defect Versus Patent Ductus Arteriosus. At the same volume of left-to-right shunt, the left ventricular systolic mechanical overload is greater with a patent ductus because of higher afterload.

Acute Versus Chronic Overloading. Although it takes a long time before contractility is seriously depressed by volume overloading, the degree of impairment ultimately exceeds that occurring with a pressure overload and is more likely to be irreversible.

DIASTOLIC MECHANICAL INHIBITION

Conditions causing a decrease in ventricular diastolic function impede venous return. In dogs and cats, pericardial disorders are the most common and significant causes. Right ventricular filling pressure normally is less than that of the left ventricle. Therefore, the right ventricle is particularly adversely affected. Right heart failure with cardiac tamponade is most commonly caused by hemopericardium produced by benign sanguineous pericarditis or by intrapericardial neoplasms. Venous return can also be impeded by conditions that stiffen the ventricular walls such as feline hypertrophic and restrictive cardiomyopathies. Each primarily affects the left ventricle.

CLINICAL MANIFESTATIONS OF HEART FAILURE
(pp. 859–861)

With the exception of generalized venous engorgement, the other physical signs associated with heart failure (Table 91–1) may have a noncardiac pathogenesis. The classic signs related to heart failure are congestion and edema. Pulmonary edema can form precipitously and rapidly become fatal. In fulminating cases of left heart failure, edema fluid accumulates in the bronchi and trachea, where it mixes with air and may appear in the nose and mouth as a blood-tinged froth. The so-called "heart failure" cough is usually caused by severe left heart enlargement with compression of the left bronchus. Consequently, a cough may draw attention to left-sided heart disease, but is not necessarily indicative of heart failure.

Dogs have a predilection for developing ascites, but in cats pleural effusion is more common. Hepatomegaly due to chronic passive congestion is a prominent and consistent finding in all cases of pure right-sided and generalized heart failure. Following successful diuresis, such patients frequently look emaciated, and it becomes apparent in retrospect that considerable tissue edema had been present. Overt pitting edema in limbs and the body wall is relatively uncommon. Tachycardia, blanched mucous membranes, and cool extremities are common signs of sympathetic overstimulation in heart failure. Signs of decompensating heart failure include cachexia, weakness, reduced urine flow, and hypotension, in addition to the side effects associated with congestion.

CLINICAL EVALUATION OF CARDIAC FUNCTION
(pp. 861–866)

It is important to remember that rather than making the physical examination obsolete, modern medical instrumentation should give us more confidence in our physical diagnostic ability by providing an

TABLE 91–1. PHYSICAL SIGNS ASSOCIATED WITH HEART FAILURE

PULMONARY SIGNS (LEFT HEART)	SYSTEMIC SIGNS (RIGHT HEART)
Rales (alveolar edema)	Generalized venous engorgement
Frothy, pink expectorant	Hepatomegaly
Shortness of breath, tachypnea	Serous effusions in body cavities
Nocturnal dyspnea (orthopnea)	Ascites
Cough	Pleural effusion
	Pericardial effusion
	Dependent peripheral edema
	Weight gain (retained fluid)

SIGNS ATTRIBUTABLE TO EITHER LEFT OR RIGHT HEART FAILURE

Weakness and fatigue (general exercise intolerance)
Exertional dyspnea
Gallop rhythm (accentuated third heart sound)
Poor peripheral perfusion
   Pale membranes
   Slow capillary refill time
   Mild cyanosis
   Cool extremities
Tachycardia
Weight loss (cachexia)

independent means of substantiating our conclusions. Reliable signs of heart disease must be identified before a diagnosis of heart failure can be justified. This requires a discerning interpretation of heart sounds and murmurs, arterial pulse quality and venous distention, cardiac rhythm, and radiographic chamber size.

VENTRICULAR FILLING PRESSURE

Central venous (CVP) and pulmonary capillary wedge (PCWP) pressures measure filling pressure of the right and left ventricles, respectively. For monitoring PCWP, a Swan-Ganz balloon-tipped catheter can be passed percutaneously under local anesthesia via a jugular vein into a peripheral branch of a pulmonary artery and left in place for several days. Normally, mean left atrial pressure will be less than 12 mm Hg, and the risk of pulmonary edema increases substantially as it nears 20 mm Hg.

EJECTION PHASE INDICES

These indices of LV contractility are the *ejection fraction*, the *per cent fractional shortening* (%FS) of the end-diastolic minor axis internal dimension, and the *velocity of circumferential fiber shortening* (V_{CF}), which is the %FS corrected for the ejection time. The fact that each can be calculated from data obtained noninvasively by M-mode echocardiography is an important practical advantage. By creating a low-impedance leak, severe mitral regurgitation lowers afterload and facilitates shortening. Therefore, unless ejection phase indices fall at or above the high normal range, depressed contractility should be suspected in cases of chronic mitral regurgitation. Dilated cardiomyopathic hearts are usually neither pressure- nor volume-overloaded. Consequently, ejection phase indices are helpful in distinguishing these hearts from normal.

The ejection phase indices provide an indication of basal contractility, but unless loading is accounted for, comparisons between individuals are tenuous. However, the indices are useful for serial comparisons. Typically, the normal range of %FS is higher for small individuals. Consequently, failure to give consideration to body size when evaluating the ejection phase indices can lead to erroneous conclusions.

Empiric evidence in humans indicates that a better correlation exists between angiographically determined EF and mitral valve E-point septal separation (EPSS) than either M-mode echocardiographic %FS or EF. EPSS is more representative of global left ventricular function than inferences drawn from M-mode measurements of ventricular chamber dimensions. Furthermore, it is unaffected by paradoxical septal motion and other wall motion abnormalities that invalidate calculations of %FS and EF. A wide EPSS is indicative of low EF due to either systolic or diastolic dysfunction.

PRESSURE-VOLUME RELATIONSHIPS

The end-systolic pressure-volume relation (ESPVR) defines the systolic properties of the left ventricular chamber. Since the ESPVR is virtually independent of preload and afterload, it provides the most objective means of comparing basal myocardial contractility in individuals and monitoring directional changes. However, due to the invasiveness of this technique, it still is impractical for routine patient evaluations.

STROKE VOLUME AND CARDIAC OUTPUT

Like the ejection phase indices, Doppler indices are influenced by ventricular loading and heart rate. However, the fact that they assess global rather than regional ventricular performance, as do M-mode indices, makes Doppler echocardiography a particularly valuable tool in experienced hands.

SYSTOLIC TIME INTERVALS (STI)

Although still useful, the STI have lost favor to the ejection phase indices and P/V relations. Heart failure increases PEP and decreases ET.

DIASTOLIC FUNCTION

Early in the course of heart disease, diastolic dysfunction may precede systolic dysfunction. No simple, direct method of assessing diastolic function exists. The diastolic pressure-volume relationship provides the most objective method. Doppler echocardiography is a convenient method of analyzing transmitral flow velocity, and it has been used extensively to assess diastolic function.

CHAPTER 92

THERAPY OF HEART FAILURE
(pages 867–892)

CLASSIFICATION AND STAGING OF HEART FAILURE
(p. 868)

The New York Heart Association (NYHA) Functional Classification, based largely on the degree of activity restriction resulting from the signs of heart failure, is probably the one most widely used in human medicine and has been adapted to veterinary use. The NYHA Functional Classification can be summarized as follows:

Class I: No limitation. Physical activity, including normal exercise, does not cause symptoms.

Class II: Slight limitation of physical activity. Ordinary physical activity results in symptoms.

Class III: Marked limitation of physical activity. Less than ordinary activity leads to symptoms.

Class IV: Inability to carry on any activity without symptoms. Symptoms present at rest.

DRUGS THAT IMPROVE CONTRACTILITY (POSITIVE INOTROPES) (pp. 868–875)

1. All positive inotropes can potentially increase the myocardial oxygen consumption (MVO_2), and all are potentially arrhythmogenic.

2. All result in increased intracellular calcium levels or in increased sensitivity of the contractile proteins to intracellular calcium.

3. None of these agents has been shown to significantly alter the underlying pathology that caused the heart to fail.

4. The efficacy of most of these drugs is uncertain in many clinical settings.

5. Most of the available positive inotropic drugs have a relatively narrow therapeutic index.

DIGITALIS

Actions. Digitalization of human patients with moderate to severe heart failure induces sustained inhibition of the sympathetic activation that characterizes the syndrome of heart failure. This inhibition precedes any measurable hemodynamic effects. Acute digitalization of human patients also normalizes the baroreceptor reflexes that are impaired in heart failure. Digitalis also has positive inotropic and supraventricular antiarrhythmic actions. These antiarrhythmic effects are caused by a combination of direct and neurally mediated effects on the heart. These properties form the basis for the use of digitalis in slowing the ventricular response to atrial fibrillation and breaking or preventing atrial or AV nodal reentrant tachycardias. They also account for the frequently observed prolongation of the P-R interval accompanying digitalis usage.

Pharmacokinetics. Digoxin is the most commonly used digitalis preparation in veterinary medicine. Digoxin elimination is heavily dependent on glomerular filtration. Animals with decreased glomerular filtration rates, whether or not they are azotemic, are thus at increased risk of digoxin toxicity. Dosage reductions for animals with compromised

---

Original chapter written by Bruce W. Keene and John E. Rush

glomerular filtration are necessary. If digoxin must be used to digitalize an azotemic patient, we recommend (1) reducing the dosage of digoxin by 50 per cent for every 50 per cent rise in the BUN and (2) monitoring serum digoxin levels beginning 8 to 12 hours after the morning dose on the third, fifth, and seventh day of maintenance digitalization.

Indications and Current Use. Considering currently available information, we use digitalis in the management of heart failure secondary to chronic valvular heart disease whenever signs attributable to congestive heart failure are present. In the therapy of cardiac diseases in which the primary pathophysiologic defect is systolic myocardial dysfunction (e.g., dilated cardiomyopathy) and in the absence of serious contraindications (e.g., ventricular arrhythmias that increase in frequency or severity with therapy), digitalization is indicated in both the dog and the cat.

Digitalis is generally contraindicated in animals with sinus node dysfunction, unless their symptoms can be shown to arise from episodes of supraventricular tachycardia. Atrioventricular nodal dysfunction more serious than first-degree AV block also represents an important contraindication to digitalis. Other conditions in which digoxin is relatively contraindicated include pericardial disease, hypertrophic cardiomyopathy, and aortic stenosis.

The dosage of digoxin should be based on lean body weight. Compensatory dosage reductions are recommended for animals with ascites. Published dosage recommendations include 0.010 mg/lb/day (0.022 mg/kg/day), 0.010 mg/lb (0.022 mg/kg) divided twice daily, these dosages multiplied by 0.75 for the elixir and by 0.85 for the tablet, and 0.22 mg/m^2 twice daily. Doberman pinschers with dilated cardiomyopathy are particularly sensitive to digitalis and prone to toxicity.

In general, cats are easily intoxicated with digitalis. Adult cats undergoing digitalization for dilated cardiomyopathy (still the most common indication) are started directly on a maintenance schedule of one-fourth of a 0.125-mg tablet every other day, and digoxin serum levels are evaluated on the seventh day.

Toxicity and Drug Interactions. Electrolyte abnormalities (most frequently, hypokalemia) significantly influence both the occurrence and severity of digitalis intoxication. Anorexia, concurrent use of diuretics, and hyperaldosteronism are the most common contributors to the development of hypokalemia. Hypercalcemia can also complicate digitalis intoxication. The use of quinidine in patients receiving digoxin should be avoided when possible, and a reduced dosage of digoxin should be used if the combination is necessary. In dogs, acute withdrawal of phenobarbital, as well as chronic phenobarbital therapy, has been associated with digoxin intoxication. Aspirin has also been shown to increase serum digoxin concentrations in the dog.

The clinical manifestations of digitalis intoxication are caused by both direct and neurally mediated actions. Signs of intoxication vary among individuals, but anorexia, depression, and/or borborygmus are frequent early complaints, followed by nausea, vomiting, and diarrhea. Cardiac arrhythmias commonly attend digitalis intoxication. Sinus bradycardia with varying degrees of AV block, ventricular bigeminy or tachycardia, junctional or supraventricular arrhythmias, and unusually slow ventricular response rates to atrial fibrillation are all signs of digitalis intoxication.

Signs of digoxin intoxication are consistently observed when serum digoxin concentrations rise above 2.5 ng/ml in normal dogs. In animals showing clinical or electrocardiographic signs of intoxication, digitalis should be discontinued pending evaluation of the serum drug concentration. The patient should receive appropriate supportive care until the clinical signs resolve. If digitalis is indicated, therapy can be reinstituted at appropriately reduced (usually 50 per cent) dosages.

Mild signs of digitalis intoxication can be managed by withdrawal of the drug for 1 to 2 days and restarting therapy with a 50 per cent dose reduction. Successful treatment of severe digitalis intoxication requires intensive care and monitoring.

CATECHOLAMINES

All of the catecholamines have short serum half-lives, usually less than 2 minutes. These drugs are usually administered intravenously and are generally useful only for the short-term management of severe heart failure. All of the catecholamines are potentially arrhythmogenic.

Epinephrine

Indications and Current Use.   Epinephrine remains the drug of choice for positive inotropic and circulatory support following cardiac arrest. The usual dosage used during resuscitation is 0.25 to 0.5 cc/10 lb (0.5 to 1.0 cc/10 kg) of 1:10,000 solution administered intravenously or intratracheally.

Isoproterenol

Indications and Current Use.   Isoproterenol is rarely used therapeutically except in the emergency treatment of high-grade or complete AV block that has proved unresponsive to anticholinergics. Infusion rates vary from 0.02 to 0.04 µg/lb/min (0.045 to 0.09 µg/kg/min).

Dopamine

Indications and Current Use.   Low doses are useful in the management of acute oliguric renal failure. Higher doses can be used for circulatory support in patients with cardiovascular depression. Dopamine may be useful at midrange dosages for the management of primary myocardial disease that has resulted in heart failure. Dopamine is rarely used as a primary drug in the management of heart failure except in cases of cardiogenic shock related to anesthesia or following cardiac resuscitation, when arterial blood pressure support becomes critical. In this setting, dopamine infusion is initiated at 0.5 µg/lb/min (1 µg/kg/min), and the patient is closely monitored. Infusion rates are then judiciously increased in increments of 1 to 3 µg/lb/min (3 to 5 µg/kg/min) approximately every 8 to 10 minutes until the desired effects are achieved or signs of toxicity occur.

Dobutamine

Beta blockers can effectively abolish the inotropic effects of dobutamine.
Indications and Current Use.   Currently, the routine clinical use of dobutamine is generally limited to veterinary patients with severe, intractable heart failure caused or complicated by myocardial failure or depression. Dobutamine is contraindicated in patients with hypertrophic subaortic stenosis or any heart disease characterized by ventricular hypertrophy that might result in outflow tract obstruction under catecholamine stimulation (e.g., hypertrophic cardiomyopathy).

Therapy should be initiated at low dosages (0.5 to 1 µg/lb/min [1 to 2 µg/kg/min] in the dog; 0.25 µg/lb/min [0.5 µg/kg/min] in the cat). Clinical improvement usually occurs at infusion rates of 1 to 5 µg/lb/min (2.5 to 10 µg/kg/min) in the dog. In patients that respond to therapy, dobutamine infusion is usually maintained for 1 to 3 days. Cats appear to be exquisitely sensitive to dobutamine and may manifest toxic signs of seizures and/or vomiting. Dobutamine is available in 250-mg vials for reconstitution, usually with 5 per cent dextrose in water.

Toxicity and Drug Interaction.   Side effects observed with dobutamine include tachyarrhythmias, vomition, nervousness, and seizures (cats). Discontinuation of the drug is usually effective in alleviating arrhythmias or other toxic manifestations.

BIPYRIDINE DERIVATIVES (pp. 875–878)

AMRINONE

Indications and Current Use. Use of amrinone should be limited to the short-term therapy of patients with severe heart failure or myocardial depression. Published dosage recommendations for the dog and cat suggest an initial bolus of 0.5 to 1.5 mg/lb (1 to 3 mg/kg), followed immediately by a constant rate infusion of 5 to 50 µg/lb/min (10 to 100 µg/kg/min).

Toxicity and Drug Interactions. Hypotension, arrhythmia, or GI distress may indicate overdosage, and the infusion rate should be promptly decreased or the drug discontinued. Amrinone must be diluted in nondextrose-containing solutions.

MILRINONE

See textbook.

DIURETICS (pp. 878–881)

Diuretics continue to be a pharmacologic mainstay of the acute therapy of heart failure.

HIGH-CEILING OR LOOP DIURETICS

The family of high-ceiling or loop diuretics includes furosemide, ethacrynic acid, and bumetanide. These are all potent diuretics that act at the thick ascending limb of the loop of Henle to inhibit active chloride transport. In general, these drugs are effective in the face of hypoalbuminemia, acid-base or electrolyte imbalances, and low glomerular filtration rates, making refractoriness to therapy unusual in the absence of severe renal failure.

Furosemide

Indications and Current Use. Furosemide is widely considered to be "first-line" therapy in the management of inappropriate fluid retention secondary to heart failure from any cause other than pericardial disease. The routine maintenance oral dosage for dogs with chronic congestive heart failure treated concurrently with an angiotensin-converting enzyme inhibitor is approximately 0.5 mg/lb (1 mg/kg) q12h. In dogs with acute, severe congestive heart failure, furosemide is usually administered parenterally at a dosage of 1 to 2 mg/lb (2 to 4 mg/kg), and that dose is often repeated in 2 to 6 hours until the animal is stable. Experience suggests that most cats respond well to lower dosages (0.5 to 1 mg/lb [1 to 2 mg/kg] q12h to q48h).

Toxicity and Drug Interactions. Concurrent use of aminoglycoside antibiotics (especially gentamycin) and furosemide is contraindicated. Hypokalemia is the most common electrolyte imbalance accompanying furosemide therapy. Hyponatremia can also be a potentially serious complication of both advanced congestive heart failure and furosemide therapy. Despite low serum sodium levels in these heart failure patients, total body sodium levels are usually normal or increased. This condition has been termed dilutional hyponatremia and represents a serious complication of advanced congestive heart failure. Dilutional hyponatremia is one of the few clinical situations in which water restriction is indicated. Further diuretic therapy is inappropriate.

Supplementation of B-complex vitamins is recommended for patients on continuous diuretic therapy.

THIAZIDE DIURETICS

The thiazide diuretics act on the proximal portion of the distal convoluted tubule to inhibit resorption of sodium and cause secretion of potassium. The thiazide diuretics are not effective in patients with compromised renal function. They are contraindicated in azotemic animals.

Indications and Current Use. Chlorothiazide and hydrochlorothiazide are the most commonly used thiazides in veterinary medicine. The usual oral dosage of chlorothiazide is 10 to 20 mg/lb (20 to 40 mg/kg) q12h. The recommended dosage of hydrochlorothiazide is 1 to 2 mg/lb (2 to 4 mg/kg) q12h.

Toxicity and Drug Interactions. In animals with normal renal function, the thiazide diuretics have little potential for toxicity. Hypokalemia is the most commonly observed electrolyte disturbance.

POTASSIUM-SPARING DIURETICS

Spironolactone and triamterene are the potassium-sparing diuretics currently used in veterinary medicine. Spironolactone is a competitive antagonist of aldosterone.

Indications and Current Use. Our most common use of spironolactone is in the management of dogs with congestive heart failure secondary to either chronic valvular heart disease or dilated cardiomyopathy that has become unresponsive to drug therapy with an angiotensin-converting enzyme inhibitor, digoxin, and furosemide. The recommended dosage in the dog is 1 to 2 mg/lb/day (2 to 4 mg/kg/day).

Toxicity and Drug Interactions. Potassium-sparing diuretics should generally not be administered concurrently with potassium supplements. The use of spironolactone in combination with angiotensin-converting enzyme inhibitors is widely assumed to increase the potential for hyperkalemia.

VASODILATORS (pp. 881–884)

Although vasodilators promise attractive potential benefits in the management of heart failure, serious drawbacks are associated with their inappropriate or overzealous use. Inappropriate use of arterial dilators may cause serious hypotension and reflex tachycardia. In consideration of the adverse effects associated with their inappropriate use, every effort to obtain a definitive diagnosis along with as much hemodynamic information as possible should be made prior to initiating vasodilator therapy.

Abrupt discontinuation of vasodilator therapy can be associated with a "rebound" phenomenon (increased systemic vascular resistance, ventricular filling pressures, and decreased cardiac output). With this in mind, vasodilator therapy that is to be discontinued is *not* stopped suddenly, but is generally tapered over a period of days.

HYDRALAZINE

Hydralazine is a direct-acting arteriolar dilator.

Indications and Current Use. Hydralazine is often beneficial in patients with chronic cough secondary to left atrial enlargement that has caused compression or collapse of the left main stem bronchus. It may be useful in any situation in which arteriolar dilation is likely to be beneficial (e.g., low output heart failure from any cause other than aortic stenosis or hypertrophic cardiomyopathy). Hydralazine may be added to a regimen of an angiotensin-converting enzyme inhibitor, digoxin, and diuretic in patients with refractory signs of congestive heart failure.

Studies have recommended an initial oral dosage of 0.5 mg/lb (1 mg/kg), to be increased by 0.5 mg/lb (1 mg/kg) to a maximum of 1.5 mg/lb (3 mg/kg), depending on the therapeutic response. The recommended therapeutic end points of hydralazine titration are a mean arterial blood pressure of 70 to 80 mm Hg and central venous oxygen tensions greater than 30 mm Hg. If arterial blood pressure and/or blood gas monitoring are unavailable, an initial hydralazine dosage of 0.25 to 0.5 mg/lb (0.5 to 1 mg/kg) q12h is recommended, and this dosage is slowly increased to a maximum of 1.5 mg/lb (3 mg/kg) over several days.

Toxicity and Drug Interactions. Hypotension is the most commonly reported complication. The drug should be discontinued for 24 hours and restarted at 50 per cent of the initial dose. Another potentially significant side effect of hydralazine is reflex tachycardia. Gastrointestinal disturbances (most commonly anorexia and vomiting) sometimes occur during hydralazine therapy.

NITROGLYCERIN AND OTHER NITRATES

Nitroglycerin and the nitrates cause direct relaxation of venous smooth muscle.

Indications and Current Use. The nitrates are used primarily for the acute treatment of cardiogenic pulmonary edema. One-quarter to one-half inch of ointment per 10 lb usually results in measurable reductions in central venous or pulmonary capillary wedge pressure within 30 minutes.

Toxicity and Drug Interactions. Overdosage with nitroglycerin can result in severely compromised cardiac output because of large reductions in preload. Some degree of lethargy and/or somnolence is often seen with nitroglycerin therapy in animals.

SODIUM NITROPRUSSIDE

Sodium nitroprusside is a balanced vasodilator that acts directly on arterial and venous vascular smooth muscle; it must be administered by constant intravenous infusion.

Indications and Current Use. The drug is most often used to improve cardiac output and reduce ventricular filling pressures (and thus pulmonary edema) in patients with severe heart failure. In the dog, the initial infusion rate used at our hospital is 0.5 µg/lb/min (1 µg/kg/min), and the rate of infusion is increased by 0.5 µg/lb/min (1 µg/kg/min) every 5 minutes until the mean arterial pressure reaches the target level of approximately 70 mm Hg.

Toxicity and Drug Interactions. Hypotension may develop rapidly and can be managed by simply reducing the infusion rate. Maximum clinical and hemodynamic benefits are usually obtained when the drug is used in combination with dobutamine. Nitroprusside is metabolized to cyanide. High doses or protracted (days) therapy with nitroprusside can theoretically result in cyanide poisoning.

PRAZOSIN

See textbook.

ANGIOTENSIN-CONVERTING ENZYME (ACE) INHIBITORS (pp. 884–886)

ACE inhibitors to function as balanced vasodilators, reducing both afterload and preload in heart failure patients. ACE inhibition can potentially prevent or at least slow the progressive myocyte hypertrophy and fibrosis that complicates many heart diseases.

CAPTOPRIL

Indications and Current Use. Captopril is rarely used because of the proven safety and efficacy of enalapril, the short pharmacodynamic half-life of captopril in the dog, and the perceived higher incidence of gastrointestinal side effects of captopril therapy. The initial dosage in the dog is usually 0.10 to 0.22 mg/lb (0.25 to 0.5 mg/kg) q8h; this dosage may be titrated upward.

Toxicity and Drug Interactions. Hypotension is a potential complication, and low initial doses with gradual dose titration are recommended to minimize this problem. Gastrointestinal disturbances, including anorexia, vomiting, and diarrhea (sometimes severe and bloody), are frequently observed. Hyperkalemia may occur with captopril therapy. Renal insufficiency has been observed in veterinary patients receiving captopril. Dosage should not exceed 1 mg/lb (2 mg/kg) administered three times daily, and the drug should be used cautiously in patients with demonstrated renal dysfunction. No more than modest dietary sodium restriction is advised. The clinically useful dosage of captopril in the cat has been reported to range from 0.5 to 1 mg/lb (1 to 2 mg/kg) administered three times daily.

ENALAPRIL

Enalapril appears to cause fewer gastrointestinal side effects than captopril in dogs, and enjoys a longer pharmacodynamic half-life in dogs.

Indications and Current Use. Enalapril is now considered a "first-choice" drug in the management of chronic congestive heart failure from a variety of causes in dogs. While still controversial, current recommendations include the use of enalapril early in the course of heart failure therapy. In the treatment of chronic canine valvular heart disease (mitral insufficiency) or dilated cardiomyopathy, we often initiate enalapril therapy as soon as significant chamber enlargement (and systolic ventricular dysfunction in the case of dilated cardiomyopathy) is documented. Enlapril is dosed at 0.22 mg/lb (0.5 mg/kg) once or twice a day. The use of enalapril in treating feline hypertrophic cardiomyopathy is controversial because of the theoretic risk of exacerbating dynamic left ventricular outflow obstruction.

Toxicity and Drug Interactions. In general, enalapril appears to have a benign side-effect profile in clinical practice.

BETA-ADRENERGIC RECEPTOR BLOCKERS
(pp. 886–888)

Because of the strong evidence that the chronic activation of the sympathetic nervous system that characterizes heart failure has long-term detrimental effects on the myocardium, interest has focused on the use of beta blockers to "up-regulate" or restore beta-adrenergic receptor numbers and sensitivity and protect the myocardium from the cellular effects of catecholamine excess in the setting of heart failure, especially that caused by dilated cardiomyopathy. The classic first-generation agents (propanolol and timolol) are nonselective (i.e., they block both β_1- and β_2-receptors) and possess no obvious ancillary cardiovascular effects. Second-generation drugs selectively block the β_1-receptor, including atenolol, metoprolol, and betaxolol. Third-generation beta blockers cause cardiovascular effects in addition to beta blockade.

PROPRANOLOL

Indications and Current Use. Propranolol is commonly used in the therapy of heart failure to slow the ventricular response to atrial fibrillation. Because the effects of propranolol depend on the base-line level of sympathetic tone, no universal dosage recommendations can be made. In the dog, propranolol is usually started at an oral dosage of 0.05 to 0.1 mg/lb (0.1 to 0.2 mg/kg) q8h, or about 10 mg q8h in a large-breed dog. This dose is gradually increased over several days until the desired heart rate response is attained. The starting dose of propranolol in cats is generally one-quarter of a 10-mg tablet q8h, to be increased over a period of weeks up to a maximum dose of 10 to 15 mg q8h, if required to control the heart rate and development of clinical signs with excitement or stress. Intravenous propranolol is rarely indicated.

Toxicity and Drug Interactions. Propranolol should not be used in animals with asthma, bradycardia, systemic thromboembolism, or heart block. Beta blockers may reduce the sympathetic compensation for hypoglycemia and may necessitate changes in insulin dosage in the diabetic patient to prevent hypoglycemia. Beta-receptor blockers should be tapered over several days if therapy is to be discontinued.

ATENOLOL

Indications and Current Use. Atenolol is a relatively specific β_1-receptor blocker that has the apparent advantage of a longer pharmacodynamic half-life. The initial dose should be low (6.25 mg/cat or small dog q12h; 6.25 to 12.5 mg/large dog q12h), gradually increasing until a dose is reached that adequately regulates the heart rate. It should be pointed out that heart rate is simply used as an easily accessible marker of efficacy.

Toxicity and Drug Interactions. Usual signs of overdosage include bradycardia, weakness, and lethargy.

CALCIUM ANTAGONISTS (pp. 888–889)

While all are potent coronary arterial dilators, verapamil is a potent negative inotrope, useful as a supraventricular antiarrhythmic. Nifedipine has insignificant negative inotropic and antiarrhythmic properties in the intact animal but is a potent arterial vasodilator, and diltiazem is intermediate in antiarrhythmic, inotropic, and vasodilating effects.

Preliminary evidence collected from a small number of cats strongly suggests that diltiazem may be superior to both verapamil and propranolol in the management of diastolic dysfunction and heart failure secondary to hypertrophic cardiomyopathy. The usual dose of diltiazem utilized in the management of hypertrophic cardiomyopathy is 7.5 mg per cat, q8h. Diltiazem is also an attractive and apparently effective alternative to the addition of a beta blocker to digoxin in the management of atrial fibrillation. The initial dose is generally 0.25 mg/lb (0.5 mg/kg), titrated upward to achieve a target ventricular response over a period of several days.

TAURINE SUPPLEMENTATION (p. 889)

Plasma taurine deficiency has been shown to be associated with dilated cardiomyopathy in most (but not all) cats with the disease. In cats with dilated cardiomyopathy, taurine should be administered at 250 mg orally twice daily.

L-CARNITINE SUPPLEMENTATION (p. 889)

The overall prevalence of myocardial carnitine deficiency and the magnitude of the potential benefit of oral carnitine supplementation in the therapy of canine dilated cardiomyopathy in the general population remain unknown at this time, although preliminary evidence suggests that a substantial portion (approximately 50 per cent) of the population may be affected.

ANCILLARY THERAPY (pp. 889–890)

Morphine. Morphine is useful in the treatment of acute cardiogenic pulmonary edema. Morphine is not generally used in cats because of the possibility of "morphine rage." The recommended dosage of morphine in dogs is 0.05 to 0.10 mg/lb (0.1 to 0.25 mg/kg) subcutaneously, repeated as necessary. Overdosing may result in marked centrally mediated respiratory depression.

Rest and Stress Management. Strict rest is used to reduce the animal's oxygen and energy requirements. Patients with acute cardiogenic pulmonary edema should be considered extremely fragile, and both stress and exercise should be kept to an absolute minimum. In the majority of cases, permanent, moderate-to-severe exercise restriction will be necessary.

Oxygen Therapy. Oxygen supplementation can be lifesaving in the patient with acute, severe pulmonary edema. Narcotic sedation followed immediately by postural drainage, endotracheal intubation, and mechanical ventilation including low levels (3 to 5 cm water) of positive end-expiratory pressure may be lifesaving.

Thoracocentesis and Abdominocentesis. Both procedures should be performed aseptically.

Fluid Therapy. Central hemodynamic monitoring (central venous pressure, pulmonary capillary wedge pressure, arterial blood pressure, and cardiac output) is extremely useful in adjusting the fluid dosage to optimize the preload under emergency, life-threatening circumstances.

As a general recommendation, we prefer low-sodium solutions, and 0.45 per cent sodium chloride with 2.5 per cent dextrose appropriately supplemented with potassium chloride is often used.

Cough Suppressants. Hydrocodenone or butorphenol are the most commonly employed narcotic cough suppressants.

CHAPTER 93

CONGENITAL HEART DISEASE
(pages 892–943)

History. Maturity is a factor when assessing the effect of pulmonary vascular resistance on the magnitude of systemic-to-pulmonary shunts. Left-to-right shunting may not be fully manifested until a number of weeks after birth. Congenital subaortic stenosis may actually develop during the first 2 months of life, and the associated cardiac murmur can actually increase in intensity as the dog grows to maturity. Breed associations with canine cardiac defects in North America and Great Britain, summarized in Table 93–1, emphasize the genetic basis of some malformations.

Physical Examination. Normal pups and kittens can exhibit innocent systolic cardiac murmurs, which must be distinguished from murmurs caused by a cardiac malformation. Hyperkinetic ("waterhammer") arterial pulsations are characteristic of lesions causing abnormal diastolic run-off of aortic blood as occurs with patent ductus arteriosus or aortic regurgitation. Hypokinetic pulses are typical of subaortic

---

Original chapter written by John D. Bonagura and Peter G. G. Darke

TABLE 93–1. BREED PREDILECTIONS IN CONGENITAL HEART DISEASE

Basset hound	Pulmonic stenosis
Beagle	Pulmonic stenosis
Bichon frise	Patent ductus arteriosus (PDA)
Boxer	Subaortic stenosis, pulmonic stenosis, atrial septal defect
Boykin spaniel	Pulmonic stenosis
Bull terrier	Mitral dysplasia, aortic stenosis
Chihuahua	PDA, pulmonic stenosis
Chow chow	Cor triatriatum dexter, pulmonic stenosis
Cocker spaniel	PDA, pulmonic stenosis
Collie	PDA
Doberman pinscher	Atrial septal defect
English bulldog	Tetralogy of Fallot, ventricular septal defect, pulmonic stenosis
English springer spaniel	PDA, ventricular septal defect
German shepherd	Subaortic stenosis, mitral and tricuspid valve dysplasia, PDA
German shorthair pointer	Subaortic stenosis
Golden retriever	Subaortic stenosis, tricuspid valve and mitral valve dysplasia
Great Dane	Mitral and tricuspid valve dysplasia, subaortic stenosis
Keeshond	Tetralogy of Fallot, PDA
Labrador retriever	Tricuspid valve dysplasia, PDA, pulmonic stenosis
Maltese	PDA
Mastiff	Pulmonic stenosis, mitral valve dysplasia
Newfoundland	Subaortic stenosis, mitral valve dysplasia, pulmonic stenosis
Poodle	PDA
Pomeranian	PDA
Rottweiler	Subaortic stenosis
Samoyed	Pulmonic stenosis, ?atrial septal defect, subaortic stenosis
Schnauzer	Pulmonic stenosis
Shetland sheepdog	PDA
Terrier breeds	Pulmonic stenosis
Weimaraner	Tricuspid dysplasia, peritoneopericardial hernia
West Highland white terrier	Pulmonic stenosis, ventricular septal defect
Yorkshire terrier	PDA

stenosis or conditions like tricuspid dysplasia, which are characterized by diminished ventricular output. Cyanosis often indicates pulmonary-to-systemic shunting. Prominent jugular pulsations may suggest an abnormality of the right side of the heart such as pulmonic stenosis or tricuspid regurgitation.

Laboratory Tests. Of note is the presence of a higher than normal PCV in a neonate with right-to-left shunting. Polycythemia is often noted with tetralogy of Fallot, reversed patent ductus arteriosus, and complex cyanotic heart disease.

CARDIAC IMAGING

Radiography. There is a tendency to overinterpret the right ventricle in neonates, in which some right ventricular dominance is normal. Aortic widening in the cranial mediastinum is typical of the post-stenotic dilatation of subaortic stenosis or the aortic anomaly sometimes noted with tetralogy of Fallot. Aneurysmal dilatation of the descending aorta is common with patent ductus arteriosus. Enlargement of the main pulmonary artery may accompany poststenotic turbulent flow from pulmonic stenosis, increased flow caused by any left-to-right shunt, or pulmonary hypertension.

Pulmonary vascularity must be assessed with caution. Right-to-left shunts, like tetralogy of Fallot, are characterized by diminished peripheral perfusion and normal-to-small lobar vessels. Vascularity can also be decreased in other conditions, such as pulmonic stenosis and severe tricuspid dysplasia. Conversely, left-to-right shunts, like atrioventricular septal defects and patent ductus arteriosus, have increased dimension of lobar arteries and veins with prominent peripheral vascular markings.

Echocardiography. A careful "echodoppler" study can replace the invasive cardiac catheterization and angiocardiogram in most instances. One important calculation that is often used in evaluation of congenital heart disease is the modified Bernoulli equation. When high-velocity flow is detected, the peak velocity can be used to estimate the pressure gradient across the obstruction or shunt as

$$\text{pressure gradient in mm Hg} = 4 \times 9 \text{ (peak velocity in m/s)}^2$$

ELECTROCARDIOGRAPHY

A normal ECG axis with increased QRS voltages is typical of patent ductus arteriosus. Persistence of a right ventricular hypertrophy pattern after the first few weeks of age in the dog is abnormal and highly suggestive of pulmonic stenosis, tetralogy of Fallot, tricuspid dysplasia, atrial septal defect, large ventricular septal defect, or pulmonary hypertension.

CAUSES, PREVALENCE, AND CLASSIFICATION OF CONGENITAL HEART DISEASE (pp. 902–903)

CAUSES OF CARDIAC MALFORMATIONS

Congenital cardiac defects may develop as a result of genetic, environmental, chromosomal, infectious, toxicologic, nutritional, and drug-related factors.

PREVALENCE OF CONGENITAL HEART DISEASE

Most surveys suggest that patent ductus arteriosus is the most common malformation in the dog, and either atrioventricular septal defect or atrioventricular valve dysplasia the most common among cats; however, subaortic stenosis is rapidly emerging as the most commonly diagnosed condition in dogs in many regions of the world.

CARDIAC MALFORMATIONS CAUSING SYSTEMIC-TO-PULMONARY SHUNTING (pp. 903–916)

PATENT DUCTUS ARTERIOSUS

While the ductus may be probe-patent in pups less than 4 days of age, it generally closes by 7 or 8 days post-whelping. In a small percentage of cases, the lumen of the PDA is so large that pulmonary vascular pressure and resistance markedly increase. This type of ductus was the most severe, and reversal of the shunt developed within the first months of life. Documentation of shunt reversal after 6 months of age is lacking.

Clinical Findings. Female dogs of certain breeds are at greatest risk for development of PDA (see Table 93–1).

Left-to-Right Shunting PDA. Arterial pulses are hyperkinetic, a continuous thrill may be palpated at the craniodorsal cardiac base, and a continuous murmur is audible. Electrocardiography usually indicates left atrial enlargement with widening of the P waves and left ventricular dilatation characterized by a normal frontal axis and increased-voltage Q waves and R waves in craniocaudal leads II, III, and aVF, and in the lower left chest leads such as V_2 and V_3. Radiography documents pulmonary overcirculation, left atrial and left ventricular enlargement, and possible dilatation of the main pulmonary artery and descending aorta. Echocardiography substantiates left-sided cardiac enlargement and dilation of the aorta and pulmonary artery. The ductus can be imaged in many cases, but Doppler studies are less ambiguous.

PDA with Pulmonary Hypertension. The symptomatic patient may exhibit shortness of breath, pelvic limb weakness or collapse, seizures, and differential cyanosis (cyanosis of the caudal mucous membranes with pink cranial membranes). Perfusion of the kidneys with hypoxemic blood leads to secondary polycythemia and hyperviscosity, with the PCV often exceeding 65 per cent. The continuous cardiac murmur is no longer present. An ejection sound, protosystolic murmur, and a loud or split second heart sound may be evident over the pulmonary artery. Right ventricular hypertrophy is evident. The thoracic x-ray film also indicates dilatation of the main pulmonary artery and proximal lobar arteries, peripheral hypoperfusion, and a "ductus bump" of the descending aorta. Contrast echocardiography, with saline injected in the cephalic vein, will lead to opacification of the descending aorta.

Clinical Management. Surgery is recommended in all cases of left-to-right shunting PDA diagnosed in dogs under 2 years of age. The optimal time for surgery has not been determined, but ductus ligation should be done early, usually between 8 and 16 weeks of age, or sooner if cardiac failure is imminent. When congestive heart failure has developed, the patient is stabilized medically with digoxin and furosemide prior to surgery.

Prognosis with surgery is excellent. Most pets are clinically normal following surgery, and overall cardiac size normalizes, although the heart and great vessels continue to be misshapen in outline. Postoperative Doppler studies may indicate a trivial residual shunt, although the murmur is absent and the clinical consequences, in the absence of surgical infection, are unimportant.

Treatment of *reversed PDA* with secondary polycythemia consists of enforced rest, limitation of exercise, avoidance of stress, and maintenance of the PCV between 62 and 68 per cent.

ATRIAL AND VENTRICULAR SEPTAL DEFECTS

Typically, blood shunts from left to right. However, conditions that increase right atrial or ventricular pressures will retard left-to-right shunting and may lead to reversed shunting.

Atrial Septal Defect. Blood preferentially shunts into the right ventricle. The resultant volume overload of the right atrium (RA), right ventricle (RV), pulmonary artery (PA), and pulmonary veins leads to enlargement of these structures. Whereas the shunting of blood per se does not generate a cardiac murmur, excessive transvalvular flow velocity can cause murmurs of relative tricuspid or pulmonic stenosis. Delayed closure of the pulmonic valve causes splitting of the second heart sound.

Ventricular Septal Defect. Owing to the higher pressure in the left ventricle than in the right, left-to-right shunting develops. With high ventricular septal defects, much of the shunt flow is pumped immediately into the pulmonary artery. Left ventricular failure can develop in situations of marked left-to-right shunt. Very large, nonrestrictive defects cause the two ventricles to behave as a common chamber, so that ventricular pressures equilibrate and RVH will be evident.

Eisenmenger's Physiology. The patient with a large septal defect and left-to-right shunt may develop high pulmonary vascular resistance leading to pulmonary hypertension. Reversed shunting (right-to-left) can then develop, leading to a situation known as "Eisenmenger's physiology." As with PDA, shunt reversal with VSD develops within 6 months of birth. Eisenmenger's physiology is an irreversible condition.

Clinical Findings. Breed predispositions for septal defects are indicated in Table 93–1. Clinical findings of the typical left-to-right *atrial septal defect* include (1) soft systolic cardiac murmurs over the pulmonic and tricuspid valves, and (2) splitting of the second heart sound. Cyanosis is unexpected.

Volume overloading of the right side of the heart is typical of ASD and is evident on thoracic radiography and by echocardiography. Pulmonary vascularity is increased. Intraventricular conduction disturbances are not uncommon with atrioventricular septal defects. Cardiac catheterization of patients with ASD is useful for evaluating the magnitude of shunting.

The clinical features of *ventricular septal defect* are variable according to shunting. Most commonly, a harsh, holosystolic murmur heard best at the cranial right sternal border will be present. Thoracic radiography in VSD demonstrates pulmonary overcirculation, left atrial and ventricular dilation, and variable degrees of right ventricular enlargement. The main and lobar pulmonary arteries often are dilated.

Electrocardiography is also variable, indicating left atrial enlargement, left ventricular dilation, and/or right ventricular hypertrophy. The frontal plane leads often demonstrate abnormal early ventricular septal activation characterized by a Q wave that is wide or contains high-frequency notching. Echocardiography successfully delineates the VSD in most cases.

If heart failure is to occur, it is most likely to develop at the time resistance fails; therefore, most pups will develop CHF before 8 weeks of age. The reality is that such pups usually die before they are examined by a veterinarian. The vast majority of dogs that live to 4 months will survive for many years.

Clinical Management. Definitive treatment of these problems requires surgery using cardiopulmonary bypass. This is rarely undertaken. Pulmonary artery banding can be used to create supravalvular pulmonary stenosis and decrease the magnitude of left-to-right shunting. This procedure is recommended for dogs and cats showing signs of left-sided congestive heart failure. When left-sided congestive heart failure is severe, arterial vasodilators may be beneficial. Prognosis for Eisenmenger's syndrome is poor and is similar to that discussed for reversed PDA.

VENTRICULAR OUTFLOW OBSTRUCTION (pp. 916–933)

PULMONIC STENOSIS

Pulmonic stenosis has a genetic basis in certain canine breeds (see Table 93–1). Anomalous development of the coronary arteries is possible, especially in brachycephalic breeds.

Clinical Findings. Dogs with PS may be asymptomatic; may develop signs related to low cardiac output, such as syncope and tiring; may manifest right-sided congestive heart failure; or may develop hypoxemia from right-to-left shunting across an atrioventricular septal defect. Typical physical examination findings include prominent jugular pulse, left basilar ejection murmur over the pulmonic valve that radiates to the left craniodorsal cardiac base, and palpable right ventricular hypertrophy (right-sided heave).

Right ventricular enlargement is often evident on the ECG, echocardiogram, and thoracic radiograph. Additional radiographic features of PS include poststenotic dilation of the main pulmonary artery and pulmonary underperfusion. Angiocardiography is especially useful for surgical cases and delineates the valvular obstruction and secondary changes in the ventricle and pulmonary artery. Coronary anomalies may be evident and influence the course of therapy.

Echocardiography demonstrates hypertrophy and enlargement of the right ventricle. Doppler studies reveal increased blood velocity just proximal to and across the stenosis and turbulence in the pulmonary artery. The degree of stenosis can be graded arbitrarily as mild (Doppler gradient up to 49 mm Hg), moderate (Doppler gradient of 50 to 125 mm Hg), or severe (Doppler gradient greater than 125 mm Hg).

Clinical Management.   Affected dogs should not be bred. If significant radiographic, ECG, and echocardiographic changes are evident, or if the patient has clinical signs of disease, the pressure gradient should be determined by Doppler echocardiography. The dog with a Doppler gradient of more than 100 to 125 mm Hg should be considered a candidate for surgery or balloon valvuloplasty.

A number of surgical procedures have been advocated for the treatment of severe PS. Valvulotomy, partial valvulectomy, patch-grafting over the outflow tract, and conduits are most popular. Hypoplasia of the pulmonary valve and single or anomalous right coronary artery should be considered contraindications to balloon valvuloplasty and may require placement of a conduit from right ventricle to pulmonary artery.

SUBAORTIC STENOSIS

Clinical Findings.   Clinical findings in pups with mild SAS are minimal. Affected dogs are asymptomatic and have a soft to moderately intense ejection murmur that can easily be confused with a functional murmur. More severely affected dogs may be presented with exertional tiring, syncope, or left-sided congestive heart failure. Sudden death, without premonitory signs, is common. The murmur may become increasingly prominent during the first months of life. Thoracic radiographs can be normal or may indicate left ventricular hypertrophy. The mediastinum may be widened. Pulmonary circulation is normal.

Echocardiography demonstrates left ventricular hypertrophy, a subvalvular fibrous ring that can involve the mitral valve, and poststenotic dilation of the aorta. The ECG may be normal, but in advanced cases it indicates left ventricular hypertrophy. Holter ECG studies often demonstrate ventricular extrasystoles. Maximal Doppler gradients of >125 to 150 mm Hg are considered severe.

Natural History.   Severe SAS is a discouraging condition, since most dogs either die suddenly or develop congestive heart failure. Dogs with a Doppler pressure gradient of less than 75 mm Hg are likely to be near-normal pets.

Clinical Management.   Dogs with mild SAS are treated normally but should not be used for breeding. Prophylaxis for bacterial endocarditis is prudent in appropriate circumstances. Dogs with moderate to severe SAS should have restricted exercise. Surgical procedures have been employed to dilate, resect, or bypass the obstruction, but such surgery is infrequently performed. Balloon catheter dilation of the subaortic area has been used to reduce the severity of obstruction. We prescribe beta-adrenergic blocking drugs such as propranolol or atenolol empirically to dogs with a history of syncope (without CHF), with gradients of more than 125 mm Hg, or with significant ST-T changes or frequent ventricular extrasystoles.

AORTIC REGURGITATION

Although isolated congenital AR appears to be rare, this condition often complicates subaortic stenosis and has also been observed with ventricular septal defects. A diastolic murmur, heard best over the left hemithorax, is typical of AR. Significant AR can lead to left ventricular failure.

DYSPLASIA OF THE ATRIOVENTRICULAR VALVES

See Chapter 94.

Clinical Findings. Presenting signs, if any, are referable to exercise intolerance or congestive heart failure. The hallmark physical examination finding is a soft to loud holosystolic murmur heard best over the affected valve area and respective apex or along the left sternal border of cats with mitral dysplasia. Right, left, or biventricular congestive heart failure may be evident from examination and radiography. Atrial arrhythmias, especially atrial fibrillation, are common.

Definitive diagnosis requires echocardiography and, less often, cardiac catheterization and angiocardiography. When significant cardiomegaly is evident, the prognosis is guarded to poor. Treatment of congestive heart failure, if present, and management of atrial fibrillation are required in advanced cases.

LESIONS CAUSING RIGHT-TO-LEFT SHUNTING: CYANOTIC HEART DISEASE (p. 933)

The term *Eisenmenger's physiology* (or syndrome) has been used to define a situation in which a left-to-right shunt reverses to right-to-left in response to marked increases in pulmonary vascular resistance. Eisenmenger's syndrome develops rapidly in small animals (almost always before 6 months of age).

CLINICAL EVALUATION OF THE CYANOTIC HEART DISEASE PATIENT (pp. 934–939)

History and Physical Examination. Presenting signs include failure to grow, cyanosis, shortness of breath, exercise intolerance, weakness, syncope, and seizures. Affected animals often gasp when stressed. Most cases are polycythemic. One important auscultatory feature of Eisenmenger's syndrome is the loud or split second heart sound of pulmonary hypertension. Cyanotic heart disease (tricuspid atresia and anomalous systemic venous return are exceptions) is characterized by right ventricular hypertrophy, which is evident on echocardiograms, ECG, and the thoracic radiograph. As a general rule, the lungs appear underperfused in cyanotic heart diseases. The main pulmonary artery and proximal lobar arteries are dilated when Eisenmenger's syndrome is the basis for reversed shunting, but are not enlarged in tetralogy of Fallot or in pulmonary or tricuspid atresia.

Echocardiography. Most large defects can be easily visualized.

Cardiac Catheterization. Cardiac catheterization can demonstrate pulmonary hypertension and outline anatomic defects, pulmonary artery size, and shunting.

TETRALOGY OF FALLOT

Components of the tetralogy are right ventricular outflow obstruction (pulmonic stenosis), secondary right ventricular hypertrophy, a subaortic ventricular septal defect, and overriding aorta.

Clinical Findings. Presenting complaints and clinical complications are similar to those previously described for cyanotic heart disease. The ejection murmur of pulmonic stenosis is the most common auscultatory abnormality. Exercise or excitement may induce cyanosis by accentuating right-to-left shunting. Radiography usually shows a normal-sized heart with rounding of the right ventricular border. The ECG usually exhibits a right axis deviation; a left or cranial axis may be found in some cats. Bubble (or Doppler) studies document right-to-left shunting at the ventricular outflow level.

Clinical Management. The defect can be tolerated for years, provided pulmonary blood flow is maintained and hyperviscosity is controlled. Sudden death is common, related to complications of hypoxia, hyperviscosity, or cardiac arrhythmia. Although definitive correction of the defect can be done under cardiopulmonary bypass, such surgery is rarely performed in animals. Surgical palliation through the creation of a systemic-to-pulmonary shunt can be rewarding. Adjunctive therapy includes phlebotomy to control the PCV between 62 and 68 per cent, and the blood volume should be replaced with crystalloid fluids to maintain cardiac output and tissue oxygen delivery. Some children with tetralogy of Fallot benefit from beta-blockade with propranolol. Drugs with marked systemic vasodilating properties should be avoided.

MISCELLANEOUS CARDIAC DEFECTS (pp. 939–940)

Endocardial fibroelastosis is probably familial in some lines of Burmese and Siamese cats. The gross anatomic findings include left ventricular and left atrial dilatation, with severe endocardial thickening. The clinical features of endocardial fibroelastosis include early development of left or biventricular failure, generally before 6 months of age. *Anomalous development of the atria* has been recognized in small animals. Cor triatriatum has been reported in a cat, and cor triatriatum dexter and saccular anomalies of the caudal right atrium have been seen in dogs and cats. *Peritoneopericardial diaphragmatic hernia* is a relatively common developmental anomaly of dogs and cats. While not representative of a true cardiac anomaly, this condition can be confused with other congenital and acquired conditions. Therapy involves surgical reduction of the hernia.

VASCULAR ANOMALIES (pp. 940–943)

AORTIC ANOMALIES

Persistent Right Aortic Arch.   The cardinal feature of these defects is regurgitation of solid food due to obstruction of the esophagus rather than circulatory dysfunction.

VENOUS ANOMALIES

See textbook.

CHAPTER 94
ACQUIRED VALVULAR HEART DISEASE
(pages 944–959)

CHRONIC MITRAL VALVE INSUFFICIENCY (CMVI)
(pp. 944–952)

This disorder is the most commonly encountered cardiovascular disorder in the dog. CMVI appears to be rare in the cat.

Clinical Signs.   CMVI is a slowly progressive disorder. Although it may begin at middle age (5 to 7 years), clinical signs related to the disorder usually are not manifest until the dogs are over 10 years of

Original chapter written by Michael R. O'Grady

age. The most common presenting complaint for progressive mitral valve disease is cough. The cough is usually deep and resonant and worse at night or with exercise. The cough may be due to left mainstem bronchial compression, pulmonary interstitial congestion, or both. Individuals with pulmonary interstitial congestion also have an increased respiratory rate (tachypnea) and effort (dyspnea) of breathing. Individuals with left mainstem bronchial compression demonstrate paroxysms of cough.

Physical Examination.　The earliest physical finding is the detection of an incidental soft left apical midsystolic murmur during the routine examination of a middle-aged dog. As the disease progresses, the murmur becomes more intense and holosystolic. With advanced CMVI, S_3 and S_4 heart sounds may be ausculted. A murmur of tricuspid valve insufficiency may be detected. If pleural effusion or cardiac tamponade is present, the heart sounds will be muffled. Abnormalities in the cardiac rhythm may be identified. These are usually due to the presence of supraventricular premature contractions, atrial flutter, or atrial fibrillation. The lung sounds vary with the severity of the disease. Jugular venous distention is noted with advanced heart failure or pulmonary hypertension. Ascites is somewhat rare in isolated CMVI. Subcutaneous edema is even more uncommon.

Radiographic Findings.　The first goal of radiography is to examine for the presence of pulmonary edema. The earliest radiographic feature of pulmonary edema is venous engorgement. In the dog, alveolar edema is most apparent and first noted in the perihilar, right caudal lung lobe and apical lung lobe. In the cat, alveolar edema occurs in the periphery of the lung fields and in a patchy distribution. Left atrial enlargement is the earliest and most consistent radiographic feature of MR. The thoracic trachea becomes elevated, and the left mainstem bronchus becomes elevated and displaced dorsal to the right bronchus.

Electrocardiographic Findings.　With the important exception of documenting and allowing one to classify an arrhythmia, the ECG is of little use in the diagnosis or management of CMVI. Supraventricular premature beats constitute the most common arrhythmia encountered with CMVI.

Echocardiographic Findings.　CMVI causes a volume overload of the left atrium and left ventricle.

Differential Diagnosis.　Bacterial endocarditis of the mitral valve, a rare disorder in dogs and cats, will cause MR and is difficult to diagnose. Whereas the presence of CMVI is not difficult to diagnose, the real challenge is to determine whether the cough is due to the CMVI or to coexistent chronic small airway disease. Both small airway disease and pulmonary interstitial congestion demonstrate a peribronchial pattern on thoracic radiographs. However, only pulmonary interstitial congestion will also demonstrate pulmonary venous engorgement.

MANAGEMENT

For the Patient with Left Mainstem Bronchial Compression Without Pulmonary Interstitial Congestion.　Arterial vasodilators may be used to reduce systemic vascular resistance. Hydralazine is the most potent of those studied in the dog. Tachycardia may develop. Hydralazine therapy is usually initiated at a dose of 0.25 mg/lb q12h PO, and the dose is increased at weekly intervals to a maintenance dose of 1 mg/lb q12h PO or until hypotension is noted. If tachycardia develops, consider adding digoxin (0.22 mg/m^2 q12h PO). Additional arterial vasodilators are available, including the angiotensin converting enzyme inhibitors. Diuretics may be useful to reduce the degree of mitral regurgitation. Digoxin may reduce the regurgitant volume.

For the Patient with Pulmonary Interstitial Congestion Secondary to CMVI. Management consists of the combination of arterial vasodilator, cardiac glycoside, and diuretic therapy. In addition, a low-sodium diet and exercise restriction are useful. The need for diuretic therapy may reduce over the initial 4 weeks of therapy as the digoxin and vasodilator therapy strengthen the heart and reduce the degree of MR. Often an initial diuretic dose of 2 mg/lb q8–12h PO of furosemide for 2 to 3 days can be followed with 2 mg/lb q24h PO for another 3 to 7 days and then reduced to a maintenance dose of 1 mg/lb q24h PO. I recommend placing canine patients with pulmonary congestion on enalapril at 0.25 mg/lb q24h PO initially. After one week, an attempt should be made to increase the dose of enalapril to 0.25 mg/lb q12h PO. I recommend the use of digoxin at 0.22 mg/m^2 q12h PO. If the patient fails to improve, consider adding another arterial vasodilator such as hydralazine.

COMPLICATIONS ASSOCIATED WITH CMVI

Right-Sided Heart Failure Due to Pulmonary Hypertension

This appears to be a common complication. The pulmonary hypertension occurs presumably secondary to the persistently elevated left atrial pressures and the pulmonary congestion-induced hypoxemia. Oxygen supplementation is indicated for cases with acute collapse. Hydralazine should be considered as the initial and primary arterial vasodilator used in the management of this type of case of CMVI. Since pulmonary interstitial congestion augments pulmonary hypertension, diuretic therapy can markedly reduce pulmonary hypertension. These patients should be restricted from even mild exercise.

Acute Exacerbation of Pulmonary Interstitial Congestion Due to Ruptured Chordae Tendineae

When the left atrium has not had the opportunity to acclimatize to the increase in left atrial volume that accompanies acute MR, the left atrial pressures rise rapidly. This rapid rise in left atrial pressure results in pulmonary edema, pulmonary artery hypertension, or right heart failure. A prolapsed mitral valve leaflet or a ruptured chordae may be observed on two-dimensional echocardiography.

Management consists of providing intensive care for 48 to 72 hours and then more conservative therapy for CMVI. Intensive care should consist of providing oxygen support. Herculean dosages of diuretics such as furosemide, 4 mg/lb IV q6h, for the first 24 hours may be required. Alternative agents include intravenous sodium nitroprusside. The concurrent use of positive inotropic agents such as dobutamine or dopamine may also be useful.

Acute Exacerbation of Pulmonary Interstitial Congestion Due to the Development of a Tachyarrhythmia

The most common significant arrhythmia encountered is that of supraventricular premature beats. Ventricular dysrhythmias are less common. The goal of therapy is to reduce the heart rate that is responsible for the deterioration. Digoxin is the ideal first drug. Should digoxin be insufficient, diltiazem or selective beta-adrenergic blockers (such as atenolol or metoprolol) should be added. These should be initiated at the lowest dose level and increased gradually.

Left Atrial Rupture and Cardiac Tamponade

Clinical Picture. Most cases with left atrial rupture and hemopericardium can be expected to develop cardiac tamponade and sudden death. Physical examination may reveal marked jugular distention, muffled heart sounds, and a very weak femoral arterial pulse. Thoracic radiographs reveal a globe-shaped heart typical of pericardial effusion. A marked left atrial bulge is observed on the lateral projection. Most cases of pericardial effusion, if not due to a left atrial tear, do not demonstrate a markedly enlarged left atrium. Echocardiography remains the ideal diagnostic tool to diagnose the presence of pericardial effusion.

Management.   Immediate pericardiocentesis is indicated. Emergency thoracotomy to attempt to remove the pericardium and locate and close the left atrial tear is indicated if bleeding continues.

TRICUSPID VALVE INSUFFICIENCY (TVI) (pp. 952–954)

Primary Tricuspid Valve Insufficiency.   Primary TVI is acquired in a form analogous to chronic mitral valve insufficiency. This disorder occurs much more commonly as a concomitant of CMVI.

Secondary Tricuspid Valve Insufficiency.   Secondary TVI occurs secondary to any process that results in right ventricular enlargement.

Clinical Signs.   Isolated tricuspid insufficiency is not expected to result in clinical signs.

Electrocardiography and Radiography.   A tall P wave will be present, particularly if pulmonary hypertension is present. However, in the presence of significant pulmonary hypertension, one should expect to find electrocardiographic evidence of both right atrial and right ventricular enlargement. In cases of moderate to severe right atrial enlargement, the trachea cranial to the carina becomes elevated.

Echocardiographic Findings.   Echocardiography is an ideal diagnostic tool to detect right atrial and ventricular enlargement.

Management.   As isolated TVI is expected to be benign, most cases with signs of right heart failure occur due to some concurrent disorder. Individuals with marked ascites may benefit from combination diuretics. Repeated abdominocentesis is often required. Digoxin is often useful if right heart failure is present.

AORTIC VALVE INSUFFICIENCY (p. 954)

See Infective Endocarditis below.

INFECTIVE ENDOCARDITIS (IE) (pp. 954–958)

The German shepherd and Boxer may be predisposed to acquiring IE. *S. aureus, E. coli,* and β-hemolytic streptococci are the most common bacteria isolated in dogs with IE. Subaortic stenosis is the most common congenital defect associated with IE. Gram-negative bacteremias tend to result in a much more fulminant clinical course than that caused by gram-positive bacteremias. In the case of aortic valve infection, the resultant aortic valve insufficiency and left heart failure are usually unresponsive to therapy. Embolic events are believed to be common in IE. The kidney and spleen are the most commonly embolized organs in the dog.

Clinical Signs.   If clinical signs are related either to the primary bacteremic event or to secondary bacteremic episodes emanating from the endocardial site of infection, nonspecific signs of fever, anorexia, lethargy, and perhaps lameness will predominate. If mitral or aortic valve insufficiency develops, signs of left-sided heart failure will occur.

Physical Examination.   Fever, heart murmur, particularly a newly developed heart murmur, and lameness are the classic signs of IE. Diastolic murmurs are extremely uncommon in veterinary medicine. Thus, the finding of a diastolic murmur can be a strong clue to the presence of aortic IE.

Blood Cultures. A positive blood culture is the critical evidence of IE. In recent years, a number of findings with respect to blood cultures have been observed in people and most likely apply as well in veterinary patients. Bacteremia is continuous; therefore, there is no advantage to obtaining cultures at any particular time or body temperature. Arterial blood samples offer no advantage over venous blood.

Echocardiographic Findings. Echocardiography has become one of the most important diagnostic tools in the assessment and management of IE. Vegetations are usually not visualized during the first 2 weeks of endocarditis.

Diagnosis. A definitive diagnosis of IE requires a positive blood culture in addition to clinical and laboratory evidence of cardiac involvement.

MANAGEMENT

In general, treatment should be immediate, aggressive, and sustained to improve chances of a favorable outcome.

Antimicrobial Therapy. Antimicrobial therapy should consist of bactericidal not bacteriostatic agents; higher than usual concentrations of drug, which can be better achieved by parenteral administration; and a prolonged therapeutic course. Intravenous therapy should be utilized for at least 5 to 10 days. Therapy is usually required for 6 to 8 weeks. Most strains of *S. aureus* have *in vitro* sensitivity to cephalosporins and aminoglycosides. Most strains of *E. coli* have *in vitro* sensitivity to aminoglycosides, cephalosporins, and fluoroquinolones. A combination of gentamicin and penicillin or cephalosporin is a reasonable choice in the absence of a laboratory isolate.

Other Therapies. Congestive heart failure should be treated as previously described for congestive heart failure with CMVI. Anticoagulant therapy appears to be of no value.

PROGNOSIS

The long-term prognosis for patients with IE is poor. Most patients can expect to die from congestive heart failure, sepsis, systemic embolization, or renal failure.

PROPHYLAXIS

Prophylactic antibiotics are usually ineffective unless the type of bacteria and its sensitivity are known. Nevertheless, in patients with underlying cardiac disease, prophylactic antibiotics are recommended for patients undergoing dental procedures, or surgical or diagnostic procedures of the urogenital, intestinal, and respiratory tracts.

CHAPTER 95

CARDIAC ARRHYTHMIAS
(pages 959–995)

THE ELECTROCARDIOGRAM (pp. 962–963)

Tables 95–1 A and 95–1 B present the normal criteria for the canine and feline ECG.

CLINICAL APPROACH TO ARRHYTHMIAS (pp. 963–964)

Electrocardiography. Six- or nine-lead electrocardiograms provide information regarding cardiac size and orientation, whereas a single lead II is usually adequate for the interpretation of arrhythmias.

TABLE 95–1A. CRITERIA FOR THE NORMAL CANINE ELECTROCARDIOGRAM

Heart rate—60 to 160 beats per minute for adult dogs; up to 180 beats per minute in toy breeds, and 220 beats per minute for puppies.
Heart rhythm—Normal sinus rhythm; sinus arrhythmia; and wandering sinoatrial pacemaker.
P wave—Up to 0.4 millivolt in amplitude; up to 0.04 second in duration; always positive in leads II and aV_F; positive or isoelectric in lead I.
P-R interval—0.06 to 0.14 second duration.
QRS complex—Mean electric axis, frontal plane, 40 to 100 degrees.
Amplitude—Maximum amplitude of R wave 2.5 to 3.0 millivolts in leads II, III, and aVF. Complex positive in leads II, III, and aVF; negative in lead V_{10}.
Duration—To 0.05 second (0.06 second in dogs over 40 lb).
Q-T—0.15 to 0.22 second duration.
S-T segment and T wave—S-T segment free of marked coving (repolarization changes).
S-T segment depression not greater than 0.2 millivolt.
S-T segment elevation not greater than 0.15 millivolt.
T wave negative in lead V_{10}.
T wave amplitude not greater than 25 per cent of amplitude of R wave.

TABLE 95–1B. CRITERIA FOR THE NORMAL FELINE ELECTROCARDIOGRAM

Heart rate—240 beats per minute maximum.
Heart rhythm—Normal sinus rhythm or, infrequently, sinus arrhythmia.
P wave—Positive in leads II and aV_F; may be isoelectric or positive in lead I; should not exceed 0.03 second in duration.
P-R interval—0.04 to 0.08 second duration (inversely related to the heart rate).
QRS complex—More variable than in the canine; the mean electric axis in the frontal plane is often insignificant. Often the QRS complex is nearly isoelectric in all frontal plane limb leads (so-called horizontal heart).
The amplitude of the R wave is usually low; marked amplitude of R waves (over 0.8 millivolt) in the frontal plane leads may suggest ventricular hypertrophy.
Less than 0.04 second in duration.
Q-T segment—0.16 to 0.18 second duration.
S-T segment and T wave—S-T segment and T wave should be small and free of repolarization changes as well as marked depression or elevation.

Original chapter written by Jenifer Lunney and Stephen J. Ettinger

Treatment. It may be necessary to treat an underlying disease as well as the cardiac arrhythmia. Attempting to treat cardiac arrhythmias without correct interpretation or complete evaluation of the patient leads only to frustration and ultimate therapeutic failure.

SPECIFIC ARRHYTHMIAS (pp. 964–987)

PREMATURE ECTOPIC BEATS

Early ectopic impulses interrupt the normal cardiac rhythm in one or more of the following manners: resetting, resetting with pause, compensatory pause, and interpolation (Fig. 95–1). Generally, resetting and

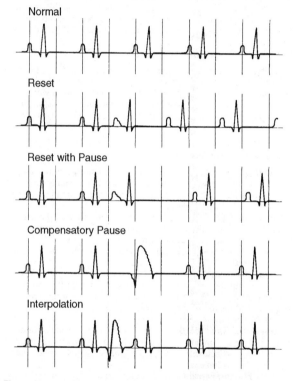

Figure 95–1. Schematic representation of normal sinus rhythm and premature complexes. *Normal sinus rhythm:* The heart rate remains constant, and the interval from P to P or from R to R does not change. *Resetting:* An atrial premature contraction (beat 3) resets the sinus rhythm, so that the period from the beginning of the premature P wave to the next normal P wave is equal to exactly one P-P interval. *Resetting with pause:* The atrial premature contraction (beat 3) followed by a pause greater than one P-P interval but less than two P-P intervals. *Compensatory pause:* The ventricular premature contraction (beat 3) is followed by a compensatory pause; that is, the period from the normal P wave in the beat preceding the ventricular premature contraction to the normal P wave of the beat following the ventricular premature contraction is equivalent to exactly two P-P intervals. The sinus P wave occurs on time, but it is not conducted through the atrioventricular node to the ventricle, which is in a refractory state due to the ventricular premature contraction. *Interpolation:* A ventricular contraction (beat 3) occurs between two normal sinus complexes without disrupting normal rhythm. Interpolated beats are unusual in dogs. (From Ettinger SJ and Suter PF: Canine Cardiology. Philadelphia, WB Saunders, 1970)

resetting with pause are associated with supraventricular premature beats. Compensatory pause and interpolation are more commonly associated with ventricular arrhythmias.

Supraventricular Premature Contractions

These cardiac beats are characterized by premature P waves that are different in configuration and/or size from the normal P wave. The QRS is usually unaffected.

Clinical Signs. Generally, animals are symptomatic for the primary disease and asymptomatic for the cardiacarrhythmia, although syncope, paroxysmal weakness, or congestive heart failure may accompany frequent premature contractions.

Treatment. If the ectopic beats are frequent enough to cause clinical signs, drugs such as the digitalis glycosides, beta blockers, or Ca^{++} channel blockers may be used to slow atrioventricular (AV) conduction.

Ventricular Premature Contractions

The QRS complex may be normal if the beat originates close to the AV junction or wide and bizarre if it has its genesis elsewhere within the ventricular myocardium. VPBs are associated with many conditions, both cardiac and noncardiac. Therapeutic indications, methods, and goals are discussed in the section under ventricular tachycardia.

TACHYCARDIAS

Supraventricular Tachycardia

Etiology. An enlarged atrium is the most common substrate for persistent or recurrent atrial tachycardias, atrial flutter, or atrial fibrillation.

Significance. The most critical determinant of the impact of the SVT is the rate of ventricular response.

Sinus Tachycardia. Excess sympathetic tone is the driving force. It may be the result of fear, apprehension, pain, hypovolemia, hypotension, hyperthermia, or anemia. Vagal maneuvers do little to slow the rate. Treatment is usually directed at correction of the underlying problem.

Atrial Tachycardias. Vagal maneuvers may transiently slow AV conduction but do not usually abolish the rhythm, as this rhythm is independent of the AV node. Automatic atrial tachycardias are often persistent and nonresponsive to treatment. Figure 95–2 shows various examples of supraventricular tachycardias.

Junctional Tachycardias. AV nodal reentrant tachycardias are thought to be a common cause of SVT. Maneuvers and drugs that increase AV conduction time or prolong the refractory period tend to abolish this arrhythmia.

Atrial Flutter/Fibrillation. Atrial fibrillation should be the first differential when encountering a rapid, irregular rhythm with normal QRS morphology. P waves are absent and irregular undulations of the base line may be noted. Quinidine has been used to convert some dogs in atrial fibrillation to a sinus rhythm. It has been most successful in large-breed dogs with an acute onset of atrial fibrillation and no evidence of underlying cardiac disease. In other cases, in which the patient is in failure or has significant cardiac disease, conversion is infrequently attempted.

Treatment of SVT. Sinus tachycardias are best alleviated by treating the underlying pathophysiologic abnormality. For other cases of SVT, agents such as the digitalis glycosides, beta blockers, and calcium channel blockers have been used. In patients with congestive heart failure, the use of negative inotropic agents such as Ca^{++} channel blockers and beta blockers must be done with careful monitoring.

Ventricular Pre-Excitation. This condition occurs when the

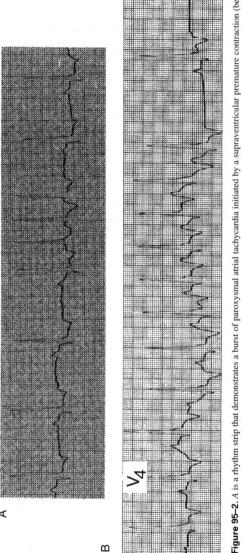

A

B

V₄

Figure 95-2. *A* is a rhythm strip that demonstrates a burst of paroxysmal atrial tachycardia initiated by a supraventricular premature contraction (beat 4). The atrial tachycardia is brief, three beats only, and then the rhythm returns to its more normal rate. During such paroxysms, the owner may be aware of weakness, staggering, or syncope in the pet. *B* is a V₄ tracing from a dog during a syncope episode. This standard poodle had dilated cardiomyopathy. The tracing demonstrates left atrial and left ventricular enlargement. The sixth beat is an atrial premature beat that begins the paroxysmal tachycardia. The tachyarrhythmia ends with an 0.84-second pause before a sinus beat occurs.

ventricle is excited prematurely via an accessory pathway capable of conducting impulses from the atria to the ventricles, partially or completely bypassing the AV node. Depending on the location of the accessory pathway and its ability to conduct antegrade, the altered pattern of ventricular excitation may be recorded as a delta wave.

Diagnosis of this condition can be difficult. Electrophysiologic mapping of the AV rim can be performed to document and isolate the location of the accessory pathway. Medical therapy can be used to slow AV conduction (vagal stimulation, beta blockers, CA^{++} channel blockers, or digitalis) or to increase the refractory period of the accessory pathway (procainamide, quinidine, disopyramide).

Ventricular Tachycardias

Ventricular tachycardia (VT) by definition means a series of three or more consecutive beats of ventricular origin. Sustained ventricular tachycardia is prolonged, whereas paroxysmal VT has short bursts of irregular rhythms that terminate spontaneously. The electrocardiographic hallmarks of ventricular tachycardia are the presence of AV dissociation, fusion beats, and capture beats (Fig. 95–3).

Supraventricular tachycardia with aberrant ventricular conduction must be distinguished from VT for therapeutic and prognostic purposes. A recently identified group of German shepherd dogs have inherited ventricular ectopy and sudden death without any defined cause. Another breed with problematic VT is Boxers.

Treatment of Ventricular Tachycardia. In veterinary patients, treatment is usually undertaken if (1) the number of VPCs is greater than 25/minute, (2) if repetitive VPCs eliciting rates greater than 130 bpm are present, (3) if the VPCs are multiform, (4) if R-on-T phenomenon exists, (5) if it is a breed at risk for sudden death, or (6) if symptoms related to the arrhythmia are present.

For life-threatening ventricular arrhythmias, lidocaine is the drug of choice. Two per cent lidocaine without epinephrine, 2 to 4 mg/lb (4 to 8 mg/kg), is given by slow bolus. If improvement is seen, constant rate infusion of 11 to 33 µg/lb/min (22 to 66 µg/kg/min) can follow. For nonresponsive cases, procainamide is often the second choice. Intravenous bolus, 1 to 10 mg/lb (2 to 20 mg/kg) over 30 minutes, may be followed by a constant rate infusion, 12 to 20 µg/lb/min (25 to 40 µg/kg/min), if the ECG reflects successful control. Third, quinidine may be used, 3 to 10 mg/lb (6.6 to 22 mg/kg) q2–4h IM or PO, until conversion or toxic side effects are observed. For reasonably stable patients, oral treatment with procainamide, quinidine, or mexiletine can be used on an outpatient basis.

Preferred therapy for cats with ventricular tachycardia includes lidocaine at a reduced dose, 0.2 to 0.5 mg/lb IV bolus then 5 to 10 µg/lb/min CRI (0.5 to 1.0 mg/kg IV bolus then 10 to 20 µg/kg/min CRI) to prevent neurologic toxicity. If the arrhythmia is refractory to lidocaine, procainamide, 0.5 to 1.0 mg/lb slow IV bolus then 5 to 10 µg/lb/min CRI (1 to 2 mg/kg slow IV bolus then 10 to 20 µg/kg/min CRI) or a beta blocker such as propranolol (0.25 to 0.5 mg slow IV bolus) are other alternatives.

Accelerated Idioventricular Rhythm. The ventricular rate varies from 70 bpm to one that approximates the sinus rate. The ventricular rate usually demonstrates a slow onset as the sinus rate slows. Owing to its slow and stable nature, suppressive therapy is often not required.

Ventricular Flutter/Ventricular Fibrillation. Hemodynamically, ventricular flutter and ventricular fibrillation are equivalent to cardiac arrest. External cardiac defibrillation should be performed immediately (<15 lbs, 1 watt sec/lb; 15 to 85 lbs, 2 watt sec/lb; >85 lbs, 2 to 5 watt sec/lb). The A,B,C,Ds of resuscitation should then follow (Chapter 15).

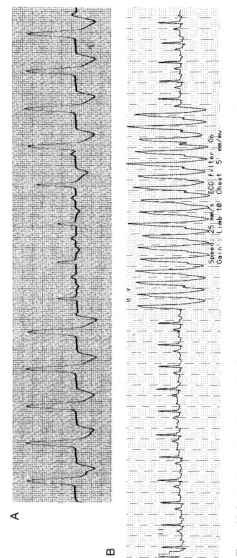

Figure 95-3. Ventricular tachycardia. *A,* As the sinus and ventricular rates approach each other, the P waves intermittently capture the rhythm (beats 6, 7, 8). Beat 9 probably represents simultaneous ventricular activation by the sinus impulse and the ectopic focus and is termed a fusion beat. *B* traces ventricular tachycardia in a Boxer. Note the left bundle branch block morphology.

BRADYARRHYTHMIAS

Wandering Pacemaker

Wandering pacemaker is a variation of sinus rhythm found in normal dogs. Wandering pacemakers require no treatment.

Sinus Arrhythmia

Sinus arrhythmia is a rhythm originating from the sinus node producing variable P-P intervals. It results from increased vagal tone and requires no treatment. Respiratory sinus arrhythmia is a frequent finding in normal dogs, especially brachycephalic breeds.

Sinus Bradycardia

In sinus bradycardia, normal P, QRS-T complexes are usually recorded at a rate less than 70 bpm. This condition can be a normal finding in large breeds or athletic, highly conditioned animals. These patients may exhibit no clinical signs. In symptomatic patients with an uncorrectable underlying cause, long-acting atropine-like drugs or permanent pacemaker implantation may be required.

SA Arrest

Intermittent sinus arrest may be a normal finding in brachycephalic breeds. Treatment is usually not required.

Atrioventricular Block

First-Degree AV Block.   In first-degree AV block, the P-R interval is greater than 140 msec in dogs and 80 msec in cats. The P waves and QRS-T complexes are otherwise normal (Fig. 95–4).

Second-Degree AV Block.   Two types are defined (Fig. 95–5). Mobitz type I (Wenckebach phenomenon) refers to a progressively lengthened P-R interval until a P wave occurs and the QRS-T is dropped. Mobitz type II is characterized by constant P-R intervals with an intermittently dropped QRS-T complex. The term *high-grade second-degree AV block* is used when two or more consecutive QRS-T complexes are consistently dropped. Type II may worsen into third-degree AV block or permit development of Stokes-Adams attacks.

Third-Degree AV Block.   Third-degree AV block indicates that no conduction occurs between the atria and the ventricles (Fig. 95–6). It is critical that these complexes be identified as escape beats and not be treated as malignant, ectopic ventricular rhythms.

Treatment of Bradyarrhythmias

Permanent pacemaker implantation is the only reliable approach to the symptomatic persistently bradycardic patient. Isoproterenol, most effective by constant rate infusion, is useful in controlling the rate in the emergency patient. In the atropine-responsive patient, long-acting oral forms of atropine-like agents have been used with variable success.

SICK SINUS SYNDROME (BRADYCARDIC-TACHYCARDIC SYNDROME)

Sick sinus syndrome is characterized by sinus bradycardia, SA block, intermittent sinus arrest, supraventricular tachyarrhythmias, or some combination of these (Fig. 95–7). Permanent pacemaker implantation affords the greatest likelihood for successful treatment.

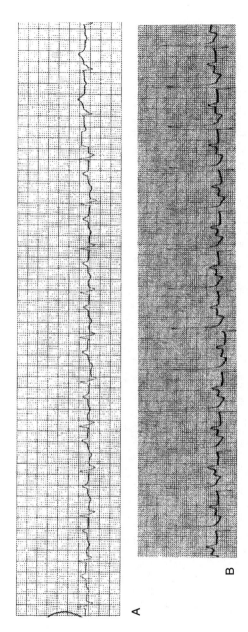

Figure 95–4. First-degree heart block. *A,* First-degree AV block in a cat. The P-R interval is 140 msec. The QRS complex is also wide. *B* is from a dog with a prolonged P-R interval, which had not been on therapy but was in heart failure and had vary large atria, accounting for the prolonged P-R interval of 0.16 second.

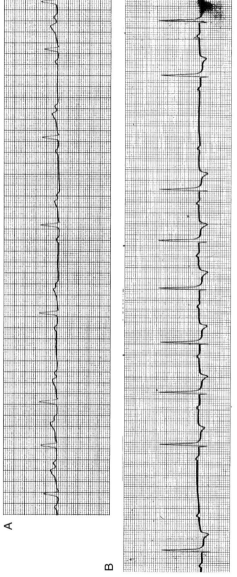

Figure 95–5. Second-degree AV block. *A,* Type I (Wenckebach) second-degree AV block is seen. The P-R interval progessively lengthens until the QRS is dropped. *B,* Type II second-degree AV block is present. The P-R interval is fairly constant until a P occurs with no following QRS.

A

B

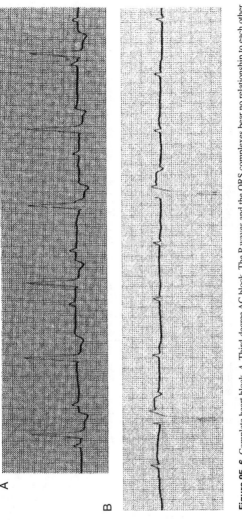

A

B

Figure 95–6. Complete heart block. *A*, Third-degree AC block. The P waves and the QRS complexes bear no relationship to each other. The regular P waves are hidden in the second, fourth, and fifth T waves. The regular upright QRS complexes represent a junctional escape rhythm. *B*, P waves are buried in both QRS complexes. The QRS orientation and rate suggest that a ventricular escape mechanism is rescuing the heart from asystole.

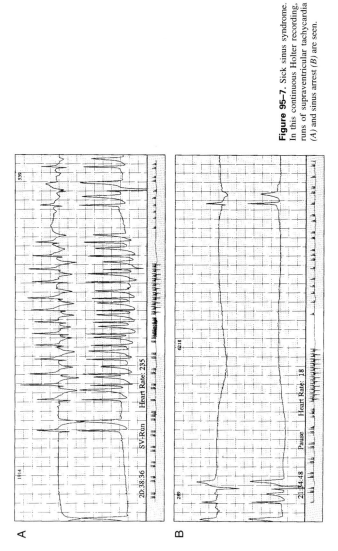

Figure 95–7. Sick sinus syndrome. In this continuous Holter recording, runs of supraventricular tachycardia (*A*) and sinus arrest (*B*) are seen.

CONDUCTION ALTERATIONS

Bundle Branch Blocks

Right bundle branch block patterns can be normal in the dog and cat. Left bundle branch block suggests severe underlying cardiac disease. It is critical to recognize the associated and preceding P wave that designates the rhythm as supraventricular (Fig. 95–8).

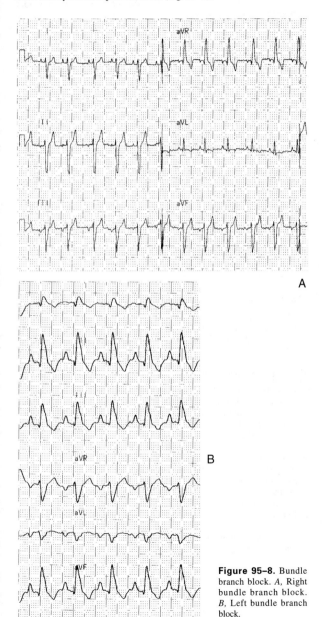

Figure 95–8. Bundle branch block. *A,* Right bundle branch block. *B,* Left bundle branch block.

THERAPY OF ARRHYTHMIAS (pp. 987–994)

CLASS I ANTIARRHYTHMICS

Class IA Drugs

Examples of drugs in this class include quinidine, procainamide, and disopyramide.

Quinidine: Quinidine is indicated for the control of supraventricular and ventricular tachyarrhythmias. Intravenous use can cause marked hypotension. Quinidine is contraindicated in third-degree AV block, digitalis intoxication, ventricular tachycardia associated with long QT intervals, myasthenia gravis, and severe hepatic failure. Principal side effects are gastrointestinal or neurologic signs.

Procainamide: Like quinidine, procainamide is used for control of APCs, VPCs, atrial fibrillation, accessory pathway, and atrial and ventricular tachycardias. Procainamide may be used in conjunction with quinidine, other class I agents, and beta blockers. Procainamide is contraindicated in the presence of third-degree AV block.

Class IB Drugs

These drugs have an affinity for diseased or ischemic tissues.

Lidocaine: Used for the acute control of life-threatening ventricular arrhythmias, lidocaine is only effective when used intravenously (see Ventricular Tachycardias, page 402, for doses). The sign of lidocaine intoxication is seizures.

Tocainide: Usual side effects are weakness, head tremor, ataxia, and head bobbing.

Mexiletine: Side effects include gastric irritation, nausea, inappetence, and tremor. Both mexiletine and tocainide appear to have synergistic properties when combined with class IA agents.

Phenytoin: Indicated for digitalis-induced arrhythmias.

Class IC Drugs

These are particularly effective in arrhythmias involving accessory pathways. They seriously depress contractility, cardiac output, and systemic blood pressure. Flecainide, encainide, and propanefone are class IC agents.

CLASS II ANTIARRHYTHMICS

Class II antiarrhythmics act through blockade of the cardiac β_1 receptors. Beta-blockade is indicated for supraventricular tachycardias, pre-excitation tachyarrhythmias, atrial flutter, and atrial fibrillation. Beta-blockade should be helpful in ventricular arrhythmias induced by sympathetic stimulation. It may be used in combination with a class I agent for refractory ventricular tachyarrhythmias in the dog or as the primary agent in the cat. Contraindications include AV block, sick sinus syndrome, and dynamic bronchial disease.

Propranolol has been the standard beta blocker used in veterinary medicine for years. As with other beta blockers, the dosage rate must be titrated individually. Intravenous therapy is reserved for acute arrhythmias, especially anesthetic- or pre-excitation-related supraventricular tachycardias. Increments of 0.25 to 0.5 mg, given every 1 to 3 minutes to a maximum of 5 mg, may be used in dogs. In cats, 0.05 to 0.1 mg is the range.

CLASS III ANTIARRHYTHMICS

See textbook.

Class IV Antiarrhythmics

Class IV drugs are the calcium channel blockers. They are indicated for the control of most supraventricular tachycardias.

Digitalis Glycosides

The primary indications for use are treatment of supraventricular tachycardias by modifying the ventricular rate response. Often a second agent in combination, such as a beta blocker or calcium channel blocker, is needed to attain adequate control. Dosing and pharmacokinetics are discussed in Chapter 92.

Adenosine

Adenosine is used in the differentiation of wide QRS tachycardias, pre-excitation syndromes, and paroxysmal supraventricular tachycardias with AV nodal reentry.

Vagal Maneuvers

Ocular pressure, snout immersion, or carotid sinus massage are the approaches more commonly used in veterinary medicine. Vagal maneuvers can be used to distinguish supraventricular and ventricular tachyarrhythmias. Many supraventricular rhythms will be slowed or even abolished.

CHAPTER 96

MYOCARDIAL DISEASES
(pages 995–1032)

PRIMARY MYOCARDIAL DISEASES OF DOGS
(pp. 996–1011)

Canine Dilated Cardiomyopathy

This disease remains primarily a disease of large and giant purebred dogs. The prevalence of DCM in male dogs (0.66 per cent) is nearly twice that in female dogs (0.34 per cent).

Clinical Manifestations

Right heart failure manifested as abdominal distention, anorexia, weight loss, and fatigue often predominates in giant breeds, whereas signs of left heart failure or syncope are more common in Doberman pinschers and Boxer dogs.

Physical Examination. A protodiastolic (S_3) gallop is an important clinical finding that is most easily appreciated in dogs in sinus rhythm. Soft and often variable regurgitant systolic murmurs, typically grades 1 to 3/6, are heard over the left and/or right AV valve regions. A variety of ventricular and supraventricular arrhythmias and conduction

---

Original chapter written by D. David Sisson and William P. Thomas

disturbances are observed. Rales/crackles and increased lung sounds may be auscultated in dogs with left heart failure and pulmonary edema. Jugular venous distention, jugular pulses, hepatomegaly, and ascites are easily detected in most dogs with right-sided heart failure.

ECG Changes. Atrial fibrillation is a common rhythm disturbance reported to be present in as many as 75 to 80 per cent of some giant-breed dogs with DCM. Other common rhythm disturbances include ventricular premature depolarizations (VPDs) and ventricular tachycardia. Ventricular rhythm disturbances are of particular concern in Boxer dogs and Doberman pinschers.

Radiographic Changes. The radiographic appearance of the heart often fails to reflect the severity of the underlying myocardial impairment.

Echocardiography. Short-axis end-systolic and end-diastolic dimensions are usually much larger in dogs with DCM than in normal dogs. The walls of the LV are usually normal in thickness or slightly thinner than normal during diastole, but there is markedly decreased inward motion and thickening during systole. Systolic ejection phase indices—such as LV fractional shortening (FS), ejection fraction (EF), and velocity of circumferential fiber shortening (VCf)—are decreased in proportion to the severity of systolic dysfunction. The distance between the mitral valve at its maximal opening (E) point in early diastole and the interventricular septum (EPSS, or E point septal separation) is also increased as a result of a low ejection fraction.

Therapy

Parenteral or oral furosemide is used to reduce plasma volume and control congestive signs (pulmonary edema, pleural effusion, ascites) in dogs with DCM. Digoxin is indicated in dogs with DCM and signs of heart failure. Digoxin is also moderately effective for slowing the ventricular rate in dogs with atrial fibrillation. Two other classes of positive inotropic drugs, beta-adrenergic agonists and phosphodiesterase inhibitors, have been used effectively to treat dogs with DCM (see Chapter 92).

Controlled clinical trials have shown that dogs with DCM treated with diuretics and digoxin benefit from the additional use of the ACE inhibitor enalapril. Combination therapy with hydralazine and a nitrate is an acceptable alternative for patients that do not tolerate ACE inhibitors.

Nitroprusside is an ultrashort-acting but extremely potent vasodilator that is primarily used to treat dogs with severe, life-threatening left heart failure and pulmonary edema.

Calcium channel and beta-adrenergic receptor blocking drugs are frequently used in dogs with DCM and atrial fibrillation when digoxin has failed to adequately control the heart rate. Calcium antagonists and beta-adrenergic blocking drugs have also been advocated for treating heart failure patients in sinus rhythm. The use of antiarrhythmic drugs to treat dogs or humans with ventricular arrhythmias secondary to DCM is controversial.

It is our current policy to treat dogs with DCM and frequent VPDs or ventricular tachycardia with a class I drug, usually procainamide. Based on limited experience, mexiletine and tocainide appear to be effective for treating some otherwise resistant ventricular arrhythmias. Dogs with infrequent VPDs on a resting ECG are not treated or are further evaluated by 24-hour ambulatory ECG recordings.

Prognosis

DCM in dogs is currently almost always a fatal disease. Most dogs with signs of heart failure die as a result of the disease within 6 months to 2 years. The response to medical therapy and the subsequent clinical

course of DCM in any individual dog is extremely variable and difficult to predict from any single finding.

HYPERTROPHIC CARDIOMYOPATHY IN DOGS

Pathology

The most consistent feature of HCM is marked concentric left ventricular hypertrophy. The hypertrophy may be symmetric or asymmetric. Obstructive and nonobstructive forms of HCM are also recognized.
In the obstructive form of the disease, abnormal systolic anterior
motion (SAM) of the mitral valve toward the interventricular septum
narrows and obstructs the outflow tract.

UNCLASSIFIED MYOCARDIAL DISEASES OF DOGS

Endocardial Fibroelastosis

Primary (congenital) EFE should probably be considered a congenital form of DCM. Secondary EFE is associated with congenital malformations of the left heart and has been observed mainly in pups with
subvalvular aortic stenosis.

Glycogen Storage Disease

Clinical signs were mainly due to profound skeletal muscular weakness and megaesophagus.

Atrioventricular Myopathy (Silent Atria, Persistent Atrial Standstill)

Studies often reveal dilated, thin, almost transparent atria with little or
no visible muscle. The most commonly affected dogs are English
springer spaniels or Old English sheepdogs. Affected dogs are usually
presented for weakness, collapse, or syncope caused by severe bradycardia. The most common ECG abnormality is persistent atrial standstill.

Duchenne-Type Cardiomyopathy (Canine X-Linked Muscular Dystrophy)

In dogs with CXMD, myocardial lesions are not grossly visible prior
to 11 weeks of age, but they become obvious by 6.5 months of age and
are extensive by 6 years of age. Clinical signs of skeletal muscular dystrophy appear at about 8 weeks of age and dominate the clinical picture
during the first few years of life. Only a few dogs have survived until 5
or 6 years of age when signs of congestive heart failure become obvious. Radiographic cardiomegaly is usually modest, but the cardiac
apex may be distinctly pointed. Signs of congestive heart failure can be
treated by traditional means.

Neoplastic Diseases of the Myocardium

Most signs reflect the presence of pericardial effusion, obstruction to
blood flow, valvular insufficiency, or cardiac arrhythmias. The most
common primary cardiac tumor in dogs is hemangiosarcoma arising
from the right atrium or auricle.

SECONDARY MYOCARDIAL DISEASES OF DOGS
(pp. 1011–1014)

NONINFECTIOUS MYOCARDIAL DISEASES

Drugs and Toxins

An increasingly common potential cause of serious cardiotoxicity is
the increased use of anticancer chemotherapeutic drugs in dogs, partic-

ularly anthracycline antibiotics such as doxorubicin (Adriamycin). Severe doxorubicin cardiac toxicity is usually progressive and fatal, even if the drug is withdrawn.

Nutritional Deficiencies

The amino acid taurine and the compound carnitine are discussed in sections on dilated cardiomyopathy.

Physical Injury

In most cases, signs of injury to other organs are more apparent initially than the myocardial injury, which may not manifest itself for 12 to 24 hours or longer. The primary clinical manifestations are electrocardiographic ST-T abnormalities and arrhythmias.

Ischemic Myocardial Disease

Macroscopic Myocardial Infarction.   Myocardial infarction ("heart attack") due to occlusion of a major coronary artery branch is an extremely rare event in the dog.
Microscopic Myocardial Infarction.   Microscopic infarction is commonly found in the hearts of older dogs. Their true clinical significance remains unknown.
Other Causes of Myocardial Ischemia/Necrosis.   Dogs with acute gastric dilation-volvulus frequently develop ventricular arrhythmias. Dogs with acute pancreatitis may also develop arrhythmias and myocardial ischemia.

Cardiac Manifestations of Systemic Disease

Included are gastrointestinal, renal, neurologic, endocrine, and metabolic conditions.

MYOCARDITIS IN DOGS

Primary bacterial, fungal, or rickettsial infection of the myocardium is rare.

Viral Myocarditis

Canine parvovirus may cause neonatal myocarditis and acute left heart failure in young pups (3 to 10 weeks old).

Trypanosomiasis (Chagas' Disease)

Acute signs of systemic infection (anorexia, weight loss, diarrhea, and lymphadenopathy) usually overshadow signs of acute cardiac involvement. Antemortem diagnosis requires demonstration of parasitemia by culture or xenodiagnosis, or serodiagnosis using complement fixation or other tests. In the chronic phase, there is cardiac chamber dilation and myocardial fibrosis, especially in the right atrium and right ventricle.

PRIMARY MYOCARDIAL DISEASES OF CATS
(pp. 1014–1023)

FELINE DILATED CARDIOMYOPATHY

Following recognition of the association between taurine depletion and DCM in cats by Pion et al. in 1987, additional taurine was added to most commercial cat foods in the United States. As a result, the number of cases of DCM in cats markedly declined. Idiopathic DCM is occasionally diagnosed in cats that show no evidence of taurine deficiency.

Clinical Manifestations

Most cats are presented for treatment following a brief (several days) history of dyspnea, inactivity, or loss of appetite. About 80 per cent of cats with DCM have a detectable gallop heart sound. About one-third of cats with DCM and low plasma taurine concentrations also exhibit central retinal degeneration. Cats with DCM and signs of heart failure are often mildly or moderately azotemic.

ECG and Radiographic Findings.　Electrocardiographic abnormalities are present in most cats with DCM and include increased QRS voltages, widened P waves, and a high prevalence of ventricular arrhythmias. Typical radiographic changes include generalized cardiomegaly and pleural effusion.

Echocardiography.　Echocardiography is the safest and most reliable method for diagnosing feline DCM. Dilation of the left atrium and left ventricle and decreased LV contractility (fractional shortening, ejection fraction) are the most obvious echocardiographic abnormalities observed in cats with DCM. Left atrial thrombi are also occasionally seen.

Therapy

If they can be medically managed for 2 to 3 weeks, there is a good chance of effecting a clinical cure in cats with taurine deficiency DCM. Because the clinical response to taurine supplementation (250 to 500 mg taurine/day) is not immediate, most cats with DCM require standard medical treatment for heart failure (e.g., digoxin, furosemide) for 1 or 2 months.

Any large pleural effusion should be at least partially removed by thoracentesis. Effective diuretic dosages in cats are generally lower (0.25 to 1.0 mg/lb [0.5 to 2.0 mg/kg] q8–24h) than those recommended for dogs. Treatment of severe low-output failure and cardiogenic shock requires intensive therapy and is often unsuccessful. In this setting, positive inotropic support can be provided using dobutamine infused intravenously at a rate of 1 to 2.2 μg/lb/min (2 to 5 μg/kg/min). Cardiac output can often be improved and congestion relieved in critically ill cats by the prudent use of vasodilators. Recommended therapies include oral hydralzaine, 0.2 to 0.4 mg/lb q12h (0.5 to 0.8 mg/kg q12h), in combination with cutaneous 2 per cent nitroglycerine paste (1/4 inch q8–12h).

FELINE HYPERTROPHIC CARDIOMYOPATHY

Neutered male cats were found to be at increased risk for HCM.

Clinical Manifestations

Physical Examination.　Many cats with HCM are initially asymptomatic and are diagnosed by echocardiographic evaluation of a heart murmur, gallop sound, or arrhythmia. A systolic murmur is heard in about two-thirds of cats with HCM. A gallop rhythm is audible in about 40 per cent and arrhythmia in about 25 per cent of affected cats.

Electrocardiography.　A variety of arrhythmias and conduction disturbances have been described with feline HCM.

Radiography and Angiography.　Thoracic radiographs of asymptomatic cats with HCM may be normal or may show mild left atrial enlargement. More obvious cardiomegaly with left atrial enlargement, pulmonary venous distention, and interstitial or alveolar pulmonary edema are observed in cats with HCM and clinical signs of respiratory distress.

Echocardiography.　Careful examination of the entire heart in both long-axis and short-axis planes by two-dimensional echocardiography is required to demonstrate the true extent of the diverse patterns of ventricular hypertrophy. An isolated finding of slightly increased septal or LV wall thickness in a cat without left atrial dilation or other clinical findings is insufficient to make this diagnosis.

Treatment

Treatment of asymptomatic cats with apparent idiopathic LV hypertrophy may not be necessary in the absence of obvious left atrial enlargement, LV outflow tract obstruction, or a serious cardiac arrhythmia. By contrast, cats presenting with acute pulmonary edema require prompt and aggressive treatment, but most can be successfully treated in the short term with IV furosemide (1.0 mg/lb [2.2 mg/kg]) and supplemental oxygen therapy. Resolution of severe pulmonary edema may be hastened by application of 1/8 to 1/4 inch of 2 per cent nitroglycerine ointment. Furosemide (6.25 to 12.5 mg q8–24h) is continued in most cats with HCM and signs of edema.

Two classes of drugs have been advocated to improve LV filling and cardiac performance in cats with HCM: calcium channel blockers and beta-adrenergic receptor blockers. There is currently no consensus regarding the choice between beta blockers and calcium channel blockers for the management of feline or human HCM. We prefer to use propranolol in cats with the obstructive form of HCM. When owner compliance is a problem, once-daily treatment with atenolol (6.25 to 12.5mg/cat q12–24h) is a convenient alternative to propranolol. In cats without evidence of dynamic obstruction, initial treatment with either propranolol (2.5 to 7.5 mg/cat q8h) or diltiazem (7.5 to 15 mg/cat q8h) is appropriate. Therapy to prevent systemic arterial embolism is probably advisable.

RESTRICTIVE AND UNCLASSIFIED CARDIOMYOPATHIES IN CATS

It has become increasingly apparent that many cats with myocardial disease are difficult to categorize, and terms such as *intermediate* or *intergrade* cardiomyopathy have evolved for this poorly defined, poorly understood group.

Clinical Manifestations

Congestive heart failure with pleural effusion and/or pulmonary edema and systemic thromboembolism are common in cats with restrictive/indeterminate forms of cardiomyopathy. Heart sounds are normal in some cats, but most have an apical systolic murmur, prominent diastolic gallop, or audible arrhythmia. When the heart is not obscured by pleural effusion, thoracic radiographs often show marked left atrial or bi-atrial enlargement.

Echocardiographic changes in cats with restrictive/indeterminate cardiomyopathy are extremely variable. The most consistent echocardiographic finding is dilation of the left atrium. The left ventricle is usually normal-sized or slightly dilated. Various patterns of regional myocardial hypertrophy are observed in the septum or LV of some cats.

Treatment and Prognosis

Because of the variability of the findings in this group, specific treatment recommendations for cats with restrictive/indeterminate myocardial diseases are difficult to make. Therapy is best formulated after performing a complete cardiac evaluation and estimating the relative contributions of systolic versus diastolic dysfunction.

OTHER UNCOMMON MYOCARDIAL DISEASES OF CATS

Increased Moderator Bands

The significance of these bands and their relationship to the concurrent heart disease is uncertain because many healthy cats also have networks of LV moderator bands.

SECONDARY MYOCARDIAL DISEASES OF CATS
(pp. 1023–1026)

HYPERTHYROIDISM

Also see Chapter 114. The resulting increased heart rate, decreased peripheral vascular resistance, and increased myocardial contractility together increase cardiac output and create a high-output (hyperdynamic) circulatory state in which the resting cardiac output is increased even in the face of congestive heart failure. Myocardial hypertrophy is a prominent feature of feline hyperthyroidism. Systemic hypertension appears to be common in hyperthyroid cats. Increased resting heart rate is one of the most consistent clinical findings in hyperthyroid cats. Some affected cats exhibit open-mouthed breathing when stressed, even in the absence of congestive heart failure. Other common findings include strong to bounding arterial pulses, mildly distended jugular veins, a jugular venous pulse, apical systolic murmur, cardiac arrhythmias, and a diastolic gallop.

A variety of arrhythmias and conduction disturbances have been reported. About one-half of cats with hyperthyroidism have mild to moderate cardiac enlargement on thoracic radiographs. Hyperthyroid cats without marked cardiomegaly and signs of heart failure do not usually require cardioactive drugs. Treatment of heart failure in hyperthyroid cats requires relief of edema with a diuretic and reduction of circulating thyroid hormones with the oral antithyroid drug methimazole.

ACROMEGALY (HYPERSOMATOTROPISM)

In 14 cases described by Peterson et al., all affected cats had insulin-resistant diabetes mellitus and enlargement of the liver, heart, kidneys, or tongue.

SYSTEMIC HYPERTENSION

Diseases of cats associated with systemic hypertension include hyperthyroidism, chronic renal disease, diabetes mellitus, acromegaly, and primary aldosteronism. The pathologic features of hypertensive cardiomyopathy have not been described in cats and may be indistinguishable from those observed in feline HCM. The frequent association of feline hypertension with renal parenchymal disease suggests that therapy should be tailored to this circumstance. Sodium retention should be reduced by means of a salt-restricted diet and a diuretic. Angiotensin-converting enzyme inhibitors may also prove useful.

INFILTRATIVE MYOCARDIAL DISEASE

Neoplastic infiltration of the heart is rare in cats. Lymphoma is the most common tumor of the feline myocardium.

DRUGS, TOXINS, AND PHYSICAL INJURY

Doxorubicin has received the most attention in cats. However, clinical signs of heart failure were not observed even after a cumulative dose of 300 mg/m^2, and no cat showed ECG abnormalities. With the possible exception of heat stroke and hypothermia, physical causes of myocardial damage are infrequently recognized in cats.

SYSTEMIC ARTERIAL THROMBOEMBOLISM
(pp. 1026–1027)

Most investigators agree that systemic thromboembolism will occur in at least 10 to 20 per cent of cats with hypertrophic or restrictive cardiomyopathy. The consequences of systemic arterial embolization depend on the site of embolization, the completeness of the obstruction, the functional patency of collateral circulation, and the duration of obstruction.

Initial diagnostic efforts are directed toward defining the site and severity of the vascular obstruction and the nature and severity of underlying heart disease. Surgical removal of aortic emboli should only be attempted in cats with complete obstructions and only within the first 12 hours of occurrence, if at all. Many cats die when surgery is attempted because of underlying heart disease. Clot dissolution with streptokinase and recombinant tissue plasminogen activator (TPA) has been attempted in cats with varying degrees of success.

Many cats with saddle thrombi, especially those with incomplete occlusions, will regain limited function of the hindlimbs with more conservative therapy. Recovery takes several weeks to months, and residual deficits (peripheral neuropathy, muscle contracture) are common. To prevent additional clot formation, heparin can be administered IV at 100 IU/lb (220 IU/kg) initially, followed by maintenance subcutaneous doses of 30 IU/lb q6h (66 IU/kg q6h). Acepromazine or hydralazine has also been recommended. Low-dose aspirin (10 mg/lb [25 mg/kg] PO) every 3 days is the most widely employed prophylactic measure.

CHAPTER 97
PERICARDIAL DISORDERS
(pages 1032–1045)

PATHOPHYSIOLOGY (pp. 1033–1035)

Because the right ventricle is affected earlier and more severely than the left as intrapericardial pressures rise, clinical signs of right heart failure, such as hepatosplenomegaly and ascites, usually predominate.

CONGENITAL DISEASES OF THE PERICARDIUM
(pp. 1035–1036)

Pericardial Defects. Partial pericardial defects are usually clinically silent. Clinical signs may occur if a portion of the heart herniates through the defect and becomes incarcerated. Peritoneopericardial diaphragmatic hernias (PPDH) have been frequently reported in dogs and cats. Clinical signs are most commonly referable to the gastrointestinal or respiratory systems. Many animals exhibit no clinical signs. In many cases, only the omentum or falciform ligament is located within the pericardial sac.

If the hernia is large and a significant amount of abdominal viscera has migrated into the pericardial sac, the abdomen may seem empty on palpation. Concurrent defects, such as sternal malformations and cranial abdominal hernias, may also be detected. In most cases, echocardiography readily identifies the presence of abdominal viscera within

Original chapter written by Matthew W. Miller and D. David Sisson the pericardial sac. Surgical correction of the hernia with replacement of viable herniated viscera is recommended in animals with clinical signs or with demonstrated compromise of a herniated organ.

Pericardial Cysts. Distortion of the cardiac silhouette, most obvious on the dorsoventral radiographic view, was observed in most of the affected dogs. Surgical removal of the cyst and subtotal pericardiectomy was curative in the five dogs in which it was attempted.

ACQUIRED PERICARDIAL DISEASES (pp. 1036–1045)

PERICARDIAL EFFUSION

Bloody effusion can result from trauma, left atrial tears, idiopathic pericarditis, or neoplasia. German shepherd and golden retriever dogs are at increased risk for hemangiosarcoma of the right atrium. Infective pericarditis is uncommon in dogs, but it has been reported secondary to bacterial and fungal infection. In cats, pericardial effusion is often associated with feline cardiomyopathy and feline infectious peritonitis (FIP) virus infection.

Diagnosis

History and Physical Examination. Animals with pericardial effusion are often presented with a vague clinical history of lethargy, weakness, exercise intolerance, and anorexia. More severely compromised animals evidence obvious abdominal distention, respiratory difficulty, or syncope. The heart sounds are usually muffled. Jugular venous distention or a positive hepatojugular reflux is almost invariably present. Measurement of central venous pressure (CVP) will document systemic venous hypertension. Measures of CVP usually exceed 10 to 12 mm Hg (normal = <6 mm Hg) if cardiac tamponade is present. Femoral arterial pulses are often abnormal (weak and abrupt).

Radiography. The cardiac silhouette typically loses its angles and waists and becomes globe-shaped when a large volume of pericardial fluid accumulates. If systemic congestion has developed, distention of the caudal vena cava, hepatomegaly, and ascites are usually evident. Deviation of the trachea or mainstem bronchi suggests the possibility of a heart base tumor.

Electrocardiography. Electrical alternans, defined as a beat-to-beat voltage variation of the QRS or ST-T complexes, may be recorded in as many as 50 per cent of patients with pericardial effusion. Reductions in QRS voltage (R < 1 mV in lead II) are commonly recorded in dogs with pericardial effusion.

Echocardiography. An anechoic space between the epicardium and pericardium is the classic echocardiographic finding in pericardial effusion. Echocardiography usually permits visualization of intrapericardiac or cardiac mass lesions. Echocardiographic findings that strongly suggest the presence of cardiac tamponade include diastolic collapse of the right atrium or right ventricle.

Laboratory Evaluation. Blood chemistry profiles typically reflect evidence of passive organ congestion (mildly elevated liver enzymes), reduced cardiac output (prerenal uremia), or dilutional changes in protein and electrolyte concentrations. Caution should be exercised when evaluating the cellular component of pericardial effusates for neoplastic cells, as false-negative and false-positive interpretations are common.

Therapy and Prognosis

Pericardiocentesis. Pericardiocentesis is indicated for initial stabilization of dogs and cats with pericardial effusion resulting in cardiac tamponade. Shave and surgically prepare a large area of the right hemithorax. Local anesthesia is usually adequate, but mild sedation is sometimes necessary. The puncture site is usually determined based on the location of the heart on thoracic radiographs. Most pericardial effusions are hemorrhagic in character and have a "port wine" appearance. Pericardial effusion can be differentiated from peripheral blood in that it rarely clots unless it is from very recent hemorrhage. Also, the packed cell volume of the effusate is usually significantly different from that of peripheral blood.

Pericardiectomy.   Pericardiectomy is advisable in dogs or cats with septic or foreign body pericarditis. Surgery is also often necessary in dogs with acute cardiac tamponade caused by a left atrial tear. In patients requiring repeated pericardiocentesis (two or more recurrences), we recommend subtotal pericardiectomy. The treatment and long-term prognosis for animals with cardiac or pericardial neoplasia vary with the specific tumor type responsible for the effusion.

Aortic body tumors have been successfully removed in a small number of dogs. When this alternative is not feasible, subtotal pericardiectomy should be considered. Aortic body tumors are slow growing and are often late to metastasize. The prognosis for dogs with cardiac hemangiosarcoma is poor. Many of these mass lesions are not amenable to surgical removal. Recent reports have suggested that percutaneous pericardial balloon dilation may be a reasonable alternative to subtotal pericardiectomy for the management of both neoplastic and recurring idiopathic effusions.

CONSTRICTIVE PERICARDIAL DISEASE

The most common owner complaint at presentation was that of abdominal enlargement. Less frequently, owners complained of dyspnea, tachypnea, weakness, syncope, and weight loss.

Diagnosis.   Ascites and jugular venous distention are the most common abnormal physical examination findings. Electrocardiographic abnormalities include prolongation of the P wave, reductions in QRS voltage amplitude, and sinus tachycardia. Dilation of the caudal vena cava is common, and pleural effusion may be evident. Central venous pressure is invariably elevated in dogs with clinical evidence of right heart failure.

Echocardiography is sometimes highly suggestive of constrictive pericardial disease. Many of the changes are subtle, and the distinction between constrictive pericardial disease and restrictive cardiomyopathy may be difficult. Flattening of the left ventricular endocardium during diastole and abnormal diastolic (early notch) and systolic septal motion are among the more consistent echocardiographic findings.

Therapy and Prognosis.   Successful treatment of constrictive pericarditis requires surgical removal of the pericardium.

CHAPTER 98

HEARTWORM DISEASE
(pages 1046–1068)

CARDIOPULMONARY DISEASE DEVELOPMENT

Life Cycle. Heartworm infection is spread by many different species of mosquitoes. Approximately 6 months after the infective larvae enter their new host, microfilaremia occurs, and their numbers usually increase markedly over the next 6 months. Subsequently, the microfilarial concentration frequently declines. Dogs with higher heartworm burdens generally have more severe pulmonary hypertension and thromboembolism. Pulmonary hypertension and the central arteriographic lesions can resolve after elimination of adult heartworms. Residual fibrosis can remain about the distal arteries, but proximal arteries return toward normalcy. The worst pulmonary disease is seen after adult heartworms have died. Coughing and dyspnea are the most common signs and are usually associated with parenchymal disease of caudal lung lobes. The increased pumping work of perfusing the diseased arterial system produces a sequence of right ventricular dilation, hypertrophy, and right-sided congestive heart failure.

PRETREATMENT EVALUATION

No tests have been found to be useful in predicting thiacetarsamide complications.

Microfilarial Detection and Differentiation. Examination of peripheral blood for microfilaria is indicated in all heartworm-infected dogs or suspect dogs, all dogs intended to receive diethylcarbamazine, and all dogs being placed on prophylaxis for the first time.

Immunodiagnostic Tests. These are the preferred means for routine screening for heartworm infection.

Radiology. Thoracic radiographs are the diagnostic procedures most useful in characterizing disease severity. Typical changes include right ventricular enlargement, increased prominence of the main pulmonary artery, enlarged lobar pulmonary arteries, enlargement of peripheral pulmonary arteries, and perivascular parenchymal disease. The diameter of the right cranial lobar artery at its intersection with the right fourth rib should not exceed the narrowest diameter of the fourth rib, and the diameter of the caudal lobar arteries at their intersection with the ninth rib should be no larger than the narrowest diameter of the ninth rib.

The Minimum Data Base. The widespread availability of accurate, cost-efficient laboratory profiles makes it reasonable for the minimum data base for all heartworm-infected dogs to include a complete blood count, a serum chemistry profile, a urinalysis, and thoracic radiographs. Thoracic radiography is the single diagnostic test that provides the most information about the severity of heartworm disease. An extended data base is indicated if abnormalities are revealed by the minimum data base. Mild to moderate prerenal azotemia is not a contraindication to heartworm treatment, but fluid therapy to resolve azotemia is required.

Liver enzyme activity (serum alanine aminotransferase and serum alkaline phosphatase) provides little value as a component of the minimum data base. Up to a tenfold increase in serum liver enzyme activity

---

Original chapter written by Clarence A. Rawlings and Clay A. Calvert

has not been associated with an increased incidence of acute thiacetarsamide sodium toxicity, mortality, or treatment failures.

CLINICAL SYNDROMES (DIAGNOSIS AND TREATMENT) (pp. 1054–1058)

Asymptomatic Patients. Dogs that are determined to be asymptomatic should be treated with an adulticide and microfilaricide soon after infection is diagnosed. We recommend no supplemental therapy beyond good nutrition and the standard adulticide and microfilaricide treatment.

Patients with Pulmonary Disease. When severe parenchymal disease produces signs prior to adulticide treatment, treatment is the same as that following adulticide treatment. The most useful diagnostic tool, after a good physical examination, is the thoracic radiograph. Thrombocytopenia is common, reflecting platelet consumption on the injured arterial surfaces and dead heartworm fragments. Many dogs with parenchymal disease produced by heartworms have occult infections.

Treatment is strict cage confinement and anti-inflammatory dosages of daily corticosteroids (prednisolone or prednisone, 0.5 to 1 mg/lb (1 to 2 mg/kg). Corticosteroid treatment seldom requires more than a week of administration. Oxygen can markedly reduce pulmonary hypertension.

Occult Heartworm Infection and Disease. The most dramatic type of "occult heartworm infection" is "occult disease" produced by immune-mediated destruction of microfilaria. This syndrome typically produces the most severely diseased conditions.

Severe Pulmonary Arterial Disease. Typical signs include coughing, exercise intolerance, syncope, weight loss, and right-sided congestive heart failure. If parenchymal disease is confirmed, corticosteroids such as prednisone, 0.5 to 1 mg/lb/day (1 to 2 mg/kg/day), are recommended until clinical and radiographic signs begin to resolve, usually in 3 to 7 days. Thrombocytopenia is common, may be severe, and is often associated with coughing, hemoptysis, and radiographic evidence of parenchymal lung disease.

There are at least three treatment approaches to the patient with severe pulmonary arterial disease. First, high heartworm burdens can be reduced surgically, thereby sparing the dog the difficulty of coping with dying and dead heartworms. A long, flexible alligator forceps is guided via the jugular vein into the right heart and pulmonary arteries. A second approach is an effort to reduce the worm burden by means of an initial and partial adulticide regimen. A third approach consists of cage confinement and antithrombotic therapy. Cage confinement and aspirin treatment (2 to 3 mg/lb/day [5 to 7 mg/kg/day]) are recommended for 2 to 3 weeks before treatment, during treatment, and for 3 to 4 weeks following treatment. Low-dosage heparinization can be used in place of aspirin. Dogs with right-sided congestive heart failure should be treated with conservative dosages of diuretics and a low-sodium diet.

Thrombocytopenia is usually associated with thromboembolic complications. Heparin (20 to 31 U/lb [50 to 70 U/kg] SC, q8h) is effective, with thrombocytopenia and hemoglobinuria typically resolving within 3 days.

Occult Heartworm Disease Pneumonitis. Coughing and dyspnea are the predominant clinical signs, but severely affected dogs may experience mild cyanosis, anorexia, and weight loss. The thoracic radiographic abnormalities associated with heartworm pneumonitis are diffuse, bilateral linear interstitial and alveolar infiltrates of the caudal lung lobes. Heartworm pneumonitis should be treated with corticosteroids. Most dogs experience rapid and complete resolution of radiographic abnormalities within 3 to 5 days of treatment. Thiacetarsamide treatment should be initiated as soon thereafter as feasible.

HEARTWORM INFECTION (pp. 1058–1060)

ADULTICIDE TREATMENT

Indications and Contraindications for Arsenical Treatment. The existence of concomitant, life-threatening diseases may be a contraindication to thiacetarsamide treatment.

Method and Effect of Arsenical Treatment. The recommended dosage of thiacetarsamide is 1.0 mg/lb (0.10 ml/lb) or 2.2 mg/kg (0.22 ml/kg) twice a day for 2 days, intravenously. When multiple injections are given at or near the same site, the possibility of extravascular drug leakage is increased.

Immature worms, especially female worms, are resistant to thiacetarsamide. It is not necessary, however, to kill 100 per cent of adult heartworms in order to produce significant resolution of pulmonary arterial disease. An antigen test can be performed 3 months following arsenical treatment to determine whether adult heartworms remain, as the antigen should be cleared by this time.

Melarsamine is given as an intramuscular injection deep into the lumbar muscles. The dosage is 1.2 mg/lb (2.5 mg/kg) given twice at a 24-hour interval. Melarsamine has proved to be more efficacious than thiacetarsamide.

Thiacetarsamide Sodium Toxicity. Most dogs that experience acute reactions to thiacetarsamide do so following the first or second dosages. The earliest laboratory sign of hepatic toxicity is bilirubinuria. Bilirubinuria is a common finding following the third and fourth injections, but it is cause for concern only if the dog is clinically sick.

There is no specific treatment for hepatotoxicity resulting in icterus other than maintenance or reestablishment of hydration, restricted activity, and a high-carbohydrate, low-fat diet. Occasionally icterus and severe illness develop several days following completion of treatment. Serum liver enzyme activity commonly increases during thiacetarsamide treatment. It is not necessary to monitor serum liver enzyme activity during treatment.

Indications to Interrupt Thiacetarsamide Treatment. Vomiting, lethargy, and anorexia are common complications of thiacetarsamide treatment. The combination of repetitive vomiting, lethargy, and anorexia is indicative of serious toxicity, and under no circumstances should treatment be continued. Icterus, an uncommon complication of thiacetarsamide toxicity, is always an indication to stop therapy. Marked bilirubinuria following the first treatment is an indication to proceed with caution, but is usually not the sole reason to abort treatment. If azotemia is discovered during the course of treatment, treatment is interrupted only if the serum urea nitrogen is moderately elevated.

MICROFILARICIDE TREATMENT

Microfilaricide treatment is given 3 to 6 weeks after thiacetarsamide treatment. Ivermectin and milbemycin are highly effective microfilaricides that are not FDA approved for this purpose. A single dosage of ivermectin (0.022 mg/lb [0.05 mg/kg]) administered 4 weeks post-thiacetarsamide rapidly reduces microfilaria numbers and eliminates microfilaria in approximately 90 per cent of the dogs. The same approach is used with milbemycin, the dosage being 0.22 mg/lb (0.5 mg/kg).

A microfilaria concentration test is performed 3 weeks after microfilaricide treatment. If microfilaremia persists, the regimen is repeated. Caution is advised in treating collies with either ivermectin or milbemycin.

PREVENTION OF HEARTWORM INFECTION
(pp. 1060–1061)

Heartworm infection can be prevented with daily diethylcarbamazine or monthly treatment with one of the macrolide antibiotics (ivermectin or milbemycin oxime). In addition, some clients apparently forget to give their dog its daily preventive dose, and these dogs can develop infections. Since diethylcarbamazine probably affects a molting stage, such as the L_3 to L_4 at 9 to 12 days after infection, it may be discontinued one month after the first frost and resumed one month prior to the spring mosquito season.

Heartworm-positive dogs should not be given diethylcarbamazine. Ivermectin has proved effective in preventing infection. The minimum dosage is 2.5 gm/lb (5.98 gm/kg). High dosages of ivermectin have produced toxicity in heartworm-positive dogs when given to collies to eliminate microfilaria.

Milbemycin is another antibiotic macrolide. The heartworm prophylactic dosage of 0.23 mg/lb (0.5 mg/kg) is also effective in controlling roundworm and hookworm infections. A similar drug, moxidectin, has proved 100 per cent effective in preventing heartworm infection, but its approval by the FDA is pending. A probable dosage will be 1.4 µg/lb (3 µg/kg), which is safe in collies and is not microfilaricidal.

Advantages of the macrolide antibiotics over diethylcarbamazine are that dogs do not need to be free of heartworms for a preventive program to be started. If ivermectin is given as a microfilaricide, infections contracted during the previous 2 months should be blocked.

FELINE HEARTWORM DISEASE (pp. 1061–1067)

Cats are assumed to be relatively resistant to heartworm infection. Adult *D. immitis* in cats appear to have a life span of 2 to 3 years, which is less than that in dogs. It appears that some cats spontaneously eliminate the worms. Aberrant migration of *D. immitis* larvae, such as to the brain or systemic arteries, are more common in the cat than in the dog.

The pathophysiologic responses of cats to heartworms are similar to those in dogs, but exaggerated. As in the dog, caudal lobar arteries are most severely affected. Radiographic changes typical of heartworm disease are present within 3 to 5 months. Changes include enlargement of the caudal pulmonary arteries, right ventricular enlargement, and both diffuse and focal areas of pulmonary parenchymal disease.

Clinical Manifestations. The most common historical findings of cats with heartworm disease are coughing and dyspnea, which are usually paroxysmal in nature. Vomiting, anorexia, lethargy, and weight loss are common nonspecific complaints. Acute pulmonary thromboembolism is a common manifestation of heartworm infection. Affected cats become severely dyspneic, weak, and tachycardic. Chronic manifestations of heartworm infection are vomiting, cor pulmonale including right-sided congestive heart failure, and relapsing PIE. Pleural effusion, often accompanied by ascites, is seen in some cats with chronic infections.

Radiography. Thoracic radiographs remain the most useful test for diagnosis of feline heartworm disease. Enlargement of the main pulmonary artery segment is not well visualized in cats. Signs include lobar pulmonary artery enlargement, right ventricular enlargement, and parenchymal lung disease. The alveolar disease produced by thromboembolism tends to have a patchy lobar distribution. Pleural effusion may occur in cats with advanced heartworm disease. The most common cause of pleural effusion in heartworm-infected cats is right-sided congestive heart failure.

Echocardiography. Cardiac ultrasonography should be considered for any cat with suspected heartworm infection.

Diagnosis of Infection. The possibility of feline heartworm disease should be considered in cats with respiratory signs, crackles, unexplained syncope, systolic heart murmurs, gallop heart rhythms, eosinophilia, basophilia, hyperglobulinemia, or vomiting.

Serologic tests usually simplify the diagnosis. The most useful serologic tests for feline heartworm disease identify *D. immitis* adult antigens. Tests are more likely to be positive when gravid females are present. False-negative test results usually occur when less than three adult female worms are present.

Most cats with naturally acquired heartworm infections do not have microfilaremia. Cardiac ultrasonography is indicated in all cats suspected or known to be infected. The use of arteriography should be considered if a cat suspected of having heartworms has equivocal radiographic signs and negative test results on microfilaria concentration tests, antigen tests, and ultrasonography.

THERAPY OF HEARTWORM INFECTION

Cats exhibiting persistent clinical signs consistent with heartworm infection, especially those with low worm burdens, should probably receive adulticide therapy. Treatment of adult *D. immitis* with thiacetarsamide (1 mg/lb [2.2 mg/kg] IV q12h, for 2 days) is somewhat effective. The appropriate dosage schedule for thiacetarsamide in the cat relative to efficacy and toxicity has not been determined. Although unproven, premedication with a soluble corticosteroid and an antihistamine prior to each injection of thiacetarsamide may reduce the risk of the acute respiratory distress syndrome. There is also a significant risk of acute, fatal thromboembolilc complications during the first 2 to 3 weeks after adulticide treatment.

Owing to the uncertain risk of peracute reactions and the high risk of thromboembolism, we do not recommend adulticide therapy in many cats. Thiacetarsamide should be reserved for cats with persistent or frequent clinical signs, especially signs of pulmonary hypertension and right-sided congestive heart failure. If a high worm burden is indicated, either by an antigen concentration test or by cardiac ultrasonography, an attempt should be made to retrieve the worms from the right heart and posterior vena cava. Microfilaricide treatment is usually unnecessary because most cats have no or only a few circulating microfilaria. When indicated, ivermectin is an effective microfilaricidal treatment.

THERAPY OF HEARTWORM DISEASE

Anti-inflammatory dosages of corticosteroids and/or heparin are given to cats with acute dyspnea due to thromboembolism following thiacetarsamide treatment. Aspirin is difficult to appropriately dose and has minimal benefit in reducing the incidence or severity of thromboembolic complications in cats.

An allergic pneumonitis resembling that seen in dogs is sometimes observed. Affected cats manifest coughing, dyspnea, and crackles. The pneumonitis usually resolves quickly with glucocorticoid therapy. Dyspnea and coughing are also signs of thromboembolic disease, and the differential diagnosis requires thoracic radiographs.

Severely affected cats should be confined to a cage and administered oxygen, glucocorticoid, and supportive fluid therapy. If the platelet count decreases below 100,000/mm^3 in a cat with a normal or slightly prolonged activated clotting time, heparin, (50 to 70 U/kg) 22 to 35 U/lb (50–75 U/kg) SC q8h should be administered until clinical signs are markedly improved, for 5 to 21 days, or until the platelet count exceeds 200,000/mm^3.

Infected cats with right-sided congestive heart failure consistently have severe pulmonary arterial disease. The treatment for these cats includes cage confinement, possibly oxygen administration, the judicious use of a diuretic, and thoracocentesis when indicated. Whether digoxin is indicated in the treatment of right-sided congestive heart failure due to heartworm disease is uncertain. In general, digoxin is ineffective for the treatment of cor pulmonale.

HEARTWORM PROPHYLAXIS

The need for a heartworm preventive program for cats is controversial. We recommend prophylaxis for cats when local feline infections have been documented. Monthly administration of both ivermectin and milbemycin oxime have proved effective. The preventive dosage for milbemycin oxime is the same as that for dogs (0.22 to 40 mg/lb [0.5 to 0.99 mg/kg]), and the reported ivermectin dosage for cats is 11 μg/lb (24 μg/kg).

CHAPTER 99

PERIPHERAL VASCULAR DISEASE
(pages 1068–1081)

OCCLUSIVE ARTERIAL DISEASES (pp. 1068–1071)

Most emboli constitute blood clots that have broken free from a site of thrombus formation (thromboemboli).

ARTERIAL THROMBOEMBOLISM IN CATS

See Chapter 96.

ARTERIAL THROMBOSIS AND THROMBOEMBOLISM IN DOGS

Thrombosis may result from a wide variety of systemic and metabolic disorders (Table 99–1).

Clinical Signs. Microthrombus formation is common, particularly after trauma or surgery. However, rapid clot lysis and abundant collateral circulation usually result in absence of outward clinical signs. Classic signs of acute arterial limb occlusion relate to seven "Ps," namely pain, paleness, paresthesia, pulselessness, polar (cold), paresis/paralysis, and prostration. Aortic thromboembolism has been reported in dogs with bacterial endocarditis, aberrant heartworm migration, and renal amyloidosis. With endocarditis, the mitral and/or aortic valves are usually affected. Bacterial embolization from these valves may cause a systemic shower of emboli, which frequently affect abdominal organs, especially the kidneys and small intestines.

Diagnosis. Acute vascular occlusion to a limb usually causes definitive clinical signs. A minimal clinical pathology data base is advised to evaluate and detect renal or hepatic disease, dirofilariasis, disseminated intravascular coagulation, and systemic and metabolic diseases. Thrombosis of internal organs and the brain may be difficult to diagnose.

Original chapter written by Peter F. Suter and Philip R. Fox

TABLE 99–1. THROMBOSIS AND THROMBOEMBOLISM: CAUSES AND PREDISPOSING FACTORS

Vascular disorders (endothelial and/or wall injury)
    Arteriosclerosis (hyalinosis, amyloidosis)
    Atherosclerotic vascular disease
    Vasculitis (angiitis), phlebitis, arteritis
    Suppurative, septicemic, or granulomatous processes
    Parasitism (aberrant dirofilariasis)
    Catheterization, indwelling catheters
    Injection of irritating or hypertonic substances
    Neoplasia
    Abscesses
Slowed or disrupted blood flow
    Hypovolemia
    Shock
    Congestive heart failure
    Bacterial endocarditis (heart valve vegetations)
    Vascular incarceration or compression
Hypercoagulability, changes in blood constituents
    Cushing's Syndrome
    Protein-losing enteropathy
    Renal amyloidosis, glomerulopathies
    DIC
    Polycythemia
    Platelet disorders, thrombocytosis
    Immune hemolytic anemia
    Dehydration and/or hyperviscosity
Thromboembolism
    Septic, nonseptic emboli
    Extraneous foreign material (hair, catheter fragments, foreign bodies)

Treatment. Therapy should be directed toward the underlying disease or cause of thrombosis. If diagnosed early, especially within 8 to 12 hours, some thrombi may be physically removed before ischemic neuromyopathy is too advanced. Analgesics must be given. Fluid therapy should be initiated to correct acid-base or electrolyte abnormalities and dehydration. Anticoagulants are usually advocated, although there is some controversy about efficacy. Heparin is most commonly chosen. Low-dose heparin is advocated (5 to 10 IU/kg constant rate IV infusion, or 75 to 150 IU/kg subcutaneously q6–8h). Monitoring by APTT is necessary to adjust this dose so that the APTT is prolonged from 1.5 to 2 times normal. Heparin can be neutralized by protamine sulfate administration.

NONOCCLUSIVE ARTERIAL DISEASES (pp. 1071–1077)

ARTERIAL ANEURYSM

See textbook.

ARTERIOVENOUS FISTULAS (ARTERIOVENOUS MALFORMATIONS)

These are reported uncommonly in dogs and rarely in cats. Communications of the cardiac chambers or great vessels may occur as a centrally located anomaly and be intracardiac (e.g., ventricular septal defect) or extracardiac (e.g., patent ductus arteriosus). These are reviewed in Chapter 93. Acquired A-V fistulas are always localized, i.e., confined to one area connecting an artery to a vein. In contrast, congenital A-V malformations are rare and consist of several poorly defined small A-V communications that seldom cause clinical problems. The most common cause of an acquired A-V fistula is blunt or penetrating trauma. Most A-V fistulas involve the extremities. They have been recorded as a complication of mass ligation of arteries and veins.

The A-V fistula creates a low-pressure conduit for systemic circulation. Fistulas with large shunts may result in arterial hypotension and reduced peripheral vascular resistance, venous hypertension, increased cardiac preload, elevated heart rate, pulmonary hypertension, and potentially high-output heart failure. Small A-V fistulas of the extremities are noticed by the owners as painless, easily compressible, warm bulges. With medium-sized or large fistulas of the extremities, a continuous palpable thrill and pulsation, along with a machinery murmur, can be detected. The leg or region distal to the fistula may be swollen and warmer or colder than the proximal area (sometimes with severe local ischemia), painful, and affected by pitting or secondary inflammatory edema.

When firm pressure is applied proximal to the A-V fistula, or if the feeding artery is compressed, the thrill and bruit disappear, and pulse and heart rate may drop as a result of diminished venous return and reduced cardiac output. This is referred to as Branham's bradycardia sign. A-V fistulas of the liver connect the hepatic artery to the portal vein and cause portal hypertension. Abdominal distention due to low protein ascites is a major clinical sign. Portosystemic collateral vessels and signs of hepatoencephalopathy may develop. Pulmonary A-V fistulas can lead to respiratory distress and cyanosis.

The absence of a normal capillary phase and premature outlining of the veins are typical arteriographic findings in shunting lesions. It is important to try to identify the barely visible distal continuation of the artery feeding the fistula. Diagnostic ultrasonography, especially color Doppler imaging, has been clinically useful in man to identify and localize A-V fistulas. The treatment of A-V fistulas is primarily surgical. The surgical reanastomosing of the affected artery to its distal normal continuation is usually not a critical factor.

ARTERIOSCLEROSIS AND ATHEROSCLEROSIS

Arteriosclerotic lesions are common in old dogs and cats. Atherosclerosis is considered a form of arteriosclerosis. The inner sections of arterial wall are thickened by deposits of plaque containing cholesterol, lipoid material, and lipophages. A predisposition for spontaneous atherosclerosis has been found in old (9 years old and older), obese dogs with atrophied thyroid glands and hypothyroidism. Atherosclerosis has not been described in cats.

Laboratory abnormalities include hypercholesterolemia, lipidemia, low T_3 and T_4 values, elevated BUN and liver enzymes, and high values for the alpha$_2$ and beta fractions in the protein electrophoresis.

VASCULITIS, ANGIITIS

Vasculitis occurs commonly in a wide variety of inflammatory and toxic conditions and can affect arteries and veins of all sizes in many locations. By definition, the etiology of secondary vasculitides is known and is thus readily classifiable. They usually result from infectious diseases such as feline infectious peritonitis, canine coronavirus infection, parvovirus infection (rare), Rocky Mountain spotted fever, leishmaniasis, and dirofilariasis. They may also occur in drug reactions and in immunopathogenic connective tissue and collagen diseases such as systemic lupus erythematosus and rheumatoid arthritis. These and other secondary vasculitides are described elsewhere in this textbook.

Hypersensitivity Vasculitis, Periarteritis, Polyarteritis

Lesions of hypersensitivity vasculitis (HV) affect mainly arterioles, capillaries, and venules and are uniform in nature. They most often result from deposition of immune complexes. The most commonly affected organ is the skin, although mucous membranes, renal glomeruli, lungs, and the central nervous system may also be involved. Skin lesions include wheals, urticaria, purpura, nodules, bullae, crusty lesions, necrosis, and ulcers. Skin and renal lesions rarely occur together in the same patient.

Lymphopenia, eosinopenia, hypoalbuminemia, hyperglobulinemia, and hyperfibrinogenemia occur commonly. Diagnostic confirmation requires histologic examination of skin, organ, or lymph node biopsies, and exclusion of other immune-mediated diseases based on a negative Coombs, ANA, and other appropriate tests. Differential diagnosis includes pemphigus vulgaris and foliaceus, bullous pemphigoid, systemic lupus erythematosus, dirofilariasis, specific infectious diseases, chronic neoplasia, and cold hemagglutination disease.

Many therapies have been advocated. Administration of all unnecessary drugs should be discontinued. In many cases immunosuppressive dosages of glucocorticoids with or without an antibiotic have been used successfully. Cyclophosphamide has been advocated if that fails.

Polyarteritis Nodosa

Target tissues include the kidneys, skin, mucous membranes, adrenals, meninges, gastrointestinal tract, connective tissue, and myocardium. The lungs are usually spared. The clinical presentation includes systemic signs (pyrexia, lethargy, reluctance to walk, vague pain, or weight loss) and a wide spectrum of organ system abnormalities (linear skin ulceration, ulceration of mucous membranes, nasal discharge, spinal pain, and signs of cardiac and/or renal failure). Diagnosis is confirmed by histologic examination of skin biopsy. Treatment includes glucocorticoids and/or cyclophosphamide.

Lymphomatoid Granulomatosis and Miscellaneous Vasculitides

Pulmonary nodular lesions of variable size due to lymphomatosis were first described in dogs. The differential diagnosis is primary or secondary neoplasia, with which this condition is often confused. Diagnosis is rarely made clinically and requires histologic examination of biopsy material. Therapy with glucocorticoids and cytotoxic immunosuppressive drugs is only temporarily effective.

DISEASES OF VEINS (p. 1077)

Diseases of the venous system are usually of minor clinical importance. Perforation or blunt trauma to veins is usually well tolerated. Even when venous occlusion or severance is severe, edema and cyanosis are usually temporary because of large collateral systems.

DISEASES OF THE PERIPHERAL LYMPHATICS (pp. 1077–1080)

INFLAMMATORY LYMPHATIC DISORDERS (LYMPHANGITIS AND LYMPHADENITIS)

Lymphangitis and lymphadenitis often occur secondary to a variety of local infections. Pyrexia, anorexia, and depression are common. Therapy consists of moist, warm, local compresses or soaks, which reduce swelling and promote drainage. Aggressive local and systemic antibiotic therapy in animals with fever and anorexia usually promote rapid recovery.

LYMPHEDEMA

Primary Lymphedema

Lymphedema due to aplasia or hypoplasia of proximal lymph channels and/or popliteal lymph nodes occurs most often in the hind limbs of young dogs. Mild cases are restricted to the hind limbs, whereas severe cases may progress to whole body edema. The edema is not usually accompanied by lameness. Growth and activity are normal. Rest and limb massage do not usually reduce the severity of edema.

The diagnosis of primary lymphedema is based on history and clinical signs. Radiographic lymphography may be needed to confirm the diagnosis in subtle cases. Primary lymphedema is characterized by lymph node aplasia and small lymphatics ending blindly. Lymphatic channel cannulation is difficult unless lymphangiectases have formed. Their identification is facilitated in milder cases by subcutaneous injection of vital dyes (e.g., 3 per cent Evans blue dye or 11 per cent patent blue violet) into the toe webs. When aplastic, lymphatics suitable for cannulation and injection of radiocontrast agent may not be found. Prognosis for resolution of congenital lymphedema is guarded.

Secondary Lymphedema

Secondary lymphedema is often due to a combination of lymphatic and venous obstruction. The most common etiologies include post-traumatic or postsurgical interruption of lymphatics, excision of lymph nodes containing neoplastic metastases, and blockage of lymph nodes and lymph vessels by compression or invasive neoplasms. The location and severity of obstruction determines the extent of edema formation. Secondary lymphedema is more common than primary lymphedema. A complete history is helpful in distinguishing between these categories.

Diagnosis is based largely on history and clinical examination. It is facilitated by diagnostic imaging, which evaluates regions where the presumptive obstruction is located. Diagnostic ultrasonography can provide valuable information about soft tissue masses and readily identifies enlarged lymph nodes and other structures. Ulceration, dermatitis, cyanosis, weeping varices, and/or fat necrosis are signs of venous obstruction rather than lymph stasis.

The prognosis of secondary lymphedema depends on the underlying primary disease. Medical options include long-term (months) heavy bandage application (e.g., Robert Jones splint), local topical skin care, and short-term drug administration including diuretics, glucocorticoids, and coumarin. Surgical options may be considered when conservative therapy fails and includes (1) procedures to facilitate lymph drainage from affected limbs (lymphangioplasty, bridging procedures, shunts, omental transposition), and (2) procedures to excise abnormal tissue.

Lymphangioma, Lymphangiosarcoma

Lymphangiomas are benign tumors of lymphatic capillaries. The lesions present as large, fluctuant masses in the subcutaneous, fascial, mediastinal, and retroperitoneal spaces. Prognosis is usually good following appropriate surgical excision or marsupialization. Lymphangiosarcoma is a rare malignant tumor in dogs and cats. Clinical signs include pitting edema of extremities, inguinal region, and axilla. Diagnosis requires biopsy including skin tissue. The prognosis is poor.

CHAPTER 100

ORAL AND SALIVARY GLAND DISORDERS
(pages 1084–1097)

ORAL NEOPLASIA (pp. 1084–1088)

Geriatric patients are predisposed in general; however, fibrosarcoma has been reported to occur more frequently in young, large breeds. Papillary SCC, virus-induced papillomatosis, and undifferentiated malignant tumors may also be included in the differential diagnosis for young dogs with oral masses. Large-breed dogs have a higher incidence of fibrosarcoma and nontonsillar SCC; small breeds have a higher incidence of malignant melanoma and tonsillar SCC. Dogs with heavily pigmented oral mucosa are predisposed to malignant melanoma.

BENIGN NEOPLASMS

Canine oral papillomas (COP) are multiple lesions of viral etiology. Grossly, COPs appear on the mucosa as pale, smooth elevations with a rough surface aging to dark gray, shriveled lesions. Complete regression requires 1 to 2 weeks with no apparent scarring.

Epulides originate from the periodontal stroma and are often located in the gingiva near incisor teeth. The epulides are separated into three types based on histologic origin: fibromatous or fibrous epulis, ossifying epulis, and squamous or acanthomatous epulis. The fibromatous and ossifying epulides are pedunculated, nonulcerating, and noninvasive masses. Acanthomatous epulis, although benign, has characteristics of malignancy including local invasiveness and bone destruction. However, acanthomatous epulis does not metastasize.

MALIGNANT NEOPLASMS

Malignant melanomas grow rapidly and are characterized by early gingiva and bone invasion. Metastasis to regional lymph nodes occurs early in the disease process, with lung the most common site for visceral metastasis. Malignant melanomas are dome-shaped or sessile, and they have varying amounts of pigmentation, ranging from black and brown through mottled, or are nonpigmented. Melanomas of the mucocutaneous junction are invariably malignant.

Original chapter written by Mark M. Smith

Squamous cell carcinoma (SCC) may project from the gingival mucosa but more commonly is an ulcerated, erosive lesion. It frequently involves the gingiva mesial to the canine teeth in dogs and ventral to the tongue in cats. Bone involvement is particularly common in dogs, with a 77 per cent occurrence rate. Metastasis to local and regional lymph nodes is common, while visceral metastasis to lung is rare and late in the disease process.

Fibrosarcoma occurs in the same oral locations as SCC, with a greater frequency along the lateral maxillary arcade between the canine and fourth premolar teeth. The neoplasm is firm and smooth with nodules that may become ulcerated. Fibrosarcomas are invasive, and recurrence following local excision is common. Regional lymphatic and visceral metastasis is unusual.

Transmissible venereal sarcoma should be treated as a metastatic form of the primary disease. Although lesions often regress spontaneously, treatment should be considered for persistent lesions, especially if they interfere with mastication or respiratory function.

ORAL NEOPLASIA: CLINICAL SIGNS, DIAGNOSIS, AND STAGING

Inability to swallow or associated pain may result in the appearance of saliva (sometimes tinged with blood) drooling from the lip commissures at inappropriate times. Severe destructive periodontal disease, halitosis, and tooth loss are potential sequelae. *Diagnosis* of oral neoplastic conditions is based on histopathologic examination. A CBC, chemistry profile, nd urinalysis, thoracic radiographs (3 views), skull radiographs, and regional lymph node evaluation are recommended.

TREATMENT

Resective surgery plus radiation and/or chemotherapy are usually well tolerated by dogs and cats, leaving conservative management for only the more debilitated and/or geriatric patients. The ideal surgical procedure is one that offers the greatest possibility of cure, restores or maintains function, and has an acceptable cosmetic result. Benign neoplasms that do not involve bone are surgically excised. Malignant neoplasms are also excised; however, an attempt to acquire tumor-free 2-cm margins is important. Hemimaxillectomy and hemimandibulectomy are procedures that maximize the removal of the entire bony component of the neoplastic process. Epulides are treated by aggressive surgical resection. Odontogenic tumors are treated by local excisional surgery requiring partial or segmental ostectomy.

Radiation therapy may be particularly indicated for stage I SCC or following resective surgery for SCC with non-free margins. *Chemotherapy* may provide short-term palliation for oral neoplasia not amenable to surgery, or for recurrence following surgical excision.

PROGNOSIS

Malignant oral neoplasms have a guarded to poor prognosis regardless of size or location in the oral cavity. The most positive prognosis for oral SCC in dogs is attained with both surgery and radiation therapy. Treatment of oral SCC in cats is strictly palliative, with no improved survival interval. Oral malignant melanoma may be resected locally with tumor-free margins; however, regional or distant metastasis usually occurs. Tumor-free margins for oral fibrosarcoma are more difficult to achieve, and local recurrence is likely.

Benign oral neoplasms, epulides, and odontogenic neoplasms have an excellent prognosis following complete surgical excision.

DISEASES OF THE LIPS, CHEEKS, AND PALATE
(pp. 1088–1091)

CONGENITAL ABNORMALITIES

Various breeds are affected by primary and secondary cleft palates, with brachycephalic breeds having about a 30 per cent risk. Clinical signs and history associated with secondary cleft palate include failure to create adequate negative pressure for nursing, coughing, gagging, sneezing, nasal reflux, tonsillitis, rhinitis, aspiration pneumonia, and poor weight gain. These problems are treated with antimicrobial therapy and nutritional support until surgical repair is feasible at approximately 6 to 8 weeks of age.

Concurrent hard and soft palate clefts may be repaired in two stages, especially for wide clefts, to minimize negative effects of tissue undermining and manipulation over an extensive area. Clefts of the primary palate usually do not cause functional problems but are repaired for aesthetic reasons. Animals with a history of primary and/or secondary cleft palate should be neutered, since the developmental anomaly may be heritable.

Lip-fold dermatitis is more commonly reported in spaniels, setters, and other breeds of dogs with pendulous upper lips and prominent lower lip lateral folds. The differential diagnosis includes periodontal disease, demodicosis, dermatophytosis, pemphigus, canine acne, juvenile pyoderma, hypopigmentation, ulcerations related to renal failure, and contact dermatitis from plastic food dishes. Dental prophylaxis for concurrent periodontal disease and daily lip fold cleansing with 2.5 per cent benzoyl peroxide shampoo improve the condition. Surgical correction permanently alleviates the problem and provides an excellent prognosis.

TRAUMA

Injury causing laceration of the cheek or lip is treated by placement of sutures for apposition of the mucosa and skin. Abscess communicating with the oral cavity is lanced and drained per os. Head injury in the cat often results in mandibular symphyseal fracture, maxillary dysfunction, and separation of the hard palate. Many cases of hard palate fracture heal spontaneously in 2 to 4 weeks with conservative management. Surgical intervention will reduce the incidence of oronasal fistula from a permanent palate defect in patients managed conservatively.

Electrical burns appear similar to thermal burns superficially; however, the pathophysiologic effects of electrical injury often progress deep into tissue along pathways of current flow. Initial therapy for chemical injury is copious lavage with water.

Patients with oral burns should receive a thorough physical examination to determine systemic effects of the agent, which may be life threatening. Airway compromise may be related to pulmonary edema from smoke inhalation or electrical exposure. Chemical ingestion may cause severe gastrointestinal alterations. Local tissue ischemia from thermal, electrical, or chemical burns results in tissue death and potential for secondary bacterial infection. These areas are generally apparent by 3 to 5 days after injury. Treatment of the systemically stable patient includes dilute chlorhexidine solution lavage, sharp/blunt debridement, and empirical antimicrobial therapy. Oral tissue defects heal by second intention. Osteonecrosis or oronasal fistula requires further surgery.

Oronasal fistula is an abnormal communication between the oral and nasal cavities and may be secondary to tooth root abscess, tooth extraction, traumatic palatal defect, irradiation, and wound dehiscence following resective oral surgery. A secondary rhinitis and sinusitis develop from food contamination of the nasal cavity. Rhinitis is treated by copious nasal irrigation with NaCl at the time of surgery followed by administration of a broad- spectrum antimicrobial for 2 weeks. Although the prognosis is good for oronasal fistula repair, multiple surgical procedures may be required for complete resolution.

ACQUIRED DISEASES

Feline eosinophilic granuloma complex (FEGC) includes eosinophilic ulcer, plaque, and linear granuloma. Clinical signs include dysphagia and/or ptyalism. Biopsy of the lesion should be performed to confirm the diagnosis and differentiate it from neoplastic disease. Ancillary tests should include a complete blood count, which usually shows an absolute eosinophilia. Concurrent or potentially causative hypersensitivity diseases should be considered during the diagnostic phase of treatment.

The mainstay of FEGC treatment is corticosteroid therapy. Progestational compounds (progesterone or medroxyprogesterone) are often used to treat FEGC but have potential side effects that make their use undesirable. Patients not responding to either corticosteroids or progestational compounds have a poor prognosis and are candidates for more aggressive therapy such as irradiation, cryosurgery, laser therapy, or immunotherapy.

Labial granuloma is reported most frequently in the oral cavity of the Siberian Husky, less than 3 years old, with lesions similar to feline linear granuloma occurring along the tongue or palatine mucosa. Oral prednisolone administration (0.25 to 1.0 mg/lb daily) usually provides resolution. Patients with lingual lesions have a 40 per cent recurrence rate and may eventually require chronic, alternate-day corticosteroid therapy.

Stomatitis is inflammation of the oral mucosa. A complete history and thorough physical examination are essential. Oral ulcerations occur in at least four different immune-mediated diseases including systemic lupus erythematosus, bullous (pemphigus) disease, idiopathic vasculitis, and toxic epidermal necrosis (Chapter 148). The many infectious diseases that are manifested by lesions in the oral cavity include feline leukemia virus, feline immunodeficiency virus, feline syncytium-forming virus, feline calicivirus, feline herpes virus, and feline infectious peritonitis (Chapter 70). Canine distemper and feline panleukopenia virus may cause stomatitis, although other organs are more severely affected. Candidiasis *(Candida albicans)* may cause severe stomatitis in dogs and cats.

Cats with chronic gingivitis/stomatitis may have ulceration and extension of granulation tissue involving the palatoglossal folds and fauces. Oral ulcerations are associated with advanced stages of uremia. Immune-mediated ulcerative gingivitis/stomatitis afflicts Maltese terriers. A prudent treatment plan includes regular teeth cleaning, oral preventative medicine at home, and intermittent or chronic provocative corticosteroid therapy. Antimicrobial therapy (metronidazole) emphasizing anaerobic pathogens may be administered on an intermittent, chronic basis.

DISEASES OF THE TONGUE (pp. 1091–1092)

CONGENITAL ABNORMALITIES

Ankyloglossia and incomplete or abnormal development of the tongue ("bird tongue") occur in small animals. Patients affected by the latter condition may die within a few days of birth from an inability to nurse, while surviving animals usually have varying degrees of difficulty in eating and drinking. Ankyloglossia occurs secondary to an inappropriate rostral attachment of the lingual frenulum. Incision of the overlong frenulum provides normal lingual motion.

TRAUMA

Injury to the tongue is relatively common secondary to burns, external trauma, self-trauma during recovery from anesthesia, plant and sharp inanimate foreign bodies, strangulation from elastic materials, and frenulum laceration from string foreign bodies. Traumatic loss of approximately one-third of the tongue is not necessarily associated with clinical signs.

ACQUIRED DISEASE

Glossitis is relatively rare in the dog and cat. Clinical signs may include blood-tinged saliva, anorexia, dysphagia, excessive tongue movements, halitosis, and drooling. The differential diagnosis for glossitis includes feline herpes, calicivirus, panleukopenia virus, and leukemia virus; azotemia; heavy metal toxicosis; vitamin deficiency; neoplasia; necrotizing stomatitis; fungal infection; and plant foreign material penetration.

NUTRITIONAL SUPPORT OF THE PATIENT WITH ORAL DISEASE (p. 1092)

See Chapter 54 for a detailed description of enteral and parenteral feeding techniques and guidelines.

ANTIMICROBIAL THERAPY FOR ORAL DISEASE (p. 1092)

The bases of antimicrobial therapy are the results of aerobic and anaerobic culture and sensitivity. Amoxicillin and/or metronidazole are antimicrobials effective against many oral pathogens or opportunistic normal flora.

DISEASES OF THE SALIVARY GLANDS (pp. 1092–1096)

The salivary system in dogs is composed of the paired parotid, mandibular, sublingual, and zygomatic glands

ACQUIRED DISEASES

Ptyalism is a rare primary disease, more commonly related to poisoning, viral diseases, intraoral pathology, congenital malformation, neuromuscular diseases affecting swallowing, and portosystemic shunt. Primary ptyalism is diagnosed in young dogs after weaning. The lips may be dry while the animal is sleeping, but copious, uncontrolled salivation occurs with excitement or feeding. Surgical ligation of the parotid salivary duct is the recommended treatment.

Xerostomia has been seen in dogs with disease similar to human Sjögren's syndrome (xerostomia, keratoconjunctivitis sicca, and rheumatoid arthritis). Recommended treatment is immunosuppressive medication.

Sialadenitis is rarely recognized as a primary disease process; however, trauma or systemic viral disease (i.e., distemper) can cause inflammation of the salivary glands. The inflammation usually resolves without specific therapy, although a fistulous tract with drainage of saliva may result if a major salivary duct is damaged. Although pathology of the zygomatic gland is rare, sialadenitis is the most common disease affecting this gland. Clinical signs may include epiphora, swelling below the eye, divergent strabismus of the affected eye, swelling lateral to the second maxillary molar, and exophthalmos. Swelling not responsive to antimicrobials would warrant paracentesis of the lesion, which may be evident caudolateral to the second maxillary molar. Retrobulbar abscess, which may occur secondary to inflammation of the zygomatic gland, is treated by ventral drainage, using a stab incision caudolateral to the second maxillary molar, and antimicrobial therapy.

Salivary gland infarction occurs in 8 per cent of salivary gland diseased dogs and cats with clinical signs of firm regional edema, fever, elevated WBC count, and anorexia. These animals may have cervical pain and be reluctant to open their mouths. Differential diagnosis includes pharyngeal or retrobulbar abscess, masticatory muscle disease, cervical disc disease, and trauma. The disease is self-limiting, resolving in 7 to 10 days with or without antimicrobial therapy.

Neoplasia involving the salivary glands is uncommon. Prevalence of salivary gland neoplasms in cats is almost twice that of dogs. The most common neoplasms affecting salivary glands in dogs and cats are carcinoma and adenocarcinoma. Total surgical excision of salivary malignant neoplasms is difficult because of invasive characteristics and the intricate neurologic and vascular anatomy of the salivary gland region. Therefore, local treatment should include radiotherapy, with or without surgical intervention, to debulk the neoplasm.

Salivary fistula may result from parotid duct injury. Affected patients have a chronic wound on the side of the head with consistent drainage of serous fluid, which increases in volume at feeding. Ligation of the duct is an effective and practical treatment option.

Mucocele is the most common clinically recognized disease of the salivary glands in dogs. A mucocele is an accumulation of saliva in the subcutaneous tissue and the consequent tissue reaction. The sublingual gland is the most common salivary gland associated with salivary mucocele. Regardless of the location of origin, mucocele usually forms near the intermandibular area (cervical mucocele). Other locations include under the tongue (sublingual mucocele), and the pharynx (pharyngeal mucocele).

A cervical mucocele is initially an acute, painful swelling resulting from an inflammatory response. A decreased inflammatory response allows for the more common presenting history of a slowly enlarging or intermittently large, fluid-filled, nonpainful swelling. Blood-tinged saliva secondary to trauma caused by eating, poor prehension of food, or reluctance to eat are clinical signs that can be associated with sublingual mucocele. The most common clinical signs associated with mucocele of the pharyngeal wall are respiratory distress and difficulty in swallowing secondary to partial obstruction of the pharynx. A visible periorbital mass is usually the presenting clinical sign of zygomatic mucocele.

Mucocele paracentesis reveals a stringy, sometimes blood-tinged fluid with low cell numbers. Sialoliths are concretions of calcium phosphate or calcium carbonate and may occur with chronic mucocele. The most common indication for sialography is to determine the location of a salivary gland/duct defect in patients with salivary mucocele.

The intimate anatomic association of the sublingual and mandibular glands and their ducts requires resection of both structures. Surgical removal of both the sublingual and mandibular salivary glands, combined with drainage of the mucocele, has been advocated for treating mucoceles. Sublingual mucocele, especially if acute or associated with known trauma, may resolve following marsupialization or oral drainage. Therefore, resective surgery of the mandibular and sublingual gland/duct complex may be reserved for recurrent lesions.

The clinical signs for zygomatic mucocele and neoplasia are similar to those described for zygomatic sialadenitis. Additional signs, such as osteolytic changes of the zygomatic arch and enlargement of the submandibular lymph node, may accompany neoplasia originating in the zygomatic gland. Surgical removal of the zygomatic gland is indicated either for neoplasia or for mucocele of zygomatic origin.

CHAPTER 101

DENTISTRY
(pages 1097–1124)

Tables 101–1 and 101–2 present dental formulas and the tooth eruption time table for dogs and cats.

FUNCTIONAL TOOTH TERMINOLOGY GLOSSARY

Alveolar process refers to the tooth-dependent bone housing the tooth roots.

Ameloblasts are the enamel-producing cells of the inner dental epithelium of the enamel organ on the unerupted tooth bud crown.

Apex refers to the terminal end of the root tip through which blood vessels, nerves, and lymphatic vessels supply the pulp.

Apical/periapical, in a directional sense, refers to the rootward direction of the tooth. The zone of hard and soft tissues surrounding the root apex is termed *periapical.*

Attached gingiva is the tough, collagen-rich, parakeratinized tissue covering the alveolar process and forms the critical collar of desmosomal attachment around the neck of each tooth (gingival epithelium).

Carnassial teeth are anatomically designated by their shearing and overlap occlusion, specifically the most caudal maxillary premolars (always assigned to the fourth premolar) and the mandibular first molars.

TABLE 101–1. DOG AND CAT DENTAL FORMULAS

Dog		
Primary	2 × (Di 3/3 Dc 1/1 Dp 3/3)	= 28
Permanent	2 × (I 3/3 C 1/1 P 4/4 M 2/3)	= 42
Cat		
Primary	2 × (Di 3/3 Dc 1/1 Dp 3/2)	= 26
Permanent	2 × (I 3/3 C 1/1 P 3/2 M 1/1)	= 30

TABLE 101–2. TOOTH ERUPTION TIME TABLE IN DOGS AND CATS

	DECIDUOUS TEETH* (Age in Weeks)		PERMANENT TEETH† (Age in Months)	
	Puppy	*Kitten*	*Dog*	*Cat*
Incisors	4–6	3–4	2–5	3.5–5.5
Canines	3–5	3–4	5–7	5.5–6.5
Premolars	5–6	5–6	4–6	4–5
Molars	—	—	5–7	5–6

*Primary, temporary, deciduous, or milk teeth.
†Secondary teeth.
Note: Eruption time is closely correlated to lifespan and breed size, i.e., the larger the breed, the shorter the lifespan, the earlier the teeth erupt.
Adapted from Evans HE: Miller's Anatomy of the Dog. 3rd ed. Philadelphia, WB Saunders, 1993, p 394, Table 7–1; and Dyce KM, et al.: Textbook of Veterinary Anatomy. Philadelphia, WB Saunders, 1987, p 377, Table 11–1 and p 379, Table 11–2.

Original chapter written by Leigh West-Hyde and Michael Floyd

Cementum is a specialized calcified connective tissue covering the tooth root and formed by cementoblasts.

Cementoenamel junction (CEJ) is the junction of the crown and root.

Cheekteeth are the premolar and molar teeth as a group.

Coronal means "toward the tooth crown."

Cusp is the pointed eminence or tip of the coronal surface of the tooth.

Dentin forms the bulk of the calcified tooth structure, is manufactured by pulpal odontoblasts, and is covered and sealed coronally by enamel and apically by cementum.

Dentinal tubules, numbering 19,000 to 45,000 per square millimeter, are arranged perpendicular to the pulp, are surrounded by the circumpulpal mineralized dentine, are occupied by an extension of the odontoblast (odontoblastic process), and contain a serous-like fluid.

Developmental grooves are important normal contours of the crown, most notably the buccal surface of maxillary carnassial teeth of the dog and cat.

Enamel covers the tooth crown, and gingival epithelium is unable to attach to it except at the CEJ.

Endodontium refers to the internal dental pulp.

Furcation is the root junction of multi-rooted teeth, either bifurcations or trifurcations.

Gingiva is the term applied to the epithelial and connective tissues that surround and attach to the tooth and alveolar process.

Gingival margin is the clinically visible crest of gingiva opposing the tooth surface.

Gingival sulcus/crevice is the niche formed by the junction of the tooth and the gingiva.

Lateral/accessory canals are vascular passages through the root dentin connecting the pulp and the periodontal space, and may occur on the lateral root, near the root apex, or in the furcation.

Mesial/distal are designations for surfaces between teeth (proximal) with reference to the central incisor of the dental arch: mesial is the tooth proximal surface closer to the midline; distal is farther from the dental midline.

Neck/cervical line refers to the constricted portion of the tooth apical to the coronal enamel bulge where the gingival epithelium normally attaches at the CEJ. The term *neck lesion* refers to the peculiar odontoclastic tooth resorption process of cat teeth.

Odontoblasts are circumpulpal, mesenchymal cells of the pulp and root canal chamber which manufacture dentin throughout life.

Odontoclasts are tooth-resorbing cells derived from multilineage hematopoietic cells.

Periodontium is the tooth attachment/support complex consisting of soft tissue (gingiva and periodontal ligament) and hard tissue (alveolar bone and tooth root cementum), all of which share developmental, topographic, and functional relationships.

Periodontal ligaments (PL) are the collagenous fiber bundles that span the space between the alveolar bone of the tooth socket and the root cemental surface, inserting to each surface via Sharpey's fibers.

Pulp is the soft tissue within the fixed internal chamber of the tooth, consisting of circumpulpal odontoblasts and a body of blood vessels, nerves, and lymphatics supported by connective tissue.

Pulp chamber/pulp horn is the coronal portion of the internal tooth space occupied by pulpal tissue and connects the pulpal root canals of multi-rooted teeth.

Root canal refers to the apical portion of the root chamber occupied by the pulp. It is also used as a therapeutic term for tooth salvage via the endodontic procedure of removal of pulpal contents, cleaning/reshaping the canal, sealing the canal, and finally filling the empty chamber with biocompatible materials.

Saliva has major dental significance because of its protective functions.

Triadan system, a method of dental designation, assigns each tooth a three-digit number that designates both tooth type and dental quadrant location.

PERIODONTAL DISEASE (pp. 1102–1107)

PREVALENCE, DEFINITION, AND SIDE EFFECTS

Periodontal disease is the most common cause of tooth loss in dogs and cats. The focus of this disease process at the tooth- crown junction is the conversion of a normal gingival sulcus to the pathologic environment of the periodontal pocket. Periodontal disease results from infectious inflammation of the gingival sulcus and affects all components of the tooth attachment apparatus. Periodontal disease is a disease spectrum encompassing gingivitis and periodontitis. Gingivitis is a completely reversible process involving inflammation of the marginal gingiva. Periodontitis is an irreversible progression of dental disease in which there is apical (toward root apex) migration of the gingival epithelial attachment to the tooth with alveolar bone resorption.

CLINICAL SIGNS OF PERIODONTAL DISEASE

Owners most frequently report nonspecific symptoms, halitosis, or behavior changes referable to chronic oral pain such as poor self-grooming, teeth chatter or teeth grinding, hesitancy to open or close mouth completely, decrease in chewing of toys/treats, pawing at mouth, facial rubbing, reluctance to perform trained bite behaviors, personality changes, prehension difficulties, head- or mouth-handling shyness, or soft food preference. Sneezing, unilateral nasal discharge, and incessant nose-licking are often noted in patients with advanced disease with oronasal fistulation. More signs of periodontal disease are mobile teeth, asymmetric facial swelling, gingival recession, mild to moderate gingival hemorrhage, and nasal discharge. Definitive oral examination may reveal periodontal or periapical abscesses, periodontal pockets, and oronasal fistulas.

PATHOPHYSIOLOGY AND DISEASE CHARACTERISTICS

Periodontal disease is a disease continuum initially involving only gingival soft tissue inflammation (reversible gingivitis) with possible progression to loss of gingival epithelial attachment and alveolar bone destruction (irreversible but controllable periodontitis). The progression of gingivitis to periodontitis is not inevitable. Plaque is 70 to 80 per cent proliferating microorganisms with epithelial cells, leukocytes, and macrophages attached to a matrix consisting of salivary glycoproteins and extracellular, bacteria-produced polysaccharides. The clinically detectable response to established gingivitis is marginal hyperemia with a variable width of edema in the attached gingiva; clinical signs of attachment loss of periodontitis is pocket formation (sulcus depth exceeds 3 mm in dog and 1 mm in cat) detected with a perioprobe, gum recession, and root furcation or cementum exposure.

Dental calculus is mineralized plaque and may be located supragingivally or subgingivally. The calcified structure of calculus is not pathogenic per se; however, calculus does form a fixed nidus for plaque accumulation and holds the plaque close to the gingiva. In this sense, calculus is a significant pathogenic factor in periodontal disease.

TRUE POCKET VERSUS PSEUDOPOCKET FORMATION

A true periodontal pocket means that there is (a) loss of epithelial attachment of the gingiva to the tooth surface at the cementoenamel junction, (b) apical migration of the junctional epithelium, and (c) transformation of the junctional epithelium into a pocket epithelium.

Clinical exploration with a periodontal probe will give an abnormal probing depth greater than 3 mm for most dogs and 1 mm for cats and small dogs. The pocket may bleed easily. Bone destruction will occur soon after attachment loss occurs.

Pseudopockets are characterized by an abnormal probing depth, but the gingival epithelial attachment is still at the cementoenamel junction. Pseudopockets are usually created when there is gingival hyperplasia. Gingival hyperplasia may occur with chronic gingival inflammation, as a breed predisposition, as a sequela to chronic mouth breathing, associated with tooth eruption, and in benign or neoplastic gingival growths.

Drugs reported to cause gingival hyperplasia in the dog are cyclosporine, some calcium channel blocking agents, and phenytoin derivatives. Generalized gingival hyperplasia is a common clinical observation in older dogs. Benign gingival hyperplasia has a breed predisposition for collies, Boxers, and other large breed dogs. Treatment is usually unnecessary. Benign or neoplastic tumors may mimic gingival hyperplasia. *Epulis* is the most common benign oral tumor of dogs (see Chapter 100).

PREDILECTION SITES AND PATTERNS OF BONE LOSS

Predilection sites for calculus deposition are related to proximity to ductal openings of salivary glands. The buccal surface of the maxillary caudal cheekteeth is the most common site. Also, the lingual surface of the mandibular incisors is more prone to calculus formation.

The dog has some specific trouble spots for periodontal disease predisposition: (1) the palatal surface of canine teeth, (2) the maxillary fourth premolar, (3) the maxillary first molar, and (4) the mesial and distal interproximal surfaces of the first mandibular molar and others.

PERIODONTAL TREATMENT PLANNING: ROOT PLANING

Periodontal therapy should not be attempted without definitive assessment of periodontal supporting tissues, i.e., full mouth perioprobe examination and dental radiographs. Extraction of a tooth may be the least desirable option for both the owner and the veterinarian; however, domestic dogs and cats are able to maintain normal food intake levels even if completely edentulous. Several patient factors have roles in periodontal therapy salvage versus extraction: age, other health problems, compliance with home care protocol, anesthetic risk, individual tooth importance, importance of dentition for animal to perform its job tasks, animal's mouth orientation, and chewing vices.

The base-line objective of periodontal therapy is to reduce or eliminate pathogenic microorganisms from the crown and root surfaces to attain and maintain "clean" crown and root surfaces via scaling and polishing. Periodontal therapy requires fastidious pocket cleaning, which consists of cemental root surface cleaning (planing) and gingival tissue curettage. Scaling (cleaning) the root surface of plaque, calculus, and necrotic cementum is called root planing. Root planing attempts to produce a "glass-like" smoothness to the root surface to discourage redeposition of plaque bacteria and subsequent plaque mineralization (calculus formation).

PERIODONTAL DISEASE IN THE CAT (p. 1107)

The cornerstones of treatment of periodontal disease in the cat are scaling, root planing, and gingival curettage and subgingival lavage. Antibiotics such as penicillin, ampicillin, clindamycin, metronidazole, and trimethoprim-sulfamethoxazole are appropriate choices for postperiodontal therapy. Periodontal disease with various patterns of stomatitis may require steroids, immunomodulation drugs, and/or nonsteroidal anti-inflammatory drugs. Whole mouth extraction or partial extraction may be the most viable option in nonresponsive and/or intractably painful stomatitis in noncompliant feline patients.

ORAL EXAMINATION (pp. 1107–1117)

A thorough and well-performed oral examination is fundamental to all dental treatment. For an oral examination to be complete, however, findings must be recorded on a dental chart ("charting"). Patients benefit by having previously unidentified dental and medical conditions diagnosed and treated. Veterinarians benefit by identifying and recording oral abnormalities so that dental treatment plans can be devised and implemented.

INITIAL ORAL EXAMINATION

The initial examination is performed on the awake animal with the client present and the examiner wearing gloves. The extraoral examination should include evaluation of facial symmetry, temporomandibular joint function, regional lymph nodes, salivary glands, lips, and perioral skin. Palpation of the temporomandibular joints during jaw movement may detect abnormalities such as crepitus, pain, locking, or laxity. Enlarged submandibular lymph nodes are often associated with oral pathology. The closed mouth occlusion of the dentition should also be examined. The intraoral examination consists of the closed occlusion and open mouth phase.

Bite Evaluation

When evaluating the bite, one must consider the placement relationships of the incisors, canines, premolars, and molars. A practical system specific for the dog classifies occlusion as normal, brachygnathic (shortened mandible), or prognathic (elongated mandible).

Brachygnathic (Overshot) Bite. This condition varies from mild to severe. In the mildest form, the lower incisors just miss touching the upper incisors, whereas in the severe form, the lower incisors can be several millimeters (even centimeters) caudal to the upper incisors. If the jaw is brachygnathic and there is palatal trauma, the mandibular canines should not be extracted.

Prognathic (Undershot) Bite. For brachycephalic breeds, such as bulldogs, Boxers, Boston terriers, and Persian and Himalayan cats, the prognathic bite is considered normal as part of the breed characteristics. The mildest form of prognathism is characterized by a level bite in which there is incisal edge to edge occlusion. Prognathic bites usually require no treatment.

Other Bite Abnormalities. See the textbook.

DEFINITIVE ORAL EXAMINATION (PATIENT ANESTHETIZED)

A perioprobe and dental explorer hand instrument is essential for evaluating the attachment status of the periodontal tissue around every tooth. Exuberant calculus deposits may need to be removed in order to access the gingival sulcus and score the gingival inflammation. Depending on the charted findings, dental radiographs may be taken to aid in the definitive treatment plan. Dental prophylaxis is the base-line therapy for all patients, with root planing of periodontal pockets and extraction of end-stage periodontally involved teeth being the next most likely procedures in the routine patient.

THE TRIADAN NUMBERING SYSTEM AND DENTAL CHARTING: CHART CODE KEY ENCYCLOPEDIA

Carious lesion refers to acid demineralization of the tooth surface secondary to sugar fermentation by plaque bacteria.

Crowding implies that the dentition has inadequate space on the alveolar bridge so that there is proximal tooth contact or overlap occurs.

Calculus or tartar is mineralized concretions of salivary calcium and phosphorus salts and tooth surface plaque, which has species-variable mineral content. Calculus hampers plaque removal. Plaque cannot be removed with rinsing but requires mechanical removal with a toothbrush or prophy paste. Calculus removal requires dental instrumentation.

Discolored tooth implies either extrinsic or intrinsic discoloration. Extrinsic stains are removable with thorough cleaning and polishing. Intrinsic stains of the tooth structure itself may arise from abnormal development before or after eruption, from acquired disease, or from iatrogenic staining secondary to a dental procedure. Excessive fluoride, iron, or drugs such as tetracycline ingested during tooth formation may cause intrinsic stains.

Enamel defect may be a focal or generalized aplasia or total absence of enamel. Enamel hypoplasia can be induced by distemper or by high fever during tooth bud formation (<5 months of age).

Epulides are considered the most common benign oral neoplasms of the dog and rare in the cat.

Furcation is the anatomic area of a multi-rooted tooth where the roots divide.

Fractured tooth refers to either crown or root fractures. The true dental emergency is a freshly fractured tooth with pulpal exposure. Maintaining an endodontically live tooth is the preferable option.

Gum recession or atrophy refers to the exposure of the root surface by an apical (toward root apex) shift in the position of the gingiva and alveolar crestal bone.

Mobility is subjectively graded by opposing the tooth between the end of two metal instruments or between a finger and a metal instrument. The ease and extent of tooth movement are classified as mild, moderate, or severe. Etiology of mobility will dictate extraction versus salvage procedures.

Neck (cervical line) lesion is a feline-specific, progressive, odontoclastic resorption of tooth structure typically beginning at the cementoenamel junction (cervical line or neck) of the tooth. Recent studies have proposed that an important intiating factor is chronic periodontal disease. Staging the severity of tooth destruction and pulpal disease will allow the logical sequence of therapy, i.e., salvage via glass ionomer restoration, endodontic procedure salvage, or extraction and alveoloplasty.

Missing teeth on an oral examination merely implies that the crown is not visible at the site at which a tooth is normally positioned.

Odontoplasty is the iatrogenic mechanical reshaping of tooth surfaces. Odontoplasty is used primarily as periodontal therapy to reduce plaque-retentive crown, furcation, or root morphology.

Pulp exposure implies direct communication between the oral environment and the pulpal contents. Every effort should be made to maintain the viability of the pulp, because endodontically dead teeth are more brittle and more prone to fracture.

Pulpitis indicates pulpal inflammation due to injury accompanied by vascular hyperemia, stasis, vascular leakage, swelling, and pain. Tooth concussion or avulsion without tooth fracture is a common cause of pulpitis.

Rotated tooth is a tooth which lies transversely across the alveolar ridge. It is most frequently observed in the shortened maxilla of brachycephalic breeds of dogs and cats or in overcrowded teeth in toy breeds.

Retained deciduous or primary teeth do not undergo the normal process of root resorption requiring the coordinated activity of odontoclasts, fibroblasts, macrophages, and neutrophils. Retained deciduous teeth result in overcrowding, increased plaque retention with secondary gingivitis, and malocclusions. Treatment consists of careful extraction.

Retained roots should always be suspected if the crown of the tooth is not present, with or without jaw enlargement. Dental radiographs should always be taken and will dictate the best surgical approach to be used.

Root canal therapy is a technique used to salvage the calcified tooth structure while removing nonviable pulpal material. The therapy is indicated when pulpal pathosis is considered irreversible, as in crown attrition with pulpal (nonvital) exposure, previously avulsed teeth that have been stabilized, and a tooth with a periapical abscess. Radiographs are an essential part of the evaluation process and the root canal procedure itself.

Restoration/amalgam is an alloy of mercury, copper, silver, zinc, tin, and other metals. Amalgam is used as a crown restorative in dogs in areas subjected to heavy wear, such as canine teeth endodontic access sites, occlusal surfaces of molar teeth, and cusps and facial surfaces of the shearing carnassial teeth.

Restoration/composite is another class of dental materials used for crown repair.

Restoration/glass ionomers are brittle and particularly prone to shear stresses compared to composite or amalgam, but have inherent properties that justify their frequent use in veterinary dentistry.

Secondary dentin (reparative/irregular/tertiary) is formed in response to chronic irritation of the pulp. The aim of this defense mechanism is to protect the pulp by preventing ingress of irritants via dentinal tubules (i.e., bacteria and their by-products). The formation of reparative dentin is a normal reparative mechanism occurring in animals with chronic crown attrition related to chewing habits.

Vital pulpotomy is an endodontic procedure aimed at maintaining a live tooth pulp by partial removal of compromised pulp tissue. Vital pulpotomies are indicated whenever there is a reasonable chance of maintaining pulpal vitality.

Worn tooth refers to excessive crown attrition due to an animal's toy chewing habits, overaggressive self-grooming ("flea-teeth"), animal use (e.g., attack-trained animals), malocclusion contact rubbing of teeth, overaggressive toothbrushing, and enamel dysplasia or hypoplasia. Slow, chronic coronal wear induces low-grade pulpitis, which stimulates the formation of reparative dentin.

Wear facet denotes crown attrition (tooth wear) or enamel defect by exact location on an individual tooth (i.e., cusp tip, occlusal surface, mesial/distal proximal surface or buccal/lingual surface).

Extracted tooth is denoted on the dental chart by a cross placed over the individual tooth on the day of extraction.

Sectioning multi-rooted teeth into single-rooted portions will greatly simplify extraction and minimize root fracture complications. Extraction complications include (1) fractured root fragments, (2) intraoperative or postoperative hemorrhage, (3) mandibular fracture, (4) osteomyelitis, osteonecrosis, or bone sequestration, (5) oronasal fistula formation, and others.

INTRAORAL DENTAL RADIOLOGY (pp. 1117–1118)

Dental intraoral radiographs should be considered an essential element of the definitive oral examination because they show what the examiner cannot see on physical oral examination: the endodontic and periodontic status of the tooth root and the calcified alveolar process of the maxilla or mandible. Dental radiographs using non-screen, intraoral dental films may be used with either a standard x-ray unit or a dental x-ray unit. Dental x-ray units are preferable.

The number of dental radiographs necessary is dictated by the findings on perioprobe exploration. Dental radiographs are indicated: (1) if the oral examination results in suspicion of periodontal, endodontic, or periapical tooth disease, (2) if the gingival sulcus depth is greater than normal (dog >3 mm; cat >1 mm), (3) to evaluate any maxillary or mandibular soft or hard tissue enlargement, crepitus, instability, or asymmetry, (4) to evaluate the origin of any intraoral or extraoral fistula, (5) before and after any tooth extraction procedure, (6) before, during, and after any endodontic or restorative procedure on a tooth, (7) when a crown or root fracture is suspected, (8) to detect the presence, absence (hypodontia), or developmental stage of unerupted permanent tooth buds, (9) to determine the extent of bony involvement of an oral neoplasm for surgical border parameters, and (10) to determine the root status of a tooth with a crown that is anomalous, supernumerary, or missing.

A methodical approach to radiographic evaluation should be followed:

1. Identify teeth by type and ascertain root numbers for each.

2. Follow the outline of each tooth and examine the periodontal space for uniformity.

3. Examine the periapical region of the tooth root for uniformity of bone density.

4. Evaluate the interalveolar bone crest level (within 1 to 2 mm of the cemento-enamel junction of the tooth).

5. Examine the trabecular bone density at the root furcation for complete filling of the interradicular space and uniformity of bone density.

6. Examine the diameter of the pulp and root chamber of the individual tooth.

DENTAL PROPHYLAXIS (pp. 1118–1121)

PROCEDURAL SEQUENCE

Veterinary dentistry must ensure that the base-line preventive cleaning procedure cleans not only the supragingival crown but also the subgingival tooth surface. Supragingival and subgingival scaling removes the plaque and calculus from tooth surfaces. Regardless of the hand or power instrumentation used, the tooth surface will be scratched by the scaling process. Polishing after coronal calculus removal finishes the cleaning process by removing the pellicle, plaque debris, and tooth discoloration caused by calculus or soft deposits. Polishing involves use of a paste with abrasive grit applied with a rotating rubber cup or use of a jet stream of water and air containing an abrasive. The two most important reasons for polishing are (1) to render the tooth surface as smooth as possible to discourage plaque reaccumulation and (2) to remove the microplaque debris and thus disrupt the bacterial cycle leading to gingivitis and periodontitis.

Antibiotics are used in dentistry either *acutely* (within hours), to control iatrogenic bacteremia and prevent anachoretic infections at predisposed sites in the body at the time of the dental procedure, or *chronically* (days to weeks), to specifically treat dental disease such as severe periodontal disease. Antibiotic use in conjunction with routine dental prophylaxis of healthy animals is not warranted.

Preexisting medical conditions that may warrant the use of antibiotics prior to dental prophylaxis are cardiac valvular disease, cardiomyopathy, heart failure, immunosuppression, endocrinopathy (especially diabetes), chronic kidney disease, obstructive pulmonary disease, and hepatic failure.

HOME CARE

Given the primary etiologic role that bacteria play in dental disease, the base-line task of any home care protocol should be plaque control at the gingival margin. Use of owner-guided aids for plaque removal are limited by pet acceptance but may include plaque-disclosing solutions, toothbrushes with appropriate dentifrice, interdental or furcation appliances, oral irrigators, and chemical plaque control. Toothbrushes are the most effective mechanical plaque removers of supragingival and subgingival marginal plaque. Pet acceptance is enhanced if the jaws are not opened and the lips are gently retracted. The pet's acceptance of toothbrushing may be increased by incremental introduction and use of interim appliances such as cotton or foam-tipped applicators, soft rubber finger brushes, or a finger wrapped in soft gauze.

The dentifrice may contain fluoride and/or antitartar compounds such as pyrophosphate. Chlorhexidine is currently considered the most efficacious and most thoroughly researched antiplaque agent. Chlorhexidine is usually reserved for use in patients with periodontal disease as an oral rinse once or twice a day or as a gel with toothbrush application. The gluconate gel is taste-acceptable to both dogs and cats.

Recommendations for clinical use of fluoride in cats and dogs must take into account that the fluoride will be internally ingested with the potential for toxicity.

CHAPTER 102

DISEASES OF THE ESOPHAGUS
(pages 1124–1142)

MOTILITY DISORDERS (pp. 1128–1132)

MEGAESOPHAGUS

Megaesophagus is a term referring to generalized esophageal dilation resulting from an aperistaltic esophagus secondary to a neuromuscular disorder.

Congenital Megaesophagus. Idiopathic congenital megaesophagus is diagnosed in young dogs shortly after weaning. This form is reported to be inherited in the fox terrier and the miniature schnauzer. An increased incidence occurs in Great Danes, German shepherds, Labrador retrievers, Newfoundlands, Chinese Shar Peis, and Irish setters. Congenital megaesophagus is perhaps infrequently diagnosed because many dogs are reported to have mild clinical signs with spontaneous recovery during maturation. Dogs more than 6 months of age without resolution of signs generally have a poor prognosis for spontaneous remission. A congenital form of megaesophagus has been suspected in several cats.

Acquired Idiopathic Megaesophagus. Acquired idiopathic megaesophagus is characterized by a large dilated esophagus resulting from a lack of both primary and secondary peristaltic contractions. It occurs spontaneously in adult dogs, most often between 7 to 15 years of age, and appears to occur more frequently in large-breed dogs. It has been described in the cat but is uncommon. The etiopathogenesis of this disease in the dog is unclear.

Secondary Megaesophagus. Any condition that causes disruption of the neural reflex controlling swallowing or affects function of esophageal muscles can be responsible for a secondary megaesopha-

---

Original chapter written by David C. Twedt

TABLE 102–1. DISEASES ASSOCIATED
WITH MEGAESOPHAGUS

Neuromuscular
    Congenital megaesophagus
    Acquired idiopathic megaesophagus
    Myasthenia gravis
    Dysautonomia
    SLE
    Polymyositis and polymyopathy
    Glycogen storage disease
    Dermatomyositis
    Giant cell axon neuropathy
    Polyradiculoneuritis
    Spinal muscle atrophy
    Bilateral vagal damage
    Familial reflex myoclonus
    Cervical vertebral instability with leukomalacia
    Brain stem lesions
    Botulism
    Tetanus
    Distemper
Toxic
    Lead
    Thallium
    Anticholinesterase
    Acrylamide
Miscellaneous
    Hypoadrenocorticism
    Hypothyroidism
    Mediastinitis
    Bronchoesophageal fistula
    Cachexia
    Pyloric stenosis
    Gastric dilation volvulus
    Gastric heterotopia
    Pituitary dwarfism
    Trypanosoma cruzi
    Thymoma

Adapted from Jones BD, et al.: Diseases of the esophagus. In Ettinger SJ (ed): Textbook of Veterinary Internal Medicine. 3rd ed. Philadelphia, WB Saunders, 1989, pp 1262.

gus. Conditions that are associated with secondary megaesophagus are listed in Table 102–1. In most cases it is only one part of the overall disease syndrome.

Trauma, degenerative or inflammatory disorders, or neoplasia involving any part of the neural pathway can cause megaesophagus. Various peripheral neuropathies include polyradiculoneuritis, polyneuritis, tetanus, heavy metal toxicity, ganglioradiculitis, and dysautonomia. Peripheral bilateral damage to the vagus nerve can result in esophageal hypomotility. Damage to only one vagus nerve innervating the esophagus will not result in a megaesophagus.

Myasthenia gravis (MG) is the most common cause of secondary megaesophagus in the dog. Megaesophagus is not a consistent feature of MG in cats, although it has been reported to have a higher incidence in Abyssinian cats. Most dogs having generalized MG and muscle weakness will have concurrent megaesophagus. Occasionally, esophageal signs from megaesophagus may precede signs of generalized muscle weakness by several weeks. The diagnosis is based on the edrophonium chloride response test, electrophysiologic testing, or demonstration of MG serum autoantibodies to nicotinic acetylcholine receptors (AChR antibodies).

There is also a large subset of dogs that have megaesophagus without detectable generalized muscle weakness but are MG AChR antibody titer–positive. These dogs are said to have focal MG with selective esophageal muscle involvement. In German shepherds and golden retrievers, the incidence appears to be higher. Cases with focal myasthenia gravis are reported to have a favorable prognosis.

Although uncommon, hypothyroidism is reported to be associated with a number of neurologic signs including megaesophagus. Hypoadrenocorticism can also be associated with transient secondary megaesophagus. The esophageal hypomotility presumably occurs due to electrolyte effects on neuromuscular function.

Clinical Signs. The most frequent clinical sign of megaesophagus is regurgitation. Salivation and halitosis may result from esophagitis and the retention of food within the esophagus. In some instances the owners describe raspy breath sounds from movement of saliva and fluid in the large dilated esophagus associated with respiration. Signs of aspiration pneumonia are often concurrently associated. Other clinical findings may reflect evidence of disease conditions causing a secondary megaesophagus.

Diagnosis. A complete diagnostic evaluation should be performed, since an accurate diagnosis is important for both treatment and prognosis. A CBC, biochemical profile, urinalysis, and survey thoracic radiographs should be performed in all cases. Generally, patients with congenital and idiopathic megaesophagus have few, if any, laboratory abnormalities. Survey thoracic radiographs usually confirm the presence of a megaesophagus. Mild dilation may not be obvious, requiring contrast studies.

Esophageal motility is best determined with dynamic contrast fluoroscopy. Liquid barium or food-barium mixtures are generally used and will demonstrate a megaesophagus. It is important to ascertain that foreign bodies or obstructions are not the cause of the esophageal dilation. Diagnostic considerations to determine the cause of a secondary megaesophagus are extensive and listed in Table 102–2. All cases of unexplained megaesophagus should have myasthenia antibody titers determined, a thyroid evaluation, and an adrenal evaluation.

TABLE 102–2. SUGGESTED DIAGNOSTIC APPROACH TO MEGAESOPHAGUS

Primary tests (should be performed in all cases to confirm and direct the diagnostic work-up)
    Laboratory data base (CBC, biochemical profile, urinalysis, and fecal analysis)
    Survey radiographs
    Barium contrast esophagram (fluoroscopy if available)
Secondary tests (should be considered for most cases of megaesophagus)
    Endoscopy ± mucosal biopsy
    Acetylcholine receptor antibody test*
    ACTH stimulation test
    TSH stimulation test
Additional tests (specialized, sometimes requiring referral)
    ANA
    CPK
    Toxicology
    Muscle biopsy
    Nerve biopsy
    Electromyography
    Distemper titer
    Esophageal manometry
    CT brain scan

*Comparative Neuromuscular Laboratory, Basic Science Building, Room B 200, University of California, San Diego, La Jolla, CA 92093-0614

Treatment. The treatment for megaesophagus is first directed at any identified underlying etiology. Patients with secondary megaesophagus that are adequately treated may show improvement. In addition to specific therapy for the secondary megaesophagus, supportive nutritional management and treatment of secondary complications such as aspiration pneumonia or esophagitis are indicated.

The patient should be fed a high-caloric diet, in small frequent meals, while in an elevated or upright position to allow gravity to assist passage of the meal through the hypomotile esophagus. The diet consistency should also be individually tailored for each patient based on the diet that causes the fewest clinical signs. Animals that cannot maintain adequate nutritional balance or are in a severe catabolic state will require tube feeding. This is accomplished by the use of gastrostomy tubes.

Aspiration pneumonia is treated with antibiotic therapy. Esophagitis should be appropriately treated (see Esophagitis). At this time there does not appear to be specific drug therapy that will improve esophageal function in dogs with acquired idiopathic or idiopathic congenital megaesophagus. The surgical treatment of idiopathic congenital or acquired idiopathic megaesophagus is controversial. The recommendations include myotomy at the LES. Anecdotal reports suggest that individual cases have improved following such a surgical procedure.

Prognosis. The prognosis for megaesophagus is variable and depends on the etiology. Congenital idiopathic megaesophagus is given a poor prognosis by some; others report that young dogs improve as they mature. Radiographic changes do not always correlate with how the animal responds clinically. Adult-onset acquired idiopathic megaesophagus has a poor prognosis, which is compounded by the presence of aspiration pneumonia, and most dogs die or undergo euthanasia because of their disease. There appears to be a small group of dogs that seem to tolerate their megaesophagus with minimal complications and a small number of dogs that spontaneously improve. The prognosis for dogs with secondary megaesophagus from myasthenia gravis is generally favorable if the underlying disease is successfully managed.

DYSAUTONOMIA

Dysautonomia is a polyneuropathy of unknown etiology that occurs in both dogs and cats. It results from a failure of the sympathetic and parasympathetic nervous system. A major part of this generalized systemic disorder is esophageal hypomotility.

Clinical Signs. Dysautonomia is most frequently observed in the younger animal, and the clinical course has a rapid onset of signs. The most frequent signs are depression, anorexia, regurgitation, vomiting, constipation, and/or diarrhea. Occasionally, fecal or urinary incontinence is noted. On physical examination the animal may have a slow heart rate, dry nose, and dry mucous membranes. Most cats have prolapsed nictitating membranes. The urinary bladder may be easily expressed, and there may be decreased anal tone.

Diagnosis. Survey thoracic radiographs delineate a dilated esophagus, and barium contrast studies show esophageal and gastric hypomotility. A Schirmer tear test may show decreased tear production. Ocular testing using parasympathetic and sympathetic autonomic drugs are useful in identifying ocular denervation (Chapter 84). Subcutaneous administration of atropine may fail to increase heart rate and intradermal histamine may fail to cause a wheal. Serum catecholamine concentrations may also be decreased.

Treatment. Therapy is only supportive, and specific considerations should be instituted as described for idiopathic megaesophagus. Bethanechol and metoclopramide is reported to provide some initial symptomatic improvement. In general, dysautonomia carries a poor prognosis for long-term survival.

INFLAMMATORY AND DEGENERATIVE DISEASES
(pp. 1132–1137)

ESOPHAGITIS

Esophagitis is the inflammation of the esophageal wall, ranging from mild mucosal inflammatory changes to severe ulceration and transmural involvement. Ingestion of caustic agents such as acids, alkalis, corrosive drugs, direct thermal burns, and radiation may cause esophagitis. Dogs with megaesophagus and the chronic retention of food will develop a secondary esophagitis. The direct physical trauma from foreign bodies or from pharyngostomy or nasogastric tube placement is also a common cause. Acute or chronic vomiting with increased contact with gastric or intestinal contents may cause esophageal mucosal damage. Gastroesophageal reflux associated with incompetence of the lower esophageal sphincter is also a common cause. The damage may be limited to the mucosa in mild cases, whereas deeper penetration involving muscular layers could lead to severe complications such as stricture formation or esophageal perforation.

Clinical Signs. Mild esophageal mucosal damage is usually self-limiting, and signs are nonexistent or mild. With extensive damage, signs of esophagitis may include anorexia, dysphagia, odynophagia, excessive salivation, and regurgitation. Complications such as aspiration pneumonia may occur. With deep ulceration, esophageal stricture formation is common. Esophageal perforation results in fever, severe depression, and/or shock.

Diagnosis. The physical examination is usually unremarkable. There may be pain on palpation of the cervical esophagus. Contrast radiography may demonstrate segmental narrowing, an irregular mucosal surface, thickening of the esophageal wall, esophageal dilation, or persistence of contrast within the lumen secondary to abnormal motility.

Endoscopy with biopsy is the most reliable means of diagnosing esophagitis. In advanced cases, the endoscopic diagnosis is quite evident. The mucosa will be hyperemic and edematous with areas of ulceration.

Treatment. Immediately following the ingestion of a known caustic compound, induction of emesis should be avoided for fear of causing further esophageal damage. Administering neutralizing compounds such as dilute vinegar for alkali, milk of magnesia for acid, or egg whites or activated charcoal to absorb other toxic agents should be performed, followed by esophageal and gastric evacuation by means of tube suction. If a patient vomits while under anesthesia, the esophagus and stomach should be aspirated; aspiration should be followed by esophageal lavage using saline or water.

Esophageal rest should be initiated by first withholding oral food and water. With severe cases, a gastrostomy feeding tube should be placed to provide adequate nutrition and to bypass the injured esophagus. Specific therapy should include use of the mucosal protectant sucralfate. Treatment for reflux esophagitis should also be initiated (see Gastroesophageal Reflux).

Additional therapy should include broad-spectrum antibiotics if esophageal perforation is suspected and for therapy of aspiration pneumonia. Animals that exhibit significant esophageal pain may be given lidocaine solution. Animals that have severe esophageal ulceration extending into the deeper submucosal and muscular layers should be given anti-inflammatory doses of corticosteroids to decrease the incidence of stricture formation.

GASTROESOPHAGEAL REFLUX

Gastroesophageal (GE) reflux is a disorder causing esophagitis as a result of esophageal mucosal contact with refluxed gastric or duodenal fluid and/or ingesta. The most common causes in small animals include factors altering LES pressure, general anesthesia, hiatal hernia disorders, and persistent vomiting. Disorders of gastric motility or increased abdominal pressure are also associated with gastroesophageal reflux. During anesthesia there is a decrease in the normal esophageal clearing mechanism and LES pressure. Moderate to severe esophagitis or even stricture formation has been associated with anesthesia-related reflux.

Clinical Signs and Diagnosis. These are similar to those of dogs with esophagitis. Laboratory evaluation and routine survey radiographs are usually unremarkable. Contrast studies may delineate segmental narrowing, an irregular mucosal surface, esophageal dilation, and persistence of contrast within the lumen. Contrast fluoroscopy is usually required to demonstrate gastroesophageal reflux. Endoscopy may reveal a large open LES in conjunction with a reddened hyperemic distal esophageal mucosa.

Treatment. GE reflux may be controlled by weight reduction in the obese patient, correction of upper airway obstructions, therapy for gastric emptying disorders, or surgical correction of hiatal hernias or incompetent LES. Therapy should begin with feeding of small, frequent meals that are high in protein and low in fat. Topical sucralfate is indicated.

Reflux esophagitis is also managed by reducing gastric acid reflux with antacids, histamine H_2-receptor antagonists, or proton pump blockers. Agents such as cimetidine, ranitidine, or omeprazole will decrease gastric acid production and subsequently reduce the amount of acid available for reflux. Gastric prokinetic agents such as metoclopramide or cisapride are prescribed in combination with drugs to block acid secretion.

DISORDERS AT THE ESOPHAGEAL HIATUS

The esophageal hiatus is the opening in the diaphragm through which the esophagus passes before it enters the stomach. A hiatal hernia is defined as an abnormal protrusion of the abdominal esophagus, gastroesophageal junction (GEJ), and/or a portion of the stomach into the thoracic cavity through the esophageal hiatus of the diaphragm. The most common type of hiatal hernia in the dog and cat is a sliding hiatal hernia, which is cranial displacement of the abdominal esophagus, GEJ, and a portion of the stomach through a large, loose esophageal hiatus. Herniation is usually intermittent. Sliding hiatal hernias may be congenital or acquired. Gastroesophageal intussusception results when the gastric cardia invaginates into the terminal esophagus. Occasionally, entrapment of the stomach in the esophagus results, with acute esophageal obstruction.

Clinical Signs. Sliding hiatal hernias occur most frequently in young dogs. There appears to be a breed predisposition in Chinese Shar Peis as well as in some brachycephalic breeds. Gastroesophageal reflux usually accompanies this condition, causing reflux esophagitis and associated signs. Signs associated with a megaesophagus and esophageal obstruction may also occur. Gastroesophageal intussusception usually occurs in large-breed dogs that are less than 3 months of age following acute episodes of vomiting. There appears to be a higher incidence in German shepherd dogs.

Diagnosis. Barium contrast studies are generally required to diagnose a sliding hiatal hernia. The diagnosis is confirmed by demonstrating cranial displacement of the gastroesophageal junction and stomach into the caudal thoracic mediastinum. Repeated studies using fluoroscopy may be required to confirm the diagnosis. Endoscopy reveals additional evidence of a sliding hiatal hernia. The finding of reflux esophagitis supports the diagnosis.

Treatment. When clinical signs do occur, medical therapy for reflux esophagitis should first be instituted. Underlying causes, such as preexisting upper airway obstructions, obesity, and other causes of increased intra-abdominal pressure, should always be treated. In severe cases, surgical intervention is indicated. The surgical management of gastroesophageal intussusception should be directed at treating shock, restoring normal anatomic position of the stomach, and surgical gastropexy.

ESOPHAGEAL DIVERTICULA

Esophageal diverticula result in disturbances of normal esophageal motility or accumulation of food and fluid within the diverticulum, both of which cause signs of esophageal disease. Esophageal diverticula are uncommon and may be either congenital or acquired in origin. Acquired diverticula are described as either pulsion or traction forms. Pulsion diverticula usually arise secondary to an esophageal foreign body and occur in the distal esophagus. Traction diverticula and occur secondary to periesophageal inflammation.

Clinical Signs. These result from impaction of food or fluid in the outpouching of the esophagus. Signs include odynophagia, retching, and regurgitation. Some diverticula may progress to severe esophageal impaction and ultimate perforation.

Diagnosis. A barium contrast esophagram and endoscopy is particularly helpful in determining the location and size of the defect.

Treatment. Esophageal diverticula should be treated surgically by diverticulectomy. Medical management includes frequent feeding of small liquid or semiliquid diets. Underlying causes should be treated appropriately.

ESOPHAGEAL FISTULA

An esophageal fistula is a fibrous tract that results in an abnormal communication between the esophagus and adjacent structures. Most esophageal fistulas extend to pulmonary tissues as either esophagotracheal, esophagobronchial, or esophagopulmonary fistulas. They may be a congenital defect or occur as an acquired lesion.

Clinical Signs. Coughing and respiratory distress occur shortly after eating. Aspiration pneumonia results.

Diagnosis. An esophagram using a small amount of liquid barium contrast quickly demonstrates the fistula. Iodinated contrast agents should be avoided.

Treatment. Surgical correction is indicated.

ESOPHAGEAL OBSTRUCTION (pp. 1137–1141)

ESOPHAGEAL FOREIGN BODIES

Obstruction by foreign material usually occurs at the thoracic inlet, base of the heart, and distal esophagus. The most common foreign bodies found in dogs are bones, whereas cats have a tendency to ingest play objects.

Clinical Signs. The onset of signs may be acute if the foreign body causes complete obstruction, whereas incomplete obstruction may have caused chronic signs for days to weeks prior to presentation. Signs include excessive salivation, restlessness, anorexia, retching, dysphagia, and respiratory distress. Respiratory signs may result.

Diagnosis. In some cases a foreign body can be palpated in the cervical esophagus. An esophageal foreign body is diagnosed radiologically. If an esophageal perforation is suspected, only iodine contrast agents should be used. Esophagoscopy should then be performed.

Treatment. Prompt removal is recommended. Attempts should first be directed at endoscopic removal. If endoscopy fails, or if there is evidence of esophageal perforation, surgery is indicated.

Various conservative measures include passing a gastric tube to dislodge the foreign body, Foley catheter–assisted removal, and esophagoscopy. Removal of large foreign bodies, such as bones, often requires a heavier, rigid, pronged grasping forceps. Bones pushed into the stomach generally can be left to undergo eventual digestion. Other materials may require removal via gastrostomy. The esophagus should be carefully evaluated. Lacerations that do not extend through the esophageal wall or small perforations may be left to heal. Full-thickness tears or large areas of necrosis often require surgical intervention.

Follow-up care requires that the patient fast for 24 to 48 hours. Esophagitis or potential reflux esophagitis should be appropriately treated. A gastrostomy feeding tube should be placed if the esophageal damage is severe. With 180-degree or greater transmucosal ulceration, use of corticosteroids should be considered in these cases to prevent stricture formation. Animals with evidence of small perforations or mediastinal contamination are treated with broad-spectrum antibiotics. Foreign bodies that cannot be removed endoscopically will require surgical removal.

ESOPHAGEAL STRICTURES

Esophageal strictures generally develop as fibrotic changes secondary to intraluminal ulcerative inflammatory processes. Severe submucosal or deeper damage produces fibrotic changes which in turn cause luminal narrowing. Strictures are commonly associated with general anesthesia and enterogastric reflux, mucosal damage, and subsequent stricture formation.

Clinical Signs.   These are similar to those of any condition causing esophageal obstruction.

Diagnosis.   This is based on the clinical history and is confirmed radiographically or endoscopically. Contrast studies using barium mixed with food will best identify segmental esophageal narrowing.

Treatment.   The appropriate therapy for esophageal strictures depends on the length, location, and amount of scar tissue in the stricture. Esophageal strictures should first be managed conservatively by mechanical dilation. Generally, multiple bougienage procedures are required. A technique using balloon catheters has been described with esophageal strictures with good results. Following stricture dilation, placement of a gastrostomy tube is indicated to bypass the esophagus and as a means of supplying nutrition. Therapy for gastroesophageal reflux should also be instituted. Corticosteroids will prevent esophageal fibrosis and should be given following dilation. Surgical resection of esophageal strictures has a reported success rate of less than 50 per cent.

VASCULAR RING ANOMALIES

Vascular ring anomalies are congenital malformations of the great vessels and/or their branches (Chapter 93). Owing to entrapment of the esophagus, signs of regurgitation will occur. As esophageal dilation becomes chronic, irreversible esophageal damage occurs, causing a loss of normal motility.

Clinical Signs.   The most common clinical sign is regurgitation occurring shortly following weaning to solid foods. Secondary aspiration pneumonia may be present.

Diagnosis.   This is routinely made when barium contrast radiographs demonstrate esophageal dilation cranial to the base of the heart. There may also be dilation of the esophagus caudal to the heart. Endoscopy is helpful in confirming the diagnosis.

Treatment.   The treatment is surgical. The key to success is early diagnosis and correction before secondary esophageal changes occur.

NEOPLASIA

Esophageal neoplasia is uncommon. Metastatic lesions appear to be the most common. They are most often associated with bronchogenic, gastric, thyroid, mammary, and squamous cell carcinomas. Periesophageal tumors cause either local esophageal invasion or direct mechanical obstruction. Leiomyomas are the most common benign tumors of the esophagus. They are usually observed as incidental findings unless they are large enough to obstruct the esophageal lumen. Squamous cell carcinoma is the most common primary malignant esophageal neoplasia in cats. The most common primary esophageal tumors in dogs are sarcomas and include fibrosarcoma and osteosarcoma. Primary fibrosarcomas are often secondary to granulomas caused by the helminth parasite *Spirocera lupi*.

Clinical Signs. Signs are usually slowly progressive and associated with esophageal obstruction or abnormalities in esophageal motility.

Diagnosis. Barium contrast radiographs are required to confirm obstructive esophageal disease or neoplastic mucosal involvement. Esophagoscopy allows for evaluation and biopsy.

Treatment. Esophageal leiomyomas generally have a good prognosis following successful surgical resection. The treatment options for malignant neoplasia are limited to chemotherapy, radiation therapy, and/or surgical resection, all of which have a poor prognosis.

CHAPTER 103

DISEASES OF THE STOMACH
(pages 1143–1168)

NORMAL FLORA OF STOMACH (pp. 1145–1146)

Despite the acidic nature of the gastric lumen, bacteria (large spirilla) exist in the canine and feline stomach.

CLINICAL EVALUATION (pp. 1146–1151)

HISTORY

Five main complaints may indicate gastric disease: vomiting (including hematemesis), melena, anorexia, abdominal distention, and/or abdominal pain. Diarrhea is rarely due to gastric disease, except for gastrinoma.

Vomiting. Vomiting may also be caused by intestinal (especially duodenal) disease or various metabolic disorders (e.g., renal failure, adrenal failure, hypercalcemia, diabetic ketoacidosis, hepatic failure, pancreatitis). Furthermore, although gastric inflammation or distention typically produces vomiting via vagal afferents, not all animals with gastric disease vomit.

When material is expelled through the mouth, the clinician must be sure that the animal is vomiting (as in gastric disease) and not regurgitating (as in esophageal or pharyngeal disease) or gagging (mild

---

Original chapter written by Michael D. Willard

abdominal contraction). Unproductive retching in a large-breed dog may indicate gastric dilation/volvulus.

Hematemesis. This is an especially important symptom, as it indicates that gastric ulceration/erosion (GUE) is likely. Hematemesis is seldom due to coagulopathy. Digested blood is more common and resembles "coffee grounds" or "dirt."

Melena. The finding of a "coal black" stool, or melena, is indicative of digested blood (often from upper gastrointestinal bleeding) or ingestion of activated charcoal or bismuth (Chapter 24). This complaint is mentioned under gastric diseases because GUE is probably the most common cause of upper gastrointestinal hemorrhage in the dog.

Anorexia. Anorexia may be the only clinical sign of gastric disease (Chapter 4).

Abdominal Distention. If abdominal distention is due to air, gastric dilation/volvulus is the first major differential diagnosis to consider. Likewise, gastric disease should be considered if the distention is due to food or similar material.

Abdominal Pain. Although abdominal pain is seldom due to gastric disease (Chapter 14), severe GUE may occasionally cause abdominal splinting or tenseness.

PHYSICAL EXAMINATION

Physical examination, while always indicated in sick patients, is often unrevealing in animals with gastric disease. Making a dog stand with its front feet on an elevated stand will cause cranial abdominal contents to fall caudally, making them easier to palpate.

CLINICAL PATHOLOGY FINDINGS

Complete Blood Counts. These studies usually offer minimal information about the stomach. Chronic gastrointestinal hemorrhage may cause a nonregenerative, iron deficiency anemia. Acute gastric hemorrhage may present like any other hemorrhagic disorder (i.e., acute, nonregenerative anemia). GUE and severe, transmural inflammatory disease may produce a neutrophilic leukocytosis, usually without a left shift.

Serum Chemistry Profiles. Hypoproteinemia may be due to gastric blood loss or inflammation severe enough to cause exudation into the gastric lumen. Electrolyte disorders are common in vomiting animals. Knowledge of such alterations are critically important in planning supportive care. Hypokalemic, hypochloremic metabolic alkalosis strongly suggests vomiting of gastric contents. If hyperkalemia is present in a vomiting animal, it strongly suggests hypoadrenocorticism, severe renal failure, or severe gastrointestinal disturbances.

Urinalysis. This metabolic alkalosis can be accompanied by a paradoxical aciduria due to renal sodium conservation at the expense of hydrogen, plus renal potassium wasting.

IMAGING

Plain Radiographs. The most common radiographic diagnoses are (1) foreign body, (2) gastric enlargement due to air, fluid, or food, (3) soft tissue mass involving the stomach, (4) displacement or malpositioning of the stomach, and (5) pneumoperitoneum. Gastric or duodenal ulceration is a relatively common cause of spontaneous pneumoperitoneum.

Contrast Radiography. Contrast studies of the stomach and duodenum are often indicated in vomiting patients if plain films are not revealing (in contrast with diarrheic patients, in which they are seldom useful). See the textbook for materials and technique. Be sure that the patient has not received drugs that alter motility (e.g., atropine, aminopentamide, ketamine, xylazine). These agents produce apparent gastroparesis and gastric retention of barium, suggestive of outlet obstruction. Contrast radiographic studies may identify (1) radiolucent foreign objects, (2) masses arising from the gastric wall, (3) gastric wall infiltration, (4) mucosal ulceration, (5) gastroparesis, or (6) failure of the stomach to empty. One may also evaluate the proximal duodenum, a relatively common site of inflammatory and obstructive lesions that cause vomiting.

Double-Contrast Gastrography. This technique allows better delineation of gastric mucosal lesions but is seldom required because endoscopy is more sensitive for evaluating the gastric mucosa. Fluoroscopy has significant advantages in the evaluation of gastric motility.

Ultrasonography. When the stomach is filled with fluid, ultrasonography can detect infiltrative lesions, especially in the region of the pylorus.

ENDOSCOPY

Gastroduodenoscopy is one of the most useful tools in evaluating the stomach and proximal duodenum in vomiting animals. With it, one can quickly and safely visualize the entire gastric mucosal surface, find lesions that are undetectable radiographically, obtain multiple biopsy samples, and remove foreign objects. Disadvantages include the need for potentially expensive equipment, the necessity of anesthesia, and the inability to obtain full-thickness biopsies of the stomach or duodenum. It is *imperative* that the endoscopist be able to enter, view, and obtain biopsies from the duodenum, as that structure (not the stomach) is the site of most inflammatory lesions that cause vomiting.

Ulcers are most often found in the antrum, lesser curvature, and pylorus. Significant histopathologic lesions may exist in a normal-appearing stomach and duodenum. If a lesion (e.g., ulcer, mass) is seen, one should attempt to obtain both abnormal and normal tissue. If the lesion is hard and infiltrated, one could easily obtain just a superficial sample of overlying mucosa, which does not represent the primary, underlying lesion.

SURGERY

Exploratory surgery is indicated if endoscopy is unavailable or insufficient, or if corrective surgery is necessary. Examples of the latter include foreign objects, focal masses, perforation, and ulceration that has been resistant to appropriate medical therapy. In general, it is best to obtain a biopsy from the stomach and duodenum, even when they appear normal.

ACUTE GASTRITIS (pp. 1151–1154)

Acute gastritis is probably the most common cause of acute vomiting in dogs and cats, other than motion sickness. Many of these animals are not seriously ill, some are depressed, and a few have life-threatening disease.

CAUSES

This syndrome has a variety of causes (Table 103–1).

PATHOPHYSIOLOGY

There are several potential mechanisms of gastric injury. Most involve an inability of the gastric mucosal barrier to protect itself, not only from normal gastric acid, but also from bile acids, hypertonic solutions, and other damaging substances (e.g., alcohol).

TABLE 103–1. CAUSES OF ACUTE GASTRITIS IN DOGS AND CATS

Diet	"Toxins"
Spoiled food	Chemicals
Bacterial toxins	Plants
Dietary intolerance	Mushrooms
Dietary allergy	Drugs
Foreign object	Organ failure
Infectious agents	
Viral	
Bacterial	
Parasitic	

DIAGNOSIS

An acute onset of vomiting with a history suggestive of one of the causes is often adequate for a presumptive diagnosis. Physical findings are typically unremarkable or are limited to nausea when the abdomen is palpated. The animal may or may not be dehydrated. Abdominal pain and fever are rare.

CLINICAL APPROACH

Most patients with acute gastritis typically recover in 1 to 5 days, and such a course helps to confirm the presumptive diagnosis of acute gastritis. Selected patients (i.e., young, small, seriously ill, or dehydrated) may need fluid, electrolyte, acid-base, and/or antiemetic therapy. If the disease does not resolve in 1 to 5 days and there is no evidence of continuing exposure to the original cause, or if the gastritis seems to be inappropriately severe, the clinician must consider whether the patient is affected with some other cause of vomiting. In such instances, additional diagnostic measures (e.g., CBC, chemistry profile, urinalysis, abdominal radiographs, and/or endoscopy) are often warranted. Do not hesitate to look for fecal parvovirus antigen early in the course of disease in a young dog with "acute gastritis."

Fluid Therapy. Animals that are only slightly dehydrated with minimal ongoing losses can often be managed by reduction of oral intake (i.e., offer small amounts of ice or iced water frequently). However, animals that are vomiting profusely or those that are severely dehydrated (i.e., ≥8 per cent) should receive parenteral fluids. Subcutaneous administration is reasonable if the patient is not in immediate need of volume replacement. One should supplement fluids with potassium chloride if the vomiting is profuse, if anorexia is prolonged, and/or if the patient is hypokalemic (e.g., <3.5 mEq/L).

Dietary Therapy. It is usually wise to withhold food until the animal has stopped vomiting for at least 24 to 36 hours. Then one can offer small amounts of water and gradually proceed to a moist food. Diets that are relatively high in nonrefined carbohydrates and low in fat are preferred, as they minimally delay gastric emptying. Moderate to lower protein content is also beneficial.

Antiemetics. These are seldom needed unless (1) the patient is vomiting so profusely that it is difficult to maintain hydration, (2) the act of vomiting is making the patient so distressed that it is best to pharmacologically inhibit the vomiting, or (3) the client expressly desires the vomiting to stop immediately. Central-acting antiemetic drugs are generally more effective than peripheral-acting drugs.

Phenothiazine Derivatives. Chlorpromazine and prochlorperazine inhibit the chemoreceptor trigger zone (they are dopamine antagonists) and perhaps the medullary vomiting center. Since phenothiazine derivatives can cause vasodilation and decrease peripheral perfusion, attention must be given to hydration status. Furthermore, they are known to lower the seizure threshold in epileptic patients.

Metoclopramide. This prokinetic agent is also a dopamine antagonist that blocks the chemoreceptor trigger zone. The drug has minimal side effects but can cause extrapyramidal effects including behavioral change. Concurrent administration of anticholinergics may negate the prokinetic effect of metoclopramide.

Miscellaneous Antiemetics. Aminopentamide is a parasympatholytic drug that is reasonably effective in stopping mild to moderate vomiting, but it is of questionable efficacy in animals with severe vomiting. Other parasympatholytic drugs (atropine, methscopolamine, probanthine) are poor in stopping vomiting, and they also tend to cause intestinal stasis, which might result in other problems.

Trimethobenzamide (Tigan) is a somewhat effective antiemetic but is seldom useful in severely ill dogs or cats. Orally administered drugs such as kaopectate and attapulgite have poor efficacy in vomiting animals. 5-HT$_3$ antagonists may be effective antiemetics. Ondansetron is the only 5-HT$_3$ antagonist currently available in the United States.

HEMORRHAGIC GASTROENTERITIS (p. 1154)

Dogs affected with HGE usually have hematemesis and diarrhea (often bloody), and they are hemo-concentrated (i.e., PCV $\geq$ 55 to 60 per cent). The classic signalment is the young to middle-aged, small-breed dog (especially schnauzer, poodle, or terrier) that is kept inside. These dogs need aggressive intravenous fluid therapy. Death is due to severe hemoconcentration and/or disseminated intravascular coagulation. Antibiotics are often administered empirically.

CHRONIC GASTRITIS (pp. 1154–1155)

DIAGNOSIS

Chronic gastritis, a form of inflammatory bowel disease, is a relatively uncommon cause of vomiting in the dog and cat. It is noteworthy that lipase is produced by canine gastric mucosa, and increased serum lipase activity, long believed to be almost pathognomonic for acute pancreatitis, may be associated with canine gastric inflammatory disease. Diagnosis requires gastric mucosal biopsy.

LYMPHOCYTIC-PLASMACYTIC GASTRITIS

Lymphocytic and/or plasmacytic infiltrates are probably most common, especially in the cat, and are probably due to chronic antigenic stimulation. Lymphocytic-plasmacytic gastric infiltrates in cats are often associated with similar intestinal inflammatory infiltrates. Therapy of moderate to severe lymphocytic-plasmacytic infiltrates usually begins with corticosteroids. Metronidazole may also be effective, either combined with prednisolone or used alone. If the patient responds well to this therapy, the dose(s) may be slowly decreased. Severe cases uncommonly require concurrent cytotoxic therapy with azathioprine. It seems appropriate to recommend hypoallergenic diets that are low in fat and refined carbohydrates (to avoid delaying gastric emptying) in case the underlying cause is a food allergy.

EOSINOPHILIC GASTRITIS

We often consider food allergy to be a likely cause; however, mechanical irritation might be responsible. Cats sometimes have a hypereosinophilic syndrome, usually characterized by circulating eosinophilia and eosinophilic infiltration of organs (bone marrow, small intestine, spleen, liver, and others). Animals with eosinophilic infiltrates should be fed a restrictive hypoallergenic (also called an elimination) diet; a large percentage of these animals respond well. If dietary therapy is not successful, prednisolone should be administered, as for lymphocytic infiltrative disease. Many cats with hypereosinophilic disease respond poorly to medications, even if cytotoxic therapy is used.

ATROPHIC GASTRITIS

Atrophic and/or fibrosing gastritis is an uncommonly recognized form of chronic gastritis in the dog and cat. Therapy is uncertain, but probably involves several small meals per day, feeding a low-fat diet rich in complex carbohydrates. Antiemetics, especially metoclopramide, which may help to prevent gastroduodenal reflux, may be useful in alleviating chronic inflammation.

MISCELLANEOUS TYPES OF CHRONIC GASTRITIS

Histiocytic and/or granulomatous infiltrates are uncommon in the dog and cat. This type of gastritis seems to have a poorer prognosis than the lymphocytic-plasmacytic types. If the lesion is focal, surgical resection should be considered. If surgery is not possible, aggressive medical management with prednisolone and azathioprine seems warranted.

GASTRIC ULCERATION/EROSION (GUE)
(pp. 1155–1159)

NONSTEROIDAL DRUGS

Probably the most common cause of GUE in dogs is administration of ulcerogenic drugs, especially the nonsteroidal anti-inflammatory drugs (NSAIDs).

Risk Factors for NSAID-induced GUE. Risk factors seem to include higher doses, longer administration times, increased gastric acidity, and co-administration of another NSAID or a corticosteroid. There appears to be substantial individual variation regarding sensitivity to NSAIDs. Some NSAIDs (i.e., indomethacin, naproxen, piroxicam, and ibuprofen) seem to be particularly dangerous for dogs. Therapy of NSAID-induced GUE involves discontinuance of NSAID administration plus use of any of several effective drugs. Misoprostol appears to be effective for preventing GUE due to NSAIDs.

CORTICOSTEROIDS

Prednisone and prednisolone by themselves, at commonly administered doses, generally do not cause GUE, although co-administration of corticosteroids with NSAIDs appears to significantly increase the risk of GUE in the dog. Administration of large dexamethasone doses has been associated with GUE.

STRESS-INDUCED ULCERATION

Stress due to hypovolemic and/or septic shock or severe neurologic disease may induce GUE.

PARANEOPLASTIC SYNDROMES ASSOCIATED WITH GUE

Mast Cell Tumors. These tumors contain histamine, a potent stimulus for gastric acid secretion. If a mast cell tumor degranulates (either spontaneously or due to tumor manipulation or cell death), increased circulating levels of histamine can produce gastric hyperacidity and GUE. These tumors are more common in dogs but have been reported in cats. The continual gastric acid secretion usually causes proximal duodenal ulceration, esophagitis (due to vomiting large volumes of acid), and diarrhea (due to gastric hypersecretion and loss of proximal intestinal villi caused by the large volumes of acid entering the proximal duodenum). Gastric rugal hypertrophy occurs owing to the trophic effects of gastrin.

Diagnosis usually centers about the history (diarrhea and/or vomiting, which *sometimes* responds to therapy with H_2 antagonists), endoscopic findings, and determination of serum gastrin concentrations. The latter are increased in dogs with gastrinomas, but may also be increased by renal failure, gastric outflow obstruction, and use of H_2 antagonists. Most gastrinomas are malignant, but the patient may be palliated for months or years with aggressive H_2 antagonist or omeprazole therapy.

INFLAMMATORY BOWEL DISEASE

Inflammatory bowel disease (IBD; lymphocytic-plasmacytic or eosinophilic gastroenteritis) may be associated with gastric or proximal duodenal ulceration.

ULCERATION ASSOCIATED WITH HEPATIC AND RENAL DISEASE

Canine GUE has also been associated with severe hepatic disease. GUE-associated bleeding may cause sudden decompensation of a patient with previously controlled chronic hepatic disease. However, GUE is not commonly a significant clinical aspect of renal disease in most dogs and cats.

ULCERATION ASSOCIATED WITH FOREIGN OBJECTS

Foreign objects rarely cause GUE. However, they may prevent an ulcer from healing. Gastric adenocarcinoma and lymphosarcoma are the most common causes of neoplastic-induced ulceration.

MISCELLANEOUS

Causes of feline GUE include abdominal mast cell tumor, gastric lymphosarcoma, inflammatory bowel disease, granulomatous disease, and *O. tricuspis* infestation. Finally, some dogs and cats have idiopathic GUE.

CLINICAL SIGNS

If an animal is symptomatic for GUE, it may present because of vomiting (with or without blood), anemia, edema (from hypoproteinemia due to alimentary hemorrhage), melena, anorexia, abdominal pain, and/or septicemia (from perforation). The worst scenario for ulcer disease is perforation and subsequent peritonitis.

DIAGNOSIS

Endoscopy performed by a competent endoscopist is the most sensitive method for diagnosing GUE. If the history strongly suggests ulceration due to NSAIDs, stress, and/or mast cell tumor, it may be reasonable to treat the patient, only resorting to endoscopy if the dog does not respond as expected. It is difficult to look at an ulcer and determine the need for surgery. Surgery can be performed to find GUE; however, one can easily miss mucosal lesions when examining the serosal surface.

THERAPY

Surgery. Surgical removal of the ulcer is indicated if the patient is at risk for exsanguination or if the patient has not responded to *appropriate* medical therapy that has been administered for at least 5 to 7 days.

Medical Therapy. The principal tenets are (1) remove the cause if possible, (2) maintain mucosal perfusion, (3) decrease gastric acidity, and (4) protect the ulcer. Mucosal perfusion is important in healing ulcers, and fluid therapy is appropriate in any ulcer patient that is dehydrated. Most GUE patients that are symptomatic (i.e., are vomiting) seem to benefit from initial restriction of oral intake of nutrition.

Oral Antacids. Orally administered antacids (i.e., aluminum hydroxide ± magnesium hydroxide) can be effective in treating ulcers, but they must be administered four to six times per day in doses sufficient to titrate the gastric acid that is being produced.

Histamine₂ Receptor Antagonists. Administered parenterally, these drugs are usually more effective than orally administered acid-titrating drugs. Cimetidine was the first commercially available H_2 antagonist. It is an effective gastric antacid but may have to be administered three to four times daily. It is also a potent inhibitor of selected hepatic P450 enzymes. Famotidine is more potent than either ranitidine or cimetidine and is usually effective if administered twice and sometimes when administered once daily. There has been some suggestion that chronic H-2 antagonist therapy can cause chronic duodenitis.

Omeprazole. Omeprazole is the most potent gastric antacid agent currently available. While effective, it is also expensive and rarely required, except in patients with nonresectable gastrinoma that are not responsive to H_2 antagonist therapy.

Sucralfate. The substance tightly adheres to the ulcerated tissue, protecting it from acid and pepsin. The main concerns about using sucralfate are that (1) it is administered orally and might be vomited, and (2) it can adsorb certain other drugs and prevent, decrease, and/or delay their absorption. Quinolone antibiotics in particular may be adsorbed by sucralfate. Absorption of H-2 antagonists can be decreased by 10 to 30 per cent by sucralfate.

Prostaglandin E Analogs. These drugs are more effective than sucralfate or H_2 antagonists in preventing NSAID-induced GUE. They might be useful in treating established ulcers, but that is uncertain. Some patients develop diarrhea, which is usually self-limiting.

MISCELLANEOUS CAUSES OF GASTRIC INFLAMMATION (pp. 1159–1160)

BILIOUS VOMITING SYNDROME

The bilious vomiting syndrome (also called reflux gastritis syndrome) refers to a situation in which an otherwise normal animal (usually a dog) tends to vomit small amounts of bile in the morning. The condition is diagnosed by eliminating other concerns. Feed the dog at least twice daily, including late at night. If this approach is inadequate, administer a prokinetic drug (i.e., metoclopramide) late at night and/or early in the morning. If these manipulations are unsuccessful, the apparent dyspepsia can sometimes be controlled with H-2 antagonist therapy.

HELICOBACTER

Bacteria may be responsible for some cases of canine and feline gastritis. There is currently no evidence to support their role as an important factor in spontaneous gastritis or GUE in dogs or cats. However, if such bacteria appeared to be associated with gastric inflammation, it might be reasonable to treat for suspected *H. pylori* infection with amoxicillin plus omeprazole or with the so-called "triple therapy."

FELINE GASTROENTEROCOLITIS

Recently, a syndrome of severe gastroenterocolitis has been reported in cats which caused degeneration, necrosis, and proliferation of gastric glandular epithelium. Neither GUE nor vomiting was reported, despite the obvious gastritis. The significance of the helix-shaped bacteria found in these cats is uncertain.

PHYSALOPTERA

Physaloptera rara (Fig. 103–14 in the textbook) has been described in dogs and cats with chronic vomiting. It is difficult to find these ova in the feces because they are fragile and small. Seeing the parasite attached to the gastric or pyloric mucosa via gastroduodenoscopy is the most common means of diagnosis. Adult parasites are easily visualized, but immature worms are 2 to 3 mm long and are easily overlooked. Physically removing the parasite via the endoscope often resolves the vomiting. Therapy with pyrantel might also be effective.

OLLULANUS GASTRITIS

Ollulanus tricuspis occurs in cats (and rarely in dogs), in which it produces gastric erosions and/or chronic fibrosing gastritis. Diagnosis is usually made by finding the nematode in the vomitus. A Baermann apparatus is probably most effective in detecting the parasites in the vomitus, although one can perform direct microscopic examinations of the material. Therapy is uncertain, but tetramisole has been reported to be effective.

MISCELLANEOUS PARASITES AFFECTING THE STOMACH

Roundworms. Roundworms occasionally cause vomiting if they migrate into the stomach. Finding the parasite in the vomitus is usually sufficient grounds for diagnosis. Therapy with an appropriate anthelmintic resolves the problem.

Gnathostomiasis. This parasitic disease is rarely identified in the United States. The parasite is typically found in a gastric mass induced by the parasite itself.

Pseudomyiasis. Pseudomyiasis can occur in animals which eat fly larvae when ingesting garbage. Removal of the larvae and preventing ingestion of garbage should be curative.

BREED-ASSOCIATED GASTRITIS

Basenji dogs have been reported to have a gastritis similar to human Ménétrier's disease associated with the immunoproliferative enteritis reported in Basenjis. The principal problem is due to the intestinal lesion.

UNUSUAL GASTRITIS

Emphysematous gastritis is a rare condition, but one that should easily be diagnosed radiographically. Although not a gastritis per se, mineralization of the stomach has been reported in beagle dogs. The cause is suspected to be due to diet and is not associated with clinical signs.

GASTRIC OUTLET OBSTRUCTION (pp. 1160–1161)

There are three main causes for this problem: (1) intraluminal masses and/or foreign objects, (2) mucosal or mural proliferative and/or infiltrative disease, or (3) compression of the outflow tract by masses and/or organs outside the stomach or malpositioning of the stomach. Diagnosis of outflow obstruction may be made radiographically (i.e., failure of barium to leave the stomach, finding a mass or object in the pyloric antrum), endoscopically, or surgically. Clinical pathology sometimes reveals a hypochloremic, hypokalemic metabolic alkalosis, which is consistent with, but not diagnostic of, this problem.

SIMPLE FOREIGN OBJECTS

Unless an object obstructs the outflow or irritates the mucosa, it can remain in the animal's stomach for months without symptoms in some cases. Pica may have resulted in the animal's eating a foreign object, thus making the foreign object the result and not the cause of the vomiting. Foreign objects may be removed surgically or endoscopically, or they may be allowed to pass through the alimentary tract and out the anus, or the animal may be given an emetic and made to vomit the object, if the veterinarian is certain that it cannot cause harm when it is forcibly propelled through the esophagus. Although some objects with sharp edges (e.g., glass, needles, and fish hooks) will pass through the intestines without a problem, it is often preferable to remove them by surgery or endoscopy to avoid the risk of intestinal perforation and peritonitis.

LINEAR FOREIGN OBJECTS

These foreign objects (such as a long piece of thread) may sometimes be diagnosed by finding one end wrapped around the base of the tongue. If the foreign object is fixed at the base of the tongue and has only been present for a short time (e.g., <2 to 3 days), and if the patient does not have evidence of peritonitis, it is reasonable to cut the object at its point of attachment to see whether it will pass through the alimentary tract without further incident. However, the patient must be monitored for signs of improvement or for development of abdominal pain or depression (which are indications for surgery). One may try to remove the object endoscopically. However, it is possible to rupture a previously intact intestine if one applies traction to a linear foreign object that has sufficiently compromised the intestine. One should not hesitate to proceed to surgery if the risk of perforation seems significant.

GASTRIC ANTRAL MUCOSAL HYPERTROPHY

Tissue proliferation may be neoplastic or non-neoplastic. Non-neoplastic obstruction of the antrum/pylorus may be due to inflammatory cell infiltration or hypertrophy of the mucosal or muscular layers of the stomach. Gastric antral mucosal hypertrophy is principally found in older male dogs of the smaller breeds. Vomiting with or without weight loss is the principal finding. Diagnosis requires that the tissue occluding the pylorus be biopsied to differentiate it from a neoplasm. Therapy consists of resecting the redundant tissue. The prognosis is excellent if there are no operative problems.

HYPERTROPHIC GASTRITIS OF THE BODY OF THE STOMACH

Inflammatory cell infiltrates are commonly seen in this condition, which has been reported in older dogs or in young Drentse patrijshond dogs with stomatocytosis, hemolytic anemia, and hepatic disease.

HYPERTROPHY OF THE MUSCULAR LAYER OF THE PYLORUS

Also called pyloric stenosis and pyloric hypertrophy, this condition is less common than gastric antral mucosal hypertrophy. Male dogs seem to be at increased risk, as do brachycephalic and smaller breeds. If pyloric hypertrophy is suspected, biopsy of the affected tissue followed by pyloroplasty is recommended to relieve the pyloric obstruction.

PYTHIOSIS

This fungal infection may affect any area of the alimentary tract, but is most often found at the pylorus or in the large intestine. It principally occurs in dogs of the southeastern United States. Vomiting and weight loss are the most common signs of pyloric involvement. Diagnosis requires histopathologic or cytologic demonstration of the organism; however, an intense inflammatory reaction with eosinophils is suggestive. Grossly, the gastric mucosa usually appears ulcerated and necrotic, often with a sharp demarcation between affected and unaffected tissue. An adequate biopsy can be obtained with rigid biopsy forceps or by a surgically performed incisional biopsy. Typically, few organisms are present and special histologic stains are needed. Therapy for pythiosis requires surgical excision, as there is no medical therapy with proven efficacy. Rarely, one may find other fungal infections of the stomach.

MISCELLANEOUS CAUSES

Cryptococcosis resulting in granulomatous gastritis mimicking carcinoma has been reported in a Doberman pinscher.

GASTRIC DILATATION/VOLVULUS (pp. 1161–1163)

PATHOPHYSIOLOGY

Primarily found in 2- to 10-year-old, deep-chested dogs (especially large and giant breeds), gastric dilation plus volvulus (GDV) is rarely reported in smaller animals. When the stomach twists, the pylorus usually passes under the stomach and finally comes to rest dorsally above the cardia, on the dog's left side.

DIAGNOSIS OF ACUTE GDV

Dogs with GDV are typically brought to a veterinarian because of nausea, nonproductive retching, depression, weakness, abdominal pain, and/or abdominal distention. Physical examination usually reveals abdominal distention with tympany (except in some very large animals) and evidence of poor perfusion and/or shock. If the signs are not clearly those of GDV, prompt abdominal radiography is the next step. A lateral radiograph of the dog in right lateral recumbency is the best view for differentiating dilatation alone from dilatation with volvulus.

THERAPY OF ACUTE GDV

Shock. Shock is the first concern after GDV has been diagnosed. One should immediately administer crystalloids (initially use approximately 100 ml/lb [200 ml/kg] over 15 min) or hypertonic saline (7 per cent saline plus 6 per cent dextran 70 at 2.3 ml/lb [5 ml/kg] over 5 min).

Alleviating Gastric Distention. The next step is alleviation of gastric distention, for which an orogastric tube is recommended. Once the tube has entered the stomach and the pressure is alleviated, lavage the stomach several times with warm water to remove all food and debris. If it is difficult to intubate the stomach, do not force the tube lest you perforate the distal esophagus. It may also help to trocarize the stomach with large-bore needles (e.g., 16- to 18-gauge), or perform a temporary gastrostomy. Antibiotic therapy with broad-spectrum drugs (e.g., ampicillin plus amikacin; ampicillin plus enrofloxacin) is controversial but reasonable considering the visceral congestion that has occurred.

Surgery. If the dog has dilatation without volvulus, one may perform surgery, but it is not crucial. Surgery in such a patient consists of performing a gastropexy to prevent volvulus in any future episodes, although recurrence has rarely been reported in such patients. However, if volvulus is present, surgery is needed to restore the stomach to its normal position (volvulus is associated with impaired gastric blood flow) and to perform a gastropexy. If the stomach is twisted, it will continue to have impaired mucosal perfusion even when deflated; therefore, surgery should only be delayed as long as is necessary to make the patient the best anesthetic risk that is reasonably possible. If the patient has blood in the gastric contents, surgery should begin as soon as the patient is capable of withstanding anesthesia because of the danger of gastric perforation due to devitalization of the gastric wall.

Cardiac Arrhythmias.   Arrhythmias usually are not present when dogs with GDV are initially presented, but often occur one-half to 3 days later. Ventricular arrhythmias secondary to myocardial ischemia and reperfusion injury are the most common. However, hypokalemia, acidosis, and hypoxia promote arrhythmias and make them resistant to antiarrhythmic therapy. Antiarrhythmic therapy is not indicated whenever there are intermittent ectopic beats; rather, such therapy should begin when the arrhythmia is severe enough to decrease cardiac output. The prognosis for dogs with GDV depends somewhat on the severity of the bloat and how quickly one initiates appropriate therapy. In general, approximately 30 to 40 per cent mortality is now expected.

CHRONIC GASTRIC VOLVULUS

Chronic gastric volvulus is less common and more difficult to recognize than acute GDV. Dogs predisposed to chronic gastric volvulus are the same breeds expected to develop acute GDV. This malpositioning may be constant or intermittent. Clinically, one usually sees intermittent vomiting with or without abdominal distention and/or pain. Multiple radiographs performed over the course of days or weeks may be necessary in order to make a diagnosis. Gastropexy is often curative.

GASTRIC HYPOMOTILITY (pp. 1163–1164)

These defects may be primary (e.g., damage to gastric innervation or muscles) or secondary (e.g., hypothyroidism, ulcer, selected drugs, radiation). Motility defects are uncommon but difficult to diagnose.

DIAGNOSIS

Typically, one first suspects this disease in the patient with chronic vomiting of gastric contents. Deficient gastric emptying is then detected radiographically. One next eliminates known causes of vomiting and gastric hypomotility (i.e., alimentary tract or abdominal inflammation, recent abdominal surgery, various diseases known to cause vomiting such as renal failure, adrenal failure, or hepatic disease). After known causes of abnormal gastric motility have been ruled out, primary gastric hypomotility is presumptively diagnosed. Evaluation of gastric myoelectrical activity is potentially useful, but is typically unavailable.

THERAPY

Prokinetic Drugs.   Prokinetic drugs are usually the primary therapy when primary gastric hypomotility is the tentative diagnosis.

Dietary Therapy.   Feed several small meals per day of a moist diet low in fat, refined carbohydrates, and fiber. Protein and complex carbohydrates should make up the majority of the diet to promote gastric emptying.

ALTERED GASTRIC SECRETION (p. 1164)

HYPOSECRETION

Gastric acid hyposecretion is poorly defined in the dog. It may be a rare disease in dogs, or it may be that difficulty in accurately measuring gastric acid secretion has prevented us from recognizing it.

HYPERSECRETION

Clinical signs were vague (e.g., vomiting, anorexia, weight loss, and eating grass) and inconsistent. Clinical improvement may have been associated with use of an anticholinergic drug.

GASTRIC NEOPLASIA (pp. 1164–1165)

Gastric neoplasia (especially malignant tumors) may cause disease by obstructing gastric overflow, by preventing normal peristalsis by infiltrating the gastric wall, by ulcerating and inflaming the gastric mucosa, or by protruding into the lumen. Vomiting (with or without blood) and weight loss are common signs, but anorexia may be the only complaint by the client.

BENIGN GASTRIC TUMORS

Polyps. These may be adenomatous or hyperplastic. They are typically clinically silent, unless they produce gastric outflow obstruction. Most such polyps are fortuitously found during gastroduodenoscopy for other problems, but all such lesions should undergo biopsy, as it can be impossible to distinguish a benign polyp from carcinoma without histopathologic study. It seems appropriate to surgically remove adenomatous polyps.

Gastric Leiomyomas. These tumors usually occur in older dogs, especially beagles. They tend to occur near the gastroesophageal junction, produce minimal impingement of the alimentary canal, and are usually asymptomatic. However, they may obstruct the lower esophageal sphincter. They should be removed, if possible, to prevent further enlargement and disease.

MALIGNANT GASTRIC TUMORS

Most gastric neoplasms are primary. The most common canine gastric malignant tumor is carcinoma, of which adenocarcinomas are the principal type and scirrhous forms are less common. Carcinomas are principally found in older animals, and more often in the antrum and pyloric areas. Gastric lymphosarcoma occurs in the dog and is the most common feline gastric malignant tumor.

DIAGNOSIS

Diagnosis of gastric neoplasia requires cytologic or histopathologic examination of a mucosal mass, a thickened area of the gastric wall, and/or an ulcer. Endoscopic biopsy may be adequate but is too superficial to diagnose tumor in some animals.

THERAPY

Therapy of benign gastric neoplasms is best accomplished by resection of the lesion. Likewise, surgery is the preferred therapy of gastric carcinoma; however, most carcinomas are not diagnosed until they are so advanced as to be inoperable. Solitary gastric lymphosarcoma may be surgically resected and then treated with chemotherapy. Diffuse lymphosarcoma may be treated with combination chemotherapy, but the prognosis for long-term remission is poor. Gastric leiomyosarcomas occur infrequently. However, if they do not involve the liver, they are often amenable to resection, and the patient may live for a year or more after surgery.

CHAPTER 104

DISEASES OF THE SMALL INTESTINE
(pages 1169–1232)

Mechanism of Absorption

Fat-soluble molecules do not need a specific mechanism to cross the brush border barrier and pass by passive diffusion by dissolving in the lipid content of the membrane. Small, uncharged water-soluble molecules that are apparently also absorbed by passive diffusion are thought to pass through "pores" in the membrane. Water-soluble molecules that are too large to pass through the so-called "pore" route, including the products of carbohydrate and protein digestion, cannot dissolve in the lipid barrier and hence must cross the brush border membrane on the specific transport or carrier proteins. This means that there is a limit to the absorptive capacity even in the normal animal, and if this is exceeded, unabsorbed molecules may pass to the distal gut, where they may retain water by osmosis and cause diarrhea.

DIGESTION AND ABSORPTION OF NUTRIENTS

Carbohydrates must be hydrolyzed into monosaccharides (glucose, galactose, fructose), for which there are specific carrier proteins. Dipeptides and amino acids cross the membrane on specific carrier proteins. Dipeptides within the enterocyte are then split by cytosolic dipeptidase activity to release free amino acids. The monoglycerides and fatty acids within the micelle cross the brush border by passive diffusion, but the conjugated bile salts remain in the lumen. Although the common dietary triglycerides must be processed in this way, triglycerides with medium- and short-chain fatty acids (<14 carbon length), such as those in coconut oil, can be absorbed without further change to enter the portal blood.

Water-Soluble Vitamins

See textbook.

Fat-Soluble Vitamins

Absorption is passive and requires bile salts.

Minerals

Signs of iron malabsorption are seldom seen in intestinal disease unless intestinal blood loss results in iron deficiency anemia. Absorption of calcium and vitamin D is decreased in intestinal disease.

Original chapter written by Colin F. Burrows, Roger M. Batt, and Robert G. Sherding

Normal Gastrointestinal Microflora

There is a relatively large population in the oral cavity which falls to a low number (10 to 10^3 colony-forming units [CFU]/ml) in the stomach. The gastric microflora is predominantly gram-positive and aerobic. The number of organisms increases to approximately 10^2 to 10^5 CFU/ml in the proximal small intestine and 10^5 to 10^9 CFU/ml in the distal small intestine of dogs. The microflora of the proximal small intestine is similar to that of the stomach. In the distal ileum, gram-negative bacteria begin to outnumber gram-positive organisms, whereas coliforms are consistently present and anaerobic bacteria such as *Bacteroides, Fusobacterium,* and *Clostridium* are found in substantial concentrations. The bacterial population increases dramatically in the large intestine. The bacterial population in the colon is also incredibly diverse.

Physiologic Mechanisms of Regulation

The major host defense against bacterial overgrowth is the peristaltic activity of the stomach and small intestine, but gastric acid, intestinal immune function, and the antibacterial activity of bile and pancreatic juice are also important. A variety of individual microbial interactions also control bacterial growth, especially in the densely populated colon.

Influence of Diet

An increase in dietary protein intake moderately increases colonic clostridial concentration. A reduction in short-chain fatty acids (SCFA) concentration results in colonic mucosal atrophy and increased susceptibility to damage.

Influence of Antibiotics

In general, the ecologic change induced by antibiotics is of little consequence, but occasionally, resistant host bacteria will set up an infection or damage the mucosa.

Metabolic Activity of Gastrointestinal Flora

Major metabolic functions of the enteric flora are listed in Table 104–4 of the textbook.

Bacterial Translocation

Perhaps the most important aspect of the intestinal flora is the ability of bacteria to leave the tract and threaten the viability of the host, a process called translocation. Not only under conditions of mucosal disruption, but also in sepsis and stress, the normal flora (including both bacteria and fungi) passes directly through the mucosa into the portal circulation.

PATHOPHYSIOLOGY OF INTESTINAL DISEASE
(pp. 1178–1185)

NATURE OF INTESTINAL DAMAGE

Although diarrhea can be an obvious sign, it is important to be aware that the absence of diarrhea does not exclude the possibility of severe small intestinal disease. Failure to grow normally or loss of body weight and condition can be a prominent feature of intestinal disease in some patients. Other clinical signs may include vomiting (especially if mucosal damage is severe), hyperphagia, and coprophagia. Most animals with chronic small intestinal disease typically show no signs of systemic disease, such as lethargy and depression.

Barriers to Macromolecular Absorption

The phenomenon of macromolecule exclusion has some nonspecific components. These include gastric acid and proteases that denature and degrade antigens, a protective coating of mucus that traps antigens at the mucosal surface, and tight junctions that minimize passage of antigens between epithelial cells. These protective mechanisms are supported by the mucosal immune system, which plays a key role in surveillance and modulation of response to a spectrum of antigens including invasive pathogens and harmless food proteins.

Barrier Function of Gut-Associated Lymphoid Tissue (GALT)

Oral tolerance represents a specific immunologic unresponsiveness on systemic exposure to an antigen previously given by the enteric route and is thought to play a key role in preventing food hypersensitivity and autoimmune disease. A defective mucosal barrier allowing abnormal penetration of the lamina propria could therefore elicit a different immunologic response, resulting in systemic priming rather than tolerance.

Barrier Function, Immunoregulation, and Intestinal Disease

Intraluminal constituents that can cause intestinal damage in individuals with no underlying abnormalities in barrier function include microbial pathogens, parasites, lectins, chemicals, and drugs, although clearly a protective local immunologic response to a foreign antigen should minimize the development of chronic disease. A further cause of intestinal damage is the possible existence of a subtle defect in the immune system, allowing recognition of the structure of certain antigens either causing or prolonging some intestinal diseases.

CLASSIFICATION OF DIARRHEA

Pathogenic mechanisms may be classified as (1) *osmotic diarrhea* due to decreased nutrient digestion or absorption resulting in an increase in intraluminal osmotic solute load, (2) *exudative diarrhea* resulting from a change in intestinal permeability and intraluminal loss of plasma proteins, (3) *secretory diarrhea* due to hypersecretion of ions, and (4) *dysmotility diarrhea* as a result of abnormal intestinal or colonic motility. However, the limitations of such a simplistic approach should be appreciated, since diarrhea in an individual case typically involves more than one mechanism.

Osmotic Diarrhea

Impaired solute absorption resulting in osmotic diarrhea typically improves with fasting. Exocrine pancreatic insufficiency is an important cause of malabsorption and is probably the best-known example of osmotic diarrhea in small animal practice. Small intestinal disease can result in osmotic diarrhea by interference with either the number or functioning of individual enterocytes. Examples of conditions with an osmotic component include acute viral enteritis and chronic enteropathies with villous atrophy, such as gluten-sensitive enteropathy.

Exudative (Permeability) Diarrhea

Acute and chronic inflammation due to a variety of causes including parasitic and bacterial infections can produce diarrhea by this mechanism. Diseases associated with increases in pore size sufficient to permit exudation of plasma protein cause the syndrome of protein-losing enteropathy. Protein can be lost through elevation of mesenteric venous pressure, obstruction of lymphatic drainage (lymphangiectasia), or lowering of plasma colloid osmotic pressure. Bloody diarrhea can occur in the syndrome of hemorrhagic gastroenteritis (HGE), severe hookworm infection, salmonellosis, parvovirus infection, and ulcerative colitis.

Secretory Diarrhea

Enteric enterotoxigenic *E. coli* (ETEC) infection, which is seen primarily in young food animals, is perhaps the best-known veterinary example of secretory diarrhea. An important aspect of this type of diarrhea is that the intestinal mucosa is histologically intact and the absorptive epithelial cells still function, a fact that is used in oral fluid replacement therapy.

Secretion is also stimulated by gastrointestinal neurohumoral peptides such as vasoactive intestinal polypeptide, inflammatory mediators such as prostaglandins, and hydroxy fatty acids (such as castor oil). Hydroxy fatty acids are an important cause of the diarrhea that occurs in bacterial overgrowth and also in conditions causing steatorrhea. Hydroxylated bile salts, which may reach high concentrations in the colon in small intestinal malabsorptive disorders, have similar negative effects on fluid absorption.

Secretory diarrhea typically does not resolve with fasting. Secretory diarrhea alone does not cause weight loss unless there is anorexia, vomiting, or associated damage to the gastrointestinal tract.

Dysmotility Diarrhea

Accelerated transit is rarely a primary cause of diarrhea. In contrast, disordered motility resulting in prolonged transit may be a primary cause of diarrhea by promoting stasis and allowing the development of small intestinal bacterial overgrowth.

DIAGNOSIS OF SMALL INTESTINAL DISEASE
(pp. 1185–1195)

Table 104–1 summarizes a stepwise approach to intestinal disease in dogs.

THE HISTORY IN INTESTINAL DISEASE

Tables 104–2 and 104–3 present a check list of questions in chronic diarrhea and a summary of the basic differences between large and small bowel diarrhea.

TABLE 104–1. STEPWISE APPROACH TO INTESTINAL DISEASE IN DOGS

History and base line investigations
    Analysis of feces, blood, and urine
    ± radiography, ultrasonography if partial obstruction suspected
    ± colonoscopy if signs of large bowel disease
Exclude exocrine pancreatic insufficiency
    Assay serum trypsin-like immunoreactivity
Indirect investigation of small intestinal damage
    Serum folate and cobalamin
    Intestinal function and permeability
    Hydrogen breath test
Direct examination of small intestine
    Endoscopy or laparotomy
    Histology of biopsies
    Culture duodenal juice

TABLE 104–2. A CHECK LIST OF QUESTIONS IN CHRONIC DIARRHEA

Duration	Weeks, months, or years; intermittent or continuous
Diet	Dietary sensitivities or idiosyncrasies, recent dietary change, access to garbage
Appetite	Normal, increased, decreased, ravenous, pica
Appearance of feces	Volume, color, blood, mucus
Flatus	Presence or absence—increase over normal suggests carbohydrate malabsorption and bacterial fermentation
Frequency of defecation	Increased over normal, "accidents" at night, urgency suggest colonic disease
Vomiting	Presence or absence, frequency, and nature; presence suggests inflammation of any part of the gastrointestinal tract
Tenesmus	Presence or absence; presence suggests distal colonic, rectal, or anal disease
Body weight and condition	Overall appearance; documented weight loss suggests nutrient malabsorption or loss; interpret in conjunction with appetite
Environment	Outdoors or indoors, working dog or pet, access to parasite-infected environment, change of environment
Character and breed	Excitable, inquisitive, or aggressive animals appear to have a higher incidence of stress-induced diarrhea. Breed-specific disease? German shepherd breed has high overall incidence of pancreatic and small intestinal disease.

Appearance of the Feces. When feces are consistently bulky, the underlying disorder usually lies in the exocrine pancreas or small intestine.

Flatus. See Chapter 27.

PHYSICAL EXAMINATION

Overt physical abnormalities are uncommon in most patients with intestinal disease. The most common findings are a loss of body weight and condition in patients with nutrient malabsorption or protein-losing enteropathy. In a animals with proteincalorie malnutrition, particularly in those with hypoproteinemia due to nutrient malabsorption and protein-losing enteropathy, it is not uncommon to find lingual and buccal ulceration. The mouth should also be examined for foreign bodies, particularly in animals presented with a history of anorexia, gagging, and ptyalism. Palpation of the laryngeal and cervical areas may reveal a mass that could be a foreign body, cervical abscess, thyroid carcinoma, or other type of tumor.

A tympanitic abdomen suggests gastric dilation or dilation-volvulus, particularly in a large- or giant-breed dog presented with signs of shock. The clinician may detect the sometimes subtle intestinal thickening, masses, clumping of the intestines, enlarged mesenteric lymph nodes, abdominal effusion, or pain. Rectal examination should be postponed for humane reasons in cats and in very small dogs until the animal is heavily tranquilized or anesthetized. In other patients, the walls of the pelvic diaphragm should be examined for uniformity on both sides, smoothness, mobility, and narrowing. The iliac nodes can be palpated in most breeds as can the prostate gland in male dogs. Finally, the anal sacs should be evacuated as the hand is withdrawn and the contents examined for signs of infection.

TABLE 104–3. DIFFERENTIATION OF SMALL INTESTINAL FROM LARGE INTESTINAL DIARRHEA

PARAMETER	SMALL INTESTINE	LARGE INTESTINE
Feces		
Volume	Markedly increased	Normal or increased
Mucus	Rarely present	Frequently present
Melena	May be present	Absent
Hematochezia	Absent except in acute hemorrhagic diarrhea	Fairly common
Steatorrhea	Present with maldigestive or malabsorptive disease	Absent
Undigested food	May be present with maldigestion	Absent
Color	Color variations occur (e.g., creamy brown, green, orange, or clay color)	Color variations rare, may be bloody
Defecation		
Urgency	Absent except in acute or very severe disease	Usually but not invariably present
Tenesmus	Absent	Frequent but not invariably present
Frequency	2 to 3 times normal for the patient	Usually greater than 3 times normal
Dyschezia	Absent	Present with distal colonic or rectal disease
Ancillary signs		
Weight loss	May occur in maldigestive or malabsorptive disease	Rare except with severe colitis, diffuse tumors, or histoplasmosis
Vomiting	May be present in inflammatory diseases	Uncommon, but occurs in up to 25% to 30% of dogs with colitis
Flatulence and borborygmus	May be reported with maldigestion and malabsorption	Absent
Halitosis in the absence of oral disease	Present with maldigestion or malabsorption	Absent

471

BASE-LINE LABORATORY INVESTIGATIONS

Hematology, Clinical Biochemistry, and Urinalysis

Findings that may contribute to subsequent investigations of small intestinal disease include eosinophilia, perhaps reflecting parasitism, eosinophilic gastroenteritis, mast cell tumor, or Addison's disease; neutrophilia in inflammatory disease; neutropenia in parvovirus infection; septicemia or endotoxemia; lymphopenia in immunodeficiency, stress, or lymphangiectasia; and panhypoproteinemia in protein-losing enteropathy. Anemia from enteric blood loss or depressed erythropoiesis is caused by systemic disease, chronic malnutrition, or chronic inflammation. FeLV, FIV infection, and hyperthyroidism should be considered in cats with weight loss and diarrhea.

Albumin and globulin are both lost into the intestinal lumen in protein-losing enteropathies because mucosal damage is sufficiently severe to let the larger globulin molecule escape into the lumen. However, globulin concentration may be normal or high, particularly in animals with intense stimulation of humoral immunity due to inflammatory bowel disease. Moderately increased ALT and AST activity (up to 500 IU/L) is common in pancreatitis and in both acute and chronic enteritis.

Fecal Examination

In addition to gross appearance, microscopic examination using a direct smear and flotation may help to detect parasites, including *Giardia,* coccidia, hookworms, and whipworms; red cells; white cells; mucus; and fat (split and unsplit). In addition, in humid tropical climates endemic for *Strongyloides tumefaciens* or *Strongyloides stercoralis,* a direct smear, sedimentation, or Baermann technique can be used to look for larvae in the feces. The cysts of small coccidia such as *Cryptosporidia* spp. are best identified by Sheather's sugar centrifugation-flotation. Specific potentially enteropathogenic bacteria, such as *Salmonella* sp. and *Campylobacter* sp., can be isolated from fresh feces by use of specialized culture media.

The diagnosis of enterotoxigenic clostridia is supported by either a positive fecal enterotoxin assay (ELISA or reverse passive latex agglutination test) or the presence of large numbers of clostridial endospores (>5 spores per high-power oil immersion field), which are larger than bacteria and have a safety pin configuration in fecal cytology specimens stained with Diff-Quik. Fungal elements *(Histoplasma, Aspergillus, Pythium, Candida)* may also be identified in cytology preparations (e.g., fecal leukocyte examination, rectal mucosal scraping) or intestinal biopsies. A test for occult blood is seldom useful unless strongly positive because of the effect of diet and intestinal parasites.

DIAGNOSTIC IMAGING

Radiography

Survey radiographs should be made of both the thorax and abdomen, especially in animals presented with the complaint of vomiting.

Ultrasonography

Abdominal ultrasonography is useful for evaluating intestinal thickness, layering, luminal contents, and peristaltic function, and for diagnosis of conditions such as intestinal foreign body, intussusception, and neoplasia.

DIAGNOSIS OF EXOCRINE PANCREATIC INSUFFICIENCY (EPI)

Canine EPI is known to be associated with changes that might otherwise be considered indicative of primary small intestinal disorders.

These changes can include apparent impairment of monosaccharide absorption, abnormal serum folate and cobalamin concentrations, bacterial overgrowth, and villous atrophy. Diagnosis of EPI in dogs can be achieved by demonstrating a low concentration of serum trypsin-like immunoreactivity (TLI), which represents a sensitive and specific test (Chapter 107).

INDIRECT ASSESSMENT OF CHRONIC SMALL INTESTINAL DISEASE

Serum Folate and Cobalamin

The principle of the test is that disease of the proximal small intestine can result in a reduced serum folate concentration (see Table 104–2 in the textbook). It is particularly important to ensure that no-boil assays are not used despite their common usage in human laboratories.

Assessment of Intestinal Absorption

Interpretation problems translate into a relatively poor return for the effort involved in performing these absorption tests (D-xylose and glucose), which have now largely been abandoned in small animals. Procedures such as quantitative fecal fat analysis and plasma tests of lipid absorption are considered to be of limited value for the evaluation of the absorptive capacity of the small intestine.

Assessment of Intestinal Permeability

Assessment of intestinal permeability provides information about the physical integrity rather than the functional capacity of the mucosa, and represents a new and extremely sensitive approach to the detection of small intestinal damage.

Miscellaneous Procedures

See textbook.

DIRECT ASSESSMENT OF SMALL INTESTINAL DISEASE

Endoscopy

Evaluation of the upper and lower portions of the gastrointestinal tract using a flexible fiberoptic or video-endoscope has revolutionized the diagnosis and treatment of patients with gastrointestinal disease. It is important to take multiple biopsies from different sites, even if the bowel looks grossly or endoscopically normal. Laparotomy is justified when there is clinical or supportive evidence of protein-losing enteropathy (particularly when endoscopy has failed to provide histologic evidence of disease), disease of the small bowel beyond the reach of the endoscope, lymphosarcoma when mucosal biopsies are equivocal, or partial obstruction due to foreign bodies, neoplasia, or intussusception.

Histologic Examination of Biopsies

However, it should be appreciated that there may be minimal or no obvious morphologic abnormalities in certain disorders, despite considerable interference with intestinal function. Potential limitations of morphologic criteria alone can be considered by reference to Table 104–4, which summarizes histologic changes in the most important small intestinal diseases in dogs and cats.

Duodenal Juice

Duodenal juice can be obtained through an aspiration tube during endoscopy or by aspiration with a wide-bore needle and syringe at laparotomy. This can then be subjected to studies, including quantita-

TABLE 104–4. SUMMARY OF HISTOLOGIC CHANGES IN CHRONIC SMALL INTESTINAL DISEASES IN DOGS

CONDITION	HISTOLOGIC CHANGES
Small intestinal bacterial overgrowth (SIBO)	Minimal or no changes in most cases; may be partial villous atrophy and/or lymphocyte and plasma cell infiltrate in lamina propria of proximal small intestine
Gluten-sensitive enteropathy (GSE)	Patchy partial villous atrophy and increased intraepithelial lymphocytes in proximal small intestine
Lymphocytic-plasmacytic enteritis	Minimal or no villous atrophy; prominent infiltrate with lymphocytes and plasma cells in lamina propria of proximal small intestine
Canine "sprue"	Severe villous atrophy with variable lymphocyte/plasma cell infiltrate in lamina propria of proximal and distal small intestine
Basenji enteropathy	Partial villous atrophy, clubbing and fusion of villi, necrosis and abscessation of crypts, extreme infiltration with lymphocytes and plasma cells; severe protein-losing enteropathy
Eosinophilic enteritis	Minimal or no villous atrophy; prominent infiltrate of intestinal wall with eosinophils, and also lymphocytes and plasma cells; may affect whole or any part of gastrointestinal tract and can be protein-losing enteropathy
Intestinal lymphangiectasia	Minimal or no villous atrophy; dilatation of lymphatics in mucosa, submucosa, and serosa; severe protein-losing enteropathy
Intestinal lymphosarcoma	Typically a severe villous atrophy; dense infiltrate of intestinal wall particularly, with lymphocytes; may affect any part of gastrointestinal tract; severe protein-losing enteropathy

tive and qualitative bacterial culture to assess intestinal colonization, and examination for giardiasis.

DIARRHEAL DISEASES (pp. 1195–1212)

Other signs frequently associated with acute diarrhea are lethargy, inappetence, and vomiting. Fever, abdominal pain, and signs of dehydration are less common, but when present suggest more severe intestinal disease.

The causes of acute diarrhea, which in most patients is small intestinal in origin, can be divided into five general groups: (1) diet-induced, (2) toxin- or drug-induced (3) infectious, (4) extraintestinal, and (5) idiopathic or unclassified (see Table 104–14 in the textbook).

DIET-INDUCED DIARRHEA

Dietary causes of diarrhea are usually identified by careful history-taking and the response to a restricted diet. Acute diet-induced diarrhea is self-limiting with fasting or by feeding a restricted diet.

DRUG- AND TOXIN-INDUCED DIARRHEA

Some common examples of therapeutic agents with which diarrhea is a relatively frequent side effect include nonsteroidal anti-inflammatory agents (aspirin, indomethacin, phenylbutazone, ibuprofen, flunixin meglumine), digitalis and other cardiac drugs, dithiazanine, magnesium-containing compounds, lactulose (used for hepatic encephalopathy), many of the antiparasitic drugs, most anticancer drugs, and many antibacterial drugs (due in part to adverse effects on normal gut flora). Hemorrhagic gastroenteritis is an important complication in dogs.

Biologic toxins such as the enterotoxin that causes staphylococcal food poisoning, as well as various chemical poisons, including heavy metals (lead, arsenic, thallium), insecticides (organophosphate dips and flea treatments), lawn and garden products (insecticides, herbicides, fungicides), and some house plants may cause diarrhea if ingested. Most poisonings are accompanied by emesis, and sometimes even dramatic extraintestinal signs (e.g., the neurologic manifestations of lead, ethylene glycol, or organophosphate toxicity).

In most patients, the diarrhea resolves with symptomatic antidiarrheal therapy, prevention of further exposure to the toxin, and simply allowing time for elimination of the substance from the body.

INFECTIOUS DIARRHEA

Parasitic Diarrhea Caused by Helminths

The common helminths that parasitize the intestinal tract of the dog and cat are listed in Table 104–14 in the textbook. The most consistent clinical signs of intestinal parasitism are diarrhea and weight loss, although the overwhelming majority of infections are asymptomatic. The diagnosis of parasitism depends on the identification of eggs, cysts, larvae, trophozoites, or proglottids in the feces. Because the appearance of parasite elements in feces can be intermittent, it is important to perform fecal examinations several times before an animal with diarrhea is regarded as free of intestinal parasites.

Ascarids

Clinical Signs. Clinical signs of ascariasis might be seen with moderate to heavy infections in young puppies and kittens, in which adult worms in the small intestine can cause diarrhea, abdominal discomfort, whimpering, groaning, pot-bellied appearance, dull haircoat, dehydration, and even stunted growth. Ascarids are also frequently expelled in vomitus or diarrhea. When an animal becomes infected, there are three types of migration patterns: (1) liver-lung migration (*T. canis, T. cati*), (2) migration within the wall of the GI tract (all three ascarids), and (3) somatic tissue migration (*T. canis, T. cati*).

Treatment and Control. Most widely used are pyrantel pamoate and fenbendazole. Because most puppies are born infected with *T. canis,* treatment should be started at 2 weeks of age, before eggs are first passed in the feces, and then repeated at 4, 6, and 8 weeks of age to kill any ascarids resulting from prenatal infection, milk-borne infection, and ingestion of infective ova.

Public Health Aspects. Puppies infected with *T. canis* are considered important public health hazards because of toxocaral visceral larva migrans (VLM), a serious disorder of humans, especially children, which results from the invasion of visceral tissues by migrating *T. canis* larvae.

Hookworms

Clinical Signs. Signs of ancylostomiasis range from inapparent infection or nonspecific diarrhea to tarry (melena) or bloody (hematochezia) diarrhea accompanied by vomiting, inappetence, pallor, weakness, emaciation, dehydration, and poor growth. Anemia (which may be severe) and eosinophilia are common hematologic findings.

Life Cycle. Hookworm infection can occur by any of five routes: prenatal, milk-borne, ingestion of infective larvae (L3), skin penetration of infective larvae, and ingestion of a paratenic host. Larvae that penetrate the skin migrate by somatic or circulatory transport to the lung before reaching the intestine. Clinical signs in neonates are sometimes seen before completion of this prepatent period and the appearance of eggs in the feces.

Treatment and Control. Pyrantel pamoate is safest in very young and severely debilitated animals. Severely anemic puppies might need whole blood transfusion, iron supplementation, and supportive fluid therapy. Because of prenatal and milk-borne routes of infection, nursing puppies should be treated at 1, 2, 4, 6, and 8 weeks of age. Treatment is usually repeated after 2 to 3 weeks, partly because the initial treatment causes migration of tissue larvae to the gut with recurrence of signs. Milbemycin (Interceptor) combines heartworm prophylaxis with control of hookworms, whipworms, and ascarids.

Strongyloides

Infection of dogs occurs when third-stage larvae penetrate the skin or oral mucosa and develop in the small intestine following migration via the circulation to the lung. The diagnosis of *S. sterocoralis* depends on finding motile first-stage larvae in fresh feces, preferably using a Baermann procedure. Feline *S. tumefaciens* infection is usually asymptomatic, but mucosal and submucosal nodular lesions of the colon can occur with signs of chronic diarrhea and debilitation. A 5-day course of fenbendazole at a dose of 25 mg/lb (Panacur, 50 mg/kg per day) is the usual treatment, although ivermectin at a dose of 400 μg/lb (800 μg/kg) was effective in eliminating infection in hyperinfected dogs.

Tapeworms

The tapeworms that commonly parasitize the small bowel of dogs and cats are relatively harmless and rarely cause clinical signs. Infection with *Spirometra* spp. causes enteritis and diarrhea in the cat. The characteristic yellow-brown, single-operculated eggs are identified in fecal flotations since, unlike other tapeworm eggs, they float well. Praziquantel (Droncit), epsiprantel (Cestex), and bunamidine HCl are the preferred drugs for treatment of cestodiasis.

Other Metazoan Parasites

Trichinosis is an uncommon cause of hemorrhagic enteritis with bloody diarrhea in the cat. The illness is self-limiting without treatment, but eosinophilia can persist for 3 months. Infection by *Heterobilharzia americana* can be asymptomatic or characterized by severe bloody-mucoid diarrhea due to the tissue reaction to massive deposition of schistosome eggs within the gut wall and liver. Diagnosis is confirmed by ova detection on direct fecal examination or tissue biopsy. The treatment of choice is praziquantel (Droncit) at 10 times the dosage used to treat cestode infections.

Parasitic Diarrhea Caused by Protozoa

Coccidia

Most enteric coccidia infections of dogs and cats are commensal and nonpathogenic.

Isospora. The principal clinical sign of coccidiosis is diarrhea that varies from soft to fluid and is occasionally mucoid or bloody. Other signs include vomiting, lethargy, weight loss, and dehydration. If clinical signs are attributed to coccidiosis, as in neonates in stressful environments, effective coccidiostats should be used for treatment, such as sulfadimethoxine (usually at 25 to 30 mg/lb per day orally for 10 days), trimethoprim-sulfa (15 mg/lb per day, orally for 10 days), quinacrine (5 mg/lb per day, orally for 5 days), or amprolium. Amprolium is not approved for use in dogs but is recommended for treating kennels.

Cryptosporidia. *Cryptosporidium parvum* is a very small coccidium that has occasionally been associated with diarrhea in cats with serious underlying disease and neonatal puppies. Careful examination of slides under oil immersion is necessary to identify the tiny oocysts, which in sugar solution appear as small pinkish bodies that contain a dark dot. Cryptosporidiosis is usually self-limiting in immunocompetent hosts, but in the severely immunocompromised the infection has a poor prognosis. Spiramycin or quinine and clindamycin have been used to treat humans, but there is no proven effective treatment for cryptosporidiosis in dogs and cats.

Giardia. Clinically apparent giardiasis occurs most frequently in young dogs and cats, and is characterized by chronic intestinal malabsorption with large volumes of foul-smelling, light-colored, watery or "cow patty–like" diarrhea, steatorrhea, and weight loss. Diarrhea, the most prominent sign, can be acute or chronic, intermittent or continuous, and self-limiting or persistent.

Diagnosis. *Giardia* cysts stain well with Lugol's 2 per cent iodine, and the most reliable method for recovery of cysts from feces is by zinc sulfate centrifugation-flotation, but they also float up quite well in sodium nitrate. Trophozoites can be identified in fresh diarrheic feces suspended in saline or stained with iodine, although they are found in feces less consistently than are cysts. The presence of *Giardia* might be temporarily masked for about a week by barium, certain antibiotics, antacids, antidiarrheals, laxatives, and enemas.

If protozoa cannot be demonstrated by repeated fecal examinations, another approach is to identify trophozoites in duodenal aspirates, brushings, mucosal impression smears, or biopsies obtained via endoscopy or laparotomy. "Occult" giardiasis (which we define as animals with three negative zinc sulfate and saline smear fecal examinations) may be indirectly diagnosed by response to a therapeutic trial.

Treatment and Prognosis. Three drugs currently available in the United States are considered effective in the treatment of *Giardia*—metronidazole (Flagyl), quinacrine HCl (Atabrine), and furazolidone (Furoxone). As many as one-third of infections are metronidazole-resistant. Albendazole (Valbazen suspension), 12.5 mg/lb (25 mg/kg) twice a day for 2 days, is reported to be an extremely effective and nontoxic treatment for *Giardia* and may be useful in the treatment of metronidazole-resistant patients. Furazolidone, 2 mg/lb (4 mg/kg) orally twice a day for 5 to 10 days, is both effective and convenient in cats because it is available in a suspension form. Quinacrine, 3.3 mg/lb (6.6 mg/kg) twice a day orally for 5 days, was highly effective in treating canine giardiasis but was associated with a high incidence of side effects (anorexia, lethargy, vomiting, fever). The prognosis for giardiasis is excellent with treatment, although some cases require a longer course of therapy than is generally recommended and others must have treatment repeated when initial treatment fails to completely eliminate the infection.

Pentatrichomonas. It is generally believed that these organisms are the result rather than the cause of diarrhea. The presence of trichomoniasis is established by identification in saline fecal smears of motile, pyriform flagellated trophozoites with distinctive wavelike motion of an undulating membrane and a constant jerking and rolling motion. Pentatrichomonads can be effectively eliminated with a 5-day course of metronidazole 12 to 15 mg/lb (25 to 30 mg/kg, twice a day) or a 3-day course of tinidazole 22 mg/lb (44 mg/kg, once a day).

Canine Parvoviral Enteritis

Clinical Signs. Parvoviral enteritis usually begins with an abrupt onset of anorexia and depression, followed within hours by vomiting and usually diarrhea, which can be profuse and hemorrhagic. In some dogs, vomiting is the predominant sign and diarrhea is minimal. Physical examination often reveals fever, dehydration, and severe depression.

Diagnosis. Increased breed susceptibility has been shown for Doberman pinschers and rottweilers. Either at initial presentation or within the next 72 hours, approximately 85 per cent of dogs with parvoviral enteritis develop severe leukopenia due to lymphopenia and granulocytopenia. Gas and fluid distention of the gut are frequent radiographic findings in parvoviral enteritis and can mimic intestinal obstruction. Fecal titers are now routinely determined using the enzyme-linked immunosorbent assay (ELISA) method. Serologic determination of an anti-CPV antibody titer (by hemagglutination-inhibition, virus neutralization, and other methods) is not sufficient for diagnosis because an estimated 75 to 95 per cent of dogs in the population have seroconverted from prior vaccination or exposure.

Treatment. The cornerstone of treatment is rehydration. In most cases, intravenous fluid and electrolyte replacement is preferred, and lactated Ringer's supplemented with potassium is suggested. Dextrose may also be added to intravenous fluids in a 2½ per cent solution when needed for management of complicating hypoglycemia. Parenteral antibiotics are indicated if secondary bacterial sepsis is present or considered to be impending because of high fever, marked leukopenia, hypoglycemia, shock, DIC, or severe loss of mucosal barrier as indicated by dysentery or hematochezia.

Additional measures include antiemetic therapy for persistent vomiting, oral bismuth subsalicylate for its nonspecific antidiarrheal activity, and plasma infusion or blood transfusion if hypoproteinemia (<4.5 gm/dl) or severe blood loss anemia occurs. Traditionally, nothing is given orally until vomiting has ceased for at least 24 hours and diarrhea is subsiding and free of gross blood; this can take 3 to 5 days in severe cases. Dogs with parvovirus shed massive amounts of virus in their feces during their illness and are highly infectious for other dogs. Elimination of the virus from infected premises is difficult because the virus is so resistant; however, disinfection with dilute (1:30) chlorine bleach is suggested.

Prognosis and Complications. Most patients with parvovirus enteritis recover if they are treated appropriately for dehydration.

Canine Coronaviral Enteritis

Most infections are subclinical, although occasional epizootics of severe enteritis have occurred, mostly associated with kennels and dog shows. Clinical signs of canine coronaviral enteritis vary from inapparent to the acute onset of anorexia and depression followed by vomiting and diarrhea. Most cases are afebrile. Fecal appearance varies from yellow-orange and mushy to watery or overtly bloody. Because coronaviral enteritis is usually nonfatal and the only treatment is supportive, definitive laboratory confirmation is not needed for effective case management except to document an epizootic outbreak.

Treatment of coronaviral enteritis consists of fluid therapy and routine antidiarrheal therapy, as described previously for acute diarrhea. Most animals recover rapidly, although a few dogs have persistent diarrhea for 3 to 4 weeks.

Canine Rotaviral Enteritis

Clinical signs of acute enteritis attributed to rotavirus are occasionally seen in young puppies. The diarrhea, which can be watery to mucoid, is usually self-limiting and of brief duration, although rare fatalities have been reported. Active rotavirus infection can be established by detection of virus in feces with a commercially available enzyme immunoassay kit. Electron microscopy and virus isolation can also detect fecal excretion of rotavirus, but these are not practical for routine clinical use. Rotaviral enteritis is treated like any other acute diarrhea, with emphasis on supportive measures such as fluid therapy and dietary restriction.

Canine Distemper Viral Enteritis

The widespread epitheliotropism of canine distemper virus can cause severe febrile gastroenteritis with diarrhea and vomiting, typically accompanied by other manifestations of distemper, such as naso-ocular discharge, pneumonia, or neurologic abnormalities.

Feline Panleukopenia Enteritis

Clinical features are similar to canine parvoviral enteritis: anorexia, profound lethargy, high fever, persistent vomiting, diarrhea, and progressive dehydration. Diagnosis of feline panleukopenia enteritis is usually presumptive and made on the basis of clinical signs and the profound panleukopenia (nadir often <500 WBC/μl) in a susceptible (unvaccinated) cat. The leukopenia is fairly consistent and usually lasts only 2 to 4 days.

The treatment of feline panleukopenia is similar to that discussed for canine parvoviral enteritis. Widespread prevention of this disease has been achieved through the availability and use of highly effective vaccines. There appears to be a 2-week critical period of susceptibility, similar to that described for canine parvovirus, resulting from the phenomenon of maternal antibody interference. Despite vaccination, kittens can be infected if exposed during this time.

Feline Enteric Coronaviral Enteritis

In young kittens, especially 4 to 12 weeks of age, feline enteric coronavirus can cause an acute but mild enteritis that can be subclinical or characterized by vomiting and diarrhea. These signs are usually mild and self-limiting, lasting 2 to 4 days.

Feline Rotaviral Enteritis

The enteropathogenic significance of rotavirus in the cat is currently unclear.

BACTERIAL AND RICKETTSIAL DIARRHEA

Invasive bacteria, such as *Salmonella, Campylobacteria, Yersinia, Shigella,* and invasive strains of *Escherichia coli,* primarily invade the mucosa of the colon and distal small bowel. Thus, invasive bacteria cause acute enterocolitis characterized by leukocyte-positive, bloody-mucoid diarrhea that is frequently accompanied by abdominal pain, tenesmus, and fever. In addition, some invasive organisms can invade the submucosa and enter lymphatics and the blood stream, producing serious systemic infection (bacteremia) as well as intestinal infection.

Enterotoxigenic bacteria elaborate enterotoxins that irreversibly bind to enterocytes and either act as secretogogues that stimulate intestinal epithelial cell secretion or as cytotoxins that directly injure the mucosal epithelium. Cytotoxin-producing enterotoxigenic bacteria, such as *Clostridium difficile,* cause inflammatory large bowel diarrhea that mimics dysentery caused by the invasive enteropathogens.

Salmonella can also stimulate concomitant hypersecretion through the release of enterotoxin and increased local synthesis of prostaglandins at the site of inflammation. Secretory diarrhea associated with staphylococcal food poisoning develops when preformed toxin is ingested with the food. Because some of these are also human pathogens, particularly *Salmonella, Campylobacter,* and *Yersinia,* pets can be an important reservoir for human infection.

Salmonellosis

Clinical Signs. Salmonella infection presents in three distinct clinical syndromes (from most common to least): (1) asymptomatic carrier state, (2) gastroenteritis, and (3) gastroenteritis with bacteremia (with or without extraintestinal localization). Most animals with acute salmonella diarrhea recover within 3 to 4 weeks, although shedding of organisms continues for as long as 6 weeks. Some cats with salmonella infection may exhibit only vague nonspecific signs, a left-shifted leukogram, and fever. Because it is often an opportunistic invader, salmonella is frequently diagnosed in animals with other underlying disorders or risk factors such as recent surgery, oral antibiotic treatment, immunosuppressive therapy, or boarding.

Diagnosis.   The diagnosis depends on isolation of *Salmonella* spp. from properly cultured fecal specimens or from blood or joint fluid cultures in septicemic patients.

Treatment.   Salmonella invasion that is confined locally to the mucosa produces enteritis that is both self-limiting and unlikely to be affected by antibacterial agents. In fact, antibacterial therapy, especially with oral nonabsorbable antibiotics, can actually prolong shedding of the organism and encourage development of a prolonged convalescent carrier state. Antibacterials are also ineffective for eliminating chronic asymptomatic carriers of salmonella. However, antibiotics are indicated whenever salmonella invasion becomes severe or complicated by septicemia or endotoxemia. Most isolates are susceptible to enrofloxacin, 2.5 mg/lb (5 mg/kg) twice a day, or to trimethoprim-sulfonamide combination, 7.5 mg/lb (15 mg/kg) twice a day. In addition to antibiotics, fluid and electrolyte replacement and detection and correction of underlying predisposing conditions are important aspects of therapy.

Campylobacteriosis

Dogs and cats can serve as reservoir hosts for the three species of *Campylobacter* that are known to cause disease in humans.

Clinical Signs.   The majority of animals that harbor these organisms are asymptomatic. Clinical disease occurs most commonly in young dogs and cats. Clinical signs associated with campylobacteriosis in dogs and cats have been attributed to superficial erosive enterocolitis and are characterized by a 5- to 15-day course of watery-mucoid diarrhea that occasionally contains blood and can be accompanied by vomiting and tenesmus. Fever is usually mild or absent. *Campylobacter* is occasionally associated with chronic diarrhea.

Diagnosis.   Confirmation of campylobacteriosis depends on isolation of the organism from feces, using special selective media.

Treatment and Prognosis.   The antibiotic of choice for human campylobacteriosis is erythromycin, which can be used to treat animals at 5 mg/lb (10 mg/kg) three times a day. Antibiotics are effective in rapidly eliminating excretion of organisms and warranted to reduces the chance of spread of infection to humans or to other animals.

Yersiniosis

On rare occasions the organism has been isolated from young dogs with enterocolitis characterized by bloody-mucoid diarrhea, increased frequency of defecation, tenesmus, and an absence of systemic signs. *Yersinia* infection of dogs might be a public health concern.

Yersinia grows best at colder temperatures, and specialized isolation methods are needed to culture the organism from feces. The infection is usually susceptible to treatment with trimethoprim-sulfonamide, tetracycline, chloramphenicol, and aminoglycosides; however, culture and antibiotic sensitivity testing are recommended.

In cats, the clinical signs are vomiting, diarrhea, weight loss, depression, fever, and icterus. Feline pseudotuberculosis is usually progressive and fatal, although clinically healthy carriers of the organism have also been found. Treatment consists of a prolonged course of an antibiotic such as trimethoprim-sulfonamide combination, tetracycline, or chloramphenicol, but the prognosis is guarded.

Bacillus Piliformis *(Tyzzer's Disease)*

Tyzzer's disease, caused by a pleomorphic, gram-negative, spore-forming, obligate intracellular bacillus called *Bacillus piliformis,* is a rare but fatal disease characterized by hemorrhagic-necrotizing entero-colitis and hepatic necrosis. Puppies and kittens are most often affected. The progression of Tyzzer's disease is rapid; most animals become moribund shortly after the initial onset of signs of anorexia, depression, and diarrhea. Death occurs rapidly, usually within 48 hours, and successful therapy has not been reported. Most cases are diagnosed by the histologic identification of typical intracellular fila-mentous bacilli at the margins of necrotic foci within liver and intesti-nal lesions using methenamine silver, Giemsa, or periodic acid–Schiff (PAS) staining.

Escherichia Coli

Invasive and enterotoxigenic strains of *E. coli* are well-established causes of host-specific, acute infectious diarrhea in many animals including humans, but the role of *E. coli* as a primary enteropathogen in small animals is unclear. Definitive assays are needed to document enteropathogenicity of *E. coli* isolates from dogs and cats with natu-rally occurring diarrhea. It appears that the incidence of enterotoxi-genic *E. coli* diarrhea is extremely low in the dog. Preliminary evi-dence suggests that enteropathogenic strains of *E. coli* are more likely to play a role in cats with diarrhea than invasive or enterotoxin-produc-ing strains.

Clostridium

Clostridium spp. constitute part of the normal intestinal flora of the dog and cat, and a role in causing diarrhea in dogs and cats is sus-pected but unproven. Diagnosis of *C. difficile* is generally based on a positive assay for the cytotoxin in feces.

C. perfringens (welchii), a large anaerobic gram-positive bacillus and part of the normal microflora of the dog, has been incriminated in a number of reports as a cause of diarrhea in dogs and cats. Presump-tive diagnosis of *C. perfringens* is based on cytologic identification of fecal leukocytes and numerous large gram-positive rods associated with endospores in the feces. Definitive diagnosis is based on detection of *C. perfringens* enterotoxin by fecal assay (Oxoid) at a titer of ≥1:20. Most cases are self-limiting or responsive to antibiotics in 2 to 3 days; however, chronic or recurrent clostridial diarrhea may require long-term antibiotics (e.g., tylosin) and a fiber-supplemented diet to prevent relapses.

Other Bacteria

Staphylococcal food poisoning has not been well documented in dogs or cats, but is a plausible cause. Even though isolated from the feces, pathogenecity has yet to be established for *Shigella* spp., *Proteus* spp., *Klebsiella* spp., or spirochetes.

Rickettsial Diarrhea *(Salmon Poisoning Disease)*

Salmon poisoning is a highly fatal systemic rickettsial infection of dogs in the Pacific Northwest caused by *Neorickettsia helminthoeca* or *N. elokominica,* two related rickettsial organisms acquired by ingestion of raw salmon that harbor the disease vector, metacercariae of a fluke called *Nanophyetus salmincola.* Signs of infection include high fever, vomiting, diarrhea, anorexia, depression, naso-ocular discharge, dehy-dration, and peripheral lymphadenopathy.

The diagnosis should be suspected when these signs are seen in a dog from an endemic area and confirmed by examination of feces for characteristic operculated fluke eggs by direct smear, sugar flotation, or wash-sedimentation methods, or by detection of purple-staining intracytoplasmic rickettsial bodies in macrophages from Giemsa-stained lymph node aspirates.

Tetracycline for 2 to 3 weeks is the treatment of choice as a specific antirickettsial agent. General supportive measures such as parenteral fluid therapy should also be considered, and the trematode vector is treated with oral fenbendazole, 25 mg/lb (50 mg/kg) per day for 10 to 14 days.

Canine Hemorrhagic Enteritis (HGE)

See Chapter 103. Failure of the animal to improve dramatically after 24 to 48 hours of intravenous fluid therapy should prompt a search for other diseases that can mimic HGE (e.g., parvovirus, GI foreign body, intussusception, or intestinal volvulus).

TREATMENT OF ACUTE DIARRHEA

Dietary Modification

Placing the intestinal tract in a state of physiologic rest by dietary restriction is perhaps the single most important aspect of acute diarrhea therapy. Access to water should not be restricted, however, if the patient is not vomiting. After 24 to 48 hours, food can be gradually reintroduced. Traditionally, the first foods recommended after restriction have been easily digestible and low in fat. If dietary modification controls diarrhea, a gradual return to the original diet can be made over several days.

Antimicrobials

Antibiotics are indicated only in the unusual and specific case of acute diarrhea associated with intestinal bacterial infection or, possibly, as parenteral therapy when mucosal damage is severe as evidenced by hemorrhagic diarrhea, leukocytosis, and fever.

Motility Modifiers

Most diarrhea ia associated with decreased, rather than increased, motility. Unfortunately, most of these compounds further depress bowel motility. However, they provide some benefit by decreasing fluid secretion from the crypt and increasing fluid absorption at the villus tip. The non-narcotic antidiarrheals have no role in the symptomatic treatment of acute diarrhea; however, these compounds may be useful in controlling gastrointestinal problems that may have an underlying psychologic defect.

Protectants and Adsorbents

Several commercial compounds that contain bismuth subsalicylate, such as Pepto-Bismol and Corrective Mixture w/Paregoric, are probably the adsorbent antidiarrheals of choice in the symptomatic treatment of acute diarrhea.

INTESTINAL OBSTRUCTION (pp. 1212–1214)

Obstruction can be acute or chronic, partial or complete, and results from three basic causes: (1) extraluminal compression, (2) mural thickening, and (3) intraluminal obstruction. Functional obstruction is a separate but rare clinical entity in which there is no luminal obstruction; the mechanism of obstruction is believed to be due to an impairment of motility with a subsequent accumulation of swallowed air and ingesta. Intestinal obstruction can be simple or strangulated. Strangulation occurs most often with intussusception, volvulus, and incarcerated hernia.

Intussusception. The most common site for an intussusception to occur in the dog is the ileocolic junction, and the majority of intussusceptions occur in animals less than one year of age.

PATHOPHYSIOLOGY OF INTESTINAL OBSTRUCTION

Intestinal obstruction causes a variety of dramatic and life-threatening events, the most important of which are fluid and electrolyte disturbances and endotoxic and septic shock.

Bacterial Flora and Toxins. The number of bacteria in the lumen proximal to the site of obstruction increases dramatically. With the increase in bacterial flora comes a concomitant increase in the amount of bacterial exotoxin and endotoxin.

HISTORY AND PHYSICAL FINDINGS

Inappetence and anorexia are common complaints, but vomiting is the predominant sign. In general, the more proximal the obstruction, the more dramatic is the vomiting and associated clinical signs. Distal intestinal obstruction can be far more subtle in its presentation. The first sign may be a gradual but progressive decrease in appetite that leads to anorexia and loss of body weight and condition. Vomiting in such patients is usually intermittent at first, but becomes increasingly severe as more and more of the intestine is distended with accumulated fluid and gas. It can sometimes be as long as 4 weeks from the onset of signs to diagnosis, by which time the animal is significantly emaciated. Other signs in such patients include dry scant feces, lethargy, and depression.

Partial intestinal obstruction can be even more insidious in its onset and clinical presentation, and is usually characterized only by chronic intermittent vomiting with no loss in body weight or condition. Intestinal obstruction associated with strangulation is far more dramatic in its clinical presentation. The course of the disease in such patients is rapid and progressive, and the animal is often presented with signs of hypovolemic and endotoxic shock. Careful abdominal palpation may reveal a mass in the small intestine, a firm tubular mass, or bunching of the intestine.

DIAGNOSTIC STUDIES

Radiographic findings that suggest obstruction include gas or fluid distention (mechanical ileus) of the bowel, delayed transit of contrast material, fixation or displacement of gut loops, luminal filling defects, or the presence of foreign objects within the lumen. The aggregation and plication of the bowel associated with linear intestinal foreign bodies produces a distinctive radiographic pattern.

Abdominal ultrasonography is also a valuable technique for identifying many intestinal foreign bodies, tumors, intussusceptions, and intestinal masses. Laboratory studies are not diagnostic but are nevertheless critical in that they can help to define the degree of hemoconcentration, inflammation, and electrolyte disturbance. Hypokalemia is a common complaint, possibly with associated hyponatremia, hypochloremia, and metabolic alkalosis in high intestinal obstruction.

TREATMENT

Ideally, the patient should be taken to surgery as soon as possible after diagnosis, but only after fluid and electrolyte deficits have been replaced and antibiotic therapy has commenced.

CHRONIC ENTEROPATHIES (pp. 1214–1225)

BACTERIAL OVERGROWTH

Clinical Signs. Small intestinal bacterial overgrowth in the proximal small intestine is emerging as an important condition in many breeds of dog and typically presents in young animals as chronic intermittent small bowel diarrhea, which may be accompanied by loss of body weight or failure to gain weight. However, clinical signs are variable, and some animals may have weight loss without diarrhea whereas others may have intermittent vomiting or signs suggestive of mild colitis.

Pathophysiology of Overgrowth. Brush border biochemical abnormalities in dogs with aerobic and anaerobic overgrowth were reversed by oral antibiotic therapy, and could be due to the direct action of bacteria or their secretions on the mucosa, or the effects of bacterial metabolites such as deconjugated bile salts and hydroxy fatty acids. The consequences of SIBO may also depend on other factors, particularly the response of the local immune system to these bacteria, and this may represent the key to the understanding of relationships between the overgrowth flora and clinical disease.

Treatment of Overgrowth. The first objective is to consider treatment of any identified underlying abnormality that could be responsible for the overgrowth, such as partial obstruction due to intussusception, tumors, or foreign bodies. Oral broad-spectrum antibiotic therapy with oxytetracycline, 5 to 10 mg/lb (10 to 20 mg/kg), repeated every 8 hours for 28 days, has been particularly successful, and may need to be continued for extended periods if clinical signs recur on withdrawal of medication. Metronidazole, 5 to 10 mg/lb (10 to 20 mg/kg) every 12 hours, and tylosin, 5 to 10 mg/lb (10 to 20 mg/kg) every 12 hours, have proved to be effective alternatives. Dietary management with a commercial or home-prepared low-fat diet may also be valuable.

DIETARY SENSITIVITY

Food intolerance represents a nonimmunologic response resulting from an inability to adequately digest the food or from metabolic, toxic, or pharmacologic responses. Dietary sensitivity is defined as intestinal damage resulting from an immunologically mediated response to specific dietary antigens.

There are clearly difficulties in establishing a definitive diagnosis. Confirmation of dietary sensitivity involves monitoring the response to dietary exclusion and subsequent challenge, using not only subjective clinical criteria but also objective criteria such as intestinal permeability and morphology. This approach has been used to document a familial gluten-sensitive enteropathy in Irish setters.

Gluten-Sensitive Enteropathy in Irish Setters

Affected dogs typically present with poor weight gain or weight loss, in most cases accompanied by chronic diarrhea, and clinical signs are often first observed at approximately 6 months of age.

Diagnosis of Dietary Sensitivity

Table 104–5 shows the steps in diagnosing dietary sensitivity in the dog and cat. Intestinal lesions such as villous atrophy or increased intraepithelial lymphocytes are not pathognomonic for dietary sensitivity, and objective assessments of intestinal damage, including intestinal permeability or histopathology, therefore need to be repeated following exclusion diet and challenge in order to make a definitive diagnosis and identify an offending antigen.

TABLE 104–5. DIAGNOSIS OF DIETARY SENSITIVITY IN THE DOG AND CAT

1. Clinical association between diet and disease
2. Exclude intestinal parasites and pathogens, partial obstruction, and systemic disease
3. Exclude exocrine pancreatic insufficiency
4. Exclude small intestinal bacterial overgrowth
5. Demonstrate intestinal damage responsive to diet:
   Indirect: intestinal permeability
   Direct: villous atrophy, cellular infiltration

Treatment of Dietary Sensitivity

An exclusion diet consisting of a selected protein source should be used as trial therapy in suspected cases of dietary sensitivity, and should be fed for a period of at least 6 weeks. Boiled white rice or potato is generally a suitable carbohydrate source, and lamb or chicken is often used as a protein source, dependent on the dietary history. Cottage cheese, horsemeat, rabbit, venison, and tofu are acceptable alternatives. It should be appreciated that some animals may be sensitive to rice protein. Oral prednisone, 0.25 to 0.5 mg/lb (0.5 to 1 mg/kg) twice daily for 2 to 4 weeks, followed with a reducing dose at 2-week intervals, may assist some cases of dietary sensitivity if the initial response to exclusion diet is disappointing.

CHRONIC IDIOPATHIC ENTEROPATHIES

Lymphocytic-Plasmacytic Enteritis

Lymphocytic-plasmacytic enteritis (LPE) is the most common form of idiopathic inflammatory bowel disease identified in dogs and cats and is the most common cause of chronic vomiting and diarrhea in these two species.

Pathogenesis. Lymphocytic-plasmacytic intestinal infiltrates may be associated with many conditions, including giardiasis, campylobacteriosis, histoplasmosis, bacterial overgrowth, dietary sensitivity, lymphangiectasia, regional enteritis, and lymphosarcoma, but in the majority of cases no obvious cause can be identified.

History and Clinical Signs. Chronic intermittent vomiting and listless behavior are the most consistent signs in cats and may occur with or without diarrhea. Signs in dogs most typically include small bowel diarrhea and weight loss. Signs are often cyclic and can present as bouts or attacks of vomiting and abdominal pain with or without diarrhea that can resemble acute pancreatitis in their severity. Vomiting is often intermittent early in the disease process and progresses to become more severe and frequent, with or without diarrhea. Severe protein-losing enteropathy and hypoproteinuria can develop in these patients.

Physical Findings. At physical examination, findings vary from unremarkable to a palpably thickened intestine, cachexia, and edema or ascites.

Diagnosis. See Table 104–1. A panhypoproteinemia with associated low calcium levels may be present in advanced and severe cases. For cats, the albumin may be low (2.0 gm/dl, with a compensatory increase in globulin). Histologic examination of intestinal biopsy specimens is needed to identify lymphocytic-plasmacytic enteritis. Mild changes may simply indicate a reactive response to intestinal parasites or bacterial overgrowth. Moderate to severe changes, on the other hand, are much more significant and determine the need for aggressive treatment. Mucosal atrophy with villous blunting may be present in moderate to severe disease, and secondary lymphangiectasia and crypt abscesses may also be reported.

Dietary Management. Attention should be given to the carbohydrate content of the diet, particularly in conditions that result in reduction in villus height or functional damage to individual enterocytes, since malabsorption of small carbohydrate molecules can lead to osmotic diarrhea. A rice-based, low-fat, good-quality protein source diet is recommended.

Deficiencies of trace elements and vitamins may also make a major contribution to the clinical consequences and recovery of intestinal disease. There are now available a variety of commercial single protein source diets for cats, with either rice or potato as the carbohydrate source. Diarrhea in some cats with plasmacytic-lymphocytic enteritis also responds to the semimoist diet Tender Vittles.

Clinical experience has shown that dietary management alone usually leads to only minimal or significant but temporary control of clinical signs in both canine and feline patients with moderate to severe plasmacytic-lymphocytic enteritis.

Medical Management. Oral prednisolone (or prednisone), 0.25 to 0.5 mg/lb (0.5 to 1.0 mg/kg) every 12 hours for a month, followed by a reducing dose, is the most important component of medical therapy. Higher doses, 0.5 to 1.0 mg/lb (1 to 2 mg/kg) q12h, are indicated when the word "moderate" or "severe" appears on the biopsy report. Azathioprine, another important drug, is given at a dose of 0.5 mg/lb (1.0 mg/kg) once a day in dogs and 0.15 mg/lb (0.3 mg/kg) once a day in cats for severe plasmacytic-lymphocytic enteritis.

If clinical improvement occurs, the prednisone dose should be reduced by 50 per cent every 2 weeks. An alternate-day regimen should be continued for 8 to 12 weeks and then cautiously withdrawn. Azathioprine takes 3 to 4 weeks to begin to exert its therapeutic effects, and treatment should be continued for 3 to 9 months. Metronidazole should be given at a dose of 5 to 10 mg/lb (10 to 20 mg/kg) twice daily. After 2 to 4 weeks, the dose can be decreased to once-daily administration. Treatment with sucralfate or an H-2 blocker should be continued until serum proteins return to normal. Parenteral fat-soluble vitamins should be part of the initial treatment plan.

Lymphocytic-plasmacytic enteritis that is initially graded as moderate to severe can usually be managed successfully and maintained in remission. The two most common reasons for treatment failure in lymphocytic-plasmacytic enteritis are (1) insufficiently aggressive therapy (i.e., prednisone dose too low), and (2) the failure to recognize concurrent gastritis, gastric motility disorder, or colitis.

Canine Sprue

Consider this as a relatively severe form of lymphocytic-plasmacytic enteritis. Affected animals have been adults with a history of severe chronic diarrhea and marked loss of body weight and condition. Treatment is the same as described for severe lymphocytic-plasmacytic enteritis, consisting of aggressive use of prednisone, azathioprine, and metronidazole. The prognosis is poor.

Basenji Enteropathy

Severe lymphocytic-plasmacytic enteritis is also part of a hereditary enteropathy of Basenji dogs that can cause severe intestinal malabsorption. There is evidence of protein-losing enteropathy and hypoalbuminemia, which is accompanied by hypergammaglobulinemia despite an anticipated loss of gamma globulin into the gut lumen, probably reflecting intense stimulation of humoral immunity. Clinical signs in affected dogs include chronic, intractable diarrhea and loss of body weight. The condition is progressive, leading to emaciation and, in some cases, death. Treatment is generally unsuccessful, but remission can be obtained if aggressive treatment, as described for severe plasmacytic-lymphocytic enteritis, is initiated early in the disease process.

Eosinophilic Enteritis

The disease may also involve other regions of the gastrointestinal tract, particularly the stomach in dogs and the colon in cats.

History and Clinical Signs. Clinically there can be chronic vomiting and small bowel diarrhea, sometimes accompanied by large bowel signs including hematochezia, particularly with colonic involvement. Some cases may show slow, progressive weight loss because of nutrient malabsorption and, possibly, protein-losing enteropathy. Eosinophilic enteritis can afflict any breed, although it has received most attention in the German shepherd. The eosinophilic infiltrate may occasionally cause segmental tumor-like thickening in the gut wall that can partially obstruct the lumen and resemble lymphosarcoma.

Diagnosis. See Table 104–1.

Treatment. Treatment of eosinophilic enteritis is predicated upon the use of prednisone at an initial dose of 1.0 mg/lb (2.0 mg/kg) b.i.d. Signs should diminish in 7 to 10 days, after which the dose can be reduced in 50 per cent decrements every 2 weeks. Methylprednisolone acetate or azathioprine may be used in some cases. It is advisable to prophylactically treat afflicted patients with fenbendazole, 25 mg/lb (50 mg/kg) twice daily for 14 days.

Intestinal Lymphangiectasia

Definition and Cause. Intestinal lymphangiectasia can result from a number of causes: (1) congenital malformation of the lymphatic system, (2) infiltration or obstruction of intestinal lymphatics due to an inflammatory, fibrosing, or neoplastic process, (3) obstruction of lymph flow through the thoracic duct, and (4) abnormal drainage and increased production of intestinal lymph resulting from the elevated central venous pressure of congestive heart failure, particularly constrictive pericarditis.

History and Clinical Signs. Hypoproteinemia can be the only apparent manifestation of intestinal disease. Presenting signs include dependent pitting edema of the subcutis and limbs, ascites, and hydrothorax that can result in respiratory distress. Chronic intermittent or persistent light-colored diarrhea of a watery to semisolid consistency may be observed. Sporadic vomiting, lethargy, weight loss, and progressive emaciation are commonly associated with longstanding protein-losing enteropathy. Signs of intestinal lymphangiectasia are often insidious in onset, tend to fluctuate in intensity, and progress slowly over a period of several months before the typical features of protein-losing enteropathy become apparent. Breeds of dogs reported to be predisposed include the soft-coated Wheatan terrier, the Lundehund, and the Basenji.

Diagnosis. The initial step in diagnosis is to exclude the nonenteric causes of hypoproteinemia—liver failure (impaired hepatic synthesis of albumin) and renal disease (protein-losing glomerulonephropathies). Definitive diagnosis is established by histologic identification of the characteristic mucosal lesion in intestinal biopsies.

Treatment. The ideal diet for the dog with lymphangiectasia should contain minimal fat and provide an ample quantity of high-quality protein. These diets should be supplemented with fat-soluble vitamins (vitamins A, D, and E by intramuscular injection, and vitamin K orally). The plasma protein loss and diarrhea of lymphangiectasia can often be reduced by anti-inflammatory doses of corticosteroids, such as oral prednisolone at an initial dosage of 0.5 to 1 mg/lb (1 to 2 mg/kg) twice daily. Once remission has been achieved, this dosage should be adjusted to a lower maintenance level. In addition to dietary management and anti-inflammatory treatment, antibiotics such as tylosin, 5 to 10 mg/lb (10 to 20 mg/kg), or metronidazole, 5 to 10 mg/lb (10 to 20 mg/kg), twice daily should be considered to control secondary bacterial overgrowth.

When lymphangiectasia occurs secondary to an identifiable anatomic lymphatic or venous obstruction, surgical intervention for relief of the obstruction should be considered. In cardiac-associated lymphangiectasia, the emphasis of therapy should be directed toward control of congestive heart failure. Pericardiectomy is usually indicated for the rare case of constrictive pericarditis. Remissions of several months' duration are not uncommon; in some patients they have been maintained for over 2 years.

INTESTINAL FUNGAL INFECTIONS (pp. 1225–1227)

INTESTINAL HISTOPLASMOSIS

History and Clinical Signs. Intestinal histoplasmosis occurs most often in young dogs and cats. Severe chronic malabsorption: profuse, intractable watery diarrhea; rapidly progressive weight loss; and melena is observed in many patients. Systemic signs such as fever, pallor, inappetence, depression, and weight loss are common. Emaciation is a consistent feature of intestinal histoplasmosis. Variable findings indicative of additional sites of dissemination include cough or dyspnea (lung involvement), icterus or hepatomegaly (liver involvement), aqueous flare or chorioretinitis (eye involvement), cutaneous nodules or fistulas (skin involvement), lameness (bone involvement), neurologic signs (CNS involvement), splenomegaly, and lymphadenopathy.

Diagnosis. Definitive diagnosis depends on identification of *Histoplasma* organisms in cytology preparations, biopsies, or cultures. Serologic tests are less reliable but can be used for presumptive diagnosis. (Additional information regarding diagnosis is contained in Chapter 71.)

Treatment. Because amphotericin must be given intravenously and is frequently nephrotoxic, the oral azoles are the first-choice antifungal drugs for treatment of histoplasmosis. Ketoconazole is given initially at a dosage of 5 to 10 mg/lb (10 to 15 mg/kg) orally twice a day until remission of the disease is achieved and then continued at a maintenance dosage of 2 to 5 mg/lb (5 to 10 mg/kg) twice a day for an additional 3 to 4 months. Alternatively, itraconazole can be given orally at a dosage of 2 mg/lb (5 mg/kg) twice a day until at least 3 to 4 months of remission. Potential side effects of azoles include inappetence, vomiting, and hepatotoxicity. Although successful treatment has been reported, treatment failures have been relatively frequent.

PHYCOMYCOSIS

In dogs, phycomycotic organisms can infect any part of the digestive tract, but lesions most commonly involve the stomach, small intestine, mesentery, and mesenteric lymph nodes, resulting in extensive granulomatous tissue reaction and clinical syndromes of chronic diarrhea, vomiting, weight loss, or all. Rare cases of phycomycosis in cats are characterized by ulcerative gastroenteritis. Phycomycosis most commonly affects young large-breed dogs. The most consistent physical findings in intestinal phycomycosis are emaciation and a palpable abdominal mass.

Diagnosis. The diagnosis depends on histologic identification of sparsely septate hyphae within biopsies of stomach, intestine, or abdominal lymph nodes.

Treatment and Prognosis. The prognosis is poor, since successful treatment of phycomycosis has rarely been reported. Surgical excision has been successful in some patients and is the currently recommended treatment, perhaps with long-term follow-up therapy with oral ketoconazole, 10 to 30 mg/kg per day.

OTHER INTESTINAL MYCOSES

Both *Aspergillus* and *Candida* cause mucosal ulceration and necrotizing ulcerations that extend into the deeper layers of the bowel wall, with resultant chronic diarrhea. The antemortem diagnosis of these intestinal mycoses is difficult, usually requiring histologic identification of the fungi in tissue specimens. Information on which to base treatment is limited.

SHORT BOWEL SYNDROME (pp. 1227–1228)

History and Clinical Signs. Short bowel syndrome follows extensive bowel resection and is manifested by progressive weight loss and chronic persistent watery diarrhea that is foul-smelling and without obvious blood or mucus. Weight loss can occur in spite of a ravenous appetite.

Diagnosis. Short bowel syndrome is suspected based on history and clinical signs. Barium contrast radiography of the upper gastrointestinal tract usually demonstrates significantly accelerated stomach-to-colon transit time.

Treatment. Animals should be returned to oral food intake as early as possible to stimulate adaptive hyperplasia. As many as six to eight small low-fat meals should be fed per day. Additional vitamin and mineral supplementation is recommended.

Partial exocrine pancreatic insufficiency is treated with pancreatic enzyme supplementation; intestinal bacterial overgrowth is controlled with appropriate antibiotics such as metronidazole or tetracycline; secondary gastric acid hypersecretion is controlled by use of an oral H-2–receptor antagonist, such as cimetidine 2 to 5 mg/lb (5 to 10 mg/kg) three times a day; rapid intestinal transit time is controlled with motility-modifying antidiarrheal drugs such as diphenoxylate or loperamide; and bile acid–mediated diarrhea in cases of ileal resection is treated with bile salt–binding agents such as cholestyramine. Synthetic somatostatin also helps reduce excessive intestinal secretion.

INTESTINAL NEOPLASIA (pp. 1228–1229)

Adenocarcinoma and lymphosarcoma are the most common intestinal tumors of dogs and cats, respectively. Clinical signs of intestinal neoplasia are typically vague, and the onset is usually slow and insidious. Anorexia and weight loss may be the only early signs, but often diarrhea, vomiting, dehydration, and anemia develop. Abdominal effusion may also occur.

INTESTINAL ADENOCARCINOMA

In the cat, adenocarcinomas most commonly occur in the jejunum and ileum, whereas canine adenocarcinomas occur more frequently in the large intestine and duodenum. Intestinal adenocarcinoma may produce a segmental thickening within the bowel wall with the effect of an expanding mass, or it may grow inward toward the lumen (especially in cats), producing an annular fibrous constricting band with minimal outward enlargement that produces signs of partial obstruction. Local invasion of the mesentery, omentum, and regional lymph nodes is common. Definitive diagnosis is usually made by surgical excision or biopsy of the affected segment of bowel. The prognosis for adenocarcinoma is poor.

INTESTINAL LYMPHOSARCOMA

Intestinal LSA has two morphologic types, the diffuse type and the nodular type. In diffuse LSA, extensive infiltration of the lamina propria and submucosa with neoplastic lymphocytes may cause malabsorption, steatorrhea, diarrhea, and weight loss. In the nodular type, a segmental thickening of the bowel, most often in the ileocolic region, may cause luminal narrowing and partial intestinal obstruction. Metastasis to regional lymph nodes is common in both forms of the disease.

Definitive diagnosis is usually made by biopsy of the affected segment of bowel, most commonly during exploratory laparotomy. In some dogs and cats, an initial biopsy is interpreted as inflammatory bowel disease (lymphocytic-plasmacytic enteritis), but later biopsy (or necropsy) prompted by progression of signs in spite of therapy is read as lymphoma. Dogs respond poorly to all types of chemotherapy, but cats can be readily placed into remission using the "COP" protocol (Chapter 73).

INTESTINAL MAST CELL TUMORS

Primary mast cell tumors occur mainly in aged cats as segmental nodular thickenings involving the small bowel. Metastases occur most frequently in mesenteric lymph nodes, liver, and spleen. Treatment consists of prednisone, cimetidine, and oral antibiotics to control small intestinal bacterial overgrowth.

ADENOMATOUS POLYPS

In contrast to dogs, in which polyps most often occur in the descending colon and rectum, feline polyps occur almost exclusively in the small intestines, mostly in the proximal duodenum within 1 cm of the pylorus and occasionally in the ileum. Polyps sometimes occur as asymptomatic incidental lesions; however, more often they cause partial intestinal obstruction, acute or chronic vomiting, hematemesis, or diarrhea. Contrast radiography or endoscopy can be used for the diagnosis of duodenal polyps. The treatment for intestinal polyps is surgical excision. The prognosis for a full recovery is excellent, although perioperative mortality can be associated with severe blood loss anemia.

DUODENAL ULCERS (p. 1229)

See Chapter 103.

CHAPTER 105

DISEASES OF THE LARGE INTESTINE
(pages 1232–1260)

NORMAL FUNCTION (pp. 1233–1235)

The major functions of the colon in the dog and cat are extraction of water and electrolytes from the ileal effluent, storage of feces, and defecation. Of less importance is microbial fermentation of organic matter that escapes digestion and absorption in the small intestine.

MOTILITY

The majority of muscular contractions arising in the proximal colon are retrograde peristaltic contractions, which are initiated in the transverse colon and propagated toward the cecum. Throughout the colon, rhythmic segmentation, originating in the circular muscle layer, moves contents short distances in both antegrade and retrograde directions, preventing rapid transit. Motility in the distal colon is characterized by spontaneous giant migrating contractions or mass movements that originate in the proximal colon and migrate in an aboral direction over a segment or the entire length of the colon, moving colonic contents toward the rectum in preparation for defecation.

The intrinsic nervous system stimulates segmental contractions and peristalsis in response to distention or through chemoreceptors within the mucosa in response to changes in luminal conditions. The major function of the extrinsic nervous system is in the distal colon, where it participates in the defecation reflex.

WATER AND ELECTROLYTE TRANSPORT

The large bowel normally absorbs a smaller quantity of water than the small intestine, but does so much more efficiently.

COLONIC MICROFLORA

Anaerobic (spore- and non-spore-forming) bacteria predominate, accounting for up to 90 per cent of the microflora. Physiologic mechanisms that maintain normal colonic microflora and prevent disease induced by bacterial overgrowth or colonization of pathologic organisms include the presence of normal colonic motility, maintenance of the mucosal barrier, and local immune factors.

DIAGNOSTIC EVALUATION OF THE LARGE INTESTINE
(pp. 1235–1239)

HISTORY AND CLINICAL SIGNS

Large bowel diarrhea often is associated with excess fecal mucus, tenesmus, or hematochezia (see Table 104-3). With most large bowel diseases, the animals remain bright, alert, and active, and maintain normal appetites. Weight loss is uncommon but, if present, may suggest concurrent involvement of the small intestine, systemic disease, metastatic neoplasia, or severe ulcerative disease or whipworm infection. Abnormally shaped stools may occur in cases of neoplasia or

---

Original chapter written by Michael S. Leib and Michael E. Matz

stricture. Rectal hemorrhage, independent of defecation, can occur in some cases of neoplasia.

In our experience, approximately 50 per cent of cases of large bowel diarrhea are associated with parasitic or dietary causes. Physical examination is usually normal. Abdominal pain may be present in irritable bowel syndrome, some cases of whipworms, regional enterocolitis, colonic perforation secondary to neurologic disorders or cecal neoplasia, and bacterial disorders. Pyrexia may indicate the presence of inflammatory bowel disease, histoplasmosis, ruptured cecal tumors, or bacterial disorders. A midabdominal mass may be present in cases of intussusception, smooth muscle tumors of the cecum, foreign body, regional enterocolitis, and eosinophilic granulomatous colitis. Rarely, animals may present with extreme weakness or collapse associated with whipworm infection, peritonitis from colonic perforation associated with neurologic disease or cecal neoplasia, salmonellosis, or severe dehydration from profuse diarrhea of any cause.

FECAL EXAMINATION

See Chapter 104.

COLONOSCOPY

Because many colonic diseases diffusely affect the large intestine, examination with a rigid endoscope, which allows visualization of the descending colon, is diagnostic in approximately 80 per cent of cases. Examination of the transverse colon, ascending colon, and cecum requires a more expensive flexible endoscope. Rigid endoscopy requires only light sedation, whereas flexible endoscopy requires heavy sedation or general anesthesia. Multiple biopsy samples should always be obtained, even if the mucosa appears normal, because histologic abnormalities can be present. Biopsy samples should be obtained as deeply as possible and ideally should include the muscularis mucosa.

RADIOGRAPHY

Survey abdominal radiographs usually provide minimal information for diagnosing disorders of the large intestine. However, some neoplastic or granulomatous masses, colonic foreign bodies, or sublumbar lymphadenopathy can be identified. A dilated feces-filled colon is present in cases of megacolon.

Colonoscopic examination has largely replaced the need to perform complete barium enema examinations. However, complete barium enema is indicated in three situations: (1) when luminal narrowing prohibits passage of an endoscope, (2) when only a rigid endoscope is available and examination of the descending colon is normal, or (3) when abdominal palpation or survey radiographs identify a mural or extramural mass associated with the colon and the mucosa is found to be normal on endoscopic examination.

Ultrasonography

Assessment of wall thickness and symmetry, identification of wall layers and intraluminal contents, and identification of regional lymph node enlargement or other abdominal organ involvement are possible by ultrasonographic examination. The limiting factor in evaluation of the large bowel is the presence of air or feces, which often limits examination.

DIARRHEA-CAUSING DISORDERS (pp. 1239–1252)

DIETARY INDISCRETION

See Chapter 104.

WHIPWORM INFECTION

Trichuris vulpis infection is one of the most common causes of acute or chronic large bowel diarrhea in dogs. Abdominal pain, inappetence, and weight loss can also occur. Occasionally, dogs may experience an acute crisis resembling hypoadrenocorticism. In these cases, severe dehydration, prerenal azotemia, hyperglycemia, hyponatremia, hyperkalemia, hypochloremia, and hypercalcemia were present. Some had metabolic acidosis. Dogs responded rapidly to intense intravenous fluid therapy. Long-term cure was provided by appropriate anthelmintics for whipworms.

Whipworm eggs can be identified by means of routine fecal flotation procedures. However, if multiple fecal examinations fail to identify eggs, treatment for whipworms should be instituted before additional diagnostic tests are performed. Therapeutic agents effective against whipworms in dogs include fenbendazole, 22.7 mg/lb (50 mg/kg) PO q24h for 3 days; butamisole, 1.1 mg/lb (2.2 mg/kg) SC; dichlorvos, 13.6 mg/lb (30 mg/kg) PO; mebendazole, 10 mg/lb (22 mg/kg) PO q24h for 3 days; febantel with praziquantel, 4.5 mg/lb (10 mg/kg) PO q24h for 3 days in adult dogs and 6.8 mg/lb (15 mg/kg) PO q24h for 3 days in puppies less than 6 months of age; or febantel without praziquantel, 4.5 mg/lb (10 mg/kg) PO q24h for 3 days or 6.8 mg/lb (15 mg/kg) PO q24h for 3 days in puppies.

Treatment should be repeated in 3 weeks and again in 3 months. Frequent disposal of feces will help to reduce reinfection. In severe, recurrent cases, heartworm prophylaxis with milbemycin oxime (0.23 mg/lb [0.5 mg/kg] PO once a month) or diethylcarbamazine/oxibendazole (2.27 mg/lb [5.0 mg/kg] PO q24h) will help to control whipworm infection. Cats are rarely infected with whipworms. Clients should be warned of the possible public health significance and instructed in the appropriate sanitary measures for the disposal of fecal material.

INFLAMMATORY BOWEL DISEASE

See Chapter 104.

History and Clinical Signs

The predominant clinical sign in dogs and cats with colitis associated with IBD is diarrhea. A moderately to severely increased frequency of defecation occurs along with reduced fecal volume per defecation. Tenesmus, hematochezia, and excess mucus often are present. Weight loss and vomiting occur less frequently and may be related to concurrent involvement of the stomach and/or small intestine and not to colonic inflammation. In the early stages of IBD, clinical signs often are mild and intermittent. As the condition progresses, diarrhea often gradually increases in frequency and intensity, and may become continuous. During severe episodes, mild pyrexia, depression, and anorexia may occur. Thickened segments of bowel may be detected during abdominal palpation if small intestinal involvement is present.

Laboratory Evaluation

No consistent or diagnostic pattern of laboratory abnormalities in animals with IBD has been identified.

Radiographic, Endoscopic, and Histopathologic Findings

The definitive diagnosis of colitis requires histopathologic evaluation of mucosal biopsy samples, which may be obtained during colonoscopy (see Chapter 104).

Therapeutic Management

Dietary Management. Because of the potential role of dietary antigens as either a primary or secondary factor in the pathogenesis of

IBD, hypoallergenic diets have been recommended as the initial treatment (see Chapter 104).

Sulfasalazine. The treatment of choice for dogs with colitis that do not respond to dietary management is sulfasalazine. The recommended dosage range for sulfasalazine in dogs is 10 to 25 mg/lb (20 to 50 mg/kg) to a maximum of 1.0 gm q8h. High dosages may be needed in chronic cases. One of the most common therapeutic mistakes is discontinuation of therapy too soon after resolution of clinical signs, which can lead to diarrhea that may be refractory to the therapy that previously controlled clinical signs. After the dog has normal feces for 4 weeks, the dosing frequency should be reduced to q12h. After an additional 4 weeks without diarrhea, maintenance dosages should be decreased by 50 per cent, still given q12h. In some dogs sulfasalazine can be discontinued, whereas in other cases, long-term therapy is required.

In dogs, only vomiting and keratoconjunctivitis sicca are common side effects. Vomiting can usually be controlled by administering medication with food or using an enteric-coated preparation. If decreased tear production is detected early, reducing the dosage or discontinuing the drug may result in increased tear production and prevent progression to keratoconjunctivitis sicca.

Corticosteroids. Corticosteroids are the drugs of choice for cats with colitis that have failed to respond to dietary management (see Chapter 104). In cats, an initial dose of prednisone or prednisolone of 0.25 to 1.0 mg/lb (0.5 to 2.0 mg/kg) q24h often will improve clinical signs within 7 to 10 days. After normal feces have been produced for approximately 4 weeks, the dosage should be decreased by 50 per cent. As long as diarrhea does not recur, the dosage can gradually be reduced until the least amount given every other day that controls clinical signs is reached. Some cats require long-term treatment, whereas in others, it is possible to discontinue prednisone within 3 to 4 months. In cats that cannot tolerate daily oral medication, injectable long-acting methylprednisone acetate, 20 mg subcutaneously, can be administered every 2 to 4 weeks. In dogs, corticosteroids can be used as a single treatment or, more commonly, to reduce the sulfasalazine dosage.

Metronidazole. Although most veterinary authors suggest that it be used in conjunction with sulfasalazine or prednisone, it can be used to manage dogs and cats with IBD as a single agent. See Chapter 104.

Other Immunosuppressive Agents. See Chapter 104.

Tylosin. Tylosin can be tried in cases that do not respond to dietary management, sulfasalazine, prednisone, or metronidazole, or when adverse effects to these medications are encountered.

EOSINOPHILIC COLITIS

See Chapter 104. As a group, affected dogs tend to be younger than those with plasmacytic lymphocytic colitis. In dogs, mucosal ulceration occurs more commonly than in other forms of IBD. Most authors consider the prognosis to be excellent. In cats, the prognosis is more guarded than in cases of plasmacytic lymphocytic colitis. Early diagnosis and aggressive therapy are necessary to control clinical signs. Cats often require long-term therapy. Response in dogs should be rapid.

NEOPLASIA

Studies of colonic tumors in dogs have revealed that approximately one-third are benign, with adenomas most common, and two-thirds malignant, with adenocarcinoma (AC) and lymphosarcoma (LSA) most common. In cats, almost all colonic tumors are malignant, and LSA is most common. The clinical signs caused by colonic neoplasia are often indistinguishable from other large bowel disorders. Rectal tumors may be associated with rectal prolapse.

Benign Neoplasia

Adenomas are the most common benign tumors found in the colon, but rarely leiomyoma, papilloma, or fibroma can occur. Masses frequently occur in the distal colon and rectum, often within 3 cm of the anus. The most common clinical sign is hematochezia. Feces may be well formed but on occasion are soft and contain excess mucus. Digital rectal examination will often identify a mass and may result in discomfort and hemorrhage. In most cases of adenoma only single masses occur, but occasionally multiple tumors are present. Many adenomas can be extruded through the anus and removed with submucosal resection. Prognosis for long-term survival is excellent, although recurrence has been reported.

Leiomyomas most often occur in the rectum. Because they do not invade the mucosa, hematochezia and excess fecal mucus are uncommon. They often become very large before compressing the colon and causing diarrhea, tenesmus, constipation, or abnormally shaped stools. Survey abdominal radiographs showed evidence of extraluminal rectal compression in 50 per cent of dogs. Endoscopic biopsy would be expected to obtain normal mucosal tissue and would not help to achieve a correct diagnosis. The tumor can be removed by blunt dissection. Prognosis is excellent, as recurrence is uncommon.

Malignant Neoplasia

Adenocarcinoma. Clinical signs include diarrhea, hematochezia, tenesmus, dyschezia, abnormally shaped stools, and rectal bleeding not associated with defecation. Hematochezia, weight loss, anorexia, diarrhea, and vomiting are common signs in cats with colonic tumors. Gross mucosal ulceration appears to be more common in colonic tumors than in small bowel tumors.

Lymphosarcoma. See Chapter 104.

Leiomyosarcoma. These tumors are rare in cats. Most occurred in old dogs of medium to large size; in two cases they were incidental findings. Clinical signs included anorexia, lethargy, fever, vomiting, collapse, and diarrhea. An abdominal mass can be palpated in approximately 50 per cent of cases. However, in all cases of LMS, dogs that survive surgery have a good long-term prognosis.

IRRITABLE BOWEL SYNDROME

In dogs, IBS is an exclusion diagnosis. The most common clinical sign is large bowel diarrhea with excess fecal mucus, dyschezia, urgency to defecate, and increased frequency of defecation. Hematochezia is infrequent. Intermittent bloating, nausea, vomiting, and abdominal pain may occur. A thorough diagnostic plan must be followed without finding evidence of any other known disorder before a diagnosis of IBS can be made.

The intermittent nature of clinical signs often makes assessment of therapy difficult. If a stress factor can be identified, removal or modification can be beneficial. Diets high in fiber are often helpful in eliminating or reducing clinical signs in dogs. Episodes of diarrhea can be controlled by administration of motility-modifying agents such as loperamide or diphenoxylate. They can often be used for several days to a week and discontinued after the diarrhea resolves (see Dietary Indiscretion).

Pain can often be relieved by antispasmodic agents, and the effects of stressors can be reduced by sedatives. Librax capsules contain the sedative chlordiazepoxide (5 mg) and clidinium bromide (2.5 mg), an anticholinergic agent. A suggested dosage is 0.05 to 0.125 mg/lb (0.1 to 0.250 mg/kg) of clidinium q8–12h. The drug can be given when the owner first notices abdominal pain or diarrhea and can usually be discontinued after a few days. Other anticholinergics such as propantheline (Pro-Banthine 0.125 mg/lb [0.25 mg/kg]), hyoscyamine (Levsin 0.0015–0.003 mg/lb [0.003–0.006 mg/kg]), or dicyclomine (Bentyl 0.075 mg/lb [0.15 mg/kg] q8–12h) have been suggested. The prognosis for IBS in dogs is guarded. Affected dogs may have intermittent clinical signs for years.

FIBER-RESPONSIVE LARGE BOWEL DIARRHEA

Diagnosis is based on exclusion of known causes of large bowel diarrhea after performing a thorough diagnostic evaluation. Good response has been seen when dogs were fed a highly digestible diet supplemented with a mean of 2 tbs/day (0.7–6.0) psyllium hydrophilic mucilloid (Metamucil). Until colonic motility studies can be performed, the relationship between IBS and fiber-responsive large bowel diarrhea (FRLBD) remains clouded. Only rarely do dogs with IBS respond to dietary fiber supplementation alone.

CLOSTRIDIUM PERFRINGENS ENTEROTOXICOSIS

The disorder occurs most commonly in dogs, but is seen occasionally in cats. Acute and chronic large bowel diarrhea occurs commonly. Vomiting, weight loss, flatulence, and abdominal pain occur less frequently. Enterotoxin has also been identified in some cases of hemorrhagic gastroenteritis syndrome, parvovirus, giardiasis, and IBD.

Diagnosis can be confirmed by identifying enterotoxin in a small fecal sample by use of a reverse latex agglutination test (PET-RPLA Kit) available at many human diagnostic laboratories. Fecal samples should be collected when clinical signs are present. Diagnosis should also be suspected when more than two or three spores per oil immersion field are found in a rectal cytology specimen.

Acute cases often resolve spontaneously. Chronic cases respond to antibiotic therapy in 3 to 5 days. Metronidazole, ampicillin, or amoxicillin is an effective treatment. Cases that show intermittent clinical signs require long-term therapy. Tylosin can be used in these cases (see Inflammatory Bowel Disease). Some cases respond to a high-fiber diet.

UNCOMMON DIARRHEA-CAUSING DISORDERS
(pp. 1252–1257)

HISTOPLASMOSIS

See Chapter 104. Intestinal histoplasmosis is the most common form of disseminated disease in dogs, whereas intestinal involvement is comparatively rare in cats. Signs of large bowel diarrhea usually predominate.

INTUSSUSCEPTION

See Chapter 104. Ileocolic intussusceptions are the most common type of intussusception involving the colon and account for the majority of all intestinal intussusceptions in dogs and cats. Colocolic and colorectal intussusceptions are rarely observed.

Inversion of the cecum into the proximal colon is uncommon, but occurs in large-breed male dogs. Cecal inversion has been associated with parasitism and typhlitis. Chronic intermittent hematochezia and soft stools develop. Cecal inversions are usually not palpable. Barium enema or endoscopy is usually diagnostic. Ultrasonographic findings have not been reported. Cecal resection is curative.

COLONIC ULCERATION SECONDARY TO NEUROLOGIC DISEASE

See Chapter 104. Surgical management of dogs with neurologic problems that are treated with corticosteroids often results in gastrointestinal hemorrhage and infrequently in colonic perforation. Perforation occurs most commonly on the antimesenteric border, near the left colic (splenic) flexure. The onset of clinical signs occurs at a mean of 5 days following surgery.

HISTIOCYTIC ULCERATIVE COLITIS

Histiocytic ulcerative colitis (HUC) is an uncommon, chronic, idiopathic large bowel disease characterized by diarrhea and progressive colonic ulceration. The disease occurs most commonly in Boxers under two years of age, with the exception of rare reports in French bulldogs and cats. Initially, the dogs retain normal body condition, but as the disease progresses, weight loss and debilitation occur as a result of chronic intestinal blood and protein loss. A corrugated, thickened mucosa, hemorrhage, or pain may be evident on digital rectal examination.

Anemia and panhypoproteinemia may be recognized. Numerous erythrocytes and neutrophils are often found on rectal cytology specimens. Colonoscopic findings are variable and include punctate to diffuse foci of mucosal hyperemia, edema, and erosion; well circumscribed ulcers; thickened irregular mucosal folds; or strictures.

Treatment is similar to that described in the section on IBD, with sulfasalazine the drug of choice. If histiocytic colitis is advanced at the time of diagnosis, treatment often does not improve clinical signs, and a poor prognosis is warranted.

BACTERIAL DISORDERS

See Chapter 104 for *salmonellosis, campylobacteriosis, yersiniosis, colibacillosis,* and *pseudomembranous colitis.*

PARASITIC DISORDERS

See Chapter 104 for *trichomoniasis* and *ancylostomiasis.*

Entamoebiasis

Entamoeba histolytica is a protozoan parasite of the large bowel which primarily infects human beings and rarely dogs. A single case of spontaneous amebiasis has recently been reported in cats. Infected animals may remain asymptomatic or may demonstrate signs ranging from mild chronic bowel diarrhea to fulminant bloody dysentery.

Balantidiasis

Clinical signs associated with *Balantidium coli* infections in the dog are uncommon and have not been reported in the cat. Most infections in dogs are associated with exposure to swine.

REGIONAL ENTEROCOLITIS

This is characterized by a transmural granulomatous inflammatory response which can involve the stomach, distal ileum, cecum, proximal colon, distal colon, and rectum. Regional enterocolitis predominantly occurs in male dogs 4 years of age or less. It is associated with weight loss and chronic large and small bowel diarrhea, which may contain frank blood and/or mucus. Discomfort and thickened bowel loops may be noted on abdominal palpation. Perianal fistulas may be present. A mild to moderate eosinophilia and panhypoproteinemia are the most common laboratory abnormalities. A biopsy is necessary for a definitive diagnosis.

When partial or complete luminal obstructive lesions occur, surgical excision of the affected region is indicated for diagnostic and therapeutic purposes. The course of the disease is usually progressive. In the majority of reported cases, the dogs died or underwent euthanasia following surgical intervention.

HETEROBILHARZIASIS

See Chapter 104.

PROTOTHECOSIS

The organism eventually disseminates via hematogenous and lymphatic routes to other tissues, such as the eyes, central nervous system, kidneys, and mesenteric lymph nodes. The majority of cases occur in female dogs, and a disproportionate number have occurred in collies. The most common clinical sign is chronic, intermittent, hemorrhagic, large bowel diarrhea. Weight loss and debilitation occur as the disease progresses. CNS or ocular abnormalities may be present.

Diagnosis of prototothecosis requires demonstration of the organism in rectal scrapings, colonic biopsies, urine sediment, or culture of vitreous humor or cerebral spinal fluid. Successful treatment of disseminated disease has not been reported.

CONSTIPATION-CAUSING DISORDERS (p. 1257)

MEGACOLON

Megacolon is an uncommon condition, seen more frequently in cats than in dogs, characterized by diffuse colonic dilation with ineffective motility. Idiopathic megacolon may be congenital, but more commonly it is acquired later in life. Mechanical obstruction secondary to malunion of pelvic fractures occurs principally in cats. Intramural and extramural masses, strictures, and rarely foreign bodies can also result in obstruction. Functional obstruction secondary to metabolic diseases (e.g., hypokalemia or hypothyroidism), trauma resulting in damage to colonic innervation, and neuromuscular disorders are infrequent causes of acquired megacolon.

Constipation is the predominant clinical sign in animals with megacolon. Tenesmus and frequent attempts to defecate are commonly observed. Passage of liquid feces, which may contain mucus or blood, may occur secondary to colonic inflammation. If intractable constipation (obstipation) develops, dehydration, weakness, and vomiting may occur.

Abdominal palpation and digital rectal examination identify a markedly distended colon, packed with firm feces. Survey abdominal radiographs confirm the presence of megacolon and may identify abdominal masses, pelvic fractures, or vertebral lesions. If only mild to moderate constipation is present, bisacodyl (Dulcolax) or docusate sodium suppositories (Colace) may be given. In most cases, the animal fails to respond, and enemas must be administered. If systemic signs are present, such as vomiting, weakness and anorexia, fluid and electrolyte balance should be restored before the stool is evacuated. In severely obstipated animals, manual removal of the feces in an anesthetized patient is usually necessary.

Following complete removal of the feces, long-term medical management consists of dietary modifications combined with laxatives and periodic administration of enemas. Cisapride is often effective orally in cats. Recurrent episodes of constipation or obstipation are common. Subtotal colectomy has been successfully used in cats and a limited number of dogs.

CHAPTER 106

PATHOPHYSIOLOGY, LABORATORY DIAGNOSIS, AND DISEASES OF THE LIVER
(pages 1261–1371)

A. Laboratory Diagnosis of Hepatobiliary Disorders
(pages 1261–1312)

HISTORICAL AND PHYSICAL SIGNS OF HEPATOBILIARY DISEASE (pp. 1266–1268)

Gastrointestinal abnormalities, including anorexia, nausea, vomiting, diarrhea, and constipation, are among the most common signs in a patient with hepatobiliary disease, and with chronicity, these lead to weight loss. Anorexia and ptyalism are especially common in cats.

The development of bleeding tendencies is expected in patients with extrahepatic bile duct occlusion. Animals with chronic intrahepatic cholestasis and/or acquired hepatic insufficiency may develop bleeding tendencies.

Jaundice rapidly develops when the major bile duct is occluded. Hyperbilirubinemia develops within 12 hours and overt jaundice within 3 days. In the cat with cholestatic liver disease, the development of hyperbilirubinemia is heralded by the presence of bilirubinuria, where, unlike the dog, bilirubinuria is abnormal at any urine specific gravity. When large quantities of bilirubin pigments are passed, feces become dark green or dark green-orange. This is most common with hemolytic or prehepatic jaundice. Pale gray or tan acholic feces may be observed when bile flow is obstructed.

Polydipsia and polyuria may be major presenting complaints in patients with serious but occult liver disease. Neurobehavioral signs of hepatic encephalopathy develop in animals with severe acquired liver insufficiency or young patients with congenital portosystemic vascular anomalies. Typical signs include ptyalism and aggression (in the cat), ataxia, lethargy, stupor, head pressing, propulsive circling, amaurosis (sudden unexplained blindness), seizures, and, in some cases, coma.

HEMATOLOGY (pp. 1269–1270)

A regenerative anemia caused by blood loss associated with gastrointestinal ulceration and/or a coagulopathy occasionally is recognized. More commonly, anemia is nonregenerative (normocytic, normochromic). Erythrocyte microcytosis is associated with both acquired and congenital portosystemic shunting in the dog and cat. Thrombocytopenia may develop.

SERUM BIOCHEMISTRY (pp. 1270–1275)

ALBUMIN

Albumin is a nonspecific marker because its concentration reflects hepatic synthesis, rate of degradation, pathologic excretion, and volume of distribution.

Original section written by Sharon A. Center

GLOBULINS

Although acute-phase proteins can contribute to an increased total serum globulin concentration, the total serum globulin concentration is not a good measure of liver synthetic function because of the large component composed of immunoglobulins derived from other sources.

LIVER ENZYMES

Many systemic conditions and medications are associated with increased serum enzyme activity in the absence of serious hepatobiliary consequences. Important and representative examples are discussed in this section and shown in Tables 106–3 and 106–5 of the textbook. Liver enzyme induction is common in the dog and is the major reason for confusion in determining the clinical significance of abnormal enzyme activity. Severe hepatic dysfunction associated with end-stage cirrhosis and congenital portosystemic vascular malformations can exist in the absence of serum enzyme abnormalities. Caution must therefore be exercised in the interpretation of quiet liver enzyme activity. Enzymes should not be used as prognostic indicators unless they are sequentially monitored and a liver biopsy has been accomplished.

Alanine Aminotransferase (ALT)

Immediate increase in serum ALT activity follows hepatocellular injury or altered cell membrane permeability. After acute, severe, diffuse hepatocellular necrosis, serum ALT activity sharply increases within 24 to 48 hours up to 100-fold normal (or higher). Extrahepatic bile duct occlusion incurs a more gradual ALT increase of lesser initial magnitude. Microsomal enzyme induction in dogs commonly causes smaller increases in ALT activity than necrosis or bile duct occlusion. In the dog, marked increases in serum ALT activity may develop in association with primary hepatic neoplasia, secondary neoplasia, and nodular hyperplasia. The serum activity of ALT in cats may be increased from 2- to 45-fold normal in hepatic necrosis, cholangitis, or cholangiohepatitis; 2- to 10-fold normal in hepatic lipidosis; and 2- to 5-fold normal in severe acute anemia, septicemia, and feline leukemia virus–associated disorders.

Aspartate Aminotransferase (AST)

Increased serum AST activity can result from altered membrane permeability, necrosis, inflammation, and, in the dog, microsomal enzyme induction. Liver disease–related AST activity parallels increased ALT activity. In some cats with liver disease, AST may be a more sensitive indicator of hepatobiliary disease than ALT.

Alkaline Phosphatase (ALP)

In the dog, ALP has high sensitivity but low specificity as a test for liver disease. In the cat, it has a lower sensitivity but is more specific. Three major ALP isoenzymes are commonly identified in canine serum: bone, liver, and corticosteroid induced. In the dog, the liver and glucocorticoid isoenzymes are primarily responsible for serum ALP activity; in the cat, the liver isoenzyme is primarily responsible.

The clinical utility of ALP in the dog is not improved by isoenzyme determination. The largest increases in serum ALP are associated with diffuse or focal cholestatic disorders, primary hepatic neoplasms, and, in the dog, enzyme induction. Many extrahepatic and hepatic conditions may promote increased production of the hepatic ALP isoenzyme, particularly in the dog. Hepatic parenchymal inflammation and systemic infection or inflammation may cause secondary intrahepatic cholestasis.

The corticosteroid isoenzyme in the dog develops in animals treated with glucocorticoids, in those with spontaneous or iatrogenic hyperadrenocorticism, in dogs with hepatic or nonhepatic neoplasia, and, most important, in dogs with many different chronic illnesses. The feline liver is, by comparison, relatively insensitive to glucocorticoids. In the dog, the serum activity of the liver ALP isoenzyme may be increased by administration of the anticonvulsants phenobarbital, primidone, and phenytoin.

Gamma-Glutamyl Transferase (GGT)

Increased serum GGT activity commonly is associated with intrahepatic or extrahepatic cholestasis or pancreatitis. Glucocorticoids and certain other microsomal enzyme-inducing drugs may stimulate GGT production similar to their influence on hepatic ALP. In the cat, GGT activity may be more markedly increased in certain hepatobiliary disorders than is ALP activity. Examples include some cats with cirrhosis, major bile duct obstruction, or intrahepatic cholestasis. It is unknown whether corticosteroids or other enzyme inducers influence serum GGT activity in the cat. Clinical experience suggests that this does not occur.

MISCELLANEOUS CAUSES OF LIVER ENZYME ABNORMALITIES (pp. 1276–1277)

GLUCOCORTICOID EFFECTS

Enzyme changes induced with glucocorticoids are dependent on individual response, dose of drug, and the particular drug used. Most dogs with enzyme induction as a result of glucocorticoid induction have not developed hepatic dysfunction.

ANTICONVULSANT MEDICATIONS

Primidone, phenytoin, and phenobarbital, administered singly or in combination, cause variable increases in liver enzyme activity in the dog. Some dogs receiving chronic anticonvulsant therapy develop morphologic liver injury and functional impairment. Continued administration of traditional anticonvulsants in a patient with compromised liver function may result in drug intoxication, somnolence, or coma.

FELINE HYPERTHYROIDISM

Hyperthyroidism usually is associated with increased serum transaminases and ALP activity. Evidence of liver dysfunction appears to be uncommon in the cat.

PASSIVE CONGESTION AND CONGESTIVE HEART FAILURE

Acute and chronic passive congestion of the liver may result in mild to moderate increases in serum ALP and transaminase activities.

HEPATIC NEOPLASIA

Increases in the transaminases, ALP, and GGT are variable.

MISCELLANEOUS METABOLIC DISORDERS

Increased liver enzyme activity, particularly of ALP, is common in dogs with hypothyroidism and in dogs and cats with diabetes mellitus and pancreatitis. Disorders associated with endotoxemia, septicemia, anoxia, hyperthermia, thromboembolism, changes in hepatic perfusion caused by hypotension, and microsomal enzyme induction in the dog may be associated with increased serum ALP, GGT, ALT, and AST activity. In most instances, the magnitudes of increase do not exceed twofold to threefold normal. Idiosyncratic drug reactions resulting in biochemical changes and hepatic pathology are discussed in Chapter 62.

CARBOHYDRATE METABOLISM (pp. 1277–1278)

Causes of hepatogenic hypoclycemia include insufficient parenchymal mass, insufficient enzymes or substrates for gluconeogenesis or glycogenolysis, glucagon resistance, portosystemic shunting, and the presence of a hepatic tumor. Hepatogenic hypoglycemia should alert the clinician to consider acute fulminant hepatic failure, decompensated end-stage chronic liver disease, or severe portosystemic shunting.

Some dogs with cirrhosis develop glucose intolerance and a unique dermatologic condition. Affected dogs develop periocular and perioral erythema, crusting, and alopecia and severe hyperkeratotic footpads that crack and cause a great deal of discomfort. This has been termed necrolytic migratory erythema (hepatocutaneous syndrome). A relation with high serum glucagon levels has not been documented.

EFFECT OF LIVER DISEASE ON PLASMA LIPIDS AND LIPOPROTEINS (pp. 1278–1279)

Cholesterol synthesis is increased in obstructive jaundice. Hypercholesterolemia may also be associated with metabolic derangements stemming from other primary disease processes such as hypothyroidism, diabetes mellitus, pancreatitis, hyperadrenocorticism, nephrotic syndrome, familial hyperlipidemia, and renal insufficiency (in the cat). In some dogs receiving anticonvulsants, a progressive hepatopathy may develop, and in these, marked hypocholesterolemia correlates with severe hepatic insufficiency.

The formation of very low-density lipoprotein (VLDL) is an important mechanism by which the liver can extract excess fatty acids from plasma and mobilize it for storage elsewhere. Abnormalities in the transport of VLDL from the liver or an imbalance resulting in a greater accumulation than dispersal of triglycerides can result in hepatic lipidosis. Affected animals have not been shown to be consistently hypertriglyceridemic, hypercholesterolemic, or diabetic.

HEMOSTASIS (pp. 1279–1281)

The liver is the origin of all the coagulation factors with the exceptions of factor VIII and calcium. Bleeding in patients with liver disease is not common and is primarily due to provocative local factor—such as gastritis, ulcers, invasive procedures, or other medical problems—rather than to spontaneous hemorrhage. The severity of coagulation abnormalities seems to depend on the degree and type of hepatocellular injury.

The prothrombin coagulant factors II, VII, IX, and X are dependent on vitamin K for activation. The vitamin K cycle must be functional if thses factors are to be normally activated. Conditions resulting in vitamin K deficiency include intestinal malabsorption, major bile duct obstruction, biliary fistula, intestinal sterilization, and antagonism by warfarin-like compounds. Prolongation of the PT is the first demonstrable abnormality of the routinely used coagulation tests after vitamin K depletion.

Fibrinogen is synthesized exclusively in hepatocytes. It may increase in response to acute or chronic liver disease or any other systemic inflammatory, infectious, or necrotizing process. It is only with acute liver failure or decompensated chronic liver disease that synthetic failure is realized. Excessive catabolism of available fibrinogen may occur when liver disease is associated with disseminated intravascular coagulation (DIC). DIC may be a sequela to various hepatic disorders as well as various viral diseases that can lead to liver disease.

The overall management of the hemostatic disorders recognized in patients with hepatobiliary disease is dependent on the patient's clinical status. Blood transfusions should be reserved for patients undergoing active hemorrhage or those with documented coagulation deficiencies that must undergo surgical manipulations. Only fresh blood should be transfused. Gastrointestinal bleeding should be addressed with H-2–receptor blockers and gastric protectants. Invasive diagnostic procedures should be minimized.

VITAMIN METABOLISM (p. 1282)

Most of the water-soluble vitamins are activated in the liver. Hepatocellular necrosis, functional insufficiency, biliary obstruction, and the nutritional and hormonal dysregulations that develop in liver disease contribute to the deprivation of active or available vitamins.

BILIRUBIN METABOLISM (pp. 1282–1283)

Bilirubin pigments are derived from hemoglobin, myoglobin, cytochromes, and other heme-containing enzymes. The processing of heme derived from hemoglobin occurs in mononuclear macrophages of the reticuloendothelial system. The heme moiety is converted to biliverdin. Biliverdin is converted to unconjugated bilirubin, which is then released in the systemic circulation. Unconjugated bilirubin is transformed into conjugated bilirubin within the hepatocyte. When bilirubin has restricted entry into the biliary tract or when excessive liberation of heme pigments overwhelms the hepatobiliary processing and excretion of bilirubin, pigments regurgitate into the systemic circulation, causing hyperbilirubinemia and jaundice.

Dogs have a so-called low renal threshold for bilirubin elimination and, thus, routinely test positive for urine bilirubin. Cats do not eliminate bilirubin in urine under normal circumstances; thus, finding urine bilirubin signals the presence of hyperbilirubinemia. After conjugation and transport into the biliary system, bilirubin is expelled into the intestines in bile. The absence of bilirubin, such as occurs in extrahepatic bile duct occlusion, results in a pale tan or gray acholic stool.

URINE UROBILINOGEN (p. 1283)

Used as a test for the detection of liver disease, urobilinogen has its best application in the jaundiced patient, where its absence implies a lack of bile duct patency.

SERUM AND URINE BILIRUBIN IN THE DIFFERENTIAL DIAGNOSES OF JAUNDICE (pp. 1284–1286)

When liver disease is responsible for jaundice, a severe diffuse cholestatic disorder or major bile duct obstruction should be suspected. The total bilirubin concentration cannot differentiate between various disorders because there is wide overlapping in the bilirubin concentrations.

Because bilirubinuria is evident before tissue jaundice, it is acknowledged as a useful screening test for liver disease. Bilirubin normally is present in the urine of dogs, albeit in small amounts. Detection of urine bilirubin at any urine specific gravity in the cat is a strong indication of either a hepatobiliary or a hemolytic disorder. Differentiating between extrahepatic and intrahepatic cholestasis cannot be accomplished on the basis of laboratory tests alone.

BILIRUBIN TOXICITY (p. 1286)

Bilirubin toxicity is a rare clinical diagnosis in the dog or cat. Renal toxicity includes formation of bile casts and pigmented droplets in tubular epithelium and glomerular mesangium. Bilirubin toxicity may interplay with bile salt toxicity in the development of hepatocellular injury resulting from cholestasis.

AMMONIA AND UREA METABOLISM (pp. 1287–1290)

The liver is of central importance in the regulation of ammonia. About 80 to 90 per cent of ammonia delivered to the liver is converted to urea in the urea cycle. In hepatic insufficiency, ammonia is not adequately detoxified and enters the systemic circulation. Although ammonia is highly neurotoxic, the exact mechanism of its role in hepatic encephalopathy remains controversial.

Urea is synthesized in the liver as the major metabolic end product of hepatic ammonia detoxification. Because of the large functional reserve and tremendous regenerative capabilities of the liver, evidence of an insufficient urea cycle is a fairly late development in acquired disease. Insufficient ammonia detoxification can result from a reduction in hepatic mass, a decline in activity of hepatocellular enzymes, or portosystemic shunting. In clinical patients, ammonia intolerance most often is encountered in those with congenital portosystemic shunts or acquired liver disease associated with intrahepatic or extrahepatic circulatory deviations.

A low blood urea nitrogen (BUN) concentration can reflect a reduced ability to synthesize urea. As a test of liver insufficiency, however, the BUN has low sensitivity and low specificity. In exceptional cases, hyperammonemia develops as a result of unusual inborn metabolic aberrations.

BLOOD AMMONIA DETERMINATIONS

Ammonia measurements have high specificity but low sensitivity for the detection of serious liver disease. Clinical laboratory determination of blood ammonia values requires laborious efforts at maintaining high quality control. Samples must be immediately stored on ice, centrifuged in a precooled environment, and assayed as soon as possible (within 1 hour is recommended). Hyperammonemia is more consistently documented after a provocative test of hepatic ammonia detoxification.

AMMONIA TOLERANCE TESTING

Ammonia tolerance testing can be accomplished using solutions of ammonium chloride (NH_4Cl) administered orally, per rectum by catheter-administered enema, or by oral administration of a powder in a gelatin capsule. The standard oral tolerance test is conducted after oral administration of 45 mg/lb (100 mg/kg) body weight of NH_4Cl in a dilute solution. A control sample from a fasted, healthy animal should be concurrently evaluated. In normal animals, blood ammonia concentrations remain unchanged or increase up to twofold greater than baseline fasting values at 30 minutes. In animals with compromised hepatic function, fasting ammonia values may be normal or up to 10-fold normal.

AMMONIUM URATE CRYSTALLURIA AND CALCULI
(pp. 1290–1291)

Ammonium biurate crystalluria and/or calculi, especially in young animals, warrants thorough investigation for a congenital portosystemic shunt. Crystals usually are golden brown, variably shaped, and commonly referred to as "thorn-apple" in configuration. Clinical management of ammonium urate urolithiasis requires that liver function be appraised first. Cystic uroliths that cause clinical signs require surgical removal. In patients that do not optimally respond to surgical management, medical intervention aimed at reduction of hyperammonemia is undertaken.

SERUM BILE ACIDS (p. 1291)

See textbook.

BILE ACIDS IN LIVER DISEASE (pp. 1293–1295)

The diagnostic efficacy of fasting and 2-hour postprandial serum bile acid values in the dog and cat has established that they are useful in the diagnosis of hepatobiliary disorders associated with histologic lesions or portosystemic shunting. The issue of whether fasting or postprandial serum bile acid values perform better remains controversial. The use of both bile acid values provides the most reliable information in clinical patients because it reduces diagnostic errors caused by gastrointestinal variables.

Serum bile acid values cannot differentiate between liver disease because of the wide overlap in values among diseases (see Fig. 106–19 in the textbook). Clinically normal animals and animals with liver disease occasionally have fasting bile acid values that exceed the postprandial value. This is attributed to spontaneous gallbladder contraction during interdigestive intervals, delayed gastric emptying, slow intestinal transit, differences from the norm in cholecystokinin release, alimentary response to cholecystokinin, or gastrointestinal tract flora.

A variety of factors may promote low serum bile acid values in the presence of hepatobiliary disease. Reduced flow of bile may occur with early or transient obstruction of the biliary tree. Intestinal malabsorption of bile acids will invalidate the test, but this usually is obvious because the patient shows evidence of diarrhea or steatorrhea. Minimal amounts of food are 2 tsp for petite patients (less than or equal to 10 lb) and 2 tbsp for larger patients. The clinician should aim for a larger ingested volume if the animal is willing.

SYSTEMIC CONSEQUENCES OF HEPATIC INSUFFICIENCY (pp. 1295–1302)

HEPATIC ENCEPHALOPATHY

The complex neurobehavioral signs referred to as hepatic encephalopathy (HE) develop in animals afflicted with severe acquired liver disease and/or systemic portosystemic shunts. Despite extensive investigations into its pathogenesis, the neurochemical basis of HE has not been clearly defined. The clinical expression of HE is variable among patients. The onset can be obvious and abrupt, or insidious. Many patients appear normal between exacerbations, but some animals are chronically lethargic and mentally dull. Clinical signs include anorexia, vomiting, polydipsia, ptyalism, lethargy, depression, disorientation, aggressive or maniacal behavior, aimless walking or propulsive pacing, circling, head pressing, amaurotic blindness, weakness, collapse, seizures, and coma.

Clinical Conditions That Promote HE

The most important is the ingestion of proteins likely to precipitate HE. The derivation of nitrogen that can be metabolized into ammonia within the alimentary canal is primarily responsible. Carnivore quality protein (meat) is the greatest offender. Constipation is of major concern in patients prone to develop HE because the colon is the most important site of toxin generation and absorption.

Gastrointestinal bleeding is a leading cause of hepatic encephalopathy. Blood is one of the most potent sources of ammonia. Veterinary patients with hepatic insufficiency may develop HE as a result of endoparasitism (hookworms, coccidia), gastrointestinal ulceration, or a coagulopathy.

The development of dehydration and azotemia is problematic for the patient prone to HE. Marginal organ dysfunction can be magnified in the circumstance of dehydration. Azotemia is deleterious because increasing concentrations of urea result in increased alimentary production of ammonia.

Hypoglycemia may augment the encephalopathic effects of ammonium chloride and increase the brain ammonia concentration. Hypoglycemia should be anticipated and monitored for in patients with impaired hepatic function because the signs of neuroglycopenia simulate those of other HE toxins. Hypokalemia seems to be synergistic with some of the cerebral toxins that generate HE.

Infection or inflammation should be avoided in a patient with HE because catabolism increases the burden of nitrogen detoxification. Caution is warranted when using drugs with known central nervous system effects or that require hepatic biotransformation or excretion in patients with hepatic insufficiency and especially in those with a history of HE. Benzodiazepines should be avoided until their involvement in HE is further clarified. Adverse reactions to antihistamines, barbiturates, phenothiazines, metronidazole, and other agents have been realized in humans and veterinary patients with hepatic insufficiency and HE.

PORTAL HYPERTENSION AND ASCITES

Posthepatic portal hypertension indicates obstruction of flow at the level of the hepatic vein tributaries up to and including cardiac, pericardial, or pulmonary outflow obstructive causes. *Hepatic portal hypertension* indicates etiologic conditions within the hepatic parenchyma that cause a diminution of sinusoidal flow, such as collagenization of the sinusoids (cirrhosis), sinusoidal collapse (postnecrotic cirrhosis), and restricted portal vein and hepatic artery acinar perfusion due to periportal inflammation or fibrosis. *Prehepatic portal hypertension* indicates the presence of restricted blood flow into or through the portal vein.

Posthepatic Portal Hypertension

Posthepatic portal hypertension develops from a variety of disorders that increase resistance to blood flow in the major hepatic veins, the caudal vena cava, or the heart. They are listed in Table 106–18 in the textbook.

Hepatic Portal Hypertension

In cirrhosis, regenerative nodules and collagen deposition distort the sinusoidal microcirculatory bed and increase vascular resistance. See Table 106–19 in the textbook.

Prehepatic Portal Hypertension

With acute portal vein obstruction, portal hypertension may lead to death associated with impaired visceral perfusion, endotoxemia, and thromboembolism. When portal vein obstruction has a more gradual or insidious development, the ensuing portal hypertension can be tolerated as a result of recruitment of portosystemic collateral circulatory pathways.

Systemic Consequences

In a patient with portal hypertension, the determining factors in the development of portosystemic collateral circulation include the rate of development of the portal hypertension, the magnitude of the hypertension, and the anatomic site of the causal factors. In the patient with cirrhosis, the development of portosystemic shunting is believed to be more common than is substantiated. Posthepatic portal hypertension does not cause portosystemic shunting. When portal hypertension is the result of an arteriovenous hepatic fistula (usually a congenital intrahepatic vascular malformation), the capacitance and vascular resistance provided by the hepatic sinusoids virtually hide the existence of the fistula from the cardiovascular system and hemodynamic consequences rarely ensue.

Ascites

The *traditional concept* of ascites formation focuses on the role of diminished effective circulating volume. Initial derangements occur with imbalance of transcapillary fluid fluxes in the hepatic sinusoids and splanchnic lymphatics. This results in excessive lymph formation, which accumulates in the peritoneal cavity. Alternative theories have been proposed and are discussed in the textbook.

Large-volume paracentesis results in dynamic adjustments in the rate of ascites formation and absorption: an increased rate of ascites formation occurs concurrent with a reduced rate of fluid absorption. These phenomena provide the rationale for avoidance of large-volume therapeutic paracentesis in the cirrhotic patient because re-formation of ascites within hours to days is guaranteed if nothing more is done therapeutically to discourage fluid accumulation.

ENDOTOXEMIA IN THE PATIENT WITH IMPAIRED LIVER FUNCTION

Endotoxemia, in the absence of gram-negative bacteremia, is believed to complicate the clinical condition of patients with hepatic insufficiency.

RADIOGRAPHIC, NUCLEAR MEDICINE, AND ULTRA-SONOGRAPHIC IMAGING OF THE HEPATOBILIARY SYSTEM (pp. 1302–1308)

RADIOGRAPHY

The most important features evident on a radiographic assessment of the liver are alterations in size, position, and shape, and variation in density. The angle of the gas pocket in the stomach can be used as an anatomic landmark. In health, the gastric gas silhouette lies parallel to the intercostal spaces. A small liver shifts the gastric gas pattern to a more upright posture with cranial displacement. Radiographic features of hepatomegaly include a rounding of the liver margins, extension of the liver lobes beyond the costal arch, caudal-dorsal leftward displacement of the stomach, and caudal medial displacement of the transverse colon. Reports have suggested more reliable methods for estimating liver size. Irregular or bumpy liver margins indicate hepatic neoplasia, regenerative nodules, hepatic cysts, or other focal lesions.

The detection of gas in the common bile duct, gallbladder, or hepatic ducts may follow recent surgical intervention involving these structures. This may also indicate infection with gas-producing organisms (anaerobes usually). Emphysematous cholecystitis, gas accumulation within the wall and lumen of the gallbladder, has been seen in dogs, some of which have had diabetes mellitus. Gas within the biliary tree is expected in patients that have patent biliary diversions (cholecystoduodenostomy,

...olecystojejunostomy). Dystrophic mineralization may appear as multifocal intrahepatic densities and may be the sequela to necrosis or be associated with granulomas, hematomas, neoplastic foci, or parasitic cysts. In addition, these may represent choleliths or mineralizations associated with the gallbladder, major ducts, or biliary ductules.

The radiographic study of the portal circulation usually is accomplished by injection of contrast media into a mesenteric (jejunal) or splenic vein. Portography is recommended before surgery for the correction of portosystemic shunts in dogs because it aids the surgeon in vessel identification. In dogs, if the caudal extent of a congenital portosystemic shunt is cranial to vertebra T13, it probably is an intrahepatic anomaly.

ULTRASONOGRAPHY

Ultrasonography is useful for initial disease identification and, subsequently, as a method for monitoring disease progression; focal and diffuse liver disorders can also be detected and differentiated. Hepatic ultrasonography is indicated in the icteric patient when differentiation of extrahepatic biliary obstruction from intrahepatic disease is imperative. Ultrasonography is helpful in determining the origin of abdominal effusion. Dilated or engorged hepatic veins may distinguish passive congestion from intrahepatic portal hypertension. Ultrasound-guided biopsy collection is now a routine procedure in many clinical settings. Before biopsy procedures are undertaken, evaluation of the patient's coagulation status and prophylactic vitamin K_1 administration should be provided.

The caudal vena cava may be visualized adjacent to the diaphragm. The portal vein can be reliably visualized ventral to the caudal vena cava. Within the parenchyma, portal veins appear bright. The normal intrahepatic biliary tree is not visible and so is not confused with vascular structures. A small liver usually is difficult to image because of its position beneath the rib cage.

Ultrasonography is helpful in making a diagnosis of acquired portosystemic shunts secondary to chronic liver disease. Portal veins near the porta hepatis become large and tortuous. Examination of the gallbladder commonly reveals the presence of sludged or particulate biliary debris. This does not correlate with disease in the dog or cat but is considered a sign of fasting, anorexia, and temporary biliary stasis. If a patient is jaundiced or has present or historical laboratory indicators of cholestatic disease, however, this observation may deserve medical attention. Choleliths within the gallbladder are easily recognized using ultrasonography.

The normal gallbladder varies in size. After a prolonged fast or in the anorectic patient, the gallbladder usually is distended. The common bile duct may be seen adjacent to the portal vein in most normal animals. The remainder of the biliary tract usually is not visualized unless it is abnormal. When the gallbladder wall becomes thickened, a double-rim effect is produced by reflections from the inner and outer margins.

LIVER BIOPSY (pp. 1308–1310)

Tissue examination is essential for definitive diagnosis of hepatobiliary disease. The only exception is the patient with a congenital portosystemic vascular anomaly. The indications and contraindications for liver biopsy should be carefully considered; they are summarized in Table 106–1.

Severe microhepatica may necessitate a transthoracic needle biopsy approach. However, a laparoscopic or laparotomy approach is preferred in this instance. Once a biopsy is collected, optimal use of the sampled tissue should include histopathologic and cytologic evaluations; cultures for aerobic, anaerobic, and fungal agents, guided by the considered differential diagnoses and cytologic information; and

TABLE 106–1. CONSIDERATIONS WHEN PROCURING HEPATIC BIOPSY

INDICATIONS	CONTRAINDICATIONS OF NEEDLE BIOPSY
Hepatic failure of unknown cause	Focal cavitary lesion seen on ultrasound
Unexplained abdominal effusion/ascites	Abscess: → abdominal contamination
Persistent abnormal liver enzyme activity	Tumor: →hemorrhage, seeding
Persistent unexplained hyperbilirubinemia	Resectable lesion via laparotomy?
Unexplained hepatic insufficiency	Suspected extrahepatic bile duct obstruc-
↑ Serum bile acids	tion: laceration: → bile peritonitis
Hyperammonemia	(biliary diversion via laparotomy)
↓ Cholesterol	Small focal lesions: < 1 cm diameter
↓ Glucose	→ lesion missed
Ammonium biurates	Lesions restricted to one liver lobe:
↓ Albumin	resectable lesion via laparotomy?
Confirm suspected hepatic lipidosis (cat)	Microhepatica: requires unconventional
Unexplained, unequivocal ↓ or ↑ hepatic	needle approach
size	Coagulopathy: institute vitamin K_1
Confirm or stage neoplasia	± transfusion
Sequentially assess disease progression	
Sequentially assess response to treatment	
Evaluate for breed-related hepatopathy	

requests for copper quantification when copper storage–associated disorders are suspected. Infectious agents (bacterial organisms especially) are more easily identified on cytologic preparations than in histopathologic sections.

B. Diseases of the Liver (pages 1313–1357)

ACUTE HEPATIC FAILURE (pp. 1313–1316)

Acute hepatic failure is a clinical syndrome and not a specific diagnosis. Clinically relevant causes of acute hepatic disease in dogs and cats are summarized in Table 106–2. In many clinical cases, the inciting cause of acute hepatic failure is not identified. Diseases of the extrahepatic biliary tract should also be considered because surgical intervention is indicated for treatment of such disorders as biliary obstruction and rupture of the biliary tract.

A drug-induced cause of acute hepatic disease should be considered whenever evidence of hepatic disease is associated with a history of recent drug administration. A clinical diagnosis of toxic hepatic injury often is made when an episode of acute hepatic injury occurs, hepatic biopsy indicates diffuse hepatic necrosis, and no other cause for liver disease can be identified. Acute pancreatitis is an important cause of increased liver enzyme activity and hyperbilirubinemia in dogs and, less commonly, cats. Hepatic injury occurs secondary to the severe inflammatory process in the pancreas. Acute hemolytic anemia can be complicated by centrilobular necrosis attributed to acute hepatocellular hypoxia or to disseminated intravascular coagulation (DIC)-induced sinusoidal thrombosis. The liver undergoes cellular necrosis in response to heatstroke. Evidence of hepatic disease in the postoperative patient can be caused by factors associated with anesthesia or surgery.

Original section written by Susan E. Johnson

TABLE 106–2. CLINICALLY RELEVANT CAUSES OF ACUTE HEPATIC DISEASE IN DOGS AND CATS

Hepatotoxins
  Drugs and anesthetics
    Acetaminophen
    Griseofulvin
    Halothane
    Ketoconazole
    Mebendazole
    Methimazole
    Methoxyflurane
    Oxibendazole-diethylcarbamazine
    Tetracycline
    Thiacetarsamide
    Trimethoprim-sulfadiazine
  Chemicals and biologic substances
    Aflatoxin
    Amanita mushrooms
    Blue-green algae
    Cycadaceae (*Zamia floridana,* Sago palms)
    Pennyroyal oil
    Heavy metals

Infectious or Parasitic Agents
  Viral
    Infectious canine hepatitis
    Feline infectious peritonitis virus
  Bacterial
    Acute bacterial cholangiohepatitis
    Leptospirosis
    Liver abscess
    Extrahepatic infections and sepsis
  Fungal: Systemic mycoses (e.g., histoplasmosis)
  Protozoal: Toxoplasmosis
  Parasitic: Postcaval syndrome of heartworm disease

Systemic or Metabolic Disorders
    Acute pancreatitis
    Acute hemolytic anemia
    Idiopathic feline hepatic lipidosis

Traumatic, Thermal, or Hypoxic Injury
    Abdominal trauma
    Diaphragmatic hernia with liver entrapment
    Heatstroke
    Surgical hypotension and hypoxia
    Liver lobe torsion

DIAGNOSIS

Clinical signs of acute hepatic failure often are nonspecific and overlap those of other systemic disorders. The signs most frequently observed include acute onset of anorexia, depression, vomiting, diarrhea, and polyuria and polydipsia. The finding of jaundice on physical examination is a more specific indicator of hepatobiliary disease, especially in the absence of anemia. With severe hepatic damage, signs of hepatic encephalopathy (HE) may predominate. Clinical evidence of a bleeding tendency is uncommon except in fulminant hepatic failure.

Laboratory findings are dependent on the underlying cause of hepatic disease. Because diffuse hepatic necrosis is the most common lesion, increased serum ALT activity is the most consistent finding, and values often are markedly increased. Increased serum alkaline phosphatase (ALP) activity also commonly occurs. Total serum bilirubin commonly is increased. Fasting and postprandial serum bile acids (SBAs) usually are increased in dogs with hepatic necrosis and parallel the severity of the hepatic injury. Hypoalbuminemia usually suggests chronic rather than acute liver disease.

An inflammatory complete blood count should suggest possible acute pancreatitis or underlying infectious disease, such as leptospirosis, cholangiohepatitis, hepatic abscess, or extrahepatic bacterial infection and sepsis. Ultrasonographically, acute hepatitis is associated with diffusely decreased hepatic echogenicity.

A liver biopsy usually is required for complete evaluation of the causes of liver failure. If a coagulopathy is documented and clinical bleeding is present, liver biopsy may be too risky. On liver biopsy, a causative diagnosis may be obtained for diseases with characteristic histopathologic lesions, such as systemic fungal infections, toxoplasmosis, feline infectious peritonitis, and feline idiopathic hepatic lipidosis. When the microscopic evaluation is not diagnostic for a specific cause, descriptive morphologic characteristics such as acute necrosis or acute hepatitis aid in classification of the disorder. Chronicity is indicated by findings of fibrosis or cirrhosis.

CHOLESTATIC HEPATOBILIARY DISEASE
(pp. 1316–1317)

Cholestatic hepatobiliary disorders are characterized biochemically by increased plasma concentrations of bilirubin, cholesterol, and bile acids, and by increased activity of ALP and γ-glutamyltransferase (GGT). The hallmark feature of cholestasis is hyperbilirubinemia or jaundice.

Cholestasis can be caused by extrahepatic or intrahepatic mechanisms. Extrahepatic cholestasis is caused by mechanical obstruction of the common bile duct or main bile ducts exiting the liver near the porta hepatis or by rupture of the biliary tract. Intrahepatic cholestasis is characterized by a problem within the liver itself, causing either abnormalities of the microscopic intrahepatic biliary system or defective hepatocyte handling of bile.

A cholestatic disorder should be suspected when laboratory features indicate increased serum ALP or GGT activity that is disproportionately large compared with the increases in the hepatocellular enzymes ALT or AST, hyperbilirubinemia, bilirubinuria, and hypercholesterolemia. Biochemical findings cannot distinguish whether cholestasis is caused by intrahepatic or extrahepatic mechanisms. Ultrasonography is a useful noninvasive technique to evaluate for extrahepatic obstruction. Cholestasis is not a typical feature of certain hepatic disorders, such as congenital portosystemic shunt and passive venous congestion of the liver.

CHRONIC LIVER DISEASE, HEPATIC FIBROSIS, AND CIRRHOSIS (pp. 1317–1319)

End-stage liver disease has been associated with chronic or repeated episodes of toxin or drug exposure (e.g., hepatic copper accumulation, anticonvulsant drug therapy), infection (experimental ICH), cholestasis (cholangiohepatitis in cats), immunologic injury (idiopathic chronic hepatitis), and hypoxia ("cardiac cirrhosis"). In most clinical cases, however, the cause of cirrhosis is not determined, and gross and microscopic features are similar, regardless of the initiating injury.

Hepatic fibrosis is a key feature of cirrhosis, but these terms are not synonymous. Fibrosis occurs as a response to hepatic injury, but in the absence of regenerative nodules, it is not called cirrhosis. The pattern of fibrosis (portal, periacinar, or diffuse hepatic fibrosis) varies with of hepatic insult. Idiopathic hepatic fibrosis (but not true cirrosis) is a disease of unknown cause that is associated with chronic hepatic failure and portal hypertension. Young dogs are primarily affected, but ages range from 4 months to 7 years. German shepherds accounted for 9 of 15 dogs in one series.

End-stage liver disease associated with severe hepatic fibrosis or cirrhosis causes generalized hepatic dysfunction; thus, the clinical signs are those of chronic hepatic failure, such as anorexia, lethargy, vomiting, polyuria and polydipsia, and weight loss. With increased severity of hepatic dysfunction, signs of overt liver failure develop, including jaundice, ascites, coagulopathy, and HE.

Laboratory evidence of liver disease usually precedes the development of cirrhosis. Serum liver enzyme (ALT and ALP) activity typically is increased in cirrhosis, although the magnitude of increase may not be dramatic. These values occasionally are normal, indicating the absence of significant inflammation or intrahepatic cholestasis, or decreased viable parenchymal mass. Postprandial SBA concentrations usually are higher than fasting values in dogs with cirrhosis and are a more sensitive indicator of hepatic dysfunction.

Mild hyperbilirubinemia is present in a majority of dogs. Hyperglobulinemia, hypoalbuminemia, decreased BUN, impaired hemostasis, and microcytosis are other potential findings. Analysis of ascitic fluid reveals a transudate or modified transudate.

Microhepatica is a common radiographic finding in dogs with cirrhosis. In contrast, most cats with biliary cirrhosis have hepatomegaly. Potential ultrasonographic findings include microhepatica, irregular hepatic margins, focal lesions representing regenerative nodules, increased parenchymal echogenicity and ascites. Splenomegaly and secondary portosystemic shunts may be detected as well. Definitive diagnosis of hepatic fibrosis or cirrhosis requires liver biopsy.

TOXIN-INDUCED LIVER INJURY (pp. 1319–1320)

Blue-Green Algae Intoxication. Algae proliferate in freshwater ponds, shallow lakes, and lagoons. Toxicity is most likely to occur in the summer. Clinical signs consist of acute onset of vomiting, diarrhea, and lethargy followed by progressive tachypnea and dyspnea, jaundice, and coma.

Amanita Mushroom Poisoning. Clinical signs occur within 10 to 16 hours after ingestion and are characterized initially by gastrointestinal signs, such as vomiting and diarrhea, followed by signs of hepatic failure, including hemorrhage, HE, and terminal coma.

Aflatoxins. Aflatoxins can cause toxic hepatitis when they contaminate dog food ingredients such as corn and peanut meal. High-dose exposure is associated with acute hepatic necrosis, jaundice, DIC, and death. Repeated exposure to low doses can lead to chronic liver disease and cirrhosis.

Diagnosis

A definitive diagnosis of toxin-induced hepatic injury seldom is possible in a clinical setting unless the owner specifically observes ingestion of a substance that is a known hepatotoxin (see Table 106–3). A clinical diagnosis often is made when an episode of acute hepatic injury occurs, biopsy indicates hepatic degeneration and necrosis, and no other cause for liver disease can be identified.

DRUG-INDUCED LIVER INJURY (pp. 1320–1326)

Many drugs have the potential to cause hepatic injury in dogs and cats (Table 106–4). For most of the drugs listed in Table 106–4, acute

TABLE 106–3. ENVIRONMENTAL AGENTS WITH POTENTIAL HEPATOTOXICITY

Biologic Substances
 Aflatoxin
 Amanita mushroom toxin
 Blue-green algae
 Cycadaceae (*Zamia floridana,* Sago palms)
 Indigofera sp.
 Pennyroyal oil
 Pyrrolizidine alkaloids

Fumigants
 Carbon tetrachloride
 Dichloropropene
 Ethylene dichloride
 Ortho-dichlorobenzene
 Para-dichlorobenzene

Fungicides
 Benomyl
 Pentachloronitrobenzene
 Terrazole

Herbicides
 Paraquat
 Phenoxy herbicides
 Silvex

Household Products
 Sodium perborate (denture cleaner)
 Trichloroethane (dry cleaning fluid)
 Methyl bromide (liquid fire extinguisher)
 Petroleum hydrocarbons (fuel oils)
 Aliphatic or aromatic hydrocarbon solvents (glues and adhesives)
 Essential oils (perfumes)
 Phenols (disinfectants)

Industrial Chemicals
 Coal tar
 Dioxin
 Dimethylnitrosamine
 Polychlorinated biphenyls
 Solvents: toluene; ethyl, isopropyl, and methyl alcohol

Metals
 Arsenic
 Copper
 Lead
 Iron
 Selenium
 Manganese

Rodenticides
 Zinc phosphide
 Phosphorus

hepatic injury is most likely. Notable exceptions include anticonvulsants and corticosteroids in dogs. For most drug-induced disorders, the diagnosis is presumptive and cannot be proved.

Anticonvulsants

The anticonvulsants primidone, phenytoin, and phenobarbital, either used alone or in combination, have been associated with chronic hepatic disease and cirrhosis in dogs. Severe hepatic dysfunction

TABLE 106–4. THERAPEUTIC AGENTS WITH POTENTIAL HEPATOTOXICITY

	DOG	CAT
Agents		
Acetaminophen*	X	X
Aspirin	O	O
Phenazopyridine	—	O
Phenylbutazone	—	O
Anticonvulsants		
Phenobarbital*	X	—
Phenytoin*	X	—
Primidone*	X	—
Antimicrobials		
Amoxicillin	O	—
Amoxicillin/clavulanate	O	—
Clindamycin	O	—
Enrofloxacin	O	—
Griseofulvin*	—	X
Itraconazole*	X	—
Ketoconazole*	X	X
Tetracycline*	X	X
Trimethoprim/sulfadiazine*	X	—
Antineoplastics: Methotrexate	O	—
Antiparasitics		
Butamisol	O	—
Diethylcarbamazine*	Xa	—
Febantel/praziquantel	O	—
Fenbendazole	O	—
Glycobiarsol	—	O
Ivermectin	O	—
Mebendazole*	X	—
Milbemycin	O	—
Oxibendazole-diethylcarbamazine*	X	—
Phthalofyne	O	—
Thiacetarsamide*	X	—
Endocrine Agents		
Anabolic steroids	O	—
Glipizide*	—	X
Glucocorticoids*	X	—
Mibolerone	O	—
Megestrol acetae	—	O
Methimazole*	—	X
Propylthiouracil	—	O
Tolbutamide	O	—
Inhalation Anesthetics		
Halothane*	X	—
Methoxyflurane*	X	—
Tranquilizers, Injectable Anesthetics		
Acepromazine	O	—
Butorphenol	O	—
Ketamine	—	O
Tiletamine/zolazepam	O	O
Miscellaneous		
Aprindine	O	—
Azathioprine	O	—
Mithramycin	O	—

Drugs listed have been suggested to be associated with hepatic injury (increased ALT or ALP activity, jaundice or hyperbilirubinemia, or histologic liver lesions) in dogs or cats by way of single cases reported in the veterinary literature or isolated reports to the Center for Veterinary Medicine of possible hepatic injury.
*Most commonly recognized or documented in the veterinary literature to cause clinically relevant hepatic injury.
X, hepatic drug reaction documented; O, hepatic drug reaction suggested but poorly documented; —, hepatic drug reaction not reported; a, hepatic reaction only in dogs with microfilaremia from *D. immitis* infection.

develops in as many as 14 per cent of dogs treated with anticonvulsants for more than 6 months. Of these three anticonvulsants, phenobarbital has traditionally been considered the anticonvulsant least likely to be hepatotoxic.

Mildly increased liver enzyme activity is not a reliable indicator of serious hepatic damage in dogs given anticonvulsant drugs. Increased fasting and postprandial SBA concentrations, increased total serum bilirubin concentration, and hypoalbuminemia are better indicators of hepatic damage in this setting. In dogs with phenobarbital-induced hepatotoxicity, serum phenobarbital concentration often exceeds 40 μg/ml. Despite the evidence for hepatotoxicity, it appears that phenobarbital is still the drug of choice for long-term control of seizures in dogs.

Anticonvulsant therapy should be modified or discontinued if possible in dogs with biochemical and histologic evidence of hepatic disease. Improvement in clinical signs can be noted within days to weeks of decreasing serum phenobarbital levels. Potassium bromide has been recommended for use in dogs with phenobarbital-associated liver disease because it does not require hepatic metabolism and hepatotoxicity has not been documented to occur.

Glucocorticoids

The hepatic effects of glucocorticoid therapy in dogs include increased serum ALP activity and development of a reversible vacuolar hepatopathy. These hepatic effects can be seen with virtually any glucocorticoid preparation. Not all dogs treated with glucocorticoids develop either biochemical or histologic changes. The hepatic effects of glucocorticoid therapy are identical to those caused by endogenous hypercortisolism from spontaneous hyperadrenocorticism. Cats do not develop increased serum ALP activity or glucocorticoid hepatopathy when treated with glucocorticoids.

In dogs, increased serum ALP activity can occur within 2 days after initiating therapy and often is striking (up to 64 times normal). In contrast, serum ALT activity often is normal or only mildly increased. Glucocorticoids also cause increased serum GGT activity that parallels the increase in serum ALP activity. Steroid hepatopathy is a benign and reversible lesion and, with rare exceptions, is not associated with clinical liver dysfunction. When hepatic biopsy suggests steroid hepatopathy and a history of glucocorticoid administration is lacking, diagnostic tests for endogenous hyperadrenocorticism should be performed. Increased serum ALP activity is the most consistent biochemical abnormality.

Steroid hepatopathy should be considered in a dog with hepatomegaly; a marked increase in serum ALP activity that is disproportionately high compared with serum ALT activity; normal serum bilirubin, albumin, and blood ammonia concentrations; and normal to mildly increased fasting or postprandial SBA. Abdominal radiographs typically reveal hepatomegaly. On ultrasonography, the liver is enlarged and hepatic echogenicity is diffusely increased. A liver biopsy is indicated if a history of glucocorticoid administration (or hyperadrenocorticism) cannot be confirmed or if clinical or laboratory features are found that are not typical for steroid hepatopathy.

Steroid hepatopathy is reversible after withdrawal of exogenous glucocorticoids or treatment of spontaneous hyperadrenocorticism.

Anthelmintics

Thiacetarsamide is widely recognized as a cause of hepatic injury. This drug is a predictable hepatotoxin with a small margin of safety. Increased serum ALT activity is a common and expected finding after treatment. Administration of the heartworm preventative diethylcarbamazine to dogs infected with *Dirofilaria immitis* that are microfilaremic results in a severe shock-like clinical reaction associated with hepatic vascular lesions. The benzimidazole anthelmintics mebendazole and oxibendazole have been incriminated as causing idiosyncratic hepatic drug reactions in dogs. Oxibendazole, which is marketed in combination with diethylcarbamazine as a hookworm-heartworm preventative (Filaribits Plus), has been associated with acute and chronic hepatic injury in dogs. Doberman pinschers may be predisposed.

Antimicrobials

Trimethoprim-sulfadiazine has been reported to cause a cholestatic hepatopathy in dogs characterized by acute onset of jaundice and increased serum liver enzyme activity. A hypersensitivity reaction is suspected. Griseofulvin therapy has been associated with mild hyperbilirubinemia and increased serum ALT activity in cats. Ketoconazole has been associated with increased serum liver enzyme activity and jaundice in dogs and cats. Cats may be more sensitive to the hepatotoxic effects than dogs. A clinically significant hepatic reaction should be suspected when enzyme elevations are accompanied by jaundice or clinical signs, and it is recommended that ketoconazole therapy be discontinued.

INFECTIOUS LIVER DISEASES (pp. 1326–1329)

INFECTIOUS CANINE HEPATITIS

See textbook.

ACIDOPHIL CELL HEPATITIS

Canine acidophil cell hepatitis has been reported in Great Britain. It is caused by a transmissible agent, most likely a virus, that is distinct from CAV-1. Most dogs are presented with signs of chronic hepatic failure.

LEPTOSPIROSIS

Canine leptospirosis is classically associated with acute renal failure and hepatic disease with jaundice.

HEPATIC ABSCESSES

Omphalophlebitis is the most likely cause of hepatic abscesses in puppies and kittens. In adult dogs, hepatic abscesses usually are associated with extrahepatic infection or regional hepatic parenchymal damage. Hematogenous spread of bacteria can occur from septic foci elsewhere in the body, such as pyelonephritis, prostatitis, pyometra, endocarditis, or pancreatitis. Hepatic trauma and neoplasia can predispose patients to hepatic abscess.

Clinical signs in animals with hepatic abscesses are attributed to sepsis, inflammation, and hepatic dysfunction, and include anorexia, depression, and vomiting. The complete blood count usually reveals a neutrophilia with left shift, but with overwhelming sepsis, a neutropenia and degenerative left shift might be found. Increased serum ALP and ALT activity are common. Laboratory abnormalities may also reflect the associated disease processes.

Abdominal radiographs may be normal or reveal hepatomegaly, hepatic mass lesion, or decreased abdominal detail or effusion associated with secondary peritonitis. With proliferation of gas-producing organisms, radiolucent areas may be seen in the liver. Ultrasonographically, a liver abscess appears as a hypoechoic or anechoic structure that may contain mixed echoes. Ultrasound-guided fine-needle aspiration of a suspected liver abscess can be performed to obtain samples for cytology and culture to confirm the diagnosis.

Treatment of hepatic abscesses consists of surgical resection or drainage; administration of appropriate antibiotics; correction of associated fluid, electrolyte, and acid-base imbalances; and identification and treatment of an underlying disease process. Antibiotic therapy should be directed toward both aerobic and anaerobic bacteria. An effective combination would be intravenous penicillin combined with an aminoglycoside, until culture results are available.

EXTRAHEPATIC BACTERIAL INFECTIONS

Extrahepatic bacterial infections that are associated with sepsis and endotoxemia can cause intrahepatic cholestasis in dogs. Total serum bilirubin concentrations as high as 30 mg/dl can be seen. Mild to moderate increases in serum ALP activity can occur. Increased serum ALT activity is a less consistent finding. The SBA concentration can be markedly increased.

Extrahepatic bacterial infection–induced hepatic damage should be considered when evidence of a cholestatic hepatopathy is found concurrently with extensive bacterial infection in other organ systems (e.g., pyometra, peritonitis) or with extrahepatic disorders likely to be associated with endotoxemia (e.g., parvoviral enteritis).

MYCOSES

See textbook.

TOXOPLASMOSIS

See textbook.

CHOLANGIOHEPATITIS COMPLEX (pp. 1329–1331)

Cholangiohepatitis is an inflammatory disorder of the bile ducts and adjacent hepatocytes. It is one of the most common hepatobiliary disorders of cats but is recognized much less frequently in dogs. The following discussion focuses on cholangiohepatitis of cats.

The cause of cholangiohepatitis complex is unknown. Ascending biliary infections usually require some predisposing factor: bile stasis, cholelithiasis, liver flukes, and anatomic abnormalities. Nonsuppurative (or lymphocytic) cholangiohepatitis is characterized by a lymphocytic plasmacytic infiltrate within and around the bile ducts. Immune-mediated mechanisms have been suspected to play a role. Nonsuppurative cholangiohepatitis may be a more chronic stage of suppurative cholangiohepatitis. Suppurative cholangiohepatitis, when treated appropriately, does not necessarily progress to nonsuppurative cholangiohepatitis. Chronic low-grade interstitial pancreatitis is a common finding in cats with either suppurative or nonsuppurative cholangiohepatitis.

The most common clinical signs are anorexia, depression, weight loss, vomiting, dehydration, fever, and jaundice. Signs may be acute or chronic, intermittent or persistent. Biochemical findings with cholangiohepatitis are variable. Hyperbilirubinemia is a common finding. Serum enzyme (ALT, ALP, GGT) activity usually is mildly to moderately increased, although the ALP activity can be normal. Fasting SBA concentrations may vary from normal to greater than 400 μmol/L. Other findings indicative of more advanced hepatic dysfunction include hypoalbuminemia, decreased BUN, and ammonia intolerance. Excess bleeding may be caused by vitamin K malabsorption or by impaired hepatic synthesis of clotting factors. Hypergammaglobulinemia can be a prominent finding with nonsuppurative cholangiohepatitis.

Radiographic features include hepatomegaly and, in some cases, cholelithiasis. Ultrasonography is useful to evaluate concurrent abnormalities of the extrahepatic biliary system. Definitive diagnosis requires liver biopsy.

Inspissation of bile within intrahepatic and extrahepatic bile ducts is a common complication. Sludging of bile can cause extrahepatic biliary obstruction. Bile sludging and biliary infections are also associated with the formation of choleliths in the gallbladder and common bile duct. Systemic antibiotics are indicated for treatment of cholangiohepatitis if a neutrophilic component is present on biopsy or if a positive bacterial culture of bile is obtained. Sometimes antibiotics are used in the initial treatment of nonsuppurative cholangitis or cholangiohepatitis, before glucocorticoid therapy is started, to eliminate any bacterial component.

Prednisolone is used empirically in the treatment of nonsuppurative cholangitis or cholangiohepatitis. Continuous or intermittent therapy may be required on a long-term basis. Corticosteroids are catabolic and may worsen signs of HE. Furthermore, exacerbation of ascites may occur because of sodium-retaining properties.

Inspissation of bile within intrahepatic and extrahepatic bile ducts is associated with a poor prognosis. Ursodeoxycholic acid may be beneficial. General supportive care consisting of fluid therapy, maintenance of nutritional intake, and vitamin supplementation is especially important in debilitated cats with hepatic disease.

CANINE CHRONIC HEPATITIS (pp. 1331–1338)

GENERAL INTRODUCTION

Chronic hepatitis is a heterogeneous group of inflammatory-necrotizing diseases of the liver. There are many potential causes of this condition in dogs (see Table 106–5). Chronic hepatitis may progress to cirrhosis and liver failure, but this is unpredictable. A liver biopsy is essential for the diagnosis. To avoid confusion, the term *chronic active hepatitis* should be abandoned in the veterinary medical field. The term *chronic hepatitis* should be used instead.

FAMILIAL CHRONIC HEPATITIS

Bedlington Terriers

Chronic hepatitis in Bedlington terriers is caused by progressive copper accumulation in the liver resulting from failure of normal biliary excretion of copper. Affected dogs can be asymptomatic or show signs of acute hepatic necrosis, chronic hepatitis, or cirrhosis. Most affected dogs that are over 1 year of age have a quantitative copper concentration that is greater than 1000 μg/gm dry weight and may be as high as 12,000 μg/gm.

TABLE 106–5. CANINE CHRONIC HEPATITIS

Familial Predisposition	*Drug-Induced*
Bedlington terrier	Anticonvulsants
Cocker spaniel	Oxibendazole-diethylcarbamazine
Doberman pinscher	
Labrador retriever (?)	*Lobular Dissecting Hepatitis*
Skye terrier	*Idiopathic Chronic Hepatitis*
Standard poodle	
West Highland white terrier	
Infectious	
Infectious canine hepatitis	
Acidophil cell hepatitis	
Leptospirosis (serogroup *grippotyphosa*)	

The clinical signs vary widely, depending on the stage of disease. Affected dogs usually fit into one of three clinical categories. The first group is composed of young adults of either sex that have an acute onset of signs associated with hepatic necrosis. Signs include depression, anorexia, lethargy, and vomiting. The clinical course can be short, and most dogs die within 48 to 72 hours. Some dogs survive and recover within a few weeks. These dogs may remain asymptomatic for years or have milder recurrent bouts. The second clinical category consists of middle-aged to older dogs with a more chronic, insidious clinical course. Signs are similar but less severe than in the first group. Chronic weight loss and deterioration of general condition frequently occur. In the advanced stages of disease, cachexia, ascites, jaundice, and HE can be present. The last group consists of clinically normal but affected dogs. These dogs are younger animals that either have not yet had an acute bout of hepatitis or are in the very early stages of the chronic progressive form. Some dogs remain asymptomatic.

Other serum biochemical abnormalities typical of hepatic dysfunction eventually develop, such as hyperbilirubinemia, bilirubinuria, hypoalbuminemia, increased SBA concentration, and prolonged PT and APTT. Acute release of copper from necrotic hepatocytes occasionally causes hemolytic anemia. Liver biopsy is indicated for definitive diagnosis and staging of the disease. Dogs should be greater than 1 year of age to be sure adequate time for copper accumulation has occurred.

Evaluating the quantitative hepatic copper concentration by liver biopsy at 5 to 7 months of age and then again at 14 to 15 months can distinguish normal, affected, and carrier dogs. Measures used to control hepatic copper accumulation include copper chelators, such as D-penicillamine or trientine; drugs to decrease intestinal copper absorption, such as zinc acetate or zinc sulfate; and a low-copper diet. Months to years of D-penicillamine therapy are required to significantly decrease hepatic copper in affected Bedlingtons.

Treatment of asymptomatic but affected dogs with copper chelators or zinc acetate may prevent acute hepatitis or progression to cirrhosis. Treatment must be lifelong. Additional measures to control the complications of liver failure, such as ascites and HE, should be instituted as needed.

West Highland White Terriers

West Highland white terriers are at increased risk to develop multifocal hepatitis, hepatic necrosis, or cirrhosis that usually is associated with increased hepatic copper content. Affected animals in the early stages usually are asymptomatic. When widespread necrosis occurs, nonspecific signs of liver disease include anorexia, vomiting, diarrhea, lethargy, and jaundice. With advanced disease, jaundice and ascites are common.

Hepatic necrosis is associated with increased serum ALT activity as the earliest biochemical abnormality. With advanced disease, findings include increased liver enzyme activity, hyperbilirubinemia, increased SBA concentrations, hyperammonemia, and hypoalbuminemia. Liver biopsy for histopathology and quantitative copper analysis is required for definitive diagnosis. General principles of therapy are similar to those described for Bedlington terriers.

Doberman Pinschers

Chronic hepatitis in Doberman pinschers is a disorder associated with histologic features of chronic hepatitis and cirrhosis. Hepatic copper concentrations are increased in most affected dogs. The significance of this remains controversial. Female dogs of any age are predominantly affected. Most dogs are diagnosed in the advanced stages of hepatic failure.

Signs include anorexia, weight loss, lethargy, polyuria and polydipsia, vomiting, diarrhea, ascites, and jaundice. Evidence of excessive bleeding may occur. Signs of HE often predominate in the terminal stages. Common physical examination findings include ascites, jaundice, and weight loss. Splenomegaly (associated with portal hypertension) is common. The liver is small and not palpable.

Definitive diagnosis requires liver biopsy. Frequent laboratory findings include increased serum ALP and ALT activity, hyperbilirubinemia and bilirubinuria, hypoalbuminemia, increased SBA concentrations, and hyperammonemia. Concurrent von Willebrand's disease should also be considered in affected dogs with a bleeding disorder.

Effective treatment has not been established. Therapy with immunosuppressant drugs such as prednisolone with or without azathioprine usually is instituted as described for idiopathic chronic hepatitis. The response is usually poor. The use of copper chelating agents in this disease remains controversial.

IDIOPATHIC CHRONIC HEPATITIS

Idiopathic chronic hepatitis (previously called chronic active hepatitis or chronic active liver disease) occurs equally in male and female dogs. Common clinical findings include anorexia, depression, weakness, polyuria and polydipsia, ascites, jaundice, weight loss, and vomiting.

The diagnosis is suggested by the clinical signs in conjunction with increased serum liver enzyme activity. The diagnosis can be confirmed only by liver biopsy. Hyperbilirubinemia and bilirubinuria are common. Fasting and postprandial SBA concentrations and ammonia tolerance frequently are abnormal. Other findings may include hypoalbuminemia, hyperglobulinemia, mild nonregenerative anemia, and abnormal hemostasis. Ascitic fluid, when present, typically is a transudate. Radiographically, the liver may appear small, and on ultrasound examination, nonspecific changes in echogenicity may be detected. With end-stage liver disease, findings are consistent with cirrhosis.

Liver biopsy is required to confirm a diagnosis. Treatment has centered around the use of immunosuppressant drugs. A large study suggested that corticosteroids are beneficial in the management of chronic hepatitis in dogs. Glucocorticoid therapy is not indicated for treatment of chronic hepatitis caused by drug therapy, primary hepatic copper accumulation, or infectious agents.

Because glucocorticoids frequently increase liver enzyme activity and can cause mild increases in SBA concentrations, follow-up liver biopsy performed 2 to 3 months after starting therapy is the best way to ensure that the disease is in remission. When prednisolone alone is ineffective, combination therapy should be considered using both azathioprine and prednisolone. Ursodeoxycholic acid may be a therapeutic consideration for dogs with a significant cholestatic component. Drugs that modify hepatic fibrosis, such as colchicine, may be indicated if cirrhosis is present. Additional supportive measures are dictated by the clinical manifestations and complications of chronic hepatitis, such as ascites and HE.

NODULAR HYPERPLASIA (p. 1338)

Nodular hyperplasia of the liver, an age-related phenomenon, is a common postmortem finding in dogs over 8 years of age. No specific cause has been identified. Hyperplastic nodules are not a pre-neoplastic finding in dogs. Nodular hyperplasia usually is not associated with clinical signs but can cause mild to moderate increases in serum ALP and ALT activity.

HEPATOBILIARY NEOPLASIA (pp. 1338–1340)

Metastatic tumors are more common than primary hepatic neoplasms. Lymphosarcoma is the most common secondary hepatic tumor in dogs. Lymphosarcoma and myeloproliferative disorders also commonly involve the liver in cats. The most common primary hepatic tumors in dogs are hepatocellular adenoma (benign) and hepatocellular adenocarcinoma (malignant). In contrast, neoplasms of the biliary system predominate in cats, and bile duct adenoma (benign) is most common.

Primary hepatic neoplasms are most common in dogs and cats that are older than 10 years of age. Male dogs are at increased risk for hepatocellular carcinoma. Female dogs, especially those that have been neutered, are at increased risk for cholangiocellular carcinoma. In contrast, most cats with cholangiocellular carcinoma or adenoma are male.

The most consistent clinical signs in dogs are anorexia, lethargy, weight loss, polydipsia and polyuria, vomiting, and abdominal distention. Signs of CNS dysfunction, such as depression, dementia, and seizures, can be attributed to HE, hypoglycemia, or CNS metastases. Anorexia and lethargy are the most common presenting signs in cats. Jaundice is a less frequent finding with hepatic tumors.

Potential hematologic findings include anemia and leukocytosis. Prolongation of the PT and APTT may be identified. Mild to marked increases in serum liver enzyme (ALT and ALP) activity are common in dogs with primary hepatic tumors but less so with metastatic neoplasia. In contrast, most cats with non-hematopoietic hepatic neoplasms have increased serum ALT or AST activity, but serum ALP activity usually is normal. Other biochemical findings are variable and include hypoalbuminemia, hyperglobulinemia, and increased SBA concentrations.

Abdominal radiographic findings include symmetric or asymmetric hepatomegaly and ascites. Thoracic radiographs should be performed to detect pulmonary metastases. Potential ultrasonographic findings include focal, multifocal, or diffuse changes in hepatic echotexture. Target lesions, consisting of an echogenic center surrounded by a more sonolucent rim, often are neoplastic.

Definitive diagnosis of hepatic neoplasia requires liver biopsy and histopathologic evaluation. Surgical removal of the affected liver lobe is the treatment of choice for primary hepatic neoplasms. When all lobes are affected, the prognosis is poor. Chemotherapy is not an effective means of control for primary liver tumors. Secondary hepatic neoplasms, such as lymphosarcoma, might temporarily respond to chemotherapeutic intervention.

HEPATIC CYSTS (p. 1340)

See textbook.

HEPATIC CIRCULATORY DISORDERS (pp. 1340–1345)

CONGENITAL PORTOSYSTEMIC SHUNTS

Portosystemic shunts (PSSs) are vascular communications between the portal and systemic venous systems that allow access of portal blood to the systemic circulation without first passing through the liver. Decreased hepatic blood flow and lack of hepatotrophic factors result in hepatic atrophy. Urate urolithiasis is an important complication.

PSSs in dogs and cats can be either congenital or acquired. Congenital PSSs are not associated with portal hypertension. Acquired PSSs, which form in response to portal hypertension, typically are multiple extrahepatic shunts. Single intrahepatic PSSs are most common in large-breed dogs. Single extrahepatic PSSs are most common in cats and small-breed dogs. Several breeds appear to be at increased risk for congenital PSSs, especially miniature schnauzers and Yorkshire terriers. In contrast, mixed-breed cats are affected more commonly than purebred cats. Most animals develop signs by 6 months of age. However, a congenital PSS should still be a diagnostic consideration in middle-aged or older dogs.

Clinical signs of HE usually predominate. The most consistent signs often are subtle, such as anorexia, depression, and lethargy. Other common findings include episodic weakness, ataxia, head-pressing, disorientation, circling, pacing, behavioral changes, amaurotic blindness, seizures, and coma. Hypersalivation is a prominent sign in cats but also occurs in dogs. Bizarre aggressive behavior appears more likely in cats. Clinical signs of HE tend to wax and wane, and often are interspersed with normal periods. Signs may be exacerbated by a protein-rich meal, gastrointestinal bleeding, or administration of methionine-containing urinary acidifiers or lipotrophic agents.

Gastrointestinal signs of intermittent anorexia, vomiting, and diarrhea are common. Many affected animals have a history of stunted growth, failure to gain weight, or weight loss. Polydipsia and polyuria are common. If urolithiasis is a complicating feature, pollakiuria, dysuria, and hematuria may occur. Physical examination may be unremarkable except for small body stature or weight loss. The neurologic examination is normal, or if overt signs of HE are present, neurologic findings are consistent with diffuse cerebral disease.

Although a congenital PSS may be highly suspected based on historical, physical, laboratory, and radiographic findings, a definitive diagnosis requires identification of a shunt by contrast radiography, rectal portal scintigraphy, ultrasonography, or exploratory laparotomy. In young animals with consistent clinical features but without a demonstrable shunt, hepatic microvascular dysplasia should be considered.

Routine hematologic and biochemical findings often are unremarkable in dogs and cats with congenital PSSs. Hematologic findings include microcytosis, target cells, poikilocytosis, and mild nonregenerative anemia. Isosthenuria or hyposthenuria frequently is detected. Ammonium biurate crystals are a common finding on urine sediment examination. Coagulation tests in dogs may show increased PTT and hypofibrinogenemia. Hepatocellular dysfunction is suggested by hypoproteinemia, hypoalbuminemia, hypoglobulinemia, hypoglycemia, decreased BUN, and hypocholesterolemia. Total serum bilirubin concentration typically is normal. Serum liver enzyme activity is normal to mildly increased, consistent with a lesion of hepatic atrophy.

Fasting SBA concentrations often are increased but can be normal. Postprandial concentrations are consistently abnormal and are a good screening test for animals suspected to have PSSs. They typically exceed 100 μmol/L. Survey abdominal radiographs often are performed to evaluate for microhepatica or presence of urinary calculi. Microhepatica, a common finding of dogs with congenital PSSs, is a less consistent finding in cats.

Ultrasonography is a useful noninvasive method to evaluate animals with suspected congenital PSSs. Intrahepatic PSSs are more reliably detected with this procedure than are extrahepatic PSSs. Positive-contrast portography is the procedure of choice to characterize the type and anatomic location of PSSs. In dogs, if the shunt is cranial to the T-13 vertebra, it is probably intrahepatic; if any part of the shunt is caudal to T-13, an extrahepatic shunt is most likely.

Medical management of dogs and cats with congenital PSSs is palliative and primarily directed at control of HE with low-protein diet, lactulose, and neomycin or metronidazole. When severe CNS depression or coma prevents the oral administration of lactulose and neomycin, these drugs are administered by way of an enema. Precipitating causes of HE, such as hypoglycemia, gastrointestinal bleeding, and hypokalemia, should be identified and corrected whenever possible. If surgical shunt correction is not feasible or is declined by the owner, long-term medical management can adequately control clinical signs for as long as 2 to 4 years in some dogs. However, most dogs managed medically on a long-term basis are not clinically normal and eventually have refractory neurologic signs.

The treatment of choice for dogs and cats with a single shunt is surgical ligation of the anomalous vessel. In general, single intrahepatic PSSs are technically more difficult to correct than single extrahepatic PSSs. If preoperative portography is performed, it is recommended that surgical correction be performed during a separate anesthetic period (at least 24 to 48 hours later) to minimize the duration of general anesthesia. Total surgical ligation of single congenital PSSs is the preferred procedure; however, in many cases, only partial ligation of the shunt can be safely performed because of the risk of portal hypertension.

Routine postoperative management consists of systemic antibiotics and fluid therapy. Oral lactulose, neomycin (or metronidazole), and a protein-restricted diet usually are continued for 2 to 4 weeks or longer, depending on the individual patient's clinical response. Hepatic function tests such as SBA concentrations often improve but usually do not return to normal, even in dogs that become clinically normal. The prognosis in dogs for resolution of signs after partial or total surgical ligation of the shunt is excellent (75 to 85 per cent success rate) if the dog survives the immediate postoperative period. A good clinical outcome is most likely in dogs less than 1 year of age. The response to surgical correction of congenital PSSs in cats appears to be less encouraging than in dogs.

HEPATIC MICROVASCULAR DYSPLASIA (pp. 1345–1350)

The term *hepatic microvascular dysplasia (HMD)* has been introduced to describe histologic vascular abnormalities of the liver in dogs and cats. Many affected animals also have congenital PSSs (defined as macroscopically identifiable shunt vessels). Clinical signs suggestive of portosystemic shunting are also seen in dogs and cats with HMD for which a congenital PSS cannot be demonstrated. The high prevalence in related Cairn terriers supports a hereditary mechanism in this breed.

The clinicopathologic features of HMD alone versus HMD accompanied by a congenital PSS are similar with the following exceptions: In animals with HMD alone, clinical signs are mild or absent, dogs usually are older at presentation, and routine hematologic and biochemical test results may be normal, and postprandial SBA concentrations are only mildly increased (40–110 μmol/L) compared with HMD/PSS (>200 μmol/L). In dogs with HMD alone, a portogram may be normal or suggest partial perfusion of the liver lobes, but no vascular shunt is identified.

It is essential to rigorously pursue the diagnosis of congenital PSS because the clinical and histologic features of HMD alone are similar to those of congenital PSS. Liver biopsy should be performed to evaluate for other causes of liver disease and to identify consistent vascular changes. Dogs with HMD alone can be successfully managed with a protein-restricted diet.

MULTIPLE ACQUIRED PORTOSYSTEMIC SHUNTS

Multiple acquired PSSs are extrahepatic collateral vessels that develop as a compensatory response to portal hypertension. Portal hypertension and multiple acquired PSSs usually are associated with chronic hepatitis, cirrhosis, and idiopathic hepatic fibrosis.

Sometimes multiple acquired PSSs are detected by portography or laparotomy in young dogs in which a single congenital PSS is initially suspected. A liver biopsy should be performed to evaluate for severe intrahepatic disease causing portal hypertension. Multiple acquired PSSs may develop after surgical ligation of a congenital PSS if portal hypertension persists for 1 to 2 months.

The clinical and laboratory findings are nonspecific. Ascites is a common clinical sign. A pattern of normal to mildly increased fasting SBA accompanied by markedly increased postprandial SBA concentrations is consistent. Ultrasonographically, features of portal hypertension, such as dilated portal veins, ascites, and splenomegaly, may be detected. Multiple acquired PSSs can be confirmed by contrast portography or at exploratory laparotomy.

Surgical ligation of multiple acquired PSSs is contraindicated, as it may result in fatal portal hypertension. Suture attenuation (banding) of the abdominal vena cava has been recommended to control signs of HE and ascites.

HEPATIC ARTERIOVENOUS FISTULAS

Hepatic AV fistulas are vascular communications between the hepatic artery and the portal vein that allow blood to bypass the hepatic sinusoidal network and flow retrograde into the portal system. The diversion of high-pressure arterial blood into the low-pressure portal system causes portal hypertension, ascites, and multiple acquired PSSs.

Hepatic AV fistulas can be either congenital or acquired. The most consistent clinical signs are acute onset of depression, lethargy, ascites, vomiting, and diarrhea. Other findings include signs of HE, failure to grow or weight loss, polyuria and polydipsia, and abdominal pain. On physical examination, a continuous murmur (bruit) may be auscultated through the abdominal wall over the area of the affected liver lobe. A systolic murmur may be auscultated in some dogs.

Hematologic and biochemical findings are similar to those found in animals with congenital PSSs. On abdominal ultrasonography, hepatic AV fistulas appear as tortuous, anechoic tubular structures in the area of the liver. Secondary PSSs may be detected. Celiac arteriography or nonselective aortography can confirm the diagnosis.

Partial hepatectomy is indicated for treatment of hepatic AV fistulas that involve one liver lobe. If multiple lobes are involved or a hepatic lobe cannot be resected, de-arterialization of the affected lobes should be performed. Hepatic function may not return to normal because of persistent shunting of portal blood through acquired PSS. Caudal vena cava banding consequently has been recommended to improve hepatic perfusion and decrease portosystemic shunting of blood.

HEPATIC VENOUS OUTFLOW OBSTRUCTION

Hepatic venous outflow obstruction caused by functional or mechanical obstruction of hepatic venous return to the heart results in passive venous congestion of the liver, hepatomegaly, portal hypertension, and ascites. Causes include congestive heart failure, pericardial disorders, intracardiac tumors, congenital heart defects (cor triatriatum dexter), and partial obstruction or compression of the caudal vena cava. Rarely, obstruction occurs in the efferent venous system within the liver (central veins, intralobular veins, hepatic veins).

Ascites is a consistent clinical feature of portal hypertension associated with hepatic venous outflow obstruction. Cats are less likely than dogs to have ascites under similar circumstances. Another consequence of portal hypertension is the development of multiple acquired PSSs, except with right-sided congestive heart failure and pericardial disorders.

Animals typically are presented for persistent abdominal distention and ascites. Clinical signs of hepatic dysfunction usually are absent. Additional clinical findings are related to the underlying cause of venous outflow obstruction. The ascitic fluid is characterized as a modified transudate with greater than 2.5 gm/dl of protein. With passive venous congestion of the liver, serum liver enzyme activity usually is normal or only mildly (two to three times) increased. Fasting and postprandial SBA concentrations typically are normal. Mild to moderate hypoproteinemia is also a common biochemical finding.

Thoracic radiographs and/or cardiac ultrasonography should be performed in the initial evaluation to detect obvious underlying disorders. Hepatic ultrasonography is useful to confirm hepatomegaly in the presence of ascites. Liver biopsy is indicated to evaluate hepatomegaly, but only if the initial workup does not identify an obvious cardiac or vena caval cause for passive venous congestion.

Specialized diagnostic procedures, such as cardiac catheterization, manometry, and angiography, are indicated when routine radiographic and ultrasonographic evaluation do not identify a cause or to further characterize the pathophysiology of an obstructive lesion. The treatment and prognosis depend on the underlying cause. Congestive heart failure is managed medically. Surgery is indicated for definitive diagnosis and for removal of obstructive or compressive lesions.

HEPATIC LIPIDOSIS (pp. 1350–1353)

Hepatic lipidosis is an excessive accumulation of fat (triglycerides) in the liver. Diabetes mellitus is a well-recognized cause of hepatic lipid accumulation in dogs and cats. Hepatic lipidosis is also a common finding in cats with acute pancreatitis. Drugs (e.g., tetracycline) or toxins (e.g., carbon tetrachloride) can cause hepatic injury in dogs and cats that is associated with varying degrees of fatty change in the liver. Severe hepatic lipidosis has been recognized in toy breed puppies that become hypoglycemic and die after prolonged anorexia or fasting (juvenile hypoglycemia).

FELINE IDIOPATHIC HEPATIC LIPIDOSIS

Idiopathic hepatic lipidosis (IHL), a disease of unknown cause, is the most common liver disease of cats. It is characterized by a variable period of anorexia, leading to massive fat accumulation, severe intrahepatic cholestasis, hepatic failure, and high mortality if left untreated. The underlying metabolic disturbances are poorly understood. Severe hepatic lipidosis most commonly develops in obese cats that are inappetant for greater than 2 weeks.

IHL has no age, breed, or gender predilection. The history may reveal precipitating causes of anorexia, such as stressful events (e.g., boarding, surgery, or a change in living arrangements), a diet change, or non-hepatic diseases. Other clinical signs include lethargy, vomiting, constipation or diarrhea, and weight loss. Weight loss can be dramatic. Overt signs of HE are uncommon. Overt bleeding is uncommon. Physical examination findings may include hepatomegaly, jaundice, pallor, and seborrhea. Severe muscle wasting with preservation of body fat stores often is noted.

Hematologic findings include nonregenerative, normocytic, normochromic anemia and stress-related mature neutrophilia and lymphopenia. Biochemical findings are characterized by hyperbilirubinemia and increased serum ALP activity. Serum GGT activity, which usually parallels or exceeds ALP activity in most feline hepatic disorders, is not as significantly increased in IHL. Fasting and postprandial SBA concentrations typically are increased. Azotemia and hypokalemia may occur secondary to vomiting and dehydration. Bilirubinuria is a common finding on urinalysis. On abdominal radiographs, the liver is normal to increased in size. Ultrasonographically, the liver is hyperechoic when compared with the falciform fat.

Liver biopsy is required to distinguish IHL from other causes of hepatic disease, such as cholangiohepatitis, FIP, and hepatic neoplasia.

Detection of concurrent acute pancreatitis also appears to be important. Fine-needle aspiration is an alternative to liver biopsy. Results occasionally can be misleading because of the small sample size. Treatment is primarily supportive. The greatest success has been with aggressive nutritional support. Identification and treatment of precipitating causes should be attempted whenever possible.

The daily caloric requirement {maintenance energy requirement in calories = 1.4 × [(30 × body weight in kilograms) + 70]} should be provided by force-feeding or by nasoesophageal or gastrostomy tube. An endoscopically or surgically placed gastrostomy tube is preferred. A balanced, high-protein, canned commercial cat food (e.g., Feline Prescription Diet p/d or c/d) is fed. A restricted protein diet (Feline Prescription Diet k/d) should be used only if hyperammonemia or overt signs of HE occur. Thiamine, taurine, arginines, L-Citrulline, and choline have been empirically recommended.

Intravenous fluid therapy with a balanced electrolyte solution supplemented with potassium chloride often is required in the initial stages of treatment. Abnormal blood coagulation test results and excess bleeding occasionally respond to vitamin K_1 therapy. A fresh blood transfusion may be required. With aggressive nutritional and supportive care, the success rate for recovery from IHL is about 65 per cent. The earlier treatment is initiated, the better the prognosis. Recurrence of IHL appears unlikely.

METABOLIC AND ENDOCRINE DISORDERS
(pp. 1353–1354)

DIABETES MELLITUS

Diabetes mellitus typically is associated with hepatic lipid accumulation in dogs and cats. Clinical evidence of liver dysfunction is rare. Marked increases in serum ALP activity are especially common in dogs with concurrent hyperadrenocorticism.

PANCREATITIS

Acute pancreatitis in dogs and cats frequently is associated with increased activity of serum liver enzymes and hyperbilirubinemia resulting from secondary hepatic injury. In cats with acute pancreatitis, hepatic lipidosis is the most consistent histologic feature. Less commonly, acute pancreatitis causes jaundice and increased liver enzyme activity because of obstruction of the common bile duct.

FELINE HYPERTHYROIDISM

Hyperthyroidism frequently is associated with mild to moderate increases in serum liver enzyme activities, especially ALP. Despite these abnormalities, liver function usually is not significantly impaired.

SUPERFICIAL NECROLYTIC DERMATITIS (HEPATOCUTANEOUS SYNDROME)

Superficial necrolytic dermatitis, a dermatologic disorder of dogs characterized by crusting lesions of the paw pads, mucocutaneous junctions, ears, and pressure points frequently is accompanied by a severe vacuolar hepatopathy with marked nodular regeneration. Serum ALP activity is moderately to markedly increased. Increased serum ALT activity is a less consistent finding. Concurrent diabetes mellitus is a common finding in dogs and usually is a late development.

HEPATIC AMYLOIDOSIS

Familial amyloidosis in Abyssinian cats is associated with asymptomatic hepatic involvement in as many as 70 per cent of cases. Hypervitaminosis A has also been associated with amyloidosis in cats. Clinical and biochemical evidence of hepatic dysfunction are rare. The disease is progressive, and treatment usually is unsuccessful.

HEPATIC ENZYME DEFICIENCIES (pp. 1354–1355)

GLYCOGEN STORAGE DISEASES

Glycogen storage diseases are inherited disorders resulting from deficiency of specific enzymes required for normal glycogen metabolism. Impaired hepatic glycogen mobilization usually is associated with fasting hypoglycemia. Three types of glycogen storage diseases have been suspected to occur in dogs: type I (von Gierke's disease), type II (Pompe's disease), and type III (Cori's disease).

Hepatic glycogen storage disease, types I and III, should be considered in young dogs with persistent or recurrent fasting hypoglycemia. Failure to increase blood glucose in response to intravenous glucagon or epinephrine supports the diagnosis of a glycogen storage disease. Definitive diagnosis of these disorders requires enzyme assay of affected tissues. Specific treatment is unavailable. Therapeutic efforts are directed at control of hypoglycemia. The prognosis is poor.

UREA CYCLE ENZYME DEFICIENCY

A congenital deficiency of a urea cycle enzyme results in hyperammonemia, protein intolerance, and HE. This diagnosis should be considered in young dogs and cats with hyperammonemia and HE in which the liver biopsy is normal and a congenital PSS has been excluded. HMD is another important differential diagnosis. Enzyme assay is required for definitive diagnosis.

C. Specific and Symptomatic Medical Management of Diseases of the Liver
(pages 1358–1371)

ACUTE HEPATOBILIARY DISEASE (pp. 1358–1362)

ACUTE HEPATIC FAILURE

The goals of treatment of AHF are to remove or reverse the inciting cause, to address the systemic derangements associated with hepatic dysfunction and to facilitate hepatic regeneration.

Antidotes

Specific antidotes are unavailable for most acute hepatotoxins, except for acetaminophen. If poisoning has occurred within 2 hours, vomiting should be induced, activated charcoal should be given and a sodium sulfate cathartic administered. If cyanosis is present, oxygen should be given. Oral or intravenous administration of *N*-acetylcysteine (NAC), should be initiated as soon as possible. Ascorbic acid should be given at the same time intervals as NAC.

Fluid, Electrolyte, and Acid-Base Abnormalities

Fluid, electrolyte, and acid-base imbalances should be addressed aggressively. Replacing, maintaining, and expanding vascular volume is a critical step. Renal excretion of toxic metabolites may also be hastened. Metabolic disturbances known to aggravate HE, such as metabolic alkalosis, hypokalemia, and hypoglycemia, must be corrected.

Hepatic Encephalopathy

Administration of locally acting agents that discourage formation of readily absorbable ammonia and hasten evacuation of the intestinal tract is indicated. Lactulose has beneficial effects in animals with HE. During early management of AHF and HE, lactulose is delivered as a retention enema. If lactulose is not available, a solution of povidone-iodine or neomycin sulfate liquid in water may be used to decrease bacterial numbers.

Cats with severe hepatic lipidosis and AHF present a special challenge. Severely affected cats should be stabilized (e.g., correct acid-base, electrolyte, and fluid imbalance; control HE) before anesthesia is considered (for hepatic biopsy and/or feeding tube placement). During the initial 3 days of hospitalization, nutritional support is provided. When the cat is stable, a more permanent feeding system is placed (pharyngostomy, tube gastrostomy).

The ideal diet for management of HE should primarily have carbohydrates as the energy source; use highly digestible protein of high biologic value; contain low levels of aromatic amino acids (AAA) and methionine and high levels of branched-chain amino acids (BCAA) and arginine; have adequate vitamins A, B, C, D, E, and K; and be supplemented with potassium, calcium, and zinc.

Many animals with HE require more than dietary protein restriction. In such cases, lactulose may be added to the treatment regimen. Many animals strongly object to the sweet taste of lactulose. An attractive alternative is lactitol. Another alternative is addition of antibacterial drugs that are effective for anaerobic (metronidazole) and gram-negative urea-splitting (neomycin sulfate) organisms. Reduction in dosage or metronidazole is recommended, considering the extensive involvement of the liver in its biotransformation.

Persistent CNS signs in animals with AHF can be the result of uncontrolled HE and/or increased intracranial pressure (ICP) and cerebral edema. Recommendations for treatment of patients with raised

TABLE 106–6. CONDITIONS THAT MAY ACCENTUATE OR PRECIPITATE HE IN DOGS AND CATS

Increased generation of ammonia in the intestine
    High-protein diet (especially red meat)
    Gastrointestinal hemorrhage
    Azotemia (increased enterohepic recirculation of urea)
    Constipation
    Infection (increased tissue catabolism and endogenous nitrogen load, decreased BCAA:AAA)
Movement of ammonia intracellularly in the brain
    Metabolic alkalosis (favors formation of readily diffusible form of the ammonia molecule: $NH_3 + H^+ \rightarrow NH_{4+}$)
    Hypokalemia (increases renal ammonia production)
Increased release of ammonia during gluconeogenesis from extrahepatic sites:
    Hyperglucagonemia secondary to hypoglycemia
Excess tranquilization (direct depressant action by heightened brain benzodiazepine and barbiturate receptor sensitivity)
Use of methionine-containing compounds (urinary acidifiers, "lipotrophic agents")
Use of stored blood for transfusion (high ammonia content)

BCAA:AAA, branched-chain amino acids:aromatic amino acids.
Conditions are listed in order of frequency in clinical observations of animals with acute or chronic hepatic failure.

ICP include elevation of the head and trunk, strict bed rest, mannitol, and furosemide. Certain conditions are known to accentuate or precipitate HE and should be avoided (Table 106–6). A summary of the steps in medical management of HE in animals is given in Table 106–7.

Bleeding Tendencies

No particular treatment is indicated for subclinical coagulopathy. If there is obvious bleeding, administration of a blood component to provide factors temporarily should be started as soon as blood specimens for coagulation tests are drawn. Additional treatment for gastrointestinal bleeding consists primarily of histamine-receptor antagonists, such as cimetidine and ranitidine. It is believed that vitamin K_1 can be quickly incorporated in prothrombin synthesis by newly regenerated hepatocytes.

Susceptibility to Infection

Human patients with serious acute and chronic hepatocellular disease have a high frequency of bacteremia. Sepsis is a common cause of death. If typical markers of sepsis (e.g., fever, leukocytosis with a left shift, toxic neutrophils) are absent but there is general clinical deterioration, blood specimens for anaerobic and aerobic culture should be collected. Treatment with a combination of antibiotics with bactericidal four-quadrant coverage and minimal nephrotoxicity is instituted. Amikacin combined with ampicillin or cephazolin is a good choice initially.

CHRONIC HEPATOBILIARY DISEASE (pp. 1362–1370)

Dietary Management

Reducing the metabolic loads on the liver can be aided by dietary therapy during recovery. Protein-restricted diets are formulated to be

TABLE 106–7. MEDICAL MANAGEMENT OF HEPATIC ENCEPHALOPATHY IN DOGS AND CATS

Acute (3 Days)
Nothing by mouth
Fluids given intravenously
   1. 0.45% saline in 2.5% dextrose with added potassium (use 20 to 30 mEq KCl per liter of administered fluids) until serum electrolyte results are available
   2. Add potassium according to serum electrolyte values and standard guidelines
Enemas q6h
   1. Warm-water cleansing enemas
   2. Retention enemas (instill into the colon with a Foley catheter; leave in place for 15 to 20 minutes). Use one of the following solutions:
      a. Lactulose (3 parts lactulose to 7 parts water at 20 ml/kg)
      b. Povidone-iodine (10%)
      c. Neomycin sulfate (10 mg/lb [22 mg/kg])
Other (no clear consensus for use)
   1. Branched-chain amino acid solutions
   2. L-dopa
   3. Bromocriptine
   4. Ion exchange resins
   5. Benzodiazepine-receptor antagonists

Chronic (Long-Term)
Protein-restricted diets (commercial or homemade)
Lactulose (dogs: 2.5 to 15 ml PO q8h, cats: 2.5 to 5 ml PO q8h)
Antibiotics (dosages are for either dog or cat)
   1. Metronidazole (3.4 mg/lb [7.5 mg/kg] PO q8h)
   2. Neomycin sulfate (10 mg/lb [22 mg/kg] PO q8h)
   3. Ampicillin (10 mg/lb [22 mg/kg] PO q8h)

highly digestible, contain high-quality protein in moderately restricted quantities, and rely on nonprotein sources for most of their calories. A balanced, high-protein maintenance diet should be fed to cats without signs of HE. For cats that are demonstrating HE, a combination of boiled rice and cottage cheese can be given short term or a protein-restricted prescription diet can be used.

Fluid Therapy

Fluid therapy may be necessary during episodes of decompensation from a previously stable state.

MEDICATIONS THAT MODIFY THE PATHOLOGIC PROCESS

Decopper

In dog breeds predisposed to copper (Cu) hepatotoxicosis, progressive liver injury will occur unless dietary Cu intake is restricted and, most important, hepatic Cu is mobilized for urinary excretion. Giving a reduced Cu diet will not remove excess hepatic Cu but will help slow further accumulation. Some prescription diets (Canine U/D) contain low concentrations of Cu, or a homemade diet can be used.

Drugs that chelate Cu and promote its removal from the liver are most useful in the management of clinically affected dogs. D-Penicillamine is the drug most often recommended. Months of treatment are needed before meaningful decreases in hepatic Cu content can be expected. Trientine may be used in animals that cannot tolerate D-penicillamine. Discouraging intestinal absorption of Cu may also be beneficial. An approach has been the use of zinc (Zn) acetate. This substance may aid in the management of affected dogs early in life, before massive accumulation of hepatic Cu occurs.

Suppress Hepatic Inflammation

Use of glucocorticoids for treatment of dogs with chronic inflammatory hepatic disease is controversial. Potential benefits of glucocorticoid treatment must be weighed against the many associated adverse effects. A favorable response would be a decrease in serum alanine aminotransferase activity and improvement in hepatic functional parameters and constitutional signs (appetite, attitude, body weight). Ideally, repeat hepatic biopsy should be done to most accurately assess response to treatment. Once improvement is established, the dosage of glucocorticoids should be tapered on an alternate-day regimen to the lowest needed to maintain remission.

If remission of clinical signs, laboratory test abnormalities, or hepatic histologic lesions has been achieved with prednisone therapy but there are unacceptable adverse effects of prednisone, azathioprine, initially given together for 7 to 10 days and then on alternate days with prednisone, can be used. Complete blood counts should be monitored. Glucocorticoids have also been reported to be advantageous in cats with lymphocytic or sclerosing cholangitis/cholangiohepatitis (CCH). The dose should be decreased when clinical and laboratory data indicate improvement. Some animals may require continued treatment or may fail to respond.

Modulate Fibrosis

Fibrogenesis is a common response to chronic hepatic injury. Many diseases have the potential to progress to the point of cirrhosis, at which point the lesion is considered irreparable. Antifibrotic agents other than prednisone are indicated for animals that have histologic evidence of fibrosis or that are intolerant or nonresponsive to prednisone. The drug used most often is colchicine. The duration of time needed to achieve benefit may be a reason why there are so few reports of dogs treated with colchicine. This medication has not been considered for use in cats.

Alter Bile Acid Dynamics

Retention of hydrophobic endogenous bile acids is an established feature of cholestatic hepatopathies. These bile acids can perpetuate cholestasis. Ursodeoxycholic acid (ursodiol) has been considered for treatment of chronic human hepatopathies. Little information is available about the clinical use of ursodiol in animals. Anecdotal reports suggest that beneficial changes in liver biochemical parameters as are observed in dogs. Dehydrocholic acid has been advocated by some as valuable adjunctive therapy for cats with CCH and sludged bile. This chemical should not be used in animals with mechanical biliary obstruction.

Eliminate Infection

Most primary chronic hepatobiliary diseases in dogs and cats are not caused by bacterial agents, except for ascending CCH. Appropriate treatment is therefore based on the results of bile and/or liver tissue culture and sensitivity testing. Good empiric antibiotic choices are ampicillin, amoxicillin–clavulanic acid, a first-generation cephalosporin, enrofloxacin, any aminoglycoside, or, if anaerobes are suspected, metronidazole or clindamycin.

Hepatic Encephalopathy

Principles for treatment of HE associated with AHF should be applied to dogs and cats with chronic hepatic insufficiency (see Table 106–6). A platform of a balanced protein-restricted diet, lactulose, and/or an antimicrobial is standard. Zinc supplementation may also be beneficial. Some have proposed vena caval bending in dogs with acquired PSSs and HE to reduce and redirect the volume of shunted portal blood to improve hepatic plasma flow and decrease signs of HE.

Ascites

Ascites is a common complication of many severe chronic hepatobiliary diseases in dogs. Treatment to control moderate to marked ascites usually is indicated chiefly to relieve respiratory embarrassment or anorexia associated with a perceived sense of fullness. Dietary sodium restriction, rest, and diuretic therapy usually are needed to blunt sodium and fluid retention. The aldosterone antagonist spironolactone is the drug of choice initially. If improvement is not noted, a loop diuretic such as furosemide should be added or substituted.

Abdominocentesis is an acceptable solution for dogs with ascites that has become refractory to dietary manipulation and pharmacologic diuresis. Removal of modest volumes of fluid should be done as infrequently as possible to avoid loss of albumin, subclinical hypovolemia, and renal hypoperfusion. If large-volume centesis is deemed necessary, albumin infusion should be given. Cats seldom develop portal hypertension and ascites, except for those animals with nonsuppurative CCH.

Gastrointestinal Ulceration

Treatment for chronic gastrointestinal hemorrhage not caused by DIC consists of an H-2–receptor antagonist and/or sucralfate. Coagulopathy from DIC in dogs with decompensated CHF should be managed with heparin therapy if sufficient plasma antithrombin (AT) III activity is present (greater than 40 per cent). Because plasma AT III may be low, fresh whole blood or fresh frozen plasma transfusion with added heparin should be given for AT III and factor replacement.

Persistent, complete major bile duct obstruction or severe cholestasis of other causes can result in vitamin K deficiency. Vitamin K_1 should be administered before surgical correction or liver biopsy. Vitamin K_1 should be included in the diet of animals with CHF of other causes.

Sepsis

Animals with CHF are at comparable risk for sepsis as those with AHF. Fever, leukocytosis, sudden hypoglycemia, azotemia, and laboratory evidence of DIC are all good clues. If no obvious source of infection is apparent, blood should be cultured aerobically and anaerobically.

CHAPTER 107

EXOCRINE PANCREATIC DISEASE
(pages 1372–1392)

DISEASES OF THE EXOCRINE PANCREAS
(pp. 1374–1390)

PANCREATITIS

Acute pancreatitis may be defined as inflammation of the pancreas with a sudden onset. Recurrent acute disease refers to repeated bouts of inflammation with little or no permanent pathologic change. Chronic pancreatitis is a continuing inflammatory disease characterized by irreversible morphologic change and possibly leading to permanent impairment of function. If an initial acute episode is not fatal, there may be complete resolution, or alternatively the inflammatory process may smolder continuously and asymptomatically.

Etiology

The inciting cause of spontaneous canine and feline pancreatitis is usually unknown. There is evidence that low-protein high-fat diets induce pancreatitis. Hyperlipoproteinemia is common in dogs with acute pancreatitis, and may develop secondary to pancreatitis as a result of abdominal fat necrosis or may be a cause of the disease.

A number of drugs may cause pancreatitis. Suspect drugs include thiazide diuretics, furosemide, azathioprine, L-asparaginase, sulfonamides, and tetracycline. Considerable controversy exists as to whether or not corticosteroids or H_2-receptor antagonists such as cimetidine may induce pancreatitis. Administration of cholinesterase inhibitor insecticides and cholinergic agonists has been associated with pancreatitis.

Obstruction of the pancreatic ducts produces inflammation, edema, atrophy, and fibrosis. Conditions that may lead to partial or complete obstruction include biliary calculi, sphincter spasm, edema of the duct or duodenal wall, tumor, parasites, trauma, and surgical interference. Surgical manipulation, automobile accidents, and falls from high buildings are potential causes of pancreatic trauma. In most cases, injury to the pancreas is probably mild or unrecognized.

Original chapter written by David A. Williams

Diagnosis

History and Clinical Signs. Dogs with acute pancreatitis are usually presented because of depression, anorexia, vomiting, and, in some cases, diarrhea. Severe acute disease may be associated with shock and collapse. Signs of pain may be elicited by abdominal palpation. An anterior abdominal mass is palpable in some cases. Most affected animals are mildly to moderately dehydrated and febrile. Affected animals are usually middle-aged or older and sometimes obese. The clinical signs of chronic pancreatitis are probably extremely variable and nonspecific, if the disease is clinically apparent at all. Clinical signs of pancreatitis in cats include lethargy, anorexia, dehydration, hypothermia, and vomiting.

Radiographic signs include increased density, diminished contrast and granularity in the right cranial abdomen, displacement of the stomach to the left, widening of the angle between the pyloric antrum and the proximal duodenum, displacement of the descending duodenum to the right, static gas pattern in or thickened walls of the descending duodenum, static gas pattern in or caudal displacement of the transverse colon, and delayed passage of barium through the stomach and duodenum. Ultrasonic imaging may reveal nonhomogeneous masses and loss of echodensity.

Laboratory Aids to Diagnosis. Leukocytosis is a common hematologic finding in acute pancreatitis. The packed cell volume may be increased. Azotemia is frequently present, usually the result of dehydration. Acute renal failure may occur. Liver enzyme activities are often increased. In some cases, particularly in cats, there is hyperbilirubinemia and sometimes clinically apparent icterus. Hyperglycemia may occur. Some affected animals are diabetic following recovery. In contrast, cats with suppurative pancreatitis often develop hypoglycemia. Hypocalcemia is usually mild to moderate and rarely associated with clinical signs of tetany. Hypercholesterolemia and hypertriglyceridemia are common, and hyperlipemia is often grossly apparent even though food has not been recently ingested.

Assays for pancreatic enzymes and zymogens include amylase, lipase, phospholipase A_2 and serum trypsin-like immunoreactivity (TLI). Serum TLI tends to increase earlier and decrease sooner than other enzymes. Serum TLI is pancreas-specific in origin whereas amylase, lipase, and phospholipase activities originate from pancreatic and extrapancreatic sources. In dogs with spontaneous disease, however, there may be elevations of one enzyme accompanied by minimal increases in another, while persistently normal activities are seen in some cases. In many cases there is a lack of correlation between the magnitude of enzyme activities and clinical severity.

Increased concentrations of circulating pancreatic enzymes may also arise secondary to reduced clearance from the plasma, as happens in renal failure. Increases more than two to three times above the upper limit of normal are unlikely to result from renal dysfunction alone. Lipase activity has been reported to be a more reliable marker for the diagnosis of pancreatitis than that of amylase. However, dexamethasone has been shown to increase canine serum lipase activity up to fivefold without histologic evidence of pancreatitis. In general, assay of serum lipase and TLI is most likely to reliably identify affected dogs. Reports of acute pancreatitis in cats are few, but increases in serum amylase and lipase concentrations are less than in dogs.

Treatment

The basis for therapy of acute pancreatitis is maintenance of fluid and electrolyte balance while the pancreas is "rested" by withholding food, and thereby allowed to recover from the inflammatory episode. If drug-induced pancreatitis is suspected, any incriminated agents should be withdrawn. Sufficient balanced-electrolyte intravenous solution should be given to replace fluid deficits and provide maintenance requirements while all oral intake is suspended for 3 or 4 days. Serum potassium should be monitored and supplemented via the IV fluids. Blind correction of suspected acid-base abnormalities should not be attempted unless documentation is provided by appropriate tests. It is common practice to give parenteral antibiotics during this supportive period, particularly when toxic changes are evident in the hemogram or when the patient is febrile.

If abdominal pain is severe, analgesic therapy should be given to provide relief. Hyperglycemia is often mild and transient, but in some cases diabetes mellitus may develop, requiring treatment with insulin. Some affected animals do not improve, and some continue to deteriorate in spite of supportive care. Transfusion of plasma or whole blood to replace α-macroglobulins may be lifesaving in these circumstances.

The use of corticosteroids in pancreatitis has been recommended, but they should be given only on a short-term basis to animals in shock associated with fulminating pancreatitis, and then in concert with fluids and plasma as described above.

Treatment of pancreatic masses (pseudocyst, abscess, phlegmon) and bile duct obstruction is controversial. It is not clear whether these animals are best managed conservatively with supportive therapy, or if surgical intervention to debride necrotic tissue and allow drainage of affected areas facilitates recovery. Generally, it is wise to avoid surgical intervention unless there is clear evidence of an enlarging mass and/or sepsis in a patient that is not responding well to medical therapy. Many patients that develop obstructive jaundice in association with acute pancreatitis recover spontaneously over 2 or 3 weeks with conventional supportive care alone.

One or 2 days after vomiting has ceased, small amounts of water should be offered, and if there is no recurrence of clinical signs, food may be gradually reintroduced. The diet should have a high carbohydrate content. Protein and fat are more potent stimulants of pancreatic secretion. If there is continued improvement, gradual introduction of a low-fat maintenance diet should be attempted. Total parenteral nutrition may be beneficial by sustaining the patient while the digestive system is rested for 7 to 10 days.

In many patients suffering a single episode of pancreatitis, the only long-term therapy recommended is to avoid feeding meals with an excessively high fat content. In other patients, repeated bouts of pancreatitis occur, and it may be beneficial to feed a moderately or severely fat-restricted diet permanently.

EXOCRINE PANCREATIC INSUFFICIENCY

Progressive loss of exocrine pancreatic acinar cells ultimately leads to failure of absorption due to inadequate production of digestive enzymes. Signs of exocrine pancreatic insufficiency (EPI) do not occur until a large proportion of the gland has been destroyed.

Etiology

Pancreatic Acinar Atrophy (PAA).   Spontaneous development of severe PAA in previously healthy adult animals appears to be uniquely common in the dog. The underlying cause of canine PAA is unknown. A high prevalence in the young German shepherd dog is recognized.

Chronic Pancreatitis.   Rarely, end-stage pancreatitis is the underlying cause of EPI in dogs and cats. However, those animals with EPI and coexistent diabetes mellitus probably fall into this category.

Diagnosis

History.   Animals with EPI usually have a history of weight loss despite a normal or increased appetite. Polyphagia is often severe. Some dogs may have periods of inappetence. Coprophagia and pica are also common. Water intake may increase in some dogs, and in chronic pancreatitis there may be polyuria and polydipsia due to diabetes mellitus.

Diarrhea often accompanies EPI, but can be variable in character. Most owners report frequent passage of large volumes of semiformed feces, although some patients have intermittent or continuous explosive watery diarrhea. There may be a history of vomiting, borborygmus, and flatulence. Young German shepherd dogs are predisposed to PAA, but this disease may occur in any breed at any age.

Clinical Signs. Mild to marked weight loss is usually seen. The haircoat is often in poor condition, and some animals may give off a foul odor.

Laboratory Aids to Diagnosis. Although replacement therapy with oral pancreatic enzymes is generally successful, response to treatment is not a reliable diagnostic approach. Routine laboratory test results are generally not helpful in establishing the diagnosis of EPI. Total lipid, cholesterol, and polyunsaturated fatty acid concentrations may be reduced. Complete blood count results are usually within normal limits.

Serum Trypsin-Like Immunoreactivity (TLI). Trypsinogen is synthesized exclusively by the pancreas, and measurement of the serum concentration of this zymogen provides a good indirect index of pancreatic function in the dog. This immunoassay detects both trypsinogen and trypsin, hence the use of the term trypsin-like immunoreactivity. Serum TLI concentration is both highly sensitive and specific for the diagnosis of canine EPI (Fig. 107–1).

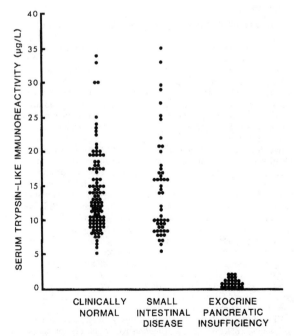

Figure 107–1. Serum trypsin-like immunoreactivity in 100 healthy dogs, 50 dogs with small intestinal disease, and 25 dogs with exocrine pancreatic insufficiency. (From Williams DA and Batt RM: Sensitivity and specificity of radioimmunoassay of serum trypsin-like immunoreactivity for the diagnosis of canine exocrine pancreatic insufficiency. JAVMA 192:195, 1988.)

Withdrawal from enzyme supplementation prior to testing of dogs that are already receiving treatment is unnecessary. Serum TLI concentrations will be normal in those rare dogs with EPI due to tumors obstructing the pancreatic ducts or to congenital deficiencies of enzymes other than trypsinogen. Equivocal serum TLI concentrations in the range 2.5 to 5.2 μg/L sometimes reflect failure to withhold food prior to collecting blood. Preliminary investigations have shown that serum TLI is subnormal in cats with EPI.

Fecal Proteolytic Activity. The reliability of this test varies widely. The widely used x-ray film digestion test is certainly unreliable. Proteolytic activity can be measured more precisely using dyed protein substrates such as azocasein, or by radial enzyme diffusion into agar gels containing casein substrate. Fecal proteolytic activity as assessed by these methods is consistently low in most dogs and cats with EPI, but because both dogs and cats with normal pancreatic function occasionally pass feces with low proteolytic activity, either repeated determinations must be made or, in dogs, the test can be performed on a single sample collected after feeding crude soybean meal for 2 days.

Other Tests. Studies have shown the bentiromide test to be relatively reliable for diagnosis of EPI in dogs, but it offers no advantages over assay of serum TLI or fecal proteolytic activity. Plasma turbidity (lipemia) after oral administration of fat is often diminished or absent in dogs with fat malabsorption, but this test and the repetition of the test after addition of pancreatic extract to the fat meal is insensitive and nonspecific for EPI.

Treatment

Enzyme Replacement. Most dogs and cats with EPI can be successfully managed by supplementing each meal with pancreatic enzymes present in commercially available dried pancreatic extracts. Numerous formulations are available, some of which are enteric-coated, and their enzyme contents and bioavailabilities vary widely. Addition of 2 teaspoonfuls of powdered nonenteric-coated preparation with each meal per 45 lb of body weight is generally an effective starting dose. This can be mixed with a maintenance dog food immediately prior to feeding. As soon as clinical improvement is apparent, owners can determine a minimum effective dose of enzyme supplement to prevent return of clinical signs.

Measures to Increase the Effectiveness of Enzyme Supplementation. Administration of pancreatic enzymes with food is generally successful. The following clinical observations have been made. Preincubation of food with enzyme powder for 30 minutes prior to feeding does not improve the effectiveness of oral enzyme treatment. The routine use of cimetidine in the treatment of EPI is not recommended. Enteric-coated preparations are often ineffective or less effective than powdered pancreatic extract or fresh pancreas.

Dietary Modification. With any individual dog it is necessary to regulate the amount of food given in order to maintain ideal body weight. Although therapy with regular maintenance dog food and appropriate enzyme replacement is usually effective, feeding of a highly digestible, low-fiber diet has been advocated. High-fiber diets probably should be avoided. Some patients may also benefit from addition of medium-chain triglycerides to the food.

Vitamin Supplementation. Dogs with EPI may have severe deficiencies of cobalamin and tocopherol which do not necessarily improve with oral pancreatic enzymes. It seems prudent to supplement these vitamins if serum concentrations are subnormal. Cobalamin must be given parenterally. Vitamin K–responsive coagulopathy has been reported concurrent with EPI.

Antibiotic Therapy. Dogs with PAA commonly have overgrowth of bacteria in the small intestine, but in most cases this is a subclinical abnormality, and affected individuals respond satisfactorily to pancreatic enzyme without antibiotics. Bacterial overgrowth can cause malabsorption and diarrhea, and in such cases antibiotic therapy may be of value. Oral oxytetracycline, metronidazole, or tylosin may be effective.

Glucocorticoid Therapy. In those few dogs that respond poorly to these treatments, oral prednisolone may be beneficial. In some such cases, lymphocytic-plasmacytic gastroenteritis coexists with EPI.

NEOPLASIA OF THE EXOCRINE PANCREAS

Pancreatic adenocarcinomas are uncommon, and they are particularly rare in cats. In both species they are seen in older animals. Adenocarcinomas are usually highly malignant tumors. Clinical signs are usually nonspecific: weight loss, anorexia, depression, and vomiting. Affected animals are often icteric because of associated obstruction of the bile ducts or widespread hepatic metastasis. Occasionally, dogs will have characteristic signs of diabetes mellitus or EPI.

Abdominal radiographs may suggest pancreatitis or indicate the presence of an anterior mass. Ultrasonographic examination may help to further define pancreatic abnormalities. There are no specific laboratory tests for pancreatic carcinoma, and results of routine tests may be misleading. Increased serum amylase and lipase activities are seen in some dogs. In most cases definitive diagnosis requires exploratory laparotomy. Chronic pancreatitis may grossly resemble pancreatic carcinoma.

PANCREATIC FLUKES IN CATS

There are several reports of infection with the pancreatic fluke, *Eurytrema procyonis,* in domestic cats. The infection is usually subclinical. Diagnosis is based on observation of characteristic eggs in the feces. Treatment with fenbendazole has been reported to be effective.

CHAPTER 108

DISEASES OF THE GALLBLADDER AND EXTRAHEPATIC BILIARY SYSTEM
(pages 1393–1398)

DIAGNOSTIC TOOLS FOR EVALUATING THE GALLBLADDER AND BILE DUCTS (pp. 1393–1394)

The CBC inconsistently reflects inflammation due to cholecystitis. Increased alanine aminotransferase (ALT) is common if inflammation ascends into the hepatic parenchyma. Increased serum alkaline phosphatase (SAP) and/or gamma-glutamyl transferase (GGT), with or without hyperbilirubinemia, is typical in partial or complete obstructions of the common bile duct. Hypercholesterolemia may be found

Original chapter written by Theresa W. Fossum and Michael D. Willard secondary to biliary tract obstruction, especially in cats. Urinalysis is helpful because marked bilirubinuria is usually seen before hyper-bilirubinemia.

Plain abdominal radiographs may reveal radiodense objects (e.g., gallstones) or air in the gallbladder. Ultrasonography is the most useful nonsurgical technique to distinguish hepatic parenchymal from biliary tract disease. Anorexic animals may have marked enlargement of the gallbladder, which can be mistaken for obstruction.

SPECIFIC DISEASES OF THE GALLBLADDER
(pp. 1395–1397)

OBSTRUCTIVE DISEASE

Pancreatic disease is the most common cause of extrahepatic biliary obstruction in dogs. Treatment initially consists of medical manage-ment of the pancreatitis. If this does not succeed, or if ascending bacte-rial infection is suspected, cholecystoduodenostomy or cholecystoje-junostomy may be considered. *Neoplasia* may also cause extrahepatic biliary obstruction. Therapy is generally unrewarding. Palliation may be achieved by cholecystojejunostomy. *Choleliths* that obstruct the common bile duct may be removed surgically.

NONOBSTRUCTIVE DISEASE

Cholecystitis is typically due to a bacterial infection of undetermined origin, although reflux of bacteria from the intestine via the common bile duct or hematogenous seeding may be the most common cause.

Bacterial cholangitis/cholangiohepatitis occurs if the infection ascends the biliary tree into the liver. *E. coli* is a relatively common cause. These animals are often presented because of icterus, anorexia, and/or vomiting. Clinical pathology data typically reveal increased serum ALT, SAP, GGT, and bilirubin. Hepatic biopsy with aerobic and anaerobic culture of bile and hepatic parenchyma are indicated. In gen-eral, β-lactam antibiotics are good initial choices until culture results are available.

Necrotizing cholecystitis occurs when a bacterial infection damages the gallbladder wall, often resulting in spillage of liquid bile into the abdomen. This usually produces a severe, generalized septic peritonitis causing anorexia, icterus, vomiting, fever, abdominal pain, and/or shock. Diagnosis is usually made by ultrasonography or at exploratory laparotomy. Treatment consists of cholecystectomy, antibiotics, and appropriate therapy for peritonitis.

Emphysematous cholecystitis occurs when the gallbladder is infected with gas-forming bacteria. Diagnosis is made by plain radiographs, and treatment consists of antibiotics. Enrofloxacin plus either amoxicillin or clindamycin is indicated.

Choleliths are often fortuitous findings at necropsy or during imag-ing with radiographs or ultrasonography. They are often clinically silent and cause no problems. If they are found in a patient with biliary tract disease, removal is indicated. *Parasites of the gallbladder and/or bile ducts* are uncommonly diagnosed. See the textbook. *Neoplasia* of the gallbladder or extrahepatic biliary tract is rare. Bile duct carcino-mas have been reported in cats and dogs.

RUPTURE OF THE GALLBLADDER OR EXTRAHEPATIC BILIARY DUCTS

Rupture may be associated with blunt abdominal trauma, cholecysti-tis, or obstruction secondary to stones, neoplasia, or parasites. *Trauma* usually causes rupture of bile ducts rather than the gallbladder. Gall-bladder rupture is more commonly associated with necrotizing chole-cystitis or cholelithiasis.

Early diagnosis of biliary tract rupture is imperative. If rupture is associated with biliary tract infection, clinical signs of bile peritonitis may develop quickly. However, in dogs with sterile bile (i.e., rupture due to trauma), clinical signs other than ascites and icterus may not be noted for several weeks. Bile in the abdominal cavity causes chemical peritonitis, which may not be associated with overt clinical signs initially. Diagnostic peritoneal lavage may assist in the early diagnosis of bile peritonitis. Surgical treatment options for rupture of the common bile duct include repair of the duct or biliary diversion.

CHAPTER 109

RECTO-ANAL DISEASE
(pages 1398–1409)

DISEASES OF THE RECTUM (pp. 1400–1405)

PERINEAL HERNIA

Perineal hernia is a condition seen almost exclusively in intact male dogs with a mean age of about 8 years. It is a less common occurrence in the cat.

History and Physical Examination. Dogs are presented with one or more of the following complaints: a reducible perineal swelling, tenesmus, dyschezia, constipation, and obstipation. The perineal swelling is usually ventrolateral to the anus on one side, but severely affected dogs may have bilateral ventral swellings. Some dogs have signs of acute urethral obstruction because of retroflexion of the urinary bladder into the perineal hernial space. Physical examination findings include a hernial sac that is palpated externally in some cases. Rectal examination reveals a defect in the pelvic diaphragm, confirming the diagnosis.

Diagnosis. Digital palpation of the rectum and anal canal will confirm the presence of unilateral or bilateral hernia. Boston terriers, Boxers, Welsh corgies, and Pekingese are all at apparent increased risk. Tenesmus resulting from prostatic disease or preexisting rectal disease might be risk factors for perineal hernia. Perineal urethrostomy and idiopathic megacolon are definite risk factors in the cat.

Therapy. Medical therapy may be attempted in mild cases. Some dogs can be maintained free of signs by the use of fecal softeners and occasional enemas. Herniorrhaphy is indicated for most cases of perineal hernia. Routine castration of all perineal hernia patients is also controversial. Since there are few contraindications to castration, it may be performed unless it unnecessarily prolongs anesthesia in a high-risk patient.

RECTAL TUMORS

The most common tumors of the rectum are benign adenomatous polyps. Occasionally, these rectal polyps invade the lamina propria and submucosa and, although they appear histologically benign, are referred to as carcinoma in situ. Colorectal adenocarcinomas tend to

Original chapter written by Robert J. Washabau and Daniel J. Brockman spread beyond the rectal wall to regional lymph nodes, liver, and lung. Most affected animals have signs of hematochezia, mucoid feces, tenesmus, and dyschezia of varying severity. Other signs depend on the tumor type and location.

Digital rectal examination typically reveals a prominent mass involving the rectal mucosa or submucosa, narrowing of the rectal lumen, pain on palpation, and blood or mucous. Survey and contrast radiography usually confirm the physical examination findings. Proctoscopy and biopsy are required for definitive diagnosis.

Tumors of the rectum, excluding lymphosarcoma, are best treated by complete surgical excision. Rectal lymphosarcomas are probably best treated initially with chemotherapy.

PROCTITIS

Proctitis infrequently occurs as a discrete entity in the dog or cat. It occurs more frequently in association with colitis or typhlocolitis. Animals with proctitis typically have signs of hematochezia, dyschezia, pain, or tenesmus. Anorectal examination in these patients frequently reveals a thickened rectal mucosa, mucohemorrhagic exudate, or blood and mucus admixed with feces. Proctoscopy and biopsy should be performed to exclude the possibility of a diffuse neoplasm.

Traumatic injuries associated with rectal foreign bodies are probably best treated by withholding food for 2 to 3 days, corticosteroid retention enemas, and/or systemic anti-inflammatory doses of corticosteroids. Other therapies include oral sulfasalazine.

RECTAL FOREIGN BODIES

Ingested sticks, bones, and metal may traverse the entire alimentary tract with only minor pathology before lodging in the rectum and causing painful obstruction. Complications include rectal fistula, colonic impaction, and perirectal abscesses if the rectal wall is compromised.

RECTAL PROLAPSE

Many animals have an antecedent history of dyschezia and tenesmus associated with anorectal or colonic inflammatory disease. On physical examination, an elongated, cylindric mass is evident with complete prolapse of the rectum. This protrusion must be carefully differentiated from a prolapsed ileocolic intussusception. Contrast radiography can be useful in differentiating these two conditions.

Incomplete prolapses are usually easily reduced manually with the aid of saline compresses or lubricants. A purse-string suture may be placed if a tendency toward recurrence seems obvious. Complete prolapses characterized by short duration and good tissue viability are probably best managed by manual reduction and placement of an anal purse-string suture. Prolapses of longer duration, in which there is substantial tissue devitalization, should instead be managed either by mucosal resection or complete resection and anastamosis. Colopexy is currently recommended for cats suffering from rectal prolapse. Postoperative management should consist of high-fiber diets and bulk or emollient laxatives to soften the feces.

RECTAL STRICTURE

Fibrosing rectal strictures result from anorectal trauma or surgery, whereas proliferative rectal strictures typically result from cancer. Most animals have dyschezia, tenesmus, and passage of a thin ribbon of feces. Digital rectal examination typically reveals a firm, circumferential fibrotic band or an asymmetric mass. Contrast radiography may be useful in identifying the proximal extent of rectal stricture. Intrarectal ultrasonography is likely to assume increasing importance in the evaluation of proliferative strictures. Biopsy and histologic examination are recommended if there is any doubt about the pathogenesis of the lesion. Mild cases of rectal stricture may respond to bougienage. Surgical correction is required in most cases.

CONGENITAL ABNORMALITIES OF THE RECTUM

Rectovaginal Fistula and Imperforate Anus

Rectovaginal fistula is a rare congenital disorder of dogs and cats that may occur with or without imperforate anus. In either case the vagina is contaminated with feces, resulting in a severe vaginitis, vulvitis, and perivulvar and perianal dermatitis. Diagnosis may be achieved either by vaginography or barium enema. The treatment is surgical correction.

DISEASES OF THE ANUS (pp. 1405–1409)

PERIANAL FISTULA

Dogs are typically presented with one or more of the following complaints: tenesmus, dyschezia, fecal incontinence, licking of the anal area, anal bleeding, constipation, and a malodorous anorectal discharge. Large-breed dogs are most commonly affected, with the highest incidence in German shepherds and Irish setters. Physical examination usually reveals single or multiple areas of ulceration, fistulous tracts, and a purulent exudate with frank hemorrhage. Anorectal palpation may reveal multiple rectocutaneous fistulas and anal stenosis. Ruptured anal sac abscess and perianal adenocarcinoma are the only important differential diagnoses.

Therapy. Suggested medical therapies have consisted of various combinations of oral antibiotics, topical antibiotics, local hydrotherapy, and topical antiseptics and anti-inflammatory agents. These therapies are not usually successful. There is little agreement as to the best method of surgical treatment. No technique is consistently curative. Further, many techniques have been associated with significant postoperative problems.

ANAL SAC IMPACTION, SACCULITIS, AND ABSCESSATION

Dogs with inflammatory lesions of the anal sacs have one or more of the following complaints: licking or biting at the anal area, tail chasing, "scooting," discomfort in sitting, perianal rubbing, painful defecation, and tenesmus. Physical examination reveals evidence of unilateral or bilateral anal sac disease. The anal sacs are often swollen and painful. Purulent or granular anal sac material, blood, unusual coloration, and turbidity are all abnormal findings.

An impacted anal sac is swollen, but usually nonpainful. The impacted anal sac contains a viscous gray to brown material that is expressed with only moderate difficulty. Anal sac abscessation is characterized by extreme perianal pain and fever. Anal sac impaction can be conservatively managed by manually expressing the anal sacs during rectal examination. Anal sacculectomy should be considered only in cases of chronic recurrence.

Anal sacculitis is best treated with topical antibiotics or antibiotic-corticosteroid combinations. This may be accomplished by duct cannulation and irrigation of the anal sac with a mild antiseptic solution, followed by instillation with an antibiotic or antibiotic-corticosteroid solution. Systemic antibiotic therapy is rarely necessary. Anal sac abscesses should be managed with open drainage. Systemic antibiotics should also be administered to dogs that are febrile or have extensive inflammation. Recurrent anal sac abscessation is probably best treated by anal sacculectomy.

ANAL SAC TUMORS

Neoplasms arising from the anal sacs are almost invariably malignant adenocarcinomas. Over 90 per cent of affected dogs have been older (>10 years) intact or spayed females. Dyschezia and a noticeable perineal swelling are the most frequent complaints. In some dogs, complaints of polyuria/polydipsia, muscular weakness, vomiting, and constipation may be made. These features are secondary to a paraneoplastic syndrome (humoral hypercalcemia of malignancy [HHM]) sometimes associated with this tumor.

Tumors are usually detected during routine anorectal examination. Most are unilateral. It is estimated that more than 50 per cent of affected dogs have physical or radiographic evidence of metastasis at the time of presentation. Surgical excision of the primary anal sac mass is the recommended treatment. Radiation therapy and immunotherapy have not proved useful.

ANAL AND PERIANAL TUMORS

Perianal Gland Adenomas

This tumor has a breed predisposition for the cocker spaniel, bulldog, beagle, and Samoyed. Eighty-five per cent of perianal gland adenomas are found in older intact male dogs. They may cause an intensely pruritic anusitis and eventually interfere with defecation. Aside from these features, perianal adenomata are neither invasive nor metastatic.

These tumors can be effectively treated by surgical excision. Radiation therapy and cryosurgery are reported to be as effective as surgery. Dogs should also be castrated because of the androgen-dependence of the tumor. Estrogen therapy could be considered if the pet owner is unwilling to accept castration.

FECAL INCONTINENCE

Reservoir incontinence occurs when there is a reduction in the reservoir capacity of the colon, best typified by total or subtotal colectomy. Sphincter incontinence occurs with denervating lesions of the external anal sphincter or with primary external anal sphincter injury. Animals are, in general, more severely and irreversibly affected with sphincter incontinence lesions. The remainder of this discussion will therefore be devoted to lesions of sphincter incontinence.

Animals affected will have an inability to control flatus, accumulate fecal material at the anal opening between defecations, involuntarily eliminate feces with excitement, or have constant anal dribbling with failure to assume even a normal defecation posture. Concurrent urinary incontinence would implicate a neural lesion. Rectal examination reveals decreased tone of the anal sphincter and rectum. Dogs with neurogenic sphincter incontinence may evidence other neurologic deficits.

A diagnosis is usually apparent from history and physical examination findings. Complete neurologic examination generally discriminates neurogenic from non-neurogenic causes of sphincter incontinence. Survey spinal radiography and myelography are indicated in the further evaluation of suspected spinal cord or cauda equina lesions.

Neurogenic and non-neurogenic sphincter incontinence are usually permanent and untreatable. It has been suggested that mild cases of incontinence may improve with empiric use of loperamide. However, most cases of external anal sphincter incompetence are unlikely to be improved by loperamide. The success rate with surgical techniques is not satisfactory. The prognosis is poor in almost all cases.

CHAPTER 110

FELINE HYPERLIPIDEMIA
(pages 1410–1414)

The hyperlipoproteinemias are disturbances of lipid transport that result from primary defects in the metabolism of lipoprotein particles and those that are secondary to an underlying metabolic abnormality such as insulin deficiency or resistance, or a deficiency of thyroid hormone.

DIAGNOSTIC TESTS (pp. 1410–1411)

Chylomicron (CM) Test. Chylomicrons (CMs) form a cream layer on the surface of the plasma sample after overnight storage at 40°F (4°C). The other lipoprotein classes remain in the infranatant.

Electrophoresis. This test does not give quantitative results, but it does indicate a shift in lipoprotein distribution.

Ultracentrifugation. This technique provides a quantitative method of measurement of cholesterol (CH), triglycerides (TGs), and apoproteins in the different lipoprotein classes.

Lipoprotein Lipase (LPL) Activity. LPL activity is measured *in vivo* after the administration of heparin, which activates the enzyme *in vivo*. Basal blood samples are collected before and ten minutes after heparin administration for LPL activity.

DIAGNOSIS OF HYPERLIPIDEMIA (p. 1411)

Three alternatives should be considered for lipemic plasma: that the sample was obtained postprandial; that the lipemia is secondary to an underlying metabolic disorder; or that the lipemia is due to a primary disorder of lipid metabolism. If the condition remains undiagnosed in spite of routine diagnostic tests, a hereditary disease should be suspected, and lipoprotein electrophoresis and/or ultracentrifugation is essential to define the nature of the defect.

SECONDARY HYPERLIPIDEMIA (pp. 1411–1412)

Nephrotic Syndrome. Plasma cholesterol concentrations are usually increased.

Diabetes Mellitus. Insulin is necessary for normal LPL activity. Thus, patients with diabetes mellitus have low LPL activity.

Drug-Induced Hyperlipemia. Diabetes mellitus has been reported in cats receiving long-term treatment with the progestogen, megestrol acetate.

PRIMARY HYPERLIPIDEMIAS (pp. 1412–1413)

Hyperchylomicronemia appears to be familial.

Clinical Signs. The most common signs observed in affected cats are xanthomas and lipemia retinalis. A common site for xanthomas is where the spinal nerves emerge through the vertebral foramina. Other common sites include bony prominences and where the sciatic nerve passes over the greater ischiatic notch. The presence of xanthomas at these sites results in pressure on the nerves and motor paral-

Original chapter written by Boyd Jones

ysis. Sensation to painful stimuli is retained. Xanthomas may occur in other organs: liver, spleen, kidney, heart, muscle, and intestines.

With severe hyperchylomicronemia (triglyceride concentration > 1000 mg/dl), lipemia retinalis can be detected by examination of the ocular fundus. Vision is not affected, and there are no apparent clinical sequelae.

Laboratory Findings. Most affected cats show a severe fasting hyperchylomicronemia. The blood has the appearance of "cream of tomato" soup. Some cats have massive elevations of plasma triglyceride (5000 to 10,000 mg/dl). In most affected cats a positive CM test is noted. Ultracentrifugation shows a significant increase in chylomicrons and a smaller increase in VLDL. HDL is decreased. Affected cats show reduced (but not absent) LPL activity in plasma. The remaining activity is due to hepatic lipase.

Therapy. Secondary hyperlipidemia should resolve if the underlying disease is adequately treated. Since hypertriglyceridemia is the major abnormality associated with primary lipid disorders, the goal of therapy is to lower serum TG levels by feeding a low-fat diet. Prescription diets (r/d Hills Pet Products) or homemade low-fat diets have been effective. *The peripheral nerve paralysis can be expected to resolve after 2 to 3 months on a low-fat diet.* Medium-chain triglyceride (MCT) oil may be considered as an alternative dietary source of lipid in cases where chylomicronemia persists despite appropriate dietary therapy. Gemfibrozil is effective in reducing TG levels in some cats.

CHAPTER 111

CANINE HYPERLIPIDEMIA
(pages 1414–1419)

In dogs, hyperlipidemia either results from a familial *(primary)* defect in lipoprotein metabolism or is an acquired disorder that develops *secondary* to a disease in which lipid metabolism is significantly altered, e.g. insulin-dependent diabetes mellitus.

THE LIPOPROTEIN CLASSES

Chylomicrons. These are the largest and least dense lipoprotein particles, and they are predominately responsible for the transport of dietary fat (triglyceride) from the intestine. Their presence is confirmed by the development of a so-called "cream layer" after the sample is allowed to stand undisturbed for 6 to 10 hours. Lipoprotein lipase hydrolyzes the triglycerides (TGs) into fatty acids, which enter adipocytes and muscle. What remains is a remnant particle that subsequently delivers cholesterol (CH) to the liver.

Very Low-Density Lipoproteins (VLDLs). Produced in the liver and containing a predominance of triglycerides, the VLDL particles are transported to tissue capillaries where they are catabolized by lipoprotein lipase.

Low-Density Lipoprotein (LDL). Subsequent to the hydrolysis of VLDL and the removal of triglycerides from its core, a short-lived intermediate-density lipoprotein is ultimately converted by the liver to LDL.

Original chapter written by Richard B. Ford

High-Density Lipoprotein (HDL). Most of the circulating CH in dogs and cats is carried in HDL.

THE HYPERLIPIDEMIC STATES (pp. 1415–1418)

Disturbances of lipid transport that culminate in excess concentrations of TG are the most important form of hyperlipidemia in veterinary medicine. Affected dogs are at risk of developing acute pancreatitis. Fasting TG concentrations in excess of 1000 mg/dl represent extreme risk. In fasted patients, serum turbidity, or *lipemia,* denotes hypertriglyceridemia. Hypercholesterolemia, on the other hand, will not cause the sample to become lipemic.

LABORATORY CONSIDERATIONS

Diagnosis of hyperlipidemia should be based on laboratory determination of serum TG and total CH. Hyperlipidemia becomes clinically important in dogs when fasting TG concentrations exceed 500 mg/dl or the CH concentration exceeds 300 mg/dl. Lipoprotein electrophoresis (LPE) appears to have limited value in the clinical evaluation of lipid disorders in the dog and cat.

The Chylomicron (CM) Test. The lipemic serum is allowed to stand undisturbed for 6 to 10 hours under refrigeration. Chylomicrons, if present, will float to the surface of the sample, forming an opaque "cream layer" over a clear infranatant. This finding suggests a disorder of CM catabolism. If the sample remains turbid, but without formation of a "cream layer," retention of VLDL, rather than chylomicrons, is suggested. In some dogs a "cream layer" may form over turbid, lipemic serum, suggesting retention of both chylomicrons and VLDL.

PRIMARY HYPERLIPIDEMIAS

Idiopathic Hyperchylomicronemia

Miniature schnauzers are predisposed to primary, or familial, hyperlipidemia.

Clinical Signs. Presenting signs most often are vomiting and diarrhea. Additional signs include nonlocalizing abdominal pain or discomfort accompanied by decreased appetite and lipemia. Affected dogs are typically 4 years of age and older. Clinical signs and history may be compatible with acute pancreatitis; however, abdominal radiographs, ultrasonograms, and laboratory evidence supporting a diagnosis of pancreatitis are typically lacking. Sustained hypertriglyceridemia is a principal risk factor for the development of acute pancreatitis.

Hypertriglyceridemia should also be considered in patients presenting with a history of seizures. The blood, and particularly the serum, is visibly lipemic and may remain so following a 24-hour or longer fast. Serum lipid determinations reveal extreme concentrations of total triglycerides (>1000 mg/dl) and moderate elevations in total CH. Dogs with a TG concentration of 500 mg/dl or higher are considered to be at risk of developing clinical signs and, as such, are candidates for dietary intervention.

Diagnosis. Idiopathic hyperchylomicronemia is confirmed in fasted dogs with lipemic serum, hypertriglyceridemia (in uncleared serum) greater than 500 mg/dl, and a positive CM test.

Therapy. Restriction of dietary fat is the first and most important line of therapy. The desired goal is a serum TG level, *in uncleared serum,* less than 500 mg/dl and a normal CH level with little or no weight loss. If the goal is reached, this diet becomes the recommended diet for life. Drug therapy for patients failing to respond to dietary fat restriction have included clofibrate, niacin, and gemfibrozil, as well as n-3 polyunsaturated fatty acids from fish oils. Indiscriminate use of these products in dogs and cats cannot be recommended until such time as dosage and efficacy are determined.

Idiopathic Hypercholesterolemia

In a limited survey of healthy adult dogs, it was suggested that primary hypercholesterolemia might occur within some families of Doberman pinschers and rottweilers. In some dogs hypercholesterolemia cannot be explained. Treatment specifically intended to lower serum CH does not appear to be warranted.

SECONDARY HYPERLIPIDEMIAS

Postprandial Hyperlipidemia. Chylomicrons will normally appear in the serum of dogs and cats within 30 minutes to 1 hour following the ingestion of a meal containing fat. This is associated with a transient (3 to 10 hours) increase in serum TG, after which levels rapidly return to base line. Physiologic hyperlipidemia is easily excluded from consideration if the patient is known to have fasted within the 12 hours prior to blood collection.

Diabetes Mellitus. In insulin-deficient states, the clearance of chylomicrons is impaired. Examination of lipid profiles reveals reveals lipemia, an increase in both chylomicrons and VLDL, and a corresponding increase in TG concentration. In some diabetic dogs, excess serum CH concentrations are present. The hyperlipidemia associated with diabetes mellitus usually improves or resolves as glycemic control is achieved. Diabetic dogs with excess serum TG concentrations appear to be at risk of developing acute pancreatitis.

Protein-Losing Nephropathy. Hyperlipidemia, characterized by increased serum CH or TG, may be detected in patients with proteinuria due to glomerulonephritis or amyloidosis.

Hyperadrenocorticism (Cushing's Disease). Hypercholesterolemia has been recognized in dogs with hyperadrenocorticism without concomitant diabetes mellitus. Affected dogs have clear serum and no discrete clinical signs specifically attributable to the excess CH concentration.

Hypothyroidism. Hypercholesterolemia is present in about two-thirds of hypothyroid dogs; atherosclerotic-type arterial lesions have occasionally been reported.

SECTION XI
THE ENDOCRINE SYSTEM

CHAPTER 112

PITUITARY-HYPOTHALAMIC DISEASE
(pages 1422–1436)

DISEASES OF THE PITUITARY GLAND (pp. 1425–1428)

PITUITARY HYPOFUNCTION (HYPOPITUITARISM) OR PITUITARY DWARFISM

Hypopituitarism is a deficiency of one (monotropic failure), several (multitropic failure), or all (panhypopituitarism) pituitary hormones. Pituitary dwarfism is most commonly seen in the German shepherd dog but has also been reported in the miniature pinscher, spitz, Carnelian bear dog, and immunodeficient Weimeraners.

Clinical signs in the young dog include a short stature compared to litter mates, a soft, woolly haircoat, bilateral symmetric alopecia sparing the head and extremities, and thin scaly skin. Musculoskeletal abnormalities include delayed closure of the epiphyseal growth plates and retention of the deciduous teeth with delayed eruption of the permanent teeth. Affected dogs may exhibit hypogonadism. Routine clinicopathologic tests usually show no significant abnormalities and are used to rule out other causes of dwarfism. Thyroid-stimulating hormone (TSH) and adrenocorticotrophic hormone (ACTH) stimulation tests are usually normal in dogs with uncomplicated hypopituitarism; however, secondary hypothyroidism or secondary hypoadrenocorticism may be seen.

Insulin response testing may support the diagnosis of growth hormone (GH) deficiency. Since GH has anti-insulin properties, patients with GH deficiency are sensitive to the hypoglycemic effects of insulin. This provacative test may cause serious hypoglycemia, and dogs undergoing the test must be closely monitored.

Definitive diagnosis requires a stimulation test utilizing the alpha-adrenergic agonist clonidine or the structurally similar sedative analgesic xylazine to stimulate the release of GH for subsequent assay. Pituitary dwarfs show little or no GH response compared to normal controls.

Therapy for hypopituitarism is GH replacement. Response to therapy may be evidenced by visible hair growth in 4 to 6 weeks. Epiphyseal closure may result soon after initiation of therapy; therefore body stature may not appreciably improve. Adverse reactions to GH therapy include diabetes mellitus and hypersensitivity reactions. Secondary hypothyroidism should be treated with thyroxine. Adrenocortical hor-

---

Original chapter written by Rhett Nichols and Leland Thompson

mone replacement therapy should be employed in dogs with secondary hypoadrenocorticism.

ACQUIRED GROWTH HORMONE DEFICIENCY

In the dog, a potential hereditary syndrome has been described in the Pomeranian, poodle, Lhasa apso, chow chow, keeshonden, Samoyed, and American water spaniel. Most dogs presented with GH-responsive dermatosis are between 1 and 5 years of age. Affected dogs usually have bilaterally symmetric truncal hair loss and hyperpigmentation. The hair loss may occur at any age but usually begins at puberty.

In dogs, routine endocrinologic testing including TSH response, ACTH response, and dexamethasone suppression testing should be performed to rule out other endocrinologic causes of alopecia. Assessment of serum GH secretion in response to clonidine, xylazine, or human GHRF have been used. Assays of canine GH are currently unavailable. Therapy is similar to that for congenital hypopituitarism.

FUNCTIONAL PITUITARY NEOPLASIA

Chromophobe adenomas are most common and may secrete excess ACTH, resulting in pituitary-dependent hyperadrenocorticism. Tumors of the pars intermedia are less common, but adenomas of the pars intermedia may cause Cushing's disease in dogs. Neoplasms of the pituitary may cause hypopituitarism due to dorsal expansion of the mass. Signs of hypopituitarism in dogs with such neoplasms include polyuria and polydipsia due to impaired antidiuretic hormone (ADH) synthesis, progressive weight loss, and atrophy of the sex organs. Derangement of osmoreceptors in the anterior hypothalamus may induce alterations in water intake ranging from adipsia to polydipsia. Hypernatremia or hyponatremia may result from abnormal water intake. Space-occupying chromophobe adenomas have been reported to induce neurologic signs such as blindness in dogs.

NONFUNCTIONAL PITUITARY NEOPLASIA

Nonfunctional neoplasms of the pituitary may also cause hypopituitarism due to expansion of the mass. Primary nonfunctional neoplasms include craniopharyngiomas and astrocytomas, whereas reported metastatic neoplasms include lymphosarcoma, malignant melanoma, and mammary carcinoma.

HYPERSOMATOTROPISM: ACROMEGALY

In cats, acromegaly usually results from the excessive secretion of GH by a pituitary adenoma. In dogs, acromegaly due to functional pituitary neoplasia is rare, and GH excess in this species more frequently arises from progestagen therapy or occurs during diestrus (progesterone phase) in the female.

Most cats with acromegaly are middle- to old-aged (8 to 14 years). Males are over-represented. Facial appearance and body size are often altered. These changes include a broadened, blunt facial structure, excessive skin folds around the face and neck, increased body weight, and enlargement of the abdomen. More distinctive findings include enlarged interdental spaces and inspiratory stridor associated with thickening of the membranes of the upper airways. Hypertrophy of internal organs such as the heart, liver, and kidneys has been described. Cardiomyopathy may occur and may progress to congestive heart failure. Polyuria and polydipsia may result from increases in glomerular filtration rate or may be secondary to diabetes mellitus (DM).

Acromegaly should be suspected in diabetic cats that are poorly responsive to insulin therapy and exhibit the characteristic signs. Computed tomography or magnetic resonance imaging of the pituitary region may demonstrate a pituitary mass. Definitive diagnosis requires demonstration of elevated circulating GH concentrations.

Symptomatic therapy should include management of DM and congestive heart failure. Specific therapy for pituitary neoplasms includes surgical excision, radiation therapy, and medical therapy. Pituitary-directed cobalt irradiation therapy is recommended as primary therapy for cats showing signs of acromegaly with evidence of a pituitary mass on computed tomography.

GROWTH HORMONE–INDUCED DIABETES MELLITUS

In the dog, DM may result from excess endogenous or exogenous GH. Initially, hyperglycemia is associated with high insulin values. As the disease progresses, pancreatic beta cell exhaustion may occur, resulting in low serum insulin concentrations. Clinical signs associated with acquired GH excess included inspiratory stridor, polyuria/polydipsia, increased soft tissue thickness, and enlarged interdental spaces. Laboratory abnormalities are typical of unregulated DM.

Definitive diagnosis would be established by demonstrating elevated circulating GH or IGF 1 concentrations or by evaluating pituitary GH response (suppression) to a glucose load. Unfortunately, there is no validated assay for GH in veterinary medicine.

Successful therapy includes withdrawal of progestagen therapy and/or ovariohysterectomy for estrus control. Close monitoring of patients following withdrawal of therapy or ovariohysterectomy is advised because insulin requirements may decrease or cease completely.

DISORDERS OF THE NEUROHYPOPHYSIS
(pp. 1428–1434)

DIABETES INSIPIDUS

Diabetes insipidus (DI) is a disorder of water metabolism characterized by polyuria, urine of low specific gravity or osmolality (so called insipid or tasteless urine), and polydipsia. It is caused by defective secretion or synthesis of ADH (central DI) or by the inability of the renal tubule to respond to this hormone (nephrogenic DI).

ETIOLOGY

The idiopathic forms of central DI are the most common in veterinary medicine. Secondary central DI usually results from head trauma or neoplasia. Congenital or primary nephrogenic DI appears to be rare in veterinary medicine. Causes of acquired (secondary) nephrogenic DI, both complete and partial, include pyelonephritis, chronic renal failure, hypercalcemia, hypokalemia, hyperadrenocorticism, hyperthyroidism, hepatic failure, and pyometra.

CLINICAL FEATURES

The physical examination in most dogs or cats with primary central and nephrogenic DI is unremarkable. Those animals with acquired central DI secondary to a growing neoplasm may have additional signs. Most dogs and cats with DI have a urine specific gravity ≤ 1.010 and an inactive sediment with trace to no proteinuria. Routine CBC, serum biochemical, and electrolyte profiles are unremarkable for central and primary nephrogenic DI. When abnormalities are present, they are usually secondary to dehydration.

The exception to the rule of normal blood work and insignificant proteinuria is the dog with central DI and concurrent pituitary-dependent hyperadrenocorticism. These animals usually have elevated serum alkaline phosphatase and cholesterol, and often have significant proteinuria scondary to glomerulonephritis.

The Modified Water-Deprivation Test. This test is designed to determine whether endogenous ADH is released in response to dehydration and whether the kidneys can respond to ADH. Since DI is an uncommon disorder, the more common causes of polyuria and polydipsia should be ruled out prior to putting a dog or cat through this procedure. Failure to recognize other polyuric syndromes may lead to an incorrect or inconclusive diagnosis or cause significant patient morbidity.

The test is performed in two stages—an abrupt water-deprivation test followed by a vasopressin response test. When more than 5 per cent of body weight has been lost, the urine is checked for specific gravity or osmolality or both. Failure to concentrate urine adequately indicates that the animal has either central or nephrogenic DI.

Following water deprivation, desmopressin acetate (DDAVP) or aqueous vasopressin may be given. Further increase in urine osmolality after administration of aqueous vasopressin or DDAVP greater than 10 per cent is suggestive of central DI or partial nephrogenic DI (Table 112–1). Increase in urine osmolality less than 10 per cent is suggestive of a vasopressin-resistant disorder (i.e., complete nephrogenic DI or psychogenic polydipsia).

To minimize the possible effects of renal medullary washout on test results, progressive water restriction prior to abrupt water deprivation is recommended by some authorities.

The ADH Trial. As an alternative to the modified water deprivation test, or in cases in which this test fails to establish a definitive diagnosis, a closely monitored therapeutic trial with DDAVP can be performed. A dramatic reduction in water intake greater than 50 per cent during the first treatment day would strongly suggest a vasopressin deficiency and a diagnosis of central DI or partial nephrogenic DI. When the polyuria is due to other causes, the decrease is seldom more than 30 per cent. It is advisable to measure water intake for 2 or more days during the DDAVP therapeutic trial.

Misdiagnosis Following Diagnostic Testing. Factors that may alter proper interpretation include renal medullary washout,

TABLE 112–1. DIFFERENTIATION OF CENTRAL DI (CDI) AND NEPHROGENIC DI (NDI) FROM PRIMARY POLYDIPSIA (PP)

PARAMETER	BEFORE WATER DEPRIVATION	AFTER WATER DEPRIVATION		
	DI and PP	CDI	NDI	PP
Urine:				
Uvol ml/24h/kg	>50	>50	>50	<50
USG	<1.010	<1.010	<1.010	<1.025
UOsm mOsm/kg	<300	<300	<300	<700
Blood:				
POsm mOsm/kg	290–310	>310	>310	±310
PNa mEq/L	<140 to >155	>155	>155	>155
PAVP pg/ml	<5.5 to >5.5	<3.0	>5.5	>5.5
UOsm/POsm	<1.0	<1.0	<1.0	2 to 3
ADH Stimulation Test:				
UOsm > POsm	±	+	–	–

Adapted from Grunbaum EG and Moritz A: The diagnosis of nephrogenic diabetes insipidus in the dog. Tierazliche Praxis 19:539, 1991.

enhanced antidiuretic response to low levels of ADH in patients with central DI, and abnormally elevated osmolar set points for ADH release. One of the most common causes of misinterpretation is the unsuspected case of hyperadrenocorticism.

OTHER TESTS USED TO DIAGNOSE DIABETES INSIPIDUS

See textbook.

TREATMENT OF DIABETES INSIPIDUS

Hormonal Replacement Therapy: Desmopressin Acetate (DDAVP)

Administration of DDAVP should completely eliminate polyuria and polydipsia, both acutely and during long-term therapy, in dogs and cats with DI. Because of individual differences, the dose required to achieve complete, around-the-clock control varies. Usually, one to four drops of the intranasal preparation administered once or twice daily in the conjunctival sac is sufficient to control signs of central DI.

The only complication of any importance is the induction of water intoxication. This complication is uncommon and results from a failure to adequately reduce water intake because of damage to the inhibitory component of the thirst mechanism. To avoid this potential problem it is recommended that subsequent doses of DDAVP be administered when polyuria recurs. If hyponatremia develops, the treatment should be stopped and the diagnosis reevaluated.

Nonhormonal Therapy

Chlorpropamide. Chlorpropamide appears to potentiate the renal tubular effects of ADH. The effectiveness of chlorpropamide in the treatment of canine central DI has been variable.

Thiazide Diuretics. Therapeutic success with nephrogenic DI and central DI has been achieved with the use of the thiazide diuretics hydrochlorothiazide and chlorothiazide. The dose of these drugs must be individualized for each patient. Side effects are rare but may include occasional hypokalemia.

Nonsteroidal Anti-Inflammatory Drugs. Renal prostaglandins have a variety of effects that impair concentrating ability. The administration of a prostaglandin inhibitor reverses these effects and probably explains the efficacy of these drugs in nephrogenic DI, whereby they can lower urine output by more than 50 per cent in some cases. NSAIDs are not recommended for use in the cat.

No Therapy. The untreated DI patient appears to survive well as long as water is always available.

SYNDROME OF INAPPROPRIATE ADH SECRETION (SIADH)

SIADH is characterized by the nonphysiologic release of ADH (not due to the usual stimuli of hyperosmolality or hypovolemia) or by impaired water excretion at a time when sodium excretion is normal. Patients with SIADH are unable to excrete a dilute urine and therefore retain ingested fluids. The hallmark of SIADH is hyponatremia due to water retention in the presence of urine osmolality above plasma osmolality.

The SIADH is produced by enhanced hypothalamic secretion, ectopic (nonhypothalamic) hormone production, the potentiation of ADH effect, or the administration of exogenous ADH. SIADH appears to be a rare disorder in veterinary medicine. Patients with SIADH may present with weight gain, weakness, lethargy, and mental confusion ultimately progressing to convulsions and coma. Laboratory features may be present, including low levels of BUN, serum creatinine, and serum albumin. The serum sodium is usually less than 130 mEq/L, and the plasma osmolality is less than 275 mOsm/kg. The urine is almost always hypertonic to plasma. Urinary sodium concentration is usually greater than 20 mEq/L.

SIADH is a diagnosis of exclusion, so all other causes of hyponatremia should initially be ruled out. Fluid restriction is the hallmark of management of SIADH. If water restriction is adequate, a steady increase in serum sodium or osmolality will occur. Patients with moderate to severe water intoxication (serum sodium concentration less than 110 mEq/L) should be treated with intravenous hypertonic saline solution. Furosemide, in large doses, is administered along with the hypertonic saline to promote renal excretion of water in excess of sodium. Sudden correction of hyponatremia may cause progressive spastic quadriplegia and death beginning 3 to 5 days after therapy.

CHAPTER 113

DISORDERS OF THE PARATHYROID GLANDS
(pages 1437–1465)

HYPERCALCEMIA (pp. 1437–1444)

The differential diagnosis of hypercalcemia is presented in Table 113–1 and in this section.

HYPERCALCEMIA OF MALIGNANCY

Malignancy-associated hypercalcemia (MAHC) is the most common cause of increased serum calcium concentrations in dogs and cats (Table 113–2). This hypercalcemia can result in renal failure, encephalopathy, coma, and death.

Lymphosarcoma. Lymphosarcoma is the most common hematopoietic tumor and the most common cause of hypercalcemia in dogs. Approximately 20 per cent of dogs afflicted with this cancer are hypercalcemic. Hypercalcemia has been documented in cats with lymphosarcoma, but at a much lower frequency than in dogs. Radiographs demonstrate an anterior mediastinal mass in approximately 40 per cent of hypercalcemic lymphoma dogs. Biopsy of the bone marrow or an enlarged organ usually reveals the diagnosis in dogs that do not have a mediastinal mass.

Multiple Myeloma. Approximately 17 per cent of dogs afflicted with this cancer are hypercalcemic.

Solid Tumors with Bone Metastasis

Primary bone tumors do not commonly result in hypercalcemia. In the dog, malignant mammary adenocarcinomas or squamous cell carcinomas are occasionally associated with bone metastasis and hypercalcemia.

Original chapter written by Edward C. Feldman

TABLE 113–1. DIFFERENTIAL DIAGNOSES OF HYPERCALCEMIA

Common
  Lymphosarcoma
  Chronic renal failure (mild hypercalcemia, when present)
  Primary hyperparathyroidism
  Hypoadrenocorticism

Less common
  Apocrine cell adenocarcinoma of the anal sac
  Multiple myeloma
  Other solid tumors
    Squamous cell carcinoma
    Thyroid adenocarcinoma
  Hypervitaminosis D (rodenticide toxicosis)

Uncommon to rare
  Malignant mammary tumors
  Nutritional secondary hyperparathyroidism
  Acute renal failure
  Blastomycosis
  Septic bone disease
  Hypothermia

Solid Tumors Without Bone Metastasis

Apocrine Cell Adenocarcinoma of the Anal Sac. Routine rectal examination reveals a space-occupying mass that may be invasive and occasionally ulcerated or the presence of sublumbar lymph node enlargement.

Other Solid Tumors. In the dog, interstitial cell tumor, squamous cell carcinoma, and thyroid adenocarcinoma may occasionally cause hypercalcemia without bone metastasis.

HYPERVITAMINOSIS D AND RODENTICIDE TOXICOSIS

Hypercalcemia and hyperphosphatemia are the anticipated electrolyte abnormalities in animals with vitamin D toxicity. The major dif-

TABLE 113–2. DIFFERENTIAL DIAGNOSIS OF HYPERCALCEMIA OF MALIGNANCY

Hematologic cancers
  Lymphosarcoma
  Lymphocytic leukemia
  Myeloproliferative disease
  Myeloma
Solid tumors with bone metastasis
  Mammary adenocarcinoma
  Nasal adenocarcinoma
  Epithelial-derived tumors
  Pancreatic adenocarcinoma
  Lung carcinoma
Solid tumors without bone metastasis
  Apocrine gland adenocarcinoma of the anal sac
  Interstitial cell tumor
  Squamous cell carcinoma
  Thyroid adenocarcinoma
  Lung carcinoma
  Pancreatic adenocarcinoma
  Fibrosarcoma

ferential diagnoses for hyperphosphatemia and hypercalcemia (see Fig. 113–2 in the textbook) are vitamin D toxicosis, renal failure (acute or chronic), and hypoadrenocorticism (Addison's Disease).

Rodenticide (cholecalciferol) toxicosis, dietary supplementation, overzealous administration of vitamin D by veterinarians to dogs or cats with hypoparathyroidism, or ingestion of *cestrum diurnum* (day-blooming jessamine). *Solanum malacoxylon* and *Trisetum flavescens* are causes of vitamin D toxicity.

HYPOADRENOCORTICISM

Serum calcium concentrations have been reported to be increased in as many as 33 per cent of dogs with adrenocortical insufficiency as well as in hypoadrenal cats. There is correlation between the degree of hyperkalemia and that of hypercalcemia. If the serum potassium concentration exceeds 6.0 to 6.5 mEq/L, a large percentage of these animals have serum calcium concentrations of 11.4 to 13.5 mg/dl. Despite the increased total serum calcium concentrations, ionized calcium levels remain in the normal range.

CHRONIC RENAL FAILURE

Incidence of Hypercalcemia. Chronic renal failure is usually associated with either normal or low serum calcium concentrations and variable degrees of hyperphosphatemia. However, as many as 10 to 20 per cent of dogs and cats with chronic renal failure have mild to moderate increases in total serum calcium concentration (11.5 to 12.5 mg/dl). Low and normal ionized calcium concentrations in renal failure are more common than would be predicted from evaluation of total serum calcium concentration. Hypercalcemic dogs with renal failure present a significant diagnostic challenge to the clinician. The question must be raised whether the hypercalcemia is resulting in renal failure or the renal failure is resulting in hypercalcemia.

In general, the worse the clinical signs, the more likely that a dog (or cat) has primary renal disease. Additionally, those unusual dogs and cats with hypercalcemia secondary to renal failure usually have serum calcium concentrations of 11.0 to 12.5 mg/dl, whereas those with primary hyperparathyroidism usually have serum calcium concentrations in excess of 13 mg/dl.

Therefore, dogs or cats with no or minimal clinical signs, persistent hypercalcemia of a magnitude greater than 13.0 mg/dl, and a serum phosphate level that is normal or low are presumed to have primary hyperparathyroidism. Those with serum calcium concentrations less than 12.5 mg/dl and hyperphosphatemia are most likely to have primary renal failure. Measurement of the serum ionized calcium concentration should help to distinguish the primary renal failure pet (normal or low) from the primary parathyroid problem (increased).

ACUTE RENAL FAILURE

Persistent hypercalcemia may develop during the diuretic phase of acute renal failure.

UNCOMMON CAUSES OF HYPERCALCEMIA

Bacterial or fungal osteomyelitis and primary or secondary tumors of bone are rare causes of hypercalcemia. Neonatal septicemia in puppies with septic emboli and lysis of bone is another rare cause of hypercalcemia. Disuse osteoporosis is a rare cause of hypercalcemia in animals immobilized due to extensive musculoskeletal or neurologic injury. Hypercalcemia has been reported to develop in severely dehydrated animals. A dog and cat have been described with severe, environmentally induced hypothermia and hypercalcemia. Reference values for total serum calcium in young dogs are approximately 11.1 ± 0.4 mg/dl (10.5 to 11.5 mg/dl), values above those observed in adults (8.8 to 11.0 mg/dl). Serum calcium values above 13.0 mg/dl are significant regardless of age.

PRIMARY HYPERPARATHYROIDISM IN DOGS
(pp. 1444–1456)

Primary hyperparathyroidism is typically diagnosed in older dogs and appears to be much less common, or at least less frequently diagnosed, in cats. Keeshonden appear to be predisposed. The gastrointestinal signs include anorexia, vomiting, constipation, and, rarely, pancreatitis. The renal signs include polyuria, polydipsia, and occasionally signs related to urinary tract calculi. Central nervous system signs include drowsiness, obtundation, and even coma. Some dogs appear asymptomatic while the other extreme includes those with severe systemic illness, usually as a result of renal failure. When clinical signs do develop in dogs, they initially tend to be mild, insidious, and nonspecific.

It is common for the physical examination to be unremarkable. Potential physical examination findings include calculi within the urinary tract and generalized muscle atrophy and/or weakness. It is usually not possible to palpate an enlarged parathyroid gland in dogs. Palpable tumors have been identified in four of eight cats.

CLINICAL PATHOLOGY

Serum Calcium

Hypercalcemia is the hallmark of primary hyperparathyroidism. The hypercalcemia is one that either remains static or slowly increases with time. Alterations in plasma albumin or protein concentration (e.g., dehydration, blood loss) may alter the total serum calcium concentration, yet the ionized (true) concentration usually remains normal. The correction formula based on the serum albumin concentration is:

$$\text{Corrected Ca (mg/dl)} = \text{Ca (mg/dl)} - \text{albumin (gm/dl)} + 3.5$$

Acidosis decreases plasma protein-binding affinity for calcium and increases ionic calcium concentrations, creating mild physiologic hypercalcemia.

Phosphorus. Low or low-normal serum phosphorus concentrations are typical (Table 113–3). When both hyperphosphatemia and azotemia are present, the clinician must rely on the history, physical examination, and other diagnostic tests to determine whether the primary problem is hypercalcemia with secondary renal failure or renal failure with secondary hypercalcemia. Dogs with renal failure and increases in total serum calcium concentration usually have mild decreases in the ionized fraction, as opposed to those with primary hyperparathyroidism, in which both the total and the ionized fractions are increased.

Blood Urea Nitrogen (BUN) and Serum Creatinine. In dogs with uncomplicated primary hyperparathyroidism, serum BUN and creatinine are usually normal. However, persistent and prolonged hypercalcemia has the potential to cause progressive nephrocalcinosis, renal damage, and uremia.

Serum Alkaline Phosphatase. In our series of hyperparathyroid dogs, only 23 per cent had any increase in SAP.

Urinalysis. The urine specific gravity may be relatively dilute (<1.015) as a result of hypercalcemia interfering with ADH action and renal concentrating ability. Isosthenuria (or hyposthenuria) may develop from any cause of hypercalcemia and is nonspecific. Hematuria, pyuria, bacteriuria, and crystalluria may be found on examination of the urine sediment if secondary bacterial cystitis or cystic calculi

TABLE 113–3. POTENTIAL CAUSES OF HYPOPHOSPHATEMIA

Decreased intestinal absorption
    Decreased dietary intake
    Malabsorption/steatorrhea
    Vomiting/diarrhea
    Phosphate-binding antacids
    Vitamin D deficiency
Increased urinary excretion
    Primary hyperparathyroidism
    Diabetes mellitus ;pm ketoacidosis
    Hyperadrenocorticism (naturally occurring/iatrogenic)
    Fanconi syndrome (renal tubular defects)
    Diuretic or bicarbonate administration
    Hypothermia recovery
    Hyperaldosteronism
    Aggressive parenteral fluid administration
    Hypercalcemia of malignancy (early stages)
Transcellular shifts
    Insulin administration
    Parenteral glucose administration
    Hyperalimentation
    Respiratory alkalosis

develop. Uroliths have been composed of calcium phosphate, calcium oxalate, or mixtures of the two salts.

Lipase. A serum lipase should be evaluated to rule out the possibility of concurrent pancreatitis, especially in dogs or cats with gastrointestinal signs. Chronic pancreatitis may be associated with primary hyperparathyroidism in dogs.

Ionized Serum Calcium Concentrations

The biologically active form of calcium within the circulation is the ionized fraction. In hypercalcemia due to primary hyperparathyroidism or secondary to malignancy, the ionized calcium concentration is increased. In chronic renal failure, most serum ionized calcium values are decreased or normal. In hypocalcemia due to hypoalbuminemia, the ionized calcium concentration will be normal, as opposed to the decreased concentration that is obtained with primary hypoparathyroidism, eclampsia, and pancreatitis.

PTH CONCENTRATIONS

The serum PTH concentration must be evaluated relative to the total and, ideally, the ionized serum calcium concentration. In dogs and cats with primary hyperparathyroidism, the serum PTH concentration is typically mid-normal to exceedingly increased. Relative to their hypercalcemia, virtually all dogs and cats with primary hyperparathyroidism have excessive concentrations of serum PTH. The serum PTH concentration in dogs with malignancy-associated hypercalcemia is typically low or undetectable. A small percentage of PTH concentrations from such dogs may be normal or increased. In dogs with both renal disease and hypercalcemia, both the serum PTH concentration and the serum calcium concentration may be increased, making it difficult to decide whether the primary disorder lies in the parathyroid glands or in the kidneys.

PARATHYROID HORMONE–RELATED PROTEIN

The PTHrP-like factor has been isolated from tumor cells obtained from hypercalcemic dogs with lymphoma and apocrine gland adenocarcinomas of the anal sac. However, renal insufficiency is associated with increased concentrations of PTHrP, without malignancy.

ULTRASONOGRAPHY

The normal parathyroid glands are not routinely visualized. Adenomas larger than 5 mm in diameter have been easily visualized. The experience of the operator and the sensitivity of the equipment must be considered.

RADIOGRAPHY

Other than calculi within the urinary system, radiographic alterations associated with primary parathyroid diseases are rare.

DIAGNOSTIC APPROACH TO THE HYPERCALCEMIC PATIENT

The list of differential diagnoses for hypercalcemia is relatively short (see Table 113–1). Of these diagnoses, the most common cause in the dog and the cat is malignancy-associated hypercalcemia (see Table 113–2). Only after diagnostic tests (e.g., CBC, chemistry panel, U/A, thoracic and abdominal radiographs, lymph node or bone marrow biopsy) have failed to identify a diagnosis should trial therapy be considered. With PTH assays and various additional new aids (e.g., PTHrP assays, ultrasonography), this dilemma is certain be become less common.

ACUTE MEDICAL THERAPY FOR THE HYPERCALCEMIC PATIENT

Symptomatic therapy for hypercalcemia is indicated when dehydration, azotemia, cardiac arrhythmia, severe neurologic dysfunction, or weakness exists (IV fluids ± furosemide) may be indicated in the relatively stable patient in which the calcium $<×>$ phosphorus product exceeds 60 to 80. With a product below 60, there is no urgent need to lower the serum calcium concentration in the stable patient, as the risk for soft tissue mineralization is not great.

Correction of fluid deficits, saline diuresis, and diuretic therapy with furosemide and corticosteroids are the most commonly used modes of therapy. Because the incidence of hypercalcemia associated with lymphosarcoma is great, glucocorticoids should not be administered unless the cause of the hypercalcemia has been identified. Less commonly used drugs include diphosphates, bisphosphates, and calcitonin.

SURGICAL THERAPY

Almost all dogs with primary hyperparathyroidism have a solitary, easily identified, parathyroid adenoma. Six of the 72 dogs in our series have had parathyroid carcinoma or primary parathyroid hyperplasia. Enlargement of all four glands would suggest either multiple adenomas or, more likely, parathyroid hyperplasia. The concern would be primary versus secondary (renal or nutritional) hyperparathyroidism. The presurgical evaluation would tend to eliminate secondary disease.

The disorder may recur after surgery, suggesting that periodic rechecks of the serum calcium concentration after stabilization would be warranted. If an enlarged parathyroid gland is not found during thorough surgery, the most likely diagnoses include hypercalcemia due to occult neoplasia, ectopic PTH production by a parathyroid tumor located in the cranial mediastinum, or the presence of a nonparathyroid tumor producing PTH.

POSTOPERATIVE MANAGEMENT

Surgical removal of the autonomous PTH source results in a rapid decline in circulating PTH concentrations and a corresponding decline in serum calcium concentrations. If the serum calcium concentrations prior to surgery are below 14 mg/dl, the risk of postsurgical hypocalcemia is relatively small. If the serum calcium concentration is maintained above 8.5 mg/dl, treatment is not recommended. Presurgically, in dogs with serum calcium concentrations persistently greater than 14 mg/dl, the recommendation is to prophylactically attempt to avoid hypocalcemia after surgery by beginning vitamin D ± calcium therapy immediately following recovery from the anesthesia.

Most dogs become hypocalcemic between the second and sixth days after surgery. The serum calcium concentration should be monitored once or twice daily. Once the serum calcium concentration is stabilized and the dog has been returned to the owner, withdrawal of the supplements may be initiated. The serum calcium concentration must remain above 8 mg/dl in order to minimize the risk of tetany.

PRIMARY HYPERPARATHYROIDISM IN CATS
(pp. 1456–1457)

In one study, the most common clinical signs detected by the owners were anorexia and lethargy. A parathyroid mass was palpable in three of the seven cats. Serum calcium concentrations were 11.1 to 22.8 mg/dl. The serum phosphorus concentration was low in two cats, normal in four cats, and slightly increased in one. None of the cats had clinical problems with hypocalcemia after surgery, although two cats became hypocalcemic.

HYPOCALCEMIA/HYPOPARATHYROIDISM
(pp. 1457–1464)

The differential diagnosis of hypocalcemia is presented in Table 113–4 and in this section. Primary hypoparathyroidism develops because of an absolute or relative deficiency in secretion of parathyroid hormone (PTH). Iatrogenic primary hypoparathyroidism can follow thyroid, parathyroid, or other surgeries of the neck. Because the incidence of hyperthyroidism in cats is high, thyroid surgery and iatrogenic hypoparathyroidism are common.

Chronic renal failure is usually associated with increased serum phosphate and normal serum calcium concentrations. However, either hypocalcemia or hypercalcemia may occur in animals with chronic renal failure. Hypocalcemia, when it is noted, is a biochemical problem and rarely, if ever, clinically significant. When it occurs in dogs with acute pancreatitis, it is usually mild and subclinical. Eclampsia is caused by extreme hypocalcemia in lactating bitches and queens. The hypocalcemia associated with the malabsorption syndromes is invariably believed to occur secondary to hypoalbuminemia. Dogs and cats fed diets containing low calcium to phosphorus ratios, such as beef heart or liver, can develop severe mineral deficiencies. Usually these animals have normal serum concentrations of both calcium and phosphorus, but skeletal disorders due to bony calcium loss develop.

Acute renal failure results in abrupt and severe increases in serum phosphate concentration. Acute increases in serum phosphate could cause reduction in serum calcium concentration. Metabolites of ethylene glycol can chelate serum calcium ions and cause tetany. Commercial phosphate-containing enemas may result in acute, marked hyperphosphatemia, which may cause a reciprocal significant decline in serum calcium.

CLINICAL FEATURES OF NATURALLY OCCURRING HYPOPARATHYROIDISM IN DOGS

In reviewing the literature, we noted that hypoparathyroidism occurs at any age, the youngest dog being 6 weeks old and the oldest being 13

TABLE 113–4. DIFFERENTIAL DIAGNOSIS OF HYPOCALCEMIA

Parathyroid-related hypocalcemia
    Primary hypoparathyroidism
        Destruction of glands
            Immune-mediated process
            Iatrogenic: surgical complication
            Any disease in neck causing damage
        Idiopathic atrophy (autoimmune process?)
    Pseudohypoparathyroidism
Chronic renal failure
Hypoalbuminemia
Acute pancreatitis
Puerperal tetany (eclampsia)
Intestinal malabsorption syndromes
Nutritional secondary hyperparathyroidism (rare cause of hypocalcemia)
Anticonvulsant therapy
Acute renal failure
Ethylene glycol toxicity
Phosphate-containing enemas
Miscellaneous diagnoses
    Laboratory error
    Use of EDTA-coagulated blood
    Vitamin D deficiency
    Transfusion using citrated blood
    Soft tissue trauma
    Medullary carcinoma of the thyroid
    Primary and metastatic bone tumors
    Cancer chemotherapy

years of age. The breeds most frequently identified were toy poodles, miniature schnauzers, Laborador retrievers, German shepherd dogs, and terriers. Most owners reported that their pet appeared abnormally tense or nervous. Intense facial rubbing was observed in 12 of 25 dogs. Additional signs included cramping, tonic spasm of leg muscles, and pain in the legs. Focal muscle twitching or generalized tremors and fasciculations or trembling were frequently observed. A stiff, stilted, hunched, or rigid gait was noted by most owners.

Grand mal convulsions were observed by the owners in 20 of the 25 dogs. Some of this seizure activity was atypical of idiopathic epilepsy in that the dogs either did not appear to lose consciousness or they were not incontinent during the episode. Other than signs related to hypocalcemia, dogs have no classic abnormalities on physical examination. However, cataracts were seen in 9 of the 25 dogs. These cataracts have been small, punctate to linear, white opacities in the anterior and posterior cortical subcapsular region.

CLINICAL FEATURES OF NATURALLY OCCURRING HYPOPARATHYROIDISM IN CATS

The clinical course for each cat was characterized by an abrupt or gradual onset of intermittent neurologic or neuromuscular disturbances, which included focal or generalized muscle tremors, seizures, ataxia, stilted gait, disorientation, and weakness. Lenticular cataracts were detected in several of these cats.

DIAGNOSTIC EVALUATION

Serum Calcium. Hypocalcemia was a serendipitous finding in each of our 25 dogs and the reported cats with primary, naturally occurring hypoparathyroidism. Each dog had a history consistent with a behavioral, neurologic, muscular, or neuromuscular disorder. Each dog was severely hypocalcemic.

Serum Phosphorus. The diagnosis of hypoparathyroidism is strongly supported if both hypocalcemia and hyperphosphatemia are found. ECG findings consistent with hypocalcemia, include (1) deep, wide T waves; (2) prolonged Q-T intervals; and (3) bradycardia.

PTH Concentrations. Undetectable serum PTH concentrations in animals that are severely hypocalcemic confirm the diagnosis of primary hypoparathyroidism. However, a low normal or low value would also not be appropriate in any hypocalcemic individual that has healthy parathyroid glands. Response to therapy, coupled with ruling out of the various differential diagnoses, have served as relatively reliable and logical methods for supporting the diagnosis of primary hypoparathyroidism.

THERAPY FOR HYPOPARATHYROIDISM AND HYPOCALCEMIA

Hypocalcemic Tetany

IV Calcium. Calcium should be administered intravenously slowly, to effect. Calcium gluconate, as a 10 per cent solution, is recommended. Electrocardiographic monitoring is advisable; if bradycardia, premature ventricular complexes, or shortening of the Q-T interval is observed, the IV infusion should be briefly discontinued. This therapy is invariably successful. However, the final dose needed to control tetany is somewhat unpredictable. Fever frequently accompanies tetany and usually dissipates rapidly with control of tetany.

Post-Tetany Short-Term Maintenance

Once tetany has been controlled with IV bolus calcium gluconate, administration of subcutaneous calcium has been effective, simple, and inexpensive. One can determine the dose of calcium gluconate that was needed for controlling tetany originally, and administer that dose SQ every 6 to 8 hours. The calcium gluconate should be diluted in an equal volume of saline. The serum calcium concentration should be maintained above 8 mg/dl. Concentrations above 9 mg/dl suggest that reducing the parenteral calcium dose is warranted.

Maintenance Therapy

The need for vitamin D therapy is usually permanent in dogs and cats with primary, naturally occurring parathyroid gland failure. Supplemental calcium ensures that vitamin D has substrate upon which to function. The aim of long-term therapy is maintaining the serum calcium concentration at mildly low to low-normal concentrations (8.0 to 9.5 mg/dl).

Vitamin D_2 (Ergocalciferol). Vitamin D_2 is a widely available, relatively inexpensive drug. Initially, large doses are required to induce normocalcemia. Vitamin D_2 has been used in cats and dogs with great success. The drawbacks of vitamin D_2 include the induction of hypercalcemia, which, if it occurs, is not easily treated. IV fluids, furosemide, and corticosteroid therapy may be required.

Dihydrotachysterol. Dihydrotachysterol raises the serum calcium concentration more quickly (in 1 to 7 days), and its effects dissipate faster when administration is discontinued compared to vitamin D_2. This product is also more potent than vitamin D_2. We have seen cats and dogs that have appeared to be resistant to the tablet and capsule forms but respond readily to the liquid. We have also seen dogs and cats fail to respond to any form of dihydrotachysterol, but respond to vitamin D_2 or calcitriol.

1,25-Dihydroxyvitamin D_3 (Calcitriol). This drug offers the advantages of rapid onset of action (1 to 4 days) and short half-life (<1 day). If hypercalcemia results from overdosage, it can be rapidly corrected by discontinuing the drug. The major disadvantages of this agent are its high cost and the potency of available capsule sizes. These dosages are usually too high for cats and small dogs.

Calcium Supplementation. Calcium carbonate is the preparation of choice. Dosage recommendations are approximate, and the primary therapy that determines stability of the serum calcium concentration is the use of vitamin D.

CHAPTER 114
HYPERTHYROID DISEASES
(pages 1466–1487)

HYPERTHYROIDISM IN CATS (pp. 1466–1484)

Hyperthyroidism (thyrotoxicosis) is a multisystemic disorder resulting from excessive circulating concentrations of the thyroid hormones thyroxine (T_4) and triiodothyronine (T_3). Functional thyroid adenomatous hyperplasia (or adenoma) involving one or both (70%) thyroid lobes is the most common pathologic abnormality. Thyroid carcinoma only rarely causes hyperthyroidism in the cat, its prevalence being approximately 1 to 2 per cent.

CLINICAL FEATURES

Only 5 per cent of hyperthyroid cats are younger than 10 years of age at time of diagnosis. Table 114–1 lists the most common historical and clinical signs. In most cats, hyperthyroidism is a slowly progressive condition, and they generally maintain a good to excellent appetite and are active (or hyperactive) for their age. These features usually make an owner feel that the cat is in good health until weight loss or other troublesome signs become obvious.

On physical examination, enlargement of one or both thyroid lobes can be detected in more than 80 per cent of cats with hyperthyroidism. However, thyroid enlargement occasionally can be detected in cats without clinical and laboratory evidence of hyperthyroidism. In hyperthyroid cats in which thyroid gland enlargement is not palpable, the possibility that the affected lobes have descended into the thoracic cavity should always be considered.

Weakness and fatigability are reported less frequently in hyperthyroid cats. In some cats, neck ventroflexion may be the only recognizable sign of weakness. In cats with severe hyperthyroidism, breathlessness is not uncommon, especially after exertion. Increased appetite and food intake together with mild to severe weight loss are relatively common signs. Other GI signs include vomiting, diarrhea, and large volumes of feces. Malabsorption with increased fecal fat excretion also develops in some cats.

The increased renal hemodynamics associated with hyperdynamic circulation may be beneficial in maintaining sustainable renal function in some cats with chronic renal failure. Deterioration of renal function, with marked rises in serum concentrations of both urea nitrogen and

---

Original chapter written by Mark E. Peterson

**TABLE 114–1. CLINICAL FINDINGS IN 202 CATS
WITH HYPERTHYROIDISM**

FINDING	NO. (%) OF CATS
Historic owner complaints	
Weight loss	177 (88%)
Polyphagia	99 (49%)
Vomiting	89 (44%)
Polyuria/polydipsia	73 (36%)
Increased activity	63 (31%)
Decreased appetite	32 (16%)
Diarrhea	30 (15%)
Decreased activity	24 (12%)
Weakness	24 (12%)
Dyspnea	20 (10%)
Panting	19 (9%)
Large fecal volume	17 (8%)
Anorexia	14 (7%)
Physical examination findings	
Large thyroid gland	167 (83%)
Thin	132 (65%)
Heart murmur	109 (54%)
Tachycardia	85 (42%)
Gallop rhythm	30 (15%)
Hyperkinesis	30 (15%)
Aggressive	20 (10%)
Unkempt	19 (9%)
Increased nail growth	13 (6%)
Alopecia	6 (3%)
Congestive heart failure	4 (2%)
Ventral neck flexion	2 (1%)

Data from (1) Broussard JD and Peterson ME: Changes in the clinical and laboratory findings in hyperthyroid cats from 1982 to 1992. J Vet Intern Med 7:112, 1993; and (2) Broussard JD et al.: Changes in the clinical and laboratory findings in hyperthyroid cats from 1982 to 1992. JAVMA (in press) 1994

creatinine as well as clinical signs of renal failure will occur after correction of the hyperthyroid state in some cats that had normal (or only slightly increased) BUN and creatinine prior to treatment of the hyperthyroidism.

Polydipsia and polyuria unrelated to renal insufficiency are relatively frequent clinical signs in hyperthyroidism in cats. Some cats will exhibit dyspnea, panting, or hyperventilation at rest. Such signs develop most commonly after the stress of travel and the restraint of a physical examination. Systolic murmurs, tachycardia, and gallop rhythm are fairly common in cats with hyperthyroidism. In addition, various arrhythmias and signs of congestive heart failure (e.g., dyspnea, muffled heart sounds, ascites) may be detected.

Hyperthyroidism can induce a secondary form of cardiomyopathy in the cat—either a hypertrophic form or, much less commonly, a dilative type. Either form may result in congestive heart failure (CHF), but severe cardiac failure develops much more frequently in hyperthyroid cats with dilated cardiomyopathy. After correction of the hyperthyroid state, the hypertrophic form of thyrotoxic cardiomyopathy is usually reversible. Apathetic or masked hyperthyroidism is a clinical entity that develops in about 5 per cent of hyperthyroid cats. In these cats, depression and weakness are the dominant clinical features. Weight loss is usually accompanied by anorexia. Ventroflexion of the neck may also be observed.

SCREENING LABORATORY TESTS

The most common routine laboratory findings are listed in Table 114–2. Mature leukocytosis, eosinopenia, and lymphopenia are common hematologic findings and appear to reflect a stress response to thyroid hormone excess. Erythrocytosis is generally mild to moderate in severity and is found in approximately half of all cats with hyperthyroidism. The most common serum biochemical abnormalities include elevation in concentrations of alanine aminotransferase (ALT), aspartate aminotransferase (AST), alkaline phosphatase (AP), and lactic dehydrogenase (LDH). The cause of the high serum activities is not clear. These enzymes normalize soon after successful treatment. Evidence of concurrent renal dysfunction is also fairly common.

THYROID FUNCTION TESTS

Resting Serum Thyroid Hormone Concentrations. High basal serum total thyroid hormone concentrations are the biochemical hallmark of hyperthyroidism. Resting serum concentrations of both T_4 and T_3 are above the normal range in the vast majority of cats with hyperthyroidism. However, determination of serum T_4 is of greater diagnostic value than determination of serum T_3.

Thyroid hormone concentrations in cats with hyperthyroidism may fluctuate considerably over time. In cats with mild hyperthyroidism, the degree of fluctuation that can occur—into the normal range in some cats—suggests that a diagnosis of hyperthyroidism cannot be excluded solely on the basis of a single normal to high-normal serum T_4 or T_3. In cats with clinical signs consistent with hyperthyroidism, more than one serum T_4 determination could be required to confirm a diagnosis. Furthermore, since severe nonthyroidal illness would be expected to decrease serum thyroid hormone concentrations into the low to undetectable range in sick cats without concurrent hyperthyroidism, concomitant hyperthyroidism should be suspected in any mid-

TABLE 114–2. ROUTINE LABORATORY FINDINGS ON 202 CATS WITH HYPERTHYROIDISM

	NO. (%) OF CATS
Complete blood count	
Erythrocytosis	106 (53%)
High MCV	63 (31%)
Leukocytosis	42 (21%)
Lymphopenia	81 (40%)
Eosinopenia	69 (34%)
Serum chemistry profile	
High ALT	167 (83%)
High SAP	165 (58%)
High LDH	118 (58%)
High AST	86 (43%)
Azotemia	47 (23%)
Hyperglycemia	45 (22%)
Hyperphosphatemia	21 (10%)
Hyperbilirubinemia	7 (4%)
Complete urinalysis	
Specific gravity >1.035	57/106 (52%)
Specific gravity <1.015	3/106 (3%)

Data from (1) Broussard JD and Peterson ME: Changes in the clinical and laboratory findings in hyperthyroid cats from 1982 to 1992. (Abstract) J Vet Intern Med 7:112, 1993; and (2) Broussard JD et al.: Changes in the clinical and laboratory findings in hyperthyroid cats from 1982 to 1992. JAVMA (in press) 1994.

TABLE 114-3. ADVANTAGES AND DISADVANTAGES OF TREATMENT MODALITIES FOR CATS WITH HYPERTHYROIDISM

	METHIMAZOLE OR CARBIMAZOLE	SURGERY	RADIOIODINE
Persistent hyperthyroidism	Low (dose-related)	Rare	Low (dose-related)
Complications			
Hypoparathyroidism	Never	Common	Never
Permanent hypothyroidism	Never	Intermediate	Rare (dose-related)
Anorexia, vomiting	Common	Rare	Never
Hematologic effects	Rare (thrombocytopenia, agranulocytosis, serum ANA)	Never	Rare (only with very high doses)
Neurologic damage	Never	Rare (vocal cord paralysis, Homer's)	Never
Hospitalization time required	None	1–3 days	1–4 weeks
Time until euthyroid	1–3 weeks	1–2 days	1–12 weeks
Relapse/recurrence	High	Intermediate	Low
Ease of treatment	Simple	Most difficult	Intermediate (not readily available)

dle- to old-aged cat with severe nonthyroidal illness and high-normal serum T_4 and T_3 concentrations, especially if signs of hyperthyroidism are also present.

When one suspects mild hyperthyroidism in a cat but the serum T_4 is not high, we suggest that the second serum T_4 determination be made at least 1 to 2 weeks later. If the result is again in the normal to high-normal range and hyperthyroidism is still suspected, provocative testing with a T_3 suppression test or thyrotropin-releasing hormone (TRH) stimulation test is recommended.

Thyroid Hormone (Triiodothyronine) Suppression Test.
Normally, administration of thyroid hormone decreases pituitary secretion of TSH, which results in reduced endogenous thyroid secretion; this can be detected by a decrease in serum T_4 concentrations. When the test is performed in cats with hyperthyroidism, even in cats with only slightly high or high-normal resting serum T_4 concentrations, minimal, if any, suppression of serum T_4 concentrations is seen. In one study, all of the cats with hyperthyroidism had post-liothyronine serum T_4 values greater than 20 nmol/L ($\approx$ 1.5 µg/dl), whereas all of the normal cats and cats with nonthyroidal disease had T_4 values less than 20 nmol/L. Serum T_3 concentrations, basal and post-liothyronine, can be used to monitor owner compliance with giving the drug.

Thyrotropin-Releasing Hormone (TRH) Stimulation Test.
Studies have shown that administration of TRH reliably and consistently stimulates secretion of thyroid hormone in normal cats. In one study, cats with mild hyperthyroidism showed little, if any, rise in serum T_4 values after administration of TRH, whereas a consistent rise of serum T_4 concentrations (approximately twofold) was observed after TRH administration in both clinically normal cats and cats with nonthyroidal disease. Results indicated that a rise in serum T_4 of less than 50 per cent was consistent with mild hyperthyroidism, whereas a value of greater than 60 per cent was only seen in normal cats or cats with nonthyroidal disease; values between 50 and 60 per cent were equivocal or borderline responses.

The major disadvantage of the TRH stimulation test in cats is that side effects (e.g., salivation, vomiting, tachypnea, and defecation) almost invariably occur immediately after administration of the TRH. Fortunately, all of the adverse side effects are transient and completely resolve by the end of the 4-hour test period.

Thyroid-Stimulating Hormone (TSH) Response Test. The TSH test cannot be recommended for confirming the diagnosis of hyperthyroidism in cats with normal T_4 concentrations.

THYROID RADIONUCLIDE UPTAKE AND IMAGING

With pertechnetate (^{99m}Tc) thyroid scanning, a one-to-one ratio usually exists between the size and intensity of the salivary glands and the two thyroid lobes. In contrast, most cats with hyperthyroidism will have obvious enlargement of one or both thyroid lobes together with an increased uptake of pertechnetate into the abnormal thyroid tissue, as compared to the salivary glands. The major usefulness of thyroid imaging, however, is in determining the extent of thyroid gland involvement and in detecting possible metastasis. With unilateral thyroid lobe involvement, the normal contralateral lobe is completely suppressed and cannot be visualized.

TREATMENT

In cats, hyperthyroidism can be treated in three ways—surgical thyroidectomy, radioactive iodine (^{131}I), or chronic administration of an antithyroid drug. The advantages and disadvantages of each form of treatment, summarized in Table 114–3, should always be considered.

Antithyroid Drugs and Medical Treatment

Methimazole. Methimazole is better tolerated and safer than propylthiouracil (PTU) in the cat and can be considered the antithyroid drug of choice for both the preoperative and long-term medical management of feline hyperthyroidism. During the first 3 months of therapy, the cats should be examined every 2 to 3 weeks in order to make necessary dose adjustments and to monitor for adverse effects. Although a few cats appear to be resistant to the effects of the drug, euthyroidism can be restored in virtually all cats if a high enough dosage (25 to 30 mg/day in a few cases) is reliably administered on a daily basis.

If methimazole is given as preoperative preparation, surgical thyroidectomy can be performed once serum T_4 concentrations decrease to normal or low values (usually within 2 to 4 weeks). In cats in which long-term methimazole treatment is planned, the goal of treatment is to maintain serum T_4 values within the low-normal range with the lowest possible daily dosage. The great majority of cats will require a dose of 7.5 to 10 mg/day, and some may continue to require dosages of 15 to 20 mg/day. Although divided doses of methimazole tend to be most effective, euthyroidism can often be maintained when the necessary dose is given only once daily.

Mild clinical side effects are relatively common and include anorexia, vomiting, and lethargy. In most cats, these adverse signs are transient and resolve despite continued administration of the drug. Self-induced excoriations of the face and neck also may develop in a few cats. Cessation of methimazole administration is usually required for complete resolution of these excoriations. Finally, hepatic toxicity is an uncommon but serious reaction that can develop during drug treatment. A variety of hematologic abnormalities, including eosinophilia, lymphocytosis, and transient leukopenia with a normal differential count, may develop. More serious hematologic reactions include severe thrombocytopenia and agranulocytosis. Immune-mediated hemolytic anemia may also develop but is extremely rare.

Carbimazole. See textbook.

Other Drugs. The β-adrenoceptor blocking drugs (e.g., propranolol or atenolol) are most useful as an adjunctive treatment in combination with an antithyroid drug or before surgery or radioiodine therapy. Both drugs block many of the cardiovascular and neuromuscular effects of excess thyroid hormone and control the tachycardia, hypertension, and hyperexcitability commonly associated with hyperthyroidism in cats. In addition, treatment with a β-adrenergic blocker helps prevent arrhythmias that commonly develop during the anesthetic period in untreated cats with hyperthyroidism.

Surgery

Although thyroidectomy is generally successful, it can be associated with significant morbidity and mortality. All hyperthyroid cats should therefore be prepared for surgery by administration of an antithyroid drug, a β-adrenoceptor blocking drug, or iodide to decrease the metabolic and cardiac complications associated with hyperthyroidism. After methimazole treatment has maintained euthyroidism for 1 to 3 weeks, most systemic complications will have improved or resolved, minimizing anesthetic and surgical complications.

Many potential complications are associated with thyroidectomy, including hypoparathyroidism, Horner's syndrome, and laryngeal paralysis. Since only one parathyroid gland is required for maintenance of normocalcemia, hypoparathyroidism develops only in cats treated with bilateral thyroidectomy. After bilateral thyroidectomy, the serum calcium concentration should be monitored on a daily basis until it has stabilized within the normal range. Spontaneous recovery of parathyroid function may occur weeks to months after surgery.

Serum thyroid hormone concentrations fall to subnormal levels for two to three months after hemithyroidectomy for unilateral involvement of the thyroid gland. However, T_4 supplementation is rarely required during this period. If bilateral thyroidectomy has been performed, T_4 should be started 24 to 48 hours after surgery. T_4 and T_3 may spontaneously increase to within normal range weeks to months postoperatively.

Radioactive Iodine

Radioiodine, like stable iodine, is concentrated by the thyroid gland after administration. Radioiodine then irradiates and destroys the hyperfunctioning tissue. However, normal thyroid tissue tends to be protected from the effects of radioiodine, since the uninvolved thyroid tissue is suppressed and receives only a small dose of radiation.

The radioisotope most frequently used is ^{131}I. The ideal goal of ^{131}I therapy is to restore euthyroidism with a single dose of radiation without producing hypothyroidism. Iodine-131 will be more effective in destroying hyperfunctioning tissue if the cat has not been treated with methimazole (or if antithyroid medication has been discontinued for at least a week).

Overall, use of radioiodine may be the optimum treatment for cats with hyperthyroidism when nuclear medicine facilities are available. A single ^{131}I treatment will restore euthyroidism in most cats, whereas cats that remain persistently hyperthyroid can be successfully re-treated with radioiodine and those that become hypothyroid can be supplemented readily with T_4. At present, the major disadvantage of radioiodine therapy is the unavailability of facilities that can safely handle ^{131}I and accurately determine the ideal dose.

HYPERTHYROIDISM AND THYROID TUMORS IN DOGS
(pp. 1484–1486)

Most canine tumors are large, invasive carcinomas that are not hyperfunctional. Because many of these tumors are malignant and have reached an advanced state at the time of diagnosis, the prognosis is often poor.

CLINICAL FEATURES

Most dogs with thyroid tumors are presented because the owner has noticed an enlargement of the neck. Most thyroid tumors in dogs are large, easily palpable, and fixed to the soft tissues of the neck. Because of the large tumor volume and high incidence of metastasis, clinical signs such as dyspnea, cough, hoarseness, dysphagia, vomiting, anorexia, and weight loss may be reported.

Of all thyroid tumors in dogs, approximately 5 to 10 per cent will be autonomous and hyperfunctional. In these dogs, the hyperthyroid state is usually the major reason for examination. Polydipsia and polyuria are usually the earliest and most predominant signs. Weight loss, despite an increase in appetite, is also common. Other signs that may develop include weakness and fatigue, heat intolerance, nervousness or restless behavior, and more frequent defecation with semiformed feces.

DIAGNOSIS

Thyroid neoplasia should be suspected in any dog with an enlarging mass in the ventral cervical region. Fine-needle aspiration cytology may be helpful in differentiating a thyroid tumor from an abscess, salivary mucocele, or enlarged lymph node. A definitive diagnosis usually requires an excisional biopsy and histopathology.

One of the major differential diagnoses for hyperthyroidism in dogs is the presence of autoantibodies to T_4, T_3, or both. These autoantibodies produce spurious results when serum or plasma T_4 or T_3 is measured by radioimmunoassay. However, these dogs commonly have clinical and laboratory evidence of hypothyroidism.

Screening laboratory tests (e.g., complete blood count, serum biochemical profile, urinalysis) should always be performed in a dog with suspected thyroid neoplasia. Thoracic radiographs should be reviewed, since about a third of these dogs have pulmonary metastasis at the time of diagnosis.

TREATMENT

Most thyroid carcinomas in dogs retain the ability to concentrate radioiodine. It appears that radioiodine treatment alone can result in palliation of clinical signs in dogs that have large unresectable primary tumors or massive thyroid metastasis. However, large, repetitive ^{131}I doses may be required for an adequate response. Although radioiodine therapy may prolong survival, this therapy is not nearly so successful as might be expected.

For most dogs with thyroid tumors (with or without associated hyperthyroidism), the initial treatment of choice is attempted surgical resection. Complete excision of large invasive carcinomas is usually difficult and may be impossible. However, debulking of the tumor mass may be beneficial in preparation for other treatment, as well as in making the dog more comfortable.

Total removal of all malignant thyroid tissue is not common. Therefore, chemotherapy (e.g., doxorubicin [Adriamycin]) becomes an important adjunctive mode of therapy when complete surgical removal is not successful, when distant metastatic lesions are identified, or when the size of the primary tumor is so large that metastasis is likely even though it cannot be identified by thoracic radiographs or other routine diagnostic tests. External beam (cobalt) irradiation also appears to be useful as adjunct therapy for thyroid carcinoma in dogs.

CHAPTER 115

HYPOTHYROID DISEASES
(pages 1487–1501)

PRIMARY HYPOTHYROIDISM

Primary acquired hypothyroidism is the most common type of hypothyroidism in the dog. It is usually the result of lymphocytic thyroiditis or thyroid atrophy. Congenital hypothyroidism is rare.

CENTRAL HYPOTHYROIDISM

Central acquired hypothyroidism is usually caused by adenohypophyseal or hypothalamic neoplasia. Central congenital hypothyroidism is rare.

CLINICAL SIGNS (pp. 1488–1491)

The most common clinical signs in hypothyroid dogs are bilateral alopecia, with or without hyperpigmentation, and a dry hair coat or seborrhea. Other clinical signs are physical lethargy, mental dullness,

Original chapter written by C. B. Chastain and David L. Panciera cold intolerance, slow heart rate, infertility in males and females, constipation, and weight gain. Myxedema of the skin may be evident on the head, particularly over the eyes and the shoulders. Physical signs in thyroidectomized cats are usually subclinical. Lethargy may be present, and seborrhea, matting of hair, and alopecia of the pinnae may also develop. Covert presentations can result from atypical clinical signs such as those associated with myopathy, neuropathy, impaired mental state, stunted growth, bleeding, and signs of concurrent endocrine diseases.

Myopathy and Neuropathy. Affected dogs may have elevated serum creatine kinase values and usually hypercholesterolemia. The most common finding in affected dogs is a metabolic dysfunction in type II fibers leading to type II fiber atrophy. Generalized peripheral neuropathy causes signs similar to those of myopathy, with lameness, dragging of the feet, tetraparesis, hearing impairment, or nystagmus.

Central Nervous System Disease Signs or Impaired Mental State. An impaired mental state resulting from associated atherosclerosis, cerebral myxedema, or a hypothalamic or hypophyseal tumor can be a presenting sign. The most dangerous possible sequela of severe hypothyroidism is myxedema coma. Most recognized cases have involved Doberman pinschers. Hypothermia, usually without shivering, is a cardinal sign of impending or current myxedema coma. Other effects are hypoventilation, hypotension, and bradycardia.

Stunted Growth (Cretinous Dwarfism). Untreated congenital or juvenile-onset hypothyroidism will result in stunted physical growth. The two most common causes are forms of primary hypothyroidism, thyroid dysgenesis and dyshormonogenesis. Severe congenital hypothyroidism causes disproportionate (short-legged) dwarfism and subnormal mentality. Other physical signs can include short-broad skull, shortened mandible, protruding tongue, lateral strabismus, exophthalmos, alopecia, hypothermia, bradycardia, muscular weakness, delayed dental eruption, and (depending on the cause) goiter.

Cardiovascular Disease. Hypothyroidism causes impaired myocardial conductivity and function. Echocardiographic evidence of left ventricular hypocontractility with altered systolic time intervals may occur. Electrocardiographic changes include sinus bradycardia and a reduction in the amplitude of the P and R waves.

Bleeding. A relationship between von Willebrand's disease and hypothyroidism has been proposed. However, there is no evidence of a direct relationship between the two diseases in the dog.

Other Concurrent Endocrine Disease Signs. In myxedema coma there can be impaired secretion of adrenocorticotropic hormone (secondary hypoadrenocorticism) and enhanced secretion of antidiuretic hormone (the syndrome of inappropriate ADH). Hyperprolactinemia is believed to occur in dogs with severe hypothyroidism and may cause inappropriate galactorrhea in up to 25 per cent of hypothyroid, sexually intact bitches.

Clinical signs of secondary hypothyroidism in juvenile dogs may be accompanied by multiple adenohypophyseal hormone deficiencies. Growth hormone deficiency is always concurrently present. Dogs with hypothyroidism caused by lymphocytic thyroiditis may also develop hypoadrenocorticism, hypoparathyroidism, primary hypogonadism, or diabetes mellitus. These concurrent endocrinopathies may represent autoimmune (lymphocytic) destruction of multiple endocrine glands. Hypothyroidism reportedly causes insulin resistance in dogs. This can result in impairment of glycemic control during insulin treatment.

DIAGNOSIS (pp. 1491–1498)

Serum Cholesterol. Of hypothyroid dogs 66 to 75 per cent have elevated levels of serum cholesterol.

Nonregenerative Anemia. Twenty-five to 40 per cent of hypothyroid dogs have a mild normochromic, normocytic nonregenerative anemia.

Serum Creatine Kinase (CK) Activity. Advanced cases of hypothyroidism with myopathy may have an increased serum CK activity.

CONFIRMING LABORATORY EXAMINATIONS

Serum T_4 and Free T_4. Base-line serum T_4 and FT_4 determinations by validated radioimmunoassays (RIA) are the preferable laboratory assessments for the diagnosis of hypothyroidism. If the serum T_4 or FT_4 level is within the mid- to high-normal range, hypothyroidism is unlikely to be present. If the baseline serum T_4 and FT_4 concentrations are abnormally low, a probable diagnosis of hypothyroidism is appropriate and a therapeutic trial is justified. Clinical signs should be consistent with hypothyroidism, and the effects of severe nonthyroidal illnesses and drug suppression of T_4 concentration need to be ruled out. Should only one or neither of the base-line hormone values be abnormally low, the possibility of hypothroidism may be pursued further by a TSH stimulation test or a carefully conducted therapeutic trial.

Fluctuations into low ranges are common in normal euthyroid sick dogs. Serum T_4 is decreased in hypothyroidism more often than serum T_3, and serum T_4 fluctuations into normal range are rare and transient in hypothyroid dogs. Most aging studies in dogs indicate there are slight decreases in basal T_4 of about 0.1 μg/dl/year.

Serum T_4 Response to TSH Stimulation. The most definitive method currently available for diagnosing hypothyroidism in dogs is exogenous TSH stimulation. Its use is limited by the expense of TSH for injection and its inconsistent availability. The best criterion for test interpretation is the absolute level of T_4 attained after TSH stimulation. Normal dogs usually have a rise of at least 2 μg/dl from the base line.

Reverse Triiodothyronine (rT_3). Serum reverse triiodothyronine (rT_3) determination can be helpful in some cases in which discordant or equivocal screening assays for serum T_4 and FT_4 have been obtained. If serum rT_3 levels are high, hypothyroidism is not present.

DIFFERENTIATING CAUSES

Repeated TSH Stimulation. Daily TSH injections of 10 units for 3 or more days may gradually stimulate a serum T_4 response if hypothyroidism is secondary or tertiary in origin. No response to TSH administration occurs from repeated TSH administration if primary hypothyroidism is present.

Antithyroglobulin Antibodies (ATGA) and Anti-T_3 or Anti-T_4 Antibodies. Damage to the thyroid often results in the development of antithyroglobulin antibodies (ATGA). Approximately half of hypothyroid dogs have been reported to have ATGA. Normal dogs may also have ATGA, so that the presence of ATGA is not a definite indication that hypothyroidism will develop.

Thyroid Biopsy. Primary and secondary hypothyroidism have characteristic histopathologic changes.

POTENTIALLY MISLEADING LABORATORY FINDINGS OR INTERPRETATIONS

Many nonthyroidal illnesses are associated with a reduction in serum T_3 and T_4 levels (Table 115–1). The majority of dogs with hyperadrenocorticism have either low serum T_4 or T_3, or both. The slope of the TSH response remains normal in most cases, but absolute pre- and post-TSH serum T_4 values are lower.

Dogs with diseases causing Horner's syndrome, facial paralysis, congestive cardiomyopathy, laryngeal paralysis, or intervertebral disc

TABLE 115–1. SOME KNOWN CAUSES OF EUTHYROID SICK SYDROME IN DOGS

Calorie or protein deficiency
Surgery (or anesthesia)
Debilitating diseases such as:
  Diabetes mellitus
  Hyperadrenocorticism
  Addison's disease
  Kidney failure
  Liver disease
  Intervertebral disc disease
  Certain neuromuscular diseases
  Pyoderma

protrusion may have lowered levels of serum T_3 or T_4. The underlying disease is usually the cause of the lowered serum thyroid hormone levels. Treatment with thyroid hormones is not beneficial and is probably detrimental in euthyroid sick syndrome. Several drugs may lower serum T_4 or T_3 levels (Table 115–2).

TREATMENT RECOMMENDATIONS (pp. 1498–1499)

Sodium levothyroxine (L-thyroxine), a synthetic product, is the treatment of choice in the dog. Triiodothyronine treatment is rarely justified. The initial dose of L-thyroxine should be decreased and the frequency increased in cases of diabetes mellitus or heart disease to allow gradual adaptation to the increased metabolic rate. If hypoadrenocorticism is also present, thyroid replacement should be preceded by adrenocortical hormone replacement therapy to preclude the risk of a hypoadrenocortical crisis.

Thyroid hormones in excess of physiologic levels are catabolic, leading to increased gluconeogenesis, protein breakdown, and nitrogen wasting. Overt signs of overdosage are uncommon but include polyuria, polydipsia, nervousness, weight loss, increased appetite, panting, weakness and fatigue, seeking cool areas, restlessness, elevated resting heart rate, and fever. Hypoglycemia can occur.

The treatment of myxedema stupor or coma must begin before the results of measuring serum T_4 levels are received. Treatment consists of intravenous L-thyroxine, intravenous administration of glucocorticoids, broad-spectrum antibiotics, passive rewarming with blankets, and mechanical respiratory support in some cases.

Post-pill testing should be reserved for patients that have received therapy for at least one month and either have shown no response or are exhibiting signs of hyperthyroidism. Peak serum T_4 concentrations,

TABLE 115–2. DRUG-INDUCED SUPPRESSION OF SERUM THYROID HORMONE LEVELS IN DOGS

Phenytoin	Thiopental and methoxyflurane
Salicylates	Furosemide
Flunixin	Fatty acids
Glucocorticoids	Ipodate
Mitotane	Phenobarbital*
Anabolic steroids	Phenylbutazone*
Halothane	

*May not be significant decrease.

expected at 4 to 8 hours after administration, should be near or slightly above the upper limit of the normal range.

MISINTERPRETATION OF THE RESPONSE TO TRIAL THERAPY

The presumptive diagnosis of hypothyroidism is ultimately validated by clinical improvement of problems attributed to hypothyroidism. In some instances, improvement does not substantiate a diagnosis of hypothyroidism. Temporary improvement in conditions such as alopecia can be a pharmacologic response to thyroid hormones. Concurrent treatment resulting in resolution of the clinical signs independent of L-thyroxine treatment may also cause an erroneous assumption that hypothyroidism is present.

CHAPTER 116

INSULIN-SECRETING ISLET CELL NEOPLASIA
(pages 1501–1509)

Insulin-secreting tumors typically occur in the middle-aged or older dog. Various breeds are suggested to have a higher incidence, including the standard poodle, boxer, fox terrier, German shepherd, and Irish setter. This remains a rare diagnosis in cats.

ANAMNESIS (pp. 1502–1503)

Clinical signs associated with an insulin-secreting tumor typically are related to neuroglycopenia (hypoglycemia) and an elevation in circulating catecholamine concentrations. One characteristic of hypoglycemic signs is their episodic nature. Seizure activity is more common than syncope or coma and appears to be self-limiting, typically lasting from 30 seconds to 5 minutes. There is a strong association between the development of clinical signs of hypoglycemia and fasting, excitement, exercise, and eating.

PHYSICAL EXAMINATION (p. 1503)

The physical examination is surprisingly unremarkable. Weight gain is evident in some dogs and probably is a result of the potent anabolic effects of insulin. Peripheral neuropathies have been reported in dogs with insulin-secreting tumors, which may produce detectable alterations on physical examination, including proprioception deficits, depressed reflexes, and muscle atrophy.

CLINICAL PATHOLOGIC ABNORMALITIES
(pp. 1503–1504)

The only consistent abnormality found in the biochemistry panel is hypoglycemia. In one study, the mean initial blood glucose concentra-

---

Original chapter written by Richard W. Nelson

tion in 71 dogs was 46 mg/dl, with a range of 15 to 78 mg/dl. Nine of the 71 (13 per cent) dogs had random blood glucose concentration greater than 60 mg/dl. Dogs with insulin-secreting tumors occasionally may have a normal blood glucose concentration on random testing. Fasting with hourly evaluations of the blood glucose should be done in these dogs. It is rare that fasts beyond 12 hours would fail to produce hypoglycemia in dogs with insulin-secreting tumors.

RADIOGRAPHY AND ULTRASONOGRAPHY (p. 1504)

Abdominal radiographs are routinely interpreted as normal. Thoracic radiographs are of limited help because β-cell tumors seldom metastasize to the lungs. Ultrasonic detection of a mass lesion in the region of the pancreas helps to confirm the suspicion of β-cell tumor. Failure to identify a mass lesion is common and does not rule out a β-cell tumor.

DIFFERENTIAL DIAGNOSIS (p. 1504)

Most of these animals have the common history of episodic weakness or seizures, which encompasses a wide variety of organic disorders (see Table 116–1). Once fasting hypoglycemia has been confirmed, careful evaluation of the history, physical findings, and routine clinical pathology usually provides clues to the underlying cause (Table 116–2).

CONFIRMATION OF AN INSULIN-SECRETING TUMOR (pp. 1504–1505)

The confirmation of an insulin-secreting tumor requires confirmation of hypoglycemia with concurrent inappropriate insulin secretion

TABLE 116–1. DISORDERS THAT MAY RESULT IN EPISODIC WEAKNESS (INCLUDES SEIZURES)

Neuromuscular Disorders
Infectious: viral encephalitis (canine distemper), cryptococcosis, toxoplasmosis
Congenital: hydrocephalus
Trauma
Acquired: myasthenia gravis, tetanus, discospondylitis, idiopathic polyradiculoneuritis (coon hound paralysis), polymyositis, polyarthritis
Neoplasia
Toxin: lead poisoning
Idiopathic epilepsy
Idiopathic polyneuropathy
Cardiovascular Disorders
Congenital: anatomic defects
Acquired: tachyarrhythmias or bradyarrhythmias, heartworm, bacterial endocarditis
Neoplasm: hemangiosarcoma
Coagulopathy (warfarin-induced)
Metabolic Disorders
Hepatic encephalopathy
Hypocalcemia
Polycythemia
Hypoadrenocorticism
Hyperviscosity syndrome
Pheochromocytoma
Hypoglycemia
Hypokalemia
Anemia

TABLE 116–2. CLASSIFICATION OF FASTING HYPOGLYCEMIA

I. Endocrine
  A. Excess insulin or insulin-like factors
    1. Insulin-producing islet cell tumors
    2. Extrapancreatic tumors producing and secreting insulin-like substances
    3. Iatrogenic-insulin overdose
  B. Growth hormone deficiency
    1. Hypopituitarism affecting several tropic hormones (i.e., ACTH, GH)
    2. Monotropic GH deficiency
  C. Cortisol deficiency
    1. Hypopituitarism
    2. Isolated ACTH deficiency
    3. Hypoadrenocorticism
II. Hepatic
  A. Congenital
    1. Vascular shunts
    2. Glycogen storage diseases
  B. Acquired
    1. Vascular shunts
    2. Chronic fibrosis (cirrhosis)
    3. Hepatic necrosis: toxins, infectious agents
III. Substrate
  A. Extrapancreatic tumors that use large quantities of glucose
  B. Fasting hypoglycemia of pregnancy
  C. Puppy hypoglycemia = ketonemia (alanine deficiency?)
  D. Uremia
  E. Severe malnutrition
  F. Severe polycythemia
IV. Miscellaneous
  A. Artifact
  B. Iatrogenic insulin overdose

ACTH, corticotropin; GH, growth hormone.

and identification of a pancreatic mass by means of ultrasonography or exploratory celiotomy. Documenting a serum insulin concentration greater than 20 μU/ml in a dog with a corresponding blood glucose concentration less than 60 mg/dl and appropriate clinical signs and clinicopathologic findings strongly supports the diagnosis. An insulin-secreting tumor is also possible with a serum insulin concentration in the high normal range (i.e., 10 to 20 μU/ml) and the low normal range (i.e., 5 to 10 μU/ml). To determine the amended insulin-glucose ratio, blood glucose and serum insulin concentration are entered into the following formula:

$$\frac{\text{plasma insulin } (\mu U/ml) \times 100}{\text{plasma glucose } (mg/dl) - 30}$$

Whenever the blood glucose is less than 30 mg/dl, the number 1 is used as the divisor. This test is not specific. Some dogs with other causes of hypoglycemia may have abnormal amended ratios.

SURGICAL THERAPY (pp. 1505–1507)

Surgical exploration is the best diagnostic, therapeutic, and prognostic tool for insulin-secreting tumors. The surgical intent should be to remove as much abnormal tissue as possible, including resectable sites of metastases. Surgery offers a chance to "cure" dogs with a resectable solitary mass. With nonresectable tumors or those with obvious metastases, removal or debulking of as much abnormal tissue as possible frequently has resulted in remission of, or at least reduction in, clinical signs and improved response to medical therapy. If surgery is performed, euthanasia is not recommended regardless of the findings at surgery. Many dogs with metastatic disease can be managed medically with minimal complications for several months to more than 1 year.

Most dogs with insulin-secreting tumors have masses that are visible to the surgeon. In a smaller group of dogs, these tumors may be detected only by palpation. If the surgeon fails to recognize a mass and the diagnosis has been confirmed by glucose and insulin measurements, the surgeon should attempt to remove at least one-half of the pancreas in the hope of removing the portion that contains the tumor.

Postoperative complications include pancreatitis, hypoglycemia, and hyperglycemia. Insulin therapy is initiated only when hyperglycemia and glucosuria persist for longer than 2 or 3 days. Diabetes mellitus usually is transient, lasting from a few days to several months.

MEDICAL THERAPY FOR AN ACUTE HYPOGLYCEMIC CRISIS (p. 1507)

If an owner reports by telephone that the pet is having a hypoglycemic seizure, the owner should be instructed to pour a sugar solution (e.g., Karo syrup) over his or her fingers and rub the syrup on the pet's buccal mucosa. Hypoglycemic dogs and cats usually respond in 30 to 120 seconds. The owner should never be instructed to place a hand or object into an animal's mouth because the person is likely to be bitten. Veterinary attention can then be sought.

In the hospital, clinical signs of hypoglycemia usually can be alleviated with the IV administration of 50% dextrose. It is imperative to avoid overstimulation of the tumor when administering dextrose IV. Overstimulation of the tumor can result in massive release of insulin into the circulation and rebound, severe hypoglycemia.

Hyperglycemia-hypoglycemia cycles can be avoided by minimizing rapid increases in the blood glucose concentration. Once the signs are controlled with judicious administration of IV dextrose, diet and glucocorticoids can then be initiated. Rarely, a hypoglycemic dog or cat with CNS signs fails to respond to glucose administration. Irreversible cerebral lesions may result from long-term, severe hypoglycemia and the resultant cerebral hypoxia.

MEDICAL THERAPY FOR CHRONIC HYPOGLYCEMIA (pp. 1507–1509)

If a constant source of calories is provided as a substrate for the excess insulin, hypoglycemic episodes can be reduced in frequency or avoided. Diets that are high in proteins, fats, and complex carbohydrates are recommended, fed in three to six small meals daily. Exercise should be limited. Simple sugars should be avoided.

Glucocorticoids should be initiated when dietary manipulations are no longer effective in preventing signs of hypoglycemia. Prednisone is most often used. If signs are not controlled on a low dosage or recur sometime later, the dose should gradually be increased until signs of hypoglycemia abate or the daily dose is 4 to 6 mg/kg/day. With evidence of hypercortisolism, the dose of prednisone should be reduced and diazoxide therapy initiated.

The goal of diazoxide therapy is to establish a dosage in which hypoglycemia and its clinical signs are reduced or absent, while avoiding hyperglycemia (greater than 180 mg/dl) and its associated clinical signs. The most common adverse reactions to diazoxide administration are anorexia and vomiting. Thiazide diuretics may potentiate the effects of diazoxide to enhance the hyperglycemic effect if diazoxide alone is not effective.

Octreotide (Sandostatin), an analog of somatostatin, can rapidly decrease serum insulin concentration in some dogs with insulin-secreting neoplasia. This drug can be well tolerated and can be used for the management of both acute and chronic hypoglycemia in some dogs with insulin-secreting neoplasia.

PROGNOSIS (p. 1509)

Because of the extremely high likelihood of metastasis the long-term prognosis, at best, is guarded to poor. The mean survival time for dogs treated medically is about 12 months from the onset of clinical signs of hypoglycemia. About one-third of dogs undergoing surgery die or are euthanized at the time of or within 1 month of surgery. An additional one-third of dogs die or are euthanized within 6 months of surgery. One-third of dogs live beyond 6 months postoperative before hypoglycemia recurs. Many of these latter dogs live well beyond 1 year after surgery.

CHAPTER 117

DIABETES MELLITUS
(pages 1510–1537)

CLASSIFICATION AND ETIOLOGY (pp. 1510–1513)

Overview of Classification. Diabetes mellitus is classified as type I and type II. Type 1 diabetes mellitus is characterized by destruction of beta cells with progressive and eventual complete loss of insulin secretion. These animals require insulin treatment from the time of diagnosis (i.e., insulin-dependent diabetes mellitus [IDDM]). Alternatively, dogs and cats may gradually lose insulin secretion as beta cells are destroyed slowly. These animals may have an initial period in which hyperglycemia may be mild or be easily controlled with small doses of insulin (i.e., non-insulin-dependent diabetes mellitus [NIDDM]); however, with time, insulin deficiency becomes absolute and IDDM develops.

Type II diabetes mellitus is characterized by insulin resistance and/or dysfunctional beta cells. Insulin secretion may be high, low, or normal, but is insufficient to overcome insulin resistance in peripheral tissues. Insulin secretion prevents ketoacidosis in most type II diabetic patients. Type II diabetics may be IDDM or NIDDM, depending on the severity of insulin resistance and the functional status of the beta cells. Type I and type II diabetes mellitus have been recognized in both dogs and cats.

Secondary diabetes mellitus includes those diabetic dogs and cats that develop carbohydrate intolerance secondary to concurrent insulin-resistant disease. Examples include the bitch in diestrus, hyperadrenocorticism, and acromegaly.

Original chapter written by Richard W. Nelson

Insulin-Dependent Diabetes Mellitus.   The most common clinically recognized form of diabetes mellitus in the dog and cat is IDDM. Clinically, pancreatitis is often seen in dogs with diabetes mellitus and has been suggested as a cause of diabetes after destruction of the islets.

Non-Insulin-Dependent Diabetes Mellitus.   Clinical recognition of NIDDM is more frequent in the cat than in the dog. Obesity, genetics, and islet amyloidosis are important factors. Clinical recognition of NIDDM is uncommon in the dog.

Transient Diabetes Mellitus.   Insulin requirements wax and wane in approximately 20 per cent of diabetic cats. Some diabetic cats may never require insulin therapy once the initial bout of insulin-requiring diabetes mellitus has dissipated; others become permanently insulin-dependent weeks to months after resolution of a prior diabetic state. Some theorize that cats with transient diabetes are subclinical until the endocrine pancreas is stressed by inflammation, systemic disease, or administration of an insulin-antagonistic drug. A transient or reversible form of IDDM is uncommon in the dog.

Diagnosis of IDDM versus NIDDM.   All dogs should be considered to have IDDM and should be treated with insulin, unless there is a strong suspicion of secondary diabetes mellitus. The significant incidence of NIDDM and transient diabetes in cats raises interesting questions concerning the need for insulin treatment. Glycemic control can be maintained in some diabetic cats with dietary treatment and oral hypoglycemic drugs. Unfortunately, the ultimate differentiation between IDDM and NIDDM is often made retrospectively, after the clinician has had several weeks to assess the response of the cat to therapy and to determine the patient's need for insulin.

SIGNALMENT (pp. 1514–1515)

Dogs with diabetes mellitus are usually 4 to 14 years old, with a peak incidence at 7 to 9 years. Females are affected about twice as frequently as males. Pulik, Cairn terriers, and miniature pinschers are breeds at higher risk along with poodles, dachshunds, miniature schnauzers, and beagles. The majority of diabetic cats have been more than 6 years of age, and predominately neutered males

ANAMNESIS (p. 1515)

The history in virtually all diabetics includes the classic alterations of polydipsia, polyuria, polyphagia, and weight loss. Occasionally an owner will present a dog because of sudden blindness caused by cataract formation or a cat because of rear limb weakness and a plantigrade posture.

PHYSICAL EXAMINATION (pp. 1515–1516)

The findings on physical examination depend on the presence and severity of diabetic ketoacidosis (DKA) and the nature of any concurrent disorders. In the nonketotic diabetic there are no classic physical findings. Many diabetic dogs and cats are obese but are otherwise in good physical condition. Dogs and cats with prolonged untreated diabetes may have lost weight but are rarely emaciated. Hepatomegaly and cataracts are common.

In the ketoacidotic diabetic dog or cat, physical findings include dehydration, depression, weakness, tachypnea, vomiting, and sometimes a strong odor of acetone on the breath. With severe metabolic acidosis, slow deep breathing (i.e., Kussmaul respiration) may be observed. Gastrointestinal signs of vomiting, abdominal pain, and distention are common in DKA.

TABLE 117–1. CAUSES OF HYPERGLYCEMIA IN THE DOG AND CAT

Diabetes mellitus*
"Stress" (cat)*
Postprandial (soft moist foods)
Hyperadrenocorticism*
Acromegaly (cat)
Diestrus (bitch)
Pheochromocytoma (dog)
Pancreatitis
Exocrine pancreatic neoplasia
Renal insufficiency
Drug therapy,* most notably glucocorticoids, progestagens, megestrol acetate
Glucose-containing fluids, esp. TPN mixtures
Laboratory error

*Common cause.

DIAGNOSIS (pp. 1516–1518)

A diagnosis of diabetes mellitus requires the presence of appropriate clinical signs (i.e., polyuria, polydipsia, polyphagia, weight loss) and documentation of persistent fasting hyperglycemia and glycosuria. The concurrent documentation of ketonuria establishes diabetic DKA. If ketonuria is not present, but DKA is suspected, the serum can be tested with Acetest tablets. Hyperglycemia differentiates diabetes mellitus from primary renal glycosuria, whereas glycosuria differentiates diabetes mellitus from other causes of hyperglycemia (Table 117–1). Hyperglycemia in the range of 300 to 400 mg/dl may occur in stressed cats. Glycosuria usually does not develop with stress hyperglycemia.

PATIENT EVALUATION

Nonketotic Diabetic. The clinician must be aware of any disease that might be causing or contributing to the carbohydrate intolerance and must identify any abnormalities that are a result of the diabetic state (e.g., infection). The minimum laboratory evaluation should include a complete blood count, biochemical panel, serum lipase, serum thyroxine (cat), and urinalysis with bacterial culture.

Ketoacidotic Diabetic. The laboratory evaluation is similar to that of the nonketotic diabetic. The healthy ketotic diabetic can usually be managed conservatively, without fluid therapy or intensive care. In contrast, ill ketoacidotic diabetic dogs and cats are critical metabolic emergencies that require a much more aggressive diagnostic and therapeutic plan.

CLINICAL PATHOLOGIC ABNORMALITIES

Hemogram. The hemogram is usually normal in the uncomplicated diabetic pet. A mild, apparent polycythemia may be present if the animal is dehydrated. An elevation of the white blood cell count may be caused by either an infectious process or severe inflammation, especially if an underlying pancreatitis is present.

Biochemical Panel. Clinical pathologic abnormalities associated with the liver, which are common in diabetic dogs and cats, are usually caused by hepatic lipidosis, pancreatitis, and, less commonly, extrahepatic biliary obstruction caused by acute severe pancreatitis. Serum alanine transaminase and, in dogs, alkaline phosphatase concentrations are commonly increased. An elevation in BUN and creatinine may be due to either primary renal failure or prerenal uremia secondary to dehydration. Hyperlipidemia and obvious lipemia are common in untreated diabetics. Hypertriglyceridemia is responsible for lipemia.

Pancreatic Enzymes. Exocrine pancreatic insufficiency and chronic and acute pancreatitis are associated with diabetes mellitus in both the dog and the cat. Animals with concomitant pancreatitis frequently have hyperlipasemia and hyperamylasemia. Chronic inflammation and renal failure are two of the nonpancreatic conditions that may increase serum pancreatic enzyme concentrations. Diabetic dogs and cats can also have histologically confirmed pancreatitis and normal pancreatic enzyme concentrations.

Urinalysis. Abnormalities include glycosuria, ketonuria, proteinuria, and bacteriuria with or without associated pyuria and hematuria. A relatively healthy diabetic may have trace to small amounts of ketones in the urine. If large amounts of ketones are present in the urine, a diagnosis of DKA should be made. Proteinuria may be the result of urinary tract infection or glomerular damage secondary to disruption of the basement membrane.

THERAPY: ILL KETOACIDOTIC DIABETIC (pp. 1518–1522)

Proper therapy does not imply forcing as rapid a return to normal as possible. If all abnormal parameters can be slowly returned toward normal (i.e., over a period of 36 to 48 hours), there is greater likelihood of success in therapy.

FLUID THERAPY

Fluid Composition and Rate. With rare exceptions, all dogs and cats with DKA have significant deficits in total body sodium, regardless of the measured serum concentration. Unless serum electrolytes dictate otherwise, the initial intravenous fluid of choice is 0.9 per cent sodium chloride with appropriate potassium supplementation (Table 117–2). Only if the osmolality is above 350 mOsm/kg should hypotonic fluids (i.e., 0.45 per cent saline) be considered. Hyperosmolality should be corrected during the initial 24 to 36 hours of treatment, but no faster, with appropriate fluid and insulin therapy.

Fluid administration should be directed at gradually replacing all deficits over a period of 24 to 48 hours. Rapid replacement is rarely indicated except if the dog or cat is in shock. A fluid rate of 1.5 to 2 times maintenance is typically chosen initially. Accurate assessment of urine output is extremely important in the severely ill ketoacidotic dog or cat. A minimum of 1.0 to 2.0 ml of urine/kg of body weight/hour should be produced following the initial phase of fluid therapy. An important aid in fluid therapy is the frequent assessment (i.e., at least twice daily) of serum sodium, potassium, and acid-base (total venous CO_2 or arterial blood gas) status.

Potassium Supplementation. During therapy for DKA the serum potassium concentration will decrease and should be addressed (see Table 117–2).

TABLE 117–2. GUIDELINE FOR POTASSIUM SUPPLEMENTATION IN IV FLUIDS*

SERUM K+ (MEQ/L)	K+ SUPPLEMENT/LITER OF FLUIDS
>3.5	20
3.0–3.5	30
2.5–3.0	40
2.0–2.5	60
<2.0	80

*Total hourly potassium administration should not exceed 0.5 mEq/kg body weight.

Phosphate Supplementation. Hypophosphatemia is not commonly identified at initial presentation, even though total body phosphorus "stores" may be severely depleted. Initiation of insulin therapy and correction of the metabolic acidosis may result in potentially severe hypophosphatemia (<1.5 mg/dl). Life-threatening hemolytic anemia is the most common problem, if not recognized and treated. Weakness, ataxia, and seizures may also be observed.

Phosphate therapy is indicated if clinical signs or hemolysis is identified or if the serum phosphorus concentration is less than 1.5 mg/dl. We recommend supplementation of intravenous fluids with phosphorus to prevent the development of severe hypophosphatemia during therapy for severe DKA

BICARBONATE THERAPY

Bicarbonate is not usually supplemented when plasma bicarbonate (or total venous CO_2) is 12 mEq/L or greater, especially if the patient is alert. When the plasma bicarbonate concentration is 11 mEq/L or less (total venous CO_2 is below 12), bicarbonate therapy should be initiated. Only a portion of the bicarbonate deficit is given initially over a 6-hour period of time.

The bicarbonate deficit is calculated as:

$$\text{mEq bicarbonate} = \text{body weight (kg)} \times 0.4 \times (12 - \text{patient's bicarbonate}) \times 0.5$$

Bicarbonate should never be given by bolus infusion. After 6 hours of therapy, the acid-base status should be reevaluated.

INSULIN THERAPY

Rapid-acting regular crystalline insulin is recommended for the treatment of DKA.

Intermittent Intramuscular Regimen. Dogs and cats with severe DKA should receive an initial regular insulin loading dose of 0.2 U/kg followed by 0.1 U/kg IM every hour thereafter. The blood glucose concentration should be measured every 1 to 2 hours. The goal of initial insulin therapy is to slowly lower the blood glucose concentration to the range of 200 to 250 mg/dl, preferably over an 8- to 10-hour period. In general, hyperglycemia is corrected in 4 to 8 hours, but ketosis takes 10 to 30 hours to resolve.

Once the initial hourly insulin therapy brings the blood glucose concentration below 250 mg/dl, hourly administration of regular insulin should be discontinued; and regular insulin given every 4 to 6 hours IM or, if hydration status is good, SC every 6 to 8 hours. The initial dose is usually 0.1 to 0.4 U/kg, with subsequent adjustments based on blood glucose concentrations. The blood glucose concentration should be maintained between 150 and 300 mg/dl (with IV dextrose, if necessary) until the patient is stable and eating. Longer-acting insulins (e.g., lente, ultralente) should not be initiated until the dog or cat is stable, eating, not vomiting, maintaining fluid balance without any intravenous infusions, and no longer acidotic, azotemic, or electrolyte-deficient.

CONCURRENT ILLNESS

Therapy for DKA frequently involves the management of concurrent, often serious, illness. Common concurrent illnesses include bacterial infection, pancreatitis, congestive heart failure, renal failure, and insulin antagonistic disorders, most notably hyperadrenocorticism and diestrus. If restriction of oral intake is necessary, insulin therapy should be continued and the blood glucose concentration maintained with intravenous dextrose infusions.

THERAPY: HEALTHY KETOACIDOTIC DIABETIC (p. 1522)

If the dog or cat initially presents "healthy," short-acting regular insulin can be administered SC three times daily until ketonuria resolves. Once the ketoacidotic state has resolved and the dog or cat is stable, eating, and drinking, insulin regulation may be initiated utilizing the long-acting insulin preparations.

THERAPY: NONKETOTIC DIABETIC (pp. 1522–1524)

DIETARY THERAPY

Appropriate dietary therapy should be initiated in all diabetic dogs and cats. Dietary therapy should correct obesity, maintain consistency in the caloric content of the meals, and furnish a diet that minimizes postprandial fluctuations in blood glucose. The diets likely to be most effective are those that contain the most fiber and digestible complex carbohydrates on a dry matter basis.

Common clinical complications from feeding high-fiber diets include constipation and hypoglycemia 1 to 2 weeks after increasing the fiber content of the diet and refusal to eat the diet. Periodic changes in types of high-fiber diets and mixtures of diets has been helpful in alleviating this problem.

Diets containing increased fiber content should be fed with caution in thin diabetic dogs and cats. For these dogs and cats, weight gain usually requires reestablishment of glycemic control through insulin therapy and the feeding of a high-caloric, lower-fiber diet.

Caloric Intake and Obesity. Weight reduction improves glucose tolerance in obese dogs, presumably via improvement in obesity-induced insulin resistance. Weight reduction should be gradual in the cat to minimize the risk of developing the hepatic lipidosis syndrome.

Feeding Schedule. Multiple small meals rather than one large meal should be fed. Cats and dogs that are "nibblers" throughout the day should be allowed free access to food. "Gluttonous" cats and dogs should be fed half of the daily caloric intake at the time of the insulin injection and the remaining half approximately 8 to 10 hours later. Dogs and cats receiving exogenous insulin twice a day are usually fed equal-sized meals at the time of each insulin injection.

Modifications in Dietary Therapy. Dietary therapy for chronic renal failure, heart failure, or recurring pancreatitis is a higher priority than dietary therapy for diabetes mellitus.

ORAL HYPOGLYCEMIC DRUGS (pp. 1524–1526)

Some endogenous pancreatic insulin secretory capacity must exist for sulfonylureas to be effective in improving glycemic control. Therefore, sulfonylurea treatment is ineffective as the sole form of treatment for IDDM. Sulfonylureas may be effective in some cats with NIDDM. No consistent parameters have been identified that allow the clinician to prospectively determine which cats will respond to glipizide therapy. Selection of diabetic cats for treatment with glipizide must rely heavily on the veterinarian's assessment of the cat's health, severity of clinical signs, presence or absence of ketoacidosis, other diabetic complications (e.g., neuropathy), and owner desires.

Glipizide is discontinued and insulin therapy initiated if (1) clinical signs continue to worsen, (2) the cat becomes ill or develops ketoacidosis, (3) blood glucose concentrations remain greater than 300 mg/dl after 1 or 2 months of therapy, or (4) the owners become dissatisfied with the treatment.

TABLE 117–3. PROPERTIES OF BEEF/PORK INSULIN PREPARATIONS USED IN DOGS AND CATS*

ROUTE OF TYPE OF INSULIN	ADMINISTRATION	ONSET OF EFFECT	TIME OF MAXIMUM EFFECT		DURATION OF EFFECT	
			Dog	Cat	Dog	Cat
Regular crystalline, semilente	IV	Immediate	½-2 hr	½-2 hr	1-4 hr	1-4 hr
	IM	10-30 min	1-4 hr	1-4 hr	3-8 hr	3-8 hr
	SQ	10-30 min	1-5 hr	1-5 hr	4-10 hr	4-10 hr
NPH (isophane)†	SQ	1-2-3 hr	2-10 hr	2-8 hr	6-24 hr	4-12 hr
PZI§	SQ	1-4 hr	4-14 hr	3-12 hr	6-28 hr	6-24 hr
Lente†	SQ	< 1 hr	2-10 hr	2-8 hr	8-24 hr	6-14 hr
Ultralente‡	SQ	2-8 hr	4-16 hr	4-16 hr	8-28 hr	8-24 hr

*Purified pork and recombinant human insulins appear to be more potent, act faster, and have a shorter duration of action than beef/pork insulins.
†Initial insulin of choice for the diabetic dog.
‡Initial insulin of choice for the diabetic cat.
§At time of this writing, not commercially available.

INSULIN THERAPY (pp. 1526–1535)

Initial Insulin Treatment for Diabetic Dogs. Intermediate-acting insulins (i.e., NPH, Lente) are the initial insulins of choice for glycemic regulation of the diabetic dog. NPH insulin frequently needs to be administered twice daily if good glycemic control is to be achieved (see Table 117–3). Dietary therapy, including a high-fiber diet, is initiated concurrently.

Initial Insulin Treatment for Diabetic Cats. Long-acting insulins (i.e., PZI, Ultralente) are the initial insulins of choice for glycemic regulation of the diabetic cat. Slow absorption of Ultralente insulin is a problem in approximately 20 per cent of our diabetic cats. In these cats, Ultralente insulin is ineffective in maintaining glycemic control despite dosages of 8 to 10 U/cat twice a day. For these cats, Lente insulin twice a day is often effective.

Adjustments in Insulin Therapy. See textbook.

Monitoring the Diabetic Dog and Cat at Home. The basic objective of insulin therapy is to eliminate the clinical signs of diabetes mellitus. Currently we rely on owner observation for recurrence of clinical signs in conjunction with periodic physical examinations and assessment of body weight, serial evaluations of blood glucose concentrations, and glycosylated hemoglobin concentration to evaluate glycemic control of the diabetic state. Most important is the owner's subjective opinion of water intake, urine output, appetite, and body weight. If these factors are normal, the diabetic dog or cat is usually well controlled. Urine monitoring for glycosuria is not recommended to our clients, nor are attempts made to adjust daily insulin dosages based on morning urine glucose measurements in diabetic dogs.

Glycosylated Hemoglobin and Fructosamine. Increased glycosylated hemoglobin or fructosamine concentrations support poor glycemic control and a need for insulin adjustments. Evaluation of serial measurements of blood glucose concentration is required to determine how to adjust insulin therapy.

Adjustments in Insulin Therapy

Interpreting the Serial Blood Glucose Curve. Insulin effectiveness, glucose nadir, and duration of insulin effect are critical parameters determined from serial blood glucose curves. If the insulin is not effective in lowering the blood glucose concentration, the clinician must consider the differentials for insulin ineffectiveness and resistance. If the glucose nadir is greater than 125 mg/dl, the insulin dosage should be increased, and if the nadir is less than 80 mg/dl, the insulin dosage should be decreased.

Alterations in the frequency of insulin administration should not be made until an acceptable glucose nadir (greater than 100 mg/dl) is established. Assessment of the duration of effect of the insulin may not be valid when the glucose nadir is less than 80 mg/dl because of the potential induction of rebound hyperglycemia. The duration of effect is roughly defined as the time from the insulin injection until the blood glucose concentration exceeds 200 to 250 mg/dl. The insulin dosage should be decreased at the time twice-daily insulin therapy is initiated if the insulin's duration of effect is greater than 12 hours.

Problems with Serial Blood Glucose Curves. See textbook.

COMPLICATIONS OF INSULIN THERAPY

Hypoglycemia. Signs of hypoglycemia include lethargy, weakness, head tilting, ataxia, and seizures. Occurrence of clinical signs is dependent on the rate of decline of plasma glucose as well as on the degree of hypoglycemia.

Insulin-Induced Hyperglycemia: The Somogyi Phenomenon. Insulin-induced hyperglycemia should be suspected when there is persistent morning glycosuria (>1 gm/dl), continued polyuria and polydipsia, symptoms of hypoglycemia, weight loss, or insulin dosages approaching 2.2 U/kg body weight. Diagnosis requires demonstration of hypoglycemia (<65 mg/dl) followed by hyperglycemia (>300 mg/dl) within one 24-hour period following insulin administration. Therapy involves reducing the insulin dose.

Short Duration of Insulin Effect. Hyperglycemia may begin as early as 6 hours following insulin administration. Diabetic dogs and cats with the problem of short duration of insulin effect will have persistent morning glycosuria, evening polyuria and polydipsia, or weight loss. A diagnosis of short duration of insulin effect is made by demonstrating significant hyperglycemia (>250 mg/dl) within 18 hours or less of the insulin injection while the lowest blood glucose concentration is maintained above 80 mg/dl. Treatment involves changing the type of insulin and/or the frequency of administration.

Insulin Ineffectiveness and Resistance

For most diabetic cats, good glycemic control can be achieved with long-acting insulin, ≤5 U/cat, given once or twice daily. Insulin resistance is suspected if the insulin dosage is above 1.5 U/kg (dog) or 6 U (cat) and all blood glucose concentrations are above 300 mg/dl. Insulin resistance is also suspected when excessive amounts of insulin (i.e., insulin dosage >2.2 U/kg) are necessary to maintain the blood glucose concentration below 300 mg/dl.

Whenever insulin resistance is suspected, problems with insulin activity or administration technique should be ruled out before a diagnostic evaluation for insulin resistance is undertaken. The Somogyi phenomenon, slow or impaired absorption of subcutaneously deposited insulin, and excessive insulin-binding antibodies are variables to consider for problems with insulin activity. There are many disorders that can interfere with insulin therapy (see Table 117–4).

TABLE 117–4. RECOGNIZED CAUSES OF INSULIN INEFFECTIVENESS OR INSULIN RESISTANCE IN THE DIABETIC DOG AND CAT

CAUSED BY INSULIN THERAPY	CAUSED BY CONCURRENT DISORDER
Inactive insulin	Diabetogenic drugs
Diluted insulin	Hyperadrenocorticism
Improper administration technique	Diestrus (bitch)
Inadequate dose	Acromegaly (cat)
Somogyi phenomenon	Infection, esp. oral cavity and urinary tract
Inadequate frequency of insulin administration	Hypothyroidism (dog)
Impaired insulin absorption, esp. Ultralente insulin	Hyperthyroidism (cat)
Anti-insulin antibody excess	Renal insufficiency
	Liver insufficiency
	Cardiac insufficiency
	Chronic pancreatitis
	Exocrine pancreatic insufficiency
	Glucagonoma (dog)
	Hyperlipidemia (?)
	Phcochromocytoma (?)

CHRONIC COMPLICATIONS OF DIABETES MELLITUS
(pp. 1535–1536)

Cataracts. Cataract formation is the most common and one of the most important long-term complications associated with diabetes mellitus in the dog but is rare in the cat. Cataract formation is an irreversible process once it begins and can occur rapidly. The blindness may be corrected by removing the abnormal lens, assuming the retina is functioning normally.

Diabetic Retinopathy. This is an uncommon clinical complication in the dog and cat. There is a close correlation between diabetic retinopathy and suboptimal glycemic control.

Diabetic Neuropathies. These are rarely reported in the dog and cat. Cats often develop a plantigrade posture with the hocks touching the ground when the cat walks. In the dog, it is primarily a distal polyneuropathy. The cause is not known. There is no specific therapy for diabetic neuropathy.

Diabetic Nephropathy. Its clinical recognition appears to be low. The pathogenic mechanism is unknown. Clinical signs are dependent on the severity of the glomerulosclerosis and the functional ability of the kidney to excrete metabolic wastes.

CHAPTER 118
HYPERADRENOCORTICISM
(pages 1538–1578)

CANINE CUSHING'S SYNDROME (pp. 1538–1573)

Canine Cushing's syndrome (CCS) is caused by a pituitary tumor synthesizing and secreting excess adrenocorticotropic hormone (ACTH) with secondary adrenocortical hyperplasia; pituitary hyperplasia and, secondarily, adrenocortical hyperplasia resulting from excesses in corticotropin releasing hormone (CRH) secretion caused by a hypothalamic disorder; primary excesses in adrenal cortisol, autonomously secreted by an adrenocortical carcinoma or adenoma; and iatrogenic causes resulting from excessive glucocorticoid medication.

The vast majority (80 to 85 per cent) of dogs with naturally occurring Cushing's syndrome have pituitary-dependent hyperadrenocorticism (PDH). More than 90 per cent of dogs with PDH have a pituitary tumor. Bilateral functioning adrenocortical neoplasia is rare in dogs, as is a simultaneous functioning adrenocortical tumor and a pituitary microadenoma.

PATHOLOGY

A significant percentage of dogs with PDH (perhaps as many as 10 to 15 per cent) have large pituitary tumors, which have the potential of compressing or invading adjacent structures. Adrenal adenomas usually are encapsulated and grossly visible, ranging in size from 1 to 6 cm. Adrenal carcinomas can become quite large and are highly vascular. Partial calcification is identified in about 50 per cent of these masses.

Original chapter written by Edward C. Feldman

The cortical tissue contiguous to a functioning adrenocortical adenoma or carcinoma and that of the contralateral gland are atrophic.

SIGNALMENT

More than 75 per cent of these dogs are older than 9 years of age. Poodle breeds, dachshunds, various terrier breeds, beagles, and German shepherd dogs are most commonly represented. PDH occurs more frequently in smaller dogs. About 45 to 50 per cent of dogs with adrenocortical tumors (adenomas or carcinomas) weigh more than 20 kg.

HISTORY

Most dogs with Cushing's syndrome are not critically ill and have signs that slowly progress. Chronic exposure to excess cortisol often results in polydipsia, polyuria, polyphagia, abdominal enlargement, alopecia, pyoderma, panting, muscle weakness, and lethargy. Normal water intake for the average dog is about 20 to 30 ml/lb/day. Owners usually report water intake in polydipsic hyperadrenal dogs that is 2 to 10 times normal. About 5 per cent of dogs with Cushing's syndrome have overt diabetes mellitus.

The potbellied or pendulous abdominal profile is present in 90 to 95 per cent of affected dogs. Exercise tolerance often is reduced. Weakness has been noted in 75 to 85 per cent of dogs with Cushing's. Chronic hypercortisolism can result in an exaggeration of anterior cruciate ligament rupture and patellar luxation lameness. Cutaneous signs are common. Classically, these problems are not associated with pruritus. Dogs may be described as pruritic because of seborrhea, calcinosis cutis, demodicosis, or pyoderma.

The hair loss may begin at points of wear (such as bony prominences) and eventually involve the flanks, perineum, and abdomen. Bilaterally symmetric alopecia has also been noted in cats with Cushing's. If hair is shaved, regrowth is poor or nonexistent. Thin skin, poor healing, and susceptibility to infection is typical of hypercortisolism in dogs and cats. Pyoderma was observed in 55 per cent of hyperadrenal dogs and is especially common along the dorsal midline and trunk.

The fragility observed with thin skin is also present in the blood vessels. Excessive bruising can follow venipuncture or other minor trauma. Wounds that do heal do so tenuously. Calcium deposition in the dermis and subcutis is an uncommon sign. These areas feel like firm plaques in or under the skin. Dogs often are noted to be short of breath or to have a rapid respiratory rate.

A male dog with Cushing's usually has bilaterally small, soft, spongy testicles. A female dog with Cushing's commonly ceases estrous cycle activity. Rarely, dogs may develop a distinct myopathy characterized by persistent active muscle contraction after cessation of voluntary effort. Pelvic limb muscle stiffness is obvious on physical examination.

PHYSICAL EXAMINATION

The physical examination on a typical dog with Cushing's reveals an individual that is stable and hydrated, has good mucous membrane color, and is not in distress. Abnormalities include abdominal enlargement, increased panting, truncal obesity, bilaterally symmetric alopecia, skin infections, and comedones (hair follicles filled with keratin and debris that usually are black and easily expressed). Hyperpigmentation, ectopic calcification, testicular atrophy, clitoral hypertrophy, hepatomegaly, and easy bruisability are common. These dogs may have a single dominant sign or 10 signs.

IN-HOSPITAL EVALUATION

Finding a large percentage of abnormalities on initial screening tests allows the veterinarian to establish a presumptive diagnosis (Table 118–1).

TABLE 118–1. HEMATOLOGIC, SERUM BIOCHEMICAL, URINE, AND RADIOGRAPHIC ABNORMALITIES TYPICAL OF HYPERADRENOCORTICISM*

TEST	ABNORMALITY
Complete blood count	Mature leukocytosis
	Neutrophilia
	Lymphopenia
	Eosinopenia
	Erythrocytosis (females)
Serum chemistries	Increased alkaline phosphatase (sometimes extremely elevated)
	Increased ALT
	Increased cholesterol
	Increased fasting blood glucose
	Increased or normal insulin
	Abnormal bile acids
	Decreased BUN
	Lipemia
Urinalysis	Urine specific gravity <1.015, often <1.008
	Urinary tract infection
	Glycosuria (<10% of cases)
Radiograph/Ultrasound	Hepatomegaly
	Excellent abdominal contrast
	Pot belly
	Distended bladder
	Osteoporosis
	Calcinosis cutis/dystrophic calcification
	Adrenal calcification (usually adrenal tumor)
	Congestive heart failure (rare)
	Pulmonary thromboembolism (rare)
	Calcified trachea and mainstem bronchi
	Pulmonary metastasis of adrenal carcinoma
Miscellaneous	Low T_4/T_3 concentrations
	Response to TSH that parallels normal but both pre and post values are low
	Hypertension

*It would be unusual for an individual animal to have all these abnormalities.

Alkaline Phosphatase

An increase in serum alkaline phosphatase (ALP) activity is the most common routine laboratory abnormality in canine hyperadrenocorticism. In dogs with hyperadrenocorticism, 70 to 100 per cent of their ALP is specifically the steroid-induced fraction (SIALP). SIALP concentrations in Cushing's are considered quite sensitive but nonspecific. SIALP may be abnormal in dogs with primary hepatopathies: iatrogenic Cushing's, diabetes mellitus, and anticonvulsant therapy.

Cholesterol and Lipemia

Ninety per cent of dogs with Cushing's have increased plasma cholesterol concentrations. Lipemia is at least as frequent.

Bile Acids

These test results frequently are abnormal in dogs with Cushing's and do not aid in separating dogs with primary liver disorders from those with Cushing's.

Urinalysis

The most frequent abnormality is the finding of dilute urine (specific gravity less than 1.013). Glycosuria has been noted in 5 to 10 per cent of cases. About 50 per cent of dogs have a urinary tract infection at the time of initial examination.

Thyroid Function Tests

About 70 per cent of dogs have decreases in basal serum T_4, free T_4, and/or T_3 concentrations.

Radiographs

See Table 118–1. Positive identification of an adrenal mass occurs infrequently. Only about 50 per cent of these can be visualized radiographically because of calcification.

Ultrasonography

If bilaterally normal-sized or large adrenals are visualized, this is considered strong evidence in favor of adrenal hyperplasia caused by pituitary-dependent disease. If either adrenal is remarkably enlarged, irregular, or invading or compressing adjacent structures and the opposite adrenal cannot be visualized, suspicion of an adrenal tumor is heightened.

ASSOCIATED MEDICAL COMPLICATIONS

Hypertension

Blindness, left ventricular hypertrophy, heart failure, and glomerulopathies may be sequelae. More than 50 per cent of dogs with Cushing's are hypertensive on random testing.

Pyelonephritis and Urinary Calculi

About 5 to 10 per cent of dogs with Cushing's syndrome have urinary calculi.

Glomerulopathies

The incidence of glomerulopathies in dogs with Cushing's exceeds 50 per cent. This protein loss seldom causes significant hypoalbuminemia and has not been related to clinical signs.

Pancreatitis

See textbook.

Diabetes Mellitus

A major dilemma is encountered when attempting to determine whether a dog or cat with established diabetes mellitus has Cushing's. The major clue used by practitioners is the presence of insulin resistance. Resistance, however, is a subjective phenomenon that has myriad differential diagnoses.

Pulmonary Thromboembolism

Most of these dogs have acute respiratory distress, orthopnea, and, less commonly, a jugular pulse. Radiographs of the thorax may reveal no abnormalities, pleural effusion, or an increased diameter and blunting of the pulmonary arteries. Arterial blood gas analysis demonstrates hypoxemia and hypoclycemia. Thrombosis may be confirmed with angiography or with a radionuclear lung scan. Therapy consists of general support, oxygen, anticoagulants, and time. The prognosis for this condition is grave.

Central Nervous System Signs

The clinical signs exhibited by dogs with macrotumors often reflect both the endocrine and the space-occupying effects of the tumor. Signs commonly reported include dullness, listlessness, and a poor appetite. The signs may progress to anorexia, restlessness, delayed response to stimuli, and brief episodes of disorientation. Other signs include altered mentation, ataxia, tetraparesis, aimless pacing, nystagmus, circling, head pressing, behavior changes, blindness, seizures, and coma. The diagnosis can be confirmed only with CT or MRI.

SPECIFIC EVALUATION OF THE PITUITARY-ADRENOCORTICAL AXIS

Endocrine Testing

Urinary Corticosteroids. The urine cortisol-creatinine (C/C) ratio has potential as a screening test for hyperadrenocorticism. The urine C/C ratio readily distinguishes between apparently healthy dogs and those with hyperadrenocorticism, but the test lacks specificity: it is abnormal in dogs with Cushing's and dogs with diabetes mellitus, diabetes insipidus, pyometra, hypercalcemia, and liver failure.

ACTH Stimulation Test. ACTH stimulation test results are abnormal in 80 to 85 per cent of dogs with PDH. Test results from dogs with PDH are not distinguishable from those of dogs with adrenocortical tumors. It is possible for chronic illness to alter adrenocortical test results. The diagnosis of hyperadrenocorticism in this situation must be supported by abnormal endocrine test results and clinical signs of Cushing's.

A dog with features of Cushing's with a low-normal base-line cortisol concentration and little or no response to exogenous ACTH is likely to have iatrogenic Cushing's syndrome. Diagnosis of dogs with signs of Cushing's syndrome that are receiving anticonvulsant medication can be confusing. Such medication can cause abnormal plasma cortisol concentrations.

Low-Dose Dexamethasone Test. Several response patterns to the low dose of dexamethasone have been identified in dogs with hyperadrenocorticism (see Fig. 118–1). Complete suppression of plasma cortisol concentrations 8 hours after dexamethasone administration does not occur in dogs with adrenocortical tumors or in dogs with PDH. Anticonvulsant medications can cause dogs to have abnormal plasma cortisol concentrations. Stress may interfere with the suppressive effects of dexamethasone. Cortisol assays may measure iatrogenic glucocorticoids (not dexamethasone).

Miscellaneous Screening Tests See textbook.

Discrimination Tests

Low-Dose Dexamethasone Test. Those dogs that demonstrate suppression at 4 hours have PDH (see Fig. 118–1). Dogs that fail to demonstrate suppression at 4 hours must be evaluated further.

Endogenous ACTH Concentrations. Endogenous ACTH concentrations less than 10 pg/ml in a dog with naturally occurring hyperadrenocorticism are strongly suggestive of a functioning adrenocortical tumor (Fig. 118–2). ACTH concentrations greater than or equal to 45 pg/ml are consistent with a diagnosis of pituitary-dependent bilateral adrenal hyperplasia. Appropriate screening tests must be used first to obtain a diagnosis of hyperadrenocorticism.

High-Dose Dexamethasone Suppression Test Administration of a high dose of dexamethasone does not result in cortisol suppression with adrenocortical tumors (Fig. 118–3 and see Fig. 118–1).

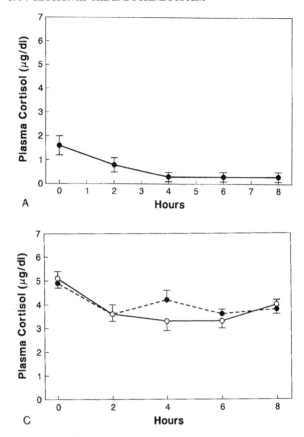

Figure 118–1. *A,* Mean plasma cortisol concentrations before and after administration of a low dose of dexamethasone in 27 normal dogs; *B,* Forty-eight dogs with adrenocortical tumors; *C,* 130 dogs with PDH; *D,* those dogs from the 178 total with Cushing's syndrome that had at least one plasma cortisol concentration less than 1.4 μg/dl after dexamethasone (total 54, each had PDH); and *E,* those dogs from the total of 178 with Cushing's syndrome with at least one plasma cortisol concentration after dexamethasone less than 50 per cent of the base-line concentration (total 95, each had PDH). Note that there are two curves for graphs *B, C, D,* and *E.* These represent the use of dexamethasone sodium phosphate (•– – –•) or dexamethasone in polyethylene glycol (○———○). There is no significant difference in results when using either of these dexamethasone products.

About 75 to 80 per cent of dogs with PDH have plasma cortisol concentrations less than 50 per cent of the base-line concentration 8 hours after administration of a high dose of dexamethasone (Fig. 118–3 and see Fig. 118–1). Dogs with naturally occurring Cushing's that suppress on the high dose have PDH. Among the dogs with Cushing's that fail to demonstrate suppression are 20 to 30 per cent of dogs with PDH and 100 per cent of dogs with adrenocortical tumors.

Computed Tomography
Adrenals. Ultrasonography is comparable for detecting adrenocortical tumors in dogs.

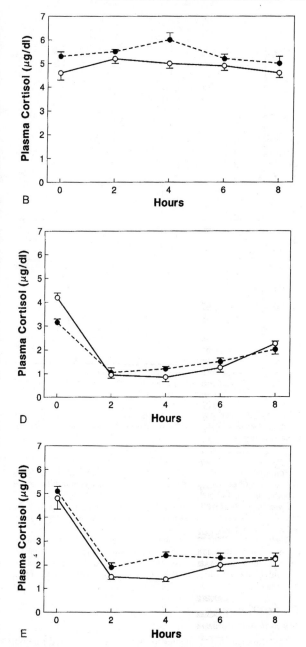

Figure 118–1. *(Continued)*

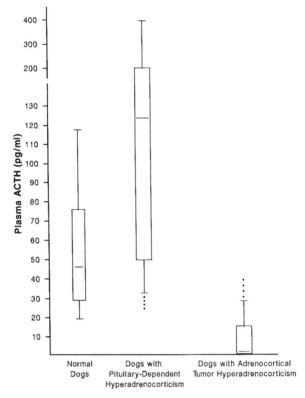

Figure 118–2. Endogenous plasma ACTH concentrations from clinically normal dogs, dogs with PDH, and dogs with functioning adrenocortical carcinomas or adenomas.

Pituitary. CT is extremely accurate for visualization of large pituitary tumors or cerebral ventricular dilation secondary to a pituitary or hypothalamic mass.

Magnetic Resonance Imaging. MRI is superior to CT in the detection of associated tumor features: edema, cysts, vascularity, hemorrhage, and necrosis.

Metyrapone Testing. If metyrapone results in a decrease in the plasma cortisol concentration and a concomitant increase in plasma 11-desoxycortisol level, a diagnosis of PDH can be made. If plasma cortisol and 11-desoxycortisol concentrations both decline, an adrenal tumor is likely.

TREATMENT—SURGERY

Adrenal Tumor

The clinician should attempt to localize the tumor and rule out metastasis. If Cushing's-related debilitation is present, treating the dog for 1 to 3 months with ketoconazole or *o,p'*-DDD could be beneficial. This time can also be used to treat other concurrent problems (infection) before surgery.

Results (Prognosis). Of 102 dogs we have diagnosed with

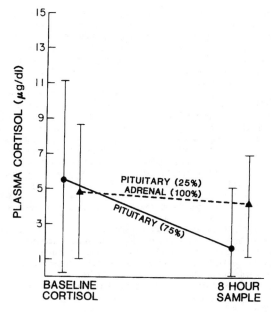

Figure 118–3. Pattern of plasma cortisol responses during high-dose dexamethsone suppression in dogs with PDH or adrenal tumor hyperadrenocorticism. Note that the suppression is diagnostic of pituitary dependency; lack of suppression included all adrenal tumor cases and 20 to 30 per cent of PDH cases.

functioning adrenocortical tumors, 41 underwent successful surgery—24 had carcinomas and 17 had adenomas. The dogs that underwent successful surgery have a good prognosis if metastasis has not occurred and if they survive the 1- to 4-week postsurgical period.

Pituitary-Dependent Hyperadrenocorticism

Hypophysectomy. This has been successfully performed in the dog.

Adrenalectomy. Because "medical adrenalectomy" is relatively easy to accomplish in dogs with o,p'-DDD, the risk of surgery seems unwarranted.

TREATMENT—o,p'-DDD

Pituitary-Dependent Hyperadrenocorticism

Initiating Therapy—Loading-Dose Phase. Therapy is begun at home. The drug must be administered immediately after the meal has been consumed to enhance absorption. Glucocorticoids are not advised, but the owner should have a small supply of prednisone tablets if an emergency should arise. o,p'-DDD administration should be stopped when the dog demonstrates reduction in appetite, the polydipsic dog consumes less than 60 ml/kg/day of water, vomiting occurs, diarrhea occurs, or the dog is unusually listless. The occurrence of any of these signs strongly indicates that the end point in therapy has been achieved.

An owner should not be provided with more than an 8-day supply of o,p'-DDD initially. The dog's appetite should be observed before each administration of o,p'-DDD. If food is rapidly consumed, medication is warranted. If food is consumed slowly or not at all, medication should be discontinued until the veterinarian is consulted. The veterinarian should see the dog 8 to 9 days after beginning therapy. At this time, a recheck of the ACTH response test is obtained. The goal of therapy is to achieve an ACTH response test result suggestive of hypoadrenocorticism. In our laboratory, this means pre- and post-ACTH plasma cortisol concentrations less than 5 µg/dl.

If the dog with Cushing's has a normal or exaggerated response to ACTH after the initial 8 to 9 days, medication should be continued. It usually is continued for 3 to 7 additional consecutive days, the shorter period being used for dogs that have shown some significant response. Repeat ACTH response tests are continued every 7 to 10 days until a low post-ACTH plasma cortisol response is achieved. Most dogs have responded during the initial 5 to 9 days of medication and almost all have responded by the 14th day of therapy. Some dogs respond in as little as 2 or 3 days, and a few have required more than 21 consecutive days.

Concomitant Glucocortoids During the Loading-Dose Phase. This is generally not recommended, but there are advantages and disadvantages with this approach.

Need for Glucocorticoids. If signs of anorexia, vomiting, diarrhea, weakness, or listlessness develop, glucocorticoid therapy is warranted. If the dog has received no glucocorticoids during the initial phase of o,p'-DDD therapy, they should be started. If the dog has been treated with glucocorticoids, the dose needs to be increased.

Planned Induction of Permanent Hypoadrenocorticism. There are several disadvantages to this protocol, and it is generally not recommended.

Need for Both Glucocorticoids and Mineralocorticoids. Electrolyte disturbances suggestive of deficient mineralocorticoids (hyperkalemia and/or hyponatremia) have resulted from o,p'-DDD administration; these dogs require both glucocorticoid and mineralocorticoid therapy (Chapter 119). This finding is extremely rare. Addison's disease in o,p'-DDD-treated dogs usually is permanent.

Time Sequence for Improvement in Signs and Biochemical Abnormalities. The most obvious and rapid response is the reduction in appetite, water intake, and urine output seen during the first 5 to 9 days of therapy. Alopecia, thin skin, acne, calcinosis cutis, and panting often take 3 to 6 months for significant improvement to be noted. The liver enzymes and cholesterol may take 6 to 18 months to improve. Six to 18 months may be required for return of normal blood pressure. Urinary tract infections may resolve quickly or linger.

Failure to Respond to o,p'-DDD. There are several reasons for apparent treatment failures. (1) A dog thought to have PDH may indeed have an adrenocortical tumor. (2) The drug itself may not be potent. (3) The drug may not be given with food. (4) A small percentage of dogs require 30 to 60 consecutive days of therapy, or 100 to 150 mg/kg/day rather than the usual initial dosage of 50 mg/kg/day. (5) The dog may have iatrogenic Cushing's syndrome. If treatment failure has occurred, the 25-day induction of hypoadrenocorticism, ketoconazole therapy, or bilateral adrenalectomy should be considered.

Therapy of Concurrent Diabetes Mellitus and Cushing's Syndrome

Most of these dogs require large doses of insulin. Attempts at extremely good control of the diabetes should not be undertaken until the Cushing's is controlled or until that diagnosis is refuted.

o,p'-DDD Dosage. These dogs should be treated in the same manner as any dog with PDH. Successful reduction in the circulating cortisol concentrations should reduce insulin requirements. About 10 per cent of these dogs require no insulin after successful therapy.

o,p'-DDD Therapy with Functioning Adrenocortical Tumors

Using similar doses of o,p'-DDD (50 mg/kg/day initially), it was demonstrated that dogs with adrenocortical tumors were relatively resistant to the adrenocorticolytic effects of the drug. Some dogs with adrenocortical tumors, however, respond to the traditional doses, and those that appear resistant often respond to higher dosages. Despite concurrent glucocorticoid therapy, some dogs suffer adverse effects sometime during treatment as a result of direct drug toxicity associated with high-dose o,p'-DDD or low cortisol concentrations or both. More than 60 per cent of the o,p'-DDD-treated dogs were considered to have a good to excellent response.

Maintenance Therapy with o,p'-DDD

Once the initial daily protocol has terminated, maintenance therapy should begin. Dogs that respond to daily o,p'-DDD therapy within 9 days or that have a post-ACTH plasma cortisol concentration less than 2 μg/dl are begun at a maintenance schedule of 25 mg/kg of o,p'-DDD every 7 days. Those that initially require more than 10 days of therapy or with a post-ACTH plasma cortisol concentration greater than 5 μg/kg receive 50 mg/kg every 7 days. The dosage is divided into two to four treatments per week.

An ACTH response test is performed 1 and 3 months after beginning the maintenance therapy. The o,p'-DDD dosage is adjusted according to these results and/or clinical signs. It is recommended that dogs be rechecked with an examination and an ACTH response test every 3 to 4 months. Overdosage with o,p'-DDD is common. In the more typical and mild forms of overdosage, the dog becomes weak, anorectic, lethargic, or ataxic, or develops vomiting and/or diarrhea. Clinical improvement in 1 to 3 hours after prednisone administration confirms an overdosage.

MEDICAL MANAGEMENT WITH KETOCONAZOLE

At high dosages, the drug affects steroid biosynthesis. The dose requirement is determined from owner opinion, physical examination results, blood chemistries, and ACTH stimulation test. The goal in ACTH stimulation results are pre- and post-cortisol concentrations less than 5 μg/kg. Eighty per cent of treated dogs have a rapid reduction in serum cortisol concentration and cortisol responsiveness to ACTH and significant improvement in their clinical condition. Signs of toxicity seldom have developed. It appears that 20 to 25 per cent of dogs fail to respond to the drug. It may be used as an alternative to o,p'-DDD in the medical management of dogs with malignant, large, or invasive adrenal tumors if surgical intervention is not an option but palliative therapy is desired. We use ketoconazole most frequently in the preoperative stabilization and improvement of surgical candidates.

TREATMENT—OTHER MEDICATIONS

See textbook.

TREATMENT—LARGE PITUITARY TUMORS (PITUITARY MACROTUMOR SYNDROME)

Conservatively, 10 to 15 per cent of dogs with PDH develop clinical problems as a result of this condition. The primary mode of treating these dogs is photon irradiation. Most dogs with CNS signs have masses much too large for safe surgical extirpation. Dogs with the subtlest signs and smallest tumors have the best response to treatment, and those with the most worrisome clinical signs and largest tumors probably should not be treated.

HYPERADRENOCORTICISM IN CATS (pp. 1573–1575)

The incidence of this condition in cats is rare. Most cats have been middle-aged or older. The most common clinical signs are polydipsia, polyuria, and polyphagia. These signs frequently are observed because the incidence of diabetes mellitus is extremely high. In most cats, Cushing's syndrome is diagnosed after documentation of insulin-resistant diabetes mellitus. A pot belly (pendulous abdomen); unkempt hair coat; thin, easily bruised, fragile, pigmented skin; and muscle wasting are also common signs. Dermatologic infections (including demodicosis) and hepatomegaly are common.

DATA BASE EVALUATION

The CBC is not contributory. More than 80 per cent of cats have hyperglycemia and glycosuria. Hypercholesterolemia and a mild increase in ALT may occur.

ESTABLISHING THE DIAGNOSIS

About 60 per cent of cats have an abnormally exaggerated response to ACTH. Dexamethasone testing is more sensitive and specific. Post-dexamethasone plasma cortisol concentrations of 1 µg/dl or greater are consistent with a diagnosis of hyperadrenocorticism. Failure to suppress on both the low- and high-dose tests is strongly consistent with a diagnosis of hyperadrenocorticism. Ultrasonography is an excellent tool.

DISCRIMINATION TESTING

High-Dose Dexamethasone Test

Post-dexamethasone plasma cortisol concentrations less than 50 per cent of base line are indicative of suppression. If the result is 1 µg/dl or greater and less than 50 per cent of base line, the interpretation would be Cushing's of pituitary origin. Lack of suppression supports the diagnosis of Cushing's but is not specific for adrenocortical tumor.

Plasma Endogenous ACTH

The endogenous ACTH test should aid in distinguishing between PDH and adrenocortical tumors. This test can only be interpreted reliably after the diagnosis has been confirmed with acceptable screening test results.

TREATMENT

Transient resolution of hyperadrenocorticism could be extremely beneficial to cats in which surgery is planned. Cats with Cushing's syndrome are prone to infection and heal poorly. These complications can be minimized by presurgical management with either *o,p'*-DDD, ketoconazole, or metyrapone.

The surgeon must be prepared to make decisions regarding removal of one or both adrenals at surgery. In cats, this disease must be considered serious, with a guarded to grave prognosis.

PRIMARY MINERALOCORTICOID EXCESS— PRIMARY HYPERALDOSTERONISM (pp. 1575–1577)

We have had experience with three dogs that have been diagnosed as having primary hyperaldosteronism. The primary owner concern in each dog was episodic weakness, and each dog had a serum potassium concentration less than 3 mEq/L. Two of the three dogs had assessment of plasma aldosterone concentrations. These concentrations were consistently extremely increased until surgical tumor removal, after which the hormone values decreased dramatically. Each dog had an adrenal tumor: one adenoma and two adenocarcinomas.

CHAPTER 119
HYPOADRENAL GLAND DISEASE
(pages 1579–1593)

ETIOLOGY (pp. 1579–1580)

PRIMARY HYPOADRENOCORTICISM

Primary hypoadrenocorticism, which is most often classified as idiopathic, is usually characterized histopathologically as bilateral adrenal atrophy with fibrosis. An immune-mediated basis for the disease is likely. Other less common causes for spontaneous primary adrenal failure include infections (coccidioidomycosis, blastomycosis, or tuberculosis), hemorrhagic infarctions, metastatic neoplasia, trauma, and amyloidosis. Iatrogenic primary hypoadrenocorticism may follow the administration of the adrenocorticolytic drug o,p'-DDD. Megestrol acetate has profound adrenal suppressive effects in cats.

SECONDARY HYPOADRENOCORTICISM

Naturally occurring secondary hypoadrenocorticism is due to a lack of normal adrenal stimulation via corticotropin-releasing hormone (CRH) or adrenocorticotropic hormone (ACTH), and implies primary hypothalamic or pituitary failure. Most of these cases are the result of inflammation, tumors, trauma, or congenital defects of the hypothalamus or pituitary gland. Iatrogenic secondary hypoadrenocorticism occurs following the administration of exogenous glucocorticoids. Adrenal atrophy may develop after the administration of virtually any glucocorticoid used by veterinarians. Long-acting depot preparations cause the most severe adrenal atrophy and result in long periods of adrenal hypofunction.

CLINICAL FINDINGS (pp. 1581–1587)

Hypoadrenocorticism is primarily a disease of middle-aged female dogs. Evidence for familial tendencies exists in standard poodles, Labrador retrievers, and Portuguese water spaniels. It is typically a disease associated with vague, nonlocalized clinical signs such as depression, lethargy, weakness, anorexia, and weight loss. In others, signs more typical of gastrointestinal (GI) diseases (vomiting, diarrhea) or renal diseases (polydipsia and polyuria) are seen.

PHYSICAL EXAMINATION FINDINGS

Depression, weakness, and dehydration are most commonly identified. Dogs in an adrenal crisis may be in shock, with bradycardia and/or weak pulses.

Original chapter written by Robert M. Hardy

TABLE 119–1. SELECTED LABORATORY VALUES IN DOGS WITH PRIMARY HYPOADRENOCORTICISM

FACTOR	NORMAL VALUE	NUMBER TESTED	MEAN	NUMBER DECREASED (%)	NUMBER INCREASED (%)	RANGE
Serum sodium	136–150 mEq/L	36	129	22(60)	0(0)	106–146
Serum potassium	3.5–5.0 mEq/L	36	7.2	0(0)	33(92)	4.7–10.8
Sodium/potassium ratio	≥27:1	36	19	35(97)	0(0)	11.2–29.1
BUN (pre-Rx)	9–25 mg/dl	36	84	0(0)	33(92)	12–223
BUN (after 24 hr Rx)	9–25 mg/dl	9	25	0(0)	4(44)	11–47
Serum calcium	8.8–11.0 mg/dl	13	11.5	0(0)	8(62)	9.3–14.4
Serum glucose	70–110 mg/dl	24	81.5	8(33)	4(17)	20–130
Serum bicarbonate	18–24 mM/L	16	14	13(81)	0(0)	9–19
Urine specific gravity	—	25	1.024	—	—	1.008–1.062

From Feldman EC: Adrenal gland disease. In Ettinger SJ (ed): Textbook of Veterinary Internal Medicine. 3rd ed. Philadelphia, WB Saunders, 1989, p 1761.

LABORATORY DIAGNOSIS

Hemogram Alterations

A mild normocytic, normochromic anemia is common in dogs. It may be masked initially by dehydration. A "nonstressed" hemogram is uncommon. Eosinophilia and lymphocytosis occur in only 10 to 15 per cent of affected dogs.

Electrolyte Abnormalities

Typically, a presumptive diagnosis of hypoadrenocorticism is made based on the presence of hyponatremia, hypochloremia, hyperkalemia, and a sodium/potassium ratio less than 27:1 (Table 119–1). Most dogs have ratios less than 20:1. Approximately 10 per cent of dogs have a normal sodium and/or a normal potassium levels. This is often due primarily to cortisol deficiency and may be caused by either primary or secondary hypoadrenocorticism. Over time, electrolyte abnormalities will develop the expected pattern. An abnormal sodium/potassium ratio is not pathognomonic for hypoadrenocorticism (see Table 119–2). Approximately one-third of dogs with hypoadrenocorticism are *hyper*calcemic when they are hyperkalemic. The range of calcium is usually 12.0 to 14.9 mg/dl.

Renal Function

Elevations in blood urea nitrogen (BUN) and creatinine and a reduction in renal concentrating ability are common. This may lead to the erroneous conclusion that primary renal failure exists. If hypotension is severe, renal ischemia may develop. Thus, a primary renal injury can be superimposed on a prerenal component. Mild to moderate degrees of metabolic acidosis exist in many dogs.

Blood Glucose

Hypoglycemia (blood glucose = <70 mg/dl) is an uncommon laboratory finding. It may be severe enough to cause weakness, tremors, and even convulsions.

Serum Albumin

A number of dogs with primary hypoadrenocorticism have mild hypoalbuminemia.

RADIOGRAPHIC FINDINGS

Thoracic radiographs may identify the presence of microcardia due to the profound hypovolemia. Megaesophagus may be noted.

ELECTROCARDIOGRAPHIC ABNORMALITIES

An EKG is a rapid tool for assessing changes in serum potassium (K^+) concentration. EKG changes tend to parallel the severity of the serum potassium concentration. Mild hyperkalemia (serum K^+ = 5.5 to 6.5 mEq/L) is generally associated with a tall, "peaked" T wave. As the K^+ concentration increases from 6.5 to 8.5 mEq/L, there is widening and flattening of the QRS complex, prolongation of the PR interval, decrease in P wave amplitude, and increase in duration of the P wave. At potassium concentrations above 8.5 mEq/L, atrial standstill, absence of P waves, and deviations of the ST segment from the base line are expected. At serum potassium concentrations of 11 to 14 mEq/L, ventricular asystole or ventricular fibrillation is common.

TABLE 119–2. DIFFERENTIAL DIAGNOSIS FOR SIGNIFICANT HYPERKALEMIA AND/OR HYPONATREMIA IN DOGS AND CATS*

   I. Hypoadrenocorticism
  II. Renal or urinary tract disease
     A. Acute primary renal failure
     B. Chronic severe oliguric or anuric renal failure (rare)
     C. Urethral obstruction
     D. Uroabdomen (ruptured ureter, bladder, or urethra)
     E. Postobstructive diuresis
     F. Nephrotic syndrome
 III. Severe liver failure
     A. Cirrhosis
     B. Neoplasia
 IV. Severe gastrointestinal diseases
     A. Parasitic infestations
       1. Trichuriasis
       2. Ascariasis
       3. Ancylostomiasis
     B. Salmonellosis
     C. Viral enteritis
       1. Parvovirus
       2. Distemper
     D. Gastric dilatation/volvulus
     E. Gastrointestinal perforation
     F. Severe malabsorption
     G. Idiopathic hemorrhagic enteritis
  V. Severe metabolic or respiratory acidosis
 VI. Congestive heart failure
VII. Massive release of potassium to the extracellular fluid
     A. Crush injuries
     B. Aortic thrombosis
     C. Rhabdomyolysis
       1. Heat stroke
       2. Exertional
     D. Massive infections
     E. Massive hemolysis (rare)
VIII. Pseudohyperkalemia
     A. The Akita breed
     B. Severe leukocytosis (>100,000 mm³)
     C. Severe thrombocytosis (>1,000,000 mm³)
 IX. Diabetes mellitus
  X. Primary polydipsia
 XI. Inappropriate ADH secretion
XII. Drug-induced
     A. Potassium-sparing diuretics
     B. Nonsteroidal anti-inflammatory agents
     C. Angiotensin-converting enzyme inhibitors
     D. Potassium-containing fluids

*Most of these diagnoses/conditions are rarely associated with abnormal electrolyte abnormalities.
Modified from Feldman EC: Adrenal gland disease. *In* Ettinger, SJ (ed): Textbook of Veterinary Internal Medicine. 3rd ed. Philadelphia, WB Saunders, 1989, p 1764.

ADRENAL FUNCTION TESTING

ACTH Stimulation Testing

Performing an ACTH stimulation test is currently the best method for confirming the diagnosis. The test is run as soon as the diagnosis is suspected, regardless of the time of day. Results in dogs and cats with hypoadrenocorticism typically have resting levels in the low normal range that fail to increase following ACTH. Some animals will have a slight increase, but in all reported cases values have been below the minimum normal post-stimulation value.

Endogenous ACTH Concentrations

Differentiating primary from secondary hypoadrenocorticism requires measurement of endogenous plasma ACTH concentrations. This is primarily of value in animals in which just glucocorticoid deficiency exists (ACTH stimulation test is nonresponsive, but electrolytes are normal). Endogenous ACTH values should be high in dogs with primary hypoadrenocorticism. Animals with pituitary failure causing their adrenal insufficiency should have low or undetectable endogenous ACTH. This is true in both naturally occurring and iatrogenic secondary hypoadrenocorticism.

THERAPY OF HYPOADRENOCORTICISM (pp. 1587–1591)

ACUTE ADRENAL CRISIS MANAGEMENT

Immediate intravenous fluid therapy is lifesaving. Normal saline (0.9 per cent sodium chloride) is the fluid of choice. The ideal fluid should be potassium-free. If the patient is found to be hypoglycemic, 50 per cent dextrose is added to the saline. Glucocorticoid replacement therapy can be delayed until a post-ACTH plasma cortisol sample is obtained. If a steroid is given during the time of ACTH stimulation testing, it should be dexamethasone. This glucocorticoid is not measured by most RIA techniques.

The ideal glucocorticoid would be hydrocortisone hemisuccinate or hydrocortisone phosphate. Prednisolone sodium succinate can be used as an alternative. There is no longer any rapid-acting parenteral mineralocorticoid preparation available. Hydrocortisone hemisuccinate or phosphate will provide adequate mineralocorticoid activity along with saline infusions to stabilize the hyperkalemia until oral daily mineralocorticoid or injectable monthly mineralocorticoids can be given.

After volume expansion and mineralocorticoid replacement, alternative strategies for controlling hyperkalemia are rarely, if ever, needed. Intravenous glucose, glucose plus regular insulin, sodium bicarbonate therapy, and intravenous 10 per cent calcium bicarbonate therapy may be considered. The metabolic acidosis seen in patients with hypoadrenocorticism is usually mild and rarely needs to be treated specifically.

MAINTENANCE THERAPY OF HYPOADRENOCORTICISM

Once patients stabilize following initial aggressive fluid, electrolyte, glucocorticoid, and acidosis therapy, maintenance therapy can be started. In most animals with primary hypoadrenocorticism, both glucocorticoid and mineralocorticoid replacement therapy will be needed for life. Prednisone may be given initially and then be gradually tapered off until the drug is discontinued entirely. The majority of dogs do well on replacement mineralocorticoid alone after the first few weeks of therapy *if* fludrocortisone acetate is used (Florinef). If dogs show signs of cortisol deficiency (anorexia, lethargy, depression), low dosages of prednisone can be started again. Fludrocortisone is a potent oral mineralocorticoid that is useful as daily replacement therapy.

Maintaining the serum potassium concentration in the high-normal range is the goal of therapy. The drug's cost and side effects (polyuria, incontinence) are limiting factors in the treatment of some dogs. In occasional animals, hyponatremia will persist in spite of normal serum potassium concentrations. In such cases, the addition of table salt to the diet should normalize the sodium concentrations. An alternative to daily oral fludrocortisone therapy is the use of injectable desoxycorticosterone pivalate (DOCP).

DOCP is useful for dogs that develop significant polydipsia and polyuria when receiving Florinef, for those that require large dosages, or for animals in which fludrocortisone appears ineffective even in large dosages. Occasionally, there are individual dosage variations with DOCP, and frequent monitoring, at least during the first few months of therapy, is of value.

Because DOCP has little or no glucocorticoid activity, it should be combined with supplemental glucocorticoid therapy, at least initially. Approximately 50 per cent of dogs do well with no supplemental glucocorticoids when maintained on DOCP alone. The owner's main disadvantages in the use of DOCP are the need to return monthly for an injection and the costs of repeated examinations and laboratory work. Recent data suggest that SC injections are as effective as IM injections, simplifying at-home management for owners.

Therapy of Secondary Hypoadrenocorticism

Animals with spontaneous or iatrogenic secondary hypoadrenocorticism need only glucocorticoids to reverse their clinical signs. In cases of iatrogenic hypoadrenocorticism, glucocorticoid dosages are gradually reduced to alternate-day therapy at low dosages until eventually no supplemental therapy is needed.

HYPOADRENOCORTICISM IN CATS (pp. 1591–1592)

Primary hypoadrenocorticism is a rare disease in cats. The cause is generally idiopathic adrenal atrophy. Spontaneous secondary hypoadrenocorticism has not been described. Iatrogenic secondary hypoadrenocorticism may occur following long-term use of either exogenous glucocorticoids or megestrol acetate.

Clinical signs are similar to those described for dogs. Physical examination findings include dehydration, weakness, and hypothermia in nearly all cases. The diagnosis is established by the same means as for dogs. ACTH stimulation testing requires a slightly different protocol. Principles of therapeutic management for cats are similar to those described for dogs. The one unique feature about treating cats is that they do not generally respond as rapidly to fluids and to glucocorticoid and mineralocorticoid replacement as dogs usually do. They may remain weak, lethargic, and depressed for 3 to 5 days after appropriate therapy is instituted.

CHAPTER 120

GASTROINTESTINAL ENDOCRINE DISEASE
(pages 1593–1602)

GASTROINTESTINAL HORMONES (pp. 1593–1595)

See textbook.

GASTRINOMA (pp. 1597–1600)

A syndrome of gastric acid hypersecretion leading to severe peptic ulceration caused by islet cell tumors (gastrinomas) has been termed *Zollinger-Ellison syndrome.*

CLINICAL FEATURES

Gastrinomas are rare. Female dogs are more often affected. Vomiting and weight loss are the most frequently reported historical complaints. Depression, lethargy, anorexia, and intermittent diarrhea are also reported. Physical examination is not remarkable in most animals. Ulceration may be associated with hematochezia, melena, hematemesis, and abdominal pain in some animals. Erosive esophagitis and esophageal ulceration may cause anorexia, regurgitation, and hematemesis in some cases.

LABORATORY FINDINGS

Regenerative anemia was present in 44 per cent of the dogs and cats with gastrinoma. Leukocytosis, neutrophilia, and increased band neutrophils were attributed to gastrointestinal inflammation. The most common biochemical abnormalities were hyperglycemia, hypoalbuminemia, hypocalcemia, hypokalemia, and increased serum alkaline phosphatase activity. Frequent vomiting was also associated with hyponatremia, hypochloremia, and metabolic alkalosis in several dogs.

RADIOGRAPHY AND ENDOSCOPY

Survey abdominal radiographs were usually normal. Contrast studies performed in six dogs revealed plaque-like defects in the fundic or small intestinal mucosa consistent with ulceration, prominent gastric rugal folds, thickened pyloric antrum, complete pyloric obstruction, intestinal thickening, and rapid small bowel transit time. Gastroesophageal endoscopy revealed esophageal inflammation or ulceration, thickened gastric rugae, gastric ulceration or hemorrhage, excessive liquid in the stomach, duodenal ulceration, and a hypertrophied pyloric antrum that impeded passage of the endoscope through the pylorus.

DIAGNOSTIC TESTS

Dogs and cats with gastrinoma have resting serum gastrin concentrations that vary from 3.5 to 100 times the highest value reported for the normal range. However, provocative testing is usually necessary to confirm the diagnosis. All animals with gastrinoma had an islet cell tumor of the pancreas. At the time of diagnosis the tumor had metastasized in 76 per cent of the cases, the liver being the most common site.

Original chapter written by Carole A. Zerbe and Robert J. Washabau

THERAPY

Gastrinomas are best treated by surgical resection. Because many gastrinomas are small, the pancreas should be carefully inspected. Since most of the tumors are located within the right lobe and body of the pancreas, we recommend a right lobe pancreatectomy if a specific tumor nodule cannot be located. If metastasis is considered too extensive for excision, a partial pancreatectomy should be performed with debulking of the primary tumor. Chemotherapy has not yet been used. However, Sandostatin, a somatostatin analogue, has been used successfully for treatment of gastrinoma in one dog.

The best therapeutic agents used for reducing gastric acid secretion include the histamine H_2-receptor antagonists, H^+, K^+-ATPase inhibitors (proton pump inhibitors), and somatostatin analogs. Cimetidine and ranitidine are the most frequently used histamine H_2-receptor antagonists. We currently recommend omeprazole for gastrinoma patients that fail to respond to treatment with histamine H_2-receptor antagonists. Sandostatin should be considered in a gastrinoma patient that has failed other medical therapies.

Treatment of ulcers includes surgical resection when appropriate, reduction of gastric acidity, and use of diffusion barriers and "cytoprotective agents" to promote ulcer healing. Sucralfate is used as a diffusion barrier to promote ulcer healing. Misoprostol has cytoprotective properties in addition to its direct acid inhibitory effect. Gastrinoma in cats and dogs appears to be highly malignant, hence the long-term prognosis is grave.

PANCREATIC POLYPEPTIDOMA (p. 1600)

Elevated plasma PP concentrations have been documented in only one dog with chronic vomiting, hypertrophic gastritis, duodenal ulceration, pancreatic adenocarcinoma, fasting hypergastrinemia, and normal serum gastrin concentrations in response to both calcium and secretin.

GLUCAGONOMA (pp. 1600–1601)

The presence of diabetes mellitus, NME, hyperglucagonemia, and a pancreatic islet cell tumor containing glucagon is diagnostic of glucagonoma. It should be emphasized that glucagonoma has not yet been rigorously documented in any veterinary species using the aforementioned criteria. Surgical resection of the pancreatic tumor is likely to be the treatment of choice. It should be noted that NME has also been documented in dogs with diabetes mellitus and hepatic cirrhosis. It is apparent that the majority of dogs with NME do not have glucagonoma.

CHAPTER 121

BREEDING MANAGEMENT OF THE BITCH
(pages 1604–1606)

Prebreeding examination should include general physical examination and evaluation of immunization status and parasite control programs. All bitches and dogs should be tested for the presence of serum *Brucella canis* antibodies.

ESTROUS CYCLE OF THE BITCH (pp. 1604–1605)

In early proestrus the vaginal cytology specimen includes noncornified (round cells with large healthy nuclei) and cornified (large angular cells with small dark pycnotic nuclei) epithelial cells, erythrocytes, and polymorphonuclear leukocytes (PMNs). By the end of proestrus, the smear is comprised completely of cornified cells (large, angular cells). The vaginal cytology specimen during estrus usually is comprised of sheets of large, angular, cornified cells. PMNs are absent until the last day or two prior to onset of diestrus. In the average bitch, ovulation occurs about 2 days after estrus onset, which is about day 12 after proestrus onset. Diestrus begins with an abrupt change in the vaginal cytology specimen from a population of predominantly cornified to predominantly noncornified epithelial cells.

TIMING OVULATION AND MATING IN THE BITCH (pp. 1605–1606)

The best reproductive performance (conception rate and litter size) in the bitch is achieved when she is bred naturally 2 to 3 days after ovulation. Prospective determination of ovulation in the bitch may be achieved by means of serum progesterone measurement, because progesterone increases in canine serum 2 to 3 days prior to ovulation.

NATURAL AND ARTIFICIAL INSEMINATION OF THE BITCH (p. 1606)

See the textbook for a review of techniques. The best performance appears to occur with frozen semen insemination 3 to 5 days following ovulation in the bitch.

Original chapter written by Shirley D. Johnston

CHAPTER 122

OVARIAN AND ESTROUS CYCLE ABNORMALITIES IN THE BITCH
(pages 1607–1613)

THE NORMAL CANINE ESTROUS CYCLE
(pp. 1607–1609)

See the textbook and Chapter 121.

VARIATIONS IN THE NORMAL CANINE ESTROUS CYCLE (p. 1609)

Delayed Puberty. Efforts at differentiating delayed puberty from an actual failure to experience reproductive cycles should be postponed until a bitch is at least 2 years old.

Silent Heat Cycles. Fastidious bitches with minimal vulvar swelling or discharge and few behavioral changes may have estrous cycles that escape detection.

Split Heat Cycles. These cycles typically occur in young bitches and are characterized by periods of bloody vaginal discharge and attracting males usually with no breeding. After a period of 2 to 10 weeks, another similar "cycle" or proestrus occurs, which may or may not proceed to estrus. The condition is not associated with reproductive pathology, and no treatment is recommended.

Management Errors. Timing of breeding, dominant bitches, and mechanical vulvar/vaginal abnormalities need to be considered.

PATTERNS OF ABNORMAL ESTROUS CYCLES
(pp. 1609–1613)

Prolonged Proestrus or Estrus. Prolonged proestrus and/or estrus most likely results from persistent secretion of estrogens. Endogenous sources of prolonged estrogen in the bitch include ovarian follicular cysts and secretory neoplasias. Follicular cysts tend to occur in bitches under 3 years of age. Vaginal bleeding secondary to infection, inflammation, or neoplasia of the genitourinary tract; a vaginal foreign body; or a coagulopathy should be differentiated from prolonged proestrus or estrus. After confirmation of naturally occurring hyperestrogenism is obtained, abdominal ultrasonography is recommended in an attempt to identify an ovarian follicular cyst or functional neoplasia.

Because follicular cysts may spontaneously undergo atresia or luteinization, not all bitches experiencing prolonged proestrus or estrus require treatment. Medical and surgical options exist for treatment of persistent follicular cysts. The use of GnRH (50 to 100 µg/bitch IM every 24 to 48 hours for up to three doses) or human placental gonadotropin (hCG; 11 IU/lb or 22 IU/kg, IM, every 24 to 48 hours) has been advocated. Medical treatment of prolonged proestrus or estrus is usually unrewarding, and surgical removal of the cyst is the most expedient means of managing the problem.

Prolonged Interestrous Intervals. An actual failure to continue to cycle must be differentiated from silent heats. Prolonged

---

Original chapter written by Autumn P. Davidson and Edward C. Feldman diestrus occurs secondary to the presence of a luteinized, progesterone secreting, ovarian cyst. Abdominal ultrasonography should identify hypoechoic structure(s) within the affected ovary(ies). Serum progesterone concentrations greater than 2 to 5 ng/ml confirm the diagnosis. Treatment with prostaglandin $F_{2\alpha}$ ($PGF_{2\alpha}$) usually causes only a transient decline in serum progesterone levels, indicating partial luteolysis. Surgical removal of the cyst(s) with histologic analysis is the recommended treatment.

Nonfunctional ovarian cysts may cause failure to cycle owing to their mass effect. Increases in plasma estrogen or progesterone will not be identified. The diagnosis, initially suspected with abdominal ultrasonography, is confirmed by histologic evaluation of surgically removed tissues. Hypothyroidism is a potential cause for failure to cycle. Glucocorticoids can feedback on pituitary gonadotrophins FSH and LH, causing a failure to cycle.

Shortened Interestrous Intervals.   Documentation of this disorder requires evaluation of serial vaginal cytologies during estrus and diestrus, and serum progesterone concentrations during the luteal phase of at least two consecutive cycles. Intervention should not take place unless the bitch is older than 3 years of age. Therapy consists of inducing anestrus through the use of mibolerone.

Hypoluteoidism.   Hypoluteoidism, primary luteal failure occurring before term gestation, is a potential but not documented cause of abortion in dogs.

Exaggerated Pseudocyesis (Pseudopregnancy).   Pseudocyesis is an exaggeration of the normal physiologic phenomena. The condition is self-limiting, usually regressing in 1 to 3 weeks, and therapy is not recommended unless the symptoms are unusually prolonged or pronounced. When it is recommended, therapy is usually directed at decreasing or eliminating lactation. Mammary stimulation—whether by licking, mothering behavior, or warm or cold compressing—should be discontinued. Mild water deprivation, for 6 to 10 hours per night, can be helpful. Alternatively, low-dose furosemide therapy, twice a day orally for up to 7 days, can be administered. Dopamine antagonists should *not* be administered.

Therapy with gonadal hormones, progesterone, estrogen, or testosterone is not recommended. Bromocriptine, 0.005 to 0.05 mg/lb/day (0.01 to 0.10 mg/kg/day) can be administered in divided doses until lactation ceases. Cabergoline, at 2.5 µg/lb/day (5.0 mg/kg/day), given once daily for 5 to 10 days, effectively reduces prolactin levels and diminishes signs of pseudocyesis with fewer side effects. Permanent avoidance of clinical pseudocyesis requires ovariohysterectomy.

CHAPTER 123

ABNORMALITIES IN PREGNANCY, PARTURITION, AND THE PERIPARTURIENT PERIOD
(pages 1614–1624)

PREGNANCY (pp. 1614–1617)

THE NORMAL PREGNANCY

See the textbook for a review of normal gestation, pregnancy diagnosis, and evaluation.

INFECTIOUS CAUSES OF FETAL DEATH AND ABORTION

Brucella canis. The most common symptom of brucellosis in the bitch is abortion of partially autolysed fetuses at about 45 to 59 days of gestation. The gray-green vaginal discharge associated with the abortion may contain a large population of organisms, and contact should be avoided. Culture of this discharge, placentas, or blood may be diagnostic. The intracellular location of the organism makes treatment failure common. Ovariohysterectomy and treatment is an option for a pet. The zoonotic potential of this infection must be considered. The current treatment of choice is a combination of minocycline, 5.7 mg/lb (12.5 mg/kg) orally every 12 hours for 2 weeks, and dihydrostreptomycin, 2.3 mg/lb (5 mg/kg) IM every 12 hours for the first week.

Canine Herpesvirus. The bitch usually appears healthy, and the diagnosis is made by histopathology of the fetus or virus isolation.

Toxoplasmosis and Neosporosis. The diagnosis is made by finding the organism in aborted fetuses or by paired serologies of the dam taken 2 weeks apart.

Feline Viral Diseases. Feline herpesvirus is common, and latent carriers may shed virus following stress, pregnancy, parturition, and lactation. Diagnosis is based on clinical signs and confirmed with virus isolation. The signs of feline panleukopenia depend on the stage of gestation at which infection occurs. Middle to late gestational infection may result in fetal mummification and/or abortion. Infection in late gestation causes CNS lesions, resulting in kittens with cerebellar hypoplasia and retinal lesions. Not all kittens are equally affected.

Feline infectious peritonitis virus (FIPV) has been associated with endometritis, fetal resorption, abortion, stillbirths, and neonatal mortality. Diagnosis is based on histopathology. Feline leukemia virus (FeLV) is a common infectious cause of fetal death, abortion, and infertility. Virus transmission occurs in utero. Reproductive failure from feline immunodeficiency virus (FIV) infection has not been fully investigated, but has been suggested. In-utero transmission is probably rare.

Endometritis and Pyometra. See Chapter 125.

ENDOCRINE DISORDERS DURING PREGNANCY

Hypoluteodism. See Chapter 122.

Gestational Diabetes. It is uncommon for the diabetic bitch to successfully carry a litter to term; abortion is common. Ovariohysterectomy of the pregnant diabetic bitch is advised.

Pregnancy Hypoglycemia and Ketonemia. This condition

Original chapter written by Melissa S. Wallace and Autumn P. Davidson is extremely rare, responds to intravenous glucose supplementation, and resolves with parturition or cesarean section.

PHYSICAL AND CONGENITAL DISORDERS DURING PREGNANCY

Iatrogenic Disorders. Many drugs and toxins are known to cause fetal death or congenital abnormalities.

Fetal Abnormalities. Fetuses may have congenital disorders that are incompatible with life.

Uterine Torsion. The diagnosis may be suspected based on signs (dystocia, sanguineous vaginal discharge, abdominal pain, and shock), radiography, and ultrasonography, but is confirmed by exploratory laparotomy.

Herniation of the Gravid Uterus. Diagnosis is made by palpation, radiography, or ultrasonography. This is often a surgical emergency.

Ectopic Pregnancy. Eventually, the inadequate blood supply results in death of the fetus and mummification. Diagnosis may be suggested by radiography or ultrasonography and is confirmed by laparotomy.

Taurine Deficiency. Cats fed taurine-deficient diets demonstrate fetal resorption, abortion, stillbirths, and low-birth-weight kittens.

PARTURITION (pp. 1617–1618)

Timing of Parturition. The rectal temperature declines to or below 99°F (37°C) 12 to 24 hours before parturition. The hypothermia is transient, resolving before or during labor. The queen has a decline in rectal temperature within 12 hours of parturition, but this sign is less reliable than in the bitch.

NORMAL PARTURITION

Stage 1. Behavior exhibited by the bitch may include restlessness, anorexia, panting, chewing, and scratching at bedding material.

Stage 2. Stage 2 labor consists of strong uterine contractions. The first puppy is normally born within 4 hours of onset of stage 2 labor, and subsequent births are 15 minutes to 2 hours apart. The queen usually has her first kitten within an hour and has another every 10 to 60 minutes.

Stage 3. The placenta from each fetus is expelled shortly after birth or within 15 minutes.

DYSTOCIA

Fetal Factors. Single-puppy pregnancies may result in an overly large fetus. Breech presentation is not an abnormality in the dog and cat.

Maternal Factors. Abnormalities that reduce the size of the pelvic canal, vagina, or vestibule can cause dystocia. Primary uterine inertia is lack of contractions or uncoordinated contractions of the myometrium. The placentas eventually separate, resulting in a green vaginal discharge. The fetuses will die unless a cesarean section is performed.

Diagnosis of Dystocia. If a bitch or queen has been in labor more than 4 hours without giving birth, or if more than 1 hour has elapsed between births with active straining, veterinary assistance is advised. If the bitch appears weak, depressed, or in shock, immediate stabilization and cesarean section are advised.

Management of Dystocia. A fetus lodged in the vaginal vault can be gently manipulated to facilitate birth. Secondary uterine inertia may be medically managed. Oxytocin is administered, 0.5 to 1 IU/lb (1 to 2 IU/kg) IM, not to exceed 20 units. If there is no improvement in contractions, 10 per cent calcium gluconate is administered slowly IV, 1 to 3 ml in the cat and 3 to 5 ml in the dog. The oxytocin may be repeated. If no birth occurs within 45 minutes of the second oxytocin dose, a cesarean section is recommended.

THE POSTPARTUM PERIOD (pp. 1618–1623)

Weaning of normal puppies and kittens usually begins by 28 to 30 days of life.

MATERNAL DISORDERS OF THE POSTPARTUM PERIOD

Rectal temperature may be mildly increased (less than 104°F [40°C]) for several days, reflecting normal postpartum inflammation. Lochia, the normal postpartum vaginal discharge, is brick red in color, has no odor, and diminishes over several weeks.

Inappropriate Maternal Behavior

See the textbook for a review of maternal behavior in the postpartum period. Occasionally, increased protective behavior or fear-induced aggression by the dam is encountered. Diazepam can be administered orally as needed—canine: 0.25 to 1.1 mg/lb (0.55 to 2.2 mg/kg); feline: 1 to 2 mg/cat.

Uterine Disorders

Uterine Prolapse.   This is an uncommon postpartum condition reported more frequently in the queen than in the bitch. Diagnosis is based on palpation of a firm, tubular mass protruding from the vulva following parturition. Laparotomy becomes necessary and ovariohysterectomy is usually indicated.

Subinvolution of Placental Sites.   The persistence of serosanguineous to hemorrhagic vaginal discharge beyond 6 to 12 weeks postpartum can indicate subinvolution of placental sites. Treatment is generally not necessary as recovery is spontaneous. Coagulopathies, trauma, neoplasia of the genitourinary tract, metritis, and proestrus should be ruled out. Treatment can be attempted with ergonovine, 0.2 mg/35 lb (0.2 mg/15 kg) IM, once. Laparotomy and ovariohysterectomy are curative if medical therapies fail.

Metritis.   Acute infection of the postpartum endometrium should be suspected if lethargy, anorexia, decreased lactation, and poor mothering occur, often accompanied by protracted fever and malodorous vaginal discharge. Therapy for acute endometritis consists of intravenous fluid and electrolyte support, antibiotics, and uterine evacuation. Ovariohysterectomy may be indicated. Medical treatments with natural prostaglandins, 0.05 to 0.125 mg/lb (0.10 to 0.25 mg/kg) given SC once daily for 3 to 5 days, can be helpful.

Puerperal Tetany

Puerperal tetany tends to occur during the first 4 weeks of lactation. Small dogs with large litters are at increased risk. Therapeutic intervention (a slow intravenous infusion of 10 per cent calcium gluconate [1 to 20 ml], given to effect) should be initiated immediately upon recognition of clinical signs, without waiting for biochemical confirmation. Cardiac monitoring for bradycardia and arrhythmias should accompany calcium administration. Corticosteroids are contraindicated. Hypoglycemia should be corrected if present. Once the immediate neurologic signs are controlled with intravenous calcium gluconate, subcutaneous infusion of an equal volume, diluted 50 per cent with saline, is given. Oral supplementation of calcium carbonate, 5 to 15 mg/lb (10 to

30 mg/kg) given every 8 hours, is initiated as soon as possible. Early weaning (at 3 weeks of age) and concurrent supplementation of the neonates with commercial milk substitutes is encouraged.

Disorders of Lactation

Agalactia. Primary agalactia is not common. Treatment for secondary agalactia includes providing necessary artificial milk supplementation to the neonates while encouraging suckling to promote milk ejection. Adequate water must be provided to the bitch.

Galactostasis. See Chapter 122.

Mastitis. The milk is commonly discolored red or brown. The diagnosis is based on physical findings. Cytologic evaluation of milk is useful in early cases without obvious signs. First-generation cephalosporins and beta-lactamase-resistant penicillins are advised. Warm compress or whirlpool therapy of the affected gland(s) followed by gentle stripping of the milk can potentially avert abscessation with rupture of the gland.

NEONATAL DISORDERS OF THE POSTPARTUM PERIOD

Postpartum Resuscitation

An airway free of amniotic fluid, placental membranes, and meconium should be established within 3 to 5 minutes of birth. Initiation of respiration can be stimulated by thoracic and facial massage with a dry, warmed towel. Immediate suckling is encouraged, as it provides colostrum, calories, and glucose. Reversal of any narcotic or barbiturate anesthetic agent used during anesthesia of the dam can improve the status of a neonate born by cesarean section. Naloxone, a narcotic antagonist, and doxapram, a respiratory analeptic, can be administered at a dose of one to two drops into the tongue or umbilical vein of the neonate. Prolonged bradycardia or cardiac standstill can be treated with epinephrine, 0.05 ml/lb (0.10 ml/kg) of a 1:10,000 solution IV, and atropine, 0.015 mg/lb (0.03 mg/kg) IM or IV.

Neonatology

Congenital Disorders. See the textbook and various sections on specific body systems of interest.

Acquired Disorders. Acquired immunodeficiencies result from failure of passive transfer of maternally derived antibodies. Neonatal malnutrition can result from poor milk production or quality, crowding, and ineffectual nursing. The birth weight should double by 12 days of age. Supplemental feedings with commercially available artificial bitch and queen milk are indicated.

Infectious disorders are generally a greater problem in weanling puppies and kittens than in neonates. Bacterial infection can cause neonatal septicemia. Early administration of an appropriate, nontoxic bactericidal antibiotic is indicated, often before a definitive diagnosis is possible. Canine herpesvirus and feline herpesvirus I infection can cause high mortality rates in 9- to 14-day-old neonates.

CHAPTER 124

REPRODUCTIVE ENDOCRINOLOGY, CONTRACEPTION, AND PREGNANCY TERMINATION IN DOGS
(pages 1625–1636)

TARGETS FOR CONTRACEPTION (pp. 1625–1628)

See the textbook for a complete review of the hormone patterns during normal ovarian cycles and pregnancy. Continuous availability of progesterone is required for initiation and maintenance of pregnancy. Treatments that prevent progesterone secretion or block progesterone action can be used to prevent or terminate unwanted pregnancies.

OPTIONS FOR CONTRACEPTION, PREGNANCY PREVENTION, AND PREGNANCY TERMINATION (pp. 1628–1629)

Ovariohysterectomy is the most obvious approach if permanent sterility is desired. In the United States, there are only two cycle-inhibiting contraceptive steroids approved and marketed for prevention of estrus in dogs, the oral progestin megestrol acetate (Ovaban, Schering Corp.) and the oral androgen mibolerone (Cheque Drops, Upjohn Co.).

MEGESTROL ACETATE ORAL CONTRACEPTION (p. 1630)

There is a tendency for progestin administration to promote the development of cystic endometrial hyperplasia and subsequent uterine infection, mammary development, and post-therapy lactation in dogs. Androgens may induce mild to severe external masculinization. Diabetes mellitus is a contraindication to the use of megestrol acetate, as are the presence of mammary tumors and uterine or liver disease.

Ovaban treatment started in proestrus, to prevent continuation of proestrus and onset of estrus, should begin during the first 3 days. Early proestrus should be verified by vaginal cytology (see Chapters 121 and 122). Bitches in early proestrus are given an Ovaban dose of 1 mg/lb (2.2 mg/kg) daily for 8 days. Suppression of proestrus occurs within 3 to 8 days after onset of treatment. Subsequent return to proestrus and estrus is expected 4 to 6 months later. If treatment is started too late in proestrus, administration of megestrol acetate or another progestin can result in stimulation of a surge release of LH, ovulation, and fertile estrus.

Anestrous Treatment with Megestrol Acetate. A longer treatment course with megestrol acetate, at a lower dose, is recommended for postponement of proestrus and estrus, 0.25 mg/lb (0.55 µg/kg) for 32 days. Initiation of treatment during anestrus should be at least 1 to 2 weeks prior to the next expected proestrus, based on previous interestrus intervals of that individual bitch.

Original chapter written by Patrick W. Concannon

MIBOLERONE ORAL CONTRACEPTION IN DOGS AND CATS (pp. 1630–1631)

Administration should begin at least 30 days prior to the next expected estrus. Return to estrus following treatment usually takes 2 to 3 months. Mibolerone side effects can be significant (see the textbook). Mibolerone should not be given to cats because of toxic side effects.

NON-APPROVED AND EXPERIMENTAL CONTRACEPTIVE STEROIDS (p. 1631)

Testosterone Injections. Weekly injections of testosterone propionate (110 mg/week) have been used to prevent estrus in greyhounds.
Depot Injectable Progestins. MPA (Depo Provera) should not be used in dogs.

NONSTEROIDAL CONTRACEPTION (pp. 1631–1632)

Devices. Intrauterine devices are not practical in dogs owing to the difficulty in cannulating the canine cervix per vagina.
Immunization. To date, no contraceptive immunization protocol for dogs has warranted large-scale clinical trials.
Long-Term GnRH Agonist Administration. A practical mode of administration poses a problem, since constant administration is required. Field trials have not been reported.

MISMATING AND POSTCOITAL, ANTINIDATORY ESTROGEN TREATMENTS (pp. 1632–1633)

Many bitches given estrogen to prevent pregnancy following mating subsequently develop cystic endometrial hyperplasia and pyometra. Therefore, postcoital estrogen administration is considered contraindicated for valuable breeding bitches. The most appropriate therapy for misalliance of bitches not intended for breeding is an ovariohysterectomy performed after the end of estrus and/or after diagnosis of early pregnancy.
Estrogen Formulations: Side Effects and Dose Selection. The need to exercise considerable caution in selecting preparations and doses is clear from reports of uterine disease, bone marrow suppression, aplastic anemia, thrombocytopenia, internal hemorrhage, and death following estrogen administration.
Estradiol Cypionate. Estradiol cypionate (EC) is not recommended for mismating. Only if a vaginal smear suggests that the bitch is truly in estrus or early diestrus should EC be considered. Treatment is limited to a single intramuscular injection of 20 µg/lb (44 µg/kg). The client should be informed of potential side effects.
Other Estrogens in Dogs. Oral DES at doses of 50 to 100 µg/lb (100 to 200 µg/kg) for 5 days is often used clinically to treat mismating in bitches.

USE OF PROSTAGLANDIN $F_{2\alpha}$ FOR TERMINATION OF PREGNANCY (pp. 1633–1634)

Administration of prostaglandin F (PGF) as an alternative to giving estrogen for mismating should probably be delayed at least until 7 to 10 days after the end of cytologic estrus and given at doses of 115 µg/lb (250 µg/kg) twice daily for 5 or more days. For all applications of PGF it would be judicious to use a dose of 25 to 50 µg/lb (50 to 100 µg/kg) for the first injection to judge the potential severity of side effects. The transient PGF side effects increase in severity with dosage and often include panting, salivation, emesis, and defecation. Bitches selected for prostaglandin therapy are preferably 25 to 35 days pregnant. Ultrasonography or radiology is useful in assessing the stage of pregnancy and viability of fetuses when uterine palpation is difficult.

$PGF_{2\alpha}$ can be administered intramuscularly or subcutaneously every 8 to 12 hours, initially at a dose of 23 µg/lb (50 µg/kg). If side effects are tolerable with a dose of 23 µg/lb (50 µg/kg), doses of 45 to 115 µg/lb (100 to 250 µg/kg) can be considered. Treatment is continued for 4 or more days until resorption (or abortion) of the last fetus is confirmed by abdominal ultrasonography. Atropine has been reported to reduce the severity of salivation, vomiting, diarrhea, and respiratory distress when administered at a dose of 23 µg/lb (50 mg/kg) IM, either at the time of $PGF_{2\alpha}$ injection or at the onset of symptoms (e.g., salivation).

USE OF OTHER AGENTS FOR TERMINATION OF PREGNANCY (pp. 1634–1635)

Glucocorticosteroids. Dexamethasone, 5 mg IM twice daily for 10 days starting on day 30, caused resorption. The same dose begun on day 45 resulted in abortion after the 10 days of treatment. In the absence of more information, the use of glucocorticoids is not justified.

Prolactin Suppression with Dopamine Agonists. Treatment with 45 µg/lb (100 µg/kg) twice daily after day 35 is likely to be routinely effective if administered until pregnancy termination is confirmed. Bromocriptine administration frequently results in emesis, lethargy, and inappetence.

Epostane in Dogs. Epostane has been shown to terminate pregnancy in dogs when given orally (50 mg/dog/day) for 7 days, starting on the first day of diestrus as determined by vaginal cytology. It will also terminate pregnancy when administered later in gestation.

CHAPTER 125

CYSTIC ENDOMETRIAL HYPERPLASIA, PYOMETRA, AND INFERTILITY
(pages 1636–1642)

CYSTIC ENDOMETRIAL HYPERPLASIA AND PYOMETRA (pp. 1636–1640)

PATHOPHYSIOLOGY

Escherichia coli is isolated in the majority of cases of canine and feline pyometra.

DIAGNOSIS

Cystic endometrial hyperplasia and pyometra is primarily a disease of middle-aged, cycling females. Pyometra is more commonly diag-

Original chapter written by Cheri A. Johnson

nosed in bitches than in queens. Most bitches and queens with pyometra have experienced estrus within the 2 months preceding the onset of clinical signs. There may be a history of previous treatment with estrogens. Vulvar discharge, abdominal distention, enlargement of the uterus, and dehydration are the most common physical findings. The most important differential diagnosis for cystic endometrial hyperplasia and pyometra is pregnancy.

The radiographic appearance of the fluid density of pyometra and that of a gravid uterus is essentially identical until fetal calcification is detectable at approximately 40 to 45 days of gestation. Ultrasonography will distinguish fetal structures from intraluminal fluid as the cause of uterine enlargement. A serum biochemical profile, complete blood count, and urinalysis are necessary to detect the metabolic abnormalities. The white blood cell count from dogs and cats with pyometra is almost always characteristic of suppurative or purulent inflammation. Increased serum alkaline phosphatase activity is observed in most bitches with pyometra.

Although azotemia is demonstrated in less than one-third of bitches with pyometra, renal function is compromised in most. Fortunately, the renal problems associated with pyometra are potentially reversible when the pyometra resolves. Vaginal cytology, white blood cell count, and clinical signs help to differentiate mucometra from pyometra.

TREATMENT

Intravenous fluid therapy is indicated to correct existing deficits, to maintain adequate tissue perfusion, and to improve renal function. A broad-spectrum, bacteriocidal antibiotic should be administered. Ovariohysterectomy is generally considered to be the treatment of choice because it is potentially curative, whereas pyometra recurs in the majority of bitches and in some queens following medical treatment.

Medical Treatment of Pyometra

Fluid and antibiotic therapy are as described above. The natural prostaglandin $F_{2\alpha}$ (Lutalyse, Upjohn) is administered to expel the uterine contents. Especially in animals in which the cervix does not promptly dilate, there is some risk that uterine contractions will cause rupture of the abnormal uterine wall. Prostaglandins are contraindicated in pregnancy, asthma and other airway disorders, sepsis, peritonitis, and other organic diseases. Systemic effects can be expected. These include panting, salivation, vomition, defecation, micturition, mydriasis, and nesting behavior.

To treat pyometra in bitches and queens with cervical patency, a recommended protocol is 0.1 to 0.25 mg/kg of $PGF_{2\alpha}$ SC once or twice daily, until the uterus is empty. At least 3 to 5 days are usually required. Abdominal radiographs or ultrasonography are extremely helpful in determining uterine size of dogs and cats. Treatment is usually considered unsuccessful if clinical signs do not resolve during 5 days of treatment or recur within several weeks. Ovariohysterectomy is usually recommended at that time. Breeding on the estrus after treatment is recommended for bitches.

INFERTILITY (pp. 1640–1641)

Infertility can result from problems with the male, with the female, with the conceptus, and/or with breeding management. Estrus cycle abnormalities are discussed in Chapter 122. Ovarian and vaginal disorders are covered in Chapters 122 and 126, respectively. Proper breeding management is discussed in Chapters 121 and 130. Male infertility is discussed in Chapter 127.

INFERTILITY AND UTERINE DISORDERS

A complete physical and reproductive tract examination should be performed. A CBC, biochemical profile, and urinalysis to assess metabolic health could reasonably be included as a routine part of evaluation for infertility. The uterus is examined by transabdominal palpation, abdominal radiographs, and ultrasonography. The normal uterus often is not identified on either. Exploratory celiotomy offers the opportunity to evaluate the uterine tubes and the uterus for structural integrity, and to obtain full-thickness biopsies and intraluminal cultures. The stage of the cycle during which the biopsy is obtained must always be considered. Abnormalities of pregnancy are discussed in Chapter 123.

CHAPTER 126
VAGINAL DISORDERS
(pages 1642–1648)

An understanding of the relationship between the vestibule and vagina anatomically and embryologically is needed to appreciate the variety of diseases affecting this area. For this, the reader is referred to the textbook.

For a discussion of hormonal effects, see textbook chapters 121, 122, 124, and 126.

EXAMINATION OF THE VESTIBULE AND VAGINA
(pp. 1643–1645)

VAGINAL CYTOLOGY

It may be desirable to use a speculum to avoid contact with the vestibule when obtaining a vaginal cytologic specimen. Parabasal and intermediate cells, seen in anestrus and early proestrus, are round cells with a relatively large nucleus. The nuclear-to-cytoplasmic ratio becomes smaller as the cells "mature." Superficial cells dominate the cytologic picture during the estrogenic (follicular) phase (late proestrus and all of estrus). An abrupt change from this cytologic pattern (back to parabasal and intermediate cells) signifies the onset of diestrus. Neutrophils in low numbers are seen normally in vaginal cytology at any time except during the peak of the estrogenic phase. Large numbers of neutrophils are seen during early diestrus. Red blood cells are seen in large numbers during early proestrus.

VISUAL AND DIGITAL EXAMINATION OF THE VAGINA AND VESTIBULE

Owing to the length of the distal reproductive tract, particularly the length of the vagina, it is impossible to digitally examine the vagina in its entirety. Vaginoscopy may be performed with an endoscope, proctoscope, or any flexible fiberoptic equipment with sufficient length (15 cm) to inspect the entire vagina.

Original chapter written by Beverly J. Purswell

VAGINAL BACTERIAL CULTURES

A positive culture for *Brucella canis* is abnormal and provides a definitive diagnosis. However, the isolation of opportunistic aerobic pathogens, anaerobic bacteria, or mycoplasmas in an asymptomatic animal does not constitute evidence of infection.

VAGINAL ABNORMALITIES (pp. 1645–1648)

VAGINITIS

Vaginal cytology will show increased numbers of neutrophils in various stages of degeneration, with or without increased numbers of bacteria. Vaginoscopy will reveal the presence and extent of hyperemia, exudate, and mucosal lesions such as vesicles, ulcers, and lymphoid follicle hyperplasia. Urinary tract problems should be ruled out as a cause for the vestibular irritation or attraction of male dogs.

Juvenile (puppy) vaginitis may respond to systemic antibacterial therapy or to topical douching, but inevitably the signs return when the treatment is discontinued. The condition will resolve naturally after the first estrous cycle, and therefore it is advisable to postpone neutering of these individuals until after the first estrus. Adult vaginitis can be caused by anatomic abnormalities. Strictures at the vagino-vestibular junction that may cause the problem can be identified by a digital examination. Foreign bodies, tumors, or uterine stump granulomas should be ruled out as predisposing causes by vaginoscopy. Contrast radiography may be helpful in identifying anatomic abnormalities, tumors, or concurrent urinary tract disease. Viral vaginitis has been described in conjunction with canine herpesvirus infections. Genital infections of canine herpesvirus result in diffuse, multifocal, raised vesicular lesions on the vaginal mucosa, no treatment is necessary.

ANATOMIC ABNORMALITIES

A persistent hymen will occur at the junction of the vagina and vestibule. Incomplete perforation of the hymen may present as an annular stricture or a vertical septum or band. Digital palpation is the preferred method for diagnosing these conditions. Digital dilation can be attempted. A vertical band is easily removed surgically. An annular stricture is more difficult to correct surgically. Infantile vulvas may be found in prepubescent bitches. The vulva is small and inverted to the point of being hidden from view. Neutering of these bitches should be postponed until after the first estrus. Eversion of the vulva normally occurs during the first estrus and the condition is self-correcting.

VAGINAL FOLD PROLAPSE; VAGINAL HYPERPLASIA; VAGINAL PROLAPSE

Under the influence of estrogen, some young bitches develop an edematous ventral fold in the distal vaginal mucosa immediately cranial to the urethral opening. Traditionally, this condition has been referred to as vaginal hyperplasia. Prolapse of a vaginal fold occurs primarily during proestrus and estrus when the bitch is under the influence of estrogen. Once this condition manifests itself, there is a tendency for recurrence at each subsequent estrus. Ovariohysterectomy resolves the condition permanently. Surgical removal of the prolapsed tissue can be attempted.

MISCELLANEOUS VAGINAL DISORDERS

A bitch that bleeds from the vulva after breeding should be examined for vaginal tears. Vaginal and vulvar neoplasia represent 2.5 to 3 per cent of all canine tumors. Seventy to 80 per cent of these tumors are benign. Leiomyomas are the most common benign tumor and are often pedunculated. Leiomyosarcoma is the most common malignant vaginal tumor. Surgical excision is the treatment of choice. Ovariohysterectomy is recommended at the time of removal.

CHAPTER 127

SEMEN ANALYSIS, ARTIFICIAL INSEMINATION, AND INFERTILITY IN THE MALE DOG
(pages 1649–1662)

SEMEN COLLECTION

See the textbook for a complete review of the techniques of semen collection.

EVALUATION METHODS AND NORMAL RANGES

Semen Volume and Sperm Motility.   Immediately after the semen sample is obtained, the volume and motility should be measured. The volume can be measured with a sterile syringe. The percentage of sperm that are moving in a progressively forward manner is estimated from several fields. Progressively forward motility in the normal ejaculate should be ≥80 per cent.

Sperm Count.   A simple method for measuring sperm count employs the Unopette system (see textbook).

There is general agreement among canine theriogenologists that 150 to 300 million sperm in an insemination is the lower limit that can be considered compatible with fertility (see Table 127–1).

Sperm Morphology.   The semen (from the second fraction) is smeared over the length of the slide, as in making a blood smear. The slide is stained with either a quick Wright's stain or a sperm morphology stain. Dry stained slides are examined under oil immersion.

TABLE 127–1. BODY WEIGHT, TOTAL SCROTAL WIDTH, AND SPERM COUNTS IN NORMAL DOGS

BODY WEIGHT (LB)	TOTAL SCROTAL WIDTH (MM)*	DAILY SPERM OUTPUT/DOG	SPERM COUNT/ EJACULATE AFTER SEXUAL REST
		(Millions, Mean ± SEM)	
10–34	33–40	287 ± 33	400 ± 110
35–59	49–52	472 ± 32	1120 ± 130
60–84	54–58	750 ± 111	1430 ± 460

*95 percent confidence interval.
Adapted from Amann RP: Reproductive physiology and endocrinology of the dog. *In* Morrow DA (ed): Current Therapy in Theriogenology 2. Philadelphia, WB Saunders, 1986, pp 536–537.

Original chapter written by Vicki N. Meyers-Wallen

Abnormal morphology includes defects of the head, midpiece, and tail, which are classified as primary or secondary defects. The percentage of sperm having normal morphology and the percentage of sperm with primary and secondary defects are recorded.

Examination of the Third Fraction of the Semen. The third fraction should be clear and colorless. Normal third fraction has a pH of 6.0 to 7.2. White and red blood cells should be rare.

ARTIFICIAL INSEMINATION (pp. 1652–1654)

BREEDING MANAGEMENT

Timing for the bitch is documented with serial vaginal cytology samples and serum progesterone levels. Normally, serum progesterone concentrations abruptly increase above baseline levels on the day of the LH peak. Using day 0 as the day of the LH peak, ovulation should occur near day 2, and the oocyte should undergo maturation between days 2 and 4.

FRESH SEMEN AIH

A minimum of two matings is recommended, on days 3 and 5, or 4 and 6, as measured from day 0.

CHILLED SEMEN AI

Chilled semen can retain motility for 2 to 4 days if properly extended and handled, whereas undiluted chilled semen has poor survival. It is preferred that the second fraction be collected separately from the first and third fractions. A minimum of two matings is recommended, on days 3 and 5 or on days 4 and 6, as measured from day 0.

For this method to be successful, it is imperative that an accurate method of predicting ovulation in the bitch is utilized. Success rates with chilled semen are higher than those obtained with frozen thawed semen.

FROZEN SEMEN AI

A decrease in the ability to achieve fertilization should be expected with frozen semen, as compared to fresh semen from the same dog. Two inseminations are recommended, on days 3 and 5, or on days 4 and 6, as measured from day 0. In general, most investigators indicate that intrauterine insemination with frozen thawed is highly preferred. Intrauterine insemination usually requires a surgical approach.

MALE INFERTILITY (pp. 1654–1661)

PHYSICAL EXAMINATION

Careful attention should be given to determining whether disease in other systems is present, such as urinary tract infection. Calipers are used to measure the total scrotal width. The results are compared to the total scrotal width expected for the body weight of the dog (see Table 127–1).

SEMEN EVALUATION

Several semen samples taken on different days are necessary to determine the average semen quality for a particular dog.

WBC Count. An estimate of white blood cell numbers in the sperm-rich sample can be obtained with the hemacytometer method, using the sample diluted for sperm count.

Sperm Agglutination. Microscopic agglutination, particularly head-to-head agglutination of sperm, has been reported after *Brucella canis* infection in the dog.

Seminal Plasma Alkaline Phosphatase Concentration.
Alkaline phosphatase in the seminal plasma is primarily of epididymal origin and is considerably higher in the second fraction than in either the first or third fractions. If the alkaline phosphatase concentration in the seminal plasma is low, this is good evidence that the second fraction was not obtained. This result may be due to the fact that the sample collected is an incomplete ejaculate, or possibly that bilateral obstruction of the excurrent ducts distal to the tail of the epididymides is present. If the alkaline phosphatase concentration in the seminal plasma is high, but no sperm are present.

Semen Cultures. A positive semen culture is not diagnostic of infertility or infection. Samples for culture can be taken from separate semen fractions or from a mixture of all three fractions of the ejaculate.

CATEGORIES OF INFERTILITY IN THE MALE DOG

The Sperm Count, Motility, and Morphology Are Within Normal Limits, but Any of the Following Is Present: Abnormal Seminal Fluid, High WBC Count, Positive Culture, Sperm Agglutination. Prostatic fluid should be clear and colorless. White blood cell counts above 2000/μl indicate that consideration should be given to cytologic evaluation and culture.

Teratozoospermia. The sperm count and motility are normal, but less than 50 per cent of the sperm are morphologically normal. There is little information directly linking specific abnormalities and the percentage of those abnormalities with infertility.

Asthenozoospermia. The sperm count is normal, but less than 25 per cent of the sperm have progressively forward motion. If few morphologic abnormalities are present, first consideration should be given to contamination of semen collection equipment with toxic agents such as urine, water, detergents, lubricants, ethylene oxide, or formalin residues.

Oligozoospermia. The sperm count is less than 200 million per ejaculate in a dog that is greater than 10 pounds.

Azoospermia. A complete ejaculate is obtained, but no spermatozoa are present in the seminal plasma. Measurement of seminal plasma alkaline phosphatase is recommended to confirm that the second fraction is present.

Aspermia. An ejaculate is not obtained.

DIFFERENTIAL DIAGNOSIS

Congenital Infertility. See textbook Chapter 129.

Acquired Infertility. Systemic diseases such as hypothyroidism and adrenal disorders should be investigated, as well as infections of the urinary or reproductive tract.

DIAGNOSTIC TESTS

Baseline Laboratory Data

Baseline laboratory data that are first recommended include complete semen evaluation, complete blood count, serum chemistry panel, urinalysis (cystocentesis sample preferred), and a test for *Brucella canis*.

Supplementary Tests

Radiographic and Ultrasound Techniques. Ultrasonography of the testes, epididymides, and prostate gland can be useful and may be indicated as a baseline test when physical examination findings are abnormal.

Evaluation of Steroid Hormones. Testosterone is the primary steroid hormone of interest, particularly in dogs with decreased libido or infertility. A single serum sample is of limited value for evaluating testosterone concentrations, since peripheral levels vary greatly over a period of hours in normal dogs. For this reason, GnRH challenge testing is recommended.

Evaluation of Gonadotropins. Repetitive sampling or GnRH challenge testing are recommended to evaluate FSH and LH concentrations. Few laboratories offer the canine FSH assay. Measurement of LH can be useful in evaluating interstitial cell function, circulating testosterone concentrations, and poor libido. When testosterone response to GnRH challenge is abnormal, the finding of normal LH concentrations supports testicular dysfunction, whereas the finding of abnormal LH concentrations supports pituitary or hypothalamic dysfunction.

Epididymal Aspiration. This invasive technique is rarely justified.

Testicular Biopsy. For dogs with oligozoospermia, a complete diagnostic evaluation, including cultures, serial semen evaluations, gonadotropin evaluations, and breeding trials to proven bitches using excellent management are recommended before testicular biopsy. Semen quality is expected to decline within 2 months of a single insult to spermatogenesis and may take 6 months or longer to improve. A wedge biopsy is the preferred technique. Proper fixation of the biopsy sample is *essential!!* Bouin's or Zenker's fluid is recommended.

DIAGNOSIS, TREATMENT, AND PROGNOSIS

The time required for a spermatogonia to form a mature sperm and to be transported to the tail of the epididymis for ejaculation is at least 2 months. Therefore semen quality is unlikely to change dramatically within 2 months of instituting a treatment, even when beneficial. A minimum of three spermatogenic cycles (6 months) is probably necessary before the results of a treatment regimen can be assessed.

Poor Semen Quality. To allow accumulation of sperm reserves, abstinence from ejaculation should be maintained for at least 4 days before the first breeding.

Hypothyroidism. This disorder is discussed at length in Chapter 115.

Hypercortisolism. See textbook Chapter 18.

Retrograde Ejaculation. Aspermia, azoospermia, or oligozoospermia may rarely be due to retrograde flow of the ejaculate into the urinary bladder (retrograde ejaculation). Retrograde ejaculation may improve with sympathomimetic drugs, such as ephedrine or phenylpropanolamine.

Toxins and Medications. Improvement may occur following withdrawal of the compound if testicular dysfunction is not severe. See textbook for a partial listing of drugs that can affect fertility.

Blockage of the Excurrent Ducts. This is diagnosed by semen evaluation and measurement of low alkaline phosphatase concentrations in the seminal plasma. Normal responses of LH, FSH, and testosterone to GnRH stimulation are expected. In humans, this condition is treated by microsurgery.

Reproductive Tract Infections. Dogs with *Brucella canis* infection should be removed from the breeding population. Successful antibiotic treatment of infections in the testes or epididymides may be followed by oligozoospermia or azoospermia. To preserve reproductive function in cases of unilateral orchitis or epididymitis, it is recommended that the ipsilateral testis and epididymis be surgically removed as soon as possible, with the hope that function of the contralateral testis and epididymis will be preserved. Treatment for chronic bacterial prostatitis is discussed elsewhere in this text (Chapter 128).

Failure in the Hypothalamic-Pituitary-Testis Axis. In older dogs, the differential diagnosis for pituitary dysfunction should include neoplasia. Repetitive sampling or GnRH challenge testing are recommended to determine whether gonadotropin and testosterone concentrations are below normal limits. Successful treatment is likely to require pulsatile LH and FSH replacement therapy.

Testicular Dysfunction. If reserve spermatogonia are no longer present in the seminiferous tubules, the prognosis for fertility is grave, regardless of the cause. Such dogs usually have testes of soft consistency or decreased total scrotal width for body weight. Normal serum testosterone concentrations, normal or elevated LH concentrations, and elevated serum FSH concentrations have been reported. Testicular biopsy will confirm that spermatogenesis is abnormal. The prognosis for return to fertility is usually poor.

CHAPTER 128
PROSTATIC DISEASES
(pages 1662–1685)

CLINICAL PROBLEMS ASSOCIATED WITH PROSTATIC DISEASE (pp. 1663–1664)

Any prostatic disease except acute prostatitis can be present without any abnormal signs being evident to the owner. Tenesmus may be caused by an enlarged prostate gland from any cause. If prostatic enlargement is marked, dysuria from urethral obstruction may result. Any disease that causes prostatic inflammation or hemorrhage can result in a urethral discharge. These include cystic hyperplasia, bacterial infection, abscessation, and neoplasia. Systemic signs of prostatic disease include fever, depression, pain in the caudal abdomen, a stiff gait in the rear limbs, and leukocytosis. Another systemic sign seen with suppurative prostatitis or prostatic abscessation is evidence of liver disease (icterus, elevated liver enzymes). Recurrent lower urinary tract infection in male dogs is often due to chronic bacterial prostatitis.

DIAGNOSTIC TECHNIQUES FOR PROSTATIC DISEASES
(pp. 1664–1673)

URINALYSIS; CBC/BIOCHEMICAL PROFILE

A urinalysis should be part of the minimum data base for all suspected cases of prostatic disease. A CBC and biochemical profile are useful.

EVALUATION OF PROSTATIC FLUID

Urethral Discharge. A urethral discharge must be distinguished from a preputial discharge. The discharge should be collected on a microscope slide, dried, stained, and examined. In general, a urethral discharge is not cultured for bacteria because of potential contamination by the normal resident bacterial flora of the distal urethra and prepuce. Prostatic fluid collected by ejaculation is preferred for culture.

Original chapter written by Jeanne A. Barsanti and Delmar R. Finco

Semen Evaluation. An ejaculate is valuable in assessing prostatic disease since prostatic fluid is the largest component of semen volume. For assessment of prostatic disease, collection of the third fraction of the ejaculate is most important. Part of the sample is used for microscopic examination and part for quantitative bacterial culture. Culturing for anaerobic bacteria is only performed if evidence for inflammatory disease is present and cultures for aerobic bacteria are negative.

Prostatic Massage. An alternative technique to collect prostatic fluid is prostatic massage. In cases of suspected prostatic neoplasia with involvement of the prostatic urethra, prostatic massage specimens are more likely to contain abnormal cells than ejaculates. The reason is that prostatic massage involves aspiration directly from the prostatic urethra. A urinary catheter biopsy or urethral brush technique can be combined with prostatic massage.

RADIOGRAPHY

In some cases, contrast cystography may be necessary to delineate the position of the bladder as a landmark for locating the prostate. Granular mineralization can be seen with inflammation or neoplasia. Marked prostatic enlargement is most often associated with abscess, cysts, and neoplasia. In order to avoid variations in technique, distention retrograde urethrocystography has been recommended as the contrast study of choice. If the prostatic urethra is markedly irregular, neoplasia is most likely. The main metastatic route for prostatic adenocarcinoma is via pelvic lymphatics to the sublumbar lymph nodes, to the vertebral bodies, and to the lungs.

ULTRASONOGRAPHY

Prostatic consistency can be evaluated better with ultrasonography than with radiography. Ultrasonography can also provide guidance for aspiration and biopsy.

PROSTATIC ASPIRATION

Needle aspiration is avoided in dogs with abscessation. If an abscess is suspected on the basis of laboratory work and ultrasonography but an aspirate is deemed necessary, the aspirate should be performed only after results of urine and/or prostatic fluid culture are available. If an abscess is aspirated, treatment with intravenous antibiotics should be started immediately.

PROSTATIC BIOPSY

Biopsy is necessary when (1) less invasive clinical findings do not indicate a probable diagnosis, (2) therapy for the suspected underlying disease is not successful, or (3) the probable diagnosis is a serious illness, such as neoplasia or abscessation, either of which requires immediate and extensive therapy. If prostatic abscessation is being considered in the differential diagnosis, aspiration should always precede a blind biopsy technique. Abscessation is a contraindication to a percutaneous biopsy. Parenchymal cystic lesions, identifiable by ultrasonography, should be aspirated rather than subjected to biopsy. The major contraindication to a prostatic biopsy is acute, septic inflammation.

PROSTATIC DISEASES (pp. 1673–1684)

BENIGN HYPERPLASIA

Hyperplasia requires the presence of the testes.

Clinical Signs. Most dogs with prostatic hyperplasia have no clinical signs. An intermittent hemorrhagic or clear light yellow urethral discharge or intermittent or persistent hematuria occurs in some dogs. The prostate gland is nonpainful and symmetrically enlarged. Semen and postmassage prostatic fluid samples may be normal or hemorrhagic. Prostatic epithelial cells, when seen, appear normal. On distention retrograde urethrocystography, the prostatic urethra may be normal or may appear narrowed and undulant without distortion or destruction. On ultrasonography, the prostate is often normal, but it may also be diffusely hyperechoic with parenchymal cavities if intra-parenchymal cysts have developed.

Diagnosis. Definitive diagnosis is only possible by biopsy. Biopsy is not recommended for confirmation of the diagnosis if the clinical signs are typical.

Treatment. Treatment is required only if related abnormal signs are present. The most effective treatment is castration. Small irregular spaces may remain after castration. If castration is not feasible, low doses of estrogens can be used. Diethylstilbestrol administered orally at 0.2 to 1 mg/day for 5 days or every few days for 3 weeks has been recommended. The potential side effects of estrogens must be weighed against their potential clinical benefit. Megestrol acetate also has anti-androgenic properties. A dose of 0.25 mg/lb/day (0.55 mg/kg/day) for 4 weeks has been recommended in dogs.   The antifungal drug keto-conazole and gonadotropin-releasing hormone analogs are also anti-androgenic. However, these drugs are essentially chemical castrators. Thus, they have no advantage over surgical castration in dogs.

SQUAMOUS METAPLASIA

Pathophysiology. Squamous metaplasia of prostatic columnar epithelium is secondary to exogenous or endogenous hyperestro-genism. The major cause is a functional Sertoli cell tumor.

Clinical Signs. With Sertoli cell tumors, the testicles may be pal-pably abnormal. With exogenous hyperestrogenism, both testicles atro-phy. Hematologic findings may reflect the toxicity of estrogens: nonre-generative anemia, thrombocytopenia, granulocytosis, or granulocytopenia. Increased numbers of squamous epithelial cells may be noted in prostatic fluid.

Diagnosis. Presumptive diagnosis is based on history, clinical signs, and, in cases of Sertoli cell tumors, histologic evaluation of the testicles. Definitive diagnosis requires prostatic biopsy.

Treatment. Treatment requires removal of the source of estrogens.

PARAPROSTATIC CYSTS

Clinical Signs. With large cysts, clinical signs may be related to encroachment on the urethra or colon resulting in dysuria or tenesmus, respectively. If the cyst is sufficiently large, abdominal distention may be seen.

Hematologic findings and urinalysis are usually normal. Fluid from a prostatic cyst can be aspirated with ultrasonographic guidance. Pro-static cyst fluid is usually yellow to serosanguineous to brown, has low numbers of WBC, has variable numbers of RBC, has variable numbers of epithelial cells, and is usually sterile. Paraprostatic cysts may miner-alize. Ultrasonography can be used to confirm the diagnosis.

Treatment. The recommended treatment for paraprostatic cysts is surgical drainage with excision or marsupialization. Castration is also recommended.

PROSTATITIS

Hyperplasia presumably does not predispose to infection. *E. coli* is the organism most frequently isolated. Lower urinary tract infections and prostatic infections are almost inseparable in dogs.

Acute Bacterial Prostatitis

Clinical Signs. Signs of systemic illness such as anorexia and lethargy are usually noted. Affected dogs are often depressed and febrile. Caudal abdominal pain may be present. A constant or intermittent urethral discharge may be present. Urine usually has blood, WBC, and bacteria present. On ultrasonography, the prostate gland may be focally to diffusely hyperechoic.

Diagnosis. A presumptive diagnosis is based on history, physical examination, hematology, urinalysis, and urine culture.

Treatment. An antibiotic should be administered for 28 days. The choice of the antibiotic should be based on urine culture and antibiotic sensitivity testing.

Chronic Bacterial Prostatitis

Clinical Signs. The prostate is not painful when palpated, and size is variable. The prostate gland may vary in symmetry and consistency.

Pyuria, hematuria, and bacteriuria on urinalysis are usually seen. The hemogram and biochemical profile are unaffected. Assessment of prostatic fluid is essential in the diagnosis. There are no specific radiographic findings. On ultrasonography, the prostate gland may be diffusely to multifocally hyperechoic. Multifocal mineralization may also be seen.

Diagnosis. Presumptive diagnosis is based on history, physical examination, hematologic findings, urinalysis, and prostatic fluid cytology and quantitative culture. Definitive diagnosis is based on prostatic tissue culture and histopathology. Culture of prostatic tissue may be negative even though infection is present.

Treatment. Chronic bacterial prostatitis is difficult to cure because the blood–prostatic fluid barrier is intact. If the causative organism is gram-positive, erythromycin, clindamycin, oleandomycin, chloramphenicol, or trimethoprim/sulfonamide can be chosen. If the organism is gram-negative, chloramphenicol, trimethoprim/sulfonamide, or enrofloxacin would be best. Antibiotics should be continued for at least 6 weeks. Urine and prostatic fluid should be recultured every 3 to 7 days and every month for 6 months after discontinuing antibiotics. Castration may be beneficial as adjunctive therapy. If oral antibiotics plus castration fail to cure the prostatic infection, only two options remain: low-dose antibiotic therapy or prostatectomy. Low-dose antibiotic therapy can be instituted to suppress the infection. Trimethoprim at 50 per cent of the usual daily dose each night is useful for this purpose. Prostatectomy will eliminate infected prostatic tissue. However, the surgical procedure is difficult and urinary incontinence is a frequent sequela.

Prostatic Abscessation

Clinical Signs. Stranguria and/or tenesmus were reported in approximately 50 per cent of cases in one survey. Clinical signs related to infection include a constant or intermittent urethral discharge. On palpation, the prostate gland is usually abnormal. The prostate gland is often asymmetric and of varying consistency. Icterus due to reactive hepatopathy may be present. A neutrophilic leukocytosis with or without a left shift is common. Urinary tract infection is often present. Prostatic fluid collected by ejaculation or massage is usually purulent and septic and may also be hemorrhagic. Prostatic enlargement, which can be asymmetric or irregular in outline, may be evident on survey radiographs. On ultrasonography, the prostate gland is usually hyperechoic with parenchymal cavities, irregular outline, and asymmetric shape.

Diagnosis. Although a presumptive diagnosis can be based on history, physical examination, hematologic findings, urinalysis, prostatic fluid cytology and culture, and imaging, the diagnosis should be confirmed by aspiration or exploratory celiotomy since the current treatment of choice is surgical drainage.

Treatment. Surgical drainage is currently the treatment of choice. There are many methods to accomplish this, including needle aspiration, tube or penrose drains, or marsupialization. With extensive prostatic involvement, removal of the prostate gland may be considered. Castration is recommended along with antibiotic and surgical therapy. Affected dogs must receive antibiotic therapy. The initial drug of choice may be chloramphenicol, trimethoprim, or a quinolone. However, the choice should be modified based on knowledge of the causative organism, its antibiotic sensitivity, and the presence or absence of bacteremia.

PROSTATIC NEOPLASIA

Prostatic neoplasia should be highest on the list of differential diagnoses in an old dog that was neutered when young and is presented with signs referable to prostatic disease or prostatic enlargement. All of the common neoplasms that affect the prostate gland are malignant.

Clinical Signs. A hemorrhagic urethral discharge may be noted. Anorexia and chronic weight loss are often present. The prostate gland may be painful on palpation and fixed to surrounding tissues. Hematuria is the predominant abnormality on urinalysis. Abnormal epithelial cells may be detected following prostatic massage. On survey abdominal radiography, asymmetric or irregular prostatic enlargement, which may be marked, may be evident. Occasional prostatic carcinomas are associated with multifocal or granular poorly defined mineral densities. Thoracic radiographs are indicated to check for metastasis to the lungs. With distention retrograde urethrocystography, periurethral asymmetry and narrowing, distortion, or destruction of the prostatic urethra may be detected. Ultrasonography usually shows focal or multifocal hyperechoic parenchyma with asymmetry and irregular prostatic outline. Echogenicity tends to be highly heterogeneous.

Diagnosis. Unless metastatic disease is evident radiographically, the diagnosis should always be confirmed by aspiration or biopsy since the prognosis is poor. If a surgical biopsy is obtained, a biopsy should also be taken from the iliac lymph nodes.

Treatment. Radiation therapy is the treatment of choice if metastatic disease is not evident. Prostatectomy is alternative therapy, but the owner must be willing to accept the probable postsurgical development of urinary incontinence. The usual goal of therapy, whether radiation or surgery, is temporary control of the tumor and amelioration of clinical signs. Cure is unlikely. In most cases, euthanasia is performed within 2 months of diagnosis because of progressive disease. Castration has had no beneficial effect in dogs.

PROSTATIC CALCULI

Prostatic calculi are usually small and smoothly marginated. These have been considered incidental findings.

CHAPTER 129

INHERITED AND CONGENITAL DISORDERS OF THE MALE AND FEMALE REPRODUCTIVE SYSTEMS
(pages 1686–1690)

EMBRYOLOGY OF THE REPRODUCTIVE ORGANS
(pp. 1686–1687)

NORMAL DEVELOPMENT

See textbook.

CAUSES OF CONGENITAL DISORDERS

Chromosomal Defects.   Chromosomal defects may be induced by environmental factors, or they may be inherited.

TYPES OF DISORDERS OF SEXUAL DEVELOPMENT
(pp. 1687–1689)

ABNORMAL CHROMOSOME NUMBERS

XXY Syndrome.   This syndrome is referred to as Klinefelter's syndrome. Cats may be of any color but are usually recognized as tricolored (calico) males.

XO Syndrome.   This syndrome is called Turner's syndrome. In dogs that have a normal female phenotype but have not cycled by 24 months of age, the XO syndrome should be considered.

XXX Syndrome.   Abnormalities of the estrous cycle and infertility are frequent findings in XXX dogs.

Chimeras and Mosaics.   *True hermaphrodites* have both ovarian and testicular tissue present in the same individual. True hermaphrodite chimeras are rare and the few reported were female in external appearance. All dogs were presented with a history of failure to cycle. *Chimeras* with testes have been reported in dogs and cats.

ABNORMALITIES OF GONADAL SEX

XX Sex Reversal.   A condition in animals in which chromosomal and gonadal sex do not agree is called sex reversal. Only XX sex reversal has been reported in the dog.

ABNORMALITIES OF PHENOTYPIC SEX

In these animals, chromosomal and gonadal sex are in agreement, but the genitalia are ambiguous.

Female Pseudohermaphrodites.   Female pseudohermaphrodites have an XX chromosome constitution and ovaries, but the internal and external genitalia are masculinized. Those animals exposed to exogenous androgens are 78,XX. The degree of masculinization ranges from mild clitoral enlargement to nearly normal male external genitalia with a prostate internally. The etiology is either androgen or progesterone administration during gestation or androgen administration to racing greyhounds.

Original chapter written by W. Duane Mickelsen and Mushtaq A. Memon

Male Pseudohermaphrodites. Male pseudohermaphrodites have an XY chromosome constitution and testes, but the internal or external genitalia are to some degree those of a female.

Hypospadias. This is an abnormality in the location of the urinary orifice, being ventral and proximal to the normal site in the glans penis. The etiology is thought to be inadequate fetal androgen production. There is a familial occurrence in the Boston terrier breed. Cryptorchidism is the most common defect found in association with hypospadias.

Cryptorchidism. Cryptorchid dogs have been shown to have an increased development of Sertoli cell tumors. Treatment of affected individuals is limited to castration. Removal of carrier parents from the breeding population should result in a decrease in the frequency of this condition.

CHAPTER 130
FELINE REPRODUCTION
(pages 1690–1705)

FEMALE REPRODUCTIVE FUNCTION (pp. 1690–1691)

THE ESTROUS CYCLE

Anestrus (about 90 days in the autumn and winter). The female is sexually inactive. Exfoliated vaginal epithelium contains predominantly parabasal and intermediate cells and small superficial cells.

Proestrus (1 to 2 days, or not shown at all). The female attracts the male by calling and rolling, but immediately rebuffs him if he approaches. Cornification of the exfoliated vaginal epithelium is not yet obvious, so that the only hint of approaching estrus may be the liquefaction of vaginal mucus.

Estrus (3 to 16 days, average 7 days). Female is attractive to males and demonstrative in her acceptance of the male. Behavior changes may precede changes in vaginal cornification, so that vaginal cytology is not a reliable tool for predicting estrus in the cat. The exfoliated vaginal epithelium is cornified. Moderate-to-scant amounts of cloudy, pink fluid exude from the vagina, but erythrocytes are not usually seen. Ovulation is induced by coitus or a comparable stimulus.

Interestrus (2 to 19 days, average 7 days). If mating does not occur or if it occurs before maturation of follicles, ovulation will not result.

Metestrus (35 to 70 days, average 45 days). The cat has ovulated but is not pregnant. It may take up to 35 additional days for the cat to show the subsequent estrus.

MALE REPRODUCTIVE FUNCTION (pp. 1691–1692)

See the textbook.

MANAGEMENT OF NATURAL BREEDING (pp. 1692)

The territoriality of the male mandates that females should be brought to the male for breeding. Females are best transported several

Original chapter written by Victor M. Shille and Nickolas J. Sojka)

weeks before the anticipated breeding to allow adaptation to the new surroundings and people, and familiarization with the male.

MANAGEMENT OF ARTIFICIAL BREEDING
(pp. 1692–1693)

SEMEN COLLECTION, EVALUATION, AND PRESERVATION

Approximately one of five male cats may be trained to have semen collected by means of an artificial vagina. Electroejaculation under anesthesia may be used in cats that cannot be trained to use the artificial vagina.

PREGNANCY AND PARTURITION (pp. 1693–1694)

EVENTS IN GESTATION

The length of gestation is variable (56 to 67 days). Hemograms of cats during pregnancy and lactation are characterized by normocytic, normochromic anemia, with a decline of about 20 per cent in erythrocyte count, hemoglobin concentration, and packed cell volume.

PREGNANCY DIAGNOSIS AND MONITORING

Pregnancy may be confirmed by abdominal palpation of the distinct gestational vesicles between the third and fourth week of gestation. After the vesicles become confluent, uterine enlargement palpated or seen in radiographs is not a reliable sign of pregnancy. Ultrasonography has been used to diagnose pregnancy. The gestational vesicles appear as round, anechoic regions, first seen 11 to 14 days postcoitus. Full skeletal ossification may be seen on radiographs after 49 days, and ossified densities in the humerus, femur, and ribs may be distinguished as early as day 38.

TERATOGENICITY OF DRUGS USED IN PREGNANCY

Virtually all drugs administered to a dam can reach the fetus.

PARTURITION

Eutocia

Stage 1 (2 to 12 hours). Restlessness, nesting, frequent grooming, tachypnea, and vocalization are observed.

Stage 2 (up to 1 hour). The fetus is entering the cervix and cranial vagina, causing strong, visible uterine and abdominal contractions. The corresponding placenta is delivered within 5 to 15 minutes.

Stage 3 (up to 6 to 12 hours or, rarely, overnight). This is the recovery stage between fetuses.

Dystocia

Since errors in fetal posture occur rarely in cats, the most common cause for obstruction is fetal oversize. Primary inertia has been reported to occur in certain family lines, suggesting a hereditary factor. Secondary uterine inertia follows exhaustion after obstructive dystocia or when delivering a large litter. Owing to the small pelvic canal, obstetric assistance is limited to treating all cats with obstructive dystocia by cesarean section. Cats with uterine inertia may benefit from administration of oxytocin (3 to 5 IU IM) and (in a separate syringe!) calcium gluconate 10 per cent (1 to 3 ml IV slowly).

GESTATIONAL DISORDERS

Ectopic Pregnancy. This condition occurs when ova are fertilized outside the uterine tubes. Vague signs of malaise and abdominal distention due to excessive peritoneal fluid suggest ectopic pregnancy. Surgical intervention will be necessary.

Postparturient Septicemia, Endometritis, and Peritonitis. Signs are a reddish-brown cloudy vaginal discharge, depression, anorexia, fever, and dehydration. Supportive therapy and aggressive use of antibiotics must be started immediately, and ovariohysterectomy may have to be done as soon as the cat's condition is stabilized.

Eclampsia. Treatment is the same as in the dog.

Fibroadenomatous Mammary Hyperplasia. This massive enlargement of mammary glands develops rapidly soon after pregnancy or during pseudopregnancy. The growth may be so rapid that skin ulcers develop. Medical therapy includes prevention of nursing by the affected cat and by other cats in the household by using stockinettes or Elizabethan collars, general care of the mammae and of the ulcerative lesions, and using antiprolactin drugs such as bromocriptin mesylate (0.25 mg once daily PO for 5 to 7 days). Mammectomy may have to be done.

Mastitis. Bacterial septicemia may develop. Vigorous antibiotic therapy and attempted evacuation of the glands with a breast pump are recommended. Neonates should continue to nurse unless they become sick.

CONTROL OF UNWANTED REPRODUCTIVE FUNCTION (pp. 1694–1695)

PERMANENT STERILIZATION

Permanent sterilization is generally achieved by ovariohysterectomy in the female and orchiectomy in the male.

TEMPORARY CONTROL OF ESTRUS

Megesterol acetate, a progestin, is used widely outside the United States for estrus control in cats, without FDA approval. Megestrol acetate may be used in males to control sexual behavior. Androgens, in particular mibolerone, are contraindicated in cats.

PREGNANCY TERMINATION

Estradiol cypionate (0.25 mg IM) given within 40 hours of copulation (but not after 5 days) delayed tubal transport and prevented implantation. Some success has been reported with the use of prostagladin $F_{2\alpha}$ when cats were treated after day 40 of gestation.

INFERTILITY IN THE FEMALE (pp. 1695–1697)

NONINFECTIOUS CAUSES OF INFERTILITY

Prolonged Anestrus. Cats fail to cycle during the winter, when days are short. Photoperiod-related anestrus may also be seen in cats kept under inadequate light conditions. Cats living beyond 12 years may show a decline in frequency, and actual cessation, of estrous periods.

Persistent Estrus. Periods of receptivity up to 45 days may occur in the presence of regular waves of follicles lasting 7 to 10 days. The waves, defined by vaginal cornification, are separated by an interestrus of 10 to 15 days. No treatment is recommended, since most of the cats will show regular cycles during the next season. Persistent estrus occurring during periods of seasonal anestrus in cats younger than 5 years of age is most likely to be associated with cystic follicular degeneration of the ovary. The recommended treatment is ovariohysterectomy. A granulosa cell tumor should be suspected in cats over 5 years of age that show chronic signs of hyperestrogenism.

Estrus in Ovariectomized Cats.   Attractiveness to males or proestrous behavior reported by owners may or may not be associated with ovarian remnants due to incomplete surgery. Elevation of E2 should be ascertained by cornification of the exfoliated vaginal epithelium. The two possible sources may be an idiopathically stimulated adrenal cortex or, indeed, an ovarian remnant. Suppressing adrenal function with a short-acting glucocorticoid results in disappearance of estrus signs within 3 to 5 days.

Ovulatory Failure.   It is recommended that cats be mated at least four times within a period of 4 to 6 hours to ensure LH release. Ovulation may be induced by administration of hCG (250 IU IM) or GnRH (25 µg IM).

Cystic Endometrial Hyperplasia.   See textbook Chapter 125. Cystic endometrial hyperplasia is usually followed by hydrometra or, if bacterial invasion and endometritis occur, by pyometra. Ovariohysterectomy is the treatment of choice unless the affected cat must absolutely be able to reproduce. In the latter case the use of antibiotics, followed in 36 to 48 hours by prostaglandin $F_{2\alpha}$ is successful in the short run. However, the condition has a tendency to recur. It is less stressful on the cat if the initial dose of prostaglandin is low (0.1 mg/kg twice a day on days 1 and 2), followed by 0.25 mg/kg twice a day on days 3, 4 and 5, and finaly, 0.3 mg/kg twice a day on days 6 and 7.

Neoplasia.   See textbook Chapter 131.

INFECTIOUS CAUSES OF INFERTILITY

Feline Panleukopenia.   See textbook Chapter 123. Depending on the gestational age at the time of exposure, the results could be infertility due to inapparent loss of embryos, abortion of mummified or macerated fetuses, or blindness, hydranencephaly, and ataxia due to retinal, cerebral, and cerebellar degeneration, respectively.

Bacterial and Other Infections.   No direct evidence of specific venereal or abortion-inducing diseases has been shown in cats.

INFERTILITY IN THE MALE (pp. 1697–1698)

NONINFECTIOUS CAUSES OF INFERTILITY

Intersex: The Calico Male Problem.   See textbook Chapter 129.

INFECTIOUS CAUSES OF INFERTILITY

Infertility in the male cat is rarely reported.

CHAPTER 131

TUMORS OF THE GENITAL SYSTEM AND MAMMARY GLANDS
(pages 1699–1704)

TUMORS OF THE MALE GENITAL TRACT
(pp. 1699–1700)

TESTICULAR TUMORS

Testicular tumors represent 5 to 15 per cent of all tumors seen in male dogs. Cryptorchid dogs and dogs with inguinal hernias are at greater risk for the development of testicular tumors.

Clinical Features

Nonpainful testicular enlargement is generally present with Sertoli cell tumors or seminomas. Interstitial cell tumors are usually small (<1 cm) and rarely of clinical significance. Feminization, due to tumor production of estrogen, can be seen in 25 to 50 per cent of dogs with Sertoli cell tumors.

Treatment and Prognosis

Surgery. Castration is the treatment of choice.
Adjunctive Therapy. Adjunctive therapy is rarely needed. Chemotherapy with vinblastine, cyclophosphamide, and methotrexate has produced measurable reduction in tumor size in dogs with metastatic Sertoli cell tumors.

PROSTATIC ADENOCARCINOMA

A comprehensive discussion of prostatic disease can be found in Chapter 128.

PENILE TUMORS

Clinical Features. Tumors of the penis are rare in dogs and cats.
Treatment. Surgical excision is the most effective treatment for penile neoplasms other than TVTs.

TUMORS OF THE PREPUCE AND SCROTUM

Mast cell tumors, squamous cell carcinomas, and melanomas are common in dogs. Tumors in this location are rare in cats. Surgical excision is usually the treatment of choice.

TUMORS OF THE FEMALE GENITAL TRACT
(pp. 1700–1701)

OVARIAN TUMORS

Ovarian tumors are uncommon in both dogs and cats owing, at least in part, to the practice of early ovario-hysterectomy.
Clinical Features. Small epithelial tumors may be found inciden-

---

Original chapter written by Deborah A. O'Keefe

tally at ovariohysterectomy. Animals with larger tumors usually present with signs referable to an abdominal mass. Tumors may be identified by abdominal ultrasonography more easily than by radiography.

Treatment.   Surgery is the mainstay of therapy for all types of ovarian tumors. Ovariohysterectomy is recommended.

TUMORS OF THE UTERUS AND CERVIX

Uterine tumors are rare in both dogs and cats. Leiomyosarcoma is the most common malignant tumor in the dog. Vaginal discharge or pyometra can sometimes accompany these tumors, and large tumors may compress adjacent structures to cause gastrointestinal or lower urinary tract signs. Chemotherapy using doxorubicin-containing protocols may be beneficial. Feline endometrial adenocarcinomas occur in cats older than 8 years. Clinical signs can include purulent, mucoid, or hemorrhagic vaginal discharge, abdominal distention, polyuria and polydipsia, and gastrointestinal disturbances. These tumors have an aggressive behavior. Ovariohysterectomy is the recommended therapy.

TUMORS OF THE VAGINA AND VULVA

The majority are benign tumors of fibrous or smooth muscle origin. These tumors may be under hormonal control in that they occur almost exclusively in older, intact females, and recurrence is higher in bitches not spayed at the time of surgical removal. Vulvar and vaginal tumors are uncommon in the cat.

Treatment.   Surgical excision, along with ovariohysterectomy, is the treatment of choice. Radiation therapy may be beneficial.

CANINE TRANSMISSIBLE VENEREAL TUMORS (p. 1701)

The transmissible venereal tumor (TVT) occurs only in dogs.

Clinical Features.   TVTs are usually found on the external genitalia of sexually intact male and female dogs. Initially, TVTs are small, raised, and hyperemic. As they enlarge, they become cauliflower-like and very friable. TVTs are immunogenic and can spontaneously regress.

Diagnosis.   TVT has a distinct cytologic appearance; the cells are round to oval with abundant pale, granular cytoplasm that characteristically contains numerous vacuoles.

Treatment.   Surgical excision may be effective for small, localized tumors. Weekly vincristine chemotherapy is the most effective treatment. Tumors that are nonresponsive to vincristine or that relapse after treatment may respond to doxorubicin. TVTs are also sensitive to radiation therapy.

CANINE MAMMARY TUMORS (pp. 1702–1703)

The development of mammary neoplasia in the dog is largely hormone-dependent.

Prognostic Factors.   Benign tumors are easily treated by surgical excision and generally carry an excellent prognosis. Sarcomas, carcinosarcomas, and inflammatory carcinomas have an extremely poor prognosis.

Clinical Features.   Both benign and malignant tumors can appear as small, firm, well-demarcated nodules so that it is impossible to differentiate the two on physical examination. Inflammatory mammary carcinoma presents as a distinct clinical entity. These tumors tend to be diffusely swollen; involve multiple, often bilateral glands; and can be both painful and warm. Fine-needle aspiration for cytologic evaluation is not recommended because it is a weak method for distinguishing benign from malignant mammary tumors.

TREATMENT

Surgery.   In the absence of metastatic disease or inflammatory carcinoma, surgery is the treatment of choice.

Chemotherapy.   There are no controlled clinical trials evaluating the effectiveness of chemotherapy. The author is currently using either doxorubicin or dactinomycin.

FELINE MAMMARY TUMORS (p. 1703)

Siamese cats are at increased risk. Approximately 80 to 90 per cent of feline mammary tumors are malignant.

Prognostic Factors.   Tumor size is the most important prognostic factor. Radical mastectomy, when compared to more conservative surgery, decreases local recurrence but does not improve survival.

Treatment.   Surgery is the recommended treatment. Chemotherapy with doxorubicin and cyclophosphamide has produced short-term complete and partial responses.

CHAPTER 132

CLINICAL APPROACH AND LABORATORY EVALUATION OF RENAL DISEASE
(pages 1706–1719)

CLINICAL APPROACH (pp. 1706–1707)

HISTORY

The history should include information about onset (acute or gradual), progression (improving, unchanging, or worsening), and response to previous therapy. Questions relating to the urinary tract include those pertaining to changes in water intake and the frequency and volume of urination. Care must be taken to distinguish dysuria and pollakiuria from polyuria and to differentiate polyuria from urinary incontinence. If hematuria is present, the owner should be questioned about its timing. Blood at the beginning of urination may indicate a disease process in the urethra or genital tract. Blood at the end of urination or throughout urination may signify a problem in either the bladder or upper urinary tract. Normal urine output ranges from 10 to 20 ml/lb/day in dogs and cats. Water intake should not exceed 40 ml/lb/day in dogs and 20 ml/lb/day in cats.

LABORATORY EVALUATION OF RENAL FUNCTION
(pp. 1707–1710)

Blood Urea Nitrogen

Renal excretion of urea occurs by glomerular filtration, and BUN concentrations are inversely proportional to GFR. However, urea clearance is not a reliable estimate of GFR, and in the face of volume depletion, decreased urea clearance may occur without a decrease in GFR.

Serum Creatinine

Creatinine is excreted by the kidneys almost entirely by glomerular filtration. Its rate of excretion is relatively constant in the steady state. *Determination of creatinine clearance provides a good estimate of GFR.* When nonrenal variables have been eliminated from consideration, an increase in BUN or serum creatinine concentration above nor-

Original chapter written by Stephen P. DiBartola

TABLE 132–1. TESTS OF GLOMERULAR FUNCTION IN DOGS AND CATS

TEST	DOG	CAT
BUN (mg/dl)	8–25	15–35
Serum creatinine (mg/dl)	0.3–1.3	0.8–1.8
Endogenous creatinine clearance (ml/min/kg)	2–5	2–5
Exogenous creatinine clearance (ml/min/kg)	3–5	2–4
^{14}C-inulin clearance (ml/min/kg)	3.3–3.8	3.0–3.5
^{3}H-tetraethylammonium clearance (ml/min/kg)	9–12	7–9
Filtration fraction	0.30–0.38	0.35–0.43
24-hour urine protein excretion (mg/kg/day)	<20	<20
U_{Pr}/U_{Cr}	<0.4	<0.4

mal implies that at least 75 per cent of the nephrons are not functioning. The BUN/creatinine ratio in prerenal and postrenal azotemia may be increased. A decrease in the BUN/creatinine ratio often follows fluid therapy and reflects decreased tubular reabsorption of urea rather than increased GFR.

Creatinine Clearance

Values for glomerular function tests in the dog and cat are presented in Table 132–1. The main indication for determination of *endogenous* creatinine clearance is the clinical suspicion of renal disease in a patient with polyuria and polydipsia but normal BUN and serum creatinine concentrations.

Radioisotopes

The advantages of these procedures are that they do not require collection of urine and are not time-consuming. The major disadvantages are the use of radioactive compounds and the need for special equipment and expertise.

Urinary Protein

Severity of proteinuria may be assessed by measuring 24-hour urine protein excretion or performing a urine protein/urine creatinine ratio (U_{Pr}/U_{Cr}). Dogs with primary glomerular disease (e.g., glomerulonephritis, glomerular amyloidosis) often have markedly increased 24- hour urine protein excretion values.

TUBULAR FUNCTION

Laboratory tests of tubular function are summarized in Table 132–2.

Urine Specific Gravity and Osmolality

Urine specific gravity (USG) or by urine osmolality (U_{Osm}) is preferable because it depends only on the number of osmotically active particles, regardless of their size.

Water Deprivation Test

This test indicated in evaluation of animals with confirmed polydipsia and polyuria, the cause of which remains undetermined after initial diagnostic evaluation. It usually is performed in animals suspected of having central or nephrogenic diabetes insipidus or psychogenic polydipsia. An animal that is dehydrated but has dilute urine has already failed the test and should not be subjected to water deprivation. The

**TABLE 132–2. TESTS OF RENAL TUBULAR
FUNCTION IN DOGS AND CATS**

TEST	DOG	CAT
Random USG	1.001–1.070	1.001–1.080
USG after 5% dehydration	1.050–1.076	1.047–1.087
Urine osmolality after 5% dehydration (mOsm/kg)	1,787–2,791	1,581–2,984
Urine-to-plasma osmolality ratio after 5% dehydration	5.7–8.9	NA
Fractional electrolyte clearance (%)		
Sodium	<1	<1
Potassium	<20	<24
Chloride	<1	<1.3
Phosphorus	<39	<73

Adapted from DiBartola SP: Clinical Evaluation of Renal Function. 16th Annual Waltham/OSU Symposium for the Treatment of Small Animal Diseases, Kal Kan Foods, Vernon, CA, 1992, p 10. NA, not available

water deprivation test also is contraindicated in animals that are azotemic. At the beginning of the water deprivation test, the bladder must be emptied and baseline data collected (body weight, hematocrit, plasma proteins, skin turgor, serum osmolality, urine osmolality, and urine specific gravity). Water then is withheld and these parameters are monitored every 2 to 4 hours. Maximal stimulation of ADH release will be present after a loss of 5 per cent of body weight. Failure to achieve maximal urinary solute concentration does not localize the level of the malfunction, and a structural or functional defect may be present anywhere along the hypothalamic-pituitary-renal axis.

Gradual Water Deprivation

This can be performed to eliminate diagnostic confusion caused by medullary solute washout. The owner can be instructed to restrict water consumption to 60 ml/lb/day 72 hours before, 45 ml/lb/day 48 hours before, and 30 ml/lb/day 24 hours before the scheduled water deprivation test. This approach should only be used in animals that are otherwise healthy on initial clinical evaluation.

Fractional Clearance of Electrolytes

The fractional clearance of sodium may be useful in the differentiation of prerenal and primary renal azotemia.

ROUTINE URINALYSIS (pp. 1711–1717)

Cystocentesis is preferred because it prevents contamination of the sample by the urethra or genital tract. In animals presented for evaluation of hematuria, however, it may be helpful first to evaluate a sample collected by voiding.

CHEMICAL PROPERTIES

pH. Urine pH varies with diet and acid base balance.

Protein. Commonly used dipstick methods for protein determination are much more sensitive to albumin than globulin. In evaluation of proteinuria, it is critical to localize the origin of the protein loss.

Glucose. Glucose is not normally present in the urine of dogs and cats.

Ketones. Causes of ketonuria include diabetic ketoacidosis, starvation or prolonged fasting, glycogen storage disease, low carbohydrate diet, persistent fever, and persistent hypoglycemia.

Occult Blood. A positive test must be interpreted in light of the urine sediment findings (i.e., presence or absence of red blood cells).

Bilirubin. Bilirubin is absent from normal feline urine. The causes of bilirubin-uria are hemolysis (e.g., autoimmune hemolytic anemia), liver disease, extrahepatic biliary obstruction, fever, and starvation.

Red Blood Cells. Occasional red blood cells are considered normal in the urine sediment.

White Blood Cells. Occasional white cells are considered normal in the urine sediment.

Epithelial Cells. These cells often are of little diagnostic significance.

Casts. The presence of casts in the urinary sediment indicates activity in the kidney itself and thus is of localizing value. Occasional hyaline and granular casts per lpf are considered normal. No cellular casts should be observed in sediment from normal urine. Small numbers of hyaline casts may be observed with fever or exercise. Coarsely and finely granular casts are suggestive of ischemic or nephrotoxic renal tubular injury. Fatty casts may be seen in nephrotic syndrome or diabetes mellitus.

Organisms. To be readily apparent microscopically, there must be $>10^4$ rods/ml urine or $>10^5$ cocci/ml urine.

Crystals. Crystals commonly are present in urine of dogs and cats and often are of little diagnostic significance. Urates are commonly observed in the urine of Dalmatian dogs and may be seen in the urine of animals with liver disease or portosystemic shunts. The presence of cystine crystals in urine of dogs and cats is abnormal and suggestive of cystinuria.

MICROBIOLOGY

Aerobic gram-negative bacteria account for the majority of UTI in dogs and cats. *Escherichia coli* is the most common. Urine samples obtained by cystocentesis from normal dogs and cats should yield no growth.

RADIOLOGY (pp. 1717–1718)

Renal size in dogs and cats can be assessed radiographically and compared to the length of vertebra L2. On the ventrodorsal view, the kidney-to- L2 ratio is 2.5 to 3.5 in dogs and 2.4 to 3.0 in cats. Excretory urography is useful in the evaluation of abnormalities in renal size, shape, or location; filling defects in the renal pelvis or ureters; certain congenital defects (e.g., unilateral agenesis); renomegaly; acute pyelonephritis; and rupture of the upper urinary tract. Excretory urography should not be performed in dehydrated patients or in those with known hypersensitivity to contrast media.

ULTRASONOGRAPHY

Renal ultrasonography is useful for differentiating solid from fluid-filled lesions and for determining the distribution of lesions within the kidney. Ethylene glycol intoxication also causes renal hyperechogenicity.

RENAL BIOPSY (pp. 1718–1719)

Renal biopsy should be considered for differentiation of protein-losing glomerular diseases, differentiation of acute renal failure from chronic renal failure, determination of the status of tubular basement membranes in acute renal failure, and establishing the response of the patient to therapy or the progression of previously documented renal disease. After renal biopsy, a brisk fluid diuresis should be initiated.

CHAPTER 133

ACUTE RENAL FAILURE
(pages 1720–1733)

Acute renal failure (ARF) is usually thought to be caused by an ischemic event or exposure to a nephrotoxicant. For an in-depth overview of the pathophysiology of ARF, see the textbook.

STAGES OF ACUTE RENAL FAILURE (pp. 1723–1724)

Acute renal failure has three distinct phases. Prompt therapeutic intervention during the induction phase may prevent progression of renal damage. The maintenance phase of ARF develops when renal tubular lesions are established. It is likely that a combination of tubular obstruction and backleak, vasoconstriction, and decreased glomerular permeability contribute to the decreased glomerular filtration of ARF. Therapeutic intervention during the maintenance phase, although often lifesaving, usually does little to diminish existing renal lesions or improve renal function. The recovery phase of ARF is associated with improved renal function.

RISK FACTORS FOR ARF (pp. 1724–1725)

Major categories of risk factors include disorders affecting renal perfusion, pre-existing renal disease, electrolyte disturbances, nephrotoxic drug administration, and dietary influences. Dehydration and volume depletion are perhaps the most significant factors that decrease renal perfusion. Concentrations of several electrolytes can affect the development of ARF. Hyponatremia potentiates contrast media-induced ARF in dogs. Hypocalcemia, hypomagnesemia, and hypokalemia are additional electrolyte abnormalities that can potentiate nephrotoxicity. Administration of potentially nephrotoxic drugs or drugs that may enhance nephrotoxicity obviously increases the risk of ARF. Furosemide potentiates gentamicin-induced nephrotoxicity. Use of NSAIDs can also increase the risk of ARF. Anesthesia, surgery, sodium and/or volume depletion, sepsis, congestive heart failure, nephrotic syndrome, and hepatic disease are conditions in which prostaglandin-induced vasodilatation becomes important and the susceptibility to NSAIDs is increased.

DIAGNOSIS OF ARF (pp. 1725–1726)

The differentiation between prerenal and renal azotemia can be difficult if urine concentrating ability is impaired in patients with prerenal azotemia. Conditions that may result in prerenal azotemia with concurrent urine concentrating defects include typical hypoadrenocorticism,

Original chapter written by Gregory F. Grauer and India F. Lane

TABLE 133–1. INDICES THAT MAY HELP DIFFERENTIATE PRERENAL AZOTEMIA FROM ARF

INDICES	PRERENAL AZOTEMIA	ARF
Urine specific gravity*	Hypersthenuric	Isosthenuric or minimally concentrated
Urine sodium (mEq/L)*	<10–20	>25
Fractional excretion of sodium (%)*	<1	>1
Urine creatinine to plasma creatinine ratio	>20:1	<10:1
Renal failure index (urine Na/urine to plasma creatinine ratio)	<1	>2

*See text for exceptions.

pyometra, liver disease, hypotonic dehydration, and administration of diuretics. Postrenal azotemia secondary to lower urinary tract obstruction should be considered if stranguria, dysuria, or complete anuria is observed. In some cases, positive contrast urethrography/cystography may be necessary to confirm a urethral obstruction. Peritoneal fluid with a creatinine concentration greater than serum creatinine is supportive of urine leakage into the abdominal cavity. Contrast radiography is the best way to confirm and localize the site of rupture. The distinction between acute and chronic renal failure is important inasmuch as the treatment objectives and prognosis vary considerably. (Table 133–2).

EARLY RECOGNITION OF RENAL DAMAGE/ DYSFUNCTION (pp. 1726–1727)

Numerous urine parameters can herald the development of ARF. Urine output should be monitored in all high-risk patients. Normal

TABLE 133–2. PARAMETERS THAT MAY HELP DIFFERENTIATE ACUTE FROM CHRONIC RENAL FAILURE

ACUTE RENAL FAILURE	CHRONIC RENAL FAILURE
History Ischemic episode or toxicant exposure	History Previous renal disease or renal insufficiency Longstanding polydipsia/polyuria Chronic weight loss, vomiting, diarrhea
Physical examination Good body flesh Smooth, swollen, painful kidneys Relatively severe clinical signs for level of dysfunction	Physical examination Poor body condition Small, irregular kidneys Relatively mild clinical signs for level of dysfunction Osteodystrophy
Clinicopathologic findings Normal or increased hematocrit Active urine sediment Normal to increased serum potassium More severe metabolic acidosis	Clinicopathologic findings Nonregenerative anemia Inactive urine sediment Normal to low serum potassium Less severe metabolic acidosis

TABLE 133–3. POTENTIAL MEASURES TO PROTECT AGAINST ARF

Fluid therapy, volume expansion, natriuresis

Use of mannitol or dopamine and furosemide (do not use furosemide in patients receiving gentamicin)

Monitor serum trough concentrations of aminoglycosides

Increasing interval between doses of gentamicin (i.e., give the same total daily dose divided twice a day rather than three times a day)

Administer cisplatin in the afternoon rather than in the morning

Use of thromboxane synthetase inhibitors?

Dietary supplementation with omega-3 fatty acids?

Dietary protein conditioning?

Use of atrial natriuretic peptide?

Use of calcium channel blockers?

---

urine output is approximately 1 to 2 ml/hr/kg body weight. Changes in urine sediment (increasing numbers of WBCs, RBCs, renal epithelial cells, or cellular or granular casts) or the acute onset of glucosuria or proteinuria may be indicative of early glomerular or tubular damage. Detection of enzymes such as gamma- glutamyl transpeptidase (GGT) and N-acetyl-beta-D-glucosaminidase (NAG) in the urine has proved to be a sensitive indicator of renal tubular damage. Enzymuria is best quantitated by 24-hour urine collection; urine enzyme/creatinine ratios may be inaccurate in the face of a changing GFR.

POTENTIAL PROTECTIVE MEASURES (pp. 1727–1728)

See Table 133–3.

MANAGEMENT OF ESTABLISHED ARF (pp. 1728–1731)

All potentially nephrotoxic drugs should be discontinued. Fluid therapy, the cornerstone of treatment for ARF, is used to correct fluid and electrolyte imbalances, improve renal hemodynamics, and induce diuresis. The large volume of fluid and rapid administration rate necessary in ARF require that fluids be given intravenously. Jugular catheters are ideal. Deficit fluid requirements should be replaced over the first 4 to 6 hours of treatment. Physiologic saline (0.9 per cent solution) is the fluid of choice. The amount of fluid required to restore extracellular fluid deficits can be calculated by multiplying the estimated per cent dehydration by the patient's body weight in kilograms. Frequent assessment of body weight, central venous pressure, packed cell volume, and plasma total solids will help to detect early overhydration. Physical manifestations of overhydration include increased bronchovesicular sounds, tachycardia, restlessness, chemosis, and serous nasal discharge. Urine production should be measured and electrolyte and acid-base status assessed. Approximately two-thirds of normal maintenance fluid needs are due to fluid loss in urine; therefore oliguric and nonoliguric patients can have large variations in their maintenance fluid needs.

Oliguric ARF patients are at risk for hyperkalemia. Moderate hyperkalemia is largely resolved with administration of potassium-free fluids (dilution) and improved urine flow (increased excretion). Sodium bicarbonate will help to correct any metabolic acidosis and lower serum potassium concentration by exchanging intracellular hydrogen ions for potassium. Glucose and insulin can also be used in emergency situations to increase intracellular shifting of potassium. Regular insulin is administered at a dosage of 0.1 to 0.25 U/kg IV, followed by a glucose bolus of

1 to 2 gm per unit of insulin given. Ten per cent calcium gluconate (0.5 to 1.0 ml/kg IV over 10 to 15 minutes) will counteract the cardiotoxic effects of excess potassium without lowering the serum potassium.

Mild to moderate metabolic acidosis also commonly resolves with fluid therapy, and specific treatment is rarely necessary unless the blood pH is less than 7.2 or total CO_2 is less than 12 mEq/L. Bicarbonate requirements can be calculated utilizing the base deficit as determined from arterial blood, or an estimated base deficit (body weight (kg) × 0.3 × base deficit = mEq bicarbonate required).

Furosemide (2 to 6 mg/kg/IV q8h) is often advocated as an initial treatment for oliguria in dogs and cats because it is easy to administer. However, an infusion of mannitol or use of a dopamine infusion in combination with furosemide is likely to be more effective. Mannitol, in a 10 or 20 per cent solution, is an excellent choice for treatment of oliguric ARF. The recommended dosage is 0.5 to 1.0 gm/kg, IV as a slow bolus over 15 to 20 minutes. Urine output should improve within one hour if the treatment is effective. A second bolus may be attempted. Hypertonic glucose (10 to 20 per cent solutions) may be used as an alternative to mannitol. The recommended infusion rate for dopamine is 1 to 5 μg/kg/min, and it is best administered with an infusion pump through a separate IV line. Adding 30 mg of dopamine to 500 ml of saline will result in a dopamine concentration of 60 μg/ml. Dopamine should not be added to alkaline fluids.

Once diuresis has been established in patients that present with oliguric ARF, or in patients with nonoliguric ARF, fluid therapy should be tailored to match urine volume and other losses, including insensible losses and continuing losses. Insensible losses are estimated at 20 ml/kg/day. In the recovery phase of potassium supplementation may be necessary.

ARF also decreases clearance of gastrin, causing hypergastrinemia and gastric hyperacidity. Secondary hemorrhagic or ulcerative gastritis leading to anorexia and vomiting is common. Vomiting may be partially controlled by administration of histamine (H_2 receptor) blockers, cimetidine (2.5 to 5 mg/kg IV or PO q8–12h) or ranitidine (2mg/kg IV or PO q8–12h), or proton pump blockers such as omeprazole (0.7 mg/kg PO q24h). Sucralfate (0.5 to 1.0 gm PO q6–8h), a gastrointestinal protectant, can also be used. Misoprostol, a synthetic prostaglandin (2 to 5 μg/kg PO q8–12h), may be used to help protect the gastric mucosa of dogs with ARF.

Vomiting also results from direct stimulation of the chemoreceptor trigger zone (CRTZ) by uremic toxins such as guanidines. This stimulation can be reduced by administration of antiemetics such as metoclopromide (0.2 to 0.5 mg/kg IV, IM, or PO q6-8h). Metoclopramide should not be used during dopamine infusion. Phenothiazine compounds, such as chlorpromazine, should be avoided unless adequate hydration and blood pressure have been restored.

Critically ill uremic patients are highly susceptible to infection. Strict aseptic techniques should be utilized in the placement of vascular and urinary catheters, the administration of parenteral medications, and the care of wounds. Protracted ARF results in a catabolic state. Some form of nutritional support is usually recommended. Caloric requirements should be met principally with carbohydrates. Further discussion of enteral and parenteral nutrition is provided in Chapter 54.

Dialytic therapy should be considered when initial fluid and diuretic therapy has not been successful. Dialysis can also be utilized to manage overhydrated patients and to hasten elimination of certain toxicants.

PROGNOSIS (pp. 1731–1732)

In general, nonoliguric ARF may have a better prognosis than oliguric ARF because typically uremia is less severe, hyperkalemia is less likely to be present, and the tendency for overhydration to occur is minimized.

CHAPTER 134

CHRONIC RENAL FAILURE
(pages 1734–1760)

CLINICAL CONSEQUENCES (pp. 1735–1742)

The onset and spectrum of clinical and biochemical events occurring in patients with chronic renal failure (CRF) may vary, depending on the nature, severity, duration, rate of progression of the underlying disease, presence of coexistent but unrelated disease, age and species of the patient. Diverse clinical and laboratory findings characterize uremia and emphasize the polysystemic nature of CRF (Table 134–1).

GASTROINTESTINAL CONSEQUENCES

Gastrointestinal complications are among the most common and prominent clinical signs of uremia. Anorexia and weight loss are common. Vomiting is a frequent but inconsistent finding in uremia. Hematemesis may occur. Severe CRF may result in uremic stomatitis characterized by oral ulcerations brownish discoloration of the dorsal

TABLE 134–1. CLINICAL FEATURES OF CHRONIC RENAL FAILURE

Historical and Physical Findings

General: Depression, fatigue, weakness, dehydration, and weight loss

Gastrointestinal: Anorexia, nausea, vomiting, diarrhea, uremic stomatitis, xerostomia, uriniferous breath, constipation

Urinary system: Polyuria, nocturia, polydipsia; palpation reveals small, often irregular kidneys

Cardiopulmonary: Arterial hypertension, heart murmurs, cardiomegaly, cardiac rhythm disturbances, dyspnea

Neuromuscular: Dullness, drowsiness, lethargy, irritability, tremors, gait imbalance, flaccid muscle weakness, myoclonus, behavioral changes, dementia, isolated cranial nerve deficits, seizures, stupor, and coma

Eyes: Scleral and conjunctival injection, retinopathy, acute-onset blindness

Skin and haircoat: Pallor, bruising, increased shedding, unkempt appearance and loss of normal sheen to coat

Laboratory Findings

Acidosis

Anemia: Usually normochromic, normocytic

Azotemia

Hyperamylasemia

Hypercalcemia or hypocalcemia

Hyperparathyroidism: Renal secondary

Hyperphosphatemia

Hypokalemia

Proteinuria

Radiology: Reduced renal size; irregular renal contours; renal mineralization; evidence of osteomalacia or osteitis fibrosa

Reduced urine concentrating ability

Renal isotope scan: Reduced renal size and function

Ultrasound: Reduced renal size, increased echogenicity

Original chapter written by David J. Polzin, Carl A. Osborne, Joseph W. Bartges, Katherine M. James, and Julie A. Churchill

surface of the tongue, necrosis and sloughing of the anterior portion of the tongue and uriniferous breath. Uremic enterocolitis, manifested as diarrhea, may occur, but it is less common than uremic gastritis. Uremic enterocolitis often is hemorrhagic. Constipation is a relatively common complication of CRF, particularly in cat.

IMPAIRED URINE CONCENTRATING ABILITY, POLYURIA, POLYDIPSIA, AND NOCTURIA

Among the earliest clinical manifestations of CRF in dogs is onset of polyuria, polydipsia, and, sometimes, nocturia caused by reduced urine concentrating ability.

ARTERIAL HYPERTENSION

Arterial hypertension is among the most common complications of CRF, reportedly occurring in 60 to 69 per cent of cats with renal failure and 50 to 93 per cent of dogs with renal failure. Organs that may be damaged by sustained arterial hypertension include the kidneys, eyes, cardiovascular system, and brain. Left ventricular hypertrophy and cardiac failure may result from sustained hypertension, although hypertension is unlikely to induce cardiac failure in a previously normal heart.

NEUROMUSCULAR CONSEQUENCES

Clinical signs of nervous system dysfunction in uremic dogs and cats may include dullness, drowsiness, lethargy, tremors, gait imbalance, myoclonus, seizures, stupor, and coma. A progressive decline in alertness and awareness occurs early in uremia. Hypokalemic polymyopathy occasionally is observed in association with CRF, primarily in cats. Hypokalemic cats may exhibit profound cervical ventroflexion and difficulty ambulating.

OCULAR CONSEQUENCES

Scleral and conjunctival injection are common manifestations of advanced uremia. Ophthalmoscopic findings may include reduced pupillary light reflexes, papilledema, retinal arterial tortuosity, retinal hemorrhage, retinal detachment, hyphema, anterior uveitis, and glaucoma.

HEMORRHAGIC CONSEQUENCES OF UREMIA

Uremia may also be characterized by a hemorrhagic tendency that typically presents as bruising, gastrointestinal hemorrhage with hematemesis or melena, bleeding from the gums, or hemorrhage subsequent to venipuncture. The bleeding time has been advocated as the best screening test.

LABORATORY FINDINGS

Acidosis

Metabolic acidosis has long been known to accompany CRF. Chronic metabolic acidosis promotes a variety of adverse clinical effect, including negative calcium balance and bone demineralization, or negative potassium balance, and protein malnutrition. Alkalinization therapy effectively reverses acidosis-associated protein breakdown. Acidosis poses an additional risk for CRF patients on protein-restricted diets.

Anemia

A progressive hypoproliferative anemia is characteristic of dogs and cats with moderate to advanced CRF. Many CRF patients have a relative, rather than absolute, erythropoietin deficiency.

Azotemia

Azotemia is an excess of urea or other nitrogenous compounds in the blood. Because these compounds are derived almost entirely from protein degradation, their production increases when dietary protein increases. BUN concentrations typically are directly related to the protein content of the diet. Because so many extrarenal factors influence BUN concentration, it is not a particularly useful measure of glomerular filtration rate in patients with CRF. Serum creatinine measurements more accurately reflect changes in renal function. The ratio of BUN to serum creatinine concentration should decline when dietary protein intake is reduced.

Hyperphosphatemia and Renal Secondary Hyperparathyroidism

Hyperphosphatemia. Hyperphosphatemia is among the most common regulatory derangements of CRF. In general, serum phosphorus concentrations parallel BUN concentrations.

Renal Secondary Hyperparathyroidism. Clinically important renal osteodystrophy is uncommon, but when it occurs, it most often is in immature patients. Bones of the skull are most severely affected ("rubber jaw" syndrome). Soft tissue calcification is another complication of renal secondary hyperparathyroidism and hyperphosphatemia. It most commonly affects the lungs, kidneys, arteries, stomach, and myocardium.

Hypokalemia

An association between polyuric renal failure and hypokalemia has been recognized in cats. In contrast, hypokalemia appears to be an uncommon manifestation of renal failure in dogs. The cardinal and most dramatic sign of hypokalemia, regardless of cause, is generalized muscle weakness. Chronic potassium depletion appears to impair renal function in cats. In many cats with CRF and hypokalemia, renal function improves after potassium supplementation. Inadequate dietary potassium intake (it should be 0.6 per cent dry matter or greater) appears to be an important factor in promoting hypokalemia in CRF.

Proteinuria

Urinary protein excretion typically is increased in dogs and cats with CRF. Proteinuria is considered a hallmark of glomerular injury and dysfunction. Presumably, reducing dietary protein intake reduces proteinuria in patients with CRF by reducing intraglomerular hypertension.

DIAGNOSTIC EVALUATION (p. 1742)

Diagnostic evaluation of patients with renal disease and renal failure is described in detail in Chapter 132.

TREATMENT (pp. 1743–1755)

Conservative medical management of CRF consists of supportive and symptomatic therapy designed to correct deficits and excesses in fluid, electrolyte, acid–base, endocrine, and nutritional balance and thereby minimize the clinical and pathophysiologic consequences of reduced renal function. It should not be expected to halt, reverse, or eliminate renal lesions responsible for CRF. Conservative medical management is intended for patients with compensated CRF; it is not intended for patients that are unable to eat or accept oral medications because of severe uremia. Clinical signs and complications of uremia should be managed as described in the section on acute renal failure (Chapter 133) before attempting conservative medical management.

AMELIORATING CLINICAL CONSEQUENCES OF EXCRETORY FAILURE

Reducing Dietary Protein Intake

We usually recommend limiting protein intake in patients with CRF when clinical signs attributable to reduced renal function develop or when serum creatinine concentration exceeds about 1.5 to 2.0 mg/dl.

We recommend that dogs with mild to moderate CRF be fed a diet that provides at least 13 per cent of gross energy as protein. We cautiously recommend that cats with CRF be fed a diet that provides at least 21 per cent of gross energy as protein. If malnutrition is detected before or after initiating diet therapy, consideration should be given to increasing dietary protein intake. If diets designed to provide the recommended protein intake fail to ameliorate the clinical and biochemical manifestations of uremia, dietary protein intake may be cautiously reduced further. Modification of diets for treatment of chronic primary polyuric failure should encompass provision of adequate non-protein calories in addition to reduction of protein.

Ameliorating Uremic Nausea and Vomiting.   As an alternative to H_2-receptor antagonists, sucralfate may be given to create a protective layer over the gastric mucosal surface. Metoclopramide may be given to minimize the action of uremic toxins on the medullary emetic chemoreceptor trigger zone.

Vitamin B Complex Deficiency.   Deficiencies of thiamine and niacin may result in anorexia. Patients with renal failure are at risk for vitamin B complex deficiency. The daily B vitamin requirement of normal cats is estimated to be six to eight times greater than that of dogs.

Enhancing Diet Palatability

It is advisable to make diet changes gradually over a period of 1 to 2 weeks. Food aversion is most likely to occur if patients are force-fed or introduced to the new diet while nauseated. Small quantities of (animal fat, butter, dehydrated cottage cheese, garlic, bouillon, clam juice) may be used to enhance the palatability of diets.

Pharmacologic Appetite Stimulants

Corticosteroids.   There is no data to support a long-term beneficial effect of glucocorticoids in uremic dogs or cats.

Benzodiazepines.   Benzodiazepine derivatives, such as diazepam and oxazepam, are at best marginally successful in renal failure patients.

Modification of Drug Dosages

Nephrotoxic drugs and drugs that require renal excretion should be avoided in patients with renal failure. If drugs that require renal excretion must be administered to patients with renal failure, dosage regimens should be adjusted to compensate for decreased organ function.

AMELIORATING CLINICAL CONSEQUENCES OF REGULATORY FAILURE

Hyperphosphatemia

Hyperphosphatemia is managed by restricting dietary phosphorus intake, oral administration of intestinal phosphorus-binding agents, or a combination of these methods. Monitoring plasma PTH activity directly is one means of measuring effectiveness of therapy. Normalization of serum phosphorus concentration has been advocated as an economically acceptable and clinically useful therapeutic end point, but such normalization should not be interpreted to indicate that plasma PTH activity is within normal limits.

Dietary Phosphorus Restriction. Because proteinaceous foods are the major dietary phosphorus sources, protein-restricted diets usually are low in phosphorus content. Serum phosphorus concentrations should be determined after the patient has been consuming the phosphorus-restricted diet for 2 to 4 weeks and should be collected after a 12-hour fast.

Intestinal Phosphorus-Binding Agents. Administration of phosphorus-binding agents should be timed to coincide with feeding. Initial doses of 30 to 90 mg/kg/day have been recommended for aluminum-based phosphorus-binding agents. The potential for toxicity of aluminum salts in dogs and cats has been confirmed, but clinical evidence of toxic accumulation of aluminum has not been reported in these species. Calcium-based phosphorus- binding agents, may be more effective than aluminum-based phosphorus-binding agents. However, calcium-based products may promote clinically significant hypercalcemia. Calcium acetate is the most effective calcium-based phosphorus- binding agent as well as the agent least likely to induce hypercalcemia.Initial doses of 60 to 90 mg/kg/day have been recommended for calcium acetate and 90 to 150 mg/kg/day for calcium carbonate. Serum calcium and phosphorus concentrations should be monitored every 4 to 6 weeks or as needed.

Hypocalcemia

In addition to their role as intestinal phosphorus-binding agents, oral calcium supplements may be used to augment the amount of calcium available for absorption. Intestinal malabsorption of calcium is common in CRF but can be overcome by increasing dietary calcium intake. Because of increased risk of inducing extraskeletal mineralization, calcium supplementation should be withheld until serum phosphorus concentrations are normalized. Calcium carbonate may be the preferred calcium supplement (as opposed to phosphate- binding agent).

Hypokalemia

Potassium replacement therapy is indicated for cats with hypokalemia (serum potassium concentrations less than 4 mEq/L). Oral administration is the safest and preferred route. Potassium gluconate is regarded as the potassium salt of choice for replacement therapy in cats. Potassium citrate solution (Polycitra-K) is an excellent alternative that has the advantage of providing simultaneous alkalinization therapy. Potassium gluconate is given initially at a dose of 2 to 6 mEq/cat/day. Routine supplementation of low oral doses of potassium (2 mEq/day) has been recommended for all cats with chronic renal disease. Diets that are acidifying and restricted in magnesium content may promote hypokalemia and should, therefore, be avoided in cats with CRF.

Metabolic Acidosis

Oral alkalinization therapy is indicated when serum bicarbonate concentration declines to or below 17 mEq/L. Oral sodium bicarbonate is the most commonly used alkalinizing agent for patients with metabolic acidosis of CRF. The suggested initial dose of sodium bicarbonate is 8 to 12 mg/kg body weight q 8 to 12 h. Prepare a solution containing about 80 mg of sodium bicarbonate per milliliter of solution (about 1 mEq/ml) by adding one-third of an 8-oz box (76 gm) of sodium bicarbonate to 1 qt (946 ml) of water. Initially, the solution is administered at a dose of 1 to 1.5 ml/10 kg of body weight. Potassium citrate is a particularly attractive alternative alkalinization agent. It may offer the advantage, at least in cats, of allowing for the simultaneous treatment of both hypokalemia and acidosis with a single drug.

Dehydration

For patients in which voluntary fluid intake is inadequate to prevent dehydration, supplemental fluids may be administered subcutaneously at home by the owner. Management of fluid needs in clinically dehydrated patients and during uremic crisis is described in Chapters 60 and 133.

Arterial Hypertension

Lowering blood pressure may reverse many of the acute ocular manifestations of hypertension. This effect remains the only established benefit of therapy for hypertension in dogs and cats.

Nonpharmacologic Therapy

Dietary Sodium Restriction. Daily sodium intake should be reduced to about 0.1 to 0.3 per cent of the diet on a dry-matter basis (10–40 mg/kg/24 h) gradually over 1–2 weeks.

Protein Restriction. Although unproved in dogs and cats, dietary protein restriction may limit or prevent renal hypertensive injury.

Pharmacologic Therapy

Angiotensin Converting Enzyme Inhibitors. Enalapril commonly is used in hypertensive renal failure. These drugs may decrease renal perfusion, causing tubular necrosis and leading to progressive renal failure. Hyperkalemia may occur in association with administration of potassium-containing drugs or potassium-sparing diuretics.

Calcium-Channel Blockers. Diltiazem commonly is used to treat arterial hypertension in dogs and cats.

Adrenergic Receptor Antagonists. β-adrenergic receptor inhibition has been associated with reduction of blood pressure in dogs and cats. The use of selective β_1-adrenergic receptor antagonists, such as atenolol and labetalol, has theoretic advantages over the use of nonselective β-adrenergic receptor antagonists.

α_1-Adrenergic receptor antagonists reduce blood pressure by peripheral arteriolar vasodilation. Prazosin appears to be moderately effective.

Arteriolar Vasodilators. Although not a first-choice antihypertensive drug for patients with CRF, hydralazine has been used to treat hypertension in dogs and cats.

Diuretics. Although thiazides, which act at the distal nephron, are effective diuretics in normal individuals, they often are ineffective in patients with renal failure. Furosemide, a loop diuretic, is more likely to be effective in reducing blood pressure in patients with hypertension associated with renal failure.

AMELIORATING CLINICAL CONSEQUENCES OF BIOSYNTHETIC FAILURE

Treating Anemia of CRF

General Guidelines for Minimizing Anemia. Often overlooked consideration is prevention of unnecessary iatrogenic blood loss. Chronic low-grade gastrointestinal blood loss can also result in severe anemia in CRF patients. Iron deficiency is a relatively common problem in patients with CRF. Determining stainable iron content in bone marrow is helpful in assessing body iron stores and may detect problems not identified by serum iron levels or transferrin saturation. Oral supplementation with iron sulfate is the preferred therapy for iron deficiency anemia. Starting doses of iron sulfate of 50 to 100 mg/day for cats and 100 to 300 mg/day for dogs have been recommended. B vitamins, folate, and niacin often can be provided as an oral supplement with iron.

Blood Transfusion. Transfusions of packed red blood cells or whole blood may be indicated for anemic CRF patients who need rapid correction of their anemia, as in preparation for surgery.

Hormone Replacement Therapy. The structure of the erythropoietin protein is well conserved across species lines, and dogs and cats can respond appropriately to rHuEPO.

Starting doses of 50 to 150 U/kg subcutaneously three times weekly are recommended. Monitoring of hematocrit is necessary to allow adjustments in dose and dosing interval. Because of the high demand for iron associated with stimulated erythropoiesis, oral supplementation is recommended for all patients receiving rHuEPO therapy.

The problem of refractory anemia is directly related to rHuEPO therapy because of the development of neutralizing anti-rHuEPO antibodies. The rHuEPO protein appears to be immunogenic in many dogs and cats, with antibody titers developing at variable times. Increased systemic blood pressure and seizures have been identified as a complication of rHuEPO therapy. Because of the high prevalence of anti-rHuEPO antibody production in both dogs and cats, the question of when to initiate rHuEPO therapy in veterinary patients with CRF is not easily answered. When hematocrit values are below 25 in dogs and 20 in cats, anemia will probably contribute to the adverse clinical signs characteristic of uremia.

Treatment of Calcitriol Deficit

Administration of vitamin D in conjunction with proportional reduction in phosphate intake has been shown to limit renal secondary hyperparathyroidism and its associated skeletal abnormalities in dogs with induced CRF. Although potentially beneficial in CRF patients, vitamin D therapy must be undertaken with great caution because hypercalcemia is a frequent and potentially serious complication of vitamin D therapy. Serum phosphate concentration must be normalized before initiating vitamin D therapy. An important advantage of calcitriol over other forms of vitamin D therapy in CRF is that calcitriol does not require renal activation for maximum efficacy. A dosage of 1.5 to 3.5 ng/kg body weight/day PO has been recommended for dogs with CRF. Vitamin D therapy may enhance intestinal absorption of calcium and phosphorus and, therefore, should not be given with meals. Continued monitoring of serum calcium, phosphate, and creatinine concentrations is necessary.

CHAPTER 135

GLOMERULAR DISEASE
(pages 1760–1775)

The major glomerular diseases of dogs and cats are immune complex glomerulonephritis and amyloidosis.

PATHOGENESIS OF GLOMERULONEPHRITIS
(pp. 1762–1763)

For a complete review of the pathogenesis of glomerulonephritis, see the textbook.

The location of the immune complexes within the glomerular capillary wall may influence the immune response.

Original chapter written by Gregory F. Grauer and Stephen P. DiBartola

TABLE 135–1. DISEASES ASSOCIATED WITH GLOMERULONEPHRITIS

DOGS	CATS
Infectious	*Infectious*
Infectious canine hepatitis	Feline leukemia virus
Bacterial endocarditis	Feline infectious peritonitis
Brucellosis	Mycoplasmal polyarthritis
Dirofilariasis	
Ehrlichiosis	
Leishmaniasis	
Pyometra	
Borelliosis	
Chronic bacterial infections	
Rocky Mountain spotted fever	
Trypanosoma	
Septicema	
Neoplasia	*Neoplasia*
Inflammatory	*Inflammatory*
Pancreatitis	Pancreatitis
Systemic lupus erythematosus	Systemic lupus erythematosus
Polyarthritis	Other immune-mediated diseases
Prostatitis	Chronic skin disease
Other	*Other*
Hyperadrenocorticism	Idiopathic
Long-term steroid therapy?	Familial
Idiopathic	Nonimmunologic—hyperfiltration?
Familial	Diabetes mellitus?
Nonimmunologic—hyperfiltration?	
Diabetes mellitus?	

If immune complexes form or are deposited closer to the capillary lumen (i.e., in subendothelial locations) there often is more histologic evidence of inflammation. Initially, glomerulonephritis results in increased glomerular permeability and proteinuria. As previously discussed, once a glomerulus has been irreversibly damaged (e.g., glomerulosclerosis), the entire nephron becomes nonfunctional. As more nephrons become involved, glomerular filtration decreases. Several infectious and inflammatory diseases have been associated with glomerular deposition or *in situ* formation of immune complexes in dogs and cats (Table 135–1).

PATHOGENESIS OF AMYLOIDOSIS (pp. 1763–1766)

For a complete review of the pathogenesis of amyloidosis, see the textbook.

Reactive (secondary) amyloidosis is a systemic syndrome characterized by tissue deposition of amyloid A protein (AA amyloid). Naturally occurring systemic amyloidosis in domestic animals as well as familial amyloidosis in the Abyssinian cat and Shar pei dog are examples. Chronic inflammation and a prolonged increase in SAA concentration are necessary prerequisites for development of reactive amyloidosis.

CLINICAL FINDINGS (pp. 1766–1767)

HISTORY

In dogs and cats, amyloid deposits in the kidneys lead to progressive renal disease, and the observed clinical signs usually are those of chronic renal failure and uremia. Ascites, edema, acute dyspnea, or blindness may be the presenting sign. Physical examination findings are variable and usually related to the presence of chronic renal failure and uremia. Many affected Shar pei dogs have a history of episodic joint swelling (usually the tibiotarsal joints) and fever that resolve within a few days, regardless of treatment.

DIAGNOSIS (pp. 1767–1769)

Urinary protein excretion should be quantitated whenever the dipstick method or sulfosalicylic acid test for proteinuria is repeatedly positive and the urine sediment examination is normal. Calculation of the urine protein-creatinine ratio in dogs accurately reflects the quantity of protein excreted in the urine over a 24-hour period. Furthermore, the magnitude of proteinuria is roughly correlated with the severity of the underlying glomerular lesion. A complete urinalysis should be obtained at the time a urine protein-creatinine ratio is evaluated because hematuria or pyuria may result in clinically significant nonglomerular proteinuria. A mean urine protein-creatinine ratio of 22.5 (range, 11.17 to 46.65) was observed in 6 dogs with amyloidosis as compared with 5.73 (range, 0.47 to 43.39) in 26 dogs with glomerulonephritis.

Proteinuria associated with hemorrhage into the urinary tract has an electrophoretic pattern similar to that of the serum, whereas early glomerular damage results primarily in albuminuria. Hypoalbuminemia occurs in many dogs and cats with glomerular disease. Isosthenuria without proteinuria is common in cats with renal medullary amyloidosis. If persistent proteinuria of renal origin is identified, a renal biopsy is indicated. A renal biopsy is necessary to differentiate glomerular amyloidosis from glomerulonephritis. This distinction is important because glomerulonephritis in dogs and cats may have a variable course characterized by clinical remission or stable renal function for an extended period, whereas amyloidosis usually is a progressive, fatal disease. In dogs other than Shar peis, amyloidosis primarily is a glomerular disease and can be diagnosed by renal cortical biopsy. Medullary amyloidosis without discernible glomerular involvement occurs in many domestic cats with amyloidosis and in many Shar pei dogs with familial amyloidosis.

TREATMENT (pp. 1769–1771)

GLOMERULONEPHRITIS

Ideally, elimination of the source of antigenic stimulation is the goal of therapy (Table 135–2).

Immunosuppressive Drugs. Routine use of corticosteroids to treat glomerulonephritis in dogs is not recommended. Treatment with corticosteroids is indicated, however, if the underlying disease process is known to be steroid-responsive (e.g., systemic lupus erythematosus).

Antiinflammatory Treatment. An extremely low dosage of aspirin (0.25 mg/lb PO once or twice a day) may selectively inhibit platelet cyclooxygenase without preventing the beneficial effects of prostacyclin formation.

Hypertension, Ascites, and Thromboembolism.

Anticoagulants. Prophylactic therapy with anticoagulants may be beneficial in patients with severe proteinuria, and measurement of antithrombin III and fibrinogen concentrations may identify those patients at greatest risk of thromboembolism.

AMYLOIDOSIS

Underlying inflammatory or neoplastic disease processes should be diagnosed and treated if possible. Aggressive cytotoxic therapy using

TABLE 135–2. TREATMENT GUIDELINES FOR GLOMERULONEPHRITIS

1. Identify and correct underlying disease processes.
2. Immunosuppressive treatment?
   a. Cyclophosphamide 2.2 mg/kg q24h for 3 or 4 days and then discontinue for 4 or 3 days, respectively
   b. Azathioprine 2 mg/kg q24–48h (dogs only)
   c. Cyclosporine 15 mg/kg q24h (dogs only)
3. Anti-inflammatory—hypercoagulability treatment
   a. Aspirin 0.5 mg/kg q12–24h
   b. Thromboxane synthetase inhibitors or thromboxane receptor antagonists
   c. Warfarin—titrate dose based on prothrombin time
4. Supportive care
   a. Dietary: sodium restriction, high-quality–low-quantity protein (Hill's prescription diets canine and feline K/D)
   b. Hypertension: dietary sodium restriction
      —Captopril 0.2–1.0 mg/kg q8–12 h
      —Enalapril 0.1–0.5 mg/kg q12–24 h
   c. Edema/ascites: dietary sodium restriction
      —Cage rest
      —Furosemide 1–2 mg/kg as needed if necessary. Caution: volume contraction and reduced GFR may results.
      —Paracentesis for patients with tense ascites and/or respiratory distress
      —Plasma transfusions?

drugs such as chlorambucil, cyclophosphamide, and methotrexate has been beneficial in some human patients with reactive amyloidosis.

Dimethylsulfoxide. We have diluted 90 per cent DMSO 1:4 with sterile water before administering it subcutaneously at a dosage of 40 mg/lb three times per week. Whether or not DMSO is beneficial in treatment of renal amyloidosis in dogs remains controversial.

Colchicine. There is no evidence that it is beneficial once amyloidosis has resulted in renal failure. It is interesting to speculate whether administration of colchicine to Shar pei dogs with recurrent fever and tibiotarsal joint swelling could prevent development of renal amyloidosis as it does in human patients with familial Mediterranean fever. It may be reasonable to consider treatment with 0.01 to 0.02 mg/lb/day colchicine in such patients.

COMPLICATIONS OF SEVERE PROTEINURIA
(pp. 1771–1773)

SODIUM RETENTION

The classic explanation for edema or ascites involves activation of the renin-angiotensin-aldosterone system.

HYPERLIPIDEMIA

Hypercholesterolemia (greater than 240 mg/dL) has been observed in 60 per cent of dogs with glomerulonephritis and 86 per cent of dogs with glomerular amyloidosis. In nephrotic patients, plasma albumin concentrations are inversely correlated with plasma cholesterol concentrations.

Hypertension. Systemic hypertension may occur in up to 84 per cent of dogs with glomerular disease. Retinal hemorrhage, detachment, and papilledema may result.

Hypercoagulability. The pulmonary arteries are the most common site for thromboembolism. Dogs with pulmonary thromboembolism usually are dyspneic and hypoxic with minimal pulmonary parenchymal radiographic abnormalities.

Clinical experience suggests that glomerulonephritis is progressive in many instances. The prognosis for dogs and cats with renal amyloidosis is uniformly poor.

CHAPTER 136
BACTERIAL INFECTIONS OF THE URINARY TRACT
(pages 1775–1788)

SIGNIFICANT BACTERIURIA

Identification of bacteria in urine is not synonymous with urinary tract infection. Quantitative urine cultures aid differentiation between bacterial pathogens and contaminants.

INFLAMMATION VERSUS INFECTION

It is essential to distinguish between inflammation and infection related to urinary tract disease. Urine culture, renal function tests, radiographic and ultrasonographic studies, endoscopy, urodynamic studies, and biopsy procedures often provide the additional information necessary to localize the disease process and establish its etiology. Detection of infection should be established by urine culture, since diagnosis based solely on recognition of inflammatory cells in urinalyses will result in overdiagnosis of infection. Conversely, absence of hematuria, pyuria, and proteinuria does not rule out the existence of infection.

CLINICAL MANIFESTATIONS

See Table 136–1.

URINALYSIS (pp. 1779–1780)

Urine sediment should be evaluated for white blood cells utilizing standard techniques. Dipstick leukocyte assays alone are unsatisfactory. Rod- shaped bacteria may be seen in unstained preparations of urine sediment if more than 10,000 bacteria/ml are present, but may not be consistently detected if their numbers are less than 10,000/ml. Cocci are difficult to detect in urine sediment if their numbers are less than 100,000/ml.

DIAGNOSTIC URINE CULTURE (pp. 1780–1782)

Urine should be cultured within 30 minutes from the time of collection. If for any reason rapid culture is not possible, the samples should be immediately refrigerated following collection.

QUANTITATIVE URINE CULTURE

Significant Bacteriuria (see Table 136–2). Quantitative urine culture includes determination of the number of bacteria (colony-form-

Original chapter written by Jody P. Lulich and Carl A. Osborne

TABLE 136–1. ABNORMALITIES THAT HELP LOCALIZE BACTERIAL URINARY TRACT INFECTIONS

SITES OF INFECTION	HISTORY	PHYSICAL EXAMINATION	LABORATORY	RADIOLOGY AND ULTRASOUND
Lower urinary tract	Dysuria, pollakiuria Urge incontinence Signs of abnormal detrussor reflex (overflow incontinence, residual urine) Gross hematuria at end of micturition Cloudy urine with abnormal odor No systemic signs of infection Recent catheterization, urethrostomy	Small, painful, thickened bladder (unless urethra obstructed) Palpable masses in urethra or bladder Flaccid bladder wall: residual urine in bladder lumen Abnormal micturition reflex ± Palpation of uroliths	Normal CBC Urinalysis = pyuria, hematuria, proteinuria, bacteriuria Urine culture (significant bacteriuria)	Kidneys usually not enlarged Structural abnormalities of lower urinary tract ± Urocystoliths and/or urethroliths ± Only thickening of bladder wall and irregularity of mucosa Rarely intraluminal gas formation (emphysematous cystitis)
Upper urinary tract	Polyuria and polydipsia ± Signs of systemic infection ± Signs of renal failure	± No detectable abnormalities ± Fever and other signs of systemic infection ± Abdominal (renal) pain Kidney is normal or increased	± Leukocytosis Urinalysis (variable) = pyuria, hematuria, proteinuria, bacteriuria WBC or granular casts Impaired concentration ± Azotemia and other abnormalities typical of renal failure	Increase in kidney size ± Abnormal kidney shape ± Nephrolithiasis ± Dilated renal pelves; dilated pelvic diverticula ± Evidence of outflow obstruction
Acute prostatitis or prostatic abscess	Urethral discharge independent of micturition Signs of systemic infection ± Reluctance to defecate or micturate	± Fever and other signs of systemic infection ± Painful prostate and/or painful abdomen ± Enlarged or asymmetric prostate	± Leukocytosis Urinalysis = pyuria, hematuria, proteinuria, bacteriuria Cytology (infectious inflammation)	± Indistinct cranial border; enlargement ± Cysts ± Reflux of contrast agent into prostate
Chronic prostatitis	Recurrent urinary tract infections Urethral discharge independent of micturition ± Dysuria	Often no detectable abnormalities ± Enlarged or asymmetric prostate	Normal CBC Similar to acute prostatitis	± Similar to acute prostatitis ± Abnormal prostatic urethra ± Mineralization

654

TABLE 136–2. INTERPRETATION OF QUANTITATIVE URINE CULTURES IN DOGS AND CATS*
(COLONY FORMING UNITS PER MILLILITER OF URINE)

	SIGNIFICANT		SUSPICIOUS		CONTAMINANT	
	Dogs	*Cats*	*Dogs*	*Cats*	*Dogs*	*Cats*
Cystocentesis	≥1000	≥1000	100 to 1000	100 to 1000	≤100	≤100
Catheterization	≥10,000	≥1000	1000 to 10,000	100 to 1000	≤1000	≤100
Voluntary voiding	≥100,000†	≥10,000	10,000 to 90,000	1000 to 10,000	≤10,000	≤1000
Manual compression	≥100,000†	≥10,000	10,000 to 90,000	1000 to 10,000	≤10,000	≤1000

*The data represent generalities. On occasion, bacterial UTI may be detected in dogs and cats with the fewer organisms (i.e., false-negative results).
†Caution: Because contamination of midstream samples may result in colony counts of 10,000/ml or more in some dogs (i.e., false-positive results), they should not be used for routine diagnostic culture of urine from dogs.

TABLE 136-3. PREDICTING SUSCEPTIBILITY OF URINARY BACTERIAL PATHOGENS TO COMMONLY USED ANTIMICROBIAL AGENTS

PATHOGEN	DRUGS OF CHOICE*	ALTERNATIVES*
Enterobacter spp.	Trimethoprim/sulfadiazine	Cephalosporins (1st and 2nd gen.) chloramphenicol, gentamicin, nitrofurantoin
Escherichia coli†	Trimethoprim/sulfadiazine, nitrofurantoin	Cephalosporins (1st, 2nd, and 3rd gen.) chloramphenicol, gentamicin
Klebsiella spp.†	Cephalosporins (1st gen.)	Amikacin, gentamicin, trimethoprim/sulfadiazine, cephalosporins (2nd and 3rd gen.)
Mycoplasma,† *Ureaplasma*	Fluoroquinolones?	Chloramphenicol, doxycycline, erythromycin, oleandomycin, tetracycline
Proteus spp.†	Ampicillin, amoxicillin, penicillin-G	Cephalosporins (1st, 2nd, and 3rd gen.), chloramphenicol, gentamicin, nitrofurantoin, trimethoprim/sulfadiazine
Pseudomonas† *aeruginosa*	Tetracycline	Carbenacillin, gentamicin, trimethoprim/sulfadiazine, cephalosporins (1st, 2nd, 3rd gen.)
Staphylococcus intermedius†	Penicillin-G, ampicillin, amoxicillin	Cephalosporins (1st gen.), chloramphenicol, nitrofurantoin, trimethoprim/sulfadiazine
Streptococcus	Penicillin-G, ampicillin, amoxicillin	Cephalosporins (1st gen.), chloramphenicol, nitrofurantoin, trimethoprim/sulfadiazine

*Enrofloxacin is highly effective in eradication of urinary tract infections caused by these pathogens. It is especially effective against life-threatening antibiotic-resistant or deep-seated gram-negative infections.
†Prior treatment with antimicrobials may alter the susceptibility of bacterial pathogens to these drugs.

ing units) per unit volume in addition to isolation and identification of bacteria. Bacterial contamination of voided and catheterized samples is more likely to occur in female than in male dogs and cats. In general, cystocentesis should be used to collect urine samples for qualitative and quantitative bacterial culture. The presence of bacteria in urine aseptically collected by cystocentesis, even in low numbers, indicates UTI.

TREATMENT (pp. 1782–1787)

ANTIMICROBIAL THERAPY

Antimicrobial Susceptibility Tests. Evaluation of the susceptibility of infecting bacteria to antimicrobial drugs is advisable as a general guide for choice of therapeutic agents because bacteria isolated from dogs and cats with UTI may vary widely in their susceptibility to specific antimicrobial agents. If UTI associated with multiple pathogens is identified, and the organisms do not have similar antimicrobial sensitivities, initial treatment of the predominant pathogen with an effective drug is recommended.

Empiric Choice of Antimicrobial Agents. To ensure adequate concentrations of the drug in the urinary tract between treatments, it is recommended that daily doses be administered shortly following micturition, and especially just prior to a period of confinement during which voiding is not permitted (such as overnight). See Table 136–3.

Duration of Therapy. Duration of therapy should be based on the elimination of UTI as defined by urine cultures in addition to amelioration of pyuria and clinical signs.

Monitoring Response to Therapy. Culture a urine sample collected by cystocentesis 3 to 5 days following initiation of therapy (so-called "test for cure").

Management of Recurrent UTI. Relapse caused by the same organism would be expected to occur shortly after cessation of antimicrobial therapy (see Table 136–4). Reinfection caused by a different organism would be expected to occur later than a relapse (see Table

TABLE 136–4. CHECKLIST OF POTENTIAL CAUSES OF PERSISTENT (RELAPSE) INFECTION WITH SAME TYPE OF BACTERIA

1. Use of improper antimicrobial susceptibility tests and/or misinterpretation of results
2. Mixed infections in which all pathogens were not eradicated by antimicrobial therapy
3. Failure to prescribe antimicrobial agents for a sufficient period to eradicate pathogens (a relapse occurs)
4. Failure to prescribe a proper dosage and/or maintenance interval for an antimicrobial agent that would otherwise be effective
5. Failure or inability of owners to administer the prescribed dosage of antimicrobial agent(s) at the proper maintenance intervals and for sufficient duration
6. Use of ineffective drugs
   a. Ineffective against uropathogens
   b. Fail to attain therapeutic concentration in urine
   c. Fail to achieve therapeutic concentrations at infection sites (especially kidneys, prostate gland, and infection-induced uroliths)
7. Failure to the patient to absorb a portion or all of an orally administered drug because of ingesta or gastrointestinal dysfunction
8. Premature assessment of therapeutic response
9. Initiation of therapy at an advanced state in the evolution of the disease
10. Formation of drug-resistant bacteria, including L-forms

TABLE 136–5. CHECKLIST OF POTENTIAL CAUSES OF REINFECTION WITH DIFFERENT BACTERIA

1. Invalid culture results caused by:
   a. Contamination of specimen during collection, transport, storage, or handling
   b. Improper technique of bacterial culture of urine
2. Continued dysfunction of host defense mechanisms (Table 136–2)
3. Failure to recognize and eliminate a predisposing cause
4. Iatrogenic infection, especially associated with catheterization
5. Sequelae to surgical techniques that have modified host defenses, especially urethrostomies and urine diversion procedures
6. Spontaneous reinfection

136–5). Detection of frequent reinfections following antimicrobial therapy is an absolute indication to evaluate the patient for a predisposing cause (see Table 136–6). Infections of the canine prostate gland are a common cause of recurrent UTI.

Prevention of Recurrent Reinfections. In some dogs with chronic UTI, elimination of predisposing causes may be impossible. The result is recurrent reinfections. In such cases it may be helpful to provide low-dose (preventive) antibacterial therapy for an indefinite period (6 months or more) with drugs primarily eliminated in urine.

ANCILLARY THERAPY

Ancillary forms of therapy include urine acidifiers, urinary antiseptics, local instillation of antimicrobial agents into the urinary bladder, altering urine volume, and use of pharmacologic agents that affect the storage and voiding phases of micturition.

CATHETER-INDUCED INFECTION (pp. 1787)

Concomitant oral or parenteral administration of antimicrobial agents during indwelling urethral catheterization of dogs and cats may

TABLE 136–6. SOME IDENTIFIABLE CAUSES OF COMPLICATED URINARY TRACT INFECTIONS AND THEIR POTENTIAL FOR CORRECTION BY THE SURGEON

I. Interference with normal micturition
   A. Mechanical obstruction to outflow
      1. Uroliths and strictures (especially of urethra)
      2. Herniated urinary bladder
      3. Prostatic cysts, abscesses, or neoplasms
      4. Obstructing urothelial neoplasms
   B. Incomplete emptying of excretory pathway
      1. Damaged innervation
         a. Vertebral fractures, luxations, subluxations
         b. Intervertebral disc disease
         c. Vertebral osteomyelitis
         d. Neoplasia
         e. Vertebral or spinal cord anomalies
         f. Reflex dyssynergia
      2. Anatomic defects
         a. Diverticula of urethra, bladder, ureters, renal pelves (especially persistent urachal diverticula
         b. Vesicoureteral reflux

TABLE 136–6. (*Continued*)

II. Anatomic defects
   A. Congenital or inherited
      1. Urethral anomalies
      2. Ectopic ureters
      3. Persistent urachal diverticula
      4. Primary vesicoureteral reflux
   B. Acquired
      1. Diseases of the urinary tract, especially lower portions
      2. Secondary vesicoureteral reflux
      3. Urethrostomy, trigonal-colonic anastomosis, and other surgical diversion procedures
III. Alteration of urothelium
   A. Trauma
      1. External force
      2. Palpation
      3. Catheterization and other instrumentation
      4. Urolithiasis
   B. Metaplasia
      1. Administration of estrogens
      2. Estrogen-producing sertoli cell neoplasms
   C. Neoplasia
   D. Urinary excretion of cytotoxic drugs such as cyclophosphamide
   E. Others
IV. Alterations in the volume, frequency, or composition of urine
   A. Decreased urine volume
      1. Negative water balance
         a. Decreased water consumption
         b. Vomiting and/or diarrhea
      2. Primary oliguric renal failure
   B. Voluntary or involuntary retention
   C. Glucosuria
   D. Formation of dilute urine*
V. Impaired Immunocompetence
   A. Diseases
      1. Congenital immunodeficiency?
      2. Acquired
         a. Hyperadrenocorticism?
         b. Uremia
   B. Corticosteroids; immunosuppressant drugs

*Formation of dilute urine predisposes the patient to lower UTI but may prevent or minimize bacterial infections of the renal medulla.

reduce the frequency of development of bacterial UTI, but alters the flora and promotes development of UTI caused by bacteria with resistance to multiple antimicrobial agents. Dog's with hyperadrenocorticism, diabetes mellitus, and uremia are at risk for iatrogenic UTI. Iatrogenic infection is least likely to occur as a consequence of a single brief catheterization. Risk of iatrogenic infection is greatest during indwelling catheterization, especially when the portion of catheter protruding from the urethra is not connected to a receptacle (i.e., it is open). In general, the risk of infection during indwelling catheterization is proportional to the duration of catheterization.

CHAPTER 137

TUMORS OF THE URINARY TRACT
(pages 1788–1796)

RENAL NEOPLASIA (pp. 1788–1791)

Primary renal neoplasia is rare in the dog and cat. Metastatic cancer to the kidney is more common. Male dogs are twice as likely as females to develop epithelial tumors (e.g., renal cell carcinoma, transitional cell carcinoma). The only breed predilection is in the German shepherd dog, in which renal cystadenocarcinoma appears to be inherited in an autosomal dominant manner. Hematuria (microscopic or gross) is present in only 10 to 33 per cent of dogs with renal tumors. More commonly, dogs with renal tumors are inappetent and depressed, and they experience significant weight loss. A palpable abdominal mass can be found in approximately half of the dogs. Anemia and azotemia are common findings. Paraneoplastic syndromes associated with renal tumors in dogs and cats include hypertrophic osteopathy, polycythemia, extreme neutrophilic leukocytosis, and cachexia.

Radiographs may reveal renomegaly or irregular outlines of the kidney(s). Frequently, the mass is so large that normal abdominal anatomy is obscured. Intravenous pyelograms increase the accuracy to over 90 per cent in confirming a mass as being renal. Intravenous pyelograms also provide a rough estimate of renal function in the contralateral kidney. Azotemia remains a relative contraindication for contrast studies. Thoracic radiographs are also recommended as pulmonary metastases are present in approximately one-third of dogs with renal carcinoma at presentation. Ultrasonography is particularly useful in identifying a mass as originating from the kidney and in evaluating the contralateral kidney and other intra-abdominal organs for metastatic neoplasia. This modality is also useful in ruling out hydronephrosis, polycystic kidney disease, and perinephric and renal cysts from consideration as causes of a renal mass. Urine cultures should be collected as secondary bacterial infection is common in animals with renal neoplasia. It is vital not to remove a kidney without evaluating the overall renal function of the patient as fully as possible using biochemical profiles, excretory urography, ultrasonography, or nuclear medicine.

Frequently, by the time of detection, the entire kidney has been invaded and destroyed. Extrarenal invasion into the epaxial musculature, adrenal gland, and vena cava is common. Renal carcinoma is considered to have a high metastatic rate. Surgery has been the mainstay of unilateral renal cancer treatment. Chemotherapy has generally been unrewarding for renal cell carcinoma. Vinblastine appears to be the most effective agent and yields response rates no greater than 10 to 15 per cent.

NEPHROBLASTOMA

Sixty per cent of the reported cases occur in dogs under one year of age. Unilateral nephrectomy is the treatment of choice.

FELINE RENAL LYMPHOMA

Renal lymphoma is the most common primary renal neoplasm in the cat. The most common clinical presentation is bilateral renomegaly in

---

Original chapter written by Alan S. Hammer and Susan LaRue

a cat with clinical signs of renal failure. Differential diagnoses should include perinephric pseudocysts, polycystic kidney disease, FIP, and pyelonephrosis or renal abscesses. Fine-needle aspirate cytology and renal biopsy are the diagnostic tests of choice. Nephrectomy is not considered a desirable treatment option. Cats with renal lymphoma test positive for FeLV approximately 50 per cent of the time. It is recommended that cytosine arabinoside be included in the chemotherapy protocols of all cats with renal lymphoma. Treatment protocols are reviewed in Chapter 73 of the textbook.

BLADDER TUMORS (pp. 1791–1794)

In contrast to the cat, in which there are almost as many mesenchymal tumors as there are epithelial, over 80 per cent of bladder tumors in the dog are transitional cell carcinoma. Another risk factor for the development of bladder cancer is obesity. Presenting complaints include incontinence, stranguria, hematuria, dysuria, pollalunis, polydipsia, and polyuria. Systemic signs of illness, such as weight loss, are less common. Urinary tract infections are common in dogs and cats with bladder tumors, and the urine should always be cultured. Paraneoplastic syndromes reported in animals with bladder tumors include hypercalcemia, hypertrophic osteopathy, hyperestrogenism, hypereosinophilia, and cancer cachexia.

Thoracic radiographs should be taken in every animal with suspected bladder neoplasia. Contrast cystography (either positive, negative, or double contrast) may reveal irregular bladder wall filling defects or diffuse thickening. In general, trigonal involvement is most likely to occur with transitional cell carcinoma. Ultrasonography is extremely useful in identifying the bladder mass, in evaluating the kidneys and ureters for hydronephrosis, and in evaluating the liver, spleen, omentum, and lymph nodes for metastatic disease.

TRANSITIONAL CELL CARCINOMA

Transitional cell carcinoma has a strong predilection for the trigone region of the bladder. Eventually, 50 per cent or more of transitional cell carcinomas will metastasize widely. Surgery remains the standard of treatment for dogs and cats with transitional cell carcinoma. It should be noted that complete resections are uncommon and usually limited to animals with tumors in the apex or fundus. Radiotherapy has been utilized as an adjunct to surgery. Systemic chemotherapy has been only partially successful. Cisplatin (40 to 60 mg/m^2) has been the drug most widely used. Cisplatin is nephrotoxic and should not be used in dogs that are azotemic; additionally, cisplatin cannot be used in cats. Protocols that may have some efficacy against transitional cell carcinoma are listed in Table 137–1.

RHABDOMYOSARCOMA

Rhabdomyosarcoma (botryoid rhabdomyosarcoma) is a relatively rare tumor of young, large-breed dogs. The Saint Bernard is the most frequent breed reported. Survival times following surgery are usually short.

URETHRAL TUMORS (pp. 1794–1795)

Primary urethral tumors are fortunately rare in dogs and even rarer in cats. There is a strong female predilection. Hematuria and stranguria are almost invariably part of the presenting complaint. Rectal and vaginal examination often reveals a firm mass or hard, corrugated urethra. Azotemia secondary to obstruction is the main laboratory abnormality.

The imaging technique of choice is contrast cystography and void-

TABLE 137–1. CHEMOTHERAPY PROTOCOLS FOR CANINE TRANSITIONAL CELL CARCINOMA

Protocol A.	Mitoxantrone, 4.5 mg/m^2 IV over 4 hours on day 1
	Cyclophosphamide, 100 mg/m^2 IV on day 8*
	5-fluorouracil, 150 mg/m^2 IV on day 15
Protocol B.	Actinomycin D, 0.7 mg/m^2 IV on day 1
	Cyclophosphamide, 100 mg/m^2 IV on day 8*
	Methotrexate, 5–10 mg/m^2 IV on day 15†
Protocol C.	Cisplatin, 40–60 mg/m^2 IV every 21 days using a saline diuresis protocol

*May substitute vincristine 0.7 mg/m^2 IV.
†Methotrexate often causes gastrointestinal toxicity and may necessitate dose reduction.

ing contrast urethrography. It is important to evaluate the sublumbar region and the vertebral bodies for evidence of metastatic disease. Aspiration biopsy could be utilized to obtain cytologic or, occasionally, histopathologic specimens. Briefly, this involves aspirating plugs of mucosa through the side ports of a flexible urethral catheter. As with bladder tumors, urinary cultures should be obtained.

Because of local invasion and the anatomic area involved, few cases will be amenable to surgical resection. At The Ohio State University, patients treated with radiotherapy often had clinical improvement, and the tumor was palpably smaller within 7 fractions. The limited vascular supply renders the colon particularly sensitive to vascular damage due to irradiation. Chemotherapy protocols used are similar to those used for bladder tumors (see Table 137–1). There is frequently no evidence of significant shrinkage of the primary tumor by chemotherapy alone.

CHAPTER 138

FAMILIAL RENAL DISEASE IN DOGS AND CATS
(pages 1796–1801)

Most familial renal diseases are progressive and ultimately fatal, and therapy usually is limited to conservative medical management of chronic renal failure (see textbook Chapter 134). The primary nature of the renal disease and its mode of inheritance, if known or suspected, are listed in Table 138–1.

HISTORY AND PHYSICAL FINDINGS (p. 1797)

The most common historical findings in dogs and cats with chronic renal failure due to familial renal disease are anorexia, lethargy, stunted growth or weight loss, polyuria and polydipsia, and vomiting. In the Pembroke Welsh corgi with renal telangiectasia, the most common

Original chapter written by Stephen P. DiBartola

client complaints are hematuria, dysuria, and apparent abdominal pain. Signs of fibrous osteodystrophy such as "rubber jaw" or pathologic fractures usually are detected in young growing dogs with renal failure. Signs of renal osteodystrophy rarely are apparent in older dogs with renal failure.

LABORATORY FINDINGS (pp. 1797–1798)

The most common laboratory findings in dogs with familial renal disease resulting in chronic renal failure are azotemia, hyperphosphatemia, isosthenuria, and nonregenerative anemia. Glucosuria is found in Norwegian elkhounds and Basenjis with primary renal tubular disorders. Juvenile renal disease in the Basenji is an animal model of Fanconi syndrome in man and is characterized by glucosuria, proteinuria, isosthenuria, and amino aciduria. In Welsh corgi dogs with renal telangiectasia, the major laboratory finding is hematuria.

PATHOLOGIC FINDINGS (pp. 1798–1800)

Selected breed peculiarities are listed below. See also Table 138–1.

Abyssinian Cat. Abyssinian cats with familial amyloidosis usually are presented between 1 and 5 years of age. Proteinuria is a variable clinical finding and reflects the severity of glomerular involvement. The principal pathologic lesions are medullary amyloid deposits.

Doberman Pinscher. Unilateral renal aplasia has been observed in some affected female Doberman pinschers.

Norwegian Elkhound. Norwegian elkhounds may also develop primary renal glucosuria that is not associated with chronic renal failure.

Samoyed. Affected male Samoyed dogs with hereditary glomerulopathy develop proteinuria, glucosuria, and isosthenuria by 2 to 3 months of age, and they develop azotemia and overt renal failure by 6 to 9 months of age. Carrier female dogs develop proteinuria at 2 to 3 months of age but remain clinically normal. Deterioration of basement membranes and onset of renal failure in affected male dogs can be delayed but not prevented by feeding a diet low in protein and phosphorus beginning at one month of age.

Soft-coated Wheaten Terrier. Numerous cystic lesions may be noted grossly in the cortex. Familial renal disease in the soft-coated Wheaten terrier may take the form of renal dysplasia or membranoproliferative glomerulonephritis. Dogs with renal dysplasia were <3 years of age when examined, whereas those with glomerulonephritis were 2 to 11 years of age.

Welsh Corgi. Welsh corgis with renal telangiectasia have red to black nodules in the kidneys. Hydronephrosis (presumably due to ureteral obstruction) occurs in almost half of all affected dogs. Similar nodular lesions may be identified in other tissues.

TABLE 138-1. FAMILIAL RENAL DISEASES OF DOGS AND CATS

BREED	DISEASE DESCRIPTION	AGE AT PRESENTATION	INHERITANCE	PROGRESSIVE RENAL FAILURE?
Abyssinian cat	Amyloidosis	1–5 yrs	Autosomal dominant (incomplete penetrance)*	Yes
Beagle	Amyloidosis	5–11 yrs	Unknown	Yes
Shar pei	Amyloidosis	1–6 yrs	Unknown	Yes
Basenji	Tubular dysfunction (Fanconi syndrome)	1–5 yrs	Unknown	Variable
Norwegian elkhound	Tubular dysfunction (renal glucosuria)	NR	Unknown	No
Beagle	Unilateral renal agenesis	Incidental finding	Unknown	No
Bull terrier	Basement membrane disorder	1–8 yrs	Autosomal dominant	Yes
Doberman pinscher	Basement membrane disorder	<1–6 yrs	Unknown	Yes
Samoyed	Basement membrane disorder	<1 yr (males)	X-linked dominant	In males
Rottweiler	Glomerular disease	≤1 yr	Unknown	Yes
Soft-coated Wheaten terrier	Glomerular disease	2–11 yrs	Unknown	Yes
Cocker spaniel	Glomerular disease (suspected)	<1–4 yrs	Unknown	Yes
Norwegian elkhound	Periglomerular fibrosis (primary lesion unknown)	<1–5 yrs	Unknown	Yes
Cairn terrier	Polycystic kidneys	6 wks	Autosomal recessive*	NR
Persian cat	Polycystic kidneys	3–10 yrs	Autosomal dominant	Yes
Chow	Renal dysplasia	<1–5 yrs	Unknown	Yes
Lhasa apso & Shih tzu	Renal dysplasia	<1–5 yrs	Unknown	Yes
Miniature schnauzer	Renal dysplasia	<1–3 yrs	Unknown	Yes
Soft-coated Wheaten terrier	Renal dysplasia	<1–3 yrs	Unknown	Yes
Standard poodle	Renal dysplasia	<1–2 yrs	Unknown	Yes
German shepherd	Multiple cystadenocarcinomas	5–11 yrs	Autosomal dominant*	Variable
Pembroke Welsh corgi	Telangiectasia	5–13 yrs	Unknown	No

NR = not reported.
*Suspected.

CHAPTER 139

RENAL TUBULAR DISORDERS
(pages 1801–1804)

RENAL GLUCOSURIA (p. 1801)

Diagnosis requires documentation of persistent glucosuria without ketonuria and with normal blood glucose concentration. There is no specific treatment.

FANCONI SYNDROME (pp. 1801–1802)

This syndrome is characterized by the presence of multiple renal tubular reabsorptive defects in Basenji dogs. Rapid progression and death may result.

Reabsorption of glucose, phosphate, and amino acids is abnormal in all affected dogs. Many dogs also have variably severe reabsorptive defects for bicarbonate, sodium, potassium, and urate. Defective urinary concentrating ability in dogs with Fanconi syndrome represents a form of nephrogenic diabetes insipidus. Proteinuria usually is mild. Metabolic acidosis is variable in severity and hyperchloremic in nature. Renal clearance studies to identify reabsorptive defects for electrolytes and amino acids are necessary to differentiate Fanconi syndrome from primary renal glucosuria. Treatment of dogs with Fanconi syndrome is limited to control of metabolic acidosis, appropriate antibiotic therapy for urinary tract infection, and conservative medical management of chronic renal failure. The clinician should strive to maintain a serum bicarbonate or total CO_2 concentration above 12 mEq/L and a serum potassium concentration of 3.5 to 5.5 mEq/L.

RENAL TUBULAR ACIDOSIS (p. 1802)

In *distal (classic or type 1) RTA,* the urine cannot be maximally acidified because of impaired H^+ ion secretion in the collecting ducts. Increased urine pH (>6.0) in the face of acidosis is the hallmark of distal RTA. Urinary tract infection by a urease-positive organism must be ruled out before the diagnosis of distal RTA is considered. In *proximal (type 2) RTA,* renal reabsorption of HCO_3^- is markedly reduced. The diagnosis of proximal RTA is made by finding acidic urine (pH <5.5 to 6.0) in the face of hyperchloremic metabolic acidosis and normal GFR, but an increased urine pH (>6.0) and increased urinary fractional excretion of HCO_3^- (>15 per cent) after plasma HCO_3^- concentration has been increased to normal. The clinical features of proximal (type 2) and distal (type 1) RTA are summarized in Table 139–1.

CYSTINURIA (p. 1803)

Cystinuria is an inborn error of metabolism. The low solubility of cystine in acidic urine predisposes to cystine stone formation. Clinical signs (e.g., dysuria, hematuria) may be related to the presence of cystic or urethral calculi or an associated urinary tract infection. Almost all dogs with cystinuria are males. Cystine crystals should be considered abnormal if observed in the urine of any dog or cat. Alkalinization of the urine using sodium bicarbonate or potassium citrate may be benefi-

Original chapter written by Stephen P. DiBartola

TABLE 139–1. CLINICAL FEATURES OF PROXIMAL AND DISTAL RENAL TUBULAR ACIDOSIS

	PROXIMAL RTA	DISTAL RTA
Hypercalciuria	Yes	Yes
Hyperphosphaturia	Yes	Yes
Urinary citrate	Normal	Decreased
Bone disease	Less severe	More severe
Nephrocalcinosis	No	Yes
Nephrolithiasis	No	Yes (calcium phosphate)
Hypokalemia	Mild	Mild to severe
Potassium wasting	Worsened by NaHCO$_3$	Improved by NaHCO$_3$
Alkali required for treatment	>5 mEq/lb/day	<2 mEq/lb/day
Other defects of proximal tubular function*	Yes	No
Reduction in plasma HCO$_3^-$	Moderate	Variable (can be severe)
FE$_{HCO_3}$ at normal plasma HCO$_3^-$ concentration†	>15%	<5%
Urine pH during acidemia	<5.5	>6.0
Urine pH after NH$_4$Cl	<5.5	>6.0

*Decreased fractional reabsorption of sodium, potassium, phosphate, urate, glucose, and amino acids.
†FE = fractional excretion.

cial in cystinuric patients. Potassium citrate may be preferable. D-penicillamine forms a disulfide with cysteine that is much more soluble and may be used at a dosage of 10 to 15 mg/lb/day divided into two daily doses. 2-Mercaptopropionylglycine has a similar mechanism of action. It has been used at a dosage of 15 to 20 mg/lb/day.

URATE TRANSPORT IN THE DALMATIAN
(pp. 1803–1804)

The liver plays the dominant role in determining the urinary excretory pattern of urate in dogs. Only a small percentage of Dalmatians develop urate stones. Furthermore, urate urolithiasis occurs in non-Dalmatian dogs and may complicate the clinical course of dogs with portosystemic shunts. The stones that form are relatively radiolucent.

Treatment of Dalmatian dogs with urate urolithiasis has included inhibition of purine metabolism, alkalinization of urine, induction of polyuria by addition of salt to the diet, and dietary changes designed to reduce purine intake. Allopurinol is used at a dosage of 5 mg/lb PO three times a day. Xanthine stones may develop in dogs receiving allopurinol. Dogs treated with allopurinol should be monitored by following urine urate/creatinine ratios. Alkalinization of urine (to pH 7.0 to 7.5) has been recommended in the preventive management. It has been recommended that polyuria be induced by addition of salt to the diet. It is unclear whether alkalinization of urine and induction of polyuria actually are beneficial. Diets low in protein also have been recommended.

NEPHROGENIC DIABETES INSIPIDUS (p. 1804)

Congenital nephrogenic diabetes insipidus is a rare disorder in small animal medicine. Affected animals are presented at a young age for severe polyuria and polydipsia. Urine osmolality and specific gravity have been in the hyposthenuric range (urine osmolality, <200 mOsm/kg;

urine specific gravity, 1.002 to 1.005). Thiazide diuretics (chlorothiazide, 10 to 20 mg/lb twice a day, or hydrochlorothiazide, 1 to 2 mg/lb twice a day) have been used to treat animals with congenital NDI. Restriction of dietary sodium and protein further reduce obligatory water loss and polyuria.

CHAPTER 140

FELINE LOWER URINARY TRACT DISEASES
(pages 1805–1832)

There are three different, but common, clinical manifestations of naturally occurring feline lower urinary tract disease: (1) nonobstructive hematuria and dysuria; (2) urolithiasis; and (3) obstruction with matrix-crystalline urethral plugs.

DIAGNOSIS AND TREATMENT OF ANATOMIC ABNORMALITIES (pp. 1808–1810)

VESICOURACHAL DIVERTICULA

Congenital and Acquired Vesicourachal Diverticula

Congenital macroscopic vesicourachal diverticula are uncommon. Persistent congenital macroscopic diverticula may predispose to urinary tract infection. In the second and most common form, microscopic remnants of the urachus located at the bladder vertex of cats remain clinically silent until lower urinary tract disease associated with increased bladder lumen pressure develops.

Diagnosis of Vesicourachal Diverticula

Feline vesicourachal diverticula are best identified by radiographic studies. Positive antegrade cystourethrography and retrograde positive contrast urethrocystography are the procedures of choice. Complete distention of the lumen of the urinary bladder with contrast media is usually recommended.

Treatment of Vesicourachal Diverticula

Most macroscopic diverticula of the bladder vertex are a sequela of lower urinary tract dysfunction. Furthermore, macroscopic diverticula may be self-limiting. If bacterial urinary tract infection is confirmed, it should be treated with appropriate antimicrobics. If a macroscopic diverticulum of the bladder vertex persists for more than 4 to 8 weeks in a cat with persistent or recurrent urinary tract infection, diverticulectomy should be considered.

Cats with acquired diverticula of the bladder vertex and sterile struvite or infection-induced struvite urocystoliths may be successfully managed by medical therapy. Because effective protocols to induce

Original chapter written by Carl A. Osborne, John M. Kruger, Jody P. Lulich, and David J. Polzin

medical dissolution of feline calcium oxalate, calcium phosphate, ammonium urate, uric acid and cystine urocystoliths have not yet been developed, surgery remains the most reliable method.

URETHRAL STRICTURES

If urethral strictures predispose to clinical signs, corrective surgery should be considered. The lower urinary tract should first be evaluated by antegrade cystourethrography or retrograde urethrocystography.

DIAGNOSIS AND TREATMENT OF INFECTIOUS AGENTS (pp. 1810–1815)

VIRAL URINARY TRACT INFECTION

The causative role of FCV in feline LUTD (feline lower urinary tract disorder) has not been conclusively shown.

Diagnosis. Exclusion of other known causes of hematuria, dysuria, and urethral obstruction should precede attempts to establish a diagnosis of viral urinary tract infection. Diagnostic criteria for viral infections include (1) isolation and identification of viral agents, (2) direct demonstration of virus particles, viral antigens, or viral nucleic acids in tissues or body fluids, and/or (3) detection and quantification of specific viral antibodies.

Treatment. Antiviral agents have not been evaluated in cats with LUTD.

BACTERIAL URINARY TRACT INFECTION

See Chapter 140 in the textbook.

When bacterial UTI has been detected in cats it frequently occurred as a secondary or complicating factor rather than as a primary etiologic factor.

Treatment. The infrequency with which bacterial uropathogens are isolated from cats with LUTD emphasizes that the routine use of antimicrobial agents in treating LUTD is unnecessary.

FUNGAL URINARY TRACT INFECTION

Fungi detected in properly collected urine samples are abnormal. Isolation of fungal organisms from two serial urine samples collected by cystocentesis should be considered significant, regardless of colony count. Flucytosine, amphotericin B, ketoconazole, itraconazole, and fluconazole have been used to treat *Candida* spp. urinary tract infection in man.

PARASITIC URINARY TRACT INFECTION

The nematode *Capillaria feliscati* is the only parasite that has been associated with clinical signs of feline LUTD. Most *C. feliscati* urinary tract infections appear to be asymptomatic. Diagnosis of *C. feliscati* is based on identification of characteristic ova in urine sediment or visualization of adult worms in the urinary bladder. Fenbendazole (11 mg/lb [25 mg/kg] q12h for 3 to 10 days) has been suggested.

DIAGNOSIS, TREATMENT, AND PREVENTION OF UROLITHS AND URETHRAL PLUGS (pp. 1815–1829)

Detection of a urolith is not always justification for surgical management. In cats, small uroliths may remain asymptomatic within the urinary tract (especially the renal pelvis and urinary bladder) for months or years. If the urolith(s) remain inactive, therapy designed to dissolve or remove them is not mandatory.

DIAGNOSIS

Uroliths. Radiographic and/or ultrasonographic evaluation of the urinary tract is required to consistently detect feline uroliths. Double-contrast cystography is usually required to detect urocystoliths less than 3 mm in diameter. Quantitative mineral analyses of representative portions of uroliths by polarizing light microscopy, infrared spectroscopy, x-ray difractometry, and energy-dispersive x-ray spectroscopy remain the diagnostic standards (Table 140–1).

AMMONIUM URATE UROLITHS

The cause of formation of most feline urate uroliths has not been established.

Treatment and Prevention. Medical protocols that consistently promote dissolution of ammonium urate uroliths in cats have not yet been developed. Surgery remains the most reliable method to remove larger, inactive uroliths. Prevention should encompass consumption of diets that are low in purine precursors (e.g., low in liver) and promote formation of less acid urine (pH ± 7) that is not highly concentrated.

TABLE 140–1. CHECKLIST OF FACTORS THAT SUGGEST PROBABLE MINERAL COMPOSITION OF FELINE UROLITHS

---

1. Urine pH
   a. Struvite and calcium apatite uroliths, usually alkaline. Sterile struvite uroliths may be observed with urine pH 6.5 or higher
   b. Ammonium urate uroliths, acid to neutral
   c. Cystine uroliths, acid*
   d. Calcium oxalate, often acid to neutral*
2. Identification of crystals in uncontaminated fresh urine sediment, preferably at body temperature
3. Type of bacteria, if any, isolated from urine
   a. Urease from bacteria, especially staphylococci and less frequently *Proteus* spp, may be associated with struvite uroliths
   b. UTI often are absent in patients with calcium oxalate, cystine, or ammonium urate
   c. Calcium oxalate, cystine, or ammonium urate uroliths may predispose to UTI; if infections are caused by urease-producing bacteria, struvite may precipitate around metabolic uroliths
4. Radiographic density and physical characteristics of uroliths
5. Serum chemistry evaluation
   a. Hypercalcemia may be associated with calcium-containing uroliths
   b. Hyperuricemia may be associated with uric acid or urate uroliths
   c. Hyerchloremia, hypokalemia, and acidemia may be associated with distal renal tubular acidosis and calcium phosphate or struvite uroliths
6. Urine chemistry evaluation
   a. Patient should be consuming a standard diagnostic diet or the diet consumed when uroliths formed
   b. Excessive quantities of one or more minerals contained in the urolith are expected. The concentration of crystallization inhibitors may be decreased
7. Breed of cat and history of uroliths in patient's ancestors or littermates
8. Drugs
   a. Corticosteroids and furosemide predispose to hypercalciuria
   b. Allopurinol predispose to xanthine
   c. Drugs containing sulfadiazine predispose to formation of uroliths containing varying quantities of sulfadiazine
9. Quantitative analysis of uroliths passed during micturition or collected via catheter technique

---

*Concomitant infection with urease-producing microbes may result in formation of alkaline urine.

CALCIUM OXALATE UROLITHS

There may be a higher prevalence of calcium oxalate uroliths in Burmese, Himalayan, and Persian breeds.

Treatment and Prevention. Medical protocols that will promote dissolution of calcium oxalate uroliths in cats are unavailable as yet. Surgery is the only practical alternative for removal of larger active calcium oxalate uroliths. However, some calcium oxalate uroliths, especially those located in the kidneys, may remain clinically silent for months to years. In cats with hypercalcemia, the cause of hypercalcemia (e.g., primary hyperparathyroidism) should be corrected.

Dietary Considerations. Humans with calcium oxalate uroliths are often advised to avoid milk and milk products as well as foods containing relatively high quantities of oxalic acid (chocolate, nuts, beans, sweet potatoes, wheat germ, spinach, and rhubarb). A diet with reduced quantities of protein, calcium, and sodium and one that does not promote formation of acidic urine (such as Prescription Diet Feline k/d, Hill's Pet Products, Topeka, KS) should be considered. Ideally, diets should not be restricted or supplemented with phosphorus or magnesium. The diet should be adequately fortified with vitamin B since vitamin B_6.

Citrate. Potassium citrate (Urocit-K, Mission Pharmaceuticals, San Antonio, Texas) recommended at a dose of 100 to 150 mg/kg/day (divided into two or three doses).

Thiazide Diuretics. Because thiazide diuretic administration can be associated with adverse affects, we cannot yet recommend their routine use.

CALCIUM PHOSPHATE UROLITHS

Calcium phosphate uroliths may occur in association with primary hyperparathyroidism.

Treatment and Prevention. Protocols designed to dissolve or prevent calcium phosphate uroliths in cats have not been studied. Surgery remains the most reliable method for removing larger active uroliths.

STRUVITE UROLITHS

Naturally Occurring Sterile Struvite Uroliths. Approximately 60 per cent of the naturally occurring uroliths removed from cats contain primarily struvite.

Naturally Occurring Infection-Induced Struvite Uroliths. Rather than being linked to urinary excretion of excessive quantities of dietary minerals, the etiopathogenesis of infection-induced struvite is linked to microbial urease that hydrolyzes urea. In cats, infection-induced struvite uroliths are far less common than sterile struvite uroliths.

Treatment. Key components in inducing dissolution of most struvite uroliths in cats appear to be (1) reduction of urine pH to approximately 6.0, and (2) reduction of urine magnesium by consumption of magnesium-restricted diets (Table 140–2). Since the feline struvitolytic diet Hills' s/d is supplemented with sodium chloride, and since it is formulated to produce aciduria, neither sodium chloride nor urine acidifiers should be concomitantly given with it. If nonacidifying diets are used, acidifiers may be mixed with them. Adequate acidification to prevent sterile struvite uroliths has been achieved with methionine (approximately 1000 mg/cat/day) or ammonium chloride (approximately 800 mg/cat/day).

Infection-Induced Struvite Uroliths. In addition to dietary therapy, it is essential to utilize antimicrobics as long as infection-induced struvite uroliths can be radiographically detected.

TABLE 140–2. SUMMARY OF RECOMMENDATIONS FOR MEDICAL DISSOLUTION OF FELINE STRUVITE UROLITHS

1. Perform appropriate diagnostic studies, including complete urinalyses, quantitative urine culture, and diagnostic radiography. Guesstimate urolith composition by evaluation of appropriate clinical data.
2. Initiate dietary management designed to reduce the urine concentration of magnesium and create a pH of approximately 6. No other food should be fed to patients consuming calculolytic diets. Monitor urine pH 4 to 8 hours after eating. Urine that is acid at this time is likely to be acid throughout the day.
3. Although attempts may be made to stimulate thirst-induced diuresis by addition of sodium chloride to the diet, it is not essential. Thirst-induced diuresis may be of benefit to patients with slowly dissolving uroliths.
4. Antimicrobic therapy
   a. Sterile struvite: Attempt to eradicate or control secondary urinary tract infections with antimicrobial agents. Although control of secondary urinary tract infection is not essential to induce sterile struvite urolith dissolution, it is warranted to prevent damage of tissues of the urinary tract by bacteria and their metabolites.
   b. Infection-induced struvite: initiate antimicrobic therapy to eradicate or control urease-positive urinary tract infections. Maintain therapy as long as uroliths can be detected by radiography.
5. Periodically (2- to 4-week intervals) monitor the size of uroliths by survey radiography. Survey radiography is preferable to retrograde contrast radiography to monitor urolith dissolution because use of catheters during retrograde radiographic studies may result in iatrogenic urinary tract infection. Alternatively, intravenous urography may be considered.
6. Periodic evaluation of urine sediment for crystalluria may be considered. *In vivo* struvite crystals should not form if therapy has been effective in promoting formation of urine that is undersaturated with magnesium ammonium phosphate.
7. Continue calculolytic diet therapy for at least 1 month following radiographic disappearance of uroliths. The rationale is to provide therapy of adequate duration to dissolve small uroliths that cannot be detected by survey radiography.
8. If uroliths increase in size during dietary management, or do not begin to decrease in size after approximately 4 to 8 weeks of appropriate medical management, alternative methods should be considered. Difficulty in inducing complete dissolution of uroliths by creating urine that is undersaturated with the suspected calculogenic crystalloid should prompt consideration that: (1) The wrong mineral component was identified (see Table 140–13 in the textbook); (2) the nucleus of the urolith is of different mineral composition than other portions of the uroliths; and (3) the owner of the patient is not complying with medical recommendations.

URETHRAL PLUGS

Treatment of Urethral Plugs

Medical Treatment. Obstructive uropathy that persists longer than about 24 hours usually results in postrenal uremia. In severe cases, initiation of supportive therapy to correct hyperkalemia, metabolic acidosis, and volume depletion should be initiated immediately after decompression of the excretory pathway by cystocentesis.

Reestablishment of Urethral Patency. Reverse flushing solutions may be effective in dissolving urethral plugs. We do not recommend use of local anesthetic agents as primary reverse flushing solutions since they may induce systemic toxicity. Short-acting barbiturates (thiamylal) that are metabolized by the liver, propofol, and/or inhalant anesthetics may be considered if general anesthesia is required. If ketamine hydrochloride is used, caution must be used since it is excreted in active form by the kidneys. Low doses (1 to 2 mg/kg/IV) have been successfully used by many clinicians. We recommend a step-by-step priority of procedures when attempting to restore urethral patency in an obstructed male cat: (1) *Gentle massage* of the penis between the thumb and fingers. Plugs located in the preprostatic (abdominal) or membranous (pelvic) urethra may occasionally be dislodged by massage of the urethra per rectum. (2) Digitally compressing the urinary bladder may, *following* urethral massage, dislodge fragments of urethral precipitates. (3) In general, *cystocentesis* should be performed if the aforementioned techniques are ineffective. In the event that patency of the urethra is not established before the bladder fills with urine again, decompressive cystocentesis should be repeated. (4) *Flushing the urethral lumen* with sterilized solutions following urethral catheterization may dislodge urethral plugs and uroliths. The general guidelines to be followed when reverse flushing feline urethras to reestablish patency are outlined in Table 140–3. (5) Inability to establish adequate urethral patency by use of catheters and reverse flushing should arouse a high index of suspicion that the underlying cause is not a urethral plug.

Immediate Aftercare. After urine flow has been reestablished by nonsurgical techniques, most of the urine should be removed from the bladder lumen. Following relief of urethral obstruction, a transitory obligatory postobstructive diuresis may develop. Therefore, it may be necessary to supplement water intake with parenteral administration of rehydrating or maintenance fluids.

Indwelling Transurethral Catheters. We do not recommend routine use of indwelling urinary catheters in cats following relief of urethral obstruction. Indwelling urinary catheters may be indicated following relief of urethral obstruction to (1) facilitate measurement of urine formation rate during intensive care of critically ill cats, (2) promote recovery of detrusor atony by maintaining an empty bladder, and (3) prevent recurrence of urethral obstruction caused by urine precipitates or mural abnormalities in high-risk patients. Sterilized catheters composed of soft pliable material are preferred. Insertion of an excessive length of catheter should be avoided. The urethral catheter should be connected to a closed sterilized drainage system when possible. Consider administration of antibiotics during indwelling transurethral catheterization only if evidence of infection is detected.

Hypotonic Urinary Bladders and Reflex Dyssynergia. Once urethral patency has been reestablished, therapy designed to maintain relatively low pressure within the bladder lumen often results in restoration of normal micturition reflex. One alternative consists of trial therapy with bethanechol, a parasympathomimetic agent. The recommended oral dosage for cats is 1.25 to 2.5 mg q8h. Bethanechol may be given in conjunction with phenoxybenzamine, an alpha-adrenergic antagonist, to facilitate relaxation of smooth muscle in the proximal urethra (oral dose = 2.5 up to 10 mg once a day). Alternatively, an indwelling catheter with its tip located within the bladder lumen may be utilized. Reflex dyssynergia may be a cause or complication of urethral outflow obstruction in male cats. The suggested treatment of this complex of neuromuscular dysfunction is administration of an alpha-adrenergic blocking agent (phenoxybenzamine). Simultaneously, the hypotonic detrusor muscle may be treated with bethanechol at the dosage described above.

Prevention of Urethral Plugs

Medical Protocols. Struvite has been the primary mineral component of most naturally occurring urethral plugs. Consult the previous sections on medical prevention of various types of feline urethral stones for details.

Surgical Protocols. Perineal urethrostomies are an effective method for minimizing recurrent obstruction contrast antegrade cystourethrography or retrograde urethrocystography should be performed to localize the site(s) of urethral obstruction before considering this technique.

TABLE 140–3. GENERAL GUIDELINES FOR REVERSE FLUSHING MALE FELINE URETHRAS OBSTRUCTED WITH INTRALUMINAL MATERIALS

1. Make every effort to protect the patient from iatrogenic complications associated with catheterization of the urethra (especially trauma, and urinary tract infection with bacteria).
2. Strive to use meticulous aseptic "feather-touch" techniques.
3. Use only sterile catheters.
4. Clean the penis and prepuce with warm water prior to catheterization.
5. Select the shortest Minnesota olive-tipped feline urethral catheter* for initial catheterization of the urethra, and attach it to a flexible IV connection set and a syringe.
6. Coat the olive tip with sterile aqueous lubricant.
7. Prior to insertion of the catheter into the external urethral orifice, the extended penis should be displaced dorsally until the long axis of the urethra is approximately parallel to the vertebral column.
8. Carefully advance the catheter to the site of obstruction. If necessary, replace the short olive-tipped Minnesota needle with a longer one. Record the site of suspected obstruction, since this information may be of value when considering use of muscle relaxants and/or when considering urethral surgery to prevent recurrent obstruction. CAUTION: Do not mistake resistance induced by curvature of the feline male urethra for a site of obstruction. In addition, never use excessive force when advancing the catheter.
9. Next, a large quantity of physiologic saline or lactated Ringer's solution (as much as several hundred ml) should be flushed into the urethral lumen and allowed to reflux out the external urethral orifice (Fig. 140–15). When possible, the catheter may be advanced toward the bladder. As a result of this maneuver, the obstructed urethral plugs may be gradually dislodged and flushed around the catheter and out of the urethral lumen. Application of steady but gentle digital pressure to the bladder wall after the urethra has been flushed with physiologic saline or lactated Ringer's solution may result in expulsion of a urethral plug or urolith from the urethral lumen. Excessive pressure should not be used because it may result in: (1) trauma to the bladder, (2) reflux of potentially infected urine into the ureters and renal pelvis, and/or (3) rupture of the bladder wall.
10. If the technique outlined in step 9 is unsuccessful, it may be necessary to attempt repulsion of suspected urethral plugs or uroliths back into the bladder lumen by occluding the distal end of the urethra around the olive tip of the catheter before injecting fluid into the urethra. By preventing reflux of solutions out of the external urethral orifice, this maneuver will tend to dilate the urethral lumen. If the obstruction persists, an attempt may be made to gently advance the suspected plug or urolith toward the bladder. *Excessive force should not be used.*
11. On occasion it is advantageous to allow the reverse flushing solution to soften the obstructing urethral plugs (this technique is ineffective for most uroliths) before attempting to propel them back into the bladder. Allowing lapse of several hours between attempts to remove firmly lodged plugs by reverse flushing has been effective.

*Minnesota feline olive-tipped urethral catheters are available from EJAY International, Inc, P.O. Box 1835, Glendora, California 91740.

IDIOPATHIC LOWER URINARY TRACT DISEASE
(pp. 1829–1831)

TREATMENT

The clinical signs of hematuria and dysuria in many untreated nonobstructed male and female cats with idiopathic lower urinary tract disease frequently subside within approximately 1 week.

Antibacterial Agents

The uselessness of antimicrobial agents in the treatment of abacteriuric cats with lower urinary tract disease has been documented.

Urinary Tract Antiseptics

At this time, the use of methenamine to treat cats with feline urinary tract disorders represents no more than an idea. Medications containing methylene blue are contraindicated in cats.

Urinary Tract Analgesics

Phenazopyridine alone or in combination with sulfa drugs is contraindicated in cats.

Smooth Muscle Antispasmodics

Many cats with inflammation of the lower urinary tract develop urge incontinence. Micturition usually occurs at a low volume of bladder filling. It is logical to consider smooth muscle antispasmodics as symptomatic treatment of urge incontinence. Propantheline may be considered to reduce the severity and frequency of urge incontinence in nonobstructed male and female cats. The suggested dose is 7.5 mg given orally approximately every 72 hours.

Anti-inflammatory Agents

Glucocorticoids. Glucocorticoids are generally contraindicated in cats with urethral obstruction and postrenal azotemia. Likewise, glucocorticoids are contraindicated in cats with bacterial UTI.

Dimethylsulfoxide (DMSO). Appropriately controlled clinical trials that are designed to evaluate the effectiveness of local instillation of DMSO into the urinary bladder of cats with signs of lower urinary tract disease have not been reported.

Urothelial Debridement

Reports of clinical experiences suggest that the technique is of little benefit. We do not recommend this procedure.

CHAPTER 141
CANINE LOWER URINARY TRACT DISORDERS
(pages 1833–1861)

LOCALIZING CLINICAL SIGNS (p. 1833)

Clinical signs localizing disease to the lower urinary tract include dysuria, pollakiuria, stranguria, hematuria, and urinary incontinence.

Original chapter written by Jody P. Lulich, Carl A. Osborne, Joseph W. Bartges, and David J. Polzin

DIAGNOSTIC TECHNIQUES FOR LOWER URINARY TRACT DISEASE (pp. 1833–1835)

EVALUATION OF URINE

Urinalysis. A complete urinalysis includes visual inspection of urine, measurement of solute concentration (usually specific gravity), evaluation of chemical constituents (reagent strip), and microscopic examination of urine sediment. We recommend collection of urine samples by cystocentesis to evaluate the urinary bladder and upper urinary tract. Urethral diseases may be best evaluated with a voided sample.

Urine Culture. The gold standard for the diagnosis of urinary tract infection is quantitative urine culture (Chapter 136).

DIAGNOSTIC IMAGING

While survey radiography is adequate for a diagnosis of radiodense uroliths or in the assessment of bladder position, contrast procedures are needed for evaluation of mucosal irregularities, diverticula, urine leakage, and radiolucent uroliths. Mucosa proliferation and blood clots are best evaluated by ultrasonography.

CYSTOURETHROSCOPY

Depending on the size of the urethra in relation to the size of the cystoscope, urethral dilation or prepubic precutaneous cystoscopy may be required.

BIOPSY OF THE LOWER URINARY TRACT

If structures can be palpated abdominally or rectally, they can be aspirated with a needle and syringe. When larger tissue samples are required, they can be obtained by catheter biopsy, by cystoscopy and pinch biopsy, or, when the urinary bladder is friable, by celiotomy and core resection.

ANATOMIC DISORDERS (pp. 1835–1837)

URETHRORECTAL FISTULA

They are uncommon. Control of secondary bacterial UTI is also an important consideration.

URETHRAL PROLAPSE

This condition occasionally occurs in brachycephalic dogs, especially English bulldogs. Physical examination typically reveals a red or purple pea- sized, doughnut-shaped lesion protruding from the end of the penis. Most cases have been managed by manual reduction combined with retention sutures, or by surgical excision of the prolapsed portion of the urethra.

PERSISTENT URACHUS

It is characterized by inappropriate loss of urine through the umbilicus during the storage phase of micturition and expulsion of urine to the exterior through the umbilicus and urethra during the voiding phase of micturition. The diagnosis of persistent urachus should be confirmed by contrast radiographic procedures. If confirmed, the canal should be surgically removed.

VESICOURACHAL DIVERTICULA

They predispose to recurrent urinary tract infection. Occasionally, a vesicourachal diverticulum develops because of increased intravesicular pressure due to obstruction of urine outflow. Vesicourachal diverticula that form as a result of urinary obstruction may heal spontaneously; those that persist should be removed surgically.

URETHRAL STRICTURE

Urethral strictures necessitating repair can be opened along the longitudinal axis then closed transversely.

URETEROCELE

Clinical signs associated with ureteroceles are variable, but may include dysuria, urinary incontinence, hematuria, chronic UTI, and urinary obstruction. Hydroureter, hydronephrosis, and impaired renal function may also be present. Confirming the diagnosis requires contrast radiography and/or ultrasonography. Clinical abnormalities are minimized or eliminated by reconstruction of the urinary tract.

URINARY TRACT TRAUMA

Clinical Signs.   Contusions and lacerations of the internal lining of the urinary bladder cause varying degrees of hematuria. Clinical signs associated with rupture of the urinary bladder are variable. Patients with ruptured urinary bladders may or may not be able to void urine. Continuous intraperitoneal extravasation of a significant quantity of urine will induce progressive signs caused by chemical and/or bacterial peritonitis within 8 to 24 hours.

Diagnosis.   The most important aspect in the diagnosis is to suspect its occurrence in all patients with a history of abdominal or pelvic injury. The location(s) and severity of trauma should be evaluated by retrograde urethrocystography. We recommend the use of a dilute solution (2.5 to 5.0 per cent) of contrast agents commonly used for intravenous urography. Abdominal paracentesis is helpful to support a diagnosis of intraperitoneal rupture of the urinary bladder. Aspirated fluid typically has a bloody appearance. Comparing the concentration of creatinine in peritoneal fluid reveals a disproportionate elevation when compared to creatinine concentration of serum sampled at the same time.

Therapy.   Surgical repair is the treatment of choice for severe trauma.

UROLITHIASIS (pp. 1837–1859)

The mere presence of uroliths in the urinary system does not always necessitate their removal; however, those resulting in clinical signs (dysuria, hematuria, urinary tract infection, incontinence, obstruction, or azotemia) should be appropriately managed.

DIAGNOSIS

One must avoid over- or underinterpreting the significance of crystalluria. In most instances, crystal formation in an anatomically and functionally normal urinary tract is harmless. Identification of crystals in such patients does not justify therapy.

Radiography.   The primary objective of radiographic or ultrasonographic evaluation of patients is to verify urolith presence, location, number, size, density, and shape. A lateral double-contrast cystogram can be performed for further verification. Compared to soft tissue density, uroliths composed of magnesium ammonium phosphate, calcium oxalate, calcium phosphate, silica, and cystine are often radiodense; those composed of urate salts may be radiolucent.

Serum Chemistry Values.   These are helpful in the identification of underlying abnormalities responsible for urolith formation.

Urine Chemistry Values. For best results, 24-hour urine samples should be collected.

Analysis of Uroliths. Because many uroliths contain more than one mineral component, it is important to examine representative portions. The nuclei of uroliths should be analyzed separately from their outer layers. In contrast to chemical methods of analysis, physical methods have proved to be far superior.

Predicting Mineral Composition Prior to Urolith Analysis (Table 141–1). Urolith dissolution may be hampered if uroliths are composed of several mineral types of differing solubility characteristics. An alternative to predicting mineral composition, small uroliths can be retrieved by means of a nonsurgical method. Small urocystoliths can also be retrieved for analysis by aspirating them into a urinary catheter. For a complete discussion of the procedure, see the textbook.

MANAGEMENT

Medical Management

Surgical Removal

Surgical candidates include patients with urolith-induced obstruction to urine outflow that cannot be corrected by nonsurgical techniques. This is especially true in patients with urinary tract infection. For dogs with certain anatomic defects of the urinary tract (persistent diverticulum or persistent urachus) that may predispose to UTI and uroliths, uroliths can be removed at the same time these abnormalities are surgically repaired.

Nonsurgical Urolith Removal

Catheter urolith retrieval and voiding urohydropropulsion permit safe and rapid removal of small to moderately sized urocystoliths.

Catheter Urolith Retrieval. Following urolith retrieval, double-contrast cystography should be performed to assess urolith status.

Voiding Urohydropropulsion. For a complete discussion of the procedure, see the textbook. Uroliths composed of magnesium ammonium phosphate, ammonium urate, or cystine that are initially too large to be voided through the urethra can be easily removed once their size is reduced by means of medical therapy.

STRUVITE UROLITHIASIS

Supersaturation of urine with magnesium ammonium phosphate is associated with urinary tract infection caused by urease-producing microbes (especially *Staphylococcus* and *Proteus* species) and alkaline urine in most dogs.

Treatment

Control of Urinary Infection. Appropriate antimicrobial agents selected on the basis of susceptibility or minimum inhibitory concentration tests should be used in therapeutic doses. Antimicrobial agents should be administered as long as the uroliths can be identified by survey radiography.

Urine Acidification. Urine acidification to a pH of approximately 6 has been effective; however, addition of urinary acidifiers often is not needed for dogs currently receiving a calculolytic diet (Hill's Prescription Diet s/d).

Calculolytic Diet. When dogs with infection-induced struvite uroliths are fed a calculolytic diet, a marked reduction in the serum concentration of urea nitrogen and slight reductions in the serum concentrations of magnesium, phosphorus, and albumin typically occur.

TABLE 141-1. PREDICTING MINERAL COMPOSITION OF UROLITHS

MINERAL TYPE	Urine pH	Crystal Appearance	Urine Culture	Radiographic Density	Radiographic Contour	Serum Abnormalities	Breed Predisposition	Gender Predisposition	Common Ages
				PREDICTORS					
Magnesium ammonium phosphate	Neutral to alkaline	4- to 6-sided colorless prisms	Urease-producing bacteria (Staphylococcus, Proteus, Enterococcus, Mycoplasma)	+ to + + + +	Smooth, round, or faceted; may assume shape of bladder or urethra	None	Miniature Schnauzer, Bichon Frise, Cocker Spaniel	Female (>80%)	2 to 8 years or younger
Calcium oxalate	Acid to neutral	Dihydrate salt, colorless envelope or octahedral shape; monohydrate salt: spindles or dumbbell shape	Negative	+ + to + + + +	Rough or spiculated (dihydrate salt); small, smooth, round (monohydrate salt); sometimes jackstone	Occasional hypercalcemia	Miniature Schnauzer, Lhasa Apso, Yorkshire Terrier, Miniature Poodle, Shih Tzu, Bichon Frise	Males (>70%)	5 to 12 years
Urate	Acid to neutral	Yellow-brown amorphous shapes or sphericals (ammonium urate)	Negative	– to + +	Smooth, round or oval	Low urea nitrogen and serum albumin in dogs with hepatic portal systemic shunts	Dalmatian, English Bulldog, Miniature Schnauzer, Yorkshire Terrier	Males (>85%)	1 to 4 years
Calcium phosphate	Alkaline to neutral (Brushite forms in acidic urine)	Amorphous, or long thin prisms	Negative	+ + to + + + +	Smooth, round or faceted	Occasional hypercalcemia	Yorkshire Terrier, Miniature Schnauzer, Cocker Spaniel	Male (>60%)	7 to 11 years
Cystine	Acid to neutral	Flat colorless, hexagonal plates	Negative	+ to + +	Smooth to slightly irregular, round to oval	None	English Bulldog, Dachshund, Basset Hound	Male (>90%)	1 to 8 years
Silica	Acid to neutral	None observed	Negative	+ + to + + + +	Round center with radial spoke-like projections (jackstone)	None	German shepherd, golden retriever, Labrador retriever, Miniature Schnauzer	Male (>90%)	4 to 9 years

These diets are designed for short-term (weeks or months) dissolution therapy rather than long-term (months to years) prophylactic therapy.

Urease Inhibitors. Acetohydroxamic acid (AHA) given orally to dogs, 25 mg/kg/day in two divided subdoses, reduces urease activity. AHA may cause reversible hemolytic anemia. AHA should not be administered to pregnant dogs.

Prevention

Infection-Induced Struvite Uroliths. Eradication or control of UTI caused by urease-producing bacteria is the most important factor in preventing recurrence. Because calculolytic diets induce polyuria, varying degrees of hypoalbuminemia, and mild alteration in hepatic enzymes and morphology, we recommend long-term use of severely protein-restricted calculolytic diets only if patients develop recurrent urolithiasis despite augmented fluid intake, urine acidification, and attempts to control infection.

Sterile Struvite Uroliths. If the urine pH of patients with sterile struvite urolithiasis remains alkaline, administration of urine acidifiers should be considered.

CALCIUM OXALATE UROLITHS

Etiopathogenesis

Hypercalciuria. Hypercalciuria has been a significant finding in dogs with calcium oxalate uroliths.

Treatment

Physical means of removing calcium oxalate uroliths remains the current method to resolve clinically active disease. In some patients, however, calcium oxalate uroliths are clinically silent.

Prevention

In dogs with hypercalcemia, the underlying cause (e.g., primary hyperparathyroidism) should be corrected.

Dietary Considerations. A diet moderately restricted in protein, calcium, oxalate, and sodium (i.e., Prescription Diet Canine u/d, Hill's, Topeka KS) may be considered in an effort to prevent recurrence. Other diets that may also be beneficial include Prescription Diet Canine w/d (Hill's, Topeka KS) and Prescription Diet Canine k/d (Hill's, Topeka KS). Ideally, diets should not be restricted or supplemented with phosphorus or magnesium.

Citrate. If persistent aciduria or hypocitriuria is recognized in dogs, therapy with wax matrix tablets of potassium citrate (Urocit- K, Mission Pharmacal) should be considered. For cats and small dogs, we commonly use a liquid product (Polycitra-K). We currently recommend a dose of 100 to 150 mg/kg/day (divided into two to three subdoses). Because Prescription Diet Canine U/D (Hill's, Topeka KS) already contains adequate quantities of potassium citrate, additional potassium citrate is often not needed.

Thiazide Diuretics. Hydrochlorothiazide may be tried (2 to 4 mg/kg q12h). Because thiazide diuretic administration can be associated with adverse effects (dehydration, hypokalemia, hypercalcemia), their use should be accompanied by appropriate clinical and laboratory monitoring.

CANINE AMMONIUM URATE AND URIC ACID UROLITHIASIS

Dalmatians. Dalmatian dogs are predisposed to urate uroliths owing to their unique metabolism of purines.

Non-Dalmatian Dogs. Non-Dalmatian breeds that appear to

have a significantly higher incidence of urate urolithiasis based on quantitative analyses are miniature schnauzers, Shih Tzus, Yorkshire terriers, and especially English bulldogs.

Portal Vascular Anomalies. A high incidence of ammonium urate uroliths has been observed in dogs with portal vascular anomalies.

Treatment

Calculolytic Diets. A purine-restricted nonacidifying diet that does not contain supplemental sodium (Prescription Diet Canine u/d, Hill's).

Xanthine Oxidase Inhibitors. Allopurinol binds to and inhibits the action of xanthine oxidase. The dosage of allopurinol is 15 mg/kg q12h. Other than formation of xanthine uroliths, adverse reactions to allopurinol are apparently uncommon in dogs.

Alkalinization of Urine. The dosage of urine alkalinizers should be individualized for each patient. Preliminary dosages of sodium bicarbonate vary from approximately 10 to 90 grains per day. Alternatively, potassium citrate in wax matrix tablets may be given (Urocit-K, Mission Pharmacal). Potassium citrate may be preferable. The goal of treatment with urine alkalinizers is to maintain a urine pH of approximately 7.0. Higher values (>7.5) should be avoided until it is determined whether they provide a significant risk factor for formation of calcium phosphate uroliths.

Eradication or Control of Urinary Tract Infection. Eradication or control of potent urease-producing microbes (staphylococci, *Proteus* spp, and *Ureaplasma*) would be especially important.

Augmenting Urine Volume. Because the calculolytic diet designed for urate urolith dissolution impairs urine concentrating capacity by decreasing renal medullary urea concentration, additional diuretic agents are not required. Excessive dietary sodium should be avoided.

Dogs with Portovascular Anomalies. It is logical to hypothesize that surgical correction of anomalous shunts would result in dissolution of uroliths composed primarily of ammonium urate.

Monitoring Response to Therapy. Ammonium urate urocystoliths have a propensity to move into the urethra of dogs. If larger, they often become lodged behind the os penis of males. Owners should be informed of this likelihood. The size of the uroliths should be periodically monitored by survey and (if necessary) double-contrast radiography. Urine pH should be monitored. Reduction of serum urea nitrogen concentration below pretreatment values (usually <10 mg/dl in previously nonazotemic patients), reduction of urine specific gravity (usually <1.020), and increase in urine pH (usually >7.0) indicate owner and patient compliance with recommendations to consume the calculolytic diet. There is no rigid therapeutic time interval after which response to dissolution therapy is unlikely.

Prevention

As a first choice, diets that are restricted in purines and that promote formation of dilute alkaline urine should be considered. If necessary, alkalinizing agents may be added to the protocol. If difficulties persist, allopurinol (approximately 10 to 20 mg/kg body weight per day) may be given.

CANINE CYSTINE UROLITHIASIS

Canine cystinuria is an inborn error of metabolism. Data contained in published pedigrees from inbred lines of dachshunds, basset hounds, and rottweilers suggest a sex-linked or autosomal recessive pattern of inheritance.

Treatment

Dietary Modification. We have successfully used a protein-restricted, alkalinizing diet (Hill's Prescription Diet Canine canned u/d).

Alkalinization of Urine. A sufficient quantity of potassium citrate or sodium bicarbonate should be given orally in divided doses to sustain a urine pH of approximately 7.5. Potassium citrate may be preferable. Hill's Prescription Diet Canine canned u/d is formulated to contain potassium citrate.

Thiol-Containing Drugs. N-(2- mercaptopropionyl)-glycine (2-MPG) decreases the concentration of cystine. Oral administration of 2-MPG (15 mg/kg q12h PO) was effective in inducing dissolution of multiple cystine urocystoliths. Two dogs developed a Coombs' positive regenerative spherocytic anemia, which resolved rapidly following withdrawal of 2-MPG. D-penicillamine has been used in the management of cystine uroliths. The most common dosage of D-penicillamine for dogs has been 15 mg/kg q12h PO. D-penicillamine administration is associated with a higher incidence of severe side effects than is 2-MPG.

Prevention

A protein-restricted, alkalinizing diet (Hill's Prescription Diet Canine canned u/d) or a combination of dietary modification combined with urine alkalinizing therapy may be initiated. If necessary, 2-MPG (15 mg/kg q12h PO) may be added.

CALCIUM PHOSPHATE UROLITHS

Pure calcium phosphate uroliths are infrequently encountered in dogs, and they are usually associated with metabolic disorders such as primary hyperparathyroidism, renal tubular acidosis, and excessive dietary calcium and phosphorus.

Treatment and Prevention

Physical means of urolith removal are often necessary to correct clinically active disease. Correction of underlying abnormalities should minimize urolith recurrence. If a specific underlying disorder is not diagnosed, we generally manage calcium phosphate uroliths similar to strategies used for calcium oxalate.

SILICA UROLITHS

The majority of submissions were from German shepherds, golden retrievers, and Labrador retrievers.

Treatment and Prevention

Effective medical protocols to induce dissolution of canine silica uroliths have yet to be developed. Our preventive recommendations include (1) change of diet (avoid diets containing substantial plant proteins) and (2) increasing urine volume (enhancing water consumption).

UNUSUAL AND RARE UROLITHS

Although crystalluria has been reported with a variety of drugs, urolith formation has only been reported with sulfonamide administration. For this reason, sulfonamide antimicrobials should not be administered to dogs with uroliths.

IDIOPATHIC GRANULOMATOUS URETHRITIS (p. 1859)

Dysuria, thickened irregular urethral wall, bacterial infection, and urinary obstruction have been described in female dogs with granulomatous urethritis. It is important to distinguish it from urethral neoplasia. It is our opinion that chronic bacterial infection plays a significant role in its development. Therapeutic recommendations for granulomatous urethritis have included prednisolone and cyclophosphamide. Cases associated with bacterial urinary tract infection or other infectious agents should be initially managed with antimicrobial drugs to eradicate infection. Only if proliferative lesions fail to regress following initial therapy should immunosuppressive drugs be considered.

DRUG-INDUCED (CYCLOPHOSPHAMIDE) CYSTITIS (p. 1859)

Sterile hemorrhagic cystitis is a common complication of cyclophosphamide administration. Once cystitis develops, the drug should be discontinued. Diuresis should be maintained and secondary UTI controlled.

COMMON MISCONCEPTIONS IN THE DIAGNOSIS AND MANAGEMENT OF CANINE LOWER URINARY TRACT DISEASE (pp. 1859–1860)

Misconception 1. Crystalluria Is an Indication for Change of Diet. Crystalluria that occurs in individuals with anatomically and functionally normal urinary tracts is usually harmless.

Misconception 2. Crystalluria Causes Hematuria and Dysuria.

Misconception 3. Cystotomy Guarantees Removal of Uroliths from the Lower Urinary Tract. Postsurgical radiography should be considered in dogs and cats with multiple uroliths.

Misconception 4. Surgery Is Needed to Manage Polypoid Cystitis. Inflammatory polyps may spontaneously resolve following eradication of infection and/or uroliths.

Misconception 5. Corticosteroids Are Indicated in the Management of Granulomatous Urethritis. Because of the potential adverse effects of immunosuppressive drugs, especially in patients with infection, prednisolone and cyclophosphamide should be reserved for refractory cases.

Misconception 6. Absence of Pyuria and Bacteriuria Is Sufficient Evidence to Rule Out Urinary Tract Infection. Bacteriuria cannot be detected by sediment examination unless concentrations of bacterial rods are greater than 10,000 organisms per milliliter, and concentrations of bacterial cocci are equal to 100,000/ml. Likewise, the degree of inflammation is variable.

Misconception 7. Persistent Alkaluria Is an Indication for Antibiotic Administration.

CHAPTER 142

ERYTHROCYTE RESPONSES AND DISORDERS
(pages 1864–1891)

ERYTHROCYTE MORPHOLOGY ON WRIGHT'S STAINED BLOOD FILMS

See the textbook (pages 1866–1870) for a review of erythrocyte morphology and staining.

RETICULOCYTE COUNTING

Counting reticulocytes is the preferred method of quantitating the regenerative response. Canine reticulocytes almost always have aggregated condensation of the organelles, making counting a relatively simple process. The cat is unique in producing at least two forms of reticulocytes, which have different interpretations and contribute to confusion during the reticulocyte count. The aggregate reticulocyte has clumped organelles that coalesce into aggregates. The punctate form has variable numbers of individual dots, which do not coalesce. The interpretation is that the aggregate form represents *active* regeneration, while the punctate form represents fairly recent *cumulative* regeneration. For this reason, it is best to include only the aggregate form in a reticulocyte count. This is important in cats because anemias, which are initially regenerative and then become nonregenerative, may have a large number of punctate forms and an absence of aggregate forms.

DETECTION OF IMMUNOGLOBULIN AND/OR COMPLEMENT ON ERYTHROCYTES

Positive Coombs' tests alone are not diagnostic of immunohemolytic disease. Positive reactions may occur with a variety of anemias and in conditions without accompanying anemia. There is documented association of Coombs' positive reactions with FeLV infection. Second, a variety of technical problems result in false-negative Coombs' reactions when overt immunohemolytic disease is present. Third, Coombs' tests done at 39°F (4°C) are overutilized and overinterpreted in veterinary medicine. Cold-reacting antibodies may be a normal finding in some dogs and cats.

Original chapter written by M. G. Weiser

ERYTHROCYTE FRAGILITY AND DEFORMABILITY

This assay measures erythrocyte resistance to lysis. It is useful for documenting immune-mediated erythrocyte injury in dogs when sphere formation is morphologically imperfect and is currently the best assay to detect erythrocyte immuno-injury in the cat. With sphere injury in immunohemolytic disease, the curve will shift to the left and the 50 per cent hemolysis point will be increased above 0.50 and 0.65 per cent saline for dogs and cats, respectively.

REFERENCE VALUES FOR CLINICAL EVALUATION OF ERYTHROCYTES (pp. 1873–1874)

Some breeds of dogs, notably the basenji, beagle, Boxer, Chihuahua, German shepherd, and poodle, can be expected to have hematocrit values in excess of 50 per cent. Some poodles may have MCV values ranging from 80 to 100 fL, a peculiarity referred to as poodle macrocytosis. Markedly regenerative anemias in dogs are usually accompanied by modest increases in MCV, whereas in cats the MCV may almost double. Prominent macrocytosis may be observed in FeLV-associated anemias whether regenerative or not. Microcytosis is a feature of iron deficiency anemia. The magnitude of reticulocytosis depends on the time of sampling during response to anemia.

NEONATAL AND JUVENILE VALUES

Dogs are born with large erythrocytes (95 to 100 fL) and relatively high hematocrit values. Hematocrit values decline to a nadir of about 30 per cent by 4 to 6 weeks, then progressively increase into the adult reference range by 4 to 6 months. Kittens are born with mean hematocrit values of about 35 per cent. Mean hematocrit values then decline to a nadir of 25 per cent by 3 to 4 weeks, then slowly increase to adult values of 35 per cent by 16 weeks.

Erythrocyte Survival.   See textbook.

Kinetics of Marrow Response to Anemia.   When marrow response mechanisms are intact, reticulocytosis will develop within 2 days of the onset of anemia and will peak at 4 to 7 days.

ANEMIA (pp. 1876–1891)

An overview of anemia and description of associated clinical findings are given in Chapter 41.

Anemia can be classified into one of four categories: hemorrhage, hemolysis, extra-marrow disease (erythropoietic depression by disease outside the marrow), and intra-marrow disease (hematopoietic disturbance by disease in the marrow space).

The first step is to determine whether the anemia is regenerative or not based on reticulocyte concentration. If regenerative, the anemia must be due to either hemorrhage or hemolysis. Plasma protein values greater than 6.5 gm/dl are probably associated with hemolysis. With hemorrhage, plasma proteins are lost proportionally with erythrocytes, and values will usually decrease below 6.0 gm/dl. If leukocytes and platelets are normal or responding in an orderly fashion, there is selective depression of erythropoiesis. This is usually due to disease outside the marrow. If there is failure to produce adequate numbers of leukocytes and/or platelets or there are abnormal circulating cells, then there is evidence of disturbed production of more than one cell line. This is usually due to disease within the marrow.

HEMORRHAGE

Pinpoint or petechial hemorrhages visible on skin and/or mucous membranes suggest thrombocytopenia. Hematomas, large subcutaneous hemorrhages, or bleeding into body cavities suggests a defect in clotting biochemistry.

Trauma/Lacerations.   With acute blood loss the hematocrit does not reflect the severity of the process. Transfusions are generally not required unless hemorrhage has occurred continuously in the face of volume replacement, resulting in hematocrits below 15 or 20 per cent.

Thrombocytopenia.   The probability of thrombocytopenia being associated with hemorrhage increases considerably as the count decreases below 50,000/μl. Almost all cases of hemorrhage not attributable to thrombocytopenia will have platelet counts in excess of 200,000/μl.

Defects in Coagulation Biochemistry.   See Chapter 145 of the textbook for a discussion of coagulation.

Iron Deficiency Anemia.   Iron deficiency anemia is important to recognize because it is a clear indication in adult dogs that chronic external blood loss has been occurring. Hematologic features of iron deficiency anemia include those of hemorrhage and erythrocyte microcytosis. Plasma proteins are decreased when the rate of blood loss is relatively high, but may be low normal with repeated loss of small blood volumes. Thrombocytosis with large platelets is a regular occurrence. Serum iron values of less than 60 μg/dl and transferrin saturation values of less than 15 per cent are guidelines for documenting iron deficiency (see Chapter 3 of the textbook). Total iron binding capacity values are not increased in dogs with iron deficiency as is commonly extrapolated from human literature. Treatment of iron deficiency should first involve correction of the cause of blood loss. This is followed by oral supplementation of iron for 30 to 60 days. In dogs with severe longstanding iron deficiency, a single injection of 5 to 10 mg/lb (10 to 20 mg/kg) of iron dextran (Imferon) should be followed by the oral supplement. Young dogs with severe anemia related to hookworm infestation may require a transfusion. Iron deficiency is rarely recognized in the adult cat.

HEMOLYSIS

Most forms of hemolytic disease in companion animals are extravascular. As a result, splenomegaly may be observed.

Immune-Mediated Hemolytic Anemias

Immunohemolytic Anemia.   Because hemolysis and development of anemia usually occur rapidly, features of acute anemia including sudden onset of exercise intolerance, pale mucous membranes, tachycardia, and hyperpnea may be present. Fever and icterus may occur. Hemoglobinuria associated with an intravascular hemolytic component is uncommon. Hematologic features usually include moderate to severe anemia, marked reticulocytosis, spherocytosis, and some degree of agglutination when blood cools to room temperature. Variable degrees of neutrophilic leukocytosis with a left shift and monocytosis are expected. Immune-mediated thrombocytopenia often occurs in conjunction with immunohemolytic anemia. Spherocytosis observed by a competent microscopist is the most definitive and reliable feature of immunohemolytic anemia. Immune-mediated agglutination is the next most convincing evidence for this disease. A positive Coombs' test is regarded as supportive of the diagnosis.

A nonregenerative form of immunohemolytic anemia is characterized by the usual hematologic features except that a complete absence of reticulocytes exists. Reticulocytopenia appears to be a result of immune-mediated consumption of developing erythroid precursors in marrow. A transfusion is more likely to be required early in treatment, and a much longer period is required for hematological improvement. To diagnose this form, it is exceedingly important to recognize sphere formation. In marrow aspirate examination there is usually a distinct maturation block at one stage.

Pure red cell aplasia may represent a special case of an immune-mediated injury to erythroid stem cells. There is an absence of erythroid cells in marrow, presumably due to destruction of committed stem cells. Immunohemolytic anemia is not recognized in cats as frequently as in dogs. Hemobartonellosis may be regarded as a form of immunohemolytic anemia. The diagnosis in cats depends on the presence of the following in decreasing order of importance: evidence of hemolytic anemia, increased fragility in hypotonic saline, agglutination, and a positive Coombs' test. Blood films from more than one bleeding should be scrutinized for hemobartonellosis.

Treatment of immunohemolytic anemia includes steroid suppression of erythrophagocytosis and supportive therapy including a transfusion if essential. Any underlying inflammatory or systemic disorder should be treated as indicated. If there is any doubt about the presence of hemobartonellosis, appropriate antibiotic therapy should be utilized. Prednisone or prednisolone, 1 to 2 mg/lb (2 to 4 mg/kg) per day, is recommended for a minimum of 2–3 weeks, then slow tapering of the drug. The guidelines for giving a transfusion are no different than for other forms of anemia. Drugs commonly utilized for more potent immunosuppressive therapy include cyclophosphamide, 50 mg/m^2 given orally for 4 consecutive days per week, or azathioprine, 1 mg/lb (2 mg/kg) given orally once per day. It is possible for the hematocrit to remain unchanged for as long as 7 to 14 days in an adequately treated patient. The predicted outcome for dealing with immunohemolytic anemia in dogs is reasonably good, but individual cases must be given a guarded prognosis when first diagnosed. The prognosis should be more guarded in cats.

Drug-related Anemia.   Levamisole (in dogs) and propylthiouracil (in cats) have been reported. Treatment of this toxicity includes cessation of drug therapy and supportive care.

Cold-agglutinin Disease.   Cold-agglutinin disease occurs rarely in dogs. Intravascular agglutination may occur in ear tips, tail tip, and feet upon exposure to cold environmental temperatures, resulting in gangrenous necrosis. Diagnosis is dependent on determining that the animal was exposed to low environmental temperature and demonstrating cold-induced agglutination *in vitro*.

Neonatal Isoerythrolysis.   This disease is considered rare in dogs and cats. It may occur when a queen with blood type B is mated with a male with blood type A. At birth, kittens from such a mating may receive anti-A antibodies from colostrum, which cause hemolysis. Because of the very low frequency of blood type B in the domestic shorthair and longhair populations, this disease is rarely a problem.

Hemolytic Anemias Due to Erythroparasitic Organisms

Hemobartonellosis.   Transmission is thought to involve blood transfer. After recovery, the cat may remain a carrier for years. In this stage, the organism can be intermittently found in small numbers on blood films and be associated with subclinical anemia. Diagnosis currently depends on finding organisms on erythrocytes using Wright's stained blood films. Experience is required to distinguish organisms from precipitated stain. A diagnosis may require examination of blood films over several days. It is extremely unlikely that organisms will be found if the cat is receiving tetracycline. Other clinical signs that occur variably include weight loss, intermittent anorexia, hyperbilirubinemia, splenomegaly, and fever. Treatment should consist of oral tetracycline. Steroids have been advocated since an immune-mediated hemolytic component is likely.

Hemobartonellosis is of less importance in dogs since it is rare and usually occurs only in splenectomized dogs. Immunohemolytic disease is an important component in canine hemobartonellosis. Treatment of canine hemobartonellosis should consist of tetracycline. Steroids may be used as in treatment for immunohemolytic anemia.

Babesiosis. An acute, severe form characterized by intravascular hemolysis indicated by hemoglobinuria, hyperbilirubinemia, dehydration, severe acidosis, fever, anorexia, depression, and collapse tends to occur in younger dogs. Subacute or chronic forms are characterized by fever, anorexia, depression, and mild to moderate anemia. The anemias are regenerative. The diagnosis is made by examination of stained blood films for intraerythrocytic pyriform bodies. A serologic test exists for establishing a diagnosis when organisms are difficult to find. It has been recommended that a serologic test for ehrlichiosis be done as part of evaluation for babesiosis. Treatment involves antiparasite drugs and appropriate supportive therapy. The two most commonly recommended drugs, diminazene aceturate and imidocarb diproprionate, are not approved for use in the United States. Considering the difficulty in obtaining these drugs, it is recommended that tetracycline be used as described for hemobartonellosis.

Cytauxzoonosis. This is a protozoal disease which occurs principally in southern states, extending from Oklahoma and Texas to Florida. It is a consistently fatal disease in domestic cats. See Chapter 66 of the textbook.

The organism's intraerythrocytic form is observed in affected cats, but the associated anemia has not been well characterized. When clinical signs first appear, a small proportion of the cells (usually less than 5 per cent) contain organisms, making diagnosis on blood films difficult, but the erythroparasitemia increases terminally.

Oxidative Injury to Erythrocytes— Hemolysis and Methemoglobinemia

Erythrocyte oxidative injury may take at least three forms including oxidation of heme iron resulting in methemoglobinemia, oxidative denaturation of hemoglobin resulting in Heinz body formation, and oxidative cross-linking of membrane proteins. Methemoglobinemia imparts a characteristic chocolate brown discoloration to blood. Membrane injury and Heinz body formation are irreversible changes. Because of slower development and a lesser proportion of hemoglobin involvement, clinical signs of anemia are usually minimal.

Canine Disease. The most common cause of Heinz body hemolysis in dogs is related to ingestion of onions. The hemolytic episode may be difficult to correlate with onion ingestion because it occurs several days later. Clinical signs are related to moderate anemia. Heinz bodies are more difficult to recognize in dogs compared to cats. Often, the most obvious finding on Wright's stained blood films are eccentrocytes. Acetaminophen toxicity results in severe methemoglobinemia and hepatocellular necrosis, which may result in death. Benzocaine-containing topical products have been reported to produce methemoglobinemia as high as 51 per cent and mild Heinz body hemolysis in dogs with ulcerated skin lesions.

Feline Disease. Unusual metabolism and unique hemoglobin structure in cats result in increased sensitivity to oxidative injury. A variety of chemical agents and drugs may induce Heinz body formation and severe hemolysis. Methylene blue-induced Heinz body hemolysis has been characterized extensively in the cat. Diagnosis of overt Heinz body hemolysis depends on observation of relatively large Heinz bodies in an appreciable proportion of erythrocytes in conjunction with a hemolysis pattern on the hemogram. Acetaminophen toxicity results in a combination of methemoglobinemia and Heinz body hemolytic anemia. Clinical signs include labored respiration and increased heart rate associated with reduced oxygen- carrying capacity, depression, hematuria, and hemoglobinuria. At the higher doses, salivation and facial edema may be observed. Markedly regenerative anemia may occur, with a hematocrit nadir and reticulocyte peak occurring about one week after drug administration. Chronic administration of low doses of acetaminophen has caused hepatic necrosis and fibrosis in cats. Other recognized causes of methemoglobinemia in cats include phenazopyridine, benzocaine, phenacetin, and DL-methionine.

Treatment of Heinz body hemolysis involves cessation of any identifiable offending drug and simple supportive care. Transfusions are not likely to be required. Severe methemoglobinemia should be treated vigorously. Methylene blue (0.45 mg/lb or 1 mg/kg given once IV) will accelerate reduction of methemoglobin back to the functional state. A blood transfusion may provide a lifesaving fraction of functional hemoglobin until methemoglobin can be reduced. Oxygen therapy is probably of little benefit. Either oral or intravenous N-acetylcysteine (65 mg/lb or 140 mg/kg q8h) and intravenous sodium sulfate (22 mg/lb or 50 mg/kg q8h) result in considerable improvement by increasing acetaminophen clearance rate and contributing to methemoglobin reduction.

Hemolytic Disease Associated with Inherited Metabolic Disorders

Several inherited enzyme deficiencies that result in variably shortened erythrocyte survival have been recognized, but are rare. There currently is no specific treatment for these disorders.

Pyruvate Kinase (PK) Deficiency. Found in basenjis and beagles, it is inherited as an autosomal recessive trait and is characterized by chronic, severe hemolysis with fairly stable kinetics. The very high reticulocyte counts make the disorder difficult to document by enzyme assays. The hematocrit is usually 15 to 30 per cent when the disease is first recognized at about 3 to 6 months of age. Thereafter, it slowly declines over the next 1 to 3 years until the affected animal becomes terminally ill. There is prominent splenomegaly. Terminal myelofibrosis may develop.

Feline Porphyria. Pigment tissue accumulation results in visible brown to reddish discoloration of teeth and bones. The degree of pigmentation, occurrence of photosensitization, and development of anemia were variable.

Miscellaneous Causes of Hemolysis

Microangiopathic Hemolytic Disease. Postcaval syndrome associated with heartworm disease (Chapter 98) and splenic torsion are examples of overt microangiopathic hemolysis.

Copper Toxicity. Intravascular hemolysis has been observed in copper-associated hepatitis in Bedlington terriers (Chapter 106). This is associated with hepatic necrosis.

EXTRA-MARROW DISEASE—SELECTIVE ERYTHROPOIETIC DEPRESSION

Clinical features of anemia are usually overshadowed by signs of the primary disease. Hematologic findings include reticulocyte counts ranging from 0 to about 20,000/μl, normocytic/normochromic indices, and unremarkable morphology.

Anemia of Chronic Disease. This is probably the most common form of nonregenerative anemia in man and dogs. It develops in association with many infectious, noninfectious, and neoplastic disorders. Hematocrit values are usually only mildly decreased, ranging from 25 to 35 per cent, unless complicated by blood loss. As a result, the anemia is rarely treated. Correction of the primary lesion is expected to result in resolution of the anemia.

Anemia of Renal Failure. Chronic renal failure with azotemia is regularly associated with nonregenerative anemia of mild to moderate magnitude.

Endocrine Failures. Mild anemia is associated with hypothyroidism and hypoadrenocorticism. The anemia is expected to slowly resolve with appropriate hormone replacement therapy.

Feline Leukemia Virus-Associated Nonregenerative Anemia. The hematologic findings in FeLV-associated anemia are extremely varied. Associated hemolytic disorders may include spontaneous Heinz body hemolysis, hemobartonellosis, and immunohemolytic anemia. The distinction between intra- and extra-marrow disease in FeLV-associated anemia should be deemphasized in the reader's mind. Simple nonregenerative anemia has been one of the more frequently recognized forms of FeLV-associated anemia. Examination of bone marrow aspirate films reveals nonspecific erythroid hypoplasia. Most FeLV positive cats, whether anemic or not, have increased erythrocyte volume and volume heterogeneity.

INTRA-MARROW DISEASE—GENERALIZED HEMATOPOIETIC DISTURBANCE

Myeloaplasia, myelodysplasia, and myeloproliferative diseases are disorders that result from injury to stem cell populations. Damage may be either to the microenvironment necessary for supporting hematopoiesis or to stem cells directly.

Myeloaplasia (Aplastic Anemia). Myeloaplasia is characterized by severe marrow depopulation and blood cytopenias including nonregenerative anemia, neutropenia, and thrombocytopenia. Examination of marrow aspirates reveals severely reduced numbers or absence of normal hematopoietic elements. A histologic section of marrow is often required to conclusively establish marrow hypoplasia or aplasia.

Feline Leukemia Virus Infection. This virus may induce aplastic anemia as one of its many sequelae in cats.

Estrogen Toxicity. Either large, repeated doses of diethylstilbestrol or single injections of the potent, long-acting estrogen estradiol cyclopentylpropionate may cause severe marrow suppression in dogs. Endogenous estrogen toxicity may occur in dogs with estrogen-secreting Sertoli cell tumors and in ferrets with prolonged estrus. Cats are apparently resistant to the development of estrogen toxicity.

Phenylbutazone Toxicity. Hematologic cytopenias with thrombocytopenic hemorrhage similar to estrogen toxicity may occur in dogs receiving phenylbutazone.

Chemotherapy. Toxicity must be anticipated even when recommended dosages of chemotherapeutic agents (see textbook Chapter 73) are used.

Canine Ehrlichiosis. In the acute form of disease there is marrow hypercellularity in the face of blood cytopenias. Marrow hypocellularity with features of aplastic anemia may develop in the chronic form of the disease.

Unknown Cause. The cause is unknown for occasional dogs with aplastic anemia. A long list of organic chemicals is established in humans and experimental animals as being capable of causing aplastic anemia. There currently is no specific treatment that results in stem cell repopulation. Broad-spectrum antibiotics and transfusions should be utilized as indicated. Steroids may be utilized to reduce thrombocytopenic hemorrhage. It is possible for stem cell repopulation to occur if intervening complications can be prevented. With intensive therapy, dogs with estrogen toxicity, phenylbutazone toxicity, and chronic ehrlichiosis have recovered within a few weeks. Most injuries related to chemotherapy are reversible. Occasional cats with FeLV-related marrow suppression may make spontaneous temporary improvements in association with steroids and other symptomatic treatment.

Myelodysplasia. In myelodysplasia, also referred to as dysmyelopoiesis, cytopenias may occur in the face of a relatively normal-appearing quantity of hematopoietic activity in marrow. This suggests that, for some unknown reason, cells are being produced but do not survive through maturation and entry into blood. The process is most frequently recognized as involving erythrocyte production, and is best recognized in the cat. Blood findings may include any combination of nonregenerative anemia, nucleated erythrocytes without reticulocytosis, increased erythrocyte volume heterogeneity, erythrocyte macrocytosis, neutropenia, hypersegmented or unusually large neutrophils, monocytosis, extremely large platelets, and thrombocytopenia. In blood and marrow, subtle morphologic changes observed in erythroid series cells may include megaloblastosis, altered synchrony of nuclear/cytoplasmic maturation, and nuclear fragmentation. A disproportionately increased number of blasts may be observed in the marrow.

Myeloproliferative Disorders.   The term myeloproliferative disorder denotes purposeless, neoplastic proliferation. Generally, marrow cytologic features include absence or severely reduced production of normal cellular elements, increased cellularity with predominance of the neoplastic cell type, and an apparent maturation arrest of the proliferating cell type. Erythremic myelosis is a specific myeloproliferative disorder comprised of neoplastic proliferation of the erythroid cell line. Treatment of myeloproliferative disorders is discouraging. Transfusions and other supportive therapy as described for aplastic anemia may provide symptomatic improvement.

Other Forms of Marrow Injury

Myelofibrosis and Osteosclerosis.   The proliferation of either fibrous or osseous elements injures the marrow space to the point that it will not support hematopoiesis. These lesions should be suspected when there is failure to obtain marrow on aspiration. They are confirmed by histologic examination of a marrow section. Extramedullary hematopoiesis is a prominent feature representing an attempt to populate blood. Myelofibrosis is also a sequela of pyruvate kinase deficiency.

Lymphoproliferative Disorders.   Lymphoma that involves marrow space, referred to as lymphocytic leukemia, may have an influence on erythropoiesis that is similar to myeloproliferative disorders. With myeloma, neoplastic marrow infiltrates are usually focal and coexist with normal or near- normal hematopoietic activity.

Chloramphenicol Toxicity.   Reversible bone marrow suppression may occur in dogs receiving doses in the range of 100 to 120 mg/lb/day (225 to 275 mg/kg/day). Cats are relatively susceptible to dose- dependent toxicity. It is currently recommended that, if used at all in the cat, chloramphenicol be limited to the smallest dose and shortest duration possible. It should not be used in dogs or cats with nonregenerative anemia.

CHAPTER 143

LEUKOCYTES IN HEALTH AND DISEASE
(pages 1892–1929)

BONE MARROW EXAMINATION

Indications for bone marrow examination associated with disorders of leukocytes include: persistent pancytopenia or neutropenia of unknown cause, suspected hematopoietic malignancy or myeloproliferative disease, leukocyte cytoplasmic and/or nuclear maturation abnormalities, assessment of lymphoproliferative disorders including documentation of multiple myeloma, and suspicion of infiltrative marrow disease secondary to neoplasia, infectious agents, or stromal proliferation. The reference intervals used for interpretation of leukocyte and bone marrow data are presented in Tables 143–1 and 143–2.

OVERVIEW OF HEMATOPOIESIS (p. 1897)

See the textbook for a review of hematopoiesis.

NEUTROPHILS (pp. 1897–1905)

Nuclear Morphologic Variations in Health

Pelger-Huët Anomaly. Pelger-Huët anomaly is a hereditary disorder of leukocyte development in which neutrophils as well as other granulocytes and monocytes have hyposegmented nuclei in the presence of a mature, coarse chromatin pattern. Megakaryocyte nuclei also are hypolobulated, suggesting a stem cell defect in the nuclear segmentation or lobulation process. Pelger-Huët anomaly is uncommon, but has been described in both dogs and cats. The anomaly is suspected when there is documentation of a persistent left shift without infection, marrow-associated neoplasia, or drug exposure. The heterozygous form of the anomaly is benign as no predisposition to infection exists. The homozygous form of the anomaly may have medical consequences including fetal death and resorption in utero, stillbirth, and possible skeletal deformities associated with chondrodysplasia.

Cytoplasmic Morphologic Variations in Health

Birman Cat Neutrophil Granulation Anomaly. Neutrophils from (autosomal receissive in Birman cats) cats contain fine pinkish-purple (azurophilic) intracytoplasmic granules in Romanowsky-stained blood smears. Although clinical and experimental evidence indicates that the Birman cat neutrophil anomaly is of little consequence, it must be differentiated from toxic granulation and mucopolysaccharidosis type VI (Morateaux-Lamy syndrome).

Nuclear Morphologic Variations in Disease

Nuclear Hyposegmentation. Nuclear hyposegmentation may indicate either immaturity of the neutrophil series or inability, on the part of a mature cell, to properly segment. Immaturity of the neutrophil series is recognized by the presence of bands, juveniles, and earlier

Original chapter written by Kenneth S. Latimer

TABLE 143–1. BLOOD AND BONE MARROW REFERENCE INTERVALS FOR DOGS

BLOOD VALUES

Cell Type	Distribution Range (%)	Absolute Range (cells/μl)
Leukocytes	—	5000–14,000
Neutrophils		
Segmenters	60–77	2900–12,000
Bands	0–3	0–450
Lymphocytes	8–30	400–2900
Monocytes	2–10	100–1400
Eosinophils	0–10	0–1300
Basophils	0–2	0–140

BONE MARROW VALUES

Cell Type	Range (%)	Mean (%)
Myeloid (granulocytic) series		
Myeloblasts	0.7–1.1	0.9
Promyelocytes	1.7–2.5	2.1
Neutrophils		
Myelocytes	5.3–7.3	6.3
Bands	9.1–13.5	11.3
Segmenters	22.2–24.8	23.5
Eosinophils		
Myelocytes	0.4–0.8	0.6
Metamyelocytes	0.4–1.0	0.7
Bands	0.8–1.6	1.2
Segmenters	0.3–1.3	0.8
Basophilic cells	0.0–0.06	0.02
Total Myeloid Cells	49.3–61.1	55.2
Erythroid series		
Rubriblasts, prorubricytes	6.1–6.9	6.5
Rubricytes, metarubricytes	23.2–32.0	27.6
Total Erythroid Cells	29.4–38.8	34.1
M:E Ratio	1.3–2.1	1.7
Other Cells		
Lymphocytes	5.5–10.9	8.2
Plasma cells	0.4–1.0	0.7
Monocytes	0.2–5.2	1.2
Macrophages	0.2–0.6	0.4
Mitotic figures	1.1–1.7	1.4

forms in the blood. These various immature neutrophil stages have finely stippled chromatin. If the neutrophil count is within the reference interval or increased, a significant left shift is indicated by the presence of 1000 or more bands per microliter of blood. In disease, mature (coarse nature chromatin pattern) hypo-segmented neutrophils are designated as pseudo-Pelger-Huët anomaly. Pseudo-Pelger-Huët anomaly occurs secondary to chronic infection, drug administration, myeloid metaplasia, and primary or metastatic neoplasia of the marrow cavity in humans. Feline leukemia virus-induced myeloid leukemia in cats also is associated with the presence of pseudo-Pelger-Huët neutrophils in the blood. In pseudo- Pelger-Huët anomaly fewer neu-

TABLE 143–2. BLOOD AND BONE MARROW REFERENCE INTERVALS FOR CATS

BLOOD VALUES

Cell Type	Distribution Range (%)	Absolute Range (cells/μl)
Leukocytes	—	5500–19,500
Neutrophils		
Segmenters	35–75	2500–12,500
Bands	0–3	0–300
Lymphocytes	20–55	1500–7000
Monocytes	1–4	0–850
Eosinophils	2–12	0–750
Basophils	0–2	0–200

BONE MARROW VALUES

Cell Type	Range (%)	Mean (%)
Myeloid (granulocytic) series		
Myeloblasts	0.0–1.8	0.4
Promyelocytes	0.6–3.8	1.2
Neutrophils		
Myelocytes	0.4–5.4	2.2
Metamyelocytes	0.6–9.6	4.2
Bands	5.0–19.4	11.0
Segmenters	17.8–38.6	27.8
Eosinophil series	0.6–7.2	3.0
Basophil series	0.0–0.4	0.2
Total Myeloid Cells	39.4–64.4	52.0
Erythroid series		
Rubriblasts	0.0–1.6	0.6
Prorubricytes, rubricytes	—	12.4
Metarubricytes	15.6–32.2	23.6
Total Erythroid Cells	24.0–48.8	36.6
M:E Ratio	0.9–2.5	1.5
Other Cells		
Lymphocytes	32.2–22.6	11.4
Plasma cells	0.0–1.2	0.2
Mitotic cells	0.0–2.0	1.0

trophils are hyposegmented than in the true congenital anomaly although exceptions do exist.

Asynchronous Nuclear Maturation. Asynchronous nuclear maturation occurs most commonly in cats during periods of intense granulopoietic activity associated with severe bacterial infection or recovery from infectious panleukopenia, but also may be a feature of myeloid leukemia.

Nuclear Hypersegmentation. Canine and feline neutrophils with five or more nuclear lobes are hypersegmented. Neutrophil hypersegmentation in blood smears from dogs and cats usually is secondary to an endogenous (prolonged stress, hyperadrenocorticism) or exogenous (iatrogenic) corticosteroid effect that prolongs the circulating half-life of neutrophils in the blood. Hypersegmented neutrophils also may be observed in granulocytic and myelomonocytic leukemia. Low numbers of normal-sized to enlarged, hypersegmented neutrophils also are seen in blood smears from miniature and toy poodles with erythrocyte macrocytosis. Nonregenerative anemia, neutropenia, and nuclear hypersegmentation of neutrophils has been described in giant schnauzers with inherited selective malabsorption of vitamin B_{12}. Affected dogs exhibit inappetence, lethargy, cachexia, and failure to thrive. Clinical signs usually are apparent by 6 to 12 weeks of age.

Cytoplasmic Morphologic Alterations in Disease

Toxic Change. These changes usually are associated with severe localized or systemic infections (septicemia), but also may occur with sterile inflammation and drug toxicity. A guarded prognosis is indicated when most neutrophils in the blood smear have toxic change. The various types of toxic change include cytoplasmic basophilia and vacuolation, the presence of Döhle (Doehle) bodies, and/or intensely stained primary granules (toxic granulation).

Intracytoplasmic Inclusions in Specific Infectious Diseases. Canine distemper inclusions are round to irregularly shaped magenta structures within leukocytes and/or erythrocytes on Romanowsky- or Diff-Quik-stained blood smears. Rickettsial inclusions are found within various leukocyte types however, certain strains of *Ehrlichia* may exhibit predisposition for infection of granulocytes. *Hepatozoon canis* gametocytes may be observed within neutrophils and/or monocytes upon examination of stained blood smears. *Histoplasma capsulatum* yeasts appear as intracytoplasmic "clusters of grapes" within neutrophils, monocytes, and/or eosinophils.

Cytoplasmic Inclusions in Congenital Diseases. In mucopolysaccharidosis type VI in cats and in mucopolysaccharidosis type VII in dogs, inclusions may be found within neutrophils that stain pinkish-purple with Romanowsky stains and metachromatically with 1 per cent toluidine blue dye. Chediak-Higashi syndrome is inherited in an autosomal recessive manner in blue smoke Persian cats with yellow-green irises, and is characterized by enlarged intracytoplasmic granules in circulating leukocytes and in melanocytes. From a clinical standpoint, it is important to identify cats with Chediak-Higashi syndrome because they bleed longer and more profusely than normal cats following venipuncture and minor surgery.

Neutrophil Cytoplasmic Changes and Inclusions in Miscellaneous Diseases. Vacuolation of the neutrophil cytoplasm occurs with drug toxicity in cats, especially after high dosages of chloramphenicol and phenylbutazone. Drug-induced changes in neutrophil morphology resemble "toxic changes." In rare instances of hemolytic disease with severe jaundice, bilirubin (hematoidin) crystals may be observed within neutrophils. Lupus erythematosus (LE) cells are leukocytes, usually neutrophils, that have phagocytized antinuclear antibody-coated DNA.

In healthy dogs, the total blood neutrophil pool is almost equally divided between the circulating neutrophil pool and the marginal neutrophil pool, producing a 1:1 ratio. In healthy cats, the circulating neutrophil pool is smaller than the marginal neutrophil pool, producing a 1:3 ratio.

NEUTROPHIL RESPONSE PATTERNS (pp. 1905–1914)

NEUTROPHILIA

Some causes of neutrophilia are listed in Table 143–3.

Physiologic Neutrophilia (Pseudoneutrophilia). Physiologic neutrophilia occurs with fear, excitement, strenuous exercise (including struggling during restraint for venipuncture), or after epinephrine injection. There is a transient shift of neutrophils from the marginal neutrophil pool into the circulating neutrophil pool without a left shift. Physiologic leukocytosis is identified by the presence of leukocytosis, neutrophilia without a left shift, lymphocytosis, and monocyte and eosinophil counts that are unaffected or elevated slightly. The lymphocytosis is frequently of greater magnitude than the neutrophilia, especially in the cat.

Corticosteroid-Associated Neutrophilia. Either endogenous release of cortisol from the adrenal cortex or exogenous administration of corticosteroids or ACTH can cause neutrophilia. Severe stress or acute disease must be present before endogenous cortisol release is sufficient to cause overt changes in the leukogram. Characteristic corticosteroid-induced changes in the leukogram include leukocytosis with neutrophilia, monocytosis, lymphopenia, and eosinopenia.

Neutrophilia Associated with Inflammation and/or Infection. Generally, the magnitude of the total neutrophil response is a reflection of the intensity of the disease process, whereas the degree of the left shift is suggestive of the severity of the disease. Neutrophilia with a left shift is considered the clinical hallmark of purulent inflammation. Exposure to endotoxin, is associated with a rapidly developing but transient neutropenia occurring over 1 to 3 hours followed by a rebound neutrophilia. In contrast, early gram-positive bacterial infection, exemplified by pneumonia, is accompanied by accelerated release of neutrophils from the bone marrow, expanded total blood neutrophil and marginal neutrophil pools, and a decreased neutrophil circulating half-life, but the neutrophil count is within the reference interval. Mild, clinically insignificant left shifts (300 to <1000 bands/μl) are associated with inflammatory disorders such as hemorrhagic cystitis, seborrheic dermatitis, tracheobronchitis, catarrhal or hemorrhagic enteritis, and granulomatous diseases in which the neutrophil is a minimal component of the exudate and/or tissue demand for neutrophils is very mild. Significant left shifts (≥1000 bands/μl) accompany pyoderma, pleuritis, peritonitis, pyometra, and abscess formation. Additionally, obscure loss of neutrophils is associated with hemorrhagic and hemolytic anemias, especially immune-mediated hemolytic anemia. Degenerative left shifts imply an intense suppurative disease and a guarded prognosis.

Leukemoid Reactions and Extreme Neutrophilic Leukocytosis. In veterinary medicine, the term leukemoid reaction suggests a total leukocyte count exceeding 75,000 cells/μl of blood with a severe left shift that may extend to myeloblasts. The term "extreme neutrophilic leukocytosis" implies a neutrophil count exceeding 100,000 cells/μl of blood with a mild left shift and no evidence of myeloid neoplasia. Although neutrophil precursors in both leukemoid reactions and granulocytic leukemia exhibit cytoplasmic basophilia, the additional presence of toxic vacuolation and Döhle bodies would favor a diagnosis of infection and leukemoid response. Extreme neutrophilic leukocytosis usually results from severe, localized pyogenic infections, especially pyometra in dogs and abscesses in cats. Cases of suspected or documented neutrophil dysfunction with secondary bacterial infection also are associated with extreme leukocytosis. Other associations with extreme neutrophilic leukocytosis in dogs include *Hepatozoon canis* infection (173,300 PMN/μl), immune-mediated hemolytic anemia, and paraneoplastic syndromes secondary to metastatic fibrosarcoma (121,800 PMN/μl), renal tubular carcinoma (128,600 and 238,800 PMN/μl), and rectal adenoma (111,400 PMN/μl).

NEUTROPENIA

Conditions associated with neutropenia in dogs and cats are listed in Table 143–3.

The major clinical consequence of neutropenia is infection.

TABLE 143–3. CAUSES OF NEUTROPHILIA AND NEUTROPENIA IN DOGS AND CATS

Neutrophilia

Physiologic response (excitement, fear)	Dog, cat
Infection	
Bacteria (various species)	Dog, cat
Rickettsia	
Rocky Mountain spotted fever	Dog
Viruses	
Canine distemper	Dog
Feline rhinotracheitis	Cat
Fungi (various species)	Dog, cat
Parasites	
Toxoplasmosis	Dog, cat
Hepatozoonosis	Dog
Immune-mediated diseases	Dog, cat
Autoimmune hemolytic anemia	
Lupus erythematosus	
Polymyositis	
Polyserositis	
Rheumatoid arthritis	
Tissue necrosis	Dog, cat
Thrombosis and infarction	
Burns	
Malignancy	
Uremia	
Drug administration	
Corticosteroids	Dog, cat
Epinephrine	Dog
Estrogen (early)	Dog
rhG-CSF (short-term neutrophilia)	Dog
rcG-CSF (long-term neutrophilia)	Dog
Paraneoplastic syndrome	
Fibrosarcoma	Dog
Rectal adenoma	Dog
Renal tubular carcinoma	Dog
Miscellaneous	Dog, cat
Acute severe stress (any cause)	
Sterile foreign body	
Hemolytic disease	
Hemorrhage	

Hematopoietic Stem Cell Death or Inhibition

Chemotherapy Drugs. Drugs such as azathioprine, cyclophosphamide, daunomycin, dimethyl myleran, doxorubicin, and 6- thioguanine induce predictable myelosuppression in dogs and cats. The nadir of leukopenia occurs within 4 to 7 days, and hematologic recovery may occur within 20 to 40 days.

Estrogen Toxicosis in Dogs. See textbook Chapter 142.

Chloramphenicol Toxicosis in Cats. See textbook Chapter 143.

Phenylbutazone Toxicosis in Dogs. See textbook Chapter 143.

Miscellaneous Drugs and Compounds. Idiosyncratic drug reactions in dogs characterized by pancytopenia or neutropenia also have been observed with trimethoprim-sulfadiazine, cephalosporin (cefazedore, cefadioxi-1) thiacetarsamide administration, and ingestion of medicated skin creme (Noxzema). Severe neutropenia also has been observed in cats with feline immunodeficiency virus when treated with griseofulvin.

Parvovirus Infection of Dogs (Parvoviral Enteritis) and Cats (Feline Panleukopenia). See textbook Chapter 143. Leukopenia is

TABLE 143–3. *(Continued)*

Neutropenia	
Infection	
Bacteria (septicemia, endotoxemia)	Dog, cat
Rickettsia	
Ehrlichia canis	Dog
Viruses	
Parvoviral enteritis	Dog
Feline panleukopenia	Cat
Feline leukemia virus	Cat
Feline immunodeficiency virus	Cat
Fungi	
Histoplasmosis (disseminated)	Dog, cat
Drug administration	
Relatively predictable	
Estrogen (overdose)	Dog
Chemotherapy agents	Dog, cat
Chloramphenicol	Cat
Idiosyncratic	
Cephalosporins	Dog, cat
Phenylbutazone	Dog
Thiacetarsamide	Dog
Noxema ingestion	Dog
Bone marrow necrosis	Dog, cat
Myelofibrosis and osteopetrosis	Dog
Neoplastic and myelodysplastic disease	
Acute granulocytic leukemia	Dog
Acute lymphoblastic leukemia	Dog
Acute myelomonocytic leukemia	Dog
Erythremic myelosis	Cat
Large granular lymphoma	Cat
Megakaryocytic myelosis/leukemia	Dog, cat
Multicentric lymphosarcoma	Dog
Myelodysplastic syndromes	Dog
Cyclic hematopoiesis	
Gray collies (congenital)	Dog
Miscellaneous dog breeds (unknown etiology)	Dog
Cyclophosphamide administration	Dog
Feline leukemia virus-associated	Cat
Immune-mediated mechanisms?	Dog, cat
Inherited malabsorption of vitamin B_{12} (giant schnauzer)	Dog
Radiation	Dog, cat

most severe approximately 5 to 8 days postinfection, and usually is accompanied by a left shift to juveniles and toxic change.

Feline Leukemia Virus Infection. Examination of blood and bone marrow data from FeLV-infected cats indicates that three patterns of neutropenia exist. The most frequent pattern is mild neutropenia with relatively normal granulopoiesis. The second pattern is moderate neutropenia with granulopoietic hypoplasia, referred to as the "panleukopenia-like syndrome." However, gastrointestinal signs may not be present. The third pattern consists of severe, persistent, insidious neutropenia with marked granulopoietic hyperplasia previously designated as subleukemic granulocytic leukemia, preleukemia, or hemopoietic dysplasia. In each of the three patterns, left shifts (sometimes severe) with toxic neutrophils may be found.

Feline Immunodeficiency Virus Infection. Neutropenia is more predictable and severe in acute viral infection, but is intermittent and of variable severity in chronic viral infection. Recent evidence suggests, however, that reappearance of leukopenia during infection coincides with the development of acquired immunodeficiency syndrome (AIDS).

Canine Ehrlichiosis. Transient leukopenia is associated with early rickettsial infection. Subclinical and chronic forms of the disease may last for years and have fewer instances of pancytopenia, thrombocytopenia, or bleeding disorders.

Reduced Hematopoietic Space

See Chapter 143 of the textbook.

Neutropenia secondary to reduced hematopoietic space is unusual but may occur with bone marrow necrosis or myelophthisic disease. In most instances, bone marrow aspiration and core biopsies will be necessary for a definitive diagnosis.

Neoplastic and Myelodysplastic Diseases. Myelophthisis maybe secondary to a variety of neoplastic or preneoplastic diseases, including erythremic myelosis, large granular lymphoma, and megakaryocytic myelosis in cats as well as acute granulocytic leukemia, acute myelomonocytic leukemia, megakaryoblastic leukemia, myelodysplastic syndromes, acute lymphoblastic leukemia, and lymphosarcoma in dogs.

Cyclic Stem Cell Input or Proliferation

Canine Cyclic Hematopoiesis. Affected collies have a diluted haircoat color (silver-grey, beige, or charcoal) and usually die prematurely. Clinical signs are related to profound, cyclic neutropenia with subsequent development of recurrent, severe, life-threatening infections. Cyclic fluctuations of leukocytes (neutrophils, monocytes, lymphocytes, and eosinophils), reticulocytes, and platelets occur approximately every 11.5 days with cycle lengths ranging from 10 to 12.4 days. With intensive antibiotic therapy and supportive care, affected dogs survive less than 3 years. Both endotoxin injections and lithium carbonate administration will eliminate cyclic neutropenia. However, endotoxin has undesirable side effects such as fever, chills, pain, and induction of shock, whereas lithium is highly toxic and must be monitored carefully.

Immune Suppression of Granulopoiesis

Although immune suppression of granulopoiesis is not well documented in animals, reports of steroid responsive neutropenias in dogs and cats suggest that this entity exists.

Reduced Survival Neutropenia

Increased Tissue Demand for Neutrophils. Neutropenia usually results from sudden, massive tissue utilization of neutrophils at a rate exceeding neutrophil replacement in the blood by the bone marrow. Clinically, neutropenia is usually secondary to localized bacterial infections of the body cavities, lung, uterus, or gastrointestinal tract, or secondary to generalized septicemia. Severe infections are associated with marked, frequently degenerative, left shifts and toxic changes.

Immune-Mediated Neutropenia. The hematologic picture of immune-mediated leukopenia is one of persistent profound neutropenia with a compensatory monocytosis. Confirmation of the diagnosis requires demonstration of antineutrophil antibodies in the serum or on neutrophils. Clinical cases of immune-mediated neutropenia have yet to be documented in dogs and cats.

Prognosis of Neutrophil Response Patterns

Response patterns that initially warrant a guarded prognosis include: any form of neutropenia, a degenerative left shift with or without toxic change or maturation abnormalities, and a leukemoid response or extreme neutrophilic leukocytosis.

Neutrophil Functional Abnormalities

Congenital abnormalities in neutrophil function should be suspected in any neonate that experiences severe, recurrent bacterial infections in the presence of a normal to markedly increased neutrophil count (Table 143–4). Furthermore, cytologic preparations from sites of infection contain few neutrophils. Unfortunately, many bioassays of cell function are subject to great variability and may not detect subtle impairments in cell function. Although specific therapy for basic defects in neutrophil function is rarely possible.

TABLE 143–4. CONDITIONS ASSOCIATED WITH DEFECTIVE NEUTROPHIL FUNCTION IN DOGS AND CATS

Adherence
    Intrinsic cell defects
        Leukocyte adhesion molecule deficiency*   Dog
          (Irish setters)
    Metabolic or nutritional disease
        Diabetes mellitus (poorly regulated)   Dog

Chemotaxis
    Abnormal chemotactic factor generation
        C3 deficiency (Brittany spaniel)   Dog
    Cellular/chemotactic factor-directed inhibitors
        Prototheocosis   Dog
    Intrinsic cellular defects
        Chediak-Higashi syndrome   Cat
        Leukocyte adhesion molecule deficiency   Dog
        Primary ciliary dyskinesia (Pointer)   Dog
    Infectious diseases
        Bacterial pyoderma   Dog
        Feline leukemia virus infection   Cat
        Feline infectious peritonitis   Cat
    Metabolic or nutritional disease   Dog
        Hyperalimentation-induced hypophosphatemia

Phagocytosis
    Intrinsic or opsonic defects
        Leukocyte adhesion molecule deficiency   Dog
        Complement deficiency (C3)   Dog
    Metabolic or nutritional disease
        Hyperalimentation-induced hypophosphatemia   Dog
    Miscellaneous conditions
        Filtration leukopheresis-collected neutrophils   Dog

Bacterial killing
    Intrinsic cellular defects
        Leukocyte adhesion molecule deficiency   Dog
        Cyclic neutropenia   Dog
        Doberman Pinscher   Dog
    Infectious diseases
        Feline leukemia virus infection   Cat
    Toxic diseases
        Lead toxicosis   Dog
        Turpentine-induced inflammation   Dog
    Metabolic or nutritional disease
        Hyperalimentation-induced hypophosphatemia   Dog

*Synonyms include canine granulocytopathy syndrome and CD11/CD18 glycoprotein deficiency.

MONOCYTES (pp. 1914–1915)

If blood smears are prepared immediately, few vacuoles are observed within monocytes. Vacuoles are observed frequently in monocytes if the blood sample stands for several hours before smears are prepared. Monocyte vacuolation, however, may be a feature of certain diseases such as sphingomyelinosis (Niemann-Pick disease) and cholesteryl ester storage disease of Siamese cats and autoimmune hemolytic anemia of dogs, wherein monocytic vacuolation may be associated with erythrophagia.

MONOCYTE RESPONSE PATTERNS (p. 1915)

MONOCYTOSIS

See Table 143–5. Both acute and chronic diseases result in monocytosis, and most of the acute conditions are trauma-related injuries. Disorders associated with suppuration, necrosis, malignancy, hemolysis, internal hemorrhage, pyogranulomatous inflammation, and immune-mediated diseases are accompanied by neutrophilia and concomitant monocytosis. Monocytosis commonly is accompanied by neutrophilia except in some unusual presentations of bacterial endocarditis and/or bacteremia in dogs, wherein monocytosis may be the only or predominant change in the leukogram.

MONOCYTOPENIA

Monocytopenia is infrequently documented and clinically unimportant.

DISORDERS OF THE MONOCYTE-MACROPHAGE SYSTEM

Hereditary disturbances of the monocyte-macrophage system in Bernese mountain dogs may present as a benign systemic histiocytosis or malignant histiocytosis.

TABLE 143–5. DISEASES ASSOCIATED WITH MONOCYTOSIS* IN DOGS AND CATS

Infectious	
Bacterial endocarditis	Dog
Bacteremia/septicemia	Dog
Suppuration, necrosis	Dog, cat
Pyogranulomatous inflammation	Dog, cat
Feline leukemia virus (cyclic hematopoiesis)	Cat
Acquired, noninfectious, non-neoplastic diseases	Dog, cat
Hemorrhage, hemolysis	
Immune-mediated diseases	
Corticosteroid treatment	
Trauma	
Neutropenia w/compensatory monocytosis	
Congenital diseases	
Cyclic hematopoiesis	Dog
Drug administration	
Corticosteroids	
rcG-CSF	Dog
Dog	
Neoplastic diseases	Dog, cat
Nonspecific malignancies	
Monocytic leukemia	
Myelomonocytic leukemia	

*Monocytosis occurs in both acute and chronic diseases.

LYMPHOCYTES (pp. 1915–1918)

Diseases involving lymphocytes per se may have minimal effects on circulating lymphocyte numbers, but alterations in cell function may be profound. Intracytoplasmic inclusions may be present within lymphocytes in canine distemper virus infection or in canine ehrlichiosis. In sphingomyelinosis (Niemann-Pick disease) and cholesteryl ester

TABLE 143–6. CONDITIONS ASSOCIATED WITH LYMPHOCYTOSIS AND LYMPHOPENIA IN DOGS AND CATS

Lymphocytosis	
Physiologic (epinephrine response)	Dog, cat
Antigenic stimulation (various etiologies)	
Blastomycosis	Dog
Chronic canine ehrlichiosis	Dog
Chronic Rocky Mountain spotted fever	Dog
Feline leukemia virus infection	Cat
Lymphoid neoplasia	Dog, cat
Lymphosarcoma	
Lymphocytic leukemia (acute and chronic)	
Thymoma	
Hypoadrenocorticism (Addison's disease)	Dog, cat
Lymphopenia	
Immunosuppressive drugs and/or radiation	Dog, cat
Corticosteroid-induced	Dog, cat
Exogenous corticosteroids or ACTH	
Endogenous corticosteroid release	
Acute stress	
Hyperadrenocorticism (Cushing's disease)	
Acute systemic infection (various etiologies)	
Canine parvovirus	Dog
Canine coronavirus	Dog
Canine distemper	Dog
Infectious canine hepatitis	Dog
Feline panleukopenia	Cat
Feline leukemia virus	Cat
Feline immunodeficiency virus	Cat
Septicemia/endotoxemia	Dog, cat
Loss of lymphocyte-rich lymph	
Chylothorax (ruptured thoracic duct)	Dog, cat
Effusion of cardiac disease	Cat
Protein-losing enteropathy	Dog
Lymphangiectasia	Dog
Ulcerative enteritis	Dog, cat
Granulomatous enteritis	Dog, cat
Alimentary lymphosarcoma	Dog, cat
Enteric neoplasms	Dog, cat
Disruption of lymph node architecture	Dog, cat
Multicentric lymphosarcoma	
Generalized granulomatous disease	
T-lymphocyte deficiency	
Acquired (neonatal infection)	
Canine distemper	Dog
Feline leukemia virus infection (FAIDS)	Cat
Feline immunodeficiency virus infection	Cat
Congenital	
Combined immunodeficiency (Basset hound)	Dog
Drug associated	
rcG-CSF	Dog
rhIL-2	Dog

storage disease of Siamese cats and in mannosidosis of Persian cats, lymphocytes may appear vacuolated. Lymphoblasts should arouse suspicion of lymphoid neoplasia when present in increased numbers on the blood smear.

PRODUCTION, RECIRCULATION, AND KINETICS

This process is discussed in detail in the textbook (pages 1916–1918).

LYMPHOCYTE RESPONSE PATTERNS (pp. 1918–1919)

Causes of lymphocytosis lymphocytosis are listed in Table 143–6. Transient lymphocytosis, a feature of physiologic leukocytosis in dogs and cats, occurs more frequently in young animals and is more dramatic in the cat.

EOSINOPHILS (pp. 1919–1920)

Primary functions of eosinophils include destruction of parasites and modulation of hypersensitivity reactions. Eosinophils also have a proinflammatory function. Greyhounds occasionally have moth-eaten, vacuolated, or degranulated eosinophils in health. Disease-associated degranulation of eosinophils, although rare, may be observed in dirofilariasis, allergic reactions, and hypereosinophilic syndromes. In Persian cats with Chediak-Higashi syndrome, eosinophil granules may appear plump or enlarged.

EOSINOPHIL RESPONSE PATTERNS (pp. 1920–1921)

Some causes of eosinophilia and eosinopenia in dogs and cats are presented in Table 143–7. Hypereosinophilic syndromes are seen most frequently in cats and are difficult, if not impossible, to distinguish from eosinophilic leukemia. As a paraneoplastic syndrome, eosinophilia is observed most frequently with mast cell neoplasia and lymphosarcoma.

TABLE 143–7. SOME CONDITIONS ASSOCIATED WITH EOSINOPHILIA AND EOSINOPENIA IN DOGS AND CATS

Eosinophilia
Hypersensitivity and/or inflammatory lesions
Alimentary tract	
Oral granuloma	Dog
Gastroenteritis (ulcerative)	Dog, cat
Gastrointestinal eosinophilic granuloma	Dog
Genitourinary tract	
Pyometra	Dog
Musculoskeletal system	
Myositis (poorly documented)	Dog
Panosteitis (rare)	Dog
Respiratory tract	
Pulmonary granulomas (heartworm-related?)	Dog
Pulmonary infiltrates with eosinophilia	Dog
Skin and special senses	
Atopy	Cat
Canine eosinophilic granuloma	Dog
Eosinophilic keratitis	Cat
Feline eosinophilic granuloma complex	Cat
Flea allergy dermatitis	Dog, cat
Food hypersensitivity	Cat
Sterile eosinophilic pustulosis	Dog

TABLE 143–7. *(Continued)*

Parasites	
Nematodes	
Aelurostrongylus abstrusus	Cat
Ascarids	Dog, cat
Coccidosis	Cat
Dipetalonema reconditum	Dog
Dirofilaria immitis	Dog, cat
Giardiasis	Cat
Hookworms	Dog
Ollulanus tricuspis	Cat
Oslerus (Filaroides) osteri	Dog
Pentastomes	Dog
Physaloptera sp	Dog
Spirocerca lupi	Dog
Toxacara canis	Cat
Trichinella spiralis	Dog, cat
Trichuris vulpis	Dog
Trematodes	
Heterobilharzia americana	Dog
Paragonimus kellicotti	Dog, cat
Platynosomum concinnum	Cat
Insects	
Fleas	Dog, cat
Trombiculosis	Cat
Protozoa	
Hepatozoon canis	Dog
Feline leukemia virus-associated	
Cyclic hematopoiesis	Cat
Leukemoid reaction/leukemia	Cat
Neoplasia-associated	
Eosinophilic leukemia	Cat
Hypereosinophilic syndrome	Dog, Cat
Myeloid leukemia	Dog
Myeloproliferative disease	Cat
Paraneoplastic syndrome	
Basal cell tumor	Cat
Fibrosarcoma	Dog
Gastric carcinoma	Cat
Lymphomatoid granulomatosis	Dog
Lymphosarcoma	Cat
Mammary carcinoma	Dog
Mast cell neoplasia (disseminated)	Dog
Myxosarcoma	Cat
Osterosarcoma	Cat
Pilomatrixoma	Cat
Renal carcinoma	Cat
Salivary carcinoma	Cat
Transitional cell carcinoma	Cat
Miscellaneous conditions	
Hyperthyroidism	Cat
Hypoadrenocorticism (unpredictable)	Dog, cat
rhIL-2 administration	Dog, cat
Eosinopenia	
Acute infection	Dog, cat
Endogenous corticosteroid release	
Acute stress (various causes)	Dog, cat
Hyperadrenocorticism	Dog, cat
Drug administration	
ACTH	Dog, cat
Corticosteroids	Dog, cat

BASOPHILS (pp. 1921–1923)

Medical technicians in human hospital laboratories fail to recognize normal cat basophils during the leukocyte differential count because of their unique tinctorial property. Morphologic distinctions between basophils and mast cells are consistent in health and disseminated, well-differentiated mast cell neoplasia, but may present difficulty in rare cases of basophilic leukemia wherein nuclear hyposegmentation of basophils is expected.

BASOPHILIA

Generally, basophilia occurs concomitantly with eosinophilia in dogs and cats. Some causes of basophilia in dogs and cats are listed in Table 143–8. The most frequent clinical cause of basophilia in dogs and cats is heartworm infestation, especially in cases of occult disease.

LEUKEMIAS AND MYELOPROLIFERATIVE SYNDROMES (pp. 1923–1927)

TERMINOLOGY AND CLASSIFICATION

Classification of the leukemia by the predominant cell type is accomplished using Romanowsky-stained blood and bone marrow smears, a battery of cytochemical stains, and electron microscopy. In addition, multiple cell lines may be involved in the neoplastic process. Common examples are myelomonocytic leukemia, in which the bipotential stem cell produces both neutrophils and monocytes, and erythroleukemia, in which both erythroid precursors and granulocytes are produced.

In addition to leukemias, hematologic dyscrasias, termed myeloproliferative syndromes, exist with cytopenias of one or more blood cell lines and no evidence of overt neoplasia in either the blood or bone marrow. However, cellular maturation abnormalities may exist. Leukemia may develop in the terminal stage of disease. In cats, leukemias are almost invariably associated with viral infection.

Clinical Signs and Physical Findings. The clinical signs

TABLE 143–8. CAUSES OF BASOPHILIA IN DOGS AND CATS

Hypersensitivity and/or inflammatory lesions	
Allergic respiratory disorders	Dog, cat
Canine cutaneous eosinophilic granuloma	Dog
Eosinophilic gastroenteritis	Dog
Feline eosinophilic granuloma complex	Cat
Pulmonary eosinophilic granuloma	Dog
Pulmonary infiltrates with eosinophilia	Dog
Parasitic diseases	
Dirofilaria immitis	Dog, cat
Dipetalonema recondium	Dog
Neoplasia	
Basophilic leukemia	Dog, cat
Essential thrombocythemia	Dog
Lymphomatoid granulomatosis	Dog
Mast cell neoplasia (disseminated)	Dog
Myeloid leukemia	Cat
Polycythemia vera	Cat
Drug administration	
Heparin	Dog
Penicillin	Dog

associated with leukemias and myeloproliferative disease are variable and vague including lethargy, anorexia, rapid weight loss, shifting limb lameness, persistent fever, dyspnea, vomiting, diarrhea, and recurrent infections. Physical findings frequently include splenomegaly, hepatomegaly, enlargement of the lymph nodes and/or tonsils, pallor of mucous membranes, fever, emaciation, and petechiae. In some instances, clinical signs may be specifically related to organ or tissue dysfunction secondary to neoplastic cell infiltration. Animals with leukemia may die as a consequence of infection, severe anemia, hemorrhage, or organ dysfunction secondary to neoplastic cell infiltration and proliferation. In addition, paraproteinemia may result, causing hemostatic problems or a hyperviscosity syndrome.

MYELOPROLIFERATIVE DISORDERS

Granulocytic (Myeloid, Neutrophilic) Leukemia. The total leukocyte count is variable, ranging from leukopenia to marked leukocytosis. Anemia usually is severe. Chronic granulocytic leukemia may present with increased numbers of more differentiated neutrophils, and must be distinguished from a leukemoid response secondary to infection.

Myelomonocytic Leukemia. Myelomonocytic leukemia is one of the more common myeloproliferative diseases in dogs and also has been reported in cats.

Monocytic Leukemia. Monocytic leukemia is uncommon in the dog and cat.

Eosinophilic Leukemia. Eosinophilic leukemia has only been reported in the cat and is difficult, if not impossible, to distinguish from hypereosinophilic syndromes. In all reported cases of leukemia, the cells were well differentiated and diagnosis was made by observation of characteristic specific (secondary) granules.

Basophilic Leukemia. Basophilic leukemia is extremely rare in both the cat and the dog. Basophilic leukemia may be difficult to distinguish from mast cell leukemia. All cases of basophilic leukemia in cats have been feline leukemia virus–test positive.

Mast Cell Leukemia. Disseminated mast cell neoplasia with a leukemic blood picture usually is associated with splenic enlargement in cats and with primary cutaneous mast cell tumors in dogs. In contrast, mast cell leukemia, which originates within the bone marrow in the absence of cutaneous or splenic neoplasms, is rare. Mast cell neoplasia should be the first diagnostic consideration in cats when large round cells containing numerous purple granules are observed on the stained blood smear.

Erythremic Myelosis. Hematopoietic malignancy involving nucleated erythrocytes (rubriblasts to metarubricytes in the absence of polychromasia) is relatively common in cats; however, this form of leukemia is rare in the dog. Feline erythremic myelosis usually is accompanied by a severe anemia with packed cell volumes ranging from 3.5 to 20 per cent. Although numerous nucleated erythrocytes may be present on the blood smear, the anemia is nonregenerative with aggregate reticulocyte counts of less than 1 per cent.

Polycythemia Vera (Polycythemia Rubra Vera, Primary Erythrocytosis). A diagnosis of polycythemia is suggested by the presence of brick-red mucous membranes, splenomegaly, and an increased packed cell volume (typically 65 to 81 per cent). Documentation of polycythemia vera requires demonstration of an expanded red cell mass in the presence of a normal PaO_2 and a decreased serum erythropoietin concentration. The diagnostic workup also should eliminate the possibility of renal cysts or tumors such as renal carcinoma, fibrosarcoma, or renal lymphosarcoma, which may produce polycythemia secondarily.

Megakaryocytic Leukemia (Myelosis). Both leukocyte and

platelet counts are variable, but megakaryoblasts may be found in the blood.

Essential Thrombocythemia.   Essential thrombocythemia is an extremely rare chronic myeloproliferative disease characterized by proliferation of megakaryocytes and persistently elevated platelet counts secondary to unregulated thrombocytopoiesis.

LYMPHOPROLIFERATIVE DISORDERS

Lymphocytic Leukemia.   Lymphocytic leukemia is one of the most common forms of leukemia in dogs and cats. Sarcomatous masses are not present in true leukemia, but are expected with lymphosarcoma. Acute lymphoblastic leukemia is characterized by immature cells in the blood and cytochemistry may be needed to identify the cell lineage. In chronic lymphocytic leukemia, the lymphocytes are small and well differentiated. This form chronic lymphocytic leukemia must be distinguished from physiologic lymphocytosis, especially in cats, and from antigenic stimulation-induced lymphocytosis as in chronic canine ehrlichiosis.

Plasma Cell Leukemia.   Plasma cell myelomas have four diagnostic features including: a monoclonal gammopathy, the presence of more than 20 per cent plasma cells within bone marrow aspirates, Bence Jones proteinuria, and radiographic evidence of osteolysis. Two of these four features are considered essential to diagnose a plasma cell myeloma.

CHAPTER 144
DISEASES OF THE LYMPH NODES AND THE SPLEEN
(pages 1930–1946)

LYMPHADENOPATHY

In the context of this chapter, the term lymphadenopathy refers to lymph node enlargement, although lymph node atrophy should also be considered a "lymphadenopathy."

Evaluation of the Patient with Lymphadenopathy

History and Physical Findings.   The presence or absence of systemic clinical signs is helpful in guiding the clinician to a diagnosis in dogs or cats with generalized lymphadenopathy, since severe systemic signs are more common in some diseases but are usually absent in dogs and cats with lymphoma or chronic leukemia. When evaluating a patient with solitary or regional lymphadenopathy, the clinician should focus attention on the area drained by those lymph nodes, since with almost certainty that is where the primary lesion will be found. Most patients with deep (intra-abdominal, intrathoracic) solitary or regional lymphadenopathy have metastatic neoplasia or systemic infectious disease (e.g., systemic mycoses). In contrast, most dogs and cats

---

Original chapter written by C. Guillermo Couto and Alan S. Hammer

with generalized lymphadenopathy have systemic fungal or rickettsial infections, idiopathic lymph node hyperplasia, or hematopoietic neoplasia. Marked lymphadenopathy (lymph node size five to ten times normal) occurs almost exclusively with lymphadenitis (e.g., lymph node abscessation, tuberculosis) and with lymphomas.

Diagnostic Studies. Two major serum biochemical abnormalities are of diagnostic value in dogs and cats with lymphadenopathy: *hypercalcemia* and *hyperglobulinemia.* Hypercalcemia is a paraneoplastic syndrome that occurs in approximately 10 to 20 per cent of dogs with lymphoma and multiple myeloma; it has also been documented in dogs with blastomycosis. Monoclonal hyperglobulinemia may occur in dogs and cats with multiple myeloma, in dogs with chronic lymphocytic leukemia (CLL), and occasionally in dogs with lymphoma, ehrlichiosis, and leishmaniasis. Polyclonal hyperglobulinemia commonly occurs in dogs and cats with systemic mycoses, in cats with feline infectious peritonitis (FIP), and in dogs with ehrlichiosis and lymphoma. In general, plain radiographs and ultrasound are beneficial in patients with deep regional lymphadenopathy involving the thoracic and abdominal cavities. Cytologic evaluation of lymph node aspirates is usually the definitive diagnostic procedure in most patients with lymphadenopathy. It is advisable not to obtain a specimen from the largest lymph node, since central necrosis usually results in a nondiagnostic sample. Also, since clinical or subclinical gingivitis is common in older dogs and cats, mandibular lymph nodes should not be aspirated routinely since they are usually reactive and they may obscure the primary diagnosis. When cytologic examination of an enlarged lymph node fails to provide a definitive diagnosis, excision of the affected node for histopathologic examination is indicated.

Selected Disorders Associated with Lymphadenopathy in Dogs and Cats

Bacterial Lymphadenitis. *Contagious streptococcal lymphadenitis* has been described in kittens. The lymph nodes in these cats were markedly enlarged and developed draining purulent lesions. Most cats responded to treatment with penicillin. *Puppy strangles* is a disorder associated with cutaneous cellulitis of the head and neck, and cervical lymphadenopathy in 4- to 12-week-old dogs. Pups usually present with fever, deep facial pyoderma, and cervical lymphadenopathy; more than one pup in the litter are commonly affected. Fine-needle aspiration of affected lymph nodes reveals purulent lymphadenitis, and staphylococcal or streptococcal organisms may be cultured. However, because of the lack of response to antibiotic therapy in a high proportion of cases, corticosteroids are usually used.

Idiopathic Lymphadenopathies. The term *distinctive peripheral lymph node hyperplasia* (DPLH) was used to describe 14 cats; eight cats were clinically normal on initial physical examination, except for the presence of lymphadenopathy; clinical signs in the other six cats included fever (five cats), lethargy (three cats), anorexia (three cats), pallor, hematuria, eczema, vomiting, and mastitis (one cat each). Therapy in affected cats included antibiotics, corticosteroids, and fluids. Based on the histologic changes and on the fact that six of the nine cats evaluated were FeLV-positive, the authors postulated that this syndrome is secondary to retroviral infection. Resolution of the lymphadenopathy was seen in all cats within 5 to 120 days; all cats were alive 12 to 84 months after initial diagnosis.

Feline Lymphoma. It is currently accepted that the majority of lymphomas in the cat are induced by FeLV.

Mediastinal Form. The average age of cats with mediastinal lymphoma is 2 to 3 years, and approximately 80 per cent of cats with mediastinal lymphoma are FeLV-positive. Clinical signs and findings

TABLE 144–1. CHEMOTHERAPY PROTOCOLS FOR CANINE AND FELINE LYMPHOMA USED AT THE OHIO STATE UNIVERSITY VETERINARY TEACHING HOSPITAL

1. Induction of remission
   - *COAP protocol (feline)*
     Cyclophosphamide (Cytoxan) 50 mg/m^2 BSA PO, 4 days a week (or every other day)
     Vincristine (Oncovin) 0.5 mg/m^2 BSA IV, once a week
     Cytosine arabinoside (Cytosar-U) 100 mg/m^2 BSA/day, IV drip or SQ, for only 2 days
     Prednisone 40 mg/m^2 BSA PO, once a day for a week; then 20 mg/m^2 BSA PO, every other day
     This protocol is used for 6 weeks; at the end of the induction phase the patient is started on maintenance therapy.
   - *CHOP protocol (feline)*
     Cyclophosphamide (Cytoxan) 100-200 mg/m^2 BSA PO, on days 15 and 16 of the cycle
     Hydroxydaunorubicin (Adriamycin) 25 mg/m^2 BSA IV, on day 1 of the cycle
     Vincristine (Oncovin) 0.5 mg/m^2 BSA IV, on days 8 and 15 of the cycle
     Prednisone 40 mg/m^2 BSA PO, once a day for a week; then 20 mg/m^2 BSA PO, every other day
     Repeat the cycle on day 22; administer a total of 3 cycles, then begin maintenance therapy.
   - *DOMAC (feline)*
     Dexamethasone 2 mg/kg SQ weekly
     Vincristine (Oncovin) 0.5 mg/m^2 BSA IV, days 8, 15, and 22
     Mitoxantrone (Novantrone) 3.5 mg/m^{2}BSA IV, days 1 and 15 over 4 hours
     Cytosine arabinoside (Cytosar-U) 200 mg/m^2 BSA IV, day 1 over 4 hours (mixed with the mitoxantrone)
     Cyclophosphamide (Cytoxan) 100–200 mg/m^2 BSA PO, days 8 and 22
     Repeat cycle on day 29; administer 3 consecutive cycles.
   - *COAP protocol (canine)*
     Cyclophosphamide (Cytoxan) 50 mg/m^2 BSA PO, 4 days a week (or every other day)
     Vincristine (Oncovin) 0.5 mg/m^2 BSA IV, once a week
     Cytosine arabinoside (Cytosar-U) 100 mg/m^2 BSA/day IV drip or SQ, for 4 days
     Prednisone 40 mg/m^2 BSA PO, once a day for a week; then 20 mg/m^2 BSA PO, every other day
     This protocol is used for 8 weeks; at the end of the induction phase the patient is started on maintenance therapy.

include dyspnea, tachypnea, regurgitation, coughing, anorexia, depression, weight loss of short duration, noncompressible anterior mediastinum, displacement of cardiac sounds dorsocaudally, absence of normal bronchovesicular sounds on the cranioventral aspect of the lungs, and dull sound on thoracic percussion. A confirmatory diagnosis can be obtained through cytologic examination of the pleural fluid (in most cases) or percutaneous fine-needle aspirates from the mass(es).

Alimentary Form. The average age of cats with alimentary lymphoma is higher than in other anatomic forms (8 years versus 2 to 5 years). Cats with alimentary lymphoma are FeLV-positive in only 30 per cent of the cases. Endoscopic biopsies of upper or lower gastrointestinal lesions are generally diagnostic.

Multicentric Form. We prefer to reserve the term multicentric for cats with solid hemolymphatic organ involvement, including deep and superficial lymph nodes, liver, spleen, and/or bone marrow. The majority (80 per cent) of cats with the multicentric form are FeLV-positive. The average age of presentation for cats with this form is 4 years.

TABLE 144–1. (Continued)

- *CHOP protocol (canine)*
  Cyclophosphamide (Cytoxan) 50 mg/m^2 BSA PO, every other day
  Hydroxydaunorubicin (Adriamycin) 30 mg/m^2 BSA IV, on day 1 of the
  cycle
  Vincristine (Oncovin) 0.75 mg/m^2 BSA IV, on days 8 and 15 of the cycle
  Prednisone 40 mg/m^2 BSA PO, once a day for a week; then 20 mg/m^2
  BSA PO, every other day
  *Repeat the cycle on day 22; administer a total of 3 cycles, then begin
  maintenance therapy.*
2. Intensification
  - *L-asparaginase* (Elspar) 10,000-20,000 IU/m^2 BSA SQ (one dose)
3. Maintenance
  - *LMP:* (canine or feline)
    Chlorambucil (Leukeran) 2 mg/m^2 BSA PO, every other day, or 20 mg/m^2
    BSA PO, every other week
    Methotrexate (Methotrexate) 2.5 mg/m^2 BSA PO, 2 to 3 times per week
    Prednisone 20 mg/m^2 PO, every other day
  - *COAP:* (canine or feline)
    Use as above every other week for 6 treatments, then every third week for
    additional 6 treatments, and try to maintain the patient on 1 treatment
    every 4th week.
4. Rescue
  - *ADIC (canine)*
    Adriamycin 30 mg/m^2 BSA IV, day 1
    Dacarbazine (DTIC) 1000 mg/m^2 BSA IV, day 1 (administered over 8
    hours)
    Repeat cycle on day 22; administer a total of 3 cycles.
  - *D-MAC (canine)*
    Dexamethasone 0.5 mg/kg SQ or PO, weekly
    Melphalan 20 mg/m^2 PO, on day 8
    Actinomycin D (Cosmegen) 0.7 mg/m^2 IV, on day 1
    Cytosine arabinoside (Cytosar-U) 200 mg/m^2 IV, on day 1 over 4 hours
    *Repeat cycle on day 15; treat continuously for a total of 8 cycles, then
    begin maintenance therapy by substituting chlorambucil 20 mg/m^2 PO for
    the melphalan.*

Marked generalized, painless lymphadenopathy is usually detected by the owner. Hepatomegaly, splenomegaly, and tonsillar enlargement are also common findings.

Leukemic Form. This form of presentation is discussed in Chapter 143.

Treatment of Cats with Lymphoma. Since lymphomas are usually systemic in nature, chemotherapy is the preferred treatment modality (see Table 144–1). If the response to the initial induction was not complete or sustained, or if the patient relapses for a second or third time, drug combinations including doxorubicin (Adriamycin) are preferred. Generally, we use COAP chemotherapy in cats with the ocular, CNS, nasal, mediastinal, renal, and multicentric forms of lymphoma. Cats with gastrointestinal lymphoma may be treated with CHOP or DOMAC. *Radiotherapy* is also effective in treating localized lymphomas, solitary extranodal masses, or lymphomatous masses that mechanically compress vital structures or organs.

Canine Lymphoma. In contrast to cats, older dogs are usually affected, and the multicentric form is by far the most common. In addition, there is a definitive breed predisposition for lymphoma, with boxers, bull mastiffs, basset hounds, Saint Bernards, and Scottish terriers being at increased risk. We also treat dogs with ocular, CNS, mediastinal, or multicentric forms of lymphoma using COAP chemotherapy (see Table 144–1). This protocol is slightly different from the one used in cats, in that we use cytosine arabinoside for 4 days (rather than 2), and we continue the induction phase for 8 weeks (rather than 6). Dogs with prior corticosteroid therapy, cutaneous involvement, or gastrointestinal lymphoma are usually treated more aggressively with CHOP chemotherapy (see Table 144–1). Following induction with COAP or CHOP, the dogs are placed on LMP maintenance therapy (see Table 144–1). Rescue protocols used in our clinic include mainly ADIC and D- MAC (see Table 144–1).

SPLEEN (pp. 1938–1945)

Extramodullary hematopoesis (EMH) may result in splenomegaly. The CBCs of dogs and cats with EMH are characterized primarily by a leukoerythroblastic reaction (presence of immature red cell and white cell precursors). EMH may be seen in association with a wide variety of primary and secondary splenic disorders.

SPLENIC MASSES (SPLENOMEGALY)

Hemangiosarcomas. Malignant vascular tumors of the spleen appear to be extremely common in dogs and are rare in cats. These neoplasms occur predominantly in older large-breed dogs, and there is an apparent predilection for males and for German shepherd dogs and golden retrievers. Clinical signs and physical findings in dogs with splenic HSA are usually vague and nonspecific, and include anorexia, weight loss, abdominal distention, weakness, pallor, and vomiting. Metastatic lesions are usually found in the liver, omentum, peritoneum, kidneys, heart, and lungs.

Hematologic findings include anemia, presence of nucleated RBCs in the blood smear, presence of acanthocytes and schistocytes, presence of Howell- Jolly bodies, thrombocytopenia, and neutrophilia. The most common hemostatic abnormality in dogs with hemangiosarcoma is thrombocytopenia, with 50 per cent of the dogs fulfilling criteria for diagnosis of DIC. Surgical resection has been the mainstay of therapy in dogs with splenic HSA. In one study, splenectomy in dogs with HSA resulted in a median survival of 65 days (mean 80 days). The median survival in dogs with HSA treated by us using a combination of vincristine (0.75 mg/m^2 IV, on days 8 and 15 of a 21- day cycle), doxorubicin (30 mg/m^2 IV, on day 1 of the cycle), cyclophosphamide (100 to 200 mg/m^2 IV, on day 1 of the cycle), and sulfadiazine trimethoprim following surgical excision was 172 days (mean 316 days).

Hemangiomas/Hematomas. Most dogs with splenic hematomas/hemangiomas are relatively healthy, do not undergo spontaneous splenic rupture and hemoabdomen, and lack significant hematologic or hemostatic abnormalities. In most dogs with hematomas, no underlying causes predisposing to intrasplenic bleeding can be found.

SPLENOMEGALY (DIFFUSE ENLARGEMENT)

As with lymph node enlargement, splenic enlargement can result from inflammatory changes (splenitis), lymphoreticular hyperplasia, congestion, or infiltration with abnormal cells or substances (e.g., amyloidosis) (Table 144–2). Common causes of portal hypertension that may lead to splenomegaly include right-sided congestive heart failure, obstruction of the caudal vena cava (e.g., due to neoplasia or heartworm disease), and intrahepatic obstruction. Splenic torsion can occur independently of the GDV syndrome. Dogs with acute splenic torsion usually present with acute abdominal pain and distention, vomiting, depression, and anorexia. Dogs with chronic splenic torsion display a wide variety of clinical signs including anorexia, weight loss, intermittent

TABLE 144–2. CLASSIFICATION OF SPLENOMEGALY IN DOGS AND CATS

TYPE	SPECIES
Inflammatory splenomegaly	
Suppurative splenitis	
Penetrating abdominal wounds	C, D
Migrating foreign bodies	C, D
Bacterial endocarditis	C, D
Septicemia	C, D
Splenic torsion	D
Toxoplasmosis	C, D
Mycobacteriosis	D, C
Infectious canine hepatitis (acute)	D
Necrotizing splenitis	
Splenic torsion	D
Splenic neoplasia	D
Infectious canine hepatitis (acute)	D
Salmonellosis	D, C
Eosinophilic splenitis	
Eosinophilic gastroenteritis	D, C?
Hypereosinophilic syndrome	C
Lymphoplasmacytic splenitis	
Infectious canine hepatitis (chronic)	D
Ehrlichiosis (chronic)	D
Pyometra	D, C
Brucellosis	D
Hemobartonellosis	D, C
Granulomatous splenitis	
Histoplasmosis	D, C
Mycobacteriosis	D, C
Leishmaniasis	D
Pyogranulomatous splenitis	
Blastomycosis	D, C?
Sporotrichosis	D
Feline infectious peritonitis	C
Hyperplastic splenomegaly	
Bacterial endocarditis	D
Brucellosis	D
Discospondylitis	D
Systemic lupus erythematosus	D
Hemolytic disorders (see text)	D, C
Congestive splenomegaly	
Pharmacologic (tranquilizers, anticonvulsants)	D, C
Portal hypertension	D, C
Splenic torsion	D
Infiltrative splenomegaly	
Neoplastic	
Acute and chronic leukemias	D, C
Systemic mastocytosis	D, C
Malignant histiocytosis	D
Lymphoma	D, C
Multiple myeloma	D, C
Metastatic neoplasia	D, C
Non-neoplastic	
Extramedullary hematopoiesis	D, C?
Hypereosinophilic syndrome	C
Amyloidosis	D

D = dog; C = cat.

TABLE 144–3. HEMATOLOGIC ABNORMALITIES IN DOGS AND CATS WITH SPLENOMEGALY

HYPERSPLENISM	HYPOSPLENISM/ASPLENIA
Regenerative anemia	Target cells
Neutropenia	Acanthocytes
Thrombocytopenia	Howell-Jolly bodies
Bicytopenias	Nucleated RBCs
Pancytopenia	Increased percentage of reticulocytes
Hypercellular bone marrow	Thrombocytosis
	Lymphocytosis?

vomiting, abdominal distention, polyuria and polydipsia, pigmenturia (due to hemoglobinuria), and abdominal pain. Ultrasonographic evaluation of these patients may reveal the presence of greatly distended splenic veins and diffuse hypoechoic splenic pattern. Hematologic abnormalities include anemia, presence of target cells, leukocytosis due to regenerative left shift, leukoerythroblastosis, and, occasionally, a positive direct Coombs' test. Disseminated intravascular coagulation appears to be a common complication. The treatment of choice for dogs with splenic torsion is splenectomy.

Evaluation of the Patient with Splenomegaly

Clinical signs in dogs and cats with splenomegaly are usually vague and nonspecific. Disorders in which the clinical signs are primarily related to the splenic enlargement are splenic torsion and primary splenic hyperplasia. Other signs associated with splenomegaly are those resulting from the hematologic consequences of the splenic enlargement and include spontaneous bleeding, pallor, and fever. The hematologic abnormalities in patients with splenomegaly are summarized in Table 144–3. Bone marrow evaluation should always be conducted prior to splenectomy in patients with cytopenias. Two-dimensional gray scale ultrasonography is extremely helpful in evaluating patients with splenomegaly or splenic masses. In addition, ultrasonographically guided fine- needle aspirates or biopsies can be easily performed.

Splenic Aspiration.   Performing transabdominal splenic FNA in patients chemically restrained with phenothiazine tranquilizers or barbiturates usually results in blood-diluted specimens.

Splenic Surgery.   Splenectomy is indicated in the following situations: (1) splenic torsion, (2) splenic rupture, (3) symptomatic splenomegaly (regardless of the cause), and (4) splenic masses. The value of splenectomy is questionable in: (1) dogs with immune-mediated blood disorders, although a recent report suggests its beneficial value; (2) dogs and cats with splenomegaly due to lymphoma in which chemotherapy failed to induce splenic remission; and (3) dogs and cats with leukemia. Splenectomy is generally contraindicated in patients with bone marrow hypoplasia in which the spleen is the main hematopoietic site.

CHAPTER 145

HEMOSTATIC DISORDERS: COAGULOPATHIES AND THROMBOSIS
(pages 1946–1963)

PHYSIOLOGY OF HEMOSTASIS

See the textbook.

LABORATORY EVALUATION OF HEMOSTASIS
(pp. 1949–1952)

Laboratory evaluation of patients with hemostatic defects requires meticulous attention to methodology and quality control procedures. At the outset it is conceded that standard clotting tests are qualitative screening tests having limited capacity to detect mild to even moderate factor deficiencies. Blood collection through any type of long catheter may activate hemostatic components. It is important that the surface of any collection, holding, or transfer containers be consistent (all plastic or all siliconized), particularly with reference to platelet function studies.

THE COMMON COAGULATION TESTS

A thorough history and physical examination of bleeding patients should attempt to resolve whether the defect involves formation of the primary or secondary hemostatic plug. Disorders of primary hemostatic plug formation include platelet dysfunction (quantitative or qualitative), von Willebrand's disease, and occasional vascular disorders (Chapter 146). Mucosal bleeding time, platelet count and function, as well as VWF levels are appropriate tests to evaluate these disorders. These patients commonly have spontaneous, immediate, short-duration bleeding causing bleeding from the nose (epistaxis) and gums, into the urine (hematuria), and, less commonly, petechiation or ecchymosis in mucous membranes. Disorders of secondary hemostatic plug formation (coagulopathies) usually involve coagulation factor deficiency, either hereditary or acquired. These patients commonly have spontaneous, delayed onset bleeding of longer duration, causing hematomas, hemarthrosis or hemorrhage into deep tissues or body cavities. Standard clotting tests (see below) are useful to compartmentalize the defect into the intrinsic, extrinsic, or common pathway. Some patients with multiple defects, as in DIC, have a variety of abnormal test results and clinical signs indicating defects in both primary and secondary hemostatic plug formation.

Activated Coagulation Time and Activated Partial Thromboplastin Time

The two tests commonly used to evaluate the intrinsic coagulation system are the activated coagulation time (ACT) and the activated partial thromboplastin time (APTT). Patients with severe thrombocytopenias (platelet counts <10,000/µl), some qualitative platelet function defects, and severe hypofibrinogenemia may have prolonged ACT tests. The APTT test is more versatile and accurate than the ACT test in

Original chapter written by Robert A. Green and Jennifer S. Thomas

detection of mild abnormalities of the intrinsic coagulation pathway. Usually the activity of a single factor must be reduced below 30 per cent of normal before the APTT test is prolonged. Determination of the specific factor deficiency in the coagulation cascade is obtained by performing APTT on 1:1 mixtures of patient plasma and test plasmas having known deficiency of a specific factor. Factor deficiencies are differentiated from effects of inhibitors such as heparin or lupus antibodies against specific hemostatic components by repeating the APTT following 1:1 dilution of the abnormal plasma with normal plasma.

One-Stage Prothrombin Time

The status of the extrinsic coagulation cascade is evaluated by the one- stage prothrombin time (OSPT). Prolonged OSPT is caused by hereditary or acquired deficiencies of factors in the extrinsic or common cascade (e.g., liver disease, vitamin K antagonism, or consumptive coagulopathies).

Thrombin Time

Prolonged TT is associated with severe hypofibrinogenemia (<100 mg/dl) and dysfibrinogenemia. Heparin or FDP may also prolong TT owing to thrombin inhibition.

Fibrinogen Assays

Hypofibrinogenemia may be associated with either decreased production or increased consumption. In chronic DIC syndromes, increased hepatic fibrinogen production may maintain fibrinogen levels within or above the normal range, despite considerable fibrinogen consumption. Acquired dysfibrinogenemia may occur secondary to hyperplasminemia or liver disease.

Fibrin(ogen) Degradation Products (FDP) Assay

FDP elevation may be due to DIC, liver disease, or primary fibrinolysis. False elevation of FDP may occur in patients receiving heparin therapy or in patients with dysfibrinogenemia. The presence of FDP impairs thrombin- mediated fibrin formation, fibrin polymerization, and, perhaps most importantly, hemostatic plug formation.

Von Willebrand's Factor Assay

The most common test for the diagnosis of von Willebrand's disease (VWD) is based on determining the patient's level of von Willebrand's factor antigen (VWF:Ag) by rocket immunoelectrophoresis.

THE COAGULOPATHIES (pp. 1953–1962)

VITAMIN K ANTAGONISM AND DEFICIENCY

Clinical Signs

The spectrum of clinical signs encountered in anticoagulant toxicoses is broad and is generally related to organ dysfunction induced by hypovolemia or hemorrhage into organ parenchyma, surrounding tissues, or body cavities. Anemia, weakness, pallor, hematemesis, epistaxis, or bloody feces are commonly seen in less acutely affected animals.

Laboratory Testing

The typical laboratory findings include marked prolongation of OSPT with moderate prolongation of APTT or ACT. The PIVKA is markedly abnormal. Platelet count, ATIII, fibrinogen, and thrombin time usually remain within normal limits.

Therapy

The three major treatment priorities are (1) correct the hypovolemia, (2) correct the coagulopathy, and (3) minimize organ dysfunction induced by accumulation of extravascular blood. Transfusion of fresh whole blood may be critical to survival in severe cases. Correction of the coagulopathy is accomplished by SQ administration of vitamin K_1 (Aquamephyton). Vitamin K_1 should not be given IV as anaphylaxis may occur. In the case of patients intoxicated by high doses of longer-acting second-generation rodenticides, vitamin K therapy needs to be extended for 3 to 6 weeks. If screening coagulation tests (OSPT, ACT) are within normal limits and remain stable for 4 days following cessation of therapy, further therapy is not required. The primary complication of vitamin K therapy at high levels (2.3 mg/lb [5 mg/kg]) is Heinz body anemia.

DISSEMINATED INTRAVASCULAR COAGULATION (DIC)

Diseases often associated with DIC include neoplasia, infections (viral, bacterial, protozoal, and parasitic), obstetric problems, shock, heat stroke, pancreatitis, immune-mediated anemia, hepatic disease, venomous snake bites, and trauma. In some cases, the clinical findings relate to the primary disease process and DIC is only detectable by means of laboratory data. In other cases, there are severe diseases associated with DIC such as multiple organ failure and bleeding. Microthrombosis leads to tissue ischemia and variable organ failure including renal failure, respiratory insufficiency, liver damage, and gastrointestinal disorders.

Laboratory Evaluation

Patients with severe, acute DIC often have multiple abnormal laboratory results whereas patients with chronic DIC may have few abnormal findings. Laboratory findings classically associated with DIC in dogs include thrombocytopenia, hypofibrinogenemia, elevated FDP, and decreased ATIII levels with prolonged OSPT and APTT. Low ATIII levels are not specific for DIC and may occur secondary to decreased production (i.e., hepatic failure) or increased loss (e.g., nephrotic failure).

Therapy

The primary focus of therapy must be resolution of the underlying disease. Fluid therapy is essential to prevent vascular stasis, restore tissue perfusion, and cause dilution of coagulation and fibrinolytic factors. Prevention of secondary complications includes correction of acid-base and electrolyte abnormalities, prevention of secondary sepsis, and maintenance of adequate tissue oxygenation. If a patient is actively bleeding, administration of fresh whole blood or plasma is recommended. In most cases of ongoing DIC, antifibrinolytic therapy is strongly contraindicated. The use of heparin to treat DIC is controversial. Heparin should not be given to actively bleeding patients until depleted factors and/or platelets have been replaced. In mild cases of DIC, the administration of mini-dose (2.3 to 4.5 IU/lb [5 to 10 IU/kg]) or low-dose (34 to 91 IU/lb [75 to 200 IU/kg]) heparin every 8 hours is recommended. In moderate to severe cases of DIC, with clinical evidence of damage due to microthrombosis, intermediate (136 to 227 IU/lb [300 to 500 IU/kg]) or high (341 to 455 IU/lb [750 to 1000 IU/kg]) doses of heparin every 8 hours may be necessary. Abrupt cessation of heparin therapy is contraindicated because of the risk of rebound effects and thrombotic complications associated with uncompensated ATIII deficiency.

PRIMARY (PATHOLOGIC) FIBRINOLYSIS

Fibrinolysis is usually associated with DIC, in which it is called secondary fibrinolysis, as an appropriate physiologic response to widespread thrombosis in the microvasculature. Primary fibrinolysis has not been documented yet in veterinary species.

LIVER DISEASE

When hepatic production or clearance mechanisms fail, the patient may manifest thrombotic, fibrinolytic, or hemorrhagic complications, depending on interrelationships between the plasma half-lives of coagulation factors and their respective inhibitors.

Laboratory Aspects

Coagulation tests, by estimating the severity of deficiency of coagulation factors, provide an accurate prognostic index in patients with acute liver failure. Generally, severe acute canine hepatopathies tend to prolong both OSPT and APTT, whereas chronic partially compensated canine hepatopathies cause slight APTT prolongation and OSPT remains within normal limits. Although liver disease is associated with deficiencies in coagulation factors, most patients express clinical bleeding only when concurrent platelet dysfunction exists.

Treatment

Fresh whole blood or platelet-rich plasma is the treatment of choice for animals with active bleeding. All icteric patients with prolonged OSPT should be given vitamin K.

HEREDITARY COAGULOPATHIES

As a general rule, deficiencies of the contact activation factors (e.g., factor XII, PK) are subclinical and only detected during coagulation testing. Deficiencies of factor VII or XI tend to cause mild disease, with bleeding problems usually occurring only when additional stress is placed on the hemostatic system (e.g., surgery, severe trauma). Patients with inherited deficiencies of factors IX and VIII of the intrinsic pathway as well as the factors X, II, and I of the common pathway have the most severe coagulopathies. Factor VIII deficiency (hemophilia A) is the most common defect, occurring in most breeds of dogs and several breeds of cats. Disease occurs almost exclusively in hemizygous males. The most common hereditary bleeding disorder is VWD. Type I VWD results from a generalized deficiency of all VWF multimers. Type III VWD is a much more severe deficiency of all VWF multimers, with no detectable VWF:Ag. Type II VWD is the rarest and is characterized by a deficiency of higher-molecular-weight multimers with severe bleeding abnormalities. It has only been identified in a family of German shorthair pointers.

Clinical Signs

Severe hemostatic abnormalities (e.g., severe hemophilia A or B) are usually associated with episodes of spontaneous hemorrhage early in life and may, in some cases, lead to a high neonatal death rate. Coagulopathies generally produce localized hemorrhage such as hematomas, hemorrhage into body cavities, or hemarthrosis. Clinical signs largely depend on the impact of hemorrhage into body cavities or organs and the related impairment of physiologic functions. Alternatively, patients with VWD have clinical signs resembling a platelet defect, including epistaxis, prolonged estrual or postpartum bleeding, and hematuria or melena due to bleeding from mucosal surfaces.

Laboratory Aspects

See Table 145–1.

Therapy

Management of animals with severe coagulation defects is largely restricted to periodic transfusion with whole blood or plasma during bleeding episodes. Unless the patient is anemic, transfusion of plasma is preferred. Fresh or fresh-frozen plasma can be administered to patients with VWD to control hemorrhage during a bleeding episode; however, administration of cryoprecipitate (a plasma concentrate rich in factor VIII, high-molecular-weight VWF, and fibrinogen) is the preferred therapy. Bleeding times shorten in most, but not all, dogs with type I VWD given DDAVP. Thyroid supplementation increased VWF:Ag levels and alleviated bleeding episodes in some dogs.

THROMBOSIS

Most thrombotic conditions of small animals are due to vascular endothelial injuries caused directly or indirectly by infectious agents (e.g., dirofilariasis, bacterial endocarditis) or vascular immune complex deposition.

Clinical Signs

The clinical signs associated with pulmonary thromboembolization in animals vary from mild subclinical effects to severe, acute dyspnea. Occasional patients may develop hemoptysis. Hematuria and sudden flank pain are often associated with renal embolization and infarction. Embolization of the central nervous system causes a variety of locomotor disturbances that can result in sudden death. Emboli commonly lodge in the aortic trifurcation of cats, causing the affected limb to become painful, cool, pulseless, paretic, and pale. Visceral arterial embolization causes sudden abdominal pain, vomiting, and bowel evacuation. Occasional patients with splenic thrombosis may present with massive splenomegaly and hemolytic anemia.

Diagnostics

Thromboembolization is visualized by sophisticated techniques, such as nuclear medicine imaging, ultrasonography, and contrast angiography, available at veterinary referral centers. In selected patients, a hypercoagulable state is suggested by modest shortening of coagulation test times (OSPT, APTT, and TT, decreased ATIII levels, platelet hypersensitivity, ad increased plasma viscosity).

Therapy

As with DIC, the best treatment for thrombosis is elimination of the predisposing cause. Every effort should be made to correct all underlying prothrombotic factors (e.g., stasis, vasculitis, sepsis, dehydration, or ATIII deficiency). Therapy to reduce the patient's pain or dyspnea during acute thrombotic attacks is also important. The therapeutic approaches that diminish thrombogenesis include the use of short-term anticoagulants (heparin), long-term anticoagulants (coumadins), and antiplatelet drugs (aspirin, dipyridamole, ticlopidine). Thrombolytic therapy using urokinase and streptokinase has been widely used to lyse existing thrombi in people. Unfortunately, laboratory parameters to accurately monitor safety and efficacy during thrombolytic therapy remain to be established in dogs and cats.

TABLE 145–1. FEATURES OF HEREDITARY COAGULATION DISORDERS IN DOGS AND CATS

FACTOR DEFICIENT	INHERITANCE PATTERN	SEVERITY OF BLEEDING DIATHESIS	AFFECTED BREEDS	COAGULATION SCREENING TESTS				DEFINITIVE TESTS
				OSPT	APTT	ACT	Bleeding Time (Mucosal)	
FVIII (Hemophilia A)	X-linked recessive	Variable	Most dog breeds, mongrels, cats	N	ABN	ABN	N*	Low FVIII:C activity; N to increased VWF:Ag
FIX (Hemophilia B)	X-linked recessive	Often severe	15 dogs breeds affected to date; variety of cats (British shorthair, domestic shorthair, Siamese mix)	N	ABN	ABN	N*	Low FIX activity
FXI	Autosomal recessive	Mild†	Springer spaniel, Great Pyrenees	N	ABN	ABN	N*	Low FXI activity
FXII (Hageman trait)	Autosomal recessive	Subclinical‡	Domestic cats Poodle	N	ABN	ABN	N	Low FXII activity
FVII	Autosomal incomplete dominance	Subclinical to mild‡	Beagle, Alaskan malamute	ABN	N	N	N	Low FVII activity
FX	Autosomal	Severe in neonates	Cocker spaniel, mongrel	ABN	ABN	ABN	N*	Low FX activity
VWF (Von Willebrand's disease)	Usually autosomal incomplete dominant; rarely autosomal recessive	Mild† to severe	Over 50 dog breeds affected to date	N	V	V	ABN	Low VWF:Ag ± low FVIII:C

*Initial primary plug formation normal. May rebleed.
†Severe bleeding may occur following major surgical procedures or trauma.
‡Usually discovered fortuitously by presurgical screening tests.
Abbreviations: N = normal; ABN = abnormal; and V = variable.

CHAPTER 146

PLATELET DISORDERS
(pages 1964–1976)

NORMAL PLATELET STRUCTURE AND FUNCTION
(pp. 1964–1969)

See the textbook.

TESTS FOR EVALUATING THE THROMBON

Quantitative Platelet Tests

Platelet Count. The most important platelet disorder is thrombocytopenia (reduced platelet numbers); consequently, the most important test for evaluating the thrombon is the platelet count. Owing to the size overlap of the feline platelet with the red blood cell, platelets cannot be counted easily with an automated electronic cell counter. In estimating platelet counts, six or seven platelets per oil immersion field is approximately $100,000/\mu l$. There is increasing evidence that for man, total platelet mass (as determined by multiplying mean platelet volume times the platelet count) is more important than circulating platelet numbers in evaluating thrombocytopenia. As a general rule, large platelets are more functional than smaller ones.

Qualitative Platelet Tests

Bleeding time is an *in vivo* test measuring platelet function. The mean buccal mucosa bleeding time for the dog and cat is 2.62 ± 0.49 and 1.9 ± 0.5 minutes respectively. The test should only be done in animals with normal or elevated platelet numbers. A normal bleeding time does not eliminate the possibility of a platelet function defect. The ability of platelets to aggregate can be measured through the use of platelet aggregometers. If platelet function is adequate, then a firm retracted clot should form in non-anticoagulated whole blood within 1 to 2 hours. As with bleeding times, clot retraction will be abnormal in cases of thrombocytopenia.

PLATELET DISORDERS (pp. 1969–1975)

DIAGNOSTIC APPROACH TO A PATIENT WITH BLEEDING DISORDER: OVERVIEW

Patients with either a quantitative or qualitative defect in platelets often have petechial or ecchymotic hemorrhages in the skin, mucous membranes, and retina, as well as epistaxis, hematuria, and bleeding into the gastrointestinal tract. The first step in the laboratory evaluation of a patient with a suspected bleeding abnormality is a complete blood count, which includes either an estimation or, ideally, an actual count of the platelets. An increase in the utilization of platelets occurs with blood loss and disseminated intravascular coagulation (DIC). Although platelets decrease in this situation, marked thrombocytopenia would not typically be seen. To rule out other causes of utilization of platelets, an activated partial thromboplastin time (APTT) and a one-stage prothrombin time (OSPT) should be run. If the APTT and OSPT tests are prolonged and there is thrombocytopenia, the animal most likely has DIC or has been exposed to a vitamin K antagonist. Once DIC or the presence of a vitamin K antagonist has been ruled out, other mechanisms of the thrombocytopenia—such as increased

Original chapter written by William J. Reagan and A. H. Rebar destruction, increased sequestration, or decreased production—must be considered. Sequestration of platelets as the primary cause usually can be confirmed by such physical findings as hepatomegaly, splenomegaly, or hypothermia. The next diagnostic step is bone marrow aspiration. If megakaryocytes are present in the bone marrow, the mechanism for the thrombocytopenia is increased destruction. Animals with qualitative platelet defects usually have normal platelet counts and normal APTT and OSPT. A bleeding time is the best screening test to determine whether a platelet function defect may be present. The most common hereditary platelet defect in the dog is von Willebrand's disease (VWD).

THROMBOCYTOPENIA

Disseminated Intravascular Coagulation. See Chapter 145.
Blood Loss. If significant thrombocytopenia (i.e., <20,000 to 40,000/μl) is identified, it is probably the cause and not a result of the hemorrhage.

Sequestration

Any disease process characterized by splenomegaly or hepatomegaly can be associated with concurrent thrombocytopenia.

Destruction: Immune-Mediated Thrombocytopenia

The laboratory diagnosis of immune-mediated thrombocytopenia is made by ruling out other causes of thrombocytopenia such as utilization and sequestration. A bone marrow aspiration should be done to distinguish between increased destruction and decreased production. Further tests for immune- mediated destruction of platelets include the platelet factor 3 (PF 3) test, the antimegakaryocyte antibody test, and measurement of platelet-associated antibody. In some studies the antimegakaryocyte antibody test has been shown to be more sensitive than the PF 3 test. Once the diagnosis of immune-mediated thrombocytopenia is made, the disease should be further classified as primary or secondary. The causes of secondary immune-mediated thrombocytopenia include drugs, neoplasia, infectious diseases, and immune-mediated diseases such as systemic lupus erythematosus. Gold compounds, cephalosporins, and estrogen have been shown to induce immune-mediated thrombocytopenia in dogs. Infectious diseases can also cause immune-mediated thrombocytopenia (see Table 146–1). Primary

TABLE 146–1. INFECTIOUS CASES OF THROMBOCYTOPENIA IN DOGS*

Viral	Bacterial
Infectious canine hepatitis	Bacteremia
Canine herpesvirus infection	Leptospirosis
Canine parvovirus infection	Salmonellosis
Canine distemper (after vaccination)	Protozoal
Rickettsial	Babesiasis
Ehrlichia canis infection	Fungal
Rocky Mountain spotted fever	Histoplasmosis
Ehrlichia platys infection	Candidiasis
Granulocytic ehrlichiosis	
Hemobartonellosis	

*Partial list of infectious diseases that can cause thrombocytopenia in the dog. Thrombocytopenia associated with disseminated intravascular coagulation may occur in the late stages of many of these diseases.
Adapted from Breitschwerdt EB: Infectious thrombocytopenia in dogs. Comp Contin Ed 10:1177, 1988.

immune-mediated thrombocytopenia is often seen concurrently with immune-mediated hemolytic anemia. Primary immune-mediated thrombocytopenia in dogs is associated with platelet counts that are very low (<20,000/µl) compared to counts associated with thrombocytopenia from other causes. Treatment includes the use of immunosuppressive agents such as corticosteroids and, in some cases, cyclophosphamide and vincristine.

Decreased Production

Although this can be a selective decrease in the megakaryocytes, it is most often associated with a decrease in one or both of the other cell lines in the bone marrow. The major causes of intramarrow disease include infections, neoplasms, drugs, and immune-mediated disorders (Chapter 142).

Miscellaneous Causes of Thrombocytopenia

Of all the infectious diseases listed in Table 146–1, ehrlichiosis and Rocky Mountain spotted fever are the two infectious diseases most likely to cause thrombocytopenia in dogs. The thrombocytopenia associated with Rocky Mountain spotted fever is generally mild compared to that associated with *E. canis* infection. In the cat, FeLV and infrequently FIV infection cause thrombocytopenia.

THROMBOCYTOSIS

Thrombocytosis Associated with Primary Bone Marrow Disease

Platelet Leukemias. Clinical signs generally are the result of a hemorrhagic tendency, which is secondary to both increases in platelet mass and functional platelet defects. Splenomegaly is common, but splenectomy is contraindicated as platelet counts may further increase following spleen removal.

Myelofibrosis. Either thrombocytosis or thrombocytopenia can occur in association with myelofibrosis. Thrombocytopenia is probably related to the elimination of marrow precursors of all cell lines. Other peripheral blood features of myelofibrosis may include profound nonregenerative anemia and leukopenia.

Polycythemia Vera (see also Chapter 43). Thrombocytosis is an occasional feature of polycythemia vera.

Secondary (Reactive) Thrombocytosis

Excitement and exercise cause thrombocytosis due to either splenic contraction or increased blood flow. Thrombocytosis also can be seen with trauma, hemorrhage, fractures, splenectomy, iron deficiency, infections, Cushing's disease, and glucocorticoid and other drug therapy. In most cases, secondary thrombocytosis is clinically insignificant.

QUALITATIVE PLATELET DISORDERS

Acquired Platelet Function Defects

Many drugs including anesthetics, antibiotics, antihistamines, antiinflammatory drugs, and heparin can potentially inhibit platelet function. One of the more common groups of drugs that inhibit platelet function include the nonsteroidal anti-inflammatory agents. Inhibition of cyclooxygenase by aspirin is irreversible, and so platelet function will not return until new platelets are synthesized and released. Some dogs with azotemia have prolonged bleeding times, possibly as a result of a primary platelet function defect. Pancreatitis has been shown to affect the function of dog platelets. Patients with liver disease can have bleeding abnormalities attributable to multiple mechanisms, including platelet dysfunction. Neoplastic disorders induce the production of abnormal platelets with subsequent functional defects or the presence of substances produced by the tumor which interfere with platelet function. The high level of paraproteins in patients with multiple myeloma probably inhibits platelet function.

Hereditary Platelet Function Defects

Von Willebrand's Disease (see also Chapter 145). Von Willebrand's disease is a common, usually mild, bleeding abnormality that has been documented in many breeds of dogs and rarely reported in the cat. Von Willebrand's disease is commonly (58 to 70 per cent prevalence) seen in Doberman pinschers. Often these dogs do not present with overt bleeding problems, but they may bleed excessively during surgical procedures. Thyroid function should be evaluated in Dobermans and other dogs with VWF deficiency. The Airedale terrier is a breed that appears to have a high prevalence of decreased VWF:Ag, but abnormal hemorrhage associated with this defect is rare.

Basset Hound Hereditary Thrombopathia. In addition to mucosal bleeding, auricular hematomas may be seen.

Chediak-Higashi Syndrome. Cats with Chediak-Higashi syndrome have platelet function defects.

CHAPTER 147

IMMUNOLOGY
(pages 1978–2002)

BASIC CONCEPTS OF THE IMMUNE SYSTEM
(pp. 1978–1979)

See the textbook for a review of the immune system.

B Cells and T Cells

There are two types of lymphocytes, B and T cells. Immunoglobulins, are produced by cells of the B cell lineage. The bulk, however, is synthesized by plasma cells derived from B cells.

T Cell Subsets

T cells do not produce immunoglobulins but act both as coordinators of the immune response and as effector cells in cell-mediated immunity. T cells have been divided into *helper T cells (Th)* and *cytotoxic T cells (Tc)*.

Biologic Properties of Immunoglobulins

IgG. In all species, IgG is the major class of immunoglobulin that is found in plasma. The major biologic function of IgG *in vivo* is to promote the removal of microorganisms and neutralize toxins.

IgA. The major biologic importance of IgA is in extravascular secretions as secretory IgA (SIgA) in the respiratory, genital, and intestinal tracts, where it is central to mucosal immunity. SIgA can neutralize toxins, adhere to bacteria and viruses, and interact with parasites and mucosal surfaces. SIgA is able to activate the alternative complement pathway.

IgM. IgM is efficient at binding antigen and producing agglutination, virus neutralization, and opsonization. In addition, IgM is a potent activator of the classic complement pathway.

IgD. IgD acts as an antigen receptor comparable to the monomeric IgM molecule.

IgE. IgE is an immunoglobulin of major importance in the effector mechanisms against parasites and in the immunopathogenesis of allergic disease. The unique nature of IgE is its ability to bind to specific receptors on the surface of mast cells and basophils. Following the cross-linking of two IgE molecules by antigen, the cells degranulate and release a number of pharmacologic mediators, including histamine, serotonin, eosinophil and neutrophil chemotactic factors,

Original chapter written by Neil T. Gorman

heparin, and an array of enzymes. A number of secondary mediators are also released, and these include the slow-reacting substance of ana-phylaxis, arachodonates, and various platelet factors. All too often the response is not against an antigen but an allergen, which is the basis of type I hypersensitivity.

REGULATION OF THE IMMUNE RESPONSE
(pp. 1993–1994)

See the textbook.

EFFECTOR MECHANISMS (pp. 1995–1996)

For a review of complement and biologic fragments (C3a and C5a) see the textbook.

HYPERSENSITIVITY (pp. 1997–2003)

Type I Hypersensitivity Reactions

Type I hypersensitivity results from an IgE response to an antigen. The IgE binds to the surface of mast and basophil cells, and on subse-quent exposure to the same antigen, degranulation of the mast cells occurs with the release of pharmacologic mediators of inflammation. The antigen responsible for such a reaction is generally termed an allergen. The reaction usually occurs within minutes, and sometimes, as with acute systemic anaphylaxis, it can be almost instantaneous. The reaction is sometimes delayed for as long as several hours.

Atopy

Atopy is defined as an inherited predisposition to develop IgE anti-bodies to environmental allergens that result in allergic disease.

Mast Cells and Mediator Release

Two major groups of mediators are released from mast cells: pre-formed and synthesized mediators. When massive and generalized mediator release occurs, systemic anaphylaxis results. The major target organ is the gut in the dog. Acute gastroenteric signs with hypovolemic shock due to the vasodilation in the gastro-intestinal tract, in particular the liver, occurs.

Type II Hypersensitivity

Type II reactions involve antibody-dependent cytotoxicity following binding of an antibody to a cell. It may also follow binding of antibody to exogenous antigen that has become associated with a cell surface or of antibody directed against a basement membrane. Examples of this are hemolytic disease of the newborn, drug hypersensitivities, autoim-mune hemolytic anemia, immune- mediated thrombocytopenia, bul-lous pemphigoid/pemphigus and some of the immune-mediated endocrinopathies.

Type III Hypersensitivity

The hallmark of type III reactions is the formation of antigen-antibody complexes, termed immune complexes, that either can exist free in the circulation or can be deposited as microprecipitates in vascular beds. The Arthus reaction is a local reaction that develops at a vessel wall and is characterized by edema, erythema, hemorrhage, and necrosis.

The term serum sickness is confined to the development of circulating immune complexes following administration of an antigen by injection. The microprecipitates form in the circulation and become deposited in basement membranes and the vascular endothelium. This can lead to a generalized vasculitis, in distinction to the localized vasculitis that is described for the Arthus reaction. The reaction is dramatically accelerated in animals that have been previously sensitized.

TYPE IV HYPERSENSITIVITY

Type IV reactions are characterized by the sensitization of a population of T cells. On subsequent challenge with the antigen, this population initiates a series of cell-mediated immunologic reactions that culminates in the influx of lymphocytes and macrophages to the site of the antigenic stimulus. This immunologic reaction is central in the immune response to Neisseria, many fungal infections, a wide range of parasitic infections and mycobacteria.

CHAPTER 148

IMMUNODEFICIENCY DISEASES
(pages 2002–2029)

IMMUNODEFICIENCY DISEASES (pp. 2002–2004)

PRIMARY (CONGENITAL) IMMUNODEFICIENCIES

Canine Cyclic Hematopoiesis

The disease is characterized by cyclic fluctuations of blood neutrophil numbers as well as all other cellular blood components. Cyclic neutropenia occurs every 8 to 12 days and persists 2 to 4 days. Clinical signs are observed only during periods of neutropenia. Signs stem from recurrent bacterial infections primarily involving the respiratory or gastrointestinal tract. The diagnosis is based on the demonstration of a cyclic neutropenia and an abnormal bactericidal assay. Treatment is focused on supportive antibiotic therapy to control infections. Affected dogs rarely survive beyond 3 years of age.

Pelger-Huët Anomaly

This is an inherited condition characterized by hyposegmentation of granulocyte nuclei. The anomaly is usually detected as an incidental finding.

Chediak-Higashi Syndrome

This is an inherited disease seen in Persian cats. The syndrome is associated with an increased susceptibility to infection, a bleeding tendency, and abnormal melanin granules that cause very pale coats and light-colored irises. The diagnosis is made by examination of a blood smear for the presence of enlarged granules in neutrophils. The finding of enlarged melanin granules in the hair shafts confirms the diagnosis. Treatment is symptomatic.

Original chapter written by James P. Thompson

Combined Immunodeficiency

The disease is characterized by B and T lymphocyte deficiencies, lymphoid hypoplasia, and thymic dysplasia. Documented cases in small animal medicine are limited to basset hound puppies.

Selective IgA Deficiency

This is characterized by decreased or absent serum concentrations of IgA. Clinical signs include recurrent upper respiratory and gastrointestinal tract infections, otitis, and dermatitis.

SECONDARY (ACQUIRED) IMMUNODEFICIENCIES

Infectious Organisms

Canine distemper virus, canine parvovirus, feline panleukopenia virus, feline leukemia virus, and feline immunodeficiency virus have each been shown to induce depression of the cell-mediated immune response. Demodicosis, ehrlichiosis, and systemic fungal disease are also closely associated with profound immunosuppression. Corticosteroids commonly induce immunosuppression. Patients with diabetes mellitus exhibit a predisposition to develop infections, as may patients with hyperestrogenism.

IMMUNE-MEDIATED DISEASES (pp. 2004–2022)

TYPE I (IMMEDIATE) HYPERSENSITIVITY

Anaphylaxis

The target organs in most animals are the splanchnic vasculature and, to a lesser extent, the smooth muscles of the lungs. Clinical signs include nausea, vomiting, diarrhea, ataxia, coldness and pallor of mucous membranes, tachypnea, and tachycardia. Anaphylaxis may also occur in localized forms, such as angioneurotic edema (swelling of the lips, eyelids, and conjunctiva) and urticarial lesions (hives). The diagnosis is usually made from a detailed history or by observing the unfolding of clinical signs. Severe anaphylactic reactions must be treated immediately. Prednisolone sodium succinate and intravenous isotonic saline should also be given.

Allergic Bronchitis

Clinical signs are usually chronic and year-round. A chronic, dry, honking type of cough is the most frequent clinical sign. Allergic bronchitis must be differentiated from other causes of chronic bronchitis. The tracheal wash is usually sterile and contains numerous eosinophils. Allergic bronchitis is usually treated with expectorants, bronchodilators, and glucocorticoids.

Allergic Pneumonitis

Allergic pneumonitis or pulmonary infiltrates with eosinophilia is common in dogs and uncommon in cats. Potential causes include a hypersensitivity reaction to allergen inhalation or to parasite migration associated with occult dirofilariasis, lung worms, and ascariasis. Clinical signs include fatigue, exercise intolerance, a soft cough, and dyspnea. Thoracic radiographs generally show a diffuse interstitial pulmonary infiltrate. Numerous eosinophils are generally present in the peripheral blood and in tracheal washes. Glucocorticoids generally induce a rapid resolution of radiographic and clinical signs.

Bronchial Asthma

Bronchial asthma has been recognized only in cats. Mild to severe attacks of wheezing, coughing, and dyspnea are the hallmark clinical signs. Asthma must be differentiated from pulmonary edema, pneumonia, pyothorax, thymic lymphoma, chylothorax, and congestive heart failure. Thoracic radiographs often show pulmonary hyperinflation and flattening of the diaphragm. Wheezing sounds are auscultated during expiration. Asthma is an intermittent disease with limited radiographic changes between attacks. Severely affected cats should not be stressed. Place the cat in an oxygen cage and immediately administer epinephrine aminophylline and prednisolone.

Atopy

Afflicted dogs typically exhibit pruritus manifested by foot licking, face rubbing, and axillary scratching. Skin changes include erythema, hyperpigmentation, lichenification, excoriation, papules, wheals, and alopecia. Seborrhea, otitis externa, and pyoderma may also be observed. The diagnosis requires intradermal skin tests and knowledge of the aeroallergens present in the environment. Critical in the diagnostic plan should be the careful ruling out of external parasites, flea allergic dermatitis, food allergy, and pelodera dermatitis. There are three methods available to treat the atopic patient: (1) avoidance of the offending allergen, (2) hyposensitization, and (3) medical therapy.

TYPE II (CYTOTOXIC) HYPERSENSITIVITY

Immune-Mediated Hemolytic Anemia

The major clinical concern in immune-mediated hemolytic anemia (IMHA) is accelerated erythrocyte destruction. Old English sheepdogs, Irish setters, and cocker spaniels are predisposed. Female dogs are affected more frequently than male dogs.

Immune-Mediated Extravascular Hemolysis. The erythrocytes characteristically become spherical (spherocytes) and, when present, are highly suggestive of IMHA.

Immune-Mediated Intravascular Hemolysis. Intravascular hemolysis is associated with hemoglobinemia and hemoglobinuria.

Cryopathic Immune-Mediated Hemolytic Anemia. This results in agglutination of erythrocytes in the cooler, peripheral vascular beds, which can lead to obstruction of small vessels, acrocyanosis, and gangrenous necrosis of the feet, ear or tail tips, and nose.

Clinical Signs. The owners generally present their animal for vague primary complaints which may include sensitivity to cold, anorexia, listlessness, weakness, and depression.

Diagnosis. The physical examination typically reveals pale mucous membranes, tachycardia, and tachypnea. Hepatomegaly or splenomegaly may be present. Icterus and fever may be observed. Peripheral lymphadenopathy may also be noted. The hemogram frequently demonstrates a leukocytosis. Usually the anemia is regenerative. The presence of spherocytes is nearly pathognomonic for IMHA. Spherocytosis is difficult to detect in the cat. The plasma fibrinogen concentration is generally elevated. The urinalysis may document hemoglobinuria or bilirubinuria. The definitive diagnosis is made by detecting antibody molecules or complement on the surface of circulating erythrocytes. The direct Coombs' test is used when anemia is demonstrated in the absence of direct agglutination. In the absence of a positive Coombs' test result, the clinician is justified in making a diagnosis of IMHA when underlying infection, neoplasia, and erythrocyte enzyme deficiencies have been eliminated. A positive reaction should be interpreted cautiously, especially when there is no clinical or laboratory evidence to support a diagnosis of IMHA. Diseases that may accompany IMHA include immune-mediated thrombocytopenia and/or systemic lupus erythematosus.

Treatment. Parenterally administered dexamethasone is preferred

TABLE 148-1. DIAGNOSTIC PARAMETERS FOR AUTOIMMUNE SKIN DISEASES

DISEASE	COMMON DISTRIBUTION	EPIDERMAL IMMUNOGLOBULIN DEPOSITION	CLEFT FORMATION	ANTINUCLEAR ANTIBODY	SYSTEMIC DISEASE
Pemphigus foliaceus	Nasal dermatitis and generalized	Intercellular	Subcorneal	–	±
Pemphigus erythematosus	Nasal dermatitis	Intercellular and basement membrane zone		Low titer	–
Pemphigus vulgaris	Mucocutaneous junctions and oral cavity	Intercellular	Suprabasilar	–	±
Pemphigus vegetans	Face and trunk	Intercellular		–	–
Bullous pemphigoid	Mucocutaneous junctions, oral cavity, and generalized	Basement membrane zone	Subepidermal	–	±
Systemic lupus erythematosus	Mucocutaneous junctions, oral cavity, and generalized	Basement membrane zone		+	+
Cutaneous lupus erythematosus	Nasal dermatitis	Basement membrane zone		Rare	–

by many clinicians in the initial management scheme. Oral prednisone or prednisolone is then used as the mainstay of glucocorticoid therapy. Danazol has been used also. Cyclophosphamide along with glucocorticoids and danazol can be used in patients that exhibit direct autoagglutination of blood or those with intravascular erythrocyte lysis. These patients also are at high risk for thromboembolic disease; heparinization is strongly recommended. It will most likely require 1 to 2 weeks before any significant benefit from cyclophosphamide will be appreciated. When blood is given, clinicians are urged to use crossmatched blood. Other therapies may include plasmapheresis and splenectomy. Cyclosporin A has also been used in the management of IMHA.

Immune-Mediated Thrombocytopenia

Female dogs are affected nearly twice as frequently as male dogs. Miniature poodles, toy poodles, and Old English sheepdogs may be predisposed. IMT may occur alone or in association with IMHA systemic lupus erythematosus and rheumatoid arthritis. Clinical signs are rarely observed until the platelet count drops below 30,000 thrombocytes/mm^3 blood. Sulfadiazine and propylthiouracil are two drugs that have been associated with acquired IMT.

Clinical Signs. Dogs are usually presented for the primary complaint of bleeding. Bleeding may be manifested most commonly by epistaxis. Mucous membrane petechiation, dermal ecchymosis, melena, hyphema, hematemesis, hematochezia, and hematuria are observed less frequently.

Diagnosis. The diagnosis of IMT is generally made by eliminating other causes of thrombocytopenia, including consumptive coagulopathy and reduced platelet production secondary to lymphoma, myeloproliferative disease, and preleukemic states. In the bleeding patient a complete coagulogram must be performed to exclude intrinsic and extrinsic coagulation system defects. Bone marrow cytology is urged to document the megakaryocytic response to the peripheral thrombocytopenia. In IMT the megakaryocytes are generally increased with a predominance of immature forms.

Treatment. Conventional therapy to reduce platelet destruction has been oral prednisone. The response to treatment is usually good, and platelet counts can return to normal in less than one week. In dogs, danazol may be used concurrently. If the platelet count remains low despite adequate glucocorticoid and danazol therapy, additional therapy with vincristine should be instituted. Dogs that receive a platelet-rich transfusion may be less likely to exhibit relapsing thrombocytopenia. Other therapies that may be valuable include splenectomy and vincristine-loaded platelet transfusion. Splenectomy is reserved for patients that exhibit refractory IMT.

Pemphigus

Diagnosis. The diagnosis of pemphigus skin diseases is generally based on histologic and immunologic examinations of skin biopsies demonstrating the presence of immunoglobulin and/or complement within the intercellular epidermal spaces (Table 148–1).

Clinical Variants

Pemphigus Foliaceus. The skin lesions appear similar in most dogs and are characterized by crusting, scaling, and alopecia. The bearded collie, Newfoundland, Akita, and schipperke appear to be at a significantly increased risk.

Nondermatologic signs include generalized lymphadenopathy, leukocytosis, and a normocytic, normochromic anemia. Some dogs may exhibit iridocyclitis and photophobia.

Pemphigus Erythematosus. The skin changes are typically confined to the face and are characterized by erythema, oozing, crusting, scaling, and alopecia.

Pemphigus Vulgaris. Pemphigus vulgaris is characterized by epidermal ulceration with a predilection for the oral mucosa and the mucocutaneous junction. Nail beds may be affected. Approximately 40 per cent of dogs can be effectively treated with corticosteroids. If improvement is not noted during the first 10 days, combination immunosuppression is recommended using prednisone and azathioprine or prednisone and cyclophosphamide. An alternative treatment choice utilizes aurothioglucose. Initial treatment should include concurrent therapy with prednisone.

Bullous Pemphigoid

Collies, Shetland sheepdogs, and perhaps Doberman pinschers may be overrepresented. The diagnosis depends on histologic and immunologic assessment of skin biopsies. The treatment is identical to that described for the pemphigus diseases.

TYPE III (IMMUNE-COMPLEX) HYPERSENSITIVITY

Systemic Lupus Erythematosus

Shetland sheepdogs, collies, Afghan hounds, beagles, Irish setters, Old English sheepdogs, poodles, and German shepherds may be overrepresented. Often the signs of disease wax and wane over considerable time. The most common clinical manifestation is a stilted gait or a shifting leg lameness from polyarthritis or polymyositis. Dermatologic changes include a symmetric to focal distribution of lesions affecting the limbs, body, head, ears, face, mucocutaneous junctions, and oral cavity. Lesions may reveal ulceration, erythema, crusting, oozing, and alopecia. Major signs include nonerosive polyarthritis, polymyositis, bullous dermatitis, proteinuria, and immune-mediated hemolytic anemia, thrombocytopenia, or leukopenia. Minor signs consist of fever, oral ulceration, pleuritis, myocarditis, pericarditis, peripheral lymphadenopathy, dementia, and seizures. Serologic tests used to support a diagnosis include the antinuclear antibody test and the lupus erythematosus cell test.

A diagnosis of SLE is made if two major signs and a positive serologic test exist or if one major sign, two minor signs, and a positive serologic test have been documented. The serum biochemistry profile may reveal hypoalbuminemia, azotemia, or creatinemia. If serum aspartate aminotransferase activity is elevated above alanine aminotransferase activity, muscle inflammation should be suspected; serum creatinine phosphokinase activity should be assessed. The urinalysis may reveal proteinuria. As many as 50 per cent of cases will exhibit evidence of glomerulonephritis. Cytologic analysis of joint fluid should reveal an increased cell count comprised predominantly of nondegenerated neutrophils and some mononuclear cells. Most immunologists agree that the ANA test is superior to the LE cell test to detect serum antinuclear antibody, *but false-negative and false-positive results may occur with each test.*

Treatment. The reduction of tissue inflammation is usually achieved through the use of prednisone or prednisolone. If improvement is not noted within 10 days, concurrent administration of azathioprine is recommended for dogs, whereas cats should receive chlorambucil. Aspirin may provide additional analgesic, antipyretic, and anti-inflammatory relief.

Cutaneous (Discoid) Lupus Erythematosus

This generally considered to be a mild or benign form of SLE. Cutaneous lupus erythematosus lacks systemic involvement and ANA tests are usually negative. The most common sign is characterized by varying degrees of depigmentation, erythema, ulceration, and erosions. Crusting and scaling of the pinnae, periorbital skin, lip, and feet are observed occasionally. Routine histopathologic examination of affected skin confirms the diagnosis. Treatment focuses on glucocorticoids. Oral administration of vitamin E has also been successful. In mild cases, topical betamethasone, topical sunscreen, and avoidance of sunlight may be adequate. Niacinamide and tetracycline may also prove effective.

Rheumatoid Arthritis

Clinical signs generally relate to morning stiffness, stiff-legged gait, pain on manipulation of joints, reluctance to exercise, and swelling of affected joints. The peripheral joints appear to be most often affected. The diagnosis should be based on criteria including morning stiffness, pain on motion of at least one joint, swelling joints, radiographic evidence of an erosive arthritis, positive rheumatoid factor test, nonseptic arthritis, and histologic evidence of a proliferative synovitis with accumulation of plasma cells and lymphocytes. Rheumatoid arthritis generally is treated with aspirin and corticosteroids. Other immunosuppressive agents such as azathioprine or cyclophosphamide may be valuable.

Feline Chronic Progressive Polyarthritis

This is associated with feline leukemia virus and feline syncytia-forming virus. The most common form of the disease is referred to as the fibrous anklyosing form and occurs exclusively in young male cats. The joints are stiff, often swollen, and show a restricted range of motion. The second form occurs more commonly in older cats and is more likely to be manifested by crepitus, joint instability, and severe joint deformity. The analysis of synovial fluid usually reveals hypersegmented neutrophils without detectable bacterial organisms. The treatment focuses on the use of corticosteroids with or without chlorambucil, cyclophosphamide, or azathioprine.

TYPE IV (DELAYED) HYPERSENSITIVITY

Allergic Contact Dermatitis

Animals with this type of allergy present with a dermatitis confined to body areas that make contact with the offending allergen. In general, haired areas of the body are not affected. Skin changes may range from mild erythema only to severely pruritic, papulovesicular lesions with secondary pigmentary changes. The diagnosis should be made by obtaining a careful history, performing a complete physical examination, evaluating patch test results, and examining skin biopsies from affected areas. Therapy should focus on removing the allergen from the immediate environment of the pet. If this is not possible, every attempt should be made to reduce the incidence of contact and the animal should be treated with prednisone or prednisolone.

DRUG HYPERSENSITIVITIES (pp. 2022–2023)

See Chapter 148 in the textbook.

PARAPROTEINEMIAS (pp. 2023–2027)

On serum electrophoresis a paraproteinemia is normally demonstrable as a sharply localized band. The presence of paraproteinemia has been documented in cases of multiple myeloma, chronic lymphocytic leukemia, plasma cell leukemia, primary (Waldenström's) macroglobulinemia, amyloidosis, benign (idiopathic) monoclonal gammopathy, and lymphoma.

CLINICAL MANIFESTATIONS OF PARAPROTEINEMIAS

Bleeding Disorders. Ecchymosis or petechiae, epistaxis, bleeding from gingival surfaces, and possible intermittent gastrointestinal bleeding may be seen.

Hyperviscosity Syndrome. A vicious cycle of pour vascular perfusion and myocardial hypoxia can be established which results in cardiac failure. CNS depression is directly related to cerebral hypoxia. Renal hypoxemia may result in renal tubule degeneration. Tubular protein may result in the development of proteinaceous casts.

CLINICAL DISEASES ASSOCIATED WITH PARAPROTEINEMIAS

Multiple Myeloma

Signs attributed to the tumor mass may include bone pain and spinal cord compression with secondary pain and/or neurologic signs. Clinical signs also result from serum hyperviscosity. The diagnosis requires the demonstration of two of the following four criteria: (1) osteolytic lesion on radiographic analysis, (2) monoclonal gammopathy, (3) plasma cells present on cytologic examination of a bone marrow aspirate, and (4) presence of Bence Jones proteinuria.

Bone marrow cytology should reveal an increase in plasma cell numbers. *Ehrlichia canis* infection can also induce plasmacytosis. The complete blood count often shows a nonregenerative anemia, a thrombocytopenia, and a leukopenia. Hypoalbuminemia, azotemia, and hypercalcemia sometimes occur. The serum globulins are usually increased, and the albumin to globulin ratio typically is ≤ 0.6. Urinalysis may reveal proteinuria.

The final laboratory test should be the quantification of each serum immunoglobulin class.

Treatment. Reduction of neoplastic plasma cells is accomplished through the use of melphalan and prednisone. The best means of decreasing serum viscosity is plasmapheresis. If the patient has adequate erythrocytes, phlebotomy may be performed and the amount of blood withdrawn replaced with isotonic saline. Reduction of hypercalcemia, if present, involves saline diuresis, furosemide, and dexamethasone, and if a significant decrease in serum calcium concentration is not observed, salmon calcitonin.

Primary (Waldenström's) Macroglobulinemia

This disorder is characterized by a neoplastic proliferation of plasma cells associated with the secretion of an IgM monoclonal gammopathy in the absence of chronic lymphoid leukemia. Clinical signs are generally attributable to the proliferation of neoplastic cells or the secretion of the immunoglobulin. Patients typically exhibit signs referable to the serum hyperviscosity syndrome. Major treatment efforts parallel those for multiple myeloma with hyperviscosity.

Benign (Idiopathic) Monoclonal Gammopathy

This is an asymptomatic plasma cell dyscrasia characterized by the presence of a paraproteinemia. The clinical presentation is benign, and by definition no clinical signs of disease are associated with this finding. Cases may progress to develop multiple myeloma.

SECTION XVI
JOINT AND SKELETAL DISORDERS

CHAPTER 149

JOINT DISEASES OF DOGS AND CATS
(pages 2032–2077)

DIAGNOSIS OF JOINT DISEASE (pp. 2034–2039)

THE HISTORY

Many joint diseases have well-documented age and breed predispositions. Examples include mucopolysaccharidoses in young Siamese or white domestic shorthaired cats, osteochondroses and hip dysplasia in immature large breeds of dog, medial patellar luxation in young, small breeds of dog, and joint neoplasia in older animals. Immune-mediated polyarthropathies may sometimes occur as a sequel to vaccination. Diet is an important factor in many joint diseases. Excesses of calories, protein, and calcium have all been associated with developmental abnormalities of joints in rapidly growing dogs. Certain systemic diseases that have consequences for the musculoskeletal system include carpal joint collapse in cats with chronic diabetes, bacterial endocarditis presenting as a polyarthropathy, and the multisystemic manifestations of systemic lupus erythematosus or rheumatoid arthritis. Polyarthritis may occur as a reaction to sulfonamides.

PHYSICAL EXAMINATION

Observation of the whole animal, both standing and in motion, is followed by palpation, manipulation, and observation of all the individual components of the musculoskeletal system, including the spine. Each limb is palpated for subtle changes in muscle symmetry, joint size, or bone contour. Following palpation, each joint is manipulated through its range of movement. Sedation or anesthesia is frequently indicated.

DIAGNOSTIC IMAGING

At least two high-quality radiographs are needed to evaluate a joint, and these should ideally be taken perpendicular to one another. More than two views are sometimes needed in evaluating the elbow or hock. Radiologic changes include articular fractures, normal or abnormal relationship of bony structures, distention of the joint capsule, loss of articular cartilage, subchondral bone sclerosis, subchondral bone ero-

Original chapter written by David Bennett and Christopher May

TABLE 149–1. GUIDELINES TO SYNOVIAL FLUID ANALYSIS IN DOGS AND CATS

PARAMETER	NORMAL JOINT	DEGENERATIVE JOINT DISEASE	IMMUNE-MEDIATED ARTHRITIS	BACTERIAL INFECTIVE ARTHRITIS
Color	Clear/pale yellow	Yellow	Yellow (+/– blood-tinged)	Yellow (+/– blood-tinged)
Clarity	Transparent	Transparent	Transparent or opaque	Opaque
Viscosity	Very high	High	Low/very low	Very low
Mucin clot	Good	Good-fair	Fair-poor	Poor
Spontaneous clot	None	+/–	Often	Often
White cells (/mm^3)	<1000	1000–5000	>5000	>5000
Neutrophils	<5%	<10%	10–95%	>90%
Mononuclear cells	>95%	>90%	5–90%	<10%
Protein (gm/dl)	2.0–2.5	2.0–3.0	2.5–5.0	>4.0
Glucose (% of serum value)	>90	N/A	N/A	<50

N/A = Not available for the dog or cat.

sions, subchondral cyst formation, calcification of periarticular or intra-articular soft tissues, and the formation of periarticular bone spurs. Distention of the joint capsule is an important sign because it is often the earliest recognizable radiographic sign. Intra-articular and periarticular soft tissue structures can be demonstrated by contrast arthrography. The apparent severity of radiographic findings does not always correlate with the severity of clinical signs. Ultrasonography can be used to assess joint effusions and the articular soft tissues. Bone scintigraphy, CT scanning, and MRI imaging are finding widespread use for assessing skeletal lesions not readily apparent on conventional radiographs.

SYNOVIAL FLUID ANALYSIS

Specific indications include investigation of articular effusions, polyarthritis, joint stiffness, joint pain, and migratory arthropathies. (See Table 149–1.) False-negative results from bacterial culture of synovial fluid can occur, especially following antibiotic therapy.

LIGAMENT, TENDON, AND MUSCLE DISEASE ASSOCIATED WITH JOINT DISEASE (pp. 2040–2042)

See the textbook.

DEVELOPMENTAL DISORDERS (pp. 2042–2049)

OSTEOCHONDROSIS

Osteochondrosis refers to an idiopathic disease characterized by disorderly endochondral ossification that affects a previously normal growth mechanism. The term osteochondrosis dissecans is used when the lesion is characterized by a separated flap of cartilage on the articular surface of a joint.

Shoulder Joint

The most common form osteochondrosis that affects the canine shoulder joint is the osteochondrosis dissecans (OCD) lesion of the humeral head. The onset of clinical signs usually occurs between 5 and 10 months of age, and males are approximately three times more frequently affected. Manipulation of the shoulder reveals pain that is evident on full extension and sometimes on full flexion. The most common radiologic finding is an irregular radiolucent subchondral defect, usually involving the caudal aspect of the humeral head. In some cases a calcified linear flap of cartilage can be seen above the subchondral defect. Surgical treatment is indicated for most cases of shoulder OCD when lameness is present and persisting and when there is pain on manipulation of the shoulder joint. Recovery is guaranteed and predictable with surgical treatment.

Elbow Joint

Osteochondrosis dissecans affects the medial humeral condyle and has been reported in several breeds. Most cases present between 4 and 8 months of age. It is usually the larger breeds that are affected, and there is a 2:1 ratio of males to females. Secondary osteoarthritis is a common sequel and can be expected to produce lameness later in life. Fragmentation of the coronoid process, although the most common lesion, is the most difficult to visualize by radiography. The diagnosis is often made from the history, the clinical features, and the presence of articular osteophytes, indicating early osteoarthritis. The OCD lesion of the medial humeral condyle is usually seen on a craniocaudal view, either as a radiolucent defect or a flattening of the articular surface of the condyle. A calcified flap of cartilage may also be seen. There is evidence to show that the conservative treatment of fragmented coronoid process and OCD of the medial epicondyle is preferable to surgery. Treatment includes regular exercise and a gradual build-up in the amount of daily exercise. Generally, by the time the dog is 12 to 18 months of age, the lameness will resolve. Surgical treatment is considered if the lameness is particularly severe or worsens with the conservative approach.

Stifle Joint

The most common manifestation is osteochondrosis dissecans of the lateral femoral condyle. Most cases present between the ages of 5 and 7 months, with a mild lameness. The disease is often bilateral. Males are more often affected than females. Both stifle joints should always undergo radiography. The lesion is seen as an irregularity or flattening in the contour of the affected condyle. The change in contour may be associated with a radiolucency of the subchondral bone, and sometimes a calcified line can be seen over the defect, representing the separated cartilage flap. Many cases remain untreated and heal spontaneously. Only those cases showing lameness should be considered for surgical treatment.

Hock Joint

Clinical signs are usually seen at about the age of 6 months, and males are most often affected. Bilateral cases are common. The lameness may be characterized by straight hindleg conformation, poor hindlimb movement, and/or a definite limp. Lateral, craniocaudal, and oblique views are often necessary to visualize the OCD lesions. In some cases, the lesions can be treated conservatively. If the clinical problem is severe, surgical exploration of the joint is advisable.

HIP DYSPLASIA

Hip dysplasia is mainly a clinical problem in the larger breeds. It is known to be an inherited disease, but it is adversely influenced by environmental factors, such as rapid growth and excessive exercise. Clinical features can be seen in the young animal or later in life when secondary osteoarthritis is the main cause of lameness. Gait abnormalities are seen in the young puppy and include a "rolling hindleg gait." The radiographic features include widening of the joint space between the femoral head and cranial acetabular wall, flattening of the cranial effective acetabular rim, and varying degrees of lateral displacement of the femoral head from the acetabulum. Osteophyte production can also be visualized, and in advanced cases, remodeling of the acetabulum, femoral head, and neck can be observed. There is often little correlation between the clinical and radiographic features of hip dysplasia. Conservative treatment can be helpful in many cases. Surgical osteotomy techniques can be used. Total hip replacement is also being regularly used. Femoral head excision is a salvage procedure for hip dysplasia and osteoarthritis.

ASEPTIC NECROSIS OF THE FEMORAL HEAD

This disease occurs commonly in the toy and small breeds of dog. These animals are usually 6 to 8 months of age and have a unilateral hindleg lameness, occasionally bilateral. Radiography normally shows the characteristic features of radiolucent defects within the femoral head. The recommended treatment is generally femoral head excision.

CONGENITAL DISORDERS (pp. 2049–2051)

CONGENITAL LUXATION/SUBLUXATION OF JOINTS

The Shoulder. Congenital shoulder luxation is most often seen in the smaller breeds. Repositioning of the joint and temporary fixation with a transarticular pin is often used for treatment.

The Elbow. Several different types of congenital elbow luxation are reported. Type I luxation, which is the most common, is characterized by posterolateral displacement of the proximal radius. Some animals can cope with the deformities, and surgery may help in some cases.

Femoropatellar Joint. Medial patellar luxation is the type most frequently seen and occurs particularly in the small toy breeds of dogs and in the cat. The problem is generally bilateral. Lameness may only be slight in some cases. There may be intermittent carriage of the limb or, if the displacement is equally severe in both stifle joints, the animal may adopt a crouched gait and posture. Palpation of the joint normally establishes the diagnosis. Surgical treatment is indicated when the clinical problem is sufficiently severe.

Temporomandibular Joint. Congenital luxation/subluxation, including dysplasia, of the temporomandibular joint is reported in the dog. Affected animals present either with the phenomenon of "open-jaw locking" or with pain on opening the mouth. Radiography will show an irregular joint space and films taken while the jaw is locked can demonstrate joint subluxation/luxation. Treatment of these cases is by partial or complete resection of the zygomatic arch on the side of contact.

CERVICAL SPONDYLOMYELOPATHY ("WOBBLER SYNDROME")

See Chapter 83 and page 644 of the textbook.

ARTHROPATHIES ASSOCIATED WITH INHERITED METABOLIC DISORDERS (pp. 2051–2052)

MUCOPOLYSACCHARIDOSIS

See also Chapters 82 and 83 and pages 617 and 675 of the textbook. The mucopolysaccharidoses are a group of diseases classed as lysosomal storage diseases. Clinical features of type VI include broadening of the maxilla, corneal clouding, pectus excavatum, and neurologic abnormalities. The epiphyseal and metaphyseal areas of the long bones are enlarged and irregularly shaped. Most cats have a chronic mucoid ocular discharge and chronic upper respiratory tract infection. Clinical signs begin at an early age. Diagnosis is confirmed by the demonstration of urinary glycosaminoglycans, identification of excessive amounts of dermatan sulfate, and confirmation of decreased arylsulfatase B activity. Examination of a blood smear will demonstrate coarse granular material in over 90 per cent of neutrophils. The clinical and radiographic features of type I are similar to those of type VI, except that long bone epiphyseal dysplasia is not a feature. The disease is characterized by the deficiency of the enzyme α- L-iduronidase. Again, there is no treatment.

NEOPLASTIC AND NEOPLASIA-LIKE ARTHROPATHIES (pp. 2052–2053)

Synovial Sarcoma. This occurs mainly in larger dogs. The stifle is by far the most commonly affected joint. Chronic lameness is usually the presenting sign. The tumor grows within the joint and will affect all the bones. Radiography of the thorax may show metastatic disease.

Other Tumors. Both lipoma and liposarcoma can affect joints. Synovial chondrosarcoma has been reported.

Tumors Eroding into Joints. Fibrosarcomas can erode into joint cavities.

Villonodular Synovitis. Two forms are described—a local nodular synovitis and a diffuse synovitis. The local form usually responds well to local resection. Radiography shows soft tissue density and bony destruction. The synovia has the characteristics of an inflammatory fluid. Excision arthroplasty has successfully been used to treat the diffuse form.

ARTHRITIS (pp. 2053–2072)

Osteoarthritis. Osteoarthritis is an inherently noninflammatory disorder of movable (synovial) joints characterized by deterioration of articular cartilage and by the formation of new bone at the joint surfaces and margins. Osteoarthritis is the most common form of joint disease affecting dogs. It is relatively uncommon in cats.

Diagnosis. Osteoarthritis most commonly presents as lameness. Stiffness after rest is a cardinal sign of joint disease and is frequently present in osteoarthritis. The stiffness usually lasts only a few minutes after rising from a period of rest. In secondary osteoarthritis, there may be clinical signs referable to the primary disease, such as a drawer sign in rupture of the cranial cruciate ligament. Osteoarthritic joints are swollen and painful on palpation. Crepitus is an inconsistent finding. Luxation or subluxation may also occur as a secondary event. Heat and redness are usually not detected. In early osteoarthritis, radiographic changes may be minimal or absent. The earliest radiographic sign is usually increased periarticular soft tissue opacity associated with synovial effusion. New bone, in the form of periarticular osteophytes, becomes radiologically apparent within a few weeks of the onset. However, osteophyte formation correlates with aging, and evidence of osteophytosis should not be used as a sole radiographic criterion for the diagnosis of osteoarthritis. Nine principal features of osteoarthritis have been identified on radiographs of dogs and cats (Table 149–2).

Treatment. The treatment of secondary osteoarthritis often requires treatment for the primary, inciting disease. However, the inciting disease may no longer be of clinical significance at the time of presentation. Therapy at this stage is palliative. In many animals, significant improvements can be made by life-style adjustments alone. Weight reduction is possibly the single most important life-style adjustment that can be made for overweight animals. A moderate exercise regimen should be maintained whenever possible. Non–weight-bearing exercise, such as swimming, may be helpful in some cases. Strict rest is indicated only during acutely painful episodes. Drugs should be used judiciously and in combination with life-style adjustments. The non-

TABLE 149–2. RADIOGRAPHIC FEATURES OF OSTEOARTHRITIS

1. Effusion and periarticular soft tissue swelling
2. Osteophyte formation
3. Subchondral bone sclerosis
4. Attrition or wearing of subchondral bone
5. Bone remodeling
6. Reduction in joint space
7. Subluxation
8. Intra-articular and periarticular soft tissue mineralization
9. Subchondral cyst formation

steroidal anti-inflammatory drugs (NSAIDs) are the most commonly used drugs in the management of osteoarthritis in dogs. All NSAIDs carry some risk of systemic side effects, particularly through damage to the gastrointestinal tract. It is good clinical practice to aim for the minimum possible dose of drug to achieve control of the disease and to attempt withdrawal of all pharmacologic support whenever feasible. The use of corticosteroids in the longterm management of osteoarthritis is limited by their systemic side effects and their effect on articular cartilage. Corticosteroid therapy in dogs should be reserved for cases with inflammatory, erosive osteoarthritis or those in which therapy with other compounds has failed. Hyaluronic acid derivatives and polysulfated glycosaminoglycans (PSGAGs) have been shown to be beneficial. Surgical options for the treatment of osteoarthritis itself include: (1) joint lavage, (2) arthodesis, (3) excision arthroplasties, and (4) replacement arthroplasties.

Traumatic Arthritis. Single episodes of acute, blunt trauma to a joint usually result in effusion, swelling, and pain with varying degrees of disruption to the cartilage, ligaments, and surrounding bone. Sprains (ligament injuries) and strains (tendon injuries) are commonly associated with traumatic arthritis. All effusions should be routinely aspirated to check for hemarthrosis as this is associated with a high incidence of intra-articular fracture or ligament rupture. The appearance of synovial fluid in traumatic arthritis is often similar to that in osteoarthritis (see Table 149–3). In the acute phases, a single episode of nondisruptive trauma should be treated by cold compresses. This is followed later by the application of a supportive dressing and/or the application of heat. Nonsteroidal anti-inflammatory or analgesic drugs may be indicated. A period of rest is followed by a graded return to normal exercise. Post-traumatic osteoarthritis describes the development of permanent joint changes that may be a sequel to trauma. Secondary osteoarthritis of this type normally develops only if the initial trauma is severe or disruptive.

INFLAMMATORY ARTHROPATHIES

Bacterial Infective Arthritis. Streptococci, staphylococci, hemolytic *Escherichia coli, Pasteurella,* and *Erysipelothrix* are the most commonly isolated bacteria from septic joints. Many dogs and cats present with bacterial infective arthritis but no evidence of a direct penetrating injury. It is believed that the route of infection is hematogenous in these cases. Preexisting joint disease predisposes the joint to opportunistic infection. In most cases there is an acute onset of lameness in a single limb. Most cases involve only a single joint. The carpus, stifle, and hock are affected most frequently. Involvement of more than two joints is most often secondary to systemic bacterial infections, such as bacterial endocarditis. Larger breeds are most often affected. The affected joint often has the cardinal signs of inflammation, being warm, swollen, and painful. Chronic or untreated cases lead to joint degeneration with associated ligament injuries. The radiographic features vary. The earliest is soft tissue swelling around the joint. A marked periosteal reaction often develops in the later stages, and there may be calcification of the periarticular soft tissues. There is often patchy sclerosis of subchondral bone. In chronic cases there is evidence of secondary osteoarthritic changes. There is an increased synovial fluid volume and the synovial fluid is usually turbid or blood tinged (see Table 149–1). The diagnosis is confirmed by culture of the organism from synovial fluid and/or synovial membrane. Systemic antibiotic therapy is continued for at least 4 to 6 weeks or for 2 weeks after the complete resolution of clinical signs. Joint lavage and drainage is indicated when the clinical signs are severe or it is an immature animal with open growth plates.

Bacterial Discospondylitis. See Chapter 83 and page 653 of the textbook. The clinical signs are mainly stiffness and spinal pain that is often localized to the site of infection. Persistent or recurring pyrexia is common. In some cases there are neurologic deficits. Glomerulonephritis and pulmonary arterial thrombi may occur as complications. The most commonly isolated organisms are staphylococci, streptococci, and coliforms. Culture of the urine may be of assistance in planning therapy. The earliest radiographic finding is narrowing of the intervertebral space. In more advanced cases there is destruction of vertebral bone on either side of the disc space. Treatment hinges on long-term systemic antibiotics and confinement. Surgical decompression, stabilization, and curettage of the lesion are indicated in some cases.

Bacterial Endocarditis and Arthritis. Several joints are usually affected. Treatment is difficult because of a poor response or because of relapses.

Lyme Arthritis. The most common presenting sign in dogs is acute lameness associated with a migratory monoarthritis or pauciarthritis. There may be pyrexia and lymphadenopathy. Analysis of synovial fluid shows changes consistent with an inflammatory arthropathy. A diagnosis of Lyme disease is difficult to establish with certainty (Table 149–3). Lyme disease is treated with (tetracyclines, penicillin derivatives, or erythromycin).

Mycoplasmal Arthritis. This is most likely to occur in debilitated or immunodepressed animals. The organisms may be seen in a synovial fluid smear. It may also be found in the cerebrospinal fluid of affected dogs and can be treated with tylosin, gentamycin, or erythromycin.

Rickettsial Arthritis. Rocky Mountain spotted fever has sequelae which include generalized central nervous signs, uveitis, sloughing of peripheral tissues affected by vasculitis, and polyarthritis. Canine ehrlichiosis may present as a polyarthritis in certain geographically restricted areas.

Viral Arthritis. A transient, sometimes protracted sterile polyarthritis can be seen following the vaccination of kittens and puppies. Calicivirus can produce an infective arthritis in the cat.

TABLE 149–3. CRITERIA FOR THE DIAGNOSIS OF LYME DISEASE IN DOGS

1. A history of potential exposure to *B. burgdorferi*
2. Seasonal incidence: associated with peaks in tick activity, particularly the nymph or adult stages, which are more likely to transmit *B. burgdorferi*
3. Appropriate clinical signs: including fever, malaise, lethargy, inappetence, lymphadenopathy, lameness, carditis (heart block), neurologic signs, and possibly glomerulonephritis
4. Laboratory/radiologic support for the diagnosis: In cases of Lyme arthritis this should include radiographic evidence of a synovial effusion and synovial fluid analysis consistent with synovitis
5. Positive serologic test for *B. burgdorferi:* Some asymptomatic animals are positive for anti-Borrelia antibodies
6. Response to antibiotic therapy
7. Identification of *B. burgdorferi* in blood, urine, synovial fluid, CSF, or tissues
8. Culture of *B. burgdorferi* from blood, urine, synovial fluid, CSF, or tissues
9. Exclusion of other possible causes of similar clinical signs: including traumatic arthritis, osteoarthritis, and the immune-mediated polyarthritides
   A diagnosis of Lyme disease in dogs should satisfy criteria 1, 3, 4, 5, and 9. Criterion 6 should subsequently be satisfied in almost all cases. Ideally, criteria 7 and 8 should also be satisfied, but this may be difficult as the organism is difficult to culture and may only be present in low numbers. Even in low numbers, the organism can be detected by sensitive molecular biology techniques such as the polymerase chain reaction or in situ hybridization, but these are not in common use for routine diagnosis at the present time.

The Immune-Based Arthritides

Immune-based arthritis is principally but not always a polyarticular disease. Immune complexes may be generated both locally within the joint and/or systemically within the circulation with secondary deposition into the joints.

The Erosive Immune-Based Arthritides

Rheumatoid Arthritis. The synovitis is caused by an immune complex reaction involving antigens complexing with specific antibody and rheumatoid factor (antibody against IgG).

Clinical Features. Lameness (often shifting in nature) is the main presenting sign, but it varies in severity. Symmetric joint involvement is typical. Affected joints are often swollen and painful on manipulation, and in advanced cases, gross deformity with abnormal motion and crepitus is apparent.

Radiographic Features. The classic feature is the presence of subchondral bone destruction visualized as an irregularity of the articular surface or as "punched out" erosions. Advanced cases may show extensive bone destruction with gross joint deformity.

Laboratory Features. Synovial fluid is often increased and usually turbid (see Table 149–1).

Treatment. High doses of analgesic and anti- inflammatory drugs can be tried. Other authorities recommend immunosuppressive therapy with prednisolone and cytotoxic drugs. Gold injections have also been tried with some success.

Periosteal Proliferative Polyarthritis (Reiter's disease). This is commonly encountered in the cat. It affects mainly the hocks and carpii, and the characteristic feature is a marked periosteal new bone often extending beyond the confines of the joint. In addition, one or more joints will show localized bony erosions. It is common in the young adult. Male castrated cats are most often affected. Affected joints are enlarged and may show pain and crepitus on manipulation. Radiographically, periosteal new bone is often the most striking feature. Bony destruction is also seen. Most cases are best treated with low doses of prednisolone. Chrysotherapy has also been used, but gold is highly toxic in cats. Euthanasia is necessary when the quality of life becomes poor.

The Nonerosive Immune-Based Arthritides

Systemic Lupus Erythematosus. Symmetric polyarthritis is regarded as the principal clinical feature.

Clinical Features. Affected animals are most often pyrexic, lethargic, and anorexic. Joints are swollen, sometimes with obvious synovial effusion and pain on manipulation. Lymphadenopathy is common. Polymyositis may concurrently occur.

Laboratory Features. SLE is characterized by the presence of circulating antinuclear antibody. However, ANA is not specific for systemic lupus erythematosus. Synovial fluid examination reveals excess, discolored, sometimes cloudy fluid, generally with a poor mucin clot. White cells are increased with a preponderance of polymorphonuclear cells (see Table 149–1).

Treatment. Corticosteroid therapy is commonly used, usually combined with cytotoxic drugs. Rest and confinement of the dog are important.

Polyarthritis/Polymyositis Syndrome. This is a nonerosive polyarthritis complicated by polymyositis. It is most often seen in the spaniel breeds. The dogs are negative for antinuclear antibody. Treatment consists of a combination of prednisolone and cytotoxic drugs.

Polyarthritis/Meningitis Syndrome. This syndrome has been seen in the Weimaraner, German shorthaired pointer, Boxer, Bernese mountain dog, and Japanese Akita. These cases present with pyrexia, stiffness, and neck pain. The arthritis is symmetric and nonerosive. Cerebrospinal fluid shows increased protein, white cells, and creatine phosphokinase levels. Some of these cases may be associated with a polyarteritis.

Familial Renal Amyloidosis in Chinese Shar Pei Dogs. These dogs present with episodes of fever and swelling of one or both hock joints, and occasionally other joints. Synovial fluid analysis will show an inflammatory synovia in one or more joints. Amyloid deposits occur in several organs, but renal amyloidosis is the most significant. Amyloidosis will eventually result in renal failure. Prognosis is poor. Colchicine treatment has been tried to control the amyloidosis.

Polyarteritis Nodosa. This is an inflammatory condition of small arteries, often of a granulomatous nature. Polyarthritis is a common feature. Occasionally meningitis and polyarthritis are both present. The animals are often pyrexic, depressed, and stiff. In some young animals (e.g., beagle) self-cure eventually occurs as the animal matures.

Idiopathic Polyarthritis. Idiopathic polyarthritis includes all those cases of inflammatory arthropathy that cannot be classified into the other groups.

Type I: Uncomplicated Idiopathic Arthritis. Many of the features of these dogs are the same as those of the rheumatoid dogs, and it might be that these idiopathic cases represent a milder or earlier form of the rheumatoid disease.

Type II: Idiopathic Arthritis Associated with Infections Remote from the Joints. The common infections are in the respiratory tract, including ocular, urinary tract, uterine, and a variety of bacterial skin infections. It is assumed that the infectious process provides an antigenic source for immune complex formation. Treatment is mainly directed toward controlling the infection.

Type III: Idiopathic Arthritis Associated with Gastrointestinal Disease. The features are similar to those of type I, but symptoms related to the gastrointestinal disease will be present.

Type IV: Idiopathic Arthritis Associated with Neoplasia Remote from the Joints. The neoplastic lesion is usually malignant, but may not be apparent by clinical assessment. Corticosteroids may help to relieve the joint inflammation.

Clinical Features. Most of these animals are presented with a bilaterally symmetric polyarthritis and fever, dullness, and loss of appetite. Most animals show swollen and painful joints and synovial effusion may be apparent.

Radiographic Features. Soft tissue swelling and/or synovial effusion may be apparent although often there is no abnormality visible. Destructive changes are rarely seen.

Laboratory Features. These dogs are usually negative for both rheumatoid factor and antinuclear antibody. Synovial fluid examination shows high levels of leukocytes with a predominance of neutrophils.

Treatment. The type I dogs usually respond well to prednisolone. If relapses occur or there is a poor response, a combination of prednisolone and cytotoxic drugs (cyclophosphamide) can be tried. Treatment of types II, III, and IV dogs is primarily directed against the infective, alimentary, or neoplastic lesion.

Miscellaneous Immune-based Arthritides

Drug-induced Arthritis. The most commonly incriminated drugs are sulfa drugs, lincomycin, erythromycin, cephalosporins, and penicillins.

Vaccination Reactions. Occasionally an immune-based polyarthritis can follow vaccine inoculations. It is usually self-limiting and clears within 2 to 3 days.

Plasmacytic-Lymphocytic Gonitis. This disease affects the stifle joints of small- and medium-sized breeds of dog. It is confined to the stifle joint. It leads to pronounced joint laxity and instability often manifested by damage to the anterior cruciate ligament. Treatment involves immunosuppressive drugs and surgical repair of the cruciate ligament in some cases.

DISEASES OF THE VERTEBRAL COLUMN
(pp. 2072–2074)

SPONDYLOSIS DEFORMANS AND ANKYLOSING HYPEROSTOSIS

Features of these diseases may be found in Chapter 83, page 690, of the textbook.

INTERVERTEBRAL DISC DISEASE.

See page 663 of the textbook.

DISEASES OF THE LUMBOSACRAL ARTICULATION (*CAUDA EQUINA* SYNDROME)

See page 673 of the textbook.

CHAPTER 150
SKELETAL DISEASES
(pages 2077–2103)

CONGENITAL BONE DISORDERS (pp. 2083–2085)

HEMIMELIA, PHOCOMELIA, AND AMELIA

In these conditions there is congenital absence of portions of the normal structures in an extremity. Hemimelia is either longitudinal (paraxial)—with absence of the ulnar, radial, or central regions in the forelimb—or transverse— with the distal portion of the limb completely absent. Radial agenesis is the most common paraxial hemimelia in cats and dogs. In phocomelia, an intercalary segment of limb is missing. In severe cases the paw with rudimentary digits is attached to the trunk like a seal flipper. Amelia is complete absence of one or more limbs. Animals affected by amelia probably die or undergo euthanasia at birth.

SYNDACTYLY

Two or more digits are fused in a bony or soft tissue union in syndactyly. This is not clinically significant in pets.

POLYDACTYLY

Polydactyly is the presence of extra digits, usually on the medial side of the paw in dogs and cats.

Original chapter written by Kenneth A. Johnson, A. D. J. Watson, and Rodney L. Page

ECTRODACTYLY

Ectrodactyly is often called split hand or lobster claw deformity. Classically, the third metacarpal bone and digit are absent. In dogs it is usually an isolated deformity without breed predilection.

DEVELOPMENTAL AND GENETIC BONE DISORDERS (pp. 2085–2089)

OSTEOPETROSIS

Defective osteoclastic resorption of bone is the principal feature of osteopetrosis. Radiographically, affected bones have a "marbled," densely homogeneous appearance. The disorder is rare and not well characterized in dogs and cats.

OSTEOGENESIS IMPERFECTA

This is characterized by excessive bone fragility, osteopenia, increased susceptibility to fracture, and secondary bone deformity. It occurs rarely in dogs and cats.

DWARFISM

Pituitary Dwarfism.   See Chapter 112 and page 1425 in the textbook.
Congenital Hypothyroidism.   See Chapter 115.

RETAINED CARTILAGE CORES

In young large- and giant-breed dogs, cartilage cores form in the metaphysis of the distal ulna. Radiographically, there is a central, radiolucent core of cartilage extending from the distal ulnar physis into the metaphyseal bone. Retarded ulnar growth causes valgus and rotation of the paw, cranial bowing of the radius, and carpal and elbow subluxation.

CRANIOMANDIBULAR OSTEOPATHY

This occurs mainly in young West Highland white, Scottish, Cairn, Boston, and other terriers. Affected pups develop mandibular swelling, drooling of saliva, prehension difficulties and/or pain on opening the mouth. The clinical course may fluctuate. Periods of pyrexia occur in some cases. Radiographic changes include irregular bony proliferation involving the mandible and tympanic bulla–petrous temporal bone areas. The diagnosis is straightforward in cases with typical clinical and radiographic features. Bone biopsy may be useful in atypical cases. Craniomandibular osteopathy is self-limiting. Anti-inflammatory drug treatment can reduce pain and discomfort. The prognosis is guarded when extensive changes occur.

MULTIPLE CARTILAGINOUS EXOSTOSES

Protuberances consist of cancellous bone and they arise in the metaphyseal region of bones. Lesions become senescent at maturity. Malignant transformation occurs rarely in aged animals. Signs include paresis due to progressive spinal cord compression (Chapter 83) and pain due to impingement of exostoses on adjacent tissues. Surgical excision of exostoses that are causing symptoms is recommended.

IDIOPATHIC BONE DISORDERS (pp. 2089–2093)

ENOSTOSIS

Enostosis (panosteitis) is a relatively common disease causing lameness in medium, large, and giant-breed dogs, especially the German shepherd dog. Two-thirds of affected dogs are male. The age of onset is 6 to 18 months. Lameness is acute in onset, not associated with trauma, and intermittent in one or more limbs. Each episode of lameness lasts 1 to 3 months, but with recurrent bouts, enostosis may persist for 2 to 9 months. In the early stages, other signs include anorexia, lethargy, pyrexia, and weight loss. On physical examination, pain is detected on deep palpation of affected bones. Bones commonly affected are the ulna, humerus, radius, femur, and tibia. Radiographically, there is granular, hazy, increased radiopacity that begins in the region of the nutrient foramen, which may extend to fill the entire medullary cavity. Although enostosis is a self-limiting disease, analgesic or nonsteroidal anti-inflammatory drugs are administered to alleviate pain and lameness.

METAPHYSEAL OSTEOPATHY

Metaphyseal osteopathy (hypertrophic osteodystrophy) is a disease of young rapidly growing dogs of the larger breeds, with onset usually at about 3 to 4 months of age. Affected pups develop metaphyseal swelling and pain, accompanied by depression, inappetence, and variable pyrexia. Some cases recover within a few days, but others have one or more relapses during the following weeks before finally recovering. Radiographic changes include an irregular radiolucent zone present in the metaphysis, separated from the normal- appearing growth plate by a dense band. Surrounding soft tissue may be swollen. Later radiographs may show metaphyseal enlargement with irregular periosteal new bone formation. There is no specific treatment. Dietary imbalances or excesses should be avoided and an anti-inflammatory analgesic given as needed to reduce pain.

SECONDARY HYPERTROPHIC OSTEOPATHY

In secondary hypertrophic osteopathy (pulmonary hypertrophic osteoarthropathy), firm nonedematous swelling develops in all four limbs, usually in response to intrathoracic disease, most often neoplasia. Other underlying associations have included pneumonitis, endocarditis, dirofilariasis, urinary rhabdomyosarcoma, and hepatic carcinoma. It is rare in cats. Signs related to limb changes often precede signs of thoracic disease. Affected animals are stiff and reluctant to move. There is swelling of all limbs, which are warm and firm and may be painful. Radiographic changes are characteristic: soft tissue swelling of the distal extremities initially, then periosteal new bone formation as either irregular nodules perpendicular to the cortex or smoother parallel deposits. Bone changes begin distally and may spread proximally to involve humerus and scapula, femur and pelvis. Ribs and vertebrae are sometimes affected. Treatment should be directed against the underlying thoracic disease. Successful resection of lung lesions can quickly remove pain, soft tissue swelling, and lameness. Relief may also follow intrathoracic vagotomy.

BONE CYST

Young dogs of larger breeds are affected most often. Bone cysts may be subclinical until they are large or fracture with trauma. The lesions occur in metaphyses. The distal radius and/or ulna are affected most often. Radiographically, the lesions are lytic and expansible, with thinned cortex and little or no periosteal reaction. Surgery has been advocated; however, cysts in some untreated dogs heal spontaneously.

NUTRITIONAL, ENDOCRINE, AND METABOLIC BONE DISORDERS (pp. 2093–2097)

NUTRITIONAL SECONDARY HYPERPARATHYROIDISM

See Chapter 113. Nutritional Secondary Hyperparathyroidism is caused by diets providing excess phosphorus and/or insufficient calcium. Affected animals have usually been fed mainly meat or organ tissue. Signs in young animals are lameness, reluctance to stand or walk, and skeletal pain. Bone fractures can follow relatively mild trauma. Effects are less dramatic in adults. Radiographically, there is decreased bone density and thin cortices, with or without fracturing. Growth plates are normal. The calcium concentration is usually within the reference range. Affected animals should be confined for the first few weeks of treatment. A good-quality, nutritionally complete commercial ration should be fed, with the addition of sufficient calcium carbonate calculated to provide a calcium:phosphorus ratio of 2:1. For severely affected cases parenteral calcium may help to reduce pain and lameness initially. The prognosis is generally good, unless skeletal deformity and disability are marked.

RENAL OSTEODYSTROPHY

See Chapters 113. Disorders of the parathyroid glands, and 134, chronic renal failure.

Changes may be most evident in the head. The mandible and maxilla may be pliable and swollen, and teeth may be malaligned, loose, or lost. Skeletal pain, fractures, and bowing of long bones can also occur. Treatment is directed against the underlying disease. Consideration can be given to administering calcium or calcitriol.

HYPERVITAMINOSIS A

Prolonged intake of excessive vitamin A supplements or ingestion of mainly liver diets can cause osteopathy. The major finding in older cats is extensive, even confluent, exostoses involving cervical and cranial thoracic vertebrae. Exostoses may also form around limb joints, especially the shoulder or elbow. The lesions are painful. Treatment necessitates avoiding the source of vitamin A. Mature cats will improve clinically. Bone growth may be retarded permanently in young animals.

NEOPLASTIC BONE DISEASE (pp. 2097–2101)

PRIMARY BONE NEOPLASIA

Osteosarcoma accounts for 85 to 90 per cent of all primary bone cancer. The most common sites are in order: distal radius, proximal humerus, distal femur, and proximal tibia. Large or giant breed dogs are particularly predisposed. The average age of occurrence is 7 years. Ninety per cent of dogs with osteosarcoma have microscopic tumor spread at the time of diagnosis even though the initial diagnostic evaluation does not detect them. The diagnosis of appendicular osteosarcoma is straight-forward. The radiographic appearance can be variable, but typical patterns are mixed osteolysis and proliferation, and periosteal reaction. A presumptive diagnosis can be made given circumstances of a large-breed dog, a preferred site, and a typical radiographic pattern. Thoracic radiologic evaluation should be obtained to screen for pulmonary metastasis. Multicentric osteosarcoma occurs in less than 5 to 10 per cent of dogs.

Therapeutic Considerations. Dogs that undergo amputation without further treatment do well for an average of 4 to 6 months. Numerous reports suggest improved survival (9–11 months) following amputation if cisplatin is administered. A preliminary report suggests that carboplatin is as effective as cisplatin in controlling osteosarcoma metastasis. If amputation is not possible, there are alternatives. Limb-sparing techniques may provide a pain-free, functional limb for dogs with tumors of the distal radius. If amputation or a limb-sparing procedure is not possible, pain relief may be achieved with palliative radiation therapy.

Nonosteogenic Primary Bone Neoplasia

Fibrosarcomas that originate in bone are rare. Radiographic appearance is similar to that of osteosarcoma, and definitive diagnosis requires biopsy. Complete surgical excision is the treatment of choice. The role of adjuvant antineoplastic drugs is unclear. Chondrosarcomas of appendicular bone are rare. The majority are reported in axial or flat bones. Treatment involves resection of the affected site. Radiation therapy may be useful if combined with surgery.

Hemangiosarcoma from bone occurs rarely in dogs and cats. The diagnosis must be confirmed by biopsy. The primary treatment considerations include management of the primary site with wide surgical excision and adjuvant doxorubicin, vincristine, and cyclophosphamide. Multilobular osteochondrosarcoma has a predilection for the skull. It produces an expansile bone lesion with characteristic radiographic pattern described as lobulated and coarsely granular. Wide surgical excision is recommended. Primary bone tumors have been rarely reported following bone fracture repair. No clear etiology has been established. Osteosarcomas account for about 90 per cent of the fracture-associated sarcomas.

Feline Bone Cancer

Osteosarcoma accounts for 90 per cent of bone cancers in cats. No clear pattern of anatomic sites exists. Survival for several years is possible following amputation. There is no recommended drug therapy for cats with nonresectable osteosarcoma. Radiation therapy may be useful for tumor control.

BONE INFECTION

Bone infection (osteomyelitis) may be bacterial, fungal or viral in origin. Beta-lactamase producing *Staphylococcus* cause approximately 50 per cent of cases of bacterial osteomyelitis. Polymicrobial infections may occur. Anaerobes are especially common in bite wound infections. Often there exists concurrent soft tissue injury, bone necrosis, sequestration, fracture instability, implanted foreign material, altered host tissue defenses, or some combination of these.

Diagnosis. Acute osteomyelitis may produce signs of systemic illness including pyrexia, inappetence, dullness, and weight loss, together with neutrophilia and left shift. Heat, pain, and swelling in muscle and periosteum surrounding the infected bone may be evident. In chronic osteomyelitis, abscessation with single or multiple sinus tracts is a prominent sign. Radiographs are essential to the diagnosis. In acute osteomyelitis, there is soft tissue swelling but no osseous changes. In chronic osteomyelitis, periosteal new bone forms early and tends to be extensive. Bone resorption produces cortical thinning, medullary lysis, and rounding of fractured bone ends. The finding of sequestra is virtually diagnostic for osteomyelitis. Isolation of bacteria from suspected bone infections should be attempted to determine the *in vitro* drug susceptibility.

Treatment. Acute osteomyelitis may be cured by 4 to 6 weeks of antibiotic therapy, provided there is limited bone necrosis and no fracture. In chronic osteomyelitis, drug treatment is invariably futile without surgical intervention to remove sequestra and debride necrotic tissue. Fractures must be stabilized and bone defects grafted with autologous cancellous bone.

INDEX

Note: Pages in *italics* indicate illustrations; those followed by t refer to tables.

APPENDIX I

LIST OF DRUGS BY TRADE AND GENERIC NAMES

TRADE NAME	GENERIC NAME
Acepromazine	Acetylpromazine
Actigall	Ursodeoxycholic acid
Adapt	Artificial tears
Adequan	Polysulfated glycosaminoglycan
Adrenalin	Epinephrine
Adriamycin	Doxorubicin
Albeta	DL-methionine
Albon	Sulfadimethoxine
Aldactazide	Hydrochlorothiazide/spironolactone
Aldactone	Spironolactone
Alkeran	Melphalan
Alternagel	Aluminum hydroxide
Ambisome	Amphotericin B
Amiglyde-V	Amikacin
Amikin	Amikacin
Aminocaproic Acid	Amicar
Amoxitabs	Amoxicillin
Amphogel	Aluminum hydroxide
Ancobon	Flucytosine
Ancotil	Flucytosine
Antirobe	Clindamycin
Apresoline	Hydralazine
Aqua-mephyton	Vitamin K_1
Asacol	Mesalamine
Asprin	Acetylsalicylic acid
Atabrine	Quinicrine
Atarax	Hydroxyzine
Augmentin	Amoxicillin/Clavulanic acid
Aureomycin	Chlortetracycline
Avlosulfon	Dapsone
Azium	Dexamethasone
Azulfidine	Sulfasalazine
Bactrim	Trimethoprim/sulfamethoxazole
Bacrovet	Sulfadimethoxine
BAL	Dimercaprol
Banamine	Flunixin meglumine
Baytril	Enrofloxacin
Benadryl	Diphenhydramine HCl
Benzapen	Penicillin G benzathine
Betadyne	Providone-iodine
Betasone	Betamethasone
Biosol	Neomycin
Brethane	Terbutaline
Buprenex	Buprenorphine HCl
Butazolidin	Phenylbutazone
Calan	Verapamil
Calcet	Calcium gluconate
Calcimar	Calcitonin
Caparsolate	Thiacetarsamide
Capoten	Captopril
Carafate	Sucralfate
Cardoxin	Digoxin
Cardizem	Diltiazem HCl
Caricide	Diethylcarbamazine
Cefa	Cephalosporin group
Centrine	Aminopentamide

LIST OF DRUGS BY TRADE AND GENERIC NAMES *(Continued)*

TRADE NAME	GENERIC NAME
Cephulac	Lactulose
Cheque	Mibolerone
Chloromycetin	Chloramphenicol
Chlor Trimeton	Chlorpheniramine maleate
Choledyl	Oxtriphylline
Chronulac	Lactulose
Cipro	Ciprofloxacin
Clavamox	Amoxicillin/clavulanic acid
Cleocin	Clindamycin
Clonopin	Clonazepam
Colace	Dioctyl sulfosuccinate
Colbenemid	Colchicine
Compazine	Prochlorperazine
Conofite	Miconazole
Corid	Amprolium
Cortrosyn	Tetracosactrin
Coscopin	Noscapine
Cuprimine	D-penicillamine
Cypip	Diethylcarbamazine
Cytomel	Liothyronine T_3
Cytosar	Cytarabine hydrochloride
Cytotec	Misoprostol
Cytoxan	Cyclophosphamide
Danocrine	Danazol
Dantefur	Nitrofurantoin
Dantrium	Dantrolene
Daranide	Dichlorphenamide
Daraprim	Pyrimethamine
Darbid	Isopropamide iodide
DDAVP	Desmopressin acetate
DDVP	Dichlorvos
DEC	Diethylcarbamazine
Decadurabolin	Nandrolone decanoate
Decholin	Dehydrocholic acid
Demerol	Mepiridine HCl
Depakene	Valproic acid
Depakote	Valproic acid
Depen	Pencillamine
Depomedrol	Methylprednisolone sodium succinate
Depo Provera	Medroxyprogesterone acetate
Depo Testosterone	Testosterone cypionate
Dermathycin	Thyrotropin/TSH
DES	Diethylstilbestrol
Dexate	Dexamethasone
Dexatrim	Phenylpropanolamine
Dexedrine	Dextroamphetamine
Diamox	Acetazolamide
Diapid	Lysine-8-Vasopressin
Dibenzyline	Phenoxybenzamine hydrochloride
Diflucan	Fluconazole
Dilantin	Phenytoin
Diprivan	Propofol
Ditrim	Trimethoprim/sulfadiazine
Diuril	Chlorothiazide
Dizan	Dithiazanine iodide
DMSO	Dimethyl sulfoxide
DNP	Disophenol
Dobutrex	Dobutamine hydrochloride
DOCA	Desoxycorticosterone acetate

LIST OF DRUGS BY TRADE AND GENERIC NAMES *(Continued)*

TRADE NAME	GENERIC NAME
DOCP	Desoxycorticosterone pivalate
DOMOSO-90	Dimethyl sulfoxide
Dopram	Doxapram
Dramamine	Dimenhydrinate
Droncit	Praziquantel
DTIC	Dacarbazine
Dycill	Dicloxacillin
Dynapen	Dicloxacillin
ECP	Estradiol cyclopenta neopropionate
Ectoral	Ronnel
Elavil	Amitriptyline
Elixophyllin	Theophylline elixir
Elspar	L-asparginase
Enacard	Enalapril maleate
Epogen	Epoetin
Eskalith	Lithium carbonate
Feldene	Piroxicam
Filaribits	Diethylcarbamazine
Flagyl	Metronidazole
Fleet	Phosphate enema
Florinef	Fludrocortisone
Flucort	Flumethasone
Follutein	Human chorionic gonadotropin
Fulvicin	Griseofulvin
Fungizone	Amphotericin B
Furoxone	Furazolidone
Garamycin	Gentamicin
Gentocin	Gentamicin
Geopen	Carbenicillin
Glucotrol	Glipizide
GoLytely	GoLytely enema
Heartguard-30	Ivermectin
Herplex	Idoxuridine
Hetacin	Hetacillin
Hycodan	Dihydrocodeinone
Hydrea	Hydroxyurea
Hydrodiuril	Hydrochlorothiazide
Hytakerol	Dihydrotachysterol
Imferon	Iron-dextran injection
Imizole	Imidocarb
Immunoregulin	Propioni bacterium acnes
Imodium	Loperamide
Imuran	Azathioprine
Inocor	Amrinone
Inderal	Propranolol
Indocin	Indomethocin
Innovar-vet	Fentanyl/droperidol
Inotropin	Dopamine hydrochloride
Interceptor	Milbemycin
Isoptin	Verapamil
Isuprel	Isoproterenol
Ivomec	Ivermectin
Jenotone	Aminopropnazine
Kaon chloride	Potassium salts

LIST OF DRUGS BY TRADE AND GENERIC NAMES *(Continued)*

TRADE NAME	GENERIC NAME
Kaon elixir	Potassium salts
Kaopectate	Kaolin/pectin
Keflex	Cephalosporin group
Kenalog	Triamcinolone
Ketaset	Ketamine HCl
Lacrilube	Artificial tears
Lanoxin	Digoxin
Lasix	Furosemide
Leukeran	Chlorambucil
Levarterenol	Norepinephrine
Levasole	Levamisole
Levophed	Norepinephrine
Levsin	Hyoscyamine
Lincocin	Lincomycin
Lithane	Lithium carbonate
Lithotabs	Lithium carbonate
Lomotil	Diphenoxylate HCl
Lopid	Gemfibrozil
Lopressor	Metoprolol
Losec	Omeprazole
Lotrimin	Clotrimazole
Lutalyse	Prostaglandin $F_{2\alpha}$
Lym DYP	Lime surfur
Lysodren	Mitotane
Macrodantin	Nitrofurantoin
Maxitrol	Dexasporin
Medrol	Methylprednisolone sodium succinate
Megace	Megestrol acetate
Mephyton	Vitamin K_1
Mestinon	Pyridostigmine bromide
Methigel	DL-methionine
Mexitil	Mexiletine
Micalcin	Calcitonin
Micro K Extencaps	Potassium salts
Milk of Magnesia	Magnesium hydroxide
Mintezol	Thiabendazole
Mitaban	Amitraz
Motrin	Ibuprofen
Mucomyst	Acetylcysteine
Mycelex	Clotrimazole
Mydriacil	Tropicamide
Mylepsin	Primidone
Nafcil	Nafcillin
Narcan	Naloxone
Nembutal	Pentobarbital
Nemex	Pyrantel pamoate
Neo-Synephrine	Phenylephrine
Neptazane	Methazolamide
Nilevar	Norethandrolone
Nipride	Nitroprusside
Nitrol	Nitroglycerine
Nizoral	Ketoconazole
Nolvasan	Chlorhexidine
Norpace	Disopyramide phosphate
Norvasc	Amlodipine
Novantrone	Mitoxantrone
Novin	Dipyrone

LIST OF DRUGS BY TRADE AND GENERIC NAMES *(Continued)*

TRADE NAME	GENERIC NAME
Numorphan	Oxymorphone
Oncovin	Vincristine
Optimmune	Cyclosporin
Ornade	Phenylpropanolamine
Orthocide	Captan powder 50%
Ovaban	Megestrol acetate
Oxydex	Benzoyl peroxide
Palosein	Orgotein
Panacur	Fenbendazole
Pentostam	Sodium stibogluconate
Pentothal	Thiopental sodium
Pepcid	Famotidine
Pepto Bismol	Bismuth subsalicylate
Percorten	Desoxycorticosterone pivalate
Periactin	Cyproheptadine
Phytonadione	Vitamin K_1
Pitocin	Oxytocin
Pitressin Tannate	Vasopressin
Platinol	Cisplatin
Pred Forte	Prednisolone ophthalmic suspension
Prilosec	Omeprazole
Primor	Sulfadimethoxine-ormetoprim
Prinivil	Lisinopril
Pro Banthine	Propantheline
Proglycem	Diazoxide
Pronestyl	Procainamide
Propagest	Phenylpropanolamine
Propulsid	Cisapride
Pro Spot	Fenthion
Prostaphlin	Oxacillin
Prostigmin	Neostigmine
Protopam	Pralidoxine
Provera	Medroxyprogesterone acetate
Prozac	Fluoxetine
Prussian Blue	Ferric Cyanoferrate
Pyoben	Benzoyl Peroxide
Pyopen	Carbenicillin
Quadrinal	Theophylline combination
Quibron	Theophylline combination
Reglan	Metoclopramide hydrochloride
Requa	Activated charcoal
Retrovir	AZT
Rheomacrodex	Dextran
Ripercol	Levamisole
Robamox	Amoxicillin
Robaxin	Methocarbamol
Robinul	Glycopyrrolate
Rocan-SR	Procainamide hydrochloride
Roferon	Interferon
Rompun	Xylazine
Sandimmune	Cyclosporine
Scolaban	Bunamidine hydrochloride
Septra	Trimethoprim-sulfamethoxazole
Serax	Oxazepam
Silvaden	Silver sulfadiazine
Solganal	Aurothioglucose

LIST OF DRUGS BY TRADE AND GENERIC NAMES *(Continued)*

TRADE NAME	GENERIC NAME
Soloxine	Levothyroxine sodium
Solu Cortef	Hydrocortisone sodium succinate
Solu Delta Cortef	Prednisolone sodium succinate
Solu Medrol	Methylprednisolone sodium succinate
Sporanox	Itraconazole
Spot On	Fenthion
Stadol	Butorphanol
Stiglin	Neostigmine
Stoxil	Idoxuridine
Strongid T	Pyrantel pamoate
Styquin	Butamisole
Sublimaze	Fentanyl
Sulfadyne	Sulfadiazine
Sulfo Dip	Lime sulfur
Surfak	Dioctyl sulfosuccinate
Surital	Thiamylal sodium
Synotic	Fluocinolone
Synthroid	Levothyroxine sodium
Syntocinon	Oxytocin
Tagamet	Cimetidine
Talwin	Pentazocine
Tapazole	Methimazole
Task	Dichlorvos
Tegison	Etretinate
Telazol	Tiletamine-zolazepam
Telmintic	Mebendazole
Temaril P	Trimeprazine and prednisone
Tenormin	Atenolol
Tensilon	Edrophonium chloride
Terramycin	Oxytetracycline
Theo Dur	Theophylline
Thorazine	Chlorpromazine
Thytropar	Throtropin TSH
Tigan	Trimethobenzamide
Timoptic	Timolol
Titralac	Calcium carbonate
Tofranil	Imipramine
Toprol-XL	Metoprolol
Torbugesic	Butorphanol
Torbutrol	Butorphanol tartrate
Tramisol	Levamisole
Triaminic	Phenylpropanolamine
Tribrissen	Trimethoprim-sulfadiazine
TUMS	Calcium carbonate
Tylan	Tylosin
Tylenol	Acetaminophen
Unipen	Nafcillin
Urecholine	Bethanechol
Urocit-K	Potassium citrate
Uroeze	Ammonium chloride
Valbazen	Albendazole
Valium	Diazepam
Vapona	Dichlorvos
Vasotec	Enalapril
Velban	Vinblastine
Veltrim	Clotrimazole
Versenate	Calcium EDTA

LIST OF DRUGS BY TRADE AND GENERIC NAMES *(Continued)*

TRADE NAME	GENERIC NAME
Veta K_1	Vitamin K_1
Vetalar	Ketamine
Vetalog	Triamcinolone
Vetinol	Noscapine
Vibramycin	Doxycycline hydrochloride
Viokase	Pancreatic enzymes
Vira-A	Vidarbine
Viroptic	Trifluridine
Vitamin B_1	Thiamine
Winstrol	Stanozolol
Wycillin	Procaine penicillin
Xylocaine	Lidocaine hydrochloride
Yomesan	Niclosamide
Zantac	Ranitidine
Zestril	Lisinopril
Zofran	Ondansetron
Zyloprim	Allopurinol
2 PAM	Pralidoxime

DRUG INDEX

Note: Drugs listed represent a compilation of the more commonly used therapeutic agents. Not all drugs are included, and some of those listed may be infrequently or never used by some. As much as possible this listing represents the more commonly used drugs in small animal practice. Drugs are listed by their generic name. Appendix I provides a listing of the trade names for many of these agents for easy cross reference purposes.

Drugs are listed by generic name with trade names in parentheses under the generic title. A brief description of the drug's actions or indications follows. Canine and feline dosage levels are given individually. The fifth column represents a "remarks" column. In this listing are commonly seen side effects, specific important remarks, or other characteristics that are particularly important to the clinician. A sixth column includes commonly available sizes and formulations. Those with HM are human labeled items; those with VM are veterinary labeled; and some are available either way. Abbreviations used in this column are: T = tablets; C = capsules; S = oral solution; I = injectable; ER = extended release oral product; O = topical ointment; OS = ophthalmic solution; OO = ophthalmic ointment; OTC = over the counter, nonprescription item.

The clinician should recheck drug dosages for accuracy as well as for specific indications, contraindications, and warnings. Drugs are listed not only by their licensed use but also by commonly practiced uses. Again the clinician should identify the specific and recommended indications for each drug.

Drug dosages, comments, and side effects are taken from the textbook. There are new and additional drugs and dosages since publication of the 4th edition of the parent textbook. Several other sources have been used including the editor's clinical experience; the *Formulary* from the Animal Medical Center, New York, NY, 1990 edition; the *Veterinary Pharmacy Formulary*, 3rd edition, by D.C. Plumb, University of Minnesota; R.W. Kirk editor, *Current Veterinary Therapy* IX, X, and XI, WB Saunders Co., Philadelphia, PA; and Dana Allen editor, *Small Animal Medicine,* J.B. Lippincott Co., Philadelphia, PA, 1991.

DRUG INDEX *(Continued)*

GENERIC NAME (Trade Name in Parentheses)	INDICATIONS	CANINE DOSE	FELINE DOSE	COMMENTS	HOW SUPPLIED	
Acemannan (Carrisyn)	Immune modulator	2 mg/kg PO, SQ, IV, SID	100 mg PO, SQ, IV, SID	Effects not well established	VM	
Acetaminophen (Tylenol)	Antipyretic Analgesic	10–20 mg/kg BID; PO	Do not use	Toxic to cats Gastric irritation Heinz body anemia	Many sizes OTC	
Acetazolamide (Diamox)	Glaucoma C.A. Inhibitor	2–10 mg/kg PO TID	2–10 mg/kg PO TID	Hypokalemia Panting	125, 250 mg HM	T
Acetylcysteine (Mucomyst)	1. Acetaminophen toxicosis in cats 2. Decrease bronchial secretion viscosity 3. Collagenase complicated corneal ulcers	1. Same as for cats 2. Nebulize as 2% soln BID 3. 1 drop 10% soln q 2–4 h in eye	70 mg/kg PO q 6 h for 3–7 treatments; may be given IV; first dose is 140 mg/kg Same	Tastes bad Conjunctivitis if prolonged use	100, 200 mg/ml HM	I
Acetylpromazine (Acepromazine)	Sedation Preanesthetic Central antiemetic	0.05–0.2 mg/kg PO, SQ, IM, IV	10–20 mg/kg PO	Oversedation causes CNS depression Do not use in patients with seizures Hypotensive agent	5, 10, 25 mg 10 mg/ml VM	T I

Drug	Indication	Dose	Dose (cat/alt)	Side effects / Notes	Supply	
Acetylsalicylic acid (Aspirin)	Analgesia Anti-inflammatory Antipyretic Post H.W. therapy DIC Antithrombotic via decreased platelet aggregation	10–25 mg/kg PO, SID–TID 5–7 mg/kg PO, SID as antithrombotic	q 48–72 h	Anorexia–Nausea G-I irritation Gastric ulcer–bleeding Platelet dysfunction	81, 300, 600 mg HM	T
ACTH Gel	Provocative agent for diagnosis of hyper- or hypoadreno-corticism	2 U/kg IM	10 U/cat	Rare allergic reaction	40, 80 IU/ml HM	I
Activated charcoal	Gastrointestinal adsorbent	1 g/5 ml water: give 10 ml of slurry/kg	1 g/5 ml water: give 10 ml of slurry/kg	1. Do not induce vomiting 2. Inhalation pneumonia 3. Follow with cathartic	HM	S
Albendazole (Valbazen)	Giardia Other endoparasites	25 mg/kg PO BID for 48 h	Same 10–21 days for *Paragonimus*	—	113.6 mg/ml VM	S
Allopurinol (Zyloprim)	Urate urolithiasis	10 mg/kg q 8 h PO, then reduce to 10 mg/kg PO daily	None	TID Rx for 30 days then SID	100, 300 mg HM	T
Aluminum hydroxide (Amphojel, AlternaGEL)	Phosphate binder Antacid	30–90 mg/kg PO SID–QID 5–10 ml/dog	Same 1–3 ml/cat	May cause metabolic alkalosis	OTC HM	S
Amikacin (Amikin) (Amiglyde-V)	1. Aminoglycoside 2. GM + and – agent	5–10 mg/kg BID, IV, IM, SQ	Same	Nephrotoxic Ototoxic Neuromuscular blockade Poor G-I absorption	50 mg/ml VM	I

DRUG INDEX (Continued)

GENERIC NAME (Trade Name in Parentheses)	INDICATIONS	CANINE DOSE	FELINE DOSE	COMMENTS	HOW SUPPLIED	
Aminocaproic acid (Amicar)	Antiprotease activity for degenerative myelopathy	15 mg/kg PO TID	—	Limited information on side effects or benefits	200 mg 250 mg/ml 250 mg/ml HM	T S I
Aminopentamide (Centrine)	Antispasmotic, cholinergic blocking agent. Similar to atropine. Useful for abdominal visceral spasm	0.02 mg/kg PO, IM, SQ q 8–12 h	0.02 mg/kg PO, IM, SQ q 8–12 h	Dryness of the mouth Atropine-like side effects	0.2 mg 0.5 mg/ml VM	T I
Aminophylline	Bronchodilator Diuretic	5–10 mg/kg PO, IV, SID–TID	2–4 mg/kg PO, SID–BID	Hyperexcitability Gastric irritation Anorexia Administer IV slowly	100, 200 mg 25 mg/ml HM	T I
Aminoproprazine (Jenotone)	Used in urethral obstructions Smooth muscle relaxant	2.2–4.4 mg/kg SID–BID IM	6.25–12.5 mg IM, SID–BID 48 h	Do not use with cystic atony	25 mg 25 mg/ml VM	T I
Amitraz (Mitaban)	Demodicosis	5 ml/gallon H_2O, dip dog; air dry; = 0.025% soln	—	Wear gloves when applying Requires multiple dips Transient pruritis noted	19.9% soln. VM	

Drug	Indication/Description	Dose		Comments	Supplied	
Amitriptyline HCl (Elavil)	Separation, anxiety-related disorders Destructive disorders Feline spraying	2.2–4.4 mg/kg PO SID	5–10 mg PO SID	Sedation Anticholinergic side effects Caution if seizure history	10, 25, 50, 75, 100, 150 mg HM	T
Amlodipine (Norvasc)	Long acting Ca channel blocking agent for hypertension	—	0.625 mg PO SID	Somnolence Hypotension	2.5, 5, 10 mg HM	T
Ammonium chloride (Uroeze)	Urinary acidifier	100 mg/kg PO BID	20 mg/kg PO BID or ¼ teaspoon powder in food	Poor palatability G-I signs	500 mg HM 400 mg VM	T T
Amoxicillin (Amoxi-tabs) (Amoxi-drops) (Robamox-V)	Penicillin class antibiotic GM + and – agent	10–20 mg/kg BID–TID PO, SQ, IM, IV	Same	Penicillin contraindications	50, 100, 150, 200, 400 mg 3; 25 g VM, HM	T I
Amoxicillin/Clavulanic acid (Clavamox) (Augmentin)	See *Amoxicillin* No penicillinase inactivation	10–20 mg/kg PO BID	Same	Penicillin sensitivity Vomiting in cats Tablets must remain in foil until used	62.5, 125, 250, 375 mg 50 mg/ml VM, HM	T S
Amphotericin B (Fungizone) (Ambisome)	Systemic mycoses	0.15 to 1 mg/kg in 5 to 20 ml of 5% dextrose in water given rapidly IV 3 times weekly for 2 to 4 months; do not exceed 2–4 mg/kg	Same	Monitor BUN Pretreat with antiemetics	50 mg/vial HM	I

DRUG INDEX (Continued)

GENERIC NAME (Trade Name in Parentheses)	INDICATIONS	CANINE DOSE	FELINE DOSE	COMMENTS	HOW SUPPLIED	
Ampicillin	Penicillin class antibiotic Routine infections	10–20 mg/kg TID PO, SQ, IM, IV	Same	Penicillin contraindications Phlebitis	125, 250, 500 mg 125 mg/5 ml 1, 3, 6 mg vials VM, HM	C S I
Amprolium (Corid)	Enteric coccidiostat	100–200 mg/kg PO in food or water (not both) for 10 days	—	Overdosage causes CNS disturbances	9.6% VM	S
Amrinone (Inocor)	Low-output heart failure Phosphodiesterase inhibitor	1–3 mg bolus IV, then 10–100 mcg/kg/min IV	—	Tachycardia Anxiety Monitor pulse and BP	5 mg/ml HM	I
Apomorphine	Induction of vomiting	¼–½ tab in third eyelid sac. Flush out with emesis 0.04–0.08 mg/kg SQ, IM, IV	Same	Do not use if decreased consciousness Periocular irritation	6 mg HM	T
Artificial tears/oint. (Adapt) (Lacrilube)	Used for insufficient tear production or with decreased blinking	1 drop in affected eye PRN	Same	Hypersensitivity	OTC HM	
Ascorbic acid (vitamin C)	Acetominophen induced methemoglobin toxicity Copper hepatotoxicity	100–500 mg PO TID	30 mg/kg QID PO, SQ, IM, IV for acetominophen toxicity	—	250 mg/ml 50, 100, 250, 500 mg, 1 g HM	I T

Drug	Indication	Dose	Feline Dose	Side Effects/Notes	Supplied	Code
(L) Asparaginase (Elspar)	Induction therapy for lymphoreticular neoplasms; Immune thrombocytopenia	400 U/kg IM, IP once or as part of a protocol; or 10,000–20,000 U/m² IM, IP, SQ	Same	Allergic symptoms; Anaphylaxis; Pancreatitis; Coagulopathies	10,000 U/vial HM	I
Atenolol (Tenormin)	B-1 Adrenergic blockade; Supraventricular tachyarrhythmias; Systemic hypertension	0.25–1.0 mg/kg PO SID–BID	⅛–¼ 25 mg tab PO SID	Hypotension; Depression; B blockade induced CHF; Inappetence, bradycardia	25, 50, 100 mg HM	T
Atropine SO$_4$	Parasympatholytic; Anticholinergic; Preanesthetic agent; Organophosphase toxicity; Supraventricular bradyarrhythmia	0.02–0.044 mg/kg IM, SQ, IV; 0.2–2.0 mg/kg IV, IM, SQ for organophosphate poisoning. Give ¼ dose IV—remainder IM, SQ	Same	Tachycardia; Mydriasis; Ileus; Photophobia; Do not use in CHF	0.5 and 2 mg/ml HM	I
Atropine sulfate ophthalmic soln./oint.	Used when pupillary dilatation is desired in the presence of inflammation of the iris and/or uveal tract	1 drop in affected eye SID–BID	1 drop in affected eye SID–BID	Atropine side effects; Contraindicated in the presence of glaucoma; Cats may salivate	0.5, 1%; 0.5, 1, 2, and 3% HM	OO OS
Aurothioglucose (Solganal)	Pemphigus complex; Autoimmune diseases	1st week: 1–5 mg IM; 2nd week: 2–10 mg IM; Then 1 mg/kg once a week IM decreasing to once a month for maintenance immunosuppression	1st week: 1 mg IM; 2nd week: 2 mg IM; Then 1 mg/kg once a week IM decreasing to once a month	Blood dyscrasias; Renal-hepatotoxicity; Neuritis-encephalitis	50 mg/ml HM	I

DRUG INDEX (Continued)

GENERIC NAME (Trade Name in Parentheses)	INDICATIONS	CANINE DOSE	FELINE DOSE	COMMENTS	HOW SUPPLIED	
Azathioprine (Imuran)	Immunosuppressive agent (SLE, RA, CAH, pemphigus, polymyositis, ITP, IHA, enteritis, etc.)	1–2 mg/kg eod–SID	0.5–1 mg/kg PO eod, SID	Monitor CBC Leukopenia Thrombocytopenia BM suppression Rarely hepatotoxic	50 mg HM	T
AZT 3'-azido-2',3'-dideoxythimidine (Retrovir)	Anti-retroviral agent	—	5 mg/kg SQ BID for 21 days	Monitor for anemia	100 mg 10 mg/ml 10 mg/ml HM	C S I
Benzoyl peroxide (Oxydex) (Pyoben)	Acne, seborrhea, pyoderma, pruritus	Shampoo p.r.n.; leave on skin for 10 minutes and rinse Gel: apply topically BID–TID	Shampoo p.r.n.; leave on skin for 10 minutes and rinse Gel: apply topically BID–TID	Bleaches fabric May be skin irritant	OTC VM, HM	
Betamethasone (Betasone)	Injectable and topical long acting steroid	0.2–0.4 mg/kg IM Topically apply TID	Topically apply TID	7–10 × potency of pred	6 mg/ml HM	I
Bethanechol (Urecholine)	Bladder atony (nonobstructive) Cholinergic agent	5–25 mg TID PO 2.5–15 mg TID SQ	2.5–5.0 mg BID PO	Do not use with obstruction or areflexic bladder	5, 10, 25, 50 mg HM	T

Drug	Indication	Dose	Dose (cat)	Side effects/Comments	Supplied	Class
Bismuth subsalicylate (Pepto Bismol)	GI tract protectant	10–30 ml every 4–6 h PO	Same with caution due to salicylate composition	Side effects: vomiting, cramping, salivation, miosis. May be treated with atropine. Causes stool to develop dark or black discoloration	OTC, HM 17, 47 mg/ml 262 mg	S T
Bunamidine (Scolaban)	*Taenia, Dipylidium, Echinococcus*	25 to 50 mg/kg PO once; fast 3 h before and after administration	Same	V/D rarely observed	100, 200, 400 mg VM	T
Buprenorphine hydrochloride (Buprinex)	Opiate agonist 1. Analgesia 2. Sedative for medical procedures	1. 0.01–0.02 mg/kg IV 2. 0.0075–0.01 mg/kg IV	0.005–0.01 mg/kg IV	Respiratory depression. Use cautiously in aged or debilitated patients. Neuroleptanalgesia when used with diazepam or acepromazine	0.324 mg/ml HM	I
Butorphanol tartrate (Torbutrol) (Torbugesic) (Stadol)	Cough suppressant Narcotic agonist/antagonist Analgesia	Analgesia 0.2–0.4 mg/kg BID-QID PO, IM, SQ, IV Antitussive 0.5–1 mg/kg BID-QID PO	Analgesia 0.1–0.4 mg/kg BID-QID SQ, IM, IV	Vomiting, sedation Possible overexcitement in cats	1, 5, 10 mg 10 mg/ml VM, HM	T I
Calcitonin (Calcimar) (Micalcin)	Reduces serum calcium in hypercalcemic states, especially cholecalciferol toxicity	4–8 IU/kg BID IV, IM, SQ	4–8 IU/kg BID IV, IM, SQ	Injections are irritating G-I upsets are a possibility	200 IU/ml HM	I
Calcium carbonate (Titralac, Tums, Calcet)	Hypocalcemia	1–4 g/day PO	Same	Could cause alkalosis	OTC, HM	

DRUG INDEX (Continued)

GENERIC NAME (Trade Name in Parentheses)	INDICATIONS	CANINE DOSE	FELINE DOSE	COMMENTS	HOW SUPPLIED	
Calcium chloride (or gluconate) (10% solution)	Ventricular asystole Hypocalcemia	0.1 ml/kg IV, IC	Same		100 mg/ml HM	I
Calcium EDTA (Versenate)	Lead and heavy metal poisoning	100 mg/kg/day, 5 days Give SQ in 4 divided doses daily Dilute in 5% dex. soln	Same	May be painful Potentially nephrotoxic	200 mg/ml HM	I
Calcium gluconate (Calcet)	Hypocalcemia Ventricular asystole	10% infusion: 0.5–2.0 ml/kg IV slowly over 15–30 minutes QID 50–150 mg Ca^{++}/kg/day in continuous IV infusion Oral: 150–250 mg/kg PO TID	Same	Arrhythmias V/D Dystrophic calcification	100 mg/ml HM	I
Captan powder 50% (Orthocide)	Dermatomycoses	Mix 2 tbsp per gallon of water, apply topically every 3–7 days. Do not rinse after applying	Same	May induce contact sensitization in humans	VM	
Captopril (Capoten)	Vasodilator, congestive heart failure Hypertension ACE inhibitor	0.5–1.5 mg/kg BID–TID PO	3.12–6.25 mg SID PO	Hypotension–depression Anorexia; V/D Could exacerbate renal failure	12.5, 25, 50, 100 mg HM	T

Drug	Description/Use	Dose	Dose 2	Comments	Supply	Class
Carbamate	Cholinesterase inhibitor for fleas, ticks, cheyletiellic mange	Use as a dip every 7–14 days; do not rinse off. Spray EOD	Same	Do not use under 4 wks old. Cholinesterase toxicity treat with atropine and bathing	VM	T I
Carbenicillin (Geopen) (Pyopen)	Serious infections. Penicillin derivative	15 mg/kg TID IM, SQ, PO	Same	See *Penicillin*	382 mg 1, 2, 5, 10, 20, 30 g HM	T I
(L) Carnitine	AA transports fatty acids into mitochondria for energy metabolism. Some cardiomyopathies	50–100 mg/kg TID PO	250–500 mg PO SID for hepatic lipidosis	Expensive. To be used with other Rx. Effects uncertain	250, 500 mg 100 mg/ml HM	T/C S
Castor oil	Irritant cathartic	8–30 ml PO	4–10 ml PO	Griping catharsis may develop. Do not use if obstructed or atonic	OTC, HM	
Cephalosporin antibiotics	Broad spectrum bacteriacidal. Less sensitive to gram + penicillinase inactivation	10–30 mg/kg BID–QID PO, SQ, IM, IV. Review each product for specific dosage, handling, and administration	Same	G-I side effects. Penicillin contraindications. Possibly nephrotoxic at high dosages or if used with aminoglycoside antibiotics	250, 500 mg 25, 50, 100 mg/cc 1, 2, 20 g vials VM, HM	C S I
Chlorambucil (Leukeran)	Lymphoreticular neoplasia. Chronic lymphocytic leukemia. Macroglobulinemia	2 mg/m2 PO SID × 3 wk beyond remission, then 1.5 mg/m² PO SID × 15 days, then q 3rd day; or 0.1 mg/kg q 48–72 h PO	1.5 mg/m2 PO SID as for dog or 0.1 mg/kg q 48–72 h PO	Bone marrow suppression. Usually a second line agent often used with pred and/or other agents	2 mg HM	T

DRUG INDEX *(Continued)*

GENERIC NAME (Trade Name in Parentheses)	INDICATIONS	CANINE DOSE	FELINE DOSE	COMMENTS	HOW SUPPLIED	
Chloramphenicol (Chloromycetin)	Broad spectrum bacteriostatic agent	30–50 mg/kg TID, PO, IV, IM, SQ	25–50 mg/kg BID. PO, IV, IM, SQ	Hepatic microsomal enzyme inhibitor	100 mg/ml 100, 250,	I T
	Mycoplasma, Rickettsia, Chlamydia and Anaerobic bacteria			May potentate some Rx-use caution	500 mg, and 1 g VM, HM	
	1% oph. oint.: Corneal ulcers and infections	Apply to eye q 4-h	Apply to eye q 4-8 h	Do not use with "cidal" agents Monitor CBC and chemistries		
	0.5% oph. soln.: Corneal ulcers and infections					
Chlorhexidine 0.5% (Nolvasan)	1. Topical antiseptic shampoo	Shampoo every 3–7 days or apply to lesions SID–BID	Same	—	OTC, HM	
	2. Topical antiseptic solution	Dilute to 1:10 and apply topically TID				
Chlorothiazide (Diuril)	Diuretic	20–40 mg/kg BID PO	Same	Hyponatremia–hypokalemia	250, 500 mg	T
	Nonhormonal Rx for CDI and NDI			Use cautiously with digitalis	50 mg/ml HM	S
Chlorpheniramine (Chlor-Trimeton)	Decongestant; antihistamine	2–4 mg PO BID–TID	1–2 mg PO BID–TID	May cause drowsiness	10 mg/ml 2 mg/ml 2, 4, 8, 12 mg HM	I S T

Drug	Clinical use	Dosage	Dosage	Comments	How supplied	
Chlorpromazine (Thorazine)	Tranquilization Antiemetic	1–3 mg/kg PO up to QID 0.5–5 mg/kg SQ, IM, IV	Same	Severe CNS depression with overdosage May potentiate seizures	10, 25, 50, 100, 200 mg 2 mg/ml 25 mg suppository 25 mg/ml HM	T S I
Cimetidine (Tagamet)	H_2 receptor antagonist Esophagitis, gastric reflux Chronic gastritis, GI tract ulceration Hypergastrinemia Effects of mast cell tumors	5 to 10 mg/kg BID–QID PO 5 mg/kg BID IV	2.5 to 5 mg/kg BID–TID PO	Hepatic microsomal enzyme inhibitor Administer slowly IV	200, 300, 400, 800 mg 50 mg/ml 150 mg/ml HM	T S I
Ciprofloxacin (Cipro)	Fluoroquinolone antibiotic Broad spectrum—"cidal" Mycoplasma	5–15 mg/kg BID PO	Same	See *Enrofloxacin*	250, 500, 750 mg HM	T
Cisapride (Propulsid)	Increases LES pressure; promotes gastric emptying	0.1–0.5 mg/kg PO BID–TID	Same	Requires adjunctive Rx as stool softener Does not ↑ gastric secretions Increases esophageal peristalsis	10 mg HM	T
Cisplatin (Platinol)	Solid carcinomas Osteosarcoma	50–70 mg/m² IV every 3–5 weeks; pretreat with IV fluids 12 h before and after Rx	None—do not use	Use anti-emetic agent BM suppression; renal insufficiency Anaphylaxis **Wear gloves**	10 and 50 mg vials HM	I

DRUG INDEX (Continued)

GENERIC NAME (Trade Name in Parentheses)	INDICATIONS	CANINE DOSE	FELINE DOSE	COMMENTS	HOW SUPPLIED	
Clindaymcin (Cleocin) (Antirobe)	Lincosamide antibiotic GM +; staphylococcus; anaerobes; bacteroides toxoplasmosis; babesiosus osteomyelitis	5–10 mg/kg BID PO Toxo: 10–40 mg/kg PO divided TID	Same Toxo: 25–50 mg/kg PO divided TID	May cause V/D and hepatotoxicity Do not use with erythromycin or chloroamphenicol	150 mg/ml 25, 75, 150 mg VM, HM	I C
Clotrimazole (Veltrim) (Lotrimin) (Mycelex)	Used topically post Aspergillosis surgery; also for Malassezia and other fungi	10 mg/kg topically	Same	—	OTC HM	
Coal tar (0.5% to 8%)	Shampoo—seborrhea, dermatitis; eczema; keratolytic	Bathe every 3 to 14 days; leave in contact with skin for 10 minutes and rinse	Same	May irritate skin	VM	
Colchicine (ColBenemid)	Chronic hepatic fibrosis	0.03 mg/kg/day PO SID–TID	No reported use	Not well described	0.5 mg HM	T
Cyclophosphamide (Cytoxan)	Lymphoreticular tumors Solid carcinomas Immune mediated disease	200 mg/m² IV weekly 50 mg/m² (or 2 mg/kg) PO 4 days on, 3 days off, or use EOD	Same	G-I signs BM suppression Hemorrhagic cystis Alopecia **Use with caution. See Chemotherapy. Wear gloves or wash after administration**	25, 50 mg 100, 200, 500 mg and 1 and 2 g vials HM	T I

Drug	Indication	Dog Dosage	Cat Dosage	Comments	Supplied	Class
Cyclosporine (Optimmune) (Sandimmune)	T lymphocyte inhibitor KCS in dogs	2% soln in oil base Use 1 drop BID both eyes until improvement occurs then SID	Do not use	May be ophthalmic irritant Monitor for infections Considered investigational	HM 4 ml olive oil and 1 ml Cyclosporine	OS
Cyproheptadine (Periactin)	H$_1$ antagonist 1. Appetite stimulant 2. Feline pica 3. Antihistamine	1. 5–20 mg PO BID 3. 1 mg/kg PO BID–TID	1. 1 mg/cat PO 2. 0.22 mg/kg PO SID	High dosages cause excitability or depression; vomiting; aggressiveness	4 mg 2 mg/5 ml HM	T S
Cytosine arabinoside (Cytosar)	Antineoplastic Lymphoma protocol	100 mg/m² daily for 2–4 days. Same SQ or IV	Same	Leukopenia—BM suppression GI toxicity Reconstituted vial good for 48 h Use along with cancer protocol	100, 200 mg 1 g and 2 g vials HM	I
Dacarbazine (DTIC)	Melanoma Sarcoma	1000 mg/m² IV q 3–4 weeks	Not recommended	G-I toxicity BM suppression	100, 200 mg vials HM	I
Danazol (Danocrine)	Modified androgen Used for ITP	5 mg/kg PO BID	Same	Adjunctive Rx for ITP and IHA	50, 100, 200 mg HM	C
Dapsone (Avlosulfon)	Antibacterial-antiinflammatory agent used for some skin disorders	1 mg/kg PO TID	50 mg BID PO	Hepatotoxicity and BM suppression may occur early in therapy	25 and 100 mg HM	T
Dehydrocholic acid (Decholin)	Used to stimulate bile flow	10 to 15 mg/kg TID PO for 7–10 days	Same	Do not use with biliary obstruction	HM	

DRUG INDEX (Continued)

GENERIC NAME (Trade Name in Parentheses)	INDICATIONS	CANINE DOSE	FELINE DOSE	COMMENTS	HOW SUPPLIED	
Desmopressin acetate (DDAVP)	1. Vasopressin analog to manage central diabetes insipidus 2. VWF disease	1–4 drops intranasally or in subconjunctival sac SID–QID (diabetes insipidus); or 1–2 mcg SQ SID–BID 1 mcg/kg SQ	Same	Hypersensitivity rkns. Use nasal spray form drops—40 × stronger than parenteral	10 mcg/spray 4 mcg/ml HM	I
Desoxycorticosterone pivalate (DOCP) (Percorten Pivilate)	Hypoadrenocorticism Each 25 mg releases 1 mg DOCA/day for 1 mo	1 cc/12 kg q 25 days; i.e., 2 mg/kg IM or SQ		Titrate dosage to effect	25 mg/ml VM	I
Dexamethasone (Azium, Dexate) (Decadron)	Potent glucocorticoid for antiinflammatory and immune suppression	0.5–2.0 mg/kg/day. Divide dosage. Dosage variable from antinflammatory to that required for immune suppression	Same	HPA axis suppression Multi organ steroid effects	0.25, 0.5, 0.75, 1, 2, 4, 6 mg 2, 8, 16 mg/ml VM, HM	T I
Dexamethasone sodium phosphate	Soluble corticosteroid Septic and hypovolemic shock Acute Rx hypoadrenocorticism	6–8 mg/kg IV	Same	HPA axis suppression Multiorgan effects LDDST = 0.01 mg/kg IV HDDST = 0.1 mg/kg IV	4, 10, 20, 24 mg/ml HM	I
Dexasporin Oph. Soln./ oint. (Maxitrol)	Neomycin, polymixin, and dexamethasone combination used for steroid responsive ophthalmic inflammation	1 drop in affected eye BID–QID	1 drop in affected eye BID–QID	Steroids are contraindicated in some specific eye diseases Systemic side effects are possible	0.05% ointment 0.1% soln HM	

	where a combined antibiotic is desirable					
Dextran (Rheomacrodex)	Hypovolemia Plasma volume expander	40–90 ml/kg IV	Same	—	10% Dextran in PSS or D5W HM	I
Dextroamphetamine (Dexedrine)	Amphetamine Narcolepsy Hyperkinesis	5–10 mg/kg PO TID 0.2–1.3 mg/kg PO PRN	—	—	5 mg 5, 10, 15 mg HM	T ER
Dextromethorphan	Antitussive	1–2 mg/kg PO TID	Same	Usually in association with other drugs, i.e., OTC cough syrup viz. Robitussin ®	OTC, HM	
Diazepam (Valium)	1. Tranquilizer 2. Anticonvulsant 3. Muscle relaxant 4. Appetite stimulant (cats) 5. Urine marking/spraying	1. Mix 2:1 with ketamine for sedation. Dose 0.1 ml/kg of mixture IV or to effect 2. 2.5–5.0 mg IV to effect. Repeat to 20 mg max 3. 2.0–10 mg PO BID–TID	1, 2. 1–5 mg IV to effect 3, 5. 1–4 mg BID PO 4. 0.1 ml IV prior to feeding	Sedation; ataxia Paradoxical excitement/aggression Class IV controlled substance	2, 5, 10 mg 5 mg/ml HM	T I
Diazoxide (Proglycem)	Hypoglycemia	10–40 mg/kg/day PO	None	Vomiting Anorexia	50 mg 50 mg/ml HM	C S
Dichlorphenamide (Daranide)	Glaucoma Carbonic anhydrase inhibitor	2–4 mg/kg q 8 h PO	2–4 mg/kg q 8 h PO	Weakness, lethargy, diarrhea Hypokalemia Hyperchloremic metabolic acidosis	50 mg HM	T

DRUG INDEX *(Continued)*

GENERIC NAME (Trade Name in Parentheses)	INDICATIONS	CANINE DOSE	FELINE DOSE	COMMENTS	HOW SUPPLIED	
Dichlorvos (Task) (Vapona) (DDVP)	Hook-, whip-, roundworms Flea collars and tags	27 to 33 mg/kg PO once 11 mg/kg PO once (puppies) Change collar every 4 months	11 mg/kg PO once Change collar every 4 months	Organophosphate toxicity Do not use with constipation; intestinal obstruction; hepatic, cardiac, or heartworm disease	10, 20 mg 68, 136, 204 mg 136, 204, 544 mg Paste VM	T C
Diethylcarbamazine (DEC) (Caricide, Cypip, Filaribits)	Heartworm prophylaxis	6–11 mg/kg SID PO, during hw season; 3 weeks pre and post season 70 mg/kg PO BID for 3 days for Crensoma	55–110 mg/kg PO for ascarids	Vomiting May decrease sperm count Anaphylaxis if micorfilaria positive dog	60, 120, 180 mg 60 mg/ml Other sizes VM, HM	T S
Diethylstilbestrol (DES)	1. Estrogen-responsive incontinence 2. Mismating 3. Perianal gland adenoma	1. 0.1–1 mg/day PO 2. 0.1–1.0 mg/day PO; begin 2–3 days after mating; continue for 5 days 3. 1 mg PO q 72 h	0.05–0.1 mg/day PO	May induce signs of estrus; decrease to lowest effective dosage High dosages may cause anemia, leukopenia, thrombocytopenia	1, 5 mg 50 mg/ml Other sizes HM	T I
Digitoxin	Positive inotropic agent Heart failure, Supraventricular tachy-arrhythmias	0.05–0.1 mg/kg/day	Not used	V/D-G-I signs Cleared via liver Less effective than digoxin	0.05, 0.1, 0.15, 0.2 mg 0.2 mg/ml HM	T I

Drug	Indications	Dosage	Notes	Supplied	
Digoxin (Lanoxin, Cardoxin)	Positive inotropic agent Congestive heart failure Supraventricular tachyarrhythmias Dilated cardiomyopathy	*Maintenance dosage* 0.22 mg/M² PO BID; or 0.022 mg/kg/day divided BID *Digitalization dosage* Double maintenance dose first 24–48 h	¼ 0.125 mg tab every other day to daily Elixir form not recommended	G-I toxicity–V/D Heart block; V. arrhythmias Decrease dosage if renal function is altered Tablets, elixir and IV dosages differ **Toxic drug—*See Chapter 92***	0.125, 0.25, 0.5 mg 0.05, 0.15 mg/ml 0.25 mg/ml VM, HM	T S I
Dihydrotachysterol (Hytakerol)	Hypocalcemia	0.03–0.06 mg/kg SID PO initially, then 0.01–0.02 mg/kg every 24–48 h PO	0.03–0.06 mg/kg SID PO initially, then 0.01–0.02 mg/kg every 24–48 h PO	Hypercalcemia Monitor serum and patient until well stabilized	0.125, 0.2, 0.4 mg 0.125 mg/ml 0.2 mg/ml HM	T C S
Diltiazem hydrochloride (Cardizem)	Calcium channel blocking agent Supraventricular arrhythmias HCM–feline	0.5–1.5 mg/kg TID PO 0.5 mg/kg IV	0.8–2.5 mg/kg BID–TID PO	Bradycardia Hypotension Anorexia	30, 60, 90, 120 mg 120, 180, 240, 320 mg 60, 90, 120, 240 mg HM	T C ER
Dimenhydrinate (Dramamine)	Motion sickness	25–50 mg q 8 h PO	12.5 mg q 8 h PO	Lethargy–drowsiness	80 mg 12.5 mg/ml 50 mg/ml HM	T S I
Dimercaprol (BAL)	Chelating agent Heavy metal toxicosis such as mercury and arsenic	2.5–5 mg/kg. IM. (Dose of 5 mg/kg used only in acute cases and only on first day.) Then: q 4 h on days 1 and 2; q 8 h on day 3; BID for next 10 days	Same	Injections sting Caution: renal insufficiency	100 mg/ml HM	I

835

DRUG INDEX (Continued)

GENERIC NAME (Trade Name in Parentheses)	INDICATIONS	CANINE DOSE	FELINE DOSE	COMMENTS	HOW SUPPLIED	
Dimethyl sulfoxide (DOMOSO) (DMSO)	Topical antinflammatory	Apply solution topically BID–TID. Use 60% otic soln. BID	None	Erythema, pruritus Investigational except as otic soln. **Wear gloves. Readily absorbed**	90% gel 90% soln. topical	VM, HM
Dioctyl sulfosuccinate (Colace, Surfak)	Stool softener	One or two 50-mg capsules q 12–24 h PO	One 50-mg capsule q 12–24 h PO	Used as enema preparation for cats and small dogs	OTC, HM	VM
Diphenhydramine HCl (Benadryl)	H₁ receptor antihistamine	2–4 mg/kg BID, TID, PO 1–2 mg/kg BID IV, IM	Same Do not use IV	Sedative Anticholinergic Antiemetic	25, 50 mg 12.5 mg/ml 10 mg/ml HM	T S I
Diphenoxylate HCl with atropine (Lomotil)	Antidiarrheal Nonanalgesic opiate	2.5–10 mg PO TID 0.1–0.2 mg/kg PO TID	0.6–1.2 mg PO BID	Sedation Constipation Ileus Use in cats with caution	2.5 mg 2.5 mg/5 ml HM	T S
Dipyrone (Novin)	Antipyretic	25 mg/kg SQ, IM, IV to TID	Same	Hypothermia BM suppression See *Chapter 26*	300 mg 500 mg/ml HM	T I
Disopyramide PO₄ (Norpace)	Ventricular dysrhythmias Type IA agent	2–5 mg/kg TID PO	None	Rarely used May be used with quinidine or procainamide	100, 150 mg 100, 150 mg HM	C ER

Dithiazanine iodide (Dizan)	Microfilaricide	6.6–11 mg/kg SID PO for 7–10 days	None	Stains stool purple V/D, anorexia	VM	I
Dobutamine HCl (Dobutrex)	Inotropic agent for cardiomyopathy, heart failure. Short term usage. B₁ agonist	2.5–20 mcg/kg/min IV Constant rate infusion	4–5 mcg/kg/min IV Constant rate infusion	Use 48 h maximum. May increase heart rate. Monitor for arrhythmias. Continue usual cardiac therapy. Cats are very sensitive to Rx and may have seizures	12.5 mg/ml HM	I
Dopamine HCl (Inotropin)	Alpha, B₁, and dopaminergic agent. Inotropic agent for heart failure. Renal vasodilator: acute renal failure. Pressor agent-hypotension	2–8 mcg/kg/min IV in LRS	Same	Tachycardia. Vasoconstriction. Requires ICU monitoring	40, 80, 160 mg/ml HM	I
Doxapram (Dopram)	Respiratory stimulant	5–10 mg/kg once IV Repeat if needed	Same	For puppy/kitten respiratory stimulation use 1–5 drops under tongue or via umbilical vein	20 mg/ml HM	I
Doxorubicin (Adriamycin)	Lymphomas. Carcinomas. Solid tumors	30 mg/m² IV once every 3 weeks, not to exceed total dose of 250 mg/m²	20 mg/m² once every 3 weeks to max. total dose of 90 mg/m²	Anaphylaxis. BM suppression. **Cardiotoxic. Severe vesicant. Wear gloves when administering**	2 mg/ml HM	I

DRUG INDEX *(Continued)*

GENERIC NAME (Trade Name in Parentheses)	INDICATIONS	CANINE DOSE	FELINE DOSE	COMMENTS	HOW SUPPLIED	
Doxycycline HCl (Vibramycin)	Tetracycline antibiotic Rickettsia, Ehrlichia, Hemobartonella, and Chlamydia	5 mg/kg (loading dose) PO then 2.5 mg/kg in 12 h, then 2.5–5 mg/kg 1–2 times a day	5 mg/kg (loading dose) PO, 2.5 mg/kg in 12 h, then 2.5 mg/kg q 24 h	Do not use in puppies, kittens, or pregnant state May cause anorexia, depression	50, 100 mg 5, 10 mg/ml HM	T/C S
Edrophonium Cl (Tensilon)	Diagnostic agent for cholinergic stimulation. Myasthenia gravis	0.11–0.22 mg/kg IV Max 5 mg	0.25–1.00 mg/cat IV	Muscarinic signs	10 mg/ml HM	I
Enalapril Maleate (Vasotec) (Enacard)	ACE inhibitor Vasodilator CHF Hypertension	0.5 mg/kg SID PO initially, then to BID if necessary	No data available	Hypotension, weakness, anorexia Avoid with renal failure Do not increase furosemide dosage when initiating or increasing enalapril dosage	1, 2.5, 5, 10, 20 mg 1.25 mg/ml VM, HM	T I
Enrofloxacin (Baytri)	Broad spectrum fluoroquinolone class antibiotic	2.5–10 mg/kg BID PO, IM	2.5–10 mg/kg BID PO, IM	Do not use in puppies or kittens. Causes cartilage pathology	5.7, 22.7, 68 mg 22.7 mg/ml VM	T I
Ephedrine	Bronchodilator	1–2 mg/kg PO BID–TID	2–5 mg BID–TID PO	Usually used in combination with sedatives and/or bronchodilators	25, 50 mg 25 mg/ml HM	C I

838

Drug	Description	Dosage	Comments	Concentration	
Epinephrine (Adrenalin)	Alpha and beta adrenergic agent used for inotropic and chronotropic support; bronchodilation; anaphylaxis; cardiac arrest	0.5–5 ml IC, IV, IT (cardiac arrest); 1:10,000 0.02 ml/kg (1:1000) SQ, IM, IV (bronchodilation)	0.1–0.2 cc IC, IV 0.1 cc SQ, IM, IV	Arrhythmogenic; Inc MVO$_2$ Vasoconstriction Avoid direct sunlight exposure Note 1:1000 and 1:10,000 solution	1:1000 1:10,000 HM	I I
Epoetin (Epogen)	Recombinant erythropoetin	100 units/kg 3 times/week SQ until RBC levels increase; then 1 time/week thereafter	Same	Anaphylaxis Hypertension G-I signs	2000, 3000, 4000 and 10,000 U/ml HM	I
Erythromycin	Macrolide antibiotic GM positive drug Campylobacter, mycoplasma, rickettsia, chlamydia	10–20 mg/kg TID PO	10 mg/kg TID PO	Hypersensitivities; G-I upsets	250, 333, 500 mg 100 mg/ml HM	T I
Estradiol cyclopentaneo-propionate (ECP)	Estradiol to terminate pregnancy	20–40 mcg/kg IM × 1 Never exceed 1 mg Use up to 3–5 days post breeding	250 mcg IM 40 hrs after copulation	May be toxic to bone marrow **Not recommended**	1, 5, 10 mg/ml HM	I
Ethanol 20%	Ethylene glycol toxicosis (inject as 20% ethanol in saline)	5.5 ml/kg IV q 4 h × 5 Rx, then q 6 h × 4 Rx	5 ml/kg IV q 6 h × 5 Rx, then q 8 h × 4 Rx	May cause or exacerbate CNS depression Monitor hydration and electrolytes	—	
Etretinate (Tegison)	Synthetic retinoid used to treat disorders of Keratinization in specific breeds (primarily cocker spaniels)	1 mg/kg PO SID	10 mg/cat PO SID	Vomiting; anemia KCS ↑ Liver enzymes	10, 25 mg HM	C

839

DRUG INDEX *(Continued)*

GENERIC NAME (Trade Name in Parentheses)	INDICATIONS	CANINE DOSE	FELINE DOSE	COMMENTS	HOW SUPPLIED	
Famotidine (Pepcid)	H_2 receptor antagonist	0.5–1 mg/kg SID IV 5 mg/kg SID PO	0.5 mg/kg SID IV 5 mg/kg SID PO	Advantage over other similar agents is once a day dosage	20, 40 mg 40 mg/5 ml 10 mg/ml HM	T S I
Fenbendazole (Panacur)	Hook-, whip-, roundworms; Taenia; paragonimus; Filaroides; Capillaria	50 mg/kg/day for 3 days; repeat in 3 weeks Whipworms; repeat in 3 months	Same Not FDA approved	Rare vomiting Safe in dogs with heartworms	222 mg/kg granules VM	
Fenthion (Prospot) (Spot-on)	Organophosphate	4–8 mg/kg. Follow instructions. Topically, not more than every 2 weeks	None	Do not use with other cholinesterase inhibiting agents. Do not use in puppies, sick, or debilitated dogs	5.6 and 13.8% soln. VM	
Ferric Cyanoferrate (Prussian Blue)	Thallium poisoning	100–200 mg/kg PO TID for 30 days		Administer in a glucose solution orally	HM	
Fluconazole (Diflucan)	Imidazole antifungal compound—especially useful for cryptococcus	2.5–5 mg/kg PO SID or divided BID	Same		50, 100, 200 mg 2 mg/ml HM	T I
Flucytosine (Ancobon) (Ancotil)	Aspergillosis Cryptococcus	100 mg/kg BID PO or ½ dose QID	Same	Renal, bone marrow, and hepatotoxicity. May cause G-I upset	250, 500 mg HM	C

Drug	Use / Description	Dosage (canine)	Dosage (feline)	Do not give to pregnant animal	Form / Concentration	
Fludrocortisone (Florinef)	Hypoadrenocorticism; Mineralocorticoid replacement therapy	0.1 mg/5 kg/SID or BI D PO; Adjust dosage by need and laboratory testing	0.1 mg/5 kg/day PO; Adjust dosage by need and laboratory testing	Hypertension	0.1 mg; HM	T
Flumethasone (Flucort)	Antiinflammatory; Corticosteroid	0.06–0.25 mg SID PO, IV, IM, SQ	0.03–0.125 mg SID PO, IV, IM, SQ	Cortisone related side effects	0.0625 mg; 0.5 mg/ml; HM	T; I
Flunixin meglumine (Banamine)	Nonsteroidal antiinflammatory analgesic agent	0.5–1.0 mg/kg SID IV; IM maximum 3 days dosage	1 mg/kg SID IV, IM	Platelet coagulopathy; Ulcerative gastritis; Use with extreme caution; Use 3–5 days only	50 mg/ml; HM	I
Fluocinolone 0.1% with 60% DMSO (Synotic)	Topical steroid plus DMSO for serious otic infection and inflammation	2–12 drops BID	2–4 drops BID		0.1% otic soln.; VM	
Fluorouracil	Chemotherapy agent for carcinoma or sarcomas	150 mg/m² IV weekly; 2–5 mg/kg IV weekly	Do not use	Part of a chemotherapy protocol	50 mg/ml; HM	I
Fluoxetine (Prozac)	Serotonin reuptake inhibitor	1–2 mg/kg SID PO		Used to treat behavioral disorders; lick granuloma; Efficacy uncertain	10, 20 mg; 4 mg/ml; HM	C; S
Furazolidone (Furoxone)	1. Amebiasis 2. Enteric coccidiosis 3. Giardiasis	1. 2.2 mg/kg TID PO 7 times 2. 8–20 mg/kg PO 7 times 3. 4 mg/kg BID PO 7 times	Same		100 mg; 50 mg/ml; HM	T; S

DRUG INDEX *(Continued)*

GENERIC NAME (Trade Name in Parentheses)	INDICATIONS	CANINE DOSE	FELINE DOSE	COMMENTS	HOW SUPPLIED	
Furosemide (Lasix)	Potent loop diuretic agent Used in acute renal failure; hypercalcemia; hypertension, CHF; ascites, and fluid retention	2–4 mg/kg BID–TID PO, SQ, IM, IV	0.5–2 mg/kg BID–TID PO, SQ, IM, IV	Use *lowest* effective dosage Monitor for hypokalemia; hyponatremia; and hypochloremic–alkalosis Caution azotemia and dehydration	12.5, 20, 40, 50, 80 mg 10 mg/ml 50 mg/ml VM, HM	T S I
Gentamicin (Garamycin) (Gentocin)	Broad spectrum aminoglycoside antibiotic	2–4 mg/kg TID, IM, SQ, IV	Same	Not effective orally Do not use in renal failure Reserved for serious identified infections only Not for anaerobic infections Nephrotoxic-ototoxic	50 mg/ml VM, HM	I
Gentamicin otic (Gentocin otic)	Ear infections Especially *Pseudomonas*, or *Proteus*	Apply TID	Apply TID	Ototoxic	3 mg/ml otic soln. VM, HM	
Gentamicin ophthalmic (Gentocin)	Conjunctival/corneal infections Especially *Psuedomonas*	Apply q 4–8 h	Apply q 4–8 h	Rarely irritating Also made with steroids. Use with extreme caution	3 mg/gm 3 mg/ml VM, HM	OO OS
Glipizide (Glucotrol)	Oral hyperglycemic agent Useful in some type II diabetes mellitus	0.25–0.5 mg/kg PO BID Generally not recommended	0.25–0.5 mg/kg PO BID	Hypoglycemia G-I effects	5, 10 mg HM	T

Drug	Indication	Dose	Alternate	Comments	Formulation	Class
Glucagon	Provocative testing agent for insulinoma, diabetes mellitus, and hyperadrenocorticism	0.03 mg/kg IV	None	May induce hypoglycemia	1 mg/ml HM	I
Glycerin suppositories	Constipation	1 suppository per rectum	Same or 3 ml liquid per rectum		OTC, HM	
Glycopyrrolate (Robinul)	Anticholinergic preanesthetic agent	0.01 mg/kg SQ, IM, IV	Same	Tachycardia, arrhythmias, intestinal ileus, mydriasis and photophobia	0.2 mg/ml VM, HM	I
GoLytely®	Large bowel evacuant	40–60 ml/kg via stomach tube	30 mg/kg by stomach tube	Withhold food Administer twice 2 hours apart prior to scope procedure	Pwdr. or conc. for dilution HM	
Goodwinol®	Demodecosis (localized)	Apply topically SID	Same	Rotenone, orthophenyl phenol and benzocaine mixture; efficacy not demonstrated	1.25% Rotenone VM	O
Griseofulvin (Fulvicin)	Dermatomycoses	50–150 mg/kg PO SID–BID	Same	Uf prep better absorbed—decrease dosage by 50% for this formulation G-I signs Teratogen Granulocytopenia	125, 250, 500 mg 125 mg/5 ml VM/HM	T S
Heparin	DIC	50–100 mcg/kg SQ TID	Same	Prolongs bleeding time Not effective for arterial thrombosis	1,000, 2000, 5000, 10,000 20,000 and 40,000 mcg/ml I HM	

843

DRUG INDEX *(Continued)*

GENERIC NAME (Trade Name in Parentheses)	INDICATIONS	CANINE DOSE	FELINE DOSE	COMMENTS	HOW SUPPLIED	
Hetacillin (Hetacin)	Similar to penicillin	10–20 mg/kg TID PO	Same	Penicillin reactions	50, 100, 200 mg VM	T
Hydralazine (Apresoline)	Arteriolar vasodilator	0.5–3 mg/kg PO BID–TID	1.25–2.5 mg/kg PO BID	Hypotension, tachycardia Malaise, depression Anorexia	10, 25, 50, 100 mg 20 mg/ml HM	T S
Hydrochlorothiazide (HydroDiuril)	Diuretic Nonhormonal therapy for CDI and NDI	2–4 mg/kg PO BID initially; then decrease by 50% or to SID	1–2 mg/kg PO BID initially; then decrease by 50% or to SID	Hypokalemia Exacerbates dig tox Dehydration	25, 50, 100 mg HM	T
Hydrochlorothiazide/spironolactone (Aldactazide)	Diuretic plus aldosterone inhibitor	Use on basis of 1 mg/kg of spironolactone SID–BID orally	Rarely used	Often used in conjunction with furosemide in severe CHF	25/25 mg 50/50 mg	T T
Hydrocodone bitartrate (Hycodan)	Narcotic antitussive	0.22 mg/kg SID–QID PO	Rarely used	Sedation C-III substance	5 mg 1 mg/ml	T S
Hydrocortisone acetate 1% cream	Topical corticosteroid for focal dermatitis	Apply topically BID–QID	Same	Prolonged usage may result in iatrogenic Cushing's syndrome	1% HM	O

Drug	Action/Indication	Dosage		Comments	Supplied	
Hydrogen peroxide	Emetic	5–10 ml (3% solution). Repeat in 15 minutes PO until emesis occurs	Same	Do not use if a caustic agent was ingested; if level of consciousness is decreased; or if unable to swallow	3% topical HM	C
Hydroxyurea (Hydrea)	Chemotherapeutic compound Bone marrow disorders, especially polycythemia vera	80 mg/kg every 3rd day or 20–40 mg/kg/day PO divided BID	Same	Anorexia, vomiting	500 mg HM	
Hydroxyzine (Atarax)	H_1 receptor antihistamine, for allergic skin disorders	1–2 mg/kg BID–TID PO	0.5–1 mg/kg BID–TID PO	Monitor CBC regularly Sedative	10, 25, 50, 100 mg 10 mg/5 ml 25, 50 mg/ml HM	T S I
Hyoscyamine (Levsin)	Inhibits acetylcholine Inhibits propulsive G-I motility	0.003–0.006 mg/kg TID PO	Same—infrequently used	Useful in IBS and functional intestinal disorders Dry mouth; urinary retention; tachycardia	0.125 mg 0.125 mg/5 ml 0.375 mg 0.5 mg/ml HM	T S ER I
Ibuprofen (Motrin)	Non-salicylate, non-steroidal antiinflammatory agent	5 mg/kg BID–TID PO	Not recommended	May cause G-I bleeding and irritation Avoid using unless absolutely necessary Renal insufficiency	OTC HM	
Idoxuridine (Herplex) (Stoxil)	Used to treat feline *herpes* keratonconjunctivitis	—	1 drop q 4 h initially; then q 6–8 h	Occasional ophthalmic irritation	0.1% HM	OS

DRUG INDEX *(Continued)*

GENERIC NAME (Trade Name in Parentheses)	INDICATIONS	CANINE DOSE	FELINE DOSE	COMMENTS	HOW SUPPLIED	
Imidocarb (Imizole)	Babesiosis Ehrlichiosis Hepatozoonosis	2–6 mg/kg IM once	—	Not available commercially in U.S.	VM	
Imipramine (Tofranil)	Serotonin inhibitor Behavioral changes, narcolepsy, cataplexy	0.5–1 mg/kg BID–TID PO	0.5 mg/kg SID–BID PO	Drowsiness; behavioral changes	10, 25, 50 mg 125 mg/ml HM	T I
Indomethacin (Indocin)	Nonsteroidal antiinflammatory	1 mg/kg divided TID PO	None	Hepatotoxicity G-I hemorrhage Not recommended for use	25, 50 mg 5 mg/ml 75 mg HM	C S ER
Insulin (Humulin R, N, U)	1. Diabetes mellitus 2. Diabetic ketoacidosis 3. Acute severe hyperkalemia	REGULAR: 0.5–1.0 U/kg initially IM or SQ; then q 4–6 h NPH: 0.5–1.0 U/kg SID SQ	1–3 U/cat SQ Usually lente and ultralente are used	**Dosage very variable—adjust and *monitor* accordingly. These are average approximate dosages. Maintain hydration. Avoid hypoglycemia and hypokalemia.** See *Chapter 117* for information about chronic use; BID Rx; additional information	100 U/ml HM	I
Interferon (Roferon)	Immune modulator with antiviral and antiproliferative effects	1 IU/10 lbs PO every 2 weeks to stimulate appetite	30 IU/cat PO 7 days on; then 7 days off	Studies uncontrolled Used mostly in +FeLV cats	3, 18, 36 million IU per vial HM	I

Drug	Indication/Action	Dose	Dose	Comments	Concentration/Availability	
Ipecac syrup	induce vomiting	1–2 ml/kg PO	Same	Do not use with activated charcoal	70 mg/ml OTC, HM	S
Iron-dextran injection (Imferon)	Iron deficiency anemia	10 mg/kg in divided doses IM 100–300 mg/day PO	Same—IM 50–100 mg/day PO	Irritating IM	Many oral OTC 50 mg/ml HM	I
Isoproterenol (Isuprel)	B-adrenergic agonist	1 mg in 250 ml 5% dextrose, IV at a rate of 0.05–0.1 mcg/kg/min or to effectuate adequate HR	0.5 mg in 250 ml 5% dextrose, IV to effect adequate HR	↑ HR ↓ BP CNS stimulation Arrhythmogenic	0.2 mg/ml HM	I
Itraconazole (Sporanox)	Antimycotic imidazole compound for blastomycosis, coccidioidomycosis, cryptococcosis; histoplasmosis	5–10 mg/kg SID–BID PO	5–13 mg/kg BID PO	Open capsules and place pellets in food if necessary	100 mg HM	C
Ivermectin (Heargard-30) (Ivomec)	GABA agonist antiparasiticide Heartworm prophylaxis; microfilaricide; sarcoptic mange; feline ear mites; Cheyletiella; Endoparasites; Demodectic mange; Sarcoptic mange and otodectes	Heartworm prophylaxis: 0.006 mg/kg PO once-monthly Microfilaricide: 0.05 mg/kg PO 1 × 2–4 weeks post adulticide Rx 200 mcg/kg PO 200–600 mcg/kg/day PO 0.3 mg/kg/PO; SQ: repeat 14 days	0.2 mg/kg SQ: repeat in 3 wks (usually under 0.1 cc) for earmites	Do not use in collies or other dogs hypersensitive to drug; CNS; vomiting; anaphylaxis	68, 136, 272 µg 10 mg/ml VM	T I
Kaolin/pectin (Kaopectate)	G-I tract protectant	1–2 ml/kg every 2 to 6 hrs PO	Same	May limit absorption of other Rx May constipate	Many OTC preparations VM; HM	T/S

847

DRUG INDEX *(Continued)*

GENERIC NAME (Trade Name in Parentheses)	INDICATIONS	CANINE DOSE	FELINE DOSE	COMMENTS	HOW SUPPLIED	
Ketamine HCl (Ketamine) (Ketaset)	Dissociative analgesic anesthetic agent Short-action 10–20 min	Used as diazepam: ketamine mixture in ratio of 1:1 or 2:1; use 1 ml/10 kg IV for sedation and minor procedures	Restraint: 11 mg/kg IM Anesthesia: 22–33 mg/kg IM or 2.2–4.4 mg/kg IV	Eyes remain open. Use ophthalmic ointment Salivation, seizures, respiratory depression, laryngospasm, hypothermia Do not use with renal failure or glaucoma	100 mg/ml VM, HM	I
Ketoconazole (Nizoral)	Antifungal agent Prototheocosis Inhibits adrenal steroid hormone synthesis	20–30 mg/kg/day divided PO Long term 10 mg/kg SID PO Cushings Rx: 15 mg/kg BID PO	10–20 mg/kg/day divided PO or SID Long term: 10 mg/kg eod	Anorexia, nausea, vomiting, constipation Hepatotoxicity Titrate upwards to avoid side effects	200 mg HM	T
Kitten Milk Replace® (KMR)	Milk replacement	—	30 ml/¼ lb BW PO daily divided into 3–6 meals	—	OTC VM	
Lactulose (Cephulac, Chronulac)	Hepatic encephalopathy Stool softener	0.1–0.5 ml/kg BID–TID PO 20 ml/kg as a retention enema; 3 parts lactulose plus 7 parts water	1–5 cc TID PO	Loosens stools; diarrhea; flatulence; cramping May use per rectum in hepatic coma patients	666 mg/ml HM	S
Laxatone	Oral mild laxative Hairball Rx	½–2 inches daily until non-constipated; then weekly or	Same	Large amounts daily could result in malabsorption	OTC VM	S

848

Drug	Indications	Dosage	Adverse effects/Precautions	How supplied	
Levamisole (Levasole) (Ripercol) (Tramisol)	Microfilaricide Immune stimulant Feline lungworms	10 mg/kg PO SID 7–14 days as a microfilaricide 2.5–5 mg/kg PO EOD for immune modulation	2.5–5 mg/kg PO EOD for immune modulation 10–20 mg/kg PO EOD for *Aleurostrongylus* and *Capillaria*	Salivation, vomiting Neurotoxic Sudden death Not FDA approved	184 mg 136 mg/ml 11.5% gel VM	T S
Levothyroxine sodium (Soloxine) (Synthroid)	Synthetic thyroid hormone replacement therapy	0.04 mg/kg SID–BID PO	0.05–0.1 mg/cat SID PO	Thyrotoxicosis	0.025, 0.05, 0.075, 0.125, 0.15 mg HM 0.1, 0.2, 0.3, 0.4, 0.5, 0.6 mg VM	T T
Lidocaine (Xylocaine)	Ventricular arrhythmias Local anesthesia	2–4 mg/kg IV over 1–2 minutes, then 0.5–2 mg/kg every 20–60 minutes, or 40–80 mcg/kg/minute constant infusion Inject SQ for local effects	0.25–1.0 mg/kg slowly IV with caution; use diluted solution as CRI 10–20 mcg/kg/minute	Give initial bolus **slowly** Seizures, hypotension Maintain current IV indwelling catheter **Use only in life threatening arrhythmias**	10, 20 mg/ml HM	I
Lime sulfur solution (Lym Dyp) (Sulfodip)	Bacterial and fungal dermatosis Sarcoptic mange	Dip weekly, let air dry; use 4–6 weeks	Same	Offensive odor Stains furniture Wear gloves to avoid hypersensitivity	2% dip VM	

849

DRUG INDEX *(Continued)*

GENERIC NAME (Trade Name in Parentheses)	INDICATIONS	CANINE DOSE	FELINE DOSE	COMMENTS	HOW SUPPLIED	
Lincomycin (Lincocin)	*Staphylococcal* and anaerobic infections Some *Mycoplasma* infections	15–25 mg/kg BID PO, IV, IM	Same	Vomiting Hepatotoxicity Do not use in combination with chloramphenicol or erythromycin	250, 500 mg HM 100, 200, 500 mg 50 mg/ml 100 mg/ml VM	T T S I
Liothyronine, T₃ (Cytobin) (Cytomel)	Synthetic thyroid hormone	4–6 mcg/kg TID PO	4.4 mcg/kg BID–TID PO 25 mcg PO TID for 8 dosages as testing agent for T₃ suppression	Thyrotoxicosis	60, 120 μg VM 5, 25, 50 μg HM	T T
Lisinopril (Zestril) (Prinivil)	Angiotensin converting enzyme inhibitor	0.4–2.0 mg/kg SID PO		Monitor BUN/CR Lethargy Anorexia	2, 10, 20, 40 mg HM	T
Lithium carbonate (Eskalith, Lithotabs)	Increased production of all cell lines by bone marrow	21–26 mg/kg/day PO	Unknown	Nausea, diarrhea, vertigo	300 mg 450 mg HM	C ER
Loperamide (Imodium)	Antidiarrheal, acute colitis	0.1–0.4 mg/kg TID PO	Same	Discontinue if not effective within 48 h	OTC 2 mg 1 mg/5 ml HM	C S

Drug	Description/Use	Dosage	Alternate Dosage	Comments	Availability	Class
Lysine-8-vasopressin (Diapid)	Central diabetes insipidus	1–2 sprays in each nostril SID–TID	Same	Rhinorrhea Irritation to nasal passages	0.185 mg/ml = 50 U HM	S
Magnesium hydroxide (Milk of Magnesia)	Antacid	5–30 ml PO SID–BID	5–15 ml PO SID–BID	Cathartic agent at 3–5 times the antacid dosage	77.5 mg/g OTC HM	I
Mannitol 20%	Osmotic diuretic used to treat acute glaucoma, cerebral edema, and oliguria-anuria	0.5–1 g/kg IV slowly over 15–20 minutes for anuria. Double dosage for acute glaucoma or cerebral edema	Same	Rehydrate patient prior to use Can repeat twice if renal output is not increased Resolubilize if crystallized before administering	200 mg/ml HM	
Mebendazole (Telmintic)	Hook-, whip-, and roundworms	22 mg/kg with food once daily for 3 days	—	Repeat as indicated V/D may develop Hepatopathies have been incriminated in a small number of cases	VM	
Medium chain triglycerides (MCT oil)	Used in protein loosing diseases—lymphangiectasia; and when long-term triglyceride intake should be reduced—chylothorax	1–2 ml/kg daily in food	Same	May be distasteful Efficacy not demonstrated	OTC HM	
Medroxyprogesterone acetate (Depo-Provera, Provera)	Long acting progesterone compound, used to decrease male dog libido and aggression, rarely as a contraceptive; in cats for psychogenic and miliary dermatitis, and spraying	10–20 mg/kg IM, SQ, every 4 months	50–100 mg/cat IM, SQ every 4 months	Overdosage may cause cystic endometritis, diabetes mellitus, adrenal hypocorticism, mammary hyperplasia/adenocarcinoma. *(see next page)*	2.5, 5, 10 mg 100, 400 mg/ml HM	T I

DRUG INDEX (Continued)

GENERIC NAME (Trade Name in Parentheses)	INDICATIONS	CANINE DOSE	FELINE DOSE	COMMENTS	NOTES
				Local alopecia may occur. Carefully weigh risks versus benefits	T
Megestrol acetate (Ovaban, Megace)	Oral progestogen used to delay estrus; treat K-9 pseudopregnancy; canine and feline behavioral modification; eosinophilic granuloma, and some chronic skin disorders	Anestrus Rx: 0.5 mg/kg PO × 32 days Proestrus Rx: 2.0 mg/kg PO × 8 days Behavior modification: 2-4 mg/kg SID PO 14 days; then decrease and stop after 6 weeks	5-10 mg SID PO × 7 days; then twice weekly. Same dose as for dog for behavioral modification	See specific diseases. Do not use in pets with reproductive problems. Avoid use with mammary tumors or hyperplasia May cause polydipsia, polyuria, polyphagia, diabetes mellitus	5, 20 mg VM 20, 40 mg HM
Melarsamine	Arsenical for treatment of adult heartworms	2.5 mg/kg SID IM for 2 doses	None	Not yet FDA approved	VM
Melphalan (Alkeran)	Multiple myeloma Lymphoreticular neoplasms Alkylating agent	0.1 mg/kg SID PO for 10 days; then 0.05 mg/kg SID PO: or 1.5 mg/m² PO SID for 7-10 days	Same	Anorexia, nausea, vomiting Leukopenia, thrombocytopenia, and anemia	2 mg HM T
Meperidine HCl (Demerol)	Narcotic analgesic with short term (2-4 hrs) effect	5-10 mg/kg IM PRN	2-4 mg/kg IM PRN	Watch for signs of narcotic overdosage, i.e., sedation, depression, seizures, hypotension Reverse with naloxone	50, 100 mg/ml 25, 50, 75, 100 mg HM I T

Drug	Description	Dosage (dog)	Dosage (cat)	Side effects / Notes	Availability	
Mesalamine (Asacol)	Inhibits prostaglandin production in the colon; Irritable bowel syndrome; ulcerative colitis	10–20 mg/kg TID PO			400 mg HM	T
Metamucil	Bulk laxative, stool softener	2–10 g SID–BID in moistened food	2–4 g SID–BID in moistened food		OTC HM	
Methimazole (Tapazole)	Feline hyperthyroidism	None	5 mg PO SID–TID	Anorexia, vomiting, and blood dyscrasias. Monitor CBC and until euthyroid	5, 10 mg HM	T
DL-Methionine (Methigel) (Albeta)	Urinary acidifier	0.2–1 g/kg TID PO	0.2–1 g SID PO	G-I irritability	75 mg/ml 200, 300, 500 mg OTC, VM, HM	S T, C
Methocarbamol (Robaxin)	Muscle relaxant	20–45 mg/kg PO BID–TID	Same	Ataxia; sedation; ptyalism; emesis	100 mg/ml 500 mg HM	I T
Methotrexate	Antimetabolite, antineoplastic agent that inhibits folic acid reductase. Used to treat some cancers or for immunosuppression	0.06 mg/kg SID PO 2.5 mg/m² once daily PO, IV, IM	Same	Leukopenia, G-I bleeding hepatoxicity. See specific cancer or disease state	2.5 mg 2.5 mg/ml HM	T I
Methylene blue	For treatment of methemoglobinemia in dogs	1–2 mg/kg IV		Use once only Can induce Heinz body hemolytic anemia	10 mg/ml HM	I

DRUG INDEX *(Continued)*

GENERIC NAME (Trade Name in Parentheses)	INDICATIONS	CANINE DOSE	FELINE DOSE	COMMENTS	HOW SUPPLIED	
Methylprednisolone acetate (Depo Medrol)	Repositol corticosteroid; for intralesional skin injections; feline asthma	1–2 mg/kg IM, SQ	Same 10–20 mg/cat for asthma	Cortisone contraindications and side effects	1, 2 mg VM	T
					2, 4, 8, 16, 24, 32 mg HM	T
					20, 40, 80 mg/ml VM, HM	I
Methyltestosterone	Anabolic drug Androgenic steroid	0.5 mg/kg PO	Same	May increase creatinine and glucose. Used in testosterone responsive incontinence	10 mg HM	C
Metoclopramide (Reglan)	Antiemetic with both central (chemoreceptor trigger zone) and peripheral (gastrointestinal) effects Increases LES pressure; promotes gastric emptying	0.2–0.5 mg/kg BID–QID PO, SQ 1–2 mg/kg given as IV infusion over 24 hours as an antiemetic	Same	Do not use with G-I obstruction, with phenothiazines or with narcotic analgesics. Atropine blocks effect. May increase seizure activity Extrapyramidal effects	5, 10 mg 1 mg/ml 5 mg/ml HM	T S I
Metronidazole (Flagyl)	Anaerobic infections of the mouth, pulmonary, G-I tract and liver. Also, *Giardia*, *Entamoeba*, *Balantidia*, *Pentatrichomonas* and *Trypanasoma* Irritable bowel disease (IBD)	10–30 mg/kg BID PO	10–25 mg/kg BID PO	Anorexia and vomiting. Neurotoxicity and hepatotoxicity may develop	250, 500 mg 500 mg/100 ml HM	T I

Drug	Action	Dosage		Notes	Forms	
Metoprolol (Lopressor) (Toprol-XL)	B_1 selective blockade	0.4–1 mg/kg BID–TID PO SID for ER formula	2–10 mg/cat SID–BID PO	Lethargy, depression Decreased HR. Use with caution with CHF	50, 100 mg 50, 100, 200 mg 1 mg/ml HM	T ER I
Mexiletine (Mexitil)	Type 1B antiarrhythmic drug used to treat ventricular arrhythmias	4–10 mg/kg BID–TID PO	—	Anorexia, depression Side effects rare	150, 200, 250 mg HM	C
Mibolerone (Cheque)	Prevent estrus (dogs only) Pseudocyesis Synthetic androgenic, anabolic steroid	1–11 kg: 30 mcg/day PO 12–22 kg: 60 mcg/day PO 23–45 kg: 120 mcg/day PO >45 kg, or German Shepherd dog (mix) 180 mcg/day PO Pseudocyesis: 10 times above dosage for 5 days PO	—	Do not use in pregnant dogs or in those with renal or hepatic disease	100 mcg/ml VM	S
Miconazole (Conofite)	Topical antifungal	Apply BID to lesion Continue after resolution of lesions for 2 weeks	Same	Contact hypersensitivity	OTC, topical cream and solution HM	
Milbemycin (Interceptor)	Anthelmintic action in heartworm prevention and hookworm control	0.5–1.0 mg/kg orally once monthly 0.5–2.3 mg/kg SID–BID PO 2–4 weeks for Demodex	—	Test for heartworms prior to initial administration	2.3, 5.75, 11.5, and 23 mg VM	T
Misoprostol (Cytotec)	Prostaglandin E₁ inhibitor. Used for ulcers due to NSAID and/or steroids	4–8 mcg/kg BID PO	—	Secretory diarrhea, vomiting, anorexia. May induce abortion in pregnant animals	100, 200 mg HM	T

855

DRUG INDEX (Continued)

GENERIC NAME (Trade Name in Parentheses)	INDICATIONS	CANINE DOSE	FELINE DOSE	COMMENTS	HOW SUPPLIED
Mitoxantrone (Novantrone)	Chemotherapeutic agent closely related to doxorubicin	5 mg/m² once every 3 weeks IV	6.25 mg/m² once every 3 weeks IV	Depression, G-I signs, leukopenia	2 mg/ml HM I
Morphine sulfate	Narcotic analgesic Acute CHF as adjunctive therapeutic agent to relieve anxiety and to vasodilate	0.25–2.0 mg/kg every 4 to 6 h IM, SQ	0.05–0.1 mg/kg every 4 to 6 hours IM, SQ	Hyperexcitability in cats Vomiting, respiratory and CNS depression. Hypotension	30 mg ER 5, 10, 20 mg suppository S 10, 20 mg/5 ml T 15, 30 mg I 2, 4, 5, 8, 10, 15 mg/ml HM
Moxidectin	Heartworm prophylaxis Macrolide antibiotic	3 mcg/kg once monthly		Safe in collies Not FDA approved	
Naloxone (Narcan)	Narcotic antagonist	0.04 mg/kg IV, IM, SC	None	The effect of the narcotic may last longer than the Naloxone. This is particularly true in end stage liver disease, porto-systemic shunts, or with drugs that are P-450 blockers	0.02, 0.4, 1 mg/ml HM I
Nandrolone decanoate (Deca-Durabolin)	Anabolic steroid and bone marrow stimulant	1 mg/kg/week IM	0.5–1.0 mg/kg/week IM	Give deep IM. Do not administer to pregnant or hepato-insufficient animals	200 mg/ml HM I

Drug	Description	Dose	Alternate Dose	Comments	Availability	Code
Neomycin (Biosol)	Aminoglycoside antibacterial used orally for G-I tract bacterial overgrowth and hepatoencephalopathy	20 mg/kg BID–TID PO	Same	In severe intestinal disease toxicity may develop. Ototoxicity and nephrotoxicity are rare with oral dosage	200 mg/ml 100, 500 mg VM, HM	S T
Neostigmine (Stiglin, Prostigmin)	Anticholinesterase agent for myasthenia gravis	0.01–0.05 mg/kg IM, SQ, PRN	Same	Muscarinic effects: vomiting, diarrhea, bradycardia are reversed by atropine	0.25, 0.5, 1 and 2 mg/ml 15 mg HM	I T
Niclosamide (Yomesan)	Tapeworm anthelmintic	154 mg/kg PO; fast 24 hours before; repeat in 2–3 weeks	Same	Occasionally soft stools	VM	T S
Nitrofurantoin (Dantefur) (Macrodantin)	Urinary tract infections Ointment for superficial wounds	4 mg/kg q 8 h PO	Same	Oral form used only for urinary tract infections	50, 100 mg 5 mg/ml 25, 50, 100 mg macro crystals HM	C
Nitroglycerin 20% ointment (Nitrol ointment)	Transdermal venodilator for reducing cardiac preload in acute CHF	Apply ¼–2 inches TID–QID topically	Apply ⅛–¼ inch TID topically	May cause hypotension. Apply *with glove* to hairless region, i.e., pinna or inguinal	2% HM	O
Nitroprusside (Nipride)	Arterial dilator Venodilator	5–7 mcg/kg/min IV CRI	1–2 mcg/kg/min IV CRI	Hypotension Cyanide toxicity Use 2–3 days IV maximum	50 mg/vial HM	I
Norepinephrine (Levophed)	B_1 and alpha agonist used to treat shock	1–2 ml in 250 ml of drip, IV to effect	None	Hypertension Tachycardia	1 mg/ml HM	I

DRUG INDEX (Continued)

GENERIC NAME (Trade Name in Parentheses)	INDICATIONS	CANINE DOSE	FELINE DOSE	COMMENTS	HOW SUPPLIED	
Omeprazole (Prilosec) (Losec)	Proton pump acid blocker; used in reflux esophagitis and hyperacidity syndromes	0.7 mg/kg SID PO		New agent—1995 Little reported clinical experience	20 mg HM	C
Ondansetron (Zofran)	5-HT₃ receptor antagonist (serotonin inhibitor) Used in conjunction with emetogenic cancer chemotherapy	0.10–0.15 mg/kg IV BID		Used before and for 48 h following specific IV cancer Rx	4, 8 mg 2 mg/ml HM	T I
O, P′–DDD (Lysodren)	Hyperadrenalcorticism. Selective necrosis of the zona fasciculata and reticularis	50 mg/kg once daily to effect (approx. 5–10 days); then 25–50 mg/kg once every 7–14 days to effect	None	Vomiting, diarrhea, weakness Mineralocorticoid deficiency	500 mg VM	T
Orgotein (Palosein)	Superoxide dismutase activity causes anti-inflammatory response	5 mg SID SQ for 7 days; then every other day or as needed		Unsubstantiated effects	5 mg/vial VM	I
Oxacillin (Prostaphlin)	Penicillin derivative used for staphloccal skin infections	22–40 mg/kg TID PO	Same	Best if not given with food	250 mg/5 ml 250, 500 mg 250, 500 mg, 1 and 2 g HM	S C I

858

Drug	Dose	Dose (alt)	Side effects / Cautions	Available forms	Code
Oxazepam (Serax)	Appetite stimulant (oral benzodiazepine agent)	0.2–1 mg/kg SID–BID PO. Rarely used in dogs	Same. Do not use long term—hepato toxicity	Overdosage results in sedation and incoordination	10, 15, 30 mg / 15 mg / HM	C / T
Oxtriphylline (Choledyl)	Bronchodilator (theophylline derivative)	4–10 mg/kg TID PO	4–10 mg/kg TID PO	Vomiting, diarrhea, hyper-excitability	100, 200 mg / 400, 600 mg / HM	T / ER
Oxymorphone (Numorphan)	Narcotic agonist for analgesia, anesthetic induction and minor procedures	Anesthesia: 0.1–0.2 mg/kg IV, IM, SQ; Analgesia: 0.03–0.2 mg/kg IV, IM, SQ, PRN	0.01–0.2 mg/kg IV, IM, SQ, PRN	Respiratory and CNS depression. Hypotension, sedation, feline hyperexcitability. Reverse with naloxone	1, 1.5 mg/ml / HM	I
Oxytetracycline (Terramycin)	Broad spectrum bacteriostatic agent. Also used for rickettsiae, mycoplasma, and spirochetes	10–20 mg/kg TID–QID PO; As o.o., apply BID–QID	Same	Do not use in pregnancy (last trimester) or in first month of life (dental staining). G-I side effects. Do not administer with antacids, dairy products, or intestinal adsorbents	50, 125 mg/ml / 250 mg / HM	I / C
Oxytocin (Pitocin, Syntocinon)	Posterior pituitary hormone used for uterine inertia; to stimulate milk flow; vasopressive effects and as an antidiuretic	Obstetrics: 5–25 U IM q 30 min or 1–2 U/kg; Milk production: 2–10 units IM; Intranasal spray	Obstetrics: 2 units/kg IM q 30 min; Milk production: 1 unit IM	Do not use if obstructed. Refrigerate vial—warm syringe before injection	10 U/ml / 40 U/ml nasal spray / HM	I

DRUG INDEX *(Continued)*

GENERIC NAME (Trade Name in Parentheses)	INDICATIONS	CANINE DOSE	FELINE DOSE	COMMENTS	HOW SUPPLIED
Pancreatic enzymes (Viokase)	Pancreatic exocrine insufficiency	½–2 tsp pwdr in 1# canned food or 2 cups moistened dry food. Allow to stand 15–30 minutes, then feed	Same	Avoid inhaling powder dust	VM, HM
Paramite dip	Organophosphate dip for fleas, ticks, and canine sarcoptic mange	2 tbls (1 oz) per gallon H_2O. Sponge on and let air dry	1 tbls (½ oz) per gallon H_2O. Sponge on and let air dry	Wear gloves to administer; use once weekly maximum. Do not use if under 8 weeks. Fever, salivation, seizures and CNS signs suggest organophophate toxicity. Use atropine injection and wash off animal	11.6% dip VM
Paregoric®	Antidiarrheal	0.05–0.06 mg/kg BID–TID PO	None	May cause constipation	OTC, HM S
Pedialyte®	Oral electrolyte maintenance soln.	Supplement to diet and fluid therapy to maintain hydration and electrolyte balance	Same		OTC, HM S
Penicillamine (Cuprimine) (Depen)	Chelating agent for lead, copper, and mercury. Also prevents cysteine urolithiasis	10–15 mg/kg PO BID		Administer on empty stomach. May cause vomiting. Monitor CBC	250 mg T 125, 250 mg C HM

Drug	Action/Use	Dose (canine)	Dose (feline)	Precautions	Availability	
Penicillin, benzathine (Benzapen)	Gm + infections; bacteriacidal	20,000–40,000 units/kg SID–BID IM, SQ	Same	Do not use with penicillin hypersensitivity. Do not use if serious infection is suspected	150,000 U/ml HM	I
Penicillin G	Gm + infections	20,000–40,000 units/kg q 6-8 h IV, IM, SQ	Same	Penicillin hypersensitivity. May contain high levels K⁺. Not very effective orally	200,000, 250,000, 400,000, 500,000, 800,000 U; 200,000 and 400,000 U/5 ml; 300,000, 500,000, 600,000, 1.2 and 2.4 million U per ml HM	T S I
Penicillin-V	Gm + infections; bacteriacidal; effective orally	10–30 mg/kg TID–QID PO	Same	250 mg = 400,000 units. Penicillin hypersensitivity	125, 250, 500 mg; 125, 250 mg/5 ml; Many other sizes HM	T S
Pentazocine (Talwin)	Narcotic agonist/antagonist used for short term analgesia	1 mg/kg IM; 2–6 mg/kg PO	2–3 mg/kg SQ, IM, IV	May cause salivation and/or sedation. Reverse with naloxone. May cause dysphoria in cats	30 mg/ml HM; Often combined with other Rx VM, HM	I
Pentobarbital (Nembutal)	Status epilepticus; Anesthesia	Anesthesia: 10–30 mg/kg IV slowly to effect; Seizures: 3–15 mg/kg IV slowly to effect	Anesthesia: 10–30 mg/kg IV slowly to effect; Seizures: 3–15 mg/kg IV slowly to effect	Respiratory depression and hypotension may develop if used with or after diazepam	50 mg/ml; Available as tablets, elixir, suppositories VM, HM	I

DRUG INDEX *(Continued)*

GENERIC NAME (Trade Name in Parentheses)	INDICATIONS	CANINE DOSE	FELINE DOSE	COMMENTS	HOW SUPPLIED	
Phenobarbital	Long acting barbiturate used for seizure control. Occasionally used as a sedative	1–2 mg/kg PO BID–TID May be given IV as a bolus of 2–15 mg/kg slowly for status epilepticus followed by 2–6 mg/hr CRI	Same	Ataxia, sedation, pu/pd. Long term (> 35 mcg/ml levels) hepatotoxicity occurs. Initial adjustment period is required. Controlled substance Available combined with phenytoin—not generally recommended	8, 16, 32, 65, 100 mg 15, 20 mg/5 ml 30, 60, 65, 130 mg/ml HM	T S I
Phenoxybenzamine HCl (Dibenzyline)	Alpha adrenergic blocking agent. Urinary incontinence due to detrussor sphincter dyssynergia	0.25–1.0 mg/kg PO BID	2.5–10 mg PO SID–BID	May result in vomiting, hypotension, rapid HR, miosis	10 mg HM	C
Phenylbutazone (Butazolidin)	Nonsteroidal antiinflammatory	10–22 mg/kg BID–TID PO	6–8 mg/kg BID PO every other week	Use lowest effective dosage. Do not exceed 800 mg/day. May cause vomiting, G-I ulceration, BM suppression	100, 400, 1000 mg VM, HM	T
Phenylephrine (Neo-Synephrine)	Post-synaptic alpha adrenergic stimulant used as nasal drops for rhinitis	1–2 drops intra-nasal pediatric soln SID–TID	Same	May cause nasal irritation chronically. Vasoconstriction and pupillary dilatation if given parenterally	10 mg/ml Oph. and intranasal OTC products HM	I

862

Drug	Indication	Dog dosage	Cat dosage	Comments	Forms	Type
Phenylpropanolamine HCl (Dexatrim, Ornade, Propagest, Triaminic)	Alpha adrenergic agonist used to treat hormone responsive urinary sphincter hypotonus (incontinence)	1 mg/kg PO TID; round up or down	12.5 mg/cat TID PO	Anxiety, dizziness, hypertension, urinary retention. If OTC drug use product without caffeine	25, 37.5 mg HM	T
Phenytoin (Dilantin)	Anticonvulsant agent	10–40 mg/kg PO TID; 5–10 mg/kg IV	Not recommended	Ataxia and vomiting. Monitor for hepatotoxicity. Metabolized very rapidly. Considered second line agent	50 mg; 30, 100 mg; 6, 25 mg/ml HM	T C S
Phosphate enemas (Fleet)	Treatment of constipation	For large dogs use one adult bottle; for medium dogs use ½ bottle or a pediatric enema. Not suggested for use in small dogs	Not recommended	May cause severe hyperphosphatemia and hypocalcemia. Do not use if dehydrated, with renal or cardiac failure or in very sick animals unless absolutely necessary	OTC, HM	
Pilocarpine Oph. Soln	Miotic agent useful in glaucoma	1. 1 drop in affected eye BID–QID 2. For KCS: 2–5 drops in food SID	Same	Ciliary spasms. Systemic signs rare when used topically. Increase strength with time and response	0.25, 0.5, 1, 2, 3, 4, 6, 8% HM	OS
Piperazine	Ascarid infection	50–110 mg/kg PO	50–100 mg/kg PO	Repeat in 3 weeks. Vomiting and diarrhea may occur at higher dosages	250 mg; 100 mg/ml VM, HM	T S
Piroxicam (Feldene)	NSAID As primary or secondary Rx for bladder TCC	0.3 mg/kg EOD or SID PO		G-I irritation Must open capsules and put in food for most animals Often, co-administered with Misoprostol	10, 20 mg HM	C

DRUG INDEX (Continued)

GENERIC NAME (Trade Name in Parentheses)	INDICATIONS	CANINE DOSE	FELINE DOSE	COMMENTS	HOW SUPPLIED	
Polysulfated Glycosaminoglycan (Adequan)	Chondroprotective agent	1–5 mg/kg IM every fourth day for 6 treatments; then as needed	Same	Approved for use in horses	100 mg/ml VM	I
Potassium bromide	Anticonvulsant	20–35 mg/kg SID PO May require an initial loading dose	Unknown	Used with phenobarbital. May potentiate side effects of sedation, incoordination Effective range 500–1500 mcg/ml Use ACS grade 25 g q.s. add to 100 ml distilled water Also available as Na$^+$ salt	250 mg/ml VM	S
Potassium chloride inj.	Treatment and prevention of hypokalemia	Add to IV fluid *per liter* based on serum K$^+$ level: Serum K: KCl 3.5–5.0 MEq = 20 MEq 3.0–3.4 = 30 2.5–2.9 = 40 2.0–2.4 = 60 <2.0 = 80	Same	Never infuse rapidly or administer over 0.5 MEq K$^+$/kg h. Monitor K$^+$ regularly	2, 10, 20, 30, 40, 60, 200, 400, 1000 MEq/ml HM	I
Potassium citrate (Urocit–K)	Inhibits Ca Oxylate crystal formation in urine Alkalinizing agent for urine	75 mg/kg BID PO 1–3 MEq/kg/day PO		Gastrointestinal irritation 5 MEq = 540 mg	5, 10 MEq HM	T

Drug	Action/Class	Large animal dose	Small animal dose	Comments	Availability/Sizes	Route
Potassium Salts (Kaon ® Elixir) (Micro K Extencaps)	Potassium supplements in various oral formulations	¼–1 tab (Tbls) (Caps) BID–TID PO	⅛–¼ tab (Tbls) (Caps) BID–TID PO	Dose according to deficit. Monitor serum K. May cause gastric irritation	Many OTC preparations different sizes VM, HM	
Povidone-iodine (Betadine)	Antiseptic–Germacide	Apply topically as indicated	Same	Available as 7.5% surgical scrub, 10% solution; cream and ointment	OTC HM	
Pralidoxime chloride (2–PAM) (Protopam Chloride)	Reactivates cholinesterase inactivated by organophosphate and other toxins	40–50 mg/kg IV over 2 min period; then q 12 h as needed (IV, IM or SQ)	20 mg/kg	Monitor patient continuously	1 g vial HM	I
Praziquantel (Droncit)	*Taenia, Dipylidium, Echinococcus, Heterobilharzia*	Use according to instructions on product according to weight	Same	Fasting not required. Do not use in puppies under 4 weeks or kittens under 6 weeks of age	23, 34 mg VM	T
Prednisolone, prednisone	Antiinflammatory— antipruritic immune system suppression	Antiinflammatory: 0.5–1 mg/kg/day oral, IM, SQ Immune suppression: 2–4.4 mg/kg/day usually orally	Same	PP/PU/PD; suppression of HPA axis—Cushing's syndrome. Taper dosage if used long term	1, 2.5, 5, 10, 20, 25, 50 mg 1 mg/ml 10, 25 mg/ml HM	T S I
Predisone ophthalmic suspension (Pred Forte)	Steroid responsive inflammation of the lids, conjunctiva, sclera, cornea and anterior segment of the eye	1 drop in affected eye BID–QID	Same	Variable strength products (0.12–1%) used as required. Do not use with purulent, viral, or fungal infection. Systemic side effects are possible but rare	0.12, 0.125, 1% HM	OS

DRUG INDEX *(Continued)*

GENERIC NAME (Trade Name in Parentheses)	INDICATIONS	CANINE DOSE	FELINE DOSE	COMMENTS	NOTES
Prednisolone sodium succinate (Solu-Delta-Cortef)	Soluble corticosteroid IV used for shock of multiple causes	11–33 mg/kg IV slow bolus Repeat up to q 6 h	Same	Causes vomiting if administered too rapidly	20 mg/ml VM, HM — I
Primidone (Mylepsin)	Anticonvulsant medication converted to phenobarbital	10–20 mg/kg/day initially; up to 50 mg/kg/day given BID–TID PO	Not recommended	Causes pu/pd/pp, sedation, and ataxia. May be hepatotoxic with prolonged use	50, 250 mg — T 50 mg/ml HM — S
Procainamide (Pronestyl; SR) (Procan–SR)	Ventricular arrhythmias	6–20 mg/kg IV slowly over 30 min then CRI 20–40 mcg/kg/min (if life threatening) 6–20 mg/kg q 4 h IM 6–20 mg/kg q 6 h PO	1–2 mg/kg bolus IV; then 10–20 mcg/kg/min CRI	Available as sustained release tablet for TID administration. This is a negative inotrope. May cause hypotension, tachycardia, and ECG changes (see *Chapter 95*)	100, 500 mg/ml — I 250, 375, 500 mg — C 250, 500, 750, 1000 mg ER HM
Prochlorperazine (Compazine)	Antiemetic	0.11–0.44 mg/kg SQ IM	Same	Sedation, hypotension. Do not use in epileptic patients. Available also in suppository formulation	5 mg/ml — I 1 mg/ml — S 5, 10, 25 mg — T 10, 15, 30 mg ER HM
Propantheline (Pro Banthine)	Anticholinergic agent used to treat diarrhea, bradycardia syndromes, and detrussor hyperreflexia	0.2 mg/kg BID–TID PO Increase to effect for bradycardia syndromes	¼–1 tab SID–BID PO	Tachycardia, dry mouth, constipation, mydriasis, ileus, urinary retention	7.5, 15 mg — T HM

Drug	Use	Dose (dog)	Dose (cat)	Comments	Supplied	
Propioni bacterium acnes (Immunoregulin)	Immune modulator potentiator	0.03–0.07 mg/kg IV at 2–3 day intervals	0.5 ml/cat IV 1–2 times a week	No controlled studies	0.4 mg/ml VM	I
Propofol (Diprivan)	Ultrashort acting anesthetic	3–6 mg/kg IV	Same	Give slowly over 1–2 min in equal dosages to effect	10 mg/ml HM	I
Propranolol (Inderal)	Beta adrenergic blocking agent used to treat supraventricular arrhythmias, some ventricular arrhythmias, and feline hypertrophic cardiomyopathy	0.25–0.5 mg IV. No more frequently than q 1–3 min to 5 mg maximum. Administer until the rate slows 0.2–1.0 mg/kg BID–TID PO, usually start low and titrate dosage	0.25–0.5 mg IV bolus slowly 2.5–5 mg/day PO, begin low and titrate dosage	Anorexia, depression, ataxia Bradycardia, negative inotropic effect Potentiates A–V nodal depression of digoxin and calcium channel blockers	10, 20, 40, 60, 80, 90 mg 60, 80, 120, 160 mg 4, 8, 80 mg/ml 1 mg/ml HM	T ER S I
Propylthiouracil (PTU)	Feline hyperthyroidism	Not used	10 mg/kg BID–TID PO	Immune mediated hemolytic anemia and thrombocytopenia. This is a second line agent. Anorexia, vomiting, and lethargy	50 mg HM	T
Prostaglandin (PGF2α) (Lutalyse)	1. Open cervix pyometra 2. Abortive agent at 31–35 days	1. 60 mcg/kg/day IM divided BID for 3–6 days 2. 0.25 mg/kg SID SQ 3–7 days (or until fetuses are expelled)	1. Same 2. 0.5–1 mg/kg SQ for 2 days only	Panting, salivation, vomiting, diarrhea, and tachycardia lasting about 30 minutes Should be given under hospital supervision	5 mg/ml VM	I
Pyrantel pamoate (Nemex, Strongid-T)	Roundworm and hookworm anthlmentic	5–10 mg/kg PO	10 mg/kg PO	Repeat in 3 weeks Safe at recommended dosages and in dogs with heartworms	22.7, 113.5 mg 2.27, 4.54, 50 mg/ml VM	T S

DRUG INDEX (Continued)

GENERIC NAME (Trade Name in Parentheses)	INDICATIONS	CANINE DOSE	FELINE DOSE	COMMENTS	HOW SUPPLIED
Pyridostigmine bromide (Mestinon)	Anticholinesterase agent used to treat myasthenia gravis	0.2–2 mg/kg BID–TID PO	0.25 mg/kg PO maximum of once daily	Available as soft tablet and syrup (60 mg/5cc). Vomiting, diarrhea, salivation, and weakness may develop	60 mg — T 180 mg — ER 60 mg/5 ml — S 5 mg/ml — I HM
Pyrimethamine (Daraprim)	Toxoplasmosis Neosporosis	0.5–1 mg/kg daily PO for 48 h; then 50%/day for 14 days	Same	Often used with sulfonamides to treat toxoplasmosis. May need to supplement with folic or folinic acid.	25 mg — T HM
Quinicrine (Atebrine)	Giardiasis Enteric coccidiosis	10 mg/kg SID PO 5–12 days	2 mg/kg SID PO 5–12 days	May cause enteric signs Considered second line agent	100 mg — T HM
Quinidine SO₄ (Quinaglute) (Quinadex)	Type 1A antiarrhythmic agent used mostly for ventricular dysrhythmias	6–20 mg/kg TID–QID PO, IM	Not recommended	Do not give IV or use with digitalis Negative inotropic agent Available in long acting tablet forms See *Chapter 95*	100, 200, 300 mg — T 275, 300, 330 mg — ER 80 mg/ml — I HM
Quibron®	Bronchodilator—expectorant combination of theophylline and guaifenesin	1 capsule BID–TID PO in large breeds only	Not recommended	Hyperexcitability; vomiting	150, 300 mg — C 300 mg — T 300 mg — ER HM

Drug	Action	Dose	Dose (2)	Comments	Formulation	Code
Rantidine HCl (Zantac)	H₂ histamine receptor antagonist	1–4 mg/kg PO SID–BID 1–2 mg/kg IV SID–BID	0.44 mg/kg PO		150, 300 mg 15 mg/ml 25 mg/ml HM	T S I
Silver sulfadiazine (Silvadene Cream)	Topical antiinfective preparation for complications of burns	Apply to burn area BID as necessary	Same	Hypersensitivity to sulfonamides	10 mg/g HM	O
Sodium bicarbonate	Metabolic acidosis	MEq/day = base deficit × 0.3 × Wt (Kg) Administer 50% quickly and recheck serum levels; then give the balance over 24 h	Same	Alkalosis, hypernatremia, CHF, hypokalemia	0.6, 1 MEq/ml 5, 10 grain HM	I T
Sodium iodide 20%	Sporotrichosis	44 mg/kg divided TID PO	Same	Monitor for iodinism: fever, ptyalism, G-I signs	20% VM	I
Sodium Stibogluconate (Pentostam)	Leishmaniasis	30–50 mg/kg SID SQ, IV		Not available in USA except through CDC		
Spironolactone (Aldactone) Spironolactone with hydrochlorothiazide (Aldactazide)	Potassium sparing diuretic; inhibits aldosterone	1–4 mg/kg BID PO	Same	Usually used with other diuretic agents. Monitor potassium	25, 50, 100 mg HM 25/25 mg	T
Stanozolol (Winstrol)	Anabolic steroid used to treat anorexia, debilitation, and anemia	0.1–0.2 mg/kg SID–BID PO 25–50 mg IM weekly	0.1–0.2 mg/kg SID–BID PO 12.5–25 mg IM weekly	Contraindicated in pregnancy	2 mg 50 mg/ml VM, HM	T I

DRUG INDEX *(Continued)*

GENERIC NAME (Trade Name in Parentheses)	INDICATIONS	CANINE DOSE	FELINE DOSE	COMMENTS	HOW SUPPLIED	
Sucralfate (Carafate)	Complexes with proteinaceous materials in stomach thereby preventing undesirable effects of acids on the gastric mucosa	¼–1 tab TID–QID PO	¼ tab BID–QID	May constipate. Interferes with absorption of many drugs administered concurrently	1 g	T
					HM	
Sulfadiazine (Suladyne)	Bacteriostatic agent used to treat toxoplasmosis and nocardiosis	90–120 mg/kg BID PO; follow by 50 mg/kg BID PO	Same	Sulfonamide precautions	500 mg	T
					HM	
Sulfadimethoxine (Bactrovet, Albon)	Bacteriostatic agent used to treat toxoplasmosis, Nocardiosis, and Coccidiosis	50 mg/kg PO day 1; then 25 mg/kg PO daily	Same	KCS, nephrotoxicity and hypersensitivity	400 mg/ml	I
					125, 250, 500 mg	T
					50, 125 mg/ml	S
					VM, HM	
Sulfadimethoxine-ormetoprim (Primor)	Potentiated sulfonamide	55 mg/kg SID PO on day 1; then 27.5 mg/kg SID thereafter for a maximum of 21 days	None	Sulfonamide contraindications	120, 240, 600, 1200 mg	T
					VM	
Sulfasalazine (Azulfidine)	Antiinflammatory effect on the colon; ulcerative and idiopathic colitis	22–55 mg/kg TID PO	10–20 mg/kg BID PO 3–5 days	KCS Avoid prolonged treatment, blood dyscrasias, vomiting	500 mg	T
					HM	
Taurine	Feline DCM Am. Cocker DCM	50 mg/kg TID PO	125–250 mg BID PO	Switch to taurine enriched diet	250 mg	T
					OTC, HM	

Drug	Use	Dose	Dose (alt)	Notes	Supply	
Terbutaline (Brethine)	Bronchodilator	1.25–5 mg BID–TID PO	1.25 mg BID PO	Excitability Vomiting	2.5, 5 mg 1 mg/ml HM	T I
Testosterone	Testosterone responsive incontinence in dogs	2.2 mg/kg IM monthly	5–10 mg/cat IM		25, 50, 100, 200 mg/ml HM	I
Tetracosactrin (Cortrosyn)	Synthetic subunit of ACTH	0.25 mg/dog IM	0.125 mg/cat IM	Measure cortisol levels one hour after administration	0.25 mg/ml HM	I
Tetracycline	Broad spectrum antibiotic; bacteriostatic. Used especially for *Brucella, Chlamydia, Mycoplasma,* and *Rickettsia;* used for pleurodesis and an an ophthalmic ointment	10–22 mg/kg TID PO for 3 weeks Pleurodesis: 20 mg/kg in 4 ml saline/kg Oph. oint: Apply TID–QID	Same	Fever, vomiting, diarrhea Do not administer with dairy products, antacids, intestinal adsorbents Do not give in last 3 wks of pregnancy or to newborns to 4 wks	100, 250, 500 25 mg/ml 250, 500 mg/vial 10 mg/g 10 mg/ml HM	T/C S I OO OS
Theophylline Elixir (Elixophyllin)	Bronchodilator	6–11 mg/kg TID PO	Rarely used at 8 mg/kg TID PO	See *Aminophylline* Restlessness, vomiting	80 mg/tbls HM	S
Thiabendazole (Mintezol)	Aspergillosis, Penicilliosis, Filaroides and feline eosinophilic granuloma complex	50 mg/kg SID PO for 3 days, repeat in 1 month	5–10 mg/kg SID PO 3 times weekly	Not licensed for feline use	500 mg 100 mg/ml VM	T S
Thiacetarsamide (Caparsolate)	Heartworm adulticide Haemobartonellosis	2.2 mg/kg BID IV for 48 h	1.1–2.2 mg/kg BID IV × 48 h Often not rec'd	Vomiting, depression, hepatotoxicity (icterus). Thromboembolic phenomena 7–14 days post-Rx Perivenous injection causes sloughing	10 mg/ml VM	I

DRUG INDEX *(Continued)*

GENERIC NAME (Trade Name in Parentheses)	INDICATIONS	CANINE DOSE	FELINE DOSE	COMMENTS	HOW SUPPLIED	
Thiamine (Vitamin B₁)	Thiamine deficiency	50–100 mg BID IM, IV, PO	50 mg BID, IM, IV, PO	Stings IM	100, 200 mg/ml 5, 10, 25, 50, 100, 250, 500 mg HM	I T
Thiamylal Na (Surital)	Ultrashort acting barbiturate anesthetic	11–17.5 mg/kg IV titrated to induction of anesthesia	Same	Respiratory and cardiac depression Avoid perivenous administration Ventricular bigeminy common	Not available 1995 May return to the market 1, 5, 10 g vials	I
Thiopental Sodium (Pentothal)	Ultrashort acting anesthetic (similar to Thiamylal Na)	13–26 mg/kg IV titrated to induction of anesthesia	Same	See Thiamylal	1, 2.5, 5 g vials HM	I
Thyrotropin TSH (thyroid-stimulating hormone) (Dermathrycin) (Thyrotropar)	Hormone used to diagnose hypothyroidism	5 U/dog to 10 kg IV, IM, SQ 10 U/dog over 10 kg IV, IM, SQ	2.5 units/cat IV	Follow protocol for testing: pre- and 6 h post-injection	5, 10 U/vial VM, HM	I
Tiletamine-zolazepam (Telazol)	Tranquilizer, dissociative combination agent used for chemical restraint	5–10 mg/kg IM	Same	Rapid onset; respiratory depression may occur quickly. Be prepared.	100 mg/ml combined VM	I

Drug (trade name)	Description / Indication	Dose	Alternate dose	Side effects / Notes	Concentration / Forms	Route
Timolol soln (Timoptic)	B blocking agent used to decrease intraocular pressures due to glaucoma	1 drop in eye BID	Same	Potentiation of beta blocking effects possible	0.25, 0.5% HM	OS
Triamcinolone (Vetalog) (Kenalog)	Intermediate acting corticosteroid used PO; by injection IM, SQ, or intralesional	0.1–0.22 mg/kg IM, SQ, PO 0.25–1.0 cc intralesional	Same	Corticosteroid effects	0.5, 1.5 mg 2 mg/ml HM; VM	T I
Trifluridine (Viroptic)	Antiherpetic viral agent		2–4 times daily in eyes		1%	OS
Triiodothyronine, T_3 (Cytomel)	Hypothyroidism: used when unable to convert thyroxine to triiodothyroxine	4–6 mcg/kg TID PO	4.4 mcg/kg BID–TID PO	Thyrotoxiosis, pu/pd/pp, nervousness, panting, tachycardia	5, 25, 50 mcg	T
Trimeprazine (Temaril-P)	Antiinflammatory-antipruritic-antitussive agent usually combined with prednisone	1/2–2 tabs BID to effect	1/4–1/2 tab SID to BID to effect	Steroid effect; drowsiness. Temaril-P contains 2 mg pred. per tablet	5 + 2 mg 3.7 + 1; 7.5 + 2 mg VM	T C
Trimethobenzamide (Tigan)	Antiemetic	3 mg/kg IM BID–TID	None	CNS reactions; hypersensitivity	100, 250 mg 100, 200 mg suppositories 100 mg/ml HM	C I
Trimethoprim/sulfadiazine (Tribrissen) (Ditrim)	Bacteriacidal broad spectrum combination agent against gram + and – bacteria, Toxoplasma, Nocardia, Pneumocystis	15–30 mg/kg BID, PO, SQ, IM Toxoplasmosis: 30 mg/kg BID PO	15–30 mg/kg BID PO, SQ, IM Toxoplasmosis: 30 mg/kg BID PO	Cats: salivation; K-9: KCS syndrome; Dobermans: polyarthropathy; ITP Hepatotoxicity and blood dyscrasias have been reported	30, 120, 480, 960 mg 60 mg/ml 24, 48% VM, HM	T S I

DRUG INDEX (Continued)

GENERIC NAME (Trade Name in Parentheses)	INDICATIONS	CANINE DOSE	FELINE DOSE	COMMENTS	HOW SUPPLIED	
Trimethroprim/ sulfamethoxazole (Bactrim) (Septra)	Same as above	Same as above	Same as above	Same as above	As above	
Tropicamide Oph. Soln. (Mydriacyl)	Mydriatic agent for eye examination	1 drop 15 min prior to ophthalmic examination	Same	Causes mydriasis and photophobia Do not use in suspected cases of glaucoma	0.5, 1% HM	OS
Tylosin (Tylan)	Macrolide antibiotic used to treat colitis	5–10 mg/kg BID PO. May increase slowly to 40 mg/kg	5–10 mg/kg BID PO	Usually used as powder with vitamins	50, 200 mg/ml 3000 mg/5 ml VM	I S
Ursodeoxycholic Acid (Actigall)	Suppresses hepatic secretion and synthesis of cholesterol Choleretic agent	10–15 mg/kg BID PO	15 mg/kg SID–BID PO	Anecdotal reports of beneficial effects in sclerosing cholangitis and biliary cirrhosis	300 mg HM	C
Valproic acid (Depakene) (Depakote)	Seizures	60–220 mg/kg TID PO	Unknown	G-I disturbances initially Hepatotoxicity with chronic use Considered third line therapeutic drug	125, 250, 500 mg 250 mg 500 mg/ml HM	T C S

Drug	Description/Use	Dose		Comments	How Supplied	
Vasopressin Vasopressin Aqueous	Diagnostic agent for central or nephrogenic diabetes insipidus	Diagnostic: 0.5 U/kg IM to maximum 5 units after 5% weight loss from water deprivation	Same	Not available as tannate in oil.	20 U ml HM	I
Verapamil (Calan) (Isoptin)	Calcium channel blocking agent used principally to treat supraventricular tachyarrhythmias	1.0–4.4 mg/kg BID–TID PO 0.06–0.14 mg/kg slowly IV	Not recommended; see *diltiazem* instead	Not suggested for IV use clinically. Negative inotropic agent; usually do not use with B blockers; may cause heart block	80, 120 mg 240 mg 5 mg/ml HM	T ER I
Vidarbine (Vira-A)	Antiherpetic viral agent	—	Apply 4–6 times daily in eyes	—	3% HM	OO
Vinblastine (Velban)	Vinca alkaloid used in cancer chemotherapy esp lymphoreticular and mast cell cancers. Also IMT	2 mg/m^2 IV weekly, or 0.05–0.1 mg/kg IV weekly	Same	See *Vincristine*	1 mg/ml HM	I
Vincristine (Oncovin)	Vinca alkaloid like vinblastine. Used also for TVT	0.025 mg/kg IV weekly or 0.5 mg/m^2 IV weekly	Same	Perivascular irritant Leukopenia Constipation Local neuropathy	1 mg/ml HM	I
Vitamin K$_1$ (Phytonadione) (Aquamephyton) (Mephyton) (Veta-K$_1$)	Coumarin and indanedione toxicity and that due to decreased levels of Vit K dependent clotting factors	Load with 2.5–3.3 mg/kg SQ multiple sites, then 1.1–3.3 mg/kg BID PO Do not give IV	Same	Anaphylaxis if given IV; 2nd generation products may require 3–4 week therapy. Use parenteral form if inhibited absorption Hepatotoxicity with chronic use	5 mg 25 mg 2, 10 mg/ml VM, HM	T C I

DRUG INDEX (Continued)

GENERIC NAME (Trade Name in Parentheses)	INDICATIONS	CANINE DOSE	FELINE DOSE	COMMENTS	HOW SUPPLIED	
Xylazine (Rompun)	Anesthetic agent with sedation and analgesia of 15–30 minutes. Emetic effect in cats	0.66–2.0 mg/kg IM 0.66–1.1 mg/kg IV	Emetic agent: 0.44–1.1 mg/kg IM	Many side effects include arrhythmias, hypotension, sensitization to halothane anesthesia	20 mg/ml VM	I
Zinc oxide	Promotes healing of irritated or abraded skin	Apply a thin film BID	Same	G-I effects and hemolytic anemia if chronically ingested in large amounts	OTC, HM	O
Zinc sulfate	Zn responsive dermatoses Copper storage disease	5–10 mg/kg BID PO	7–10 mg/kg SID PO for hepatic lipidosis	G-I irritability—administer with food	66, 110, 200, 220 mg 1 mg/ml HM	T I

CONVERSION TABLE OF WEIGHT IN KILOGRAMS TO BODY SURFACE AREA IN SQUARE METERS FOR DOGS*

KG	M^2	KG	M^2
0.5	0.06	26.0	0.88
1.0	0.10	27.0	0.90
2.0	0.15	28.0	0.92
3.0	0.20	29.0	0.94
4.0	0.25	30.0	0.96
5.0	0.29	31.0	0.99
6.0	0.33	32.0	1.01
7.0	0.36	33.0	1.03
8.0	0.40	34.0	1.05
9.0	0.43	35.0	1.07
10.0	0.46	36.0	1.09
11.0	0.49	37.0	1.11
12.0	0.52	38.0	1.13
13.0	0.55	39.0	1.15
14.0	0.58	40.0	1.17
15.0	0.60	41.0	1.19
16.0	0.63	42.0	1.21
17.0	0.66	43.0	1.23
18.0	0.69	44.0	1.25
19.0	0.71	45.0	1.26
20.0	0.74	46.0	1.28
21.0	0.76	47.0	1.30
22.0	0.78	48.0	1.32
23.0	0.81	49.0	1.34
24.0	0.83	50.0	1.36
25.0	0.85		

*Table 73–2, p. 478, of parent textbook